Health in the Americas

2007 VOLUME II–COUNTRIES

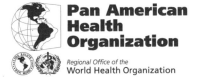

Pan American
Health
Organization

Regional Office of the
World Health Organization

PAN AMERICAN HEALTH ORGANIZATION
Pan American Sanitary Bureau, Regional Office of the
WORLD HEALTH ORGANIZATION
525 Twenty-third Street, N.W.
Washington, D.C. 20037, U.S.A.

2007

Also published in Spanish (2007), as:
Salud en las Américas, 2007
Publicación Científica y Técnica No. 622
ISBN 978 92 75 31622 8 (Obra completa, dos volúmenes)
ISBN 978 92 75 31627 9 (Volumen II–Países)

PAHO Library Cataloguing-in-Publication Data

Pan American Health Organization
    Health in the Americas: 2007
Washington, D.C.: PAHO, © 2007—2v.
(PAHO Scientific and Technical Publication No. 622)

ISBN 978 92 75 11622 9 (Two volume set)
ISBN 978 92 75 11627 X (Volume II–Countries)

I. Title   II. (Series)
III. Author

1. HEALTH STATUS INDICATORS
2. PUBLIC HEALTH ESSENTIAL FUNCTIONS
4. EQUITY IN HEALTH CONDITIONS
4. HEALTH CARE REFORM
5. SUSTAINABLE DEVELOPMENT
6. AMERICAS

NLM WA 110

The Pan American Health Organization welcomes requests for permission to reproduce or translate its publications, in part or in full. Applications and inquiries should be addressed to the Publications Area, Pan American Health Organization, Washington, D.C., U.S.A., which will be glad to provide the latest information on any changes made to the text, plans for new editions, and reprints and translations already available.

CONTENTS

PREFACE

The Secretariat of the Pan American Health Organization has a constitutional responsibility to report to the Pan American Sanitary Conference on health conditions and trends in the Region. Such is the principal purpose of this 2007 edition of *Health in the Americas*. It offers an updated, comprehensive presentation of the health situation throughout the hemisphere generally and specifically in the 46 countries and territories of the Americas, and it describes and analyzes the progress, constraints, and challenges of PAHO Member States in their efforts to improve the health of the peoples of the Region.

As a health agency, our core discipline is epidemiology, which enables us to measure, define, and compare health problems and conditions and their distribution from the perspectives of population, geography, and time. This publication addresses the issue of health as a human right, taking into account both the individual and community contexts, and examines various critical determinants of health, including those of a biological, social, cultural, economic, and political nature. That examination reveals the existence of gaps, disparities, and inequities that persist in our Region, especially those related to access to basic services, health, nutrition, housing, and adequate living conditions as well as to the lack of opportunities for human development—all of which contribute to the greater vulnerability to diseases and health risks of some population groups.

Therefore, in addition to the Secretariat's institutionally specific remit to describe and analyze health problems and the response of the health sector to those problems, we have chosen to frame our analysis in the context of the universal commitment to the Millennium Development Goals of reducing hunger and poverty, promoting gender equity in opportunities for education, preventing and controlling diseases, managing and furthering cooperation among countries, and creating and strengthening subregional and intersectoral partnerships between governments and civil society—as necessary conditions to achieve better health for the peoples of the Americas.

Production of this publication has been a major and complex undertaking of more than 500 of the Secretariat's staff members. In the course of their work, they have consulted countless sources, both official and unofficial, to compile this compendium of information; consequently, some discrepancies in the presentation of data may have occurred. It bears noting, moreover, that the quality of information from the countries varies considerably and that it was impossible to obtain from some of them within-country disaggregations of data that would enable measurement of disparities in the health status of specific population groups. Nonetheless, this regional panorama expresses our commitment to work with the countries to address the unfinished agenda of unnecessary, preventable deaths of mothers, children, and other vulnerable population groups; to continue and renew efforts to sustain achievements in health, such as the elimination of diseases preventable by immunization; and to tackle ongoing and future challenges such as, among others, HIV/AIDS, multiresistant tuberculosis, juvenile violence, and new forms of bioterrorism.

In our determination to add value to the information we provide our readers, this edition of *Health in the Americas* offers some new features such as individual highlights of each country's efforts to deal with a specific national health problem, and several other features described in the note to our readers (see next page). And, in our continuing attempts to broaden the reach of our information and to capitalize on changing technologies for the benefit of our readers, we are publishing this edition of *Health in the Americas* in print, online, and other digital platforms.

Along with the description and analysis of regional health conditions, this edition provides the perspectives of 10 internationally renowned experts regarding the "Health Agenda for the Americas, 2008-2017," an initiative of the countries of the Region launched on the occasion of the XXXVII General Assembly of the Organization of American States (Panama City, 3 June 2007), the aim of which is to pursue over the coming decade an integrated, collective enterprise to attain the health goals of the Region.

In closing, we aver that this latest in a series of 14 editions of our flagship publication gathers facts and presents intelligence with regard to health in the Americas, by providing analysis, perspectives, and context as accurately, fairly, and authoritatively as possible. We hope that our readers will bear in mind that behind every number and every statistic in this publication is the life of a girl, a boy, a woman, or a man living in some corner of the Region. We further hope that the 2012 edition of the publication will bring news of the countries' great progress in their common covenant to attain better health and longer, fuller, more fruitful lives for all the peoples of the Americas, especially those who thus far have been excluded from the benefits of development.

Mirta Roses Periago
Director

NOTE TO OUR READERS

This edition of *Health in the Americas* introduces a number of changes to previous editions.

The Regional Volume includes an opening chapter that provides an overview of health in terms of the Millennium Development Goals; of the health status continuum—the unfinished agenda, the protection of health gains, and the confrontation of emerging threats; and of the national and international health sector response to that health status. Also added is a final chapter that contemplates a vision of the future of public health in the Region in the context of the Health Agenda for the Americas, 2008-2017, with commentaries from a number of distinguished international experts. Each of the intervening chapters commences with an introductory summary, which is set off from the main text with a different format. Color is used throughout the volume to assure the clarity of graphic material. Finally, as one of the main purposes of the series *Health in the Americas* is to trace regional trends in health conditions and health systems over time, complementing this edition are quotations from the Directors of the Organization—from Hugh S. Cumming in the 1920s to Mirta Roses Periago in the 21st century—that are germane to the subjects of the various chapters.

The Country Volume presents maps of each country and territory, as well as short notices that highlight a specific health challenge and the response of the national health sector to that challenge.

Throughout both volumes, text boxes are introduced to provide additional material; figures and tables are inserted as close as possible to their in-text mention; and bibliographic references are included.

We hope that these editorial enhancements will serve both to interest and to enlighten you, our readers.

CONTRIBUTORS

COUNTRY VOLUME

Anguilla: Serene Carter-Davis (Coordinator), Byron Crape, Margaret Hazlewood, Bonnie Richardson-Lake, Thomas Yerg • **Antigua and Barbuda:** Rhonda Sealey-Thomas (Coordinator), Byron Crape, Margaret Hazlewood, James Knigth, Thomas Yerg • **Argentina:** Enrique Vázquez (Coordinator), José Luis Castro, Hugo Cohen, Luis Roberto Escoto, Carla Figliolo, María Angélica Flores, Salvador García, Caty Iannello, José Antonio Pagés, Celso Rodríguez, Luis Eliseo Velásquez, Marcelo Vila, Claudia Vivas • **Aruba:** Alejandro López (Coordinator), Gregory Fung-a-Fat, Renato Gusmao, Sharline Kolman-Weber, Patricia L. Ruiz, Thomas Yerg • **Bahamas:** Yitades Gebre (Coordinator), Charlene Bain, Byron Crape, Merceline Dahl- Regis, Camille Deleveaux, Pearl   McMillan, Linda Rae-Campbell, Thomas Yerg • **Barbados:** Pascal Frison (Coordinator), Veta Brown, Reeshemah Cheltenham Niles, Samuel Deane, César Gattini, Alejandro Giusti, Margaret Hazlewood, Carol Boyd-Scobie, John Silvi, Thomas Yerg • **Belize:** Guillermo Troya (Coordinator), Diana Beverly-Barnett, Emir Castaneda, Englebert Emmanuel, Margaret Hazlewood, Kathleen Israel, Sandra Jones, Ricardo Luján, Rony Maza, Nancy Naj, John Silvi, Lorraine Thompson, Thomas Yerg • **Bermuda:** Jacqueline Gernay (Coordinator), J. Cann, E. Casey, Janice Chang, Byron Crape, Ernest Pate, Marion Pottinger, John Silvi, Ana Treasure, Godfrey Xuereb, Thomas Yerg • **Bolivia:** Carlos Ayala (Coordinator), Dora Caballero, María del Carmen Daroca, Christian Darras, Percy Halkyer, Susana Hannover Saavedra, Henry Hernández, Martha Mejía, Juan Pablo Protto, Olivier Ronveaux, Diddie Schaaf, Ivelise Segovia, Marco F. Suárez, Jorge Terán • **Brazil:** José Antonio Escamilla (Coordinator), Zuleica Albuquerque, Paola Barbosa Marchesini, Roberto Becker, Maria Lúcia Carneiro, Luciana de Deus Chagas, Mauro Rosa Elkhoury, Rubén Figueroa, James Fitzgerald, Alejandro Giusti, Diego González, Adriana Maria P. Marques, Roberto Montoya, Marcia Moreira, José Paranaguá de Santana, João Baptista Risi Junior, Luis Fernando Rocabado, Rodolfo Rodriguez, Patricia L. Ruiz, Celsa Sampson, Rosa Maria Silvestre, Orenzio Soler, Valeska Stempliuk, Julio Manuel Suárez, Horacio Toro, Cristiana Toscazo, Enrique Vázquez, Matias Villatoro, Zaida Yadón • **British Virgin Islands:** Irad Potter (Coordinator), Byron Crape, Ronald Georges, Margaret Hazlewood, Tracia Smith-Jones, Thomas Yerg, Fernando Zacarías • **Canada:** Nick Previsich (Coordinator), Mara Brotman, Stephanie Blondin, Byron Crape, Kate Dickson, Jennifer Rae, John Silvi, Thomas Yerg • **Cayman Islands:** Jacqueline Garnay (Coordinator), E. Casey, Janice Chang, Margaret Hazlewood, Kiran Kumar, Timothy McLaughlin-Munroe, Ernest Pate, Marion Pottinger, Linda Rae-Campbell, Ana Treasure, Godfrey Xuereb, Thomas Yerg • **Chile:** Alejandro Giusti (Coordinator), Oscar Arteaga, Paula Bedregal, Paula Margozzini, Juan Manuel Sotelo • **Colombia:** Roberto Sempértegui Ontaneda (Coordinator), Pier Paolo Balladeli, Sergio Calderón, Patricia de Segurado, Jose Pablo Escobar, Bertha Gómez, Susana Helfer-Vogel, María Cristina Latorre, Juan Guillermo Orozco, Magda Palacio, Rafael Pardo, Desiree Pastor, José Ruales, Isabel Cristina Ruiz, Martha Idalí Saboya • **Costa Rica:** Humberto Montiel Paredes (Coordinator), Rosa María Borrell, Xinia Bustamante, Miryan Cruz, Catty Cuellar, Roberto Del Águila, Gerardo Galvis, Leonardo Hernández, Wilmer Marquito, Sandra Murillo, Shirley Quesada, Mayra Rodríguez, Carlos Samayoa, Javier Santacruz • **Cuba:** José Gómez (Coordinator), Adolfo Álvarez Blanco, Osvaldo Castro, Antonio González Fernández, Idalis González Polanco, Lea Guido, Gilda Marquina, Néstor Marimón Torres, Rolando Miyar, Gabriel Montalvo, Mario Pichardo, Daniel Purcallas, Ana María Sánchez Calero, Maritza Sosa, Rosa María Torres Vidal • **Dominica:** David Johnson (Coordinator), Byron Crape, Margaret Hazlewood, Paul Ricketts, Thomas Yerg • **Dominican Republic:** Celia Riera (Coordinator), Gerardo Alfaro, F. Rosario Cabrera, Pedro Luis Castellanos, Dalia Castillo, Maria Antonieta González, Rosario Guzmán, Cecilia Michel, Raúl Montesano, Carlos Morales Castillo, Cristina Nogueira, Oscar Suriel, Selma Zapata • **Ecuador:** Miguel Machuca (Coordinator), Víctor Aráuz, Caroline Chang, Luis Codina, Delmin Cury, Jean Marc Gabastou, Carlos Roberto Garzón, Edmundo Granda, Irene Leal, Jorge Luis Prosperi, Ana Quan, Rocío Rojas, Ángel Valencia, Diego Victoria • **El Salvador:** Gerardo de Cosío (Coordinator), Julio Armero Guardado, Eduardo Guerrero, Lucio Isaí Sermeño Hernández • **French Guiana, Guadeloupe and Martinique:** Henrietta Chamouillet (Coordinator), Chloé Chiltz, Thierry Cardozo, Jean-Pierre Diouf, Pascal Frison, Alejandro Giusti, Claire Lietard, Sylvie Merle, Michelle Ooms, Georges Para, Annick Vezolles, Fernando Zacarías • **Grenada:** Gabriel Clements (Coordinator), Carlene Radix, Tessa Stroude • **Guatemala:** Enrique Gil Bellorin (Coordinator), Fernando Amado, Rosario Castro, Isabel Enriquez, América de Fernández, Maggie Fischer, Daniel Frade, Federico Hernández, Jaime Juárez, Hilda Leal, Joaquín Molina, Rodrigo Rodríguez, Juanita de Rodríguez • **Guyana:** Tephany Griffith (Coordinator), Enias Baganizi, Keith Burrowes, Byron Crape, Debra Francis, Hedwig Goede, Margaret Hazlewood, Kathleen Israel, Tamara Mancero, Teofilo Monteiro, Renee Franklin Peroune, Vaulda Quamina-Griffith, Luis Seoane, Bernadette Theodore-Gandi, Luis Valdes, Thomas Yerg • **Haiti:** Michelle Ooms (Coordinator), Philippe Emmanuel Allouard, Gabriel Bidegain, Jean-Philippe Breux, Beatrice Bonnevaux, Vivianne Cayemites, Henriette Chamouillet, Philippe Doo-Kingue, Hélène Duplan-Prudhon, Karoline Fonck, Pascal Frison, Neyde Gloria Garrido, Alejandro Giusti, Carlos Gril, María Guevara, Marie-Charleine Hecdivert, Donna Isidor, Vely Jean-François, Siullin Clara Joa, Johann Julmiste, François Lacapère, Elsie Lafosse, Gerald Lerebours, Roc Magloire, Frantz Metellus, Christian Morales, José Moya, Françoise Ponticq, Jacques Hendry Rousseau, Patricia L. Ruiz, Malhi Cho Samaniego, Elisabeth Verluyten, Thomas Yerg, Fernando Zacarías • **Honduras:** Guillermo Guibovich (Coordinator), José Fiusa Lima, Raquel Fernández Pacheco, Lillian Reneau-Vernon • **Jamaica:** Jacqueline Garnay (Coordinator), Roberto Becker, E. Casey, Janice Chang, Jacqueline Duncan, Sydney Edwin, Denise Eldemire–Shearer, Donna Fraser, Andriene Grant, Margaret Hazlewood, Erica Hedmann, Maureen Irons-Morgan, Everton G. Kidd, Peter Knight, Karen Lewis Bell, Andre McNab, Valerie Nam, Ernest Pate, Marion Pottinger, Lundie Richards, Ana Treasure, Earl Wright, Godfrey Xuereb, Thomas Yerg • **Mexico:** José Moya (Coordinator), Gustavo Bergonzoli, Angel Betanzos, Verónica Carrión, Luis Castellanos, Jacobo Finkelman, Guilherme Franco Netto, Sergio Garay, Ivonne Orejel, Juan de Dios Reyes • **Montserrat:** Pascal Frison (Coordinator), Byron Crape, Lyndell Creer, Alejandro Giusti, Dorothea Hanzel, Margaret Hazlewood, Thomas

Yerg, Fernando Zacarías • **Netherlands Antilles:** Renato Gusmao (Coordinator), Sonja Caffe, Byron Crape, Izzy Gerstenbluth, Thomas Yerg • **Nicaragua:** Marianela Corriols (Coordinator), Reynaldo Aguilar, Sylvain Aldighieri, Mario Cruz, Maria A Gomes, Socorro Gross, Silvia Narváez, Eduardo Ortiz, Cristina Pedreira • **Panama:** Guadalupe Verdejo (Coordinator), Jorge Jenkins, Percy Minaya, Jorge Rodríguez, José Luis San Martín, Ángel Valencia, Gustavo Vargas • **Paraguay:** Marcia G. Moreira (Coordinator), Maria Almirón, Gladys Antonieta de Arias, Javier Espíndola, Julio Galeano, Gladys Cecilia Ghisays, Epifania Gómez, Bernardo Sánchez, Isabel Sánchez, Carmen Rosa Serrano, Sonia Tavares, Javier Uribe • **Peru:** Fernando Gonzáles Ramírez (Coordinator), Maria Edith Baca, Gaby Caro, Rigoberto Centeno, Miryan Cruz, Miguel Dávila, Adrián Díaz, Luis Gutiérrez, Mario Martínez, Mónica Padilla, Manuel Peña, Germán Perdomo, Homero Silva, Hugo Tamayo, Washington Toledo, Mario Valcárcel, Gladys Zarate • **Puerto Rico:** Raúl Castellanos (Coordinator), Dalidia Colón, Byron Crape, Raúl Figueroa Rodríguez, Patricia L. Ruiz, Migdalia Vázquez González, Thomas Yerg • **Saint Kitts and Nevis:** Patrick Martin (Coordinator), Andrew Skerritt , Thomas Yerg • **Saint Lucia:** Pascal Frison (Coordinator), Adelaide Alexander, Dwight Calixto, Xista Edmund, Margaret Hazlewood, Alinda Jaime, Kerry Joseph • **Saint Vincent and the Grenadines:** Roger Duncan (Coordinator), Severlina Cupid, Kari da Silva, Anne de Roche, Sandra Grante, Margaret Hazlewood, Nykieska Jackson, Thomas St Clare, Anneke Wilson • **Suriname:** Elwine VanKanten (Coordinator), Roberto Becker, Gustavo Bretas, Byron Crape, Alma Catharina Cuellar, Margaret Hazlewood, Stephen Simon, Thomas Yerg • **Trinidad and Tobago:** Gina Watson (Coordinator), Roberto Becker, Carol Boyd-Scobie, Alma Catharina Cuellar, Byron Crape, Marilyn Entwistle, Margaret Hazlewood, James Hospedales, Leah-Mari Richards, John Silvi, Avril Siung-Chang, Thomas Yerg • **Turks and Caicos Islands:** Yitades Gebre (Coordinator), Tashema A. Bholanath, Cheryl Ann Jones, Jackurlyn Sutton, Rufus W. Swing, Thomas Yerg • **United States of America:** MaryLou Valdéz (Coordinator), Mark A. Abdoo, Roberto Becker, Byron Crape, Alicia Díaz, Ruth Katz, Ch'uya H. Lane, Sam Notzon, Thomas Yerg • **Uruguay:** Alejandro Gherardi (Coordinator), Mónica Col, Alejandro Giusti, Elizabeth Jurado, Patricia L. Ruiz, Roberto Salvatella, Enrique Vázquez • **Venezuela:** Alejandro López Inzaurralde (Coordinator), Oswaldo Barrezueta Cobo, Renato Gusmao, Natasha Herrera, Marcelo Korc, Miguel Malo Serrano, Soledad Pérez Évora • **United States-Mexico Border Area:** Kam Suan Mung (Coordinator), Lorely Ambriz, Maria Teresa Cerqueira, Byron Crape, Sally Edwards, Luis Gutiérrez, Piedad Huerta, Guillermo Mendoza, Rosalba Ruiz, Patricia L. Ruiz, Thomas Yerg.

REGIONAL VOLUME

Overview: Judith Navarro (Coordinator), Byron Crape, Anabel Cruz, Andrea DiPaola, Oscar Mujica, Alfonso Ruiz, Patricia L. Ruiz, John Silvi, Fernando Zacarías • **Chapter 1:** Sofíaleticia Morales (Coordinator), Marco Akerman, Alfredo Calvo, Rafael Flores, Saúl Franco, Guilherme Franco Netto, Alejandro Giusti, Elsa Gómez, Jorge Iván González, Antonio Hernández, Lilia Jara, Fernando Lolas, Jesús López Macedo, Enrique Loyola, Rocío Rojas, Maria Helena Romero, Patricia L. Ruiz, Rubén Suárez, Cristina Torres, Javier Vázquez • **Chapter 2:** Gabriela Fernández (Coordinator), Raimond Armengol, Steven Ault, Alberto Barceló, Roberto Becker, Yehuda Benguigui, Keith Carter, Carlos Castillo Solórzano, Carolina Danovaro, Mirta del Granado, Amalia del Riego, Chris Drasbek, John Ehrenberg, Rainier Escalada, Saskia Estupiñán, Daniela Fernandes da Silva, Ricardo Fescina, Érika García, Andrea Gerger, Alejandro Giusti, Thomas Harkins, James Hospedales, Ithzak Levav, Marlo Libel, Silvana Luciani, Chessa Lutter, Miguel Machuca, Matilde Maddaleno, Sara Marques, Christina Marsigli, Rafael Mazín, Oscar Mujica, Monica Palak, Marta Peláez, Pilar Ramon-Pardo, Jorge Rodríguez, Rocío Rojas, Alba María Ropero, Roberto Salvatella, Roxane Salvatierra, Celsa Sampson, José Luis Sanmartin, Cristina Schneider, Juan Carlos Silva, John Silvi, Cristina Torres Parodi, Ciro Ugarte, Armando Vásquez, Enrique Vega • **Chapter 3:** Samuel Henao, Enrique Loyola y Cristina Schneider (Coordinators), Adriana Blanco, María Teresa Cerquelra, Alberto Concha-Eastman, Vera Luiza Da Costa Siva, Diego Daza, Hernan Delgado, Luiz A. Galvão, Genaro Garcia, Diego González, Eduardo Guerrero, Josefa Ippolito-Shepherd, Fernando Leanes, Jorge López, Mildred Maisonet, Maristela Monteiro, Sofialeticia Morales, José Naranjo, Mireya Palmieri, Mauricio Pardón, Enrique Pérez, Emilio Ramírez, Marilyn Rice, Eugenia Rodrigues, Celso Rodríguez, Alfonso Ruiz, Henry Salas, Rosa Sandoval, Víctor Saravia, Kerstin Schotte, Heather Selin, Homero Silva, Luz Maritza Tennassee, Ricardo Torres • **Chapter 4:** Cristina Puentes-Markides (Coordinator), Gisele Almeida, Jorge Bermúdez, Jaume Canela Soler, Regina Castro, María de los Angeles Cortés, José Ramiro Cruz, Rafael Flores, Amparo Gordillo Tobar, Pablo Jiménez, Eduardo Levcovitz, Ramón Martínez, Carme Nebot, Abel Packer, Daniel Purcallas, Priscilla Rivas-Loria, Patricia L. Ruiz, Rubén Suárez Berenguela, América Valdés, Fernando Zacarías • **Chapter 5:** Rebecca de los Ríos y Hugo Prado (Coordinators), Carlos Arosquipa, Alfredo Calvo, Mariela Canepa, Paul Mertens, Patricia L. Ruiz, Ciro Ugarte, Fernando Zacarías • **Chapter 6:** Judith Navarro (Coordinator), George A.O. Alleyne, Stephen Blount, Paulo Buss, Nils Kastberg, Gustavo Kourí, Jay McAuliffe, Sylvie Stachenko, Muthu Subramanian, Ricardo Uauy, Marijke Velzeboer-Salcedo.

Inter Programmatic Working Group for Health in the Americas 2007: Fernando Zacarías (Coordinator), Patricia L. Ruiz (Technical Secretary), Gustavo Bergonzoli, Carlos Castillo Solórzano, Anabel Cruz, Gerardo de Cosio, Amalia del Riego, Ricardo Fescina, Samuel Henao, Branka Legetic, Eduardo Levcovitz, Marlo Libel, Chessa Lutter, Miguel Machuca, Mildred Maisonet, Humberto Montiel, Hernán Montenegro, Sofialeticia Morales, Oscar Mujica, Judith Navarro, Armando Peruga, Cristina Puentes-Markides, Alba María Ropero, Alfonso Ruiz, Cristina Schneider, Javier Uribe, Enrique Vázquez, Gina Watson.

Editing and production: Anabel Cruz (Coordinator), Leslie Buechele, Patricia De los Ríos, Andrea DiPaola, Mariesther Fernández, Judith Navarro, Roberta Okey, Lucila Pacheco, Cecilia Parker, Alfonso Ruiz, Haydée Valero • **Promotion:** José Carnevali, Daniel Epstein, Mylena Pinzón, Evelyn Rodríguez, Eleana Villanueva • **Graphic Design:** Gilles Collete, Guenther Grill, Ajibola Oyeleye • **Web site:** Marcelo D'Agostino, Erico Pérez-Neto.

General Coordinator: Fernando Zacarías • **Technical Coordinator:** Patricia L. Ruiz.

We would like to thank the personnel of the ministries of health and other governmental institutions, international agencies, nongovernmental organizations, and other entities for so generously supplying the data and information used for this publication. In spite of the fact that great efforts have been made to include all contributors, we apologize for any possible errors or omissions that may have occurred.

ANGUILLA

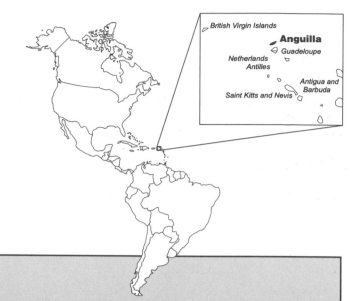

Sombrero

Dog Island

Scrub Island

The Valley ★

Anguilla

0   5   10   Miles

Anguilla, a small (35 square miles), low-lying, limestone island in the Eastern Caribbean, is part of the Leeward Islands in the British West Indies. It stretches for 16 miles from tip to tip and spans 3 miles across its widest point. It is surrounded by several offshore cays. Its highest point is Crocus Hill, which rises 65 m above sea level. The territory has a tropical climate, with average temperatures ranging between 27°C and 30°C.

GENERAL CONTEXT AND HEALTH DETERMINANTS

Anguilla is prone to hurricanes and has recently suffered from violent storms, the last being in November of 1999, when Hurricane Lenny, a category 4 hurricane, damaged the island's coastline. The estimated direct total cost incurred by damage caused by this hurricane was US$ 65.8 million. Damages to the social sector amounted to US$ 7.7 million and to the health sector was US$ 410,410.

Social, Political, and Economic Determinants

The territory has no distinct urban and rural settlements. According to the Ministry of Finance's Statistical Unit, the estimated population in 2005 was 13,000, about evenly distributed between males (49.2%) and females (50.8%). (See Figure 1.) The capital, The Valley, is the most densely populated area. All major settlements are easily accessible by the main road and a network of paved and unpaved roads.

The growth in vehicular traffic has called for improvements and expansions in the road network. Roads were resurfaced in 2003, and Anguilla's only highway officially opened in 2004.

There are two seaports and one airport. Expansion of Wallblake Airport, which began in 2003, increased the facility from 3,600 feet to 5,440 feet: the terminal and air traffic control system were upgraded and the fire and security services were improved before the airport reopened in 2005. The main seaport is located at Sandy Ground and handles commercial shipping lines that operate from Miami and Puerto Rico. The second seaport at Blowing Point handles a daily ferry and freight service that serves the St. Martin/St. Maarten-Anguilla route. There is no public transportation system; taxis and rentals are used as a means of public transportation.

Anguilla is a British overseas territory. As such, the Governor and the Deputy Governor are appointed by Her Majesty the Queen. The Governor is responsible for foreign affairs, defense, internal security, and international financial services. The territory is governed as a Westminster-style parliamentary democracy. Of the 12 members of the unicameral House of Assembly, 7 are elected by direct popular vote. General elections were last held in 2005.

The Governor presides over the Executive Council, which comprises the Chief Minister, who is the head of government; three ministers; and two ex-officio members, namely the Deputy Governor and the Attorney General. The Executive Council is responsible for the government's political, fiscal, and administrative functions; it reports to the House of Assembly. Policies are developed at the various ministries of government, based on assessed needs of their various departments.

The Government of Anguilla's mission for 2005 and beyond is to promote a society in which there is justice and equity for all; to provide universal and equitable access to a basic package of quality social and community services; to manage the environment so as to achieve long-term sustainability; and to foster a robust and sustainable economic development as a foundation for the community's social development.

Anguilla's economic activity continued to expand, moving from −0.3% in 2000 to 3.3% in 2003. The gross domestic product (GDP) in 1990 constant prices remained unchanged at US$ 69 million in 2000 and 2002, and US$ 70 million in 2001. There are no direct forms of taxation in Anguilla. In addition there are no exchange controls and the official currency, which is the Eastern Caribbean dollar, is pegged to the United States dollar at EC$ 2.68. With the exception of 2000, the economy of Anguilla has performed well, with real GDP growing at an average of about 5% in 1997–2001.

Anguilla's 2000–2005 United Front Manifesto has identified tourism as the main driver of economic development. Impressive developments occurred in the tourist industry, including construction of a five-star resort and an entertainment complex. These developments have important implications for the territory, because there is a labor shortage that calls for a careful strategy if negative social impacts and a significant increase in the inflation rate are to be avoided. The hotel and restaurant industry represented roughly 30% of the GDP (US$ 37,542,435). GDP per capita was US$ 7,646 in 2001 and US$ 7,498 in 2002. The hotel and restaurant industry employs 36% of the total labor force.

FIGURE 1. Population structure, by age and sex, Anguilla, 1990 and 2005.

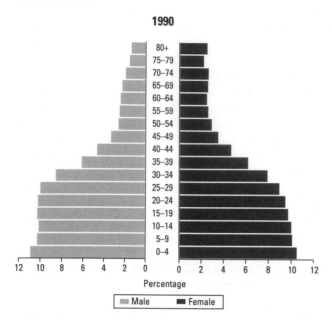

1990

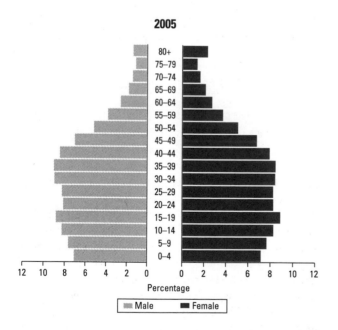

2005

The financial service sector focused on incorporating and managing internal business corporations. As a share of GDP, the finance sector contributed about 16% and construction 12% in 2005. Agriculture, mining, and manufacturing together only accounted for 7% of GDP. After tourism, the financial sector was the second most important contributor to the territory's overall economic activity, contributing US$ 17.28 million. The Government employed 29% of the labor force; the financial services industry accounted for less than 7%.

Commercial banking, accounting firms, law firms, company managers, stockbrokers, trust companies, and overseas agents make up the directory of the Anguilla financial services. However, most financial assets are concentrated in the domestic banking sector. There are four licensed domestic banks and, until recently, two offshore banks. According to the International Monetary Fund's 2003 Country Report, bank deposits in the domestic sector at the end of 2002 totaled US$ 292 million, reflecting a significant increase from the US$ 182 million in 1999. The relatively large proportion of foreign currency and nonresident deposits contributed to the decision for some banks to establish offshore subsidiaries to which these deposits are being transferred. It is intended that only foreign currency deposits held by nonresidents will be transferred to the offshore banks.

The company services sector has seen the fastest growth rate in Anguilla's offshore industry. Anguilla is attractive because it offers administrative ease and flexibility of incorporation, as well as imposing no taxes. In 2002, there were 29 licensed company managers and 12 trust companies. As of 2002, 4,642 companies and partnerships were registered. Trusts are not required to register. There is one entity engaged in securities business on the Island and one unit trust that operates a trust license.

The last national housing and population census was conducted in 2001; it recorded 3,787 households, representing a 44.6% increase since 1992. The average number of persons per household in 2001 was 3.1. The population density is 134 persons per km², as estimated in the Government of Anguilla Statistical Report of 2001.

A Poverty Assessment Survey conducted in 2002 showed that the unemployment rate had increased slightly, rising from 6.7% in 2001 to 7.8% in 2002. Among women, the unemployment rate rose from 7.0% in 2001 to 7.8% in 2002; among males, the rate held at 6% in both years.

In 2001, there were 100 dwelling units built entirely of wood, and 98 built of wood and concrete. In 1992, there were 151 homes built entirely of wood. Most dwelling units are built of concrete, which is also used as roofing material on slightly more than three-quarters of all dwellings (one-fifth of dwellings have metal or galvanized roofs).

The 1992 census found that the only public water supply sources were standpipes or public wells or tanks. Private sources that year were cisterns and piped water. At that time 12.2% of dwellings used public sources, compared to 4.7% in 2001.

In 2001, 41% of households drew their water primarily from private catchments piped into the dwellings; 33% drew their water from cisterns not piped into the home; and the remaining households relied on public water supply either piped into their yard or into their dwelling. Each hotel has its own desalination plant. The Government also operates a desalination plant that produces water for the island, at a cost. Because all government wells have been closed, the population does not rely on groundwater.

According to the 2001 census, 93% of the population had flush toilets. Of a total 3,787 households, 144 had pit latrines. Indoor bathing facilities were available in 171 households, and 153 households shared bathing facilities with another household. Electricity was available in 96.6% of homes and 3% used kerosene for lighting. Most houses have access to radio and television.

Formal education is delivered through a structured education system that covers pre-primary to postsecondary levels. Anguilla's educational system is compulsory through age 17 years. The territory has 11 private preschools, 10 of which receive a Government subsidy to facilitate access to them. There were 467 students enrolled in preschools in 2004/2005.

There are six public primary schools and two private ones distributed throughout the island. There are two special education centers attached to two of the larger primary schools. Student enrollment in public and private primary schools remained much the same in each academic year in the 2000–2005 period (1,489 students enrolled in 2000/2001, 1,427 in 2001/2002, 1,462 in 2002/2003, 1,437 in 2003/2004, and 1,473 in 2004/2005), as did the teacher:student ratio (1:19, 1:17, 1:15, 1:14, and 1:14 for the same years). Females accounted for 49.8% of students in primary school during 2005.

Secondary education in Anguilla is provided at the Albena Lake Hodge Comprehensive School, which is located in the Valley. The curriculum caters to academic, technical, and vocational subject areas. Secondary school enrollment was 1,085 in 2004/2005.

The University of the West Indies Distance Education Center and the Department of Education's Adult and Continuing Education Unit provide tertiary education. The Adult and Continuing Education Unit offers primary and secondary teacher training programs. The Distance Education Center offers a range of distance education programs. Government scholarships and loans facilitate access to tertiary education.

The adult literacy rate is 95.4%, with no differences between the sexes. According to the 1999 Labor Force Survey, 12% of the labor force (population 15 years and older) had attained university education, and 21% had tertiary education. More than half of those aged 20–34 years had obtained at least a General Certificate in Education or a Caribbean Examination Council qualification.

According to data from Anguilla's Police Force, there were five murders in 2001–2005, two each in 2002 and 2003, and one in 2004. In 1996–2000, two murders were recorded. There were no reported cases of rape or manslaughter.

There were 62 reported cases of indecent assault and 90 cases of wounding and assault.

Demographics, Mortality, and Morbidity

The average annual population growth rate was 2.5% in 2005. The average annual rate of natural increase for 2001–2005 was 0.6%. Life expectancy at birth is 74.3 years for males and 80.3 years for females. The fertility rate in 2005 was 1.7 children per woman.

The crude birth rate was 14.3 per 1,000 population in 2005, with an average of 153 live births in 2001–2005.

The number of annual live births fluctuated some, going from 182 in 2001, to 169 in 2002, 141 in 2003, 164 in 2004, and 167 in 2005. There were 35 births to teenage mothers (15–19 years old). There appears to be a downward trend of birth to teenagers in the period: 35 in 2001, 30 in 2002, 22 in 2003, 25 in 2004, and 21 in 2005.

Anguilla has experienced an increase in immigration, particularly from elsewhere in the English-speaking Caribbean. According to the 2001 census, these immigrants represented 15% of the population, compared to 10% in 1992. United States citizens are the next largest group migrating to the territory, representing 6% of the population in 2001, compared to 5% in 1992. Most of these non-Anguillians are working-age adults and children.

Between 2001 and 2005, the broad causes of mortality were diseases of the circulatory system (112 deaths, for 30.6% of all deaths); malignant neoplasms (42, for 11.5%); endocrine, nutritional, and metabolic diseases (27, for 7.9%); and external causes (14, for 3.1%).

In 2001–2005, there were 294 deaths, 173 males and 121 females. A breakdown of deaths by age group in the period shows that 2% of deaths (6 deaths) were among children under 1 year of age, 0.6% (2) were in the 1–19-year-old group, 9.2% (27) were among 20–39-year-olds, 15.6% (46) were among 40–59-year-olds, 29.2% (86) were among 60–79-year-olds, and 43.2% (127) were among the age group 80 years old and older.

HEALTH OF POPULATION GROUPS

Children under 5 Years Old

According to the 2001 census, children 0–4 years old accounted for 18.9% of the total population. There were 829 deliveries in 2001–2005; 10 stillbirths were recorded. All births take place at the Princess Alexandra Hospital and are attended by trained health care professionals. There were six deaths among children under age 1 year in 2001–2005 (two each in 2002, 2003, and 2005 and none in 2001 and 2004). Of these, four were due to conditions originating in the perinatal period, one was due to congestive heart failure, and one due to smoke inhalation and burns. Most infant deaths occur in the neonatal period. There was one death among children 1–4 years old in the period.

Infant and child health services monitor growth and development, and the nutritional status of children under 5 years of age. These services are provided at the five primary health care facilities on the island.

Children 5–9 Years Old

According to the 2001 census, children 5–9 years old accounted for 17.6% of the population. A school health assessment program evaluates the health status of children 5–9 years old. Children entering primary school for the first time undergo vision, hearing, and dental screenings, as well as height and weight

5

measurements. Children are screened again in the third grade, and another follow-up is done in the sixth grade. Routine blood analysis is also carried out, and children with hemoglobin levels at or under 10.5mg/dl are referred to the doctor and treated. An eye specialist from St. Martin conducts weekly clinics to which children are referred.

Adolescents 10–14 and 15–19 Years Old

Early onset of sexual activity, teenage pregnancy, alcoholism, and drug abuse are major concerns in these age groups. According to a 2002 National Adolescent Survey conducted with 1,225 primary- and secondary-school students, 21% were sexually active. Sexual activity in girls began at the age of 14 years and for boys, 10 years or younger. Forced sex appears to have played an important role in this young age of initiation of sexual activity for both boys and girls. According to the survey, adolescents used alcohol, cigarettes, and marijuana most often. The adolescents who regularly used these substances were somewhat more likely to have parents who had problems with alcohol, drugs, violence, or mental health. There was also a fairly strong correlation between using alcohol and/or marijuana on a regular basis and skipping school.

Of the adolescents surveyed, 14% reported that they have carried a weapon; gang involvement also was associated with carrying a weapon.

Of the students interviewed, 8% reported having been physically abused; most of the perpetrators were adults who lived with the youths. In addition, 6% reported that they had been sexually abused, with most of the perpetrators being adults outside the household. The study also showed that 65% suffered from depression and 20% had attempted suicide. Data from Anguilla's Statistical Unit, however, showed that there had only been two cases of reported child abuse in 2001–2005, one in 2002 and one in 2003.

The Ministry of Social Development established the Anguilla Probation Service in 2005, with the mandate to develop juvenile care programs. The service began accepting youth 10–17 years old as of June of 2005.

In 2001–2005, 15.8% of all births were to mothers 13–19 years of age. The Family Life Education Program that began in secondary schools in the late 1970s includes peer counseling and skills training. Family planning services also are available to adolescents at this school. The number of births to mothers under age 15 years were one each in 2001, 2002, and 2004; three in 2005; and none in 2003.

Adults 20–59 Years Old

There were 74 deaths among adults during the period 2001–2005, 49 males and 25 females. The leading causes of death were diseases of the circulatory system, malignant neoplasms, and external causes.

There was one maternal death in 2002. Prenatal care is conducted by public health trained nurses and by a resident obstetrician/gynecologist in the district health centers for the duration of pregnancy. Approximately 30% of pregnant women attending prenatal clinics enroll before the 12th week of pregnancy. Vitamins, iron, and folic acid supplements are routinely distributed. In 2005, 22% of mothers attending prenatal clinics had hemoglobin levels below 11 mg/dl, an increase from the 6.8% figure in 2004.

According to data provided by the family planning services offered at the health centers, there were 870 registered clients in 2005; 65.4% used oral contraceptives, 24% used injectables, and 8.7% used condoms. There were 80 new family planning acceptors, accounting for 9.1% of registered clients. In 2001–2005, there were eight intrauterine devices inserted. These statistics do not cover private clinic visits.

Pap smears are available at health centers but coverage was sporadic—7 examinations conducted in 2003, 24 in 2004, and 48 in 2005. Data available from the Princess Alexandra Hospital revealed that 132 cervical examinations were conducted in 2000, 67 in 2001, 102 in 2002, 113 in 2003, 70 in 2004, and 78 in 2005. Pap smears done in the private sector are not included in these numbers.

Older Adults 60 Years Old and Older

According to the 2001 census, 450 males and 508 females (8.4% of the population) were between the ages of 60 and 79 years old. In 2005, there were 13 deaths in this age group (9 males and 4 females). The main causes of death for older adults were ischemic heart disease, hypertensive disease, diabetes mellitus, and cancer of the prostate.

According to the same census, 100 males and 118 females (2% of the population) were older than 80 years old. There were 37 deaths in persons over 80 years old (23 males and 14 females) in 2005, with the main causes of death being cerebrovascular accidents, diabetes mellitus, cancer of the stomach and prostate, and acute myocardial infarction.

Primary health care providers offer routine monitoring and nursing care to home-bound elderly. The Social Security Board provides old-age pension to persons older than 65 years old, based on past contributions. Through a special arrangement with the Department of Social Development, the Social Security Board provides non-contributory pensions to persons 69 years and older who never contributed to a pension scheme. A needs assessment is conducted to ensure that the person qualifies for this pension. Free or partially subsidized medical assistance to persons in this age group is provided by the Social Welfare Department through the Medical Assistance Program.

The Miriam Gumbs Senior Citizens Home provides institutionalized care to the elderly and the destitute. In addition, a private six-bed facility became operational in 2004.

The Family

The 2002 Poverty Assessment found that slightly higher proportions of men live in poor households. In contrast, the proportion of female heads of household is higher for poor households—42% compared to 33% in not-poor households. The proportion of poor households with no adult men also is higher—25% compared to 20% in non-poor households. Poverty affects women to a much greater extent than men. Workers from poor households are more likely to be employed in the tourism sector and manual and service occupations, and these jobs tend to be amongst the lowest paid. Poor families have a greater incidence of diabetes and hypertension. Teenage pregnancies are higher among poor households.

Family health, one of the priority areas in Anguilla's National Strategic Plan for Health, intends to improve health and quality of life through comprehensive programs such as reproductive health, healthy child development, adolescent and youth health development, health of the elderly, and vulnerable populations, by addressing actual and potential health needs of the population. These services are accessible through both the public and private health care system.

Workers

The Labor Department is responsible for monitoring and investigating workers' accidents and injuries and enforcing legislation regarding the workers' health. As of December 2004, there were 11,025 employees registered with the Social Security Board, 5,979 males (54%) and 5,046 females (46%). The Social Security Board paid US$ 386,944.64 in sickness benefits in 2004 and US$ 449,904.79 in 2005. There were 2,076 and 2,573 claims in 2004 and 2005, respectively, including injury claims.

Persons with Disabilities

There are no special services available for the physically disabled but wheelchairs and other devices are procured by the family or provided by the Anguilla Red Cross in limited amounts. There is also a daily transportation service operated by the Anguilla Red Cross that takes the disabled to clinic sessions, recreational functions, and shopping.

According to the 2001 census, 601 people stated that they suffered from long-standing disability: 305 males and 296 females. The main types of disabilities are impairment of lower limb, 108 (18%); impairment of upper limb, 51 (8.4%); behavioral, 50 (8.3%); neck or spine impairments, 33 (5.4%); speech impairments, 32 (5.3%); hearing impairments, 29 (4.8%); and learning disability, 12 (2.0%).

HEALTH CONDITIONS AND PROBLEMS

COMMUNICABLE DISEASES

Vector-borne Diseases

There were 49 cases of dengue in 2001–2005; one case of **dengue hemorrhagic fever** was identified during the reporting period. Dengue type 3 was isolated in 2001, 2002, and 2003; dengue type 2 was isolated in 2002 as well.

The *Aedes aegypti* mosquito, the vector for **dengue**, is highly prevalent on the island, breeding in cisterns and rock holes; it poses a constant threat of dengue and dengue hemorrhagic fever outbreaks.

According to the Princess Alexandra Hospital's Medical Laboratory, there were no reported cases of **malaria, yellow fever, plague, Chagas' disease, schistosomiasis,** or **lymphatic phylariasis** in the reporting period.

Vaccine-preventable Diseases

Immunization coverage for the population under 1 year of age was 100% for BCG and polio in 2001–2004 and 94% in 2005; 100% for the pentavalent vaccine in 2001–2004 and 97% in 2005; and 100% for MMR in 2001–2004 and 97% in 2005. Immunization week is celebrated annually in the month of April.

There were no confirmed cases of **poliomyelitis, tetanus, whooping cough, rubella, diphtheria,** or **measles** in 2000–2005.

All pregnant women are immunized against tetanus and diphtheria.

Intestinal Infectious Diseases

According to statistics from the Health Information Unit at the Princess Alexandra Hospital, there were no reported cases of **typhoid fever, paratyphoid fever, shigellosis, food poisoning,** or **amebiasis** over the period under review. According to Princess Alexandra Hospital's Medical Laboratory, there were six cases of **necatoriasis**, three cases of **ascariasis**, four cases of **tapeworm**, three cases of **trichuriasis**, no cases of **ancylostomiasis** (hookworm) in 2001–2005.

Chronic Communicable Diseases

There were no reported cases of **tuberculosis** or **leprosy** in 2002–2005.

Acute Respiratory Infections

There were no deaths due to acute respiratory infections reported for the period under review. However, there were 12 deaths due to diseases of the respiratory system and the ages ranged from 27 years to 100 years.

HIV/AIDS and Other Sexually Transmitted Infections

According to the Medical Laboratory at the Princess Alexandra Hospital, there have been 30 cases of HIV/AIDS since the virus was first detected in Anguilla in 1988. Blood investigations revealed 11 HIV-positive cases in 2001–2005, 6 males and 5 females. All were in the age group 20–60 years of age. There were no deaths that occurred from AIDS in the period.

Zoonoses

Agricultural reports indicated that there were no reported cases of **hantavirus**, **rabies**, **Venezuelan equine encephalitis**, **bovine spongiform encephalopathy** (mad-cow disease), or **foot-and-mouth disease** in 2000–2005.

NONCOMMUNICABLE DISEASES

Metabolic and Nutritional Diseases

There were 21 deaths in adults due to **diabetes mellitus** and 2 due to **protein-energy malnutrition** in the period under review.

Cardiovascular Diseases

Ischemic heart disease (24 deaths), **cerebrovascular disease** (18 deaths), **cardiac arrest** (8 deaths), and **hypertensive disease** (7 deaths) were among the leading causes of death in 2001–2005.

Malignant Neoplasms

There were 58 deaths due to malignant neoplasms in 2001–2005, representing an increase of 23 deaths over the 1996–2000 period. The main cancer sites were the prostate (17.2%), the stomach (8.6%), the breast (6.8%), the rectum (5.1%), and the colon (3.4%).

Mental Health

The prevalence of mental disorders for 2003–2005 was 147 cases. These included 79 cases of schizophrenia, 22 of depression, 17 each of anxiety disorder and of bipolar disorder, and 6 cases of Alzheimer's disease.

There were 26 new cases of mental disorders in the period, 9 in males and 17 in females. These included 11 cases of anxiety disorder, 6 cases related to substance abuse, 2 cases of eating disorders, 1 case of personality disorder, and 3 cases of schizophrenia.

OTHER HEALTH PROBLEMS AND CONDITIONS

Oral Health

Screening for oral health and treatment takes place at the Dental Unit and as of 2004 at the Welches Polyclinic. The number of visits at these two facilities ranged from 8,533 in 2001 to 9,525 in 2005; the latter number represents a slight increase since 1997–2000, when visits ranged from 9,030 to 9,369. The number

of tooth extractions dropped slightly from 827 in 2001 to 802 in 2005. The ratio of tooth extractions to fillings was 5.5:1 in 2005.

RESPONSE OF THE HEALTH SECTOR

Health Policies and Plans

In 2003, the Government of Anguilla approved the 2003–2008 National Strategic Plan for Health, which is guided by a vision of a "Nation of Healthy and Productive Individuals, Families, and Communities." To attain this vision, the Government has identified ten priority areas—health system development, health services, human resource development and management, family health, food and nutrition and physical activity, chronic noncommunicable diseases, HIV/AIDS, communicable diseases, health and the environment, mental health, and substance abuse. These priority areas mirror those established in the Caribbean Cooperation in Health, Phase II. The Plan establishes strategic goals, objectives, expected results, and indicators for dealing with the priority areas.

In 2002, the Government of Anguilla embarked on an ambitious health sector reform program. In an effort to make the health system more efficient, the Health Authority of Anguilla was established by law in 2003 to take responsibility for the provision and efficient management of primary and secondary health care, the Miriam Gumbs Senior Citizens Home, the primary health care units, including the dental unit, the mental health unit, all health centers, and the health promotion unit. The Act also provides for the establishment and payment of health service fees and charges and personal care fees and charges. The Health Authority began to function in January 2004: it is governed by a board of directors who have the responsibility for the operational delivery of all health services, and its operations are guided by the 2003–2008 National Strategic Plan for Health. The 11 essential public health functions are addressed in the Health Authority's work programs.

The Health Authority is charged with providing the population with quality health care that is affordable, efficient, equitable, sustainable, and accessible. This mandate is specified in an annual services agreement between the Ministry of Health and the Health Authority, whereby financial resources are delegated to the Authority so it can discharge its functions. This structured approach to service planning allows resources to be allocated according to the health priorities established by the Ministry of Health. The Government planned to introduce a National Health Fund in 2006, and the first draft of the Manual of Intentions and Procedures has been circulated.

According to the 1999 United Kingdom Overseas Territories White Paper, environmental issues are the responsibility of local governments with the Government of the United Kingdom supporting local efforts. In line with this policy, the United Kingdom

Minister for Overseas Territories and Anguilla's Chief Minister signed the territory's Environment Charter in 2001.

The Department of Environment was established in 2005, under the direction of the Office of the Chief Minister. Its mandate is to provide the legal and institutional framework for conservation of biodiversity and environmental management by providing leadership for Anguilla's management of its resources and addressing the impact of rapid growth on all sectors.

Since its establishment, the Department has commissioned the drafting of four key pieces of legislation, namely the Environmental Protection Act, National Biodiversity and Cultural Heritage Act, the International Trade and Endangered Species Act, and the Conservation Easement Act. It has also developed the National Environmental Management Strategy (NEMS), which is a long-term strategic approach to achieving sustainable development in Anguilla. The other environmental legislation that are being revised are the National Trust Act and the Fisheries Management and Conservation Act and Regulation.

A Health Professions Act is being drafted. The future legislation will regulate health professions and their conduct, establish a health professions council, and provide for the registration and the annual licensing of health professionals. Also, a piece of legislation that will accredit health professionals and health facilities is pending, as is the drafting of a national communicable disease surveillance manual. The Public Health Act has been revised and renamed the Environmental Health Act. Relatively few regulations apply to the private sector.

Organization of the Health System

The Minister of Health has the overall responsibility for the population's health. As such, the Minister is charged with formulating policy, setting standards and protocols for health care, conducting monitoring and evaluation, and determining technical procedures for regulating public and private health facilities. The Department of Health Protection assesses, supervises, issues standards, monitors, and coordinates the work of other health system components and other sectors on matters related to environmental protection, basic sanitation, food hygiene, vector control, and port health. The Ministry of Health retains the Environmental Health Unit (renamed the Department of Health Protection in 2005), the Water Laboratory, and the Quality Assurance Unit (renamed the Directorate of Health Services Quality Management).

The public and private sector collaborate closely in providing health care, but the responsibility for public health care lies with the Ministry of Health. Since the inception of the Health Authority of Anguilla, the Ministry of Health is composed of the Department of Social Development, Her Majesty's Prison, the Anguilla Probation Service, the Department of Health Protection, the Water Laboratory, the Office for National AIDS Coordination, and the Directorate of Health Services Quality Management.

Under the authority of the Permanent Secretary and the Social Development Planner, each department is responsible for its own daily operations.

Private health care is provided by general physicians and specialists to those who have the capacity to pay either directly to the provider or through private insurance companies. One private health facility has its own medical laboratory and a subsidiary of the only private pharmacy on the island commenced operation at this facility in 2001.

In 2003, the Government of Anguilla set three main goals for implementing a national health insurance scheme: equity of access, cost containment, and sustainability. A manual of intentions and procedures was drafted in 2005.

According to Anguilla's existing insurance scheme the Government grants insurance benefits to all civil servants, and health benefits cover expenses in and outside of Anguilla. To be able to cover the large number of non-citizen workers employed in the hotel sector, three of the major hotels provide health insurance for their employees. Two of them use insurance companies registered in the territory and the third uses a company registered in St. Kitts and Nevis.

A national HIV/AIDS Program Office was established in 2005. In addition, a national policy for reducing mother to child transmission of HIV is currently being implemented.

Public Health Services

The Government of Anguilla is committed to relying on primary health care as the key for attaining health for all. The first point of contact with Anguilla's health care system is the primary health care physician who prescribes drugs or diagnostic tests, recommends admissions, and refers patients to specialists. To organize primary health care, the island has been divided into three health districts since 2005. Each health district is managed by a center manager who is a public health trained nurse. Moreover, to increase health care access for hotel employees, many of whom are immigrants, the Health Authority has created an additional three health zones and has introduced more clinic sessions in the western zone where most of the hotels are located. Non-citizen immigrant workers receive health care, but pay twice as much for every kind of treatment except for medication and intravenous fluids.

The HIV/AIDS coordination office within the Ministry of Health organizes public awareness campaigns and conducts seminars and workshops. The office also distributes condoms as part of the HIV/AIDS prevention and control program. Other areas for disease prevention and control are noncommunicable diseases such as diabetes, hypertension, and cancer.

Surveillance of communicable diseases is the responsibility of the surveillance officer, the environmental health officers, and the public health nurse who work in the three health districts. Medical officers are required to report all communicable disease cases to the Ministry of Health. The surveillance officer ensures that data from the public and the private sector are provided in a timely manner. The surveillance officer reports the number of cases of fever and respiratory symptoms, fever and neurological symptoms, fever and hemorrhagic symptoms, gastroenteritis, and fever with no other symptoms to the Caribbean Epidemiology Center (CAREC) on a weekly basis.

Vector control activities focus on controlling rodents and the *Aedes aegypti* mosquito. Mosquito-control activities involve stocking cisterns and water-storage facilities with larvicidal fish, conducting house inspections, and providing treatment. A mosquito awareness month supplements this effort with activities geared to all schools, from pre-primary to secondary.

The Ministry of Health's Environmental Health Unit has a vector-control program that aims at maintaining an annual *Aedes aegypti* household index at less than 5% by inspecting and abating all actual and potential mosquito breeding sites; inspections are supported by fogging and educational sessions.

Rodent control is ongoing, with baiting at food premises, schools, and public institutions.

The Ministry of Health's Water Laboratory monitors water quality for the territory, including that of the major hotels located along the coast on the western side of the island. Water is obtained from deep wells and then is desalinated. As discussed in this chapter's first section, all government wells—where much of the population got their water—have been shut down due to contamination. The Government desalinates water and distributes it at a cost. Those who cannot afford it must get their water from cisterns or catchments.

Each pleasure yacht that docks in Anguilla has its own agent on the island that is responsible for contracting a garbage collector to dispose of its waste.

Potable water is supplied by the Anguilla Water Department, which is responsible for the planning, construction, operation, and maintenance of the water supply. Anguilla has no central sewerage system; sewage is disposed of by septic tank soakaways.

The Department of Health Protection is responsible for Anguilla's solid waste management. For solid waste management purposes, since 2001 the island has been divided into four zones and household waste collection has been contracted out to private providers. In each zone, the contractor also is responsible for collecting waste from government establishments and waste generated at the beaches in the zone. The Department of Health Protection also collects and disposes of clinical waste from the hospital and the health centers, as well as bio-hazardous waste and bulky waste that accumulates around the trash bins. Hotels, business, and commercial establishments are responsible for removing their own waste to the landfill site. The Roadside Cleaning Program remained with the Department of Health Protection, and over the years, the volume of roadside litter has decreased considerably.

Anguilla does not have the technical capacity to monitor air quality, and there are no laws in place to prevent or control air quality.

The Labor Department and the Department of Health Protection are responsible for health and safety in Anguilla. As such, they receive and investigate reports of industrial accidents. Anguilla has no legislation on health and safety, but the Labor Department relies on CARICOM's Model Law on Occupational Safety and Health and the Working Environment for guidance.

Since 2004, the Health Authority has been pursuing hospital accreditation with the Canadian Council of Health Services Accreditation.

Occupational health and safety has been addressed through an assessment of the working environment, and many areas have been improved since the assessment was carried out.

The Anguilla Water Department works in collaboration with the Aqua Design Desalination Plant to provide the island with safe, reliable, and potable drinking water. The department is also responsible for the territory's water infrastructure and for protecting water resources. There is no central sewerage system on the island, but the Department of Health Protection works closely with the Chief Minister's Planning Unit to ensure that new residential building sites have the required sewerage systems (septic tank soakaways) and that government and commercial buildings have sewage package plants.

The Corito Landfill site is due to be revamped. Corito's lifespan was shortened from 18 to 2 years after excavations were done there in connection with WallBlake Airport's expansion. It has been recommended that an alternate landfill site be identified; the present site is to be temporarily improved.

The Water Laboratory monitors the coastal water around the island for fecal streptococci and issues advisories as needed. There is no monitoring for persistent organic contaminants in fish. Guidelines for pesticide use issued by the Department of Agriculture are adhered to. A Pesticide Board is planned for 2006.

Since 2003, the Food Handler's Education Certification Procedure has played an important role in the Food Safety Program. Food premises are encouraged to have food handler's registers, as a means of enabling environmental health officers to verify that workers have received the necessary food safety training, and they must ensure that their food handlers have valid permits. The Environmental Health Unit regularly monitors all food establishments. All first-time food handlers are required to participate in a training session and must pass an Environmental Health Unit examination before receiving a permit. Food handlers also must attend an educational session biannually to have their permits renewed.

The Environmental Health Unit's food handler's educational program includes sessions in personal hygiene, temperature control, cleaning and sanitation, and cross-contamination. Each food handler also must have stool tests for ova, cysts, and parasites.

Anguilla's Drinking Water

Traditionally, much of Anguilla's population drew their water from Government wells. Now, these wells have been contaminated. The Government shut down the wells to protect the population from drinking contaminated water. To fill the gap left by this water source, the Anguilla Water Department, which is responsible for the planning, construction, operation, and maintenance of the water supply, has partnered with the Aqua Design Desalination Plant to provide Anguillians with safe, reliable, and potable drinking water, at a cost.

Routine inspections of the food market and meat, poultry, and seafood products are carried out in collaboration with the Agricultural Department. Food handling premises are inspected to determine sanitary status; establish the wholesomeness of foods stored, handled, prepared, or manufactured; and ensure that food handlers have current permits.

Press releases, radio talks, and television interviews are used to inform and educate both consumers and food handlers.

In collaboration with major supermarkets and restaurants on the island, the Department of Social Development provides food vouchers to families and individuals who may need assistance. Children who are identified as needing assistance have meals provided for them through the school system. The Department also has identified the need for a meals-on-wheels program, and is currently collaborating with the Red Cross and other stakeholders to put it in place; a project proposal in this regard has been submitted to the Ministry of Health for approval. Through the Health Authority, the Senior Mental Health Nurse ensures that mentally challenged persons are provided with one cooked meal each day.

The Health Authority collaborates with the Departments of Environment and Health Protection in drafting policies that address the prevention of diseases that can be transmitted from animals to humans.

In October 2004, a five-year Comprehensive Disaster Management Strategy was developed to address various hazards—hurricanes, earthquakes, tsunamis, and human induced or technological hazards such as mass transport accidents, hazardous materials, and explosions—that could threaten Anguilla's sustainable development and the well-being of the population. A National Disaster Management Office was subsequently established in 2005. It seeks to provide an effective organization of preparedness, management, and mitigation of response to and recovery from emergencies and disasters. The Disaster Management Act also was passed in 2005.

In 2005, a national surveillance policy to detect influenza in birds and humans was developed. There were no reported cases of avian influenza.

Individual Care Services

There are four health centers and one polyclinic spread among the three health districts. All the health centers are within easy access to the entire population. The health teams providing services in the health centers encompass district medical officers, public health nurses, staff nurse-midwives, staff nurses, community health aides, and clinic aides. The core services provided at the health centers include maternal and child health, immunization, family planning, nutrition counseling, daily medical clinics that are conducted by a medical doctor, chronic disease management, and health education. Since 2005, pharmacy services have been provided at a health center in two of the health districts. Patients go from the health centers to Princess Alexandra Hospital for laboratory and x-ray services.

In addition to a resident doctor, the polyclinic has a dental unit, a physiotherapist unit, and a pharmacy. Physiotherapy, dental, and ophthalmic services are offered every week. A full range of child health services, including growth and nutritional monitoring, developmental assessment, and treatment of common childhood illnesses, also are offered.

Dental services are supplemented by a mobile unit that brings dental care to primary schools. Three dental surgeons, three dental auxiliaries, and three dental assistants are employed at the Dental Unit. There is also a private dental facility that offers a full range of services. The Dental Unit has introduced a tooth brushing program at each primary school. Oral health talks are given from preschool to secondary school. An annual Dental Health Awareness Week has been introduced to make the general public more aware of their oral health. In 2005, a sealant program began and a fluoride excretion survey was carried out, which found that fluoride levels were below optimal concentrations. A salt fluoridation programme was planned for 2006.

The maternal and child health program emphasizes prenatal care, birth attendance by trained midwives, and monitoring of child health and development. The Expanded Program on Immunization (EPI) is part of the 2003–2008 National Strategic Plan for Health; the program is a priority for the Ministry of Health.

The Department of Education employs two school health nurses to ensure the daily care of students. A monthly meeting to discuss school health issues is held between the pediatrician employed by the Health Authority of Anguilla and the school health team. School health services offer hearing and vision screening, monitor nutritional status, and make referrals for treatment.

The 36-bed Princess Alexandra Hospital is the only public hospital on the island. Its services include accident and emergency treatment, inpatient and outpatient services, surgery, obstetric and gynecology, pediatric, internal medicine, radiology, hemodialysis, and pathology. Since 2004, prenatal care services have been transferred to the health centers; prenatal care starts at 36 weeks gestation and goes up to the time of delivery.

The main pharmacy is located at the hospital and serves both the public and private sector. Anguilla has no tertiary-level care facility; patients needing such care are transferred to St. Maarten, Barbados, Trinidad and Tobago, or other Caribbean islands. According to the medical records at the Princess Alexandra Hospital, there were 164 persons transferred during the reporting period; according to the Ministry of Health, the estimated cost of these transfers to the government in 2005 was US$ 95,760. As a United Kingdom overseas territory, Anguilla is granted care for patients annually in the United Kingdom. Institutionalized care for the elderly and the destitute is provided by the Miriam Gumbs Senior Citizens Home, a 16-bed geriatric care facility, and by a 6-bed private sector facility.

There is no public health laboratory in Anguilla, but Princess Alexandra Hospital has a medical laboratory and there is a private medical laboratory at the Hughes Medical Center. Samples requiring testing beyond the public laboratory's capability are sent to a private laboratory in Saint Lucia or to CAREC.

Laboratory services provide diagnostic testing for the public and private facilities, surveillance, and patient management. The medical laboratory at the hospital ensures that reagents are available and advises the Health Authority on the purchase and maintenance of equipment. The laboratory's services include routine hematology, clinical chemistry, blood banking, and microbiology that includes parasitology, bacteriology, and serology. Cytology and virology specimens are referred overseas. All blood donations are screened for HIV, hepatitis B, and syphilis. Of 150 blood donors who were tested in 2001, there was 1 (0.7%) case of hepatitis B. In 2002 there were 226 donors and 3 (1.3%) tested positive for syphilis. In 2003 there were 303 blood donors and 4 (1.3%) tested positive for syphilis and 2 (0.7%) for hepatitis B. In 2004, 238 blood donors were tested and 1 (0.4%) tested positive for hepatitis B, and in 2005, 232 donors were tested and 1 (0.7%) tested positive for syphilis. Throughout 2001–2005, blood investigations also revealed that there were 15 cases of hepatitis B and 26 cases of syphilis, a significant increase over 1997–2000, when 19 cases of syphilis were detected.

Physiotherapy services began to be offered at the hospital in 1998. After Anguilla's Health Authority was established in 2005, this service was transferred to the polyclinic.

Mental health services are provided primarily through the community nursing service by a team of trained mental health nurses. Mental health emergencies are referred to a district medical officer and acute mental health care is offered at Princess Alexandra Hospital. Patients with severe mental disorders are held in Her Majesty's Prison and are visited weekly by a doctor and a member of the mental health nursing team. Patients requiring specialized hospital care are referred to neighboring Caribbean islands at the Government's expense. A visiting psychiatrist reviews patient care every three months.

A Mental Health Association has been established to serve as an advisory board to the Ministry of Health. A mental health policy was drafted in 2003; it includes a set of values, principles, and objectives that will guide the development of the Mental Health Act.

Construction of a mental health facility began in 2004 with financial assistance from the British Government through the Department for International Development.

The Ministry of Health has committed itself to strengthen mental health programs; establish a framework for providing mental health services; mitigate the impact of mental health disorders; sensitize the general public about mental health issues; establish an information system for mental health program and delivery; and reduce substance abuse. Improvements have been achieved through alcohol and drug education and counseling, home visits, tracking defaulters, education and training of mental health personnel, general counseling sessions for individuals and families with mental health disorders, and monitoring and evaluation. In 2003–2005 marijuana abuse counseling was offered to four clients, alcohol abuse counseling to three, and crack-cocaine base counseling to two.

A renal dialysis unit with four dialysis machines was commissioned at the hospital in 2002. Clients from Saint Kitts and Nevis are treated, as are visitors from the United States. A nephrologist who joined the health team in 2002 oversees the medical aspects of the dialysis unit.

Reproductive health services are offered through community clinics, family planning clinics, and an adolescent health clinic. A peer helper group designed to counsel secondary school peers on sexual health and reproduction was formed through Anguilla's Family Panning Association. Twenty-five students were trained as peer helpers in a collaborative effort of Family Planning Association members and school guidance counselors.

Radiological equipment is located at Princess Alexandra Hospital and serves both the public and private facilities. Mammograms are provided by the private sector. Patients must travel to St. Maarten, Puerto Rico, or the United States of America for CT and MRI scans.

Health Promotion

The Health Authority's Health Promotion Unit collaborates with the Ministry of Health and other government agencies, such as the Ministry of Education and the Department of Youth and Culture, as well as with health-related nongovernmental organizations to plan, implement, and evaluate health education, and promote health and wellness activities. Alliances have been formed with Anguilla's various media outlets and daily programs disseminate health information.

A health and family life education program has been introduced in primary and secondary schools. It addresses personal hygiene, sex education, substance abuse, HIV/AIDS and other sexually transmitted infections, and nutrition; sessions on domestic violence also are included. A healthy snack day was introduced in primary schools as a way to teach healthy eating to children.

Community leaders participated in the development of the 2003–2008 National Strategic Plan for Health.

Furthermore, the Health Authority's management team held meetings in 2004 and 2005 in several communities as a way to get feedback to them. Finally, in the preparatory process towards accreditation that began in 2004, community leaders were included on self-assessment teams of the health service, and participated in focus-group discussions with those assessing the quality of the health service.

Human Resources

The number of health personnel has increased since Anguilla's Health Authority was established. According to the Health Authority's Human Resource Department, there were 12 doctors, 3 dentists, 40 registered nurses, 4 pharmacists, 3 laboratory technologists, 2 radiographers, 10 emergency medical technicians, 1 physiotherapist, 1 nutritionist, 1 dietitian, 2 health educators, and 3 dental therapists working in Anguilla in 2005.

In 2005, permanent staff at the Hughes Medical Center were three doctors, five registered nurses, two laboratory technologists, and one pharmacist. Care at the facility also is provided by nine visiting specialists, seven males and two females, as well as a visiting nurse anesthetist.

The Department of Environmental Health employed five environmental officers (four males and one female); of the four vector-control officers, two are female.

Anguilla has seven doctors working in private practice; two are females.

Training of health personnel is determined by staffing needs of the Ministry of Health and the Health Authority, with support by the Government of Anguilla. Training is offered to public- and private-sector personnel. Because there are no training institutions for health personnel in the territory, training is obtained in various Caribbean islands, the United Kingdom, and the United States of America.

Continuing education is provided locally through the Ministry of Health, the Health Authority, professional organizations, and regional and international agencies. The Pan American Health Organization offers fellowships.

Both the public and private sectors attract health professionals from around the world. Non-nationals are offered two-year, renewable contracts. Turnover is high, especially among foreign physicians.

Health Supplies

Drugs are obtained through the Organization of Eastern Caribbean States' Pharmaceutical Procurement Services (formerly the Eastern Caribbean Drug Service). Anguilla's pharmacy is guided by the Pharmaceutical Procurement Services' regional formulary. In 2005, a national drug formulary was developed and implemented using the Procurement Services' formulary. In 2004, a Pharmaceutics and Therapeutic Committee was established to review and maintain adequate stocks, and monitor essential and necessary drugs. Drugs that are not on the regional formulary are procured mainly from an outlet in Barbados.

Vaccines for Anguilla's Expanded Program on Immunization are purchased through PAHO/WHO's Revolving Fund. Standards and protocols for the immunization program are stringently adhered to.

All reagents are obtained from various companies in the Caribbean and the United States of America.

Most laboratory supplies and equipment are purchased from companies in Puerto Rico or the United States of America. Preventive maintenance for equipment at the hospital, dental unit, the health centers, and the water laboratory is contracted out. Laboratory personnel are trained on how to use equipment by the company that sells the equipment.

Health Research and Technology

In 2004, the Health Authority purchased new hardware and Internet access for its Health Information Unit. There is no health research legislation. The Health Information Unit collaborates closely with the Statistical Unit, the Medical Records Unit, and the surveillance officer to provide necessary data for research. Anguilla participated in an adolescent health survey in 2002 and in an AIDS awareness survey in 2003. A reproductive health survey sponsored by the National Family Planning Association was conducted in 2003. A patient satisfaction survey and a dental fluoride survey were conducted in 2004. Every effort is made to implement recommendations issued in the surveys.

Health Sector Expenditures and Financing

The public health sector falls under the Ministry of Social Development. In 2005, the Ministry was allocated US$ 8,478,051, of which the public health sector received around US$ 6,962,644, or 82%. In 2005, the Health Authority received US$ 5,415,129 for its recurrent budget in 2005.

According to the Health Authority's Financial Department, public expenditure on community services amounted to US$ 817,219 in 2005; expenditures on ambulatory and hospital services amounted to US$ 2,592,881. Expenditures on drugs and other medical supplies amounted to US$ 610,332, or 11.2% of the Health Authority's budget. Expenditure for health care overseas was US$ 146,810.67 or 2.1%.

Financing for capital expenditure in the health sector is retained within the Ministry of Social Development, and equipment for the Health Authority is paid out of the capital budget. In 2005, US$ 2,996,310 was allotted to the health sector, and equipment for the Health Authority accounted for US$ 230,625, or 7.6% of the capital budget.

The health care system is financed through several mechanisms, namely insurance companies, the government insurance scheme for public servants, and patients who pay fees for service. The Health Authority is paid by the Department of Social Development for services rendered to patients who are deemed unable to pay and for the residents of the Miriam Gumbs Senior Citizens Home. Her Majesty's Prison pays for prisoners, and the Education Department pays for services rendered under the School Health Program.

Nongovernmental organizations do not provide health financing, but they may provide health services such as family planning and education on diabetes.

Technical Cooperation and External Financing

The Caribbean Environmental Health Institute (CEHI), the Caribbean Epidemiology Center (CAREC), the Pan American Health Organization (PAHO), the Caribbean Food and Nutrition Institute (CFNI), and the Caribbean Disaster Emergency Response Agency (CDERA) assist in developing policies and model legislation and in providing training.

In 2002, the United Kingdom's Department for International Development, in collaboration with PAHO, provided technical assistance to the Government of Anguilla for developing systems and mechanisms for the Anguilla Health Authority; costing of services and the development of a fee structure; and legislation for the operational regulations and the completion of the National Strategic Plan for Health. In 2005, the Department for

International Development provided financial assistance to build a Water Laboratory and an acute care mental facility on the grounds of the Princess Alexandra Hospital. PAHO provides technical assistance as well as training.

Bibliography

Anguilla, Department of Primary Health Care; Pan American Health Organization. National Strategic Plan for Health in Anguilla 2003–2008.

Anguilla Financial Services. Anguilla Commercial Online Registration Network; 2005.

Anguilla, Ministry of Finance, Statistics Department. Anguilla Census; 2001.

Anguilla, Ministry of Social Development, Anguilla Probation Service. Probation Service Report; 2005.

Anguilla, Primary Health Care Department. National Adolescent Health Survey; 2002. Found at: http://www.gov.ai/statistics/images/Adolescent%20Health%20Survey%20Summary%20Report.pdf

Anguilla United Front. Manifesto; 2005.

Caribbean Cooperation in Health Secretariat. Caribbean Cooperation in Health Phase II: A New Vision for Caribbean Health. Office of Caribbean Program Coordination, Pan American Health Organization; 1999.

Caribbean Development Bank; Government of Anguilla. Country Poverty Assessment: Anguilla. London; 2002.

Hope-Ross, Penny. A Strategic Plan for the Statistical System of Anguilla, 2005–2009. Anguilla Statistics Department; 2004.

Pan American Health Organization. Health in the Americas (2002 ed). Washington, DC; 2002. (Scientific and Technical Publication No. 587; 2 vols.).

Pan American Health Organization. Health Situation in the Americas. Basic Indicators. Washington, DC; 2005.

Policy on reducing mother to child transmission of HIV in Anguilla; 2005.

Summary of Hospital Obstetrical Statistics; 1990–2005.

ANTIGUA
AND BARBUDA

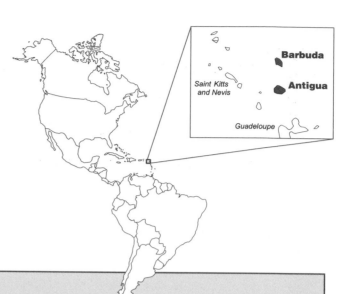

Barbuda

Saint Kitts and Nevis

Saint John's

Antigua

Redonda

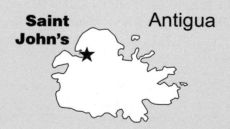

0   10   20   Miles

Montserrat

The nation of Antigua and Barbuda includes the islands of Antigua, Barbuda, and the small uninhabited rocky island of Redonda, which lie at the center of the Eastern Caribbean's Leeward Islands. The country's total area is approximately 440 km^2, with Antigua measuring 280 km^2 and Barbuda, 160 km^2; Redonda measures 1.6 km^2.

GENERAL CONTEXT AND HEALTH DETERMINANTS

Antigua, a volcanic-origin island, has rolling limestone hills and valleys to the north and east, flat central plains, and mountainous terrain to the southwest; the island's highest point is Boggy Peak, which rises 402 m. Barbuda is made up mainly of limestone and is relatively flat. Antigua boasts having 365 beaches, one for each day of the year.

Without any high mountains and after deliberate cutting down of trees to plant sugarcane during the colonial era, both islands have very low rainfall, approximately 40–42 inches annually. Droughts occur every 3 to 7 years, with the last one recorded in 2001, when only 30.9 inches of rain was reported. There are few streams and no rivers. The low rainfall was requires that Antigua and Barbuda rely heavily on desalination plants for its water supply.

Social, Political, and Economic Determinants

Antigua and Barbuda became independent from Great Britain in 1981, and the country developed its own system of government based on the Westminster model. It is governed by an elected Parliament with majority and opposition parties. The island is divided into 17 administrative constituencies, including Barbuda. Executive authority is vested in a Cabinet, headed by a Prime Minister, and comprises 18 ministers. Barbuda's affairs are administered mainly by the Barbuda Council, which was set up by an Act of Parliament in 1976. The Council consists of 11 members and 2 ex-officio members.

In 2003, the economy grew by 3.2%, compared with 2.1% growth in 2002 and 1.5% in 2001. Per capita gross domestic product (GDP) at market prices rose from EC$ 24,859 in 2001 to EC$ 27,575 in 2004. Nominal GDP at market prices (in millions of EC$) was EC$ 1,918 in 2001, EC$ 1,938 in 2002, EC$ 2,036 in 2003, EC$ 2,210 in 2004, and EC$ 2,362 in 2005.

The economy depends heavily on tourism for foreign exchange, employment, and government revenue. Following years of decline, tourism showed signs of recovery, and in 2002 tourism-related activities grew by 2.1%, following reductions of 7.6% and 0.9% in 2001 and 2000, respectively. In 2001–2005,

tourism accounted for about 12% of the GDP. In 2005, tourism grew by 7% reflecting the impact of the English cricket tour, as well as increased air transportation from the United States and the United Kingdom.

According to a 2006 United Nations report, the expansion in the tourist industry in 2002 was reflected in the number of stay over visitors, which increased by 1.7% following a 3.7% drop in 2001. The increase in cruise-ship passenger arrivals stimulated an upsurge in tourist-related activities (hotel occupancy and use of restaurants, for example) and contributed largely to the marginal increase in economic growth. It is estimated that the tourism sector employs approximately 25% of the active labor force, accounting for about 85% of the foreign exchange earnings.

There was a 2% increase in agricultural output in 2003, despite a reduction in crop production caused by an extended dry period in the first half of that year. The manufacturing sector rose by 4% in 2003—the production of beverages, construction materials, and furniture for domestic consumption accounted for this growth. Offshore financial services were a key economic diversification strategy. To attract offshore businesses, a 30-year tax exemption is applied to most forms of dividend, interest, and royalty income paid by and to foreign investors. Efforts to regulate the sector resulted in a drop in the number of registered offshore banks. Other major contributors to the economy include construction, wholesale trade, retail trade, and government services.

The International Monetary Fund Interim Index indicated that the inflation rate was near zero in 2000. In 2004, real economic output grew by 5.2%. This positive level of growth was mainly due to robust economic activity in tourism and related services, transportation services, and banking and insurance services. Among the sources of economic growth for 2005 was the continued expansion of construction, banking, insurance, and manufacturing sectors. In 2005, the government instituted a personal income tax system to ensure improvement in the nation's economic situation.

The total adult literacy rate in 2005 was 88.5% (88% for males and 90% for females). Education is free and compulsory for ages 5 to 16 years old. The quality of tertiary level education continued to improve. In 2000, the School of Nursing and the School of Pharmacy were integrated into the Antigua State College. The local center for the University of the West Indies, an institution jointly operated by the English-speaking Caribbean governments, provided continuing education. The American University of Antigua and Barbuda College of Medicine, which opened in 2003, prepares students for the United States Medical Licensing Examination (USMLE) and provides a foundation for graduate studies. The university is required to offer a small number of scholarships to Antiguan students. In 2003, the Antigua and Barbuda Hospitality Institute, a public institution providing training for the hotel and restaurant industry, was set up. The Antigua and Barbuda Institute of Continuing Education was established in September 2005 through a merger of the Youth Skills Training Project, the Evening Institute, and the Golden Opportunity Program. The Institute, whose mission is to enhance education and training of adults to ready them for participation in the labor force, encompasses the Division of Continuing Education, the Division of General Education, and the Division of Industry and Commerce.

According to the 2001 Population and Housing Census, there were 36,233 persons employed in the country in 2000. The hotel and restaurant industry had the most employed persons, 5,081, or 14% of all employed persons. There were 4,846 persons, or 13.4% of the labor force, employed in wholesale and retail trade; 4,376, or 12.2%, in public administration and defense; 3,122, or 8.6%, in construction activities; and 2,808, or 7.7%, in transport, storage, and communication. Males (18,199) slightly outnumbered females (18,046) in the labor force. The percentage of working-age persons (15–24 years old) in the population increased from 61.3% in 2002 to 64.8% in 2005.

Antigua's and Barbuda's susceptibility to drought, coupled with an unreliable water supply, require residents to collect and store potable water in cisterns, drums, and tanks during the rainy season. These practices encourage mosquito breeding, which with it accompanying health problems. Moreover, the unreliable water supply endangers hygiene and increases vulnerability to water-borne diseases. The 2001 Population and Housing Census showed that of 20,437 households, 75% had household piped water connections. The remaining households relied on standpipes, wells, water tanks, or unpiped private catchments to get their water. Flush toilets were linked to a sewer system in only 2.4% of the households; 70.2% had flush toilets linked to septic systems; 25.3% had pit latrines; and 2.1% had unknown types of toilet facilities.

In 2005, Antigua and Barbuda produced 83,988,429 kg of solid waste, including waste from cruise ships (634,720 kg, or 0.76%). Most of the collected waste was disposed of at the Cook's landfill. A site in Saint Peter parish is used sparingly to dispose of special waste, such as expired pharmaceuticals, hazardous chemicals, and lead acid batteries. In 2005, a state-of-the art sanitary landfill facility was constructed at Plantation in Barbuda.

The government is aware of the hazards associated with unsanitary food handling conditions, especially by street vendors during annual celebrations when the country attracts large numbers of visitors. In the years between 2001 and 2005, there were 195, 209, 243, 244, and 210 annually reported cases of food-borne diseases, respectively.

Antigua and Barbuda can experience hurricanes from June to November. There were no hurricanes or flood-related problems in 2001–2005.

Demographics, Mortality, and Morbidity

Mid-year revised estimates for 2001–2005 showed a steady rise in the size of the population, from 76,886 in 2001 (36,109 males and 40,777 females) to 82,786 in 2005 (see Figure 1). In 2001, there were 16,397 immigrants in Antigua and Barbuda, representing 21.3% of the population. Most came from Guyana (5,410, or 7.0% of the total population), Dominica (3,966, or 5.2%), Jamaica (3,335, or 4.3%), United States of America (2,194, or 2.9%), and the Dominican Republic (1,492, or 1.9%). Antigua and Barbuda attract many migrants looking for work. And due to the steady inflow of immigrants, measures must be put in place for managing this population.

The population growth rate was 1.9% in 2002 and 2003; it was 2.0% and 4.5% in 2004 and 2005, respectively. The estimated resident population for 2010 is projected to be 90,801 (approximately 42,642 males and 48,159 females).

The population lives in six parishes: Saint John, Saint George, Saint Peter, Saint Phillip, Saint Paul, and Saint Mary. Saint John's, the capital, is divided into two major population areas: St. John's City, home to 32% of the population, and St. John's Rural, with 27%. Barbuda's population is 1,325 persons (2% of the total population), representing a slight increase from the figure of 1,252 in the 1990–1991 census.

The population density was 175 inhabitants per km^2 in 2002 and 188 inhabitants per km^2 in 2005. In 2005, the population density of Antigua was 291 persons per km^2 and the population density of Barbuda was 8 persons per km^2.

In 2005, life expectancy at birth was 71.9 years (69.5 for males and 74.4 for females). The crude birth rate per 1,000 population averaged 15.7 between 2002 and 2004, decreasing to 14.7 in 2005. The crude death rate per 1,000 population was 5.8 (444 deaths), 5.8 (454 deaths), 6.4 (516 deaths), and 5.9 (485 deaths) for the years between 2002 and 2005. The infant mortality rate decreased from 22 infant deaths per 1,000 live births in 2004 to 16 in 2005. This decrease is attributed to improved prenatal and child care services. Fertility rates were 61.6, 62.6, 58.6, and 55.1 births per 1,000 females aged 15–49 years for the years between 2002 and 2005. There were no reported maternal deaths in 2002–2005. The dependency ratio was 38.7% from 2002 to 2003 and 35.1% from 2004 to 2005.

An analysis of the health situation and trends in 2001–2005 showed that noncommunicable diseases, such as malignant neoplasms, heart disease, diabetes mellitus, hypertensive disease, and cerebrovascular disease, and accidental and intentional injuries were among the leading causes of morbidity and mortality.

FIGURE 1. Population structure, by age and sex, Antigua and Barbuda, 1991 and 2001.

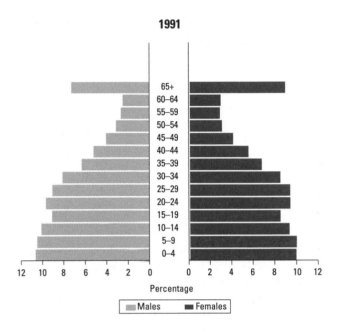

1991

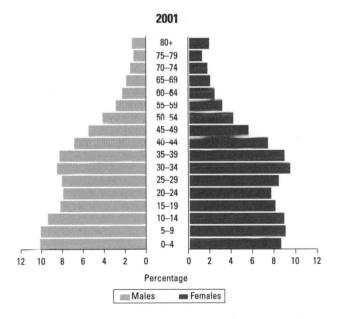

2001

ported cases of scabies. There were also 725 cases of influenza reported between 2001 and 2003.

In 2002, there were 444 deaths, 431 of which were defined by cause. The ten leading causes of death for the general population in 2002 were malignant neoplasms, with 77 deaths, or 17.9% of total deaths defined by cause; heart diseases, with 68, or 15.8%; diabetes mellitus, with 52, or 12.1%; hypertensive diseases, with 38, or 8.8%; cerebrovascular diseases, with 37, or 8.6%; accidental and intentional injuries, with 25, or 5.8%; diseases of the digestive system, with 24, or 5.6%; diseases of the respiratory system, with 22, or 5.1%; certain conditions originating in the perinatal period, with 18, or 4.2%; and HIV/AIDS, with 9, or 2.1%.

In the years from 2001 to 2004, infant mortality rates were 17.5, 14.5, 21.6, and 16.1 infant deaths per 1,000 live births, respectively. Early neonatal (under 7 days old) death rates in 2002–2005 were 11.7, 10.5, 15.1, and 9.5 neonatal deaths per 1,000 live births, respectively. The decrease between 2004 and 2005 was probably due to improved prenatal and child care services. The annual number of deliveries in the years between 2002 and 2005 were 1,222, 1,255, 1,287, and 1,246, respectively; the number of stillbirths were 21, 14, 15, and 28 for those same years. The five leading causes of mortality in 2004 were the same as those in 2002.

HEALTH OF POPULATION GROUPS

Children under 5 Years Old

According to the 2001 Population and Housing Census, children under 5 years old accounted for 9.4% of the total population. There were 1,201 live births in 2002; of these, 91.8% were delivered at Holberton Hospital, Antigua's only general hospital. That same year, 7.3% of births occurred at Adelin Medical Center, the only private hospital on the twin-islands. Only 0.8% of births were delivered outside of the medical care system. In 2003, there were 1,241 live births. Of these, 93% were delivered at Holberton Hospital, 6% at Adelin Medical Center, and only 0.9% were born outside the medical care system. Between 2001 and 2004, the annual number of stillbirths was 21, 14, 15, and 29, respectively. Hospital data show that the prevalence of low birthweight (under 2,500 g) ranged from 5.3% to 7.5% in 2001–2004.

Neonatal deaths comprised 59% to 72% of all infant deaths between 2002 and 2005, with a median of 14 neonates dying annually. Infant deaths for each of these years were 21, 18, 33, and 22, respectively. In 2002 in children 0–4 years old, there were 18 deaths due to certain conditions originating in the perinatal period; two due to diseases of the central nervous system; one due to diseases of pulmonary circulation and other forms of heart disease; and one each due to pneumonia, congenital abnormality, and accidental/intentional injury. Of 18 deaths by known causes in 2003, 12 were due to certain conditions originating in the perinatal period, five to congenital anomalies, and one to diseases of the digestive system. Health center data show that the

Certain conditions originating in the perinatal period was among the leading causes of mortality among children.

The five leading communicable diseases in 2002 were acute respiratory tract infections, gastroenteritis, ciguatera poisoning, chickenpox, and food-borne illness. In 2003, they were acute respiratory infections, gastroenteritis, influenza, ciguatera poisoning, and food-borne illness. In 2001–2005, there were 230 re-

percentage of infants exclusively breast-fed at 6 weeks was approximately 36% in 2001–2004. The proportion of mothers partially breast-feeding at 3 months after birth was more than twice that of mothers exclusively breast-feeding in the same period.

Child Health Services are provided for children under 5 years of age at various health centers throughout the country, including monitoring of growth, development, and nutritional status as well as prevention of childhood diseases through immunization.

Immunization coverage against DPT, measles, and polio was high in 2001–2005: for DPT and measles it ranged from 97% to 99%; polio coverage ranged from 93% to 99%.

Food and nutrition indicators show that in 2002, 5.3% of children 0–5 years old had anemia. In 2004, 2.7% had anemia. In 2001–2004, the percentage of underweight (weight-for-age) remained stable, at around 1.3%. In the same time period, the number of cases of gastroenteritis in children under 5 years old averaged 713 cases annually; it declined to 440 cases in 2005.

In 2001, the number of pediatric admissions to Holberton Hospital was 471.

No infants born to HIV-positive mothers (15–25 years old) in 2001–2005 tested positive for HIV infection.

Children 5–9 Years Old

The 2001 Population and Housing Census showed that children in this age group accounted for 9.6% of the total population in 2001. In 2000–2002, there were only three deaths in children 5–9 years of age.

Adolescents 10–14 and 15–19 Years Old

Adolescents 10–14 years old accounted for 9.2% of the total population in 2001; 15–19-year-olds accounted for 8.2%. In the age group 15–19 years old, 0.4% had disabilities. In 2002, there were 170 live births in the age group 13–19 years old: of these, 14, or 8.3%, were to women 13–15 years old; 43, or 25%, were to women 16–17 years old; and 113, or 67%, were to women 18–19 years old. Births to teenagers are considered high-risk births, particularly those in young women 13–16 years old. In 2003, live births peaked among 13–19-year-olds, at 209. This was due to a marked increase in the number of live births to females 16–18 years old.

Adults 20–59 Years Old

Persons in this age group accounted for 54.2% of the total population in 2001, with males accounting for 45.9% and females for 54.1%. Persons with disabilities represented 0.9% in this age group. Leading causes of mortality for defined causes among 20–59-year-olds in 2000–2002 were AIDS, with 30 deaths (9.8%

of all deaths in this age group); diabetes, with 19 deaths (6.2%); female breast cancer, with 15 deaths (4.9%); hypertensive diseases, with 15 deaths (4.9%); and heart failure and complications, with 15 deaths (4.9%). Women outnumbered men among HIV-positive persons aged 25–29 years old by a ratio of 5 to 4. Another issue of concern was the impact of HIV/AIDS on the working age population and in youth attending school. In 2002, 1.65% of the adult population was living with HIV/AIDS, and of an estimated 1,128 persons living with HIV/AIDS, 99.7% were between 15 and 49 years old.

There were 427 women who had made at least four visits to prenatal clinics up to the 32nd week of gestation in 2002 and 489 in 2003. Based on United Nations estimates of 1,528 live births in Antigua and Barbuda in 2000, about one-third of pregnant women attended government prenatal clinics that year. The country has set a target of having at least 90% of pregnant women reaching full term with hemoglobin levels at or higher than 11 g/dl, indicating the absence of anemia. In 2001–2005, fewer than 3% of pregnant women tested showed hemoglobin readings below 11 g/dl at term.

Maternal and child health data indicate that oral contraceptives were the most frequently used birth control method; other methods included condoms, injectable contraceptives, and the intrauterine contraceptive device.

The number of overweight persons (BMI greater than 25) increased from 424 in 2002 to 549 in 2004. The number of obese persons (BMI greater than 30) increased from 450 in 2002 to 739 in 2004.

The 2006 report of the United Nations Development Program stated that there were evident gender disparities in tertiary education: at the University of the West Indies School of Continuing Studies, only 20 of the 191 students enrolled for the 2003–2004 academic year were male.

Older Adults 60 Years Old and Older

According to the 2001 Population and Housing Census, there were 7,218 persons 60 years old and older; 44.2% were males and 55.8% were females. In the age group 90–94 years old, there were 123 females, and only 60 males; in the age group 94 years old and older, women (22) far outnumbered men (8).

Retirement age in government service and in many private institutions is set at 60 years old. Retired government officers are given a gratuity and/or pension, but many seek employment after the age of 60 in order to supplement this income. In 2001, 28.2% of the population aged 60 years old and over were gainfully employed. Of the older adult population, 6% was considered disabled; hemiplegia and blindness due to cataracts, glaucoma, and diabetes were common causes of disability among the elderly.

The Family

Reports from the Child and Family Guidance Center indicate that in 2001–2005 there were 31 reported cases of sexual molestation; notably, 29 of the victims were 3 to 14 years old. In the same period, there were 22 attempted suicides, 5 of which were among 3–14-year-olds. In 2003–2005, the most common cases seen at the Child and Family Guidance Center were sexual molestation cases, behavioral issues, attention deficit hyperactivity disorder/ attention deficit disorder (ADHD/ADD), and hyperactivity.

A United Nations Development Assistance Framework report indicated that women far outnumber men in the teaching profession. In 2003–2004, of the 458 teachers working in government primary schools, 401 (88%) were female; of 37 principals, 33 were female.

Statistics from the Directorate of Gender Affairs indicated that in 2001–2005 there were 1,180 calls to hot line services regarding domestic violence. Women represented 82% of all calls received; emotional abuse was the most common complaint.

Workers

In collaboration with the AIDS Secretariat, public and private-sector organizations, and the workers' union, in 2001 the government developed an HIV/AIDS policy for the workplace. The policy established the employer's position and practices as they relate specifically to HIV-infected employees and/or family members.

HEALTH CONDITIONS AND PROBLEMS

COMMUNICABLE DISEASES

Vector-borne Diseases

There were two imported cases of **malaria** in 2001 and in 2005; all four were in males. In 2001, there were nine cases of **dengue fever**, four in 2002, and none between 2003 and 2005.

Vaccine-preventable Diseases

Between 2002 and 2005, annual reported cases of **hepatitis B** ranged from 2 to 24 cases. There was one reported case of **measles** in 2001 and one in 2004.

There were no reported cases of **acute flaccid paralysis**, **non-neonatal tetanus**, **fever with rash**, or **mumps** in the reporting period. Yellow fever vaccines are available to persons traveling to areas where the disease is endemic. There were no reported cases of **poliomyelitis**.

Intestinal Infectious Diseases

In the years between 2001 and 2005, there were 284, 240, 276, 255, and 192 reported cases of ciguatera poisoning, respectively. In 2002–2003, **ciguatera poisoning** ranked third and fourth among leading causes of communicable diseases. The number of reported cases of **gastroenteritis** among those 5 years old and older continued to decline, from a peak of 1,067 cases in 2002 to 923 in 2005. Reported cases of **food-borne illnesses** totaled 1,101 in 2001–2005, including 53 cases of salmonellosis and 24 cases of shigellosis that occurred in 2001. There were no reported cases of cholera.

Between 2000 and 2001, there were six cases of **typhoid fever**.

Chronic Communicable Diseases

In 2001–2005, there were 16 cases of **tuberculosis**, 5 of which were in HIV-positive persons. Reported cases of tuberculosis increased between 2004 and 2005: there was one case in 2001, four in 2002, one in 2003, four in 2004, and six in 2005. In 2004, there was one reported case of **leprosy** (Hansen's disease), which was successfully treated.

Acute Respiratory Infections

The number of reported acute respiratory infections decreased from 19,175 in 1995–2000 to 16,056 in 2001–2005. Acute respiratory infections ranked first among the leading communicable diseases in 2002 and 2003, with 5,888 and 6,115 reported cases, respectively. In 2002 there were 275 infants diagnosed with acute respiratory infections; in 2003, there were 259. In children 1–4 years old, new reported cases of acute respiratory infections totaled 494 in 2002 and 689 in 2003. Among the population older than 5 years old, the number of reported cases peaked at 5,200 in 2001. Reported cases of acute respiratory infections in 2003–2005 fluctuated from 3,239 in 2003; to 3,099 in 2004; and to 4,202 in 2005. In 2004, a hotel reported one case of Legionnaire's disease.

HIV/AIDS and Other Sexually Transmitted Infections

The first case of AIDS was diagnosed in Antigua and Barbuda in 1985, in a homosexual male. In 1985–2005, the cumulative total was 553 confirmed cases. Heterosexual transmission is the leading mode of transmission. Of the 205 new AIDS cases in 2001–2005, 55.1% were in males and 44.9% in females. The number of new AIDS cases increased from 32 in 2001 to 62 in 2005. By the end of 2003, the Caribbean Epidemiology Center (CAREC) and the United States Centers for Disease Control and Prevention estimated that 702 persons were living with HIV/ AIDS in the country. In 2001–2005, there were 50 deaths due to AIDS—the highest number of deaths (15) occurred in 2001. Of the 10 deaths in 2004, 5 were males and 5 females—all 25 years old and older. Of the 10 deaths in 2005, 8 were males and 2 were females—all in persons 20 years old and older. As part of the effort to prevent the mother-to-child transmission of HIV/AIDS, 99% of pregnant women were tested for HIV; those testing positive received antiretroviral drugs free of cost. In addition, these women were given infant formula and encouraged not to breast-feed. Of the 553 cumulative confirmed cases of HIV infection at the end of 2005, 22 were in children 0–9 years old.

In 2005, Antigua and Barbuda's Ministry of Health, Sports, and Youth Affairs; Her Majesty's Prison; and CAREC conducted a two-day survey on HIV seroprevalence among male inmates in the prison. In addition to determining the HIV prevalence rate, the survey aimed to provide evidence to support the development of expanded, confidential, voluntary counseling and testing; prevention education; and care and treatment for incarcerated HIV-positive males. Of 163 male inmates, 100 (61%) participated in the survey. The mean age of the participants was 32 years, with the youngest being 15 years and the oldest 66 years. Three inmates tested positive for HIV for a prevalence rate of 3.0%.

Clinic data showed that in 2001–2003, the three leading sexually transmitted infections were syphilis (195), candidiasis (117), and gonococcal infection (111).

Zoonoses

There were no cases of zoonotic diseases in 2001–2005.

NONCOMMUNICABLE DISEASES

Metabolic and Nutritional Diseases

Clinic statistics showed that there were 898 new cases of diabetes mellitus and its complications in persons 20 years old and older in 2002 and 1,009 in 2003.

Cardiovascular Diseases

In 2003, there were 4,822 first-reported cases of hypertension and 214 cases of heart disease.

Malignant Neoplasms

In 2002, there were 58 incident cases of malignant neoplasms. Males accounted for 56% (33) of all incident malignant neoplasms. The leading sites were prostate (19), stomach (5), colon (2), and 1 each of esophagus, liver, and bladder. Of the 25 (44%) incident cases of malignant neoplasms in females, the leading sites were breast (8), colon (4), liver (3), esophagus (2), and 1 each in lung and bladder. In 2003, there were 59 cases of neoplasms—males accounted for 61% and females 39%. Of the 36 incident cases among men, neoplasm of the prostate accounted for 50% and for females, neoplasm of the breast and cervix accounted for 26% each.

OTHER HEALTH PROBLEMS OR ISSUES

Mental Health and Addictions

In 2004, there were 184 persons admitted to the Mental Hospital (123 males and 61 females), compared to 153 in 2005 (95 males and 58 females). Hospital statistics for 2001 showed 176

admissions, of which 30% (52) were for substance abuse and psychosis. The number of new patients aged 20 years and older first admitted for drug and alcohol abuse in 2003 was 25.

RESPONSE OF THE HEALTH SECTOR

Health Policies and Plans

The Government of Antigua and Barbuda considers that access to health care is a fundamental right of every Antiguan and Barbudan. In 2004, the government introduced a multi-sector "Agenda for Change." Under the rubric "Quality Health For All," the Agenda plans to introduce a national health insurance plan, build a public nursing home to upgrade the current geriatric Fiennes Institute, introduce a disability assistance grant, and significantly reduce taxes on many over-the-counter pharmaceutical products. The Agenda also includes a plan to provide a pension for all senior citizens, eradicate poverty and improve the quality of life of the poor and needy, provide equal opportunity for the physically challenged, and deliver improved public services.

The 2001–2004 period was distinguished by major health developments, such as the commissioning of four new health centers. The 2005 Cricket World Cup Projects (Incentives) Act was enacted to stimulate investments and construction in anticipation of the country's hosting the 2007 Cricket World Cup. It is expected that the resulting increase in tourists will generate employment, but it also will overburden the country's health infrastructure.

Organization of the Health System

The Minister of Health, Sports, and Youth Affairs provides leadership in public health care, health regulations, and service delivery. Technical and administrative staff assist the Permanent Secretary in achieving the government's goals and objectives. The Chief Medical Officer is the chief technical advisor to the Ministry and is responsible for coordinating health services in hospitals and health centers.

The Ministry of Health is the primary provider of public sector health care services. Holberton Hospital, a 141-bed hospital in Antigua, is the main provider of public, inpatient, and outpatient services. The Adelin Medical Center, a 21-bed facility, is the only private inpatient hospital in Antigua. Health services in Barbuda are provided at the eight-bed Hannah Thomas facility; there also is the 100-bed geriatric Fiennes Institute.

The national health system is financed through public taxation and levies supporting the Medical Benefits Scheme, which provides medication coverage for diseases such as asthma, diabetes, glaucoma, hypertension, cardiovascular disease, heart disease, sickle-cell anemia, leprosy, and certified lunacy. Beneficiaries are contributors, persons under 16 years old, and persons 60 years old and older. Some employees are enrolled in personal

Antigua and Barbuda Strikes Back at HIV/AIDS

The economically active population in Antigua and Barbuda is being hardest hit by the country's HIV/AIDS epidemic. Of the estimated 1,128 persons living with HIV/AIDS, almost all are between 15 and 49 years old. Moreover, women outnumber men among HIV-positive persons 25 to 29 years old. In response, the Government has joined hands with public and private stakeholders to develop an effective HIV/AIDS policy for the work place. The policy sets out the practices employers must follow in dealing with HIV-infected employees and their families. In addition, to help prevent mother-to-child transmission of HIV/AIDS, 99% of pregnant women have been tested, and those testing positive are provided free antiretroviral drugs.

or private insurance schemes. Medical care and compensation to workers injured on the job are the responsibilities of employers and the Social Security Department.

Public Health Services

Primary health care services in the districts include maternal and child health, health education, environmental sanitation, community mental health, nutrition, diabetic and hypertension screening and care, communicable disease control and surveillance, and home visitations. In 2001–2004, four new health centers became operational. Health centers use a team approach to deliver health care services. The team includes a resident medical officer, environmental health officers, family nurse practitioners, public health nurses, district nurse midwives, and clinic aides. These clinics also offer pharmacy services.

In 2001, the Government introduced a National HIV/AIDS Care, Treatment, and Prevention Policy. The policy encompasses the guiding principles that determine the protocols, practices, and services to be provided. The Government has prepared a Strategic Plan for the National Response to HIV/AIDS, 2002–2005 to guide the country's response to the increasing AIDS epidemic. The Plan acknowledges that prior efforts have been centered around the health sector and that the solutions for reducing the spread and the impact of the disease go beyond health. In 2004, the Government initiated voluntary counseling and testing for HIV/AIDS patients. In 2005, a Care and Treatment Manual and a Procedure Manual were developed by the AIDS Secretariat to ensure that all groups providing care for and treatment to persons living with HIV/AIDS used a standardized protocol. In 2005, the AIDS Secretariat appointed a Clinical Care Coordinator as the main provider of HIV/AIDS treatment, as a way to coordinate reporting activities and provide training on HIV/AIDS and the use of antiretrovirals. In 2001–2005, seven health facilities initiated voluntary counseling and testing for HIV/AIDS patients—all health centers and Holberton Hospital in Antigua, and the Hannah Thomas Hospital in Barbuda. Other initiatives conducted in 2003–2005 included a social marketing program on condoms, school-based AIDS education for youth, programs to ensure safe injections in health care settings, programs for men who have sex with men, CD4 count testing every three months, and public education to address the issues of stigma and discrimination.

The Directly Observed Treatment, Short Course (DOTS) program continues to be an integral part of the community health services for the treatment of tuberculosis. Contact tracing of TB patients is actively pursued.

In 2003, a multisectoral team was established for developing a plan for coping with severe acute respiratory syndrome (SARS). In 2005, the team drafted a plan for addressing a potential influenza pandemic.

The Ministry of Health's Information Unit, which is responsible for collecting, analyzing, and disseminating public health information, continues to require strengthening and upgrading. Disease surveillance activities are carried out by a national epidemiologist attached to the Ministry's Medical Division. There is active surveillance for vaccine-preventable diseases. There is one public health laboratory and four private ones on the island.

The National Solid Waste Management Authority (NSWMA) is responsible for the storage, collection, transportation, and disposal of waste in Antigua and Barbuda; it is comprised of four major program areas: administration, collections, disposal, and public education. The Authority conducts regular public awareness campaigns that include active collaboration with nongovernmental and community-based organizations to implement waste management projects. Antigua and Barbuda will continue to face challenges such as an increasing population, higher waste generation per household, and limited land space to dispose of solid waste. The Government continued to seek financing for a central sewerage system.

Efforts to ensure the safety of food served in hotels and by itinerant vendors include certification, health promotion, and education programs. Intensive education campaigns are conducted prior to major events such as carnival, sailing week, and cricket season. Sanitary inspectors from the Ministry of Health are responsible for periodic visits to the food and beverage departments in the hotel industry and restaurants for quality assurance assessments. In 2005, the government drafted legislation dealing with food safety, animal health, and plant health.

Individual Care Services

Holberton Hospital provides general and specialized services, including internal medicine, surgery, orthopedics, obstetrics and gynecology, radiology, and pathology. The private sector and foreign specialists provide services in nephrology, ophthalmology, neurology, and oncology. Rehabilitation services at Holberton Hospital include physiotherapy, occupational therapy, speech and language therapy, and respiratory therapy; the hospital also provides emergency medical services. Adelin Medical Center provides both outpatient and inpatient care. Barbuda residents are served by the Hannah Thomas Hospital, which mainly operates as an outpatient facility.

Some health specialty services such as radiotherapy are not accessible on the island, and patients must travel to neighboring islands or the United States for tests such as magnetic resonance imaging and for a variety of treatment options, including radiotherapy and chemotherapy. There are 26 health clinics and these make referrals to the Holberton Hospital. These clinics also hold specialized clinics for the management of diabetes, hypertension, prenatal services, child health, and birth control. There is no organizational framework for program development and implementation in the area of mental health. Consequently, the government continues to seek external assistance to upgrade and strengthen its mental health services. Institutional care for the elderly is provided at the 100-bed Fiennes Institute, which will be upgraded in the future.

Health Promotion

There are two separate systems for oral health care for Antigua and Barbuda. In Barbuda, the Barbuda Council is responsible for dental care, and it has organized an active fluoride rinse program for primary schoolchildren between the ages of 6 and 10 years. There is a fluoride varnish program for children between the ages of 3 and 5 years. The Council has contracted a private dentist to organize these programs and provide basic dental care such as filling cavities, cleaning teeth, extracting teeth, and performing root canals for the general population.

In Antigua, the central government is responsible for dental care in the public sector. A fluoride rinse program was implemented in public and private primary schools in 2002. Basic dental services including fillings, cleanings, extractions, and fluoride treatments are carried out at St. John's Health Center for schoolchildren 17 years old and younger and for persons 60 years old and older. Emergency services, extractions, and x-rays are provided for persons between 18 and 59 years of age.

Human Resources

The Ministry of Health, Sports, and Youth Affairs is responsible for human resources working in public health. There is a shortage of medical personnel in the public sector and, among other initiatives, the Government is addressing this through technical cooperation agreements with the government of Cuba, whereby a cadre of health personnel (anesthetists, radiologists, internists, an oncologist, nurses, pharmacists, and laboratory technologists) from that country is deployed to Antigua and Barbuda on fixed-term assignments to complement national health personnel. Table 1 shows the number and breakdown of health sector personnel.

Health Supplies

The Ministry of Health is responsible for the regulation and control of pharmaceutical services and general medical supplies. The Government continues to receive assistance from the Eastern Caribbean Drug Service. Vaccines are procured by the government through the Pan American Health Organization's Revolving Fund. There is a National Drug Formulary and a National Formulary Committee that regulate the purchase and use of pharmaceuticals.

Health Research and Technology

The renal dialysis unit at Holberton Hospital has five dialysis machines. There were 21 persons on dialysis in 2005. The only intensive care unit is located at that hospital; in 2004, it received new ventilators and cardiac monitors. In 2004 a magnetic resonance imaging (MRI) machine was obtained in the private sector. This reduced the number of persons who had to travel overseas for this diagnostic service. In 2004, the Holberton Hospital received a Doppler ultrasound unit, a new general ultrasound unit, and a spiral CT scanner.

Health Sector Expenditures and Financing

In 2001–2005, the total expenditure on health averaged 12.6% of the national budget. According to Antigua and Barbuda estimates of recurrent revenue and expenditure, the recurrent expenditure in health in 2004 was US$ 27.9 million and the estimated recurrent expenditure in health was US$ 24.5 million. Of the latter amount, 38% was allocated to Holberton Hospital, 21% to the Central Board of Health (environmental health), and 14% to the Medical General Division (primary health care).

Technical Cooperation and External Financing

International, non-governmental, and national agencies provide technical cooperation in Antigua and Barbuda through grants, loans, and technical cooperation in the health sector. They include international agencies such as the United Kingdom's De-

TABLE 1. Public health sector personnel categories and persons covered, by type of health worker, 2005.

Category	Total	Persons covered
Physicians	53	1,302
Dental surgeons	3	23,000
Anesthetists	2	34,500
Nutritionists/dietitians	2	34,500
Trained nurses	175	394
Ward assistants	44	1,568
Medical technologists	5	13,800
Phlebotomists	1	69,000
Laboratory assistants	2	34,500
Laboratory technicians	2	34,500
Physiotherapists	1	69,000
Radiographers	7	9,857
Pharmacists	6	11,500
Emergency medical technicians	13	5,308
First responders	3	23,000

partment for International Development (DFID), the Clinton Foundation HIV/AIDS Initiative, UNAIDS, United States Agency for International Development, U.S. Centers for Disease Control and Prevention, the United Nations Assessment Assistance Program, the Pan American Health Organization, regional health institutions, and the International Labor Organization. National groups include the Antigua and Barbuda Red Cross, special-interest groups, and service clubs.

ARGENTINA

1 Tucumán
2 Santiago del Estero
3 San Luis

Bolivia

Paraguay

Brazil

Jujuy

Salta

Formosa

Catamarca

1

2

Chaco

Misiones

Chile

La Rioja

Santa
Fe

Corrientes

San Juan

Córdoba

Entre
Ríos

Uruguay

3

Mendoza

Buenos
Aires

★ Federal District

La Pampa

Buenos Aires

Neuquén

Río
Negro

Chubut

Santa
Cruz

Tierra del Fuego

0   250   500   Miles

Argentina extends for 2,791,810 km² on the American continent; it also claims sovereign rights over 969,464 km² in Antarctica. From north to south, the country measures 3,694 km, and spans 1,423 km across at its widest point. Argentina's Atlantic coast is 4,725 km long, and its border with Chile, Bolivia, Paraguay, Brazil, and Uruguay is 9,376 km.

GENERAL CONTEXT AND HEALTH DETERMINANTS

Argentina is governed as a federal republic with a presidential system, and is ruled by its 1853 Constitution; the Constitution was last amended in 1994. The Executive, Legislative, and Judicial branches function independently; administrations serve for four years. The country is divided into five regions: Northwest, Northeast, Cuyo, Central or Pampan, and South, which encompass 24 jurisdictions (23 provinces and the autonomous city of Buenos Aires, seat of the National Government). Each province has its own constitution and elects its governing officials.

Social, Political, and Economic Determinants

In the second half of the 1990s, changes in the country's productive structure and successive external crises caused an increase in unemployment and poverty and led to a greater income distribution inequality that had never been seen in Argentina. In 1998, as a result of a drop in the gross domestic product (GDP), poverty and inequality worsened; the ensuing financial crisis led to the annulment of the currency board agreement and the devaluation of the Argentine peso early in 2002. Annual per capita income dropped from US$ 7,470 in 2000 to US$ 3,670 in 2003, falling further to US$ 3,580 in 2004 (1). These economic difficulties notwithstanding, the country was able to preserve its high human development index (HDI) rating (0.849), which has continued to gradually increase since 1975, when it was 0.784 (2).

Data on poverty and indigence in the population come from measures gathered by the National Institute of Statistics and Census (INDEC, by its Spanish acronym). The number of households and individuals below the poverty line come from the Household Survey (EPH, by its Spanish acronym), which was first conducted in 1972 and, since 2003, has been conducted quarterly by INDEC. Since 2006, EPH has been conducted in 31 urban clusters (28 up until 2005), which include the 23 provincial capitals that are representative of six of the country's areas: Metropolitan, Pampan, Northwest, Northeast, Cuyo, and Patagonian. Household income is used to determine whether members are able to satisfy essential food and other needs, relying on a "basic basket" of essential food, goods, and services (clothing, transport, education, health, etc.) as a benchmark. To calculate the percentage of poor households, the number whose income cannot cover the cost of the basic basket (including food, goods, and services) is divided by the total number of households; to calculate the percentage of indigent households the number whose income cannot cover the cost of the basket (including food, but excluding goods and services) is divided by the total number of households. The population living below the extreme poverty line (indigence) increased moderately during the second half of the 1990s: from 7.9% in 1995 to 9.6% in 2000. After the unprecedented 2001 economic crisis, which affected the living conditions of vast population sectors, the figure catapulted to more than 25% in 2002, according to estimates by the Regional Office of the World Bank in Argentina, which defines "extreme poverty" as income under US$ 1 per person per day, a level never seen in Argentina. This spike in the percentage of indigence was due to a rise in the ranks of unemployed persons and families without any earnings (which skyrocketed from 6.1% to 21.5% between 1990 and 2002) and to the decreased purchasing power of the very poorly remunerated employed.

Within the context of an extraordinary trade surplus, the restoration of order to the fiscal accounts, the normalization of the financial system, and foreign exchange intervention, the economy's extreme volatility was brought under control beginning in 2003. Signs of economic improvement include several consecutive quarters showing growth, a revaluation of the Argentine peso (ARS) (ARS 2.9 = US$ 1 in August 2005), a reduction of unemployment levels from 15.4% in the second half of 2003 to 12.5% in the first half of 2005 (EPH data), and a 14% decrease in poverty between the second half of 2003 and the second half of 2005. During this period, poverty declined for men and women and in all age groups, decreasing more in the population living below the indigence line in comparison with the non-indigent population living below the poverty line (Table 1). Changes in unemployment and poverty also are indications of economic improvement that is in the consolidation phase, considering the country's yearly growth rate of approximately 9%.

Poverty and indigence are distributed highly unequally in the country, with disparities among and within provinces that reveal a very uneven level of protection of the social and economic rights of Argentineans. In Northwest and Northeast regions,

TABLE 1. Population of 28 urban clusters, by poverty status, sex, and age group, Argentina, second half of 2003 and 2005.

Sex and poverty status	Total		Age group							
			0–13 years old		14–22 years old		23–64 years old		65 years old and older	
	2003	2005	2003	2005	2003	2005	2003	2005	2003	2005
Total (thousands)	23,163	23,410	5,870	5,553	3,585	3,669	11,054	11,735	2,654	2,453
	%	%	%	%	%	%	%	%	%	%
Not poor	52.2	66.2	36.6	50.5	42.2	58.1	58.3	72.3	74.4	84.4
Poor	47.8	33.8	63.4	49.5	57.8	41.9	41.7	27.7	25.6	15.6
Not indigent	27.3	21.7	33.4	29.0	31.9	26.8	25.0	18.6	17.4	12.1
Indigent	20.5	12.2	30.1	20.5	25.9	15.1	16.7	9.1	8.2	3.6
Women (thousands)	12,213	12,314	2,892	2,752	1,768	1,845	5,942	6,225	1,611	1,492
	%	%	%	%	%	%	%	%	%	%
Not poor	53.5	66.8	37.0	49.8	44.3	59.8	58.4	72.0	75.2	85.5
Pooor	46.5	33.2	63.0	50.2	55.7	40.2	41.6	28.0	24.8	14.5
Not indigent	26.5	21.1	33.0	28.8	31.0	25.8	24.7	18.6	16.6	11.2
Indigent	19.9	12.1	29.9	21.4	24.7	14.4	16.9	9.4	8.1	3.3
Men (thousands)	10,950	11,096	2,978	2,801	1,817	1,824	5,113	5,510	1,043	961
	%	%	%	%	%	%	%	%	%	%
Not poor	50.6	65.4	36.1	51.3	40.2	56.4	58.2	72.6	73.1	82.6
Poor	49.4	34.6	63.9	48.7	59.8	43.6	41.8	27.4	26.9	17.4
Not indigent	28.2	22.3	33.7	29.1	32.6	27.7	25.3	18.6	18.6	13.4
Indigent	21.2	12.3	30.2	19.6	27.2	15.9	16.5	8.8	8.4	4.0

Source: INDEC, Permanent Household Survey.

urban clusters have poverty rates that are much higher than the national average for both households and individuals (Figure 1).

The income-distribution inequality is a factor that plays an important role in the social deterioration, and works relatively independently of trends in poverty and indigence. In the first quarter of 2006, INDEC began publishing data on per capita family income (that is, the average income per person in the household). Results show that 20% of the population can spend between ARS 0 and ARS 140 pesos (US$ 45) per month. The poorest 10% of the population would have an average income of ARS 50 (US$ 16), and the wealthiest 10% would have an average income of ARS 1,823 (US$ 590), for an income gap of 36 between the poorest and the wealthiest segments of the population (this measure is arrived at by dividing the income of the wealthiest 10% of the population by that of the poorest 10%). Table 2 shows the changes in the income gap in 2003–2005.

Research conducted between 1992 and 2005 by the Center for Distribution, Labor, and Social Studies (CEDLAS, by its Spanish acronym) at the National University of La Plata showed that the Gini coefficient of per capita family income increased from 0.45 to 0.50, according to data for the first half of 2005. The poorest quintile's share of national income, on the other hand, decreased in the same period, from 4.8% to 3.1%; that of the wealthiest quintile increased from 50.6% to 54.7% (3). In considering these two measurements in the context of improvements in the percentages for poverty and indigence, it becomes clear that inequality is one of the most important social questions to be resolved.

In 2003, the Government gave human rights policy a central position within the work agenda. Thus, it began to tackle the repeal of impunity laws, created the Investigation Unit of the National Commission for the Right to Identity, launched "Memory Space" in what had been the headquarters of the Navy's Mechanics School (ESMA, by its Spanish acronym), and reactivated the investigation regarding the fate of the thousands of disappeared victims of State terrorism. The country still faces situations that affect the human rights of specific population groups, however, such as children and youth who break criminal laws and institutionalized psychiatric patients; there also are still cases of child exploitation and reports of torture and other mistreatment of persons detained in police stations or prisons.

The country also has advanced in terms of gender equality. Noteworthy at the institutional level is the incorporation of all human rights treaties dealing with gender equality into the National Constitution, including the Convention on the Elimination of All Forms of Discrimination against Women (CEDAW). In 2006, the National Congress ratified the Optional Protocol, whereby Argentinean women now can bring complaints regarding the infringement of their rights to an international and impartial tribunal of experts. The National Congress also enacted legislation dealing with surgical contraception (Law No. 26,130) and with comprehensive sexual education (Law No. 26,150). The National Law on Quotas No. 24,012/91 made it possible to increase the number of women in elective positions in the Legislative Branch, from 1.4% in the National Senate in 1998, to 34.7%

FIGURE 1. Poverty and indigence incidence, total urban population covered by the Housing Survey and by statistical region, Argentina, second semester of 2005.

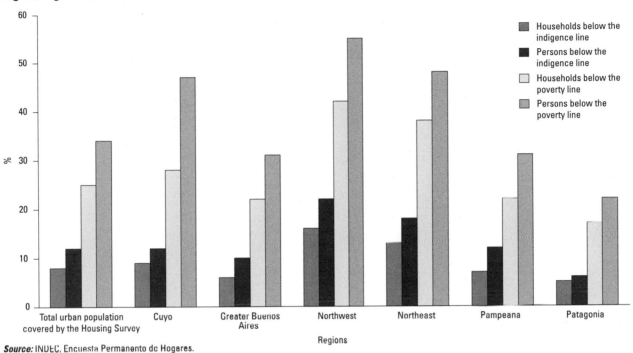

Source: INDEC, Encuesta Permanente de Hogares.

in 2001, and to 41.7% in 2003. Most provinces also have approved local laws that echo substantive aspects of the national law. Thus, female participation in provincial legislatures increased from 22.2% in 2000 to 26.6% in 2004.

In October 2003 the Government reiterated its commitment to achieving the Millennium Development Goals (MDGs). After a slow start marked by the restructuring of the unit responsible for coordinating MDGs, in 2005 the Government completed an evaluation on the process and redefined certain goals. Meanwhile, the various objectives were prioritized at the sector level. Thus, MDG 5 (improve maternal health), 6 (combat HIV/AIDS and other diseases), 7 (ensure environmental sustainability), and 8 (develop a global partnership for development) are clearly spelled out in the Ministry of Health's agenda and in the 2004–2007 Federal Health Plan. Moreover, interest in the MDGs emerged at the sub-national level, and provinces such as Tucumán, Mendoza, La Rioja, and

San Juan set or are in the process of setting their own objectives for achieving the MDGs (see Table 3).

The country is close to achieving MDG 2 (universal primary education), as indicated by the net enrollment rate in primary school (98.1%), the rate of those who remain in school in the fifth year/grade (90.7%), and the literacy rate among 15–24-year-olds (98.9%) (4). According to INDEC (1991 and 2001 censuses), the percentage of illiterates decreased from 3.7% in 1991 to 2.6% in 2001, with equal percentages for men and women, but some provinces continue to lag in certain indicators. In the northeast (Chaco, Formosa, Corrientes, and Misiones) illiteracy rates are higher than 6%. Among individuals over 64 years old nationwide, the illiteracy rate is 6.2%, a rate that trebles in the aforementioned provinces (20.2%, 20.7%, 18.8%, and 16.3%, respectively). There also is a gap of 2 to 3 percentage points between women and men, with men lagging.

TABLE 2. Income gaps by median and average per capita family income, 28 urban clusters (trimesters without Christmas bonus), Argentina, 2003–2005.

	2003	2004		2005	
	4th qtr.	2nd qtr.	4th qtr.	2nd qtr.	4th qtr.
10th decile median/1st decile median	31	29	27	27	24
10th decile average/1st decile average	47	41	38	37	32

Source: Permanent Household Survey.

TABLE 3. Selected Millennium Development Goals, indicators and targets, Argentina, 2007, 2011, and 2015.

Indicator	Reference data		Most recent available data		Targets		
	Year	Value	Year	Value	2007	2011	2015
Improve maternal health (MDG 5)							
Maternal mortality rate per 100,000 live births	1990	52.0	2004	40	3.7		1.3
% of live births delivered by a doctor or midwife	1990	96.9	2004	99.0	99.0		99.0
Gini coefficient for maternal mortality rate	1990	0.346	2004	0.303	0.344		0.311
Combat HIV/AIDS, Chagas' disease, TB, and malaria (MDG 6)							
Prevalence of HIV in pregnant women 15–24 years old (%)	2000	0.64	2003	0.39	0.35		0.32
Prevalence of condom use in youths 15–24 years old (%)			2003	61.0	67.0		75.0
Mortality rate from HIV/AIDS (per 100,000 population)	1990	0.9	2003	4.2	3.8		3.5
Incidence rate of HIV/AIDS (per 100,000 population)	1990	17.0	2003	49	42.0		37.0
Morbidity rate for TB (per 100,000 population)	1990	38.1	2003	32.0			23.1
Mortality rate for TB (per 100,000 population)	1990	4.26	2003	2.4	2.1		1.21
% of TB cases detected and cured with DOTS	1989	64.6	2003	77.6	82.0		90.0
Mortality rate for malaria (per 100,000 population)	1990	0.0	2004	0.0	0.0		0.0
% of population in areas at risk for malaria that apply effective prevention and treatment measures	1990	100.0	2004	100.0	100.0		100.0
Annual parasite index (per 1,000 population)	1990	0.765	2004	0.057	< 0.1		< 0.1
% of endemic provinces that certified interruption of vector transmission of Chagas' disease	2001	21.1	2004	26.3	42.1		100.0
Ensure a sustainable environment (MDG 7)							
Surface area covered with native forest (%)			2002	11.60	11.2	11.3	
Total surface area in the country protected to maintain biodiversity (%)			2003	6.30	7.3	8.3	> 10
Equivalent tons of petroleum to generate US$ 1,000 of GDP			2003	0.2	0.2	0.2	—
Share of renewable sources in the TPES (Total Primary Energy Supply) (%)			2003	9.90	9.9	> 10	> 10
Population with access to publicly supplied drinking water (%)					80.8	82.4	> 84
Population with sewerage coverage (%)					47.9	51.5	> 55
Deficient housing with irregular ownership (%)			2005	6.4	5.6	4.8	3.9

In 2001, about 6% of the total population had completed a university degree, two percentage points higher than in 1991. Among the population over 15 years old, men have higher percentages at intermediate or low educational levels (incomplete primary, complete primary, and incomplete secondary), while the women surpass men in complete secondary and incomplete and complete university levels. According to data from the 2001 National Population Census developed by INDEC's Sectoral Statistics Directorate, 8.7% of the population over 15 years old completed university studies (7.0% of the men and 10.3% of the women). According to EPH data, in the second half of 2004 the educational levels of men and women in urban clusters were more even, with the exception of completion of university education, in which the 3-percentage-point difference in favor of women remained the same. Data from INDEC's Sectoral Statistics Directorate based on the 2004 National Teacher Census of the Ministry of Education, Science, and Technology show that 821,726 teachers worked in formal educational establishments in 2004, that is, 25.3% more than in 1994. The 2005 National Health

and Nutrition Survey showed that 32.2% of the 311,000 households surveyed received some type of food assistance, with percentages ranging from 0.1% in the province of San Luis to 50.3% in Chaco.

Of the households included in the 2001 National Population and Housing Census, 96.6% used water from the water supply system; of these, 84.1% had water supplied to the home and the remaining 12.5% had water supplied somewhere on their property. The lack of a safe water supply is of great concern throughout the country. Even in the Buenos Aires Metropolitan Area there are major deficiencies (5) that go beyond marginalized, poor areas, extending to residential areas that have no publicly supplied water or have water supplied that may not be sanitary. Such is the case with the high levels of nitrate in the publicly supplied water, whose use by nursing mothers, children, and pregnant women is not recommended. Various toxic substances also are present in the aquifers used for human consumption: for example, long-term intake of arsenic in the water may cause chronic endemic hydroarsenicism. It has been established that 34% of the inhabitants of the province of Chaco are at risk for hydroarsenicism, 45% in La Pampa, 34.5% in San Luis, 24% in Santiago del Estero, and 26.5% in Santa Fe (6).

According to the Ministry of Justice, Security, and Human Rights' National Directorate of Criminal Policy, the crime rate (including any crime, be it sex crimes; crimes against individuals, property, liberty, the State, or the community; or crimes involving narcotics or other special laws) showed a rising trend over the past decade, although there was a decline from 2002 to 2003 (350.2 per 10,000 as compared with 369.7 per 10,000). The same source indicated that the prison population has been rising steadily since 1999, reaching 9,246 in 2003. The 2005 Amnesty International report calculates that there is a prison population of 62,500 in Argentina, which would mean that there is severe overcrowding.

Demographics, Mortality, and Morbidity

Argentina's projected population for 2005 was 38,592,150. The growth rate has been declining steadily in recent five-year periods: 1.3% in 1990–1995, 1.1% in 1995–2000, and 0.9% in 2000–2005. In the latter two five-year periods, the net migration rate decreased (dropping from 0.06% to 0.05%). Between 1980 and 2005 there was a gradual aging of the population: the aging index (population over 65 years old divided by the population under 15 years old, multiplied by 100) increased from 26.6 to 37.9. Conversely, the Fritz index (population 0–19 years old divided by the population 30–49 years old, multiplied by 100) declined from 161 to 143. This translated into changes in Argentina's population structure, whereby the mature population has increased in relation to the young population. The active population structure (population 40–64 years old divided by the population 15–39 years old, multiplied by 100), on the other hand, was younger in 2005 than in 1980 (active population structure indices of 63.5 and 67.2, respectively).[1]

The average annual birth rate per 1,000 population declined steadily from 1980–1985 (23.1) to 2000–2005 (18.0), and this trend is expected to continue at least until 2010–2015. The general mortality rate per 1,000 inhabitants also declined slightly between 1980–1985 (8.5) and 2000–2005 (7.9). The average number of children per woman decreased from 3.2 in 1980–1985 to 2.4 in 2000–2005, while the general fertility rate dropped from 97.0 per 1,000 women to 72.2 in the same period. It is estimated that in 2010–2015, the number of children per woman will decrease to 2.2 and the general fertility rate will be approximately 66 per 1,000 women.

Life expectancy at birth has increased in the past 25 years. In 1980–1985 it was 70.2 years (66.8 for men and 73.7 for women), while in 2000–2005 it averaged 74.3 (70.6 for men and 78.1 for women).

---

[1]The source of the basic data for this entire section is INDEC; based on them, the demographic indices presented here were developed.

In 2001–2005, the Federal Capital and the provinces of Buenos Aires, Catamarca, Córdoba, La Pampa, La Rioja, Neuquén, Salta, San Juan, San Luis, Santa Cruz, and Tierra de Fuego experienced internal migration. In the same period, international migration resulted in the net loss of 70,000 men and 30,000 women. The 2001 census enumerated 1,531,940 foreigners in Argentina (699,555 men and 832,385 women). More than 900,000 came from bordering countries, most (325,046) from Paraguay, followed by Bolivia (233,464). Italians and Spaniards were the most numerous among European immigrants, although they came to Argentina as part of a long-standing process, and most of them are older than 65 years old. According to INDEC data for 2005, the indigenous peoples with the highest populations are the Mapuche in Patagonia; the Kolla in Jujuy and Salta; the Toba in Chaco, Formosa, and Santa Fe; and the Wichi in Chaco, Formosa, and Salta. These four peoples represent 53% of the 402,921 persons included in the national survey. The rest of the population was divided among 17 other indigenous peoples. At least one member in 2.8% of the country's households identified him- or herself as belonging to or having descended from an indigenous group.

The general age-adjusted mortality rates are slightly higher in the most depressed regions, especially for women. The adjusted mortality rates due to malignant neoplasms are higher in the provinces and regions with higher socioeconomic levels, which is the reverse of the situation for infectious diseases. Upon analyzing the standardized mortality rate for 1999–2001, statistically significant higher rates were seen in the departments of the Northeast for infectious diseases and external causes in both sexes, and for cancer of the uterus in women. Malignant neoplasms have statistically significant higher rates in certain departments of the provinces of Buenos Aires and Entre Ríos, as does suicide in certain departments in the country's central and southern regions (7).

In 2004, mortality from diseases of the circulatory system was 247.2 per 100,000 inhabitants in men and 229.0 per 100,000 in women. The sharp decline in cardiovascular diseases between 1990 and 2004 and the increase in mortality from "other causes" are noteworthy. National experts who were consulted agree that, while a decline in real mortality from cardiovascular diseases has been observed, much of the difference is due to a change in medical certification practices, which has led to an increase in the certification of respiratory insufficiency, which in this report falls under "other causes." This practice, then, masks an important number of ill-defined causes, a problem which the health authorities are addressing. (See Table 4.)

The mortality rate from malignant tumors remained stable in both men and women, as can be seen by comparing the 2004 and 1990 rates. Death rates from external causes decreased in both sexes in 2004 as compared to 1990, but mortality from infectious diseases increased during the period. Mortality from conditions originating in the perinatal period dropped by almost half between those two years. "Other causes" did increase during the

TABLE 4. Mortality by broad groups of causes, by age group, Argentina, 2004.

| | Total | | Age group | | | | | | | | | |
| | | | 0–4 | | 5–9 | | 10–19 | | 20–59 | | 60 and older | |
	No.	%	No.	%	No.	%	No.	%	No.	%	No.	%
1. Circulatory system	90,993	31	171	1	37	4	179	6	11,798	22	78,660	35
2. Malignant tumors	54,956	19	126	1	126	15	298	9	13,558	25	40,742	18
3. External causes	18,094	6	803	7	320	39	1,851	57	9,757	18	5,273	2
4. Childhood diseases	13,343	5	536	4	51	6	114	4	3,241	6	9,364	4
5. Perinatal	5,538	2	5,538	45	—	—	—	—	—	—	—	—
6. Other	89,374	30	4,367	36	262	32	685	21	12,024	22	71,834	32
7. Ill-defined	21,753	7	681	6	35	4	122	4	3,408	6	17,394	8

period, as did "ill-defined causes." The leading cause of death in 2002–2004 was cardiac insufficiency, followed by ischemic heart disease in men and cerebrovascular disease in women. The two causes responsible for most of the potential years of life lost (PYLL) in both sexes were perinatal causes and congenital anomalies. The third leading cause in men was traffic accidents; in women, it was cerebrovascular disease.

A report by a working group on mortality (still subject to review and not yet published) analyzed the pace of change in potential years of life lost (PYLL) between 0 years old and 75 years old in 1997–2003. In men, PYLL due to ischemic heart disease and cardiac insufficiency decreased by 4.3% and 6.2% per year, respectively. An overall increase in mortality from septicemia, diabetes, acute respiratory infections, urinary tract diseases, and especially, self-inflicted injuries (7.2% per year) and assaults (5.7% per year) has been noted. In women, PYLL due to malignant tumors of the breast and of the uterus decreased 2.5% and 3.6% per year, respectively. In both sexes, PYLL due to malnutrition decreased by more than 3% per year.

The leading natural or human-caused threats to which the country is exposed are floods (75%), storms (15.9%), urban fires (7.4%), snowfall (5.2%), and forest or vegetation fires (3.8%), as well as earthquakes, volcanic activity, and technological disasters. The most severe floods occur in the River Plate Basin, which includes the Paraná, Paraguay, Iguazú, and Uruguay rivers and their leading tributaries and minor outlets, and they affect the provinces of Misiones, Corrientes, Entre Ríos, Formosa, Chaco, and Santa Fe, as well as the Pampa plains, where they affect the provinces of Buenos Aires, La Pampa, the southern part of Santa Fe, and the southern part of Córdoba.

HEALTH OF POPULATION GROUPS

Children under 5 Years Old

There are 3,349,278 children in this age group, representing 9.2% of the country's population. Between 1990 and 2004, infant

mortality decreased 43.8%. Although deaths from avoidable causes have declined, in 2000 they still accounted for nearly two of every three infant deaths. In 2003, 53% of infant deaths were due to conditions originating in the perinatal period, 22% to congenital malformations, 10% to conditions of the respiratory system, 5% to infectious and parasitic diseases, and 3% to accidents. In 2004, 57% of postneonatal mortality was avoidable with prevention and appropriate treatment, and 56% of neonatal mortality was avoidable with timely diagnosis and treatment during pregnancy and childbirth, and with diagnosis and treatment of the newborn. In that same year, differences were observed among provinces, with infant mortality rates ranging from 25.1 per 1,000 live births in Formosa (Northeast Region) and 21.8 in Catamarca (Northwest Region) to 4.1 in Tierra de Fuego and 8.7 in the Federal Capital (8). The Northeast Region had the highest infant mortality rate in 2004 (20.0 per 1,000 live births), and Patagonia Region had the lowest (12.2 per 1,000 live births). The uneven distribution of infant mortality among the provinces, using the Gini index, increased between 1990 and 2002, decreasing again starting in 2002. A study classified infant mortality trends at the departmental level in 1994–2003 into five categories: markedly declining, moderately declining, indefinite, moderately increasing, and markedly increasing (9). Even wider gaps are seen when infant mortality is analyzed by the mother's level of education. In fact, during 2002–2004, the relative risk to infants born to illiterate mothers in comparison with infants born to mothers who had completed university training was 15.1 (infant mortality rate of 97.6 per 1,000 live births in illiterate mothers and 6.5 per 1,000 live births in university-educated mothers). Based on data from the Ministry of Health's National Directorate of Health Statistics, it is possible to conclude that the relative risk between these two groups in 1995–1997 was 10. The concentration coefficient in 2004, using the percentage of unmet basic needs (UBN) as a socioeconomic variable, was −0.103.

Argentina's infant mortality goal is the internationally established MDG of reducing the 1990 infant mortality rate by two-thirds by 2015; it is possible that the country will achieve it before the target date. The 2005 infant mortality rate of 13.3 per 1,000 live births was published in August 2006, showing progress toward achieving the goal.

Mortality in children under 5 years old also has decreased in the past 15 years. Between 1990 and 2004, it dropped from 29.6 deaths per 1,000 live births to 16.6 per 1,000 (or from 622.5 per 100,000 population to 365.9 per 100,000 population). In this case, the Gini coefficient also showed an increased inequality among jurisdictions, from 0.113 in 1990 to 0.132 in 2002, slightly decreasing to 0.120 in 2003. The Government took on an additional goal when it signed on to the MDG to reduce inequalities among jurisdictions in infant mortality and in mortality in children under 5 years old by 10% between 1990 and 2015, as measured by the Gini coefficient.

In 2004, conditions arising in the perinatal period and congenital anomalies were responsible for 53% and 22% of deaths in this age group, respectively; influenza and pneumonia were responsible for 4.0% and 4.2%, respectively.

Children 5–9 Years Old

According to the 2001 census, this population group totaled 3,471,217 (9.6% of the total population). In 2004 there were 831 deaths of children 5–9 years old, for a specific rate of 23.9 per 100,000 population, considerably lower than the 33.5 per 100,000 rate seen in 1990. External causes continue to rank as the leading cause of death, representing 38.5% of all causes; 43.1% for males. Traffic accidents were the leading cause of death in this group for both females and males, followed by congenital malformations in females and malignant neoplasms of the lymphatic tissue in males.

Adolescents 10–14 and 15–19 Years Old

The 10–14-year-old group totaled 3,427,200 in 2001, and the 15–19-year-old group totaled 3,188,304 (9.5% and 8.8% of the total population, respectively). That year, a total of 3,249 deaths were recorded (1,003 in the group 10–14 years old and 2,246 in the group 15–19 years old), with specific rates of 0.29 and 0.67, respectively, and a male/female ratio of 2.1:1. In the group 10–14 years old, external causes were responsible for 40.7% of all deaths, and for 63.5% in the group 15–19 years old. The suicide rate was 16.65 per 100,000 population among males 15–19 years old. For the group as a whole (10–19 years old), the leading cause of death in males in 2002–2004 was homicide, and in females, traffic accidents; the second leading cause in both sexes was suicide. As of December 2005 there were 1,671 cases of HIV/AIDS recorded in the country among 13–19-year-olds, with a male/female ratio of 1.96:1 for diagnoses of AIDS and 0.8:1 for HIV-positive diagnoses.

In 2004, the lifetime prevalence of alcoholic beverage consumption in youths 12–15 years old was 38.7%; the lifetime prevalence of tobacco use was 11.2%. With regard to the use of illegal substances, the prevalence was 0.8%; marijuana was far and away the drug of choice for youths who consume these substances (0.6%). Prevalences in the year prior to the survey were 34.0% for alcohol, 8.7% for tobacco, and 0.7% for illegal substances. In terms of consumption in the month prior to the survey, percentages were 15.2%, 6.4%, and 0.2%, respectively (10).

Among adolescents 14–19 years old, 61.4% reported that they had had sexual relations at least once (68.4% among males and 54% among females). The average age at the time of first relations is 15 years old (15.1 in females and 14.8 in males). Some 73.3% of adolescents used a condom the first time they had sexual relations (11).

In 2004 there were five deaths among adolescents 10–14 years old due to problems related to childbirth and 24 in the group 15–19 years old; the number of live births for mothers 10–14 years old was 2,629, and 103,809 in the group 15–19 years old. Of live births in 2004, 14.6% had mothers under 20 years old.

Adults 20–59 Years Old

In 2001, there were 17,952,174 persons aged 25–59 years (49.5% of the total population). Between 1990 and 2004 there was a decline in mortality rates due to malignant neoplasms in men and women in this age group, and an increase in mortality from infectious diseases. The leading cause of death in men in 2002–2004 was ischemic heart disease and in women, malignant neoplasm of the breast; the second leading cause for both sexes was cerebrovascular disease. In 2005, 72.7% of women 18–59 years old with unmet basic needs (UBN) had only public health service coverage; among men in this age group, the percentage was 67.8%. Among women without schooling, 68.5% had only public health service coverage, as compared with 9.8% of women who had completed university studies; in men the percentages were 64.8% and 9.6%, respectively. The prevalence of tobacco use among poor women with UBN was nearly the same as that of women whose basic needs are met (30.4% and 29.4%, respectively), but they had much lower rates of giving up tobacco use (7.9% and 13.9%, respectively); this difference is accentuated when the proportion of former smokers among uneducated women (4.3%) is compared to that of university graduates (17.3%). In men, the proportion of smokers among the poor (48.1%) is higher than among those whose basic needs are met (37.5%). In both groups, the proportions of former smokers were 15.1% and 17.6%, respectively. Among men, the significant difference in the proportion of former smokers by level of education (13.0% of those without formal schooling and 23.8% of those with university degrees) remained the same. Just 19.6% of the poorest women had ever had a mammogram, as compared to 44.9% of those whose basic needs are met. The proportion of uneducated women who had had this test was 17.5%, as compared to 64.4% of those with university degrees. In terms of prevention of cervical cancer, 62% of women with UBN had had a Papanicolaou test as compared with 78.1% of those whose basic needs were met. Some 57.2% of uneducated women had had a Papanicolaou test, while 90.8% of women with university degrees had had one.

The proportion of uneducated women who fail to protect themselves during sexual relations was 39%, while the proportion of those with university degrees was 29%. For males, behavior in terms of protection during sexual relations is similar to that of women (28.7% with UBN and 26.9% with basic needs met), but it is markedly worse when considering the level of education (55.4% among those without formal education and 31.5% among those with university degrees) (12).

Maternal mortality has changed little in the past decade (see Table 3), and the national rate was approximately 40 deaths per 100,000 live births. Nevertheless, there are differences among the provinces, with much higher figures seen in the Northeast and Northwest (Corrientes 104, La Rioja 136, and Jujuy 131); the figure in the Federal Capital was 20 in 2004. The Gini coefficient was 0.303 that year, which indicates a marked inequality in the distribution of maternal mortality among the Argentine provinces. The concentration coefficient in 2004, using the percentage of UBN as a socioeconomic variable, was –0.234 (8).

Older Adults 60 Years Old and Older

The percentage of persons older than 60 years old in 2001 was 13.4% (4,871,957); the percentage of those older than 65 years old was 9.9%, and the percentage of persons older than 80 years old was 2.1%. Between 1990 and 2004, mortality from infectious diseases increased and mortality from external causes decreased for men and women in this age group. Cardiac insufficiency was the leading cause of death in men and women; the second leading cause was ischemic heart disease in men and cerebrovascular disease in women. Life expectancy at 65 years old in men was 14 years and in women it was 19 years, while for individuals 80 years old it was four years in men and six in women.

In 2001, 19.6% of persons 65 years old and older lived alone, 44.6% lived in nuclear family households (just the couple or one or both partners with unmarried children), 34.9% lived in extended- or blended-family households, and 0.9% lived in nonfamily households, a category that may include old-age homes and residences for the elderly not identified as such. In May 2002, 30.3% of older adults who lived in urban areas lived below the poverty line. In 2001, 81.3% of the population over 65 had health coverage through social security, a health insurance plan, or mutual insurance. According to the National Survey of Risk Factors for Noncommunicable Diseases, in 2005, among women over 60 years old with UBN, 52.7% did not have social security coverage, as opposed to 11.3% of women whose needs were met; 54.4% of the former perceived their overall health as average or poor, as opposed to 40% of the latter (12). Of persons over 65 years old living in urban areas, 46.6% were members of the National Insti-

tute for Social Security for Retired People and Pensioners (PAMI, by its Spanish acronym), 12.5% were not enrolled in any plan (neither PAMI, social security, prepaid health insurance plan, nor mutual insurance), and the rest were covered by some other social security plan or mutual insurance plan (a combination of PAMI and social security or private health insurance plans). Between 2001 and 2005 there was a 6.2% increase in health coverage of one type or the other for older adults, although in 2001 the information came from the census and in 2005 it came from a survey. Of this population group, 12.7% needed assistance from third parties to carry out activities of daily living or instrumental activities of daily living (or everyday activities such as the ability to make purchases, prepare food, do housework, handle finances).[2] In the group 65–69 years old, 5.4% needed assistance from third parties; this figure increased to 9.6% in the group 70–79 years old and to 30.9% among those older than 80 years old.

Workers

Insurers of occupational risks, who provide health coverage to workers, reported 494,847 accidents in 2004, 19.4% more than in 2003; 83.5% were accidents in the workplace; 0.16% of them ended in death (12% more than in 2003). The highest accident rates are in the construction industry, with an incidence index of on-the-job accidents and occupational illnesses (II AT/EP, by its Spanish acronym) of 165; the index reflects the number of workers injured because of work or while working in a one-year period, for every 1,000 workers covered. Manufacturing industries rank second, with an II AT/EP of 116, and agriculture, third, with an II AT/EP of 113. If one considers the index of incidence of decedents (IIf), however, which reflects the number of injured workers who die because of work or while working in a one-year period, for every million workers covered, the activities with the highest numbers of deaths are mining and quarrying (IIf 600.6), with construction coming in second (IIf 317.1), and agriculture, third (IIf 286.9). The highest index of on-the-job accidents is found in small and midsized enterprises (13).

Because of the 2001 crisis, many formal-sector workers lost their jobs and joined the ranks of those working in the informal labor sector, with 446,686 workers leaving the Insurers of Occupational Risk coverage system (13). Consequently, a high percentage of the population was left without health coverage and had to rely on overextended public health services, and this crisis was aggravated by the lack of medical supplies.

Urban trash recyclers became entrenched as a result of the crisis. Work and sanitary conditions for this group, which operated outside the formal employment systems, deserve special attention. There are many children and adolescents who work this way

---

[2]This functionality in the elderly is measured with the IADL scale developed by M. P. Lawton and E. M. Brody and that evaluates independence, partial dependence, and total dependency levels.

in the country's cities (50% of all recyclers in the autonomous city of Buenos Aires) (*14*), and they are exposed to infectious agents and toxic substances, and run the risk of accidents, cuts, and skin problems.

It was estimated that in 2001, 4.7% of children 5–14 years old (6.6% of males and 2.9% of females) worked and that 3.6% worked fairly regularly. There were considerable differences by age and sex, however. In the group 10–14 years old, 7.8% worked, while in the group 5–9 years old, 1.7% worked; 65% of these children helped their parents, relatives, or neighbors, and 35% worked outside their immediate social circle. One of the principal consequences of child labor is that children drop out of school or must repeat grades. Of the children who worked during the year, 7.1% did not attend school, a threefold rate than that for the group of children who did not work (2.1%) (*4*).

A 2005 study on the behavior of sex workers in Argentine cities (*15*) showed that the average age for starting this line of work was 20.9 years, three years younger for men and transvestites. Financial need, along with the impossibility of obtaining other work, were the main reasons for entering sex work; according to the same study, the need to acquire money to acquire drugs was not an important reason for entering this type of work. Of those surveyed, 93.8% reported that they always used a condom during vaginal sex, 90.3% during anal sex, and just 8.5% during oral sex. Of those surveyed, 88.9% said they had had the HIV test at some point; the percentage dropped to 78.4% among men.

Persons with Disabilities

In 2002–2003, 7.1% of the population that lived in localities of more than 5,000 inhabitants had some type of disability; 20.6% of the households in these localities included at least one person with a disability. In the Cuyo (8.9%), Pampan (7.9%), and Northwest (7.6%) regions, the percentage of the population with a disability was higher than the national average. Of the population 65 years old and older, 28.3% had some type of disability. Some 73.9% of persons with disabilities had just one disability, 20.2% had two, and 5.9% had three or more. About 32% were motor disabilities, 14% were visual disabilities, 12% were auditory disabilities, and 12% were mental disabilities. Some 38.4% of persons with disabilities did not have any social security coverage and just 14.6% had a disability certificate (*16*).

Ethnic Groups

Argentina's health statistics are not broken down by ethnic group, and that impedes having the necessary information for a precise diagnosis of the health status of the country's indigenous peoples. The Ministry of Health implemented the National Health Program for Indigenous Peoples, aimed at taking actions based on respect for cultural diversity. The provinces in which this program is being carried out are Chaco, Formosa, Jujuy, Misiones, Salta, and Tucumán. The program seeks to strengthen the role of the health promoters; promote the creation of intercultural opportunities; generate cultural awareness among health teams; foster environmental improvement, care, and protection; implement health education activities; improve food and nutritional safety; and coordinate actions with other ministerial programs and entities (*17*). The report on the HIV/AIDS situation in 2005 included the results of a study of behavior and knowledge about the disease among native peoples (*18*). HIV is seen as an "external problem," a "white problem;" ignorance about the disease and failure to use condoms are widespread in this population (*19*).

HEALTH CONDITIONS AND PROBLEMS

COMMUNICABLE DISEASES

Vector-borne Diseases

No cases of **yellow fever** have been recorded in the country since 1966; since 1998, serologic studies conducted on samples that tested negative for dengue and other arboviruses also have tested negative for yellow fever. In July 2001, the National Epidemiologic Surveillance System issued a warning about the existence of an epizootic that had begun two months earlier in howler monkeys in land bordering the state of Rio Grande do Sul, Brazil. Well-defined ecological niches, the absence of adequate surveillance, and low coverage with yellow fever vaccine were seen as warranting fear of a jungle yellow fever risk scenario similar to that experienced in 1966. In addition, high indices of *Aedes aegypti* in large cities near the border increased the risk, because of the possibility of urbanization of yellow fever. In response, vaccination was stepped up, and 98.9% coverage was achieved in the risk areas. The house indices of *A. aegypti* infestation fell below 2% in the communities in the risk area.

Between 1997 and late 2005 there were 2,799 cases of **dengue** and five outbreaks, in 1998, 2000, 2002, 2003, and 2004; there were 1,522 cases reported in 2004. The provinces of Salta, Jujuy, Formosa, and Misiones reported autochthonous cases; 72.5% of the cases during that period were in the province of Salta. The 34 cases reported in 2005 were considered to be imported from neighboring countries. In 1998–2004, serotypes DEN-1, 2, and 3 circulated; in 1998, DEN-2; in 2000 and 2002, DEN-1; in 2003 DEN-1, 2, and 3 (in the province of Salta); and in 2004, DEN-3. In April 2006, an outbreak of dengue was declared in the provinces of Misiones, Formosa, Salta, and Jujuy, with almost 300 suspected and 56 confirmed cases; the outbreak concentrated in Puerto Iguazú, with serotype DEN-3 being identified.

In terms of controlling the transmission of *Trypanosoma cruzi* as a way to combat **Chagas' disease**, there are very different situations in the country, ranging from zones where transmission has been interrupted to zones with reliable proof of vector transmission through reporting of acute cases requiring vigorous control actions. It is estimated that approximately 4,810,000 persons in 962,000 homes in 19 provinces live in endemic zones, albeit concentrated in periruban and rural areas. The poorest sectors are the most affected.

The provinces have been classified into the following categories: seven provinces are considered to be at high risk (Formosa, Chaco, Santiago del Estero, Córdoba, La Rioja, San Juan, and Mendoza); seven are considered to be at moderate risk (Salta, Tucumán, Catamarca, San Luis, Santa Fe, Corrientes, and Misiones); five are considered to be at low risk (Jujuy, Entre Ríos, La Pampa, Neuquén, and Río Negro), in which interruption of vector transmission has been certified; and the rest are considered only at risk for non-vector transmission. In 2004, the indices of house infestation by *Triatoma infestans* in high-risk provinces ranged from 5% to 26%. Coverage of control in blood banks was increased, and a prevalence of 3.2% (1%–13%) was found. The identification of infected pregnant women has not been optimal, and just 15% of the 1,500 potentially infected and treatable newborns are detected each year. The leading impact indicator—prevalence in children under 5 years old—was 4.2% as measured in 13 provinces. Future goals for the Chagas' control program are shown in Table 3.

At this writing, Argentina's endemic region for **malaria** consists of a moderate-risk zone that includes the departments of Orán and San Martín, province of Salta, encompassing some 28,000 km², with an annual parasite index of less than 1%. The low-risk zone includes the rest of the province of Salta and the provinces of Jujuy, Misiones, and Corrientes. In 2000, there were 440 positive samples, 215 in 2001, 125 in 2002, 124 in 2003, 116 in 2004, and 215 in 2005. Between 50% and 75% of cases are imported.

Under the framework of the Argentina/Bolivia Agreement for Bilateral Technical Cooperation, surveillance and control activities have been undertaken with personnel from the National Coordinating Office for Vector Control in slightly more than 140 Bolivian border localities since 1996. In 2006 there was an outbreak of malaria in the Puerto Iguazú area, province of Misiones, near the border with Paraguay and Brazil; the outbreak was concurrent with an outbreak of classical dengue in the area, and 14 cases of malaria were detected. The surveillance and control actions carried out by the national and provincial programs included vector control through spatial spraying of insecticides and actively searching for undetected cases in the population.

Since **hantavirus** was first detected in Argentina in 1992, 714 cases have been confirmed. Reports of cases are on the rise—in 2002, 89 were reported. Several species and types of hantavirus that cause disease in humans have been described in the country: Andes virus; three Andes-like viruses (Hu39694, Lechiguanas, and Orán); Laguna Negra-like virus; and Bermejo virus. Three endemic regions have been identified: Salta and Jujuy in the northern region; Buenos Aires, Santa Fe, and Entre Ríos in the central region; and Neuquén, Río Negro, and Chubut in the southern region. The hantavirus increase mostly occurred in the central region, which had 60% of the reported cases; the southern

and northern regions remained stable. Variations in the behavior of rodent populations in each risk area result in differences in the dynamic of the disease from region to region that, in turn, make case emergence seasonally specific to each region. Cases increase between April and June in the south and center regions, and between October and December in the northern region. For the timely identification of cases, surveillance of nonspecific febrile syndrome was implemented as an initial measure in provinces that had seen cases. In 2004 and 2005 new areas were identified, such as along the Uruguay River in Entre Ríos, the northern stretch of the Paraná River in Misiones, and the city of Santa Fe.

In 1993–2005, 1,747 cases of **Argentine hemorrhagic fever** were reported, and 641 were confirmed. After a spike in 1998, reports of cases steadily dropped until 2005, when a new increase was recorded. The original fatality rate of Argentine hemorrhagic fever, which exceeded 50%, was reduced to 30% after maintenance therapy was standardized, and then fell to 2%–12% with the availability of the specific treatment (immune plasma). The development of the attenuated live Junín virus vaccine (Candid #1), and its administration to the population at highest risk, was an important achievement in decreasing the incidence of the disease: comparing pre-vaccine and post-vaccine 10-year periods, on average cases decreased from 9.8 per 100,000 population to 2.6.

The **Saint Louis encephalitis virus** has been recognized in Argentina since 1963. Retrospective serologic analyses conducted on temperate-zone patients showed the appearance of acute febrile illnesses associated with this virus in 0.9% to 1.8% of subjects. Just seven cases were reported between 2002 and 2004. In January 2005, an outbreak was declared in the province of Córdoba, with 55 cases (mainly in the capital and Greater Córdoba) and nine deaths. The virus was isolated in a batch of *Culex quinquefasciatus* mosquitoes captured in the homes and surrounding area of the cases. In 2006, cases were reported in the provinces of Córdoba, Santa Fe, and Entre Ríos.

Vaccine-preventable Diseases

Argentina remains free of **poliomyelitis** and **measles**. The last recorded case of poliomyelitis from wild poliovirus was seen in 1984, and the last case of measles was reported in 2000. Regional surveillance indicators established by PAHO are, for the most part, being satisfactorily met and, since 1995, vaccination coverage has exceeded 90%, although both the indicators and the cover-age vary somewhat from province to province. For example, in 2004 the coverage for DPT-Hib (diphtheria, pertussis, tetanus, and *Haemophilus influenzae* type b) reached a national average of 95.3%, but two jurisdictions (autonomous city of Buenos Aires and San Juan) had coverage under 90%. For the triple viral vaccine (measles, mumps, and rubella), the national average was 100%, but the province of Chubut only reached an 88% coverage.

Neonatal tetanus is no longer a public health problem as defined by PAHO (less than 1 case per 1,000 live births); cases of tetanus in all ages decreased from 220 in 1980 to 14 in 2005.

With the exception of **pertussis**, practically all the vaccine-preventable diseases have shown a marked decline in the past since the mid-1990s (1996–2005). Only pertussis outbreaks were observed in 2003–2005 in at least four provinces: Catamarca and Neuquén in 2004, and Salta and Tucumán in 2005. The highest attack rates were recorded in children under 5 years old, and they were concentrated in children under 1 year old, although cases also have been reported in adolescents and adults.

The **rubella** vaccine was introduced into the national vaccination system in 1998, with two doses of the triple viral vaccine (at one year and upon starting school). In 2003, use of the MR vaccine (measles and rubella) was initiated for all women immediately after delivery or immediately after abortion, and at the age of 11 for all children who had not had at least two doses after the age of 1. Coverage achieved since the introduction of the vaccine were between 90% and 100%. To eliminate **congenital rubella syndrome**, a national rubella vaccination campaign targeting all women 15–39 years old (estimated at 7,400,000) and at-risk men was proposed for September and October 2006.

Argentina is surrounded by countries with moderate endemicity and foci of high endemicity for **hepatitis A**. As a result, the hepatitis A vaccine was introduced into the national vaccination system in 2005; all children are administered a single dose at 12 months of age. An evaluation is planned to measure the effect of this strategy and help decide whether a second dose is needed. According to data from the National Epidemiologic Surveillance System, 63,006 cases of hepatitis A and non-specific hepatitis were reported (173.8 per 100,000 inhabitants) in 2004. This indicated an increase with respect to 2003 (139 per 100,000 inhabitants). In 2004 the Northwest and Cuyo regions had rates higher than the national rate (251 and 201, respectively).

With PAHO support, Argentina initiated surveillance of **rotavirus diarrhea** in sentinel centers in 2004. Partial results indicate that rotavirus disease is an important public health problem in the country. Several studies have been conducted to analyze the burden of rotavirus disease (*20, 21, 22*). The National Regulatory Authority has registered the rotavirus vaccine; it has been administered in the private sector since early 2006, but its inclusion in the national system over the short term is not expected.

Intestinal Infectious Diseases

There are little data on the prevalence of **intestinal parasitosis** in Argentina. A 2002 study conducted in extremely poor areas in Santa Fe showed a prevalence of ascaridiasis in schoolchildren in excess of 80% (*23*).

Chronic Communicable Diseases

New cases of **tuberculosis** in all its forms have been decreasing, with 38.1 per 100,000 population in 1990 and 29.1 per 100,000 in 2005. That same year, the provinces with the highest rates were Salta (79.4 per 100,000 population), Jujuy (70.5), and Chaco

(48.2); those with the lowest were Mendoza (7.9), San Juan, and La Rioja (8.7 in each case).

In 2003–2004, the concentration coefficient, using unmet basic needs (UBN) of Argentina's departments as a socioeconomic variable, was 0.22. Approximately 35% of tuberculosis cases were seen in 20% of persons living in departments with higher percentages of UBN. In 2005, 85.3% of tuberculosis cases were pulmonary, 13.3% affected children under 15 years old, and, among the pulmonary cases in individuals over 15 years old, 72.6% were bacteriologically confirmed. That same year, eight cases of tuberculous meningitis were reported in children under 5 years old, seven of whom lived in the province of Buenos Aires.

In 2005, 3.9% of persons living with AIDS were co-infected with tuberculosis (445 cases of tuberculosis in 11,242 AIDS cases), a similar figure as seen in 2003 and 2004 and lower than that recorded in 2001, when the highest percentage, 6.4%, was reached. The mortality rate from tuberculosis fell from 3.6 to 2.2 cases per 100,000 population, for a drop of 39.8% between 1990 and 2004. The provinces with the highest mortality rates in 2003–2004 were Jujuy (9.0 per 100,000 population), Formosa (7.1), and Chaco (6.1); those with the lowest mortality rates were La Pampa (0.6), La Rioja (0.7), and Neuquén (0.9).

In 2003, information was collected on treatment results of 78.5% of tuberculosis patients with positive bacilloscopy. Among them, the success rate was 76.6%, the abandonment rate, 10.8%, and the mortality rate, 6.9%. There were five jurisdictions with abandonment rates higher than the national average, including the province of Buenos Aires and the autonomous city of Buenos Aires, which had 39% of the evaluated cases with positive bacilloscopy, with abandonment rates of 14.4% and 12.8%, respectively. The provinces of Formosa, Mendoza, and Corrientes had abandonment rates of 13.5%, 15.1%, and 26.3%, respectively. Of patients with positive bacilloscopy, 57.8% received Directly Observed Treatment, Short Course (DOTS), with variations from 0% to 100%, depending on the jurisdiction. In eight jurisdictions, DOTS coverage exceeded 95%: the five jurisdictions of the southern region (Tierra del Fuego, Santa Cruz, Chubut, Río Negro, and Neuquén), Chaco, Santa Fe, and Córdoba. Yet, four jurisdictions had DOTS coverage below 40%: the autonomous city of Buenos Aires (33.9%), the province of Buenos Aires (31.3%), Misiones (23.6%), and Santiago del Estero (0%). Progress toward the MDG pertaining to tuberculosis is shown in Table 3.

Leprosy, which is endemic in Argentina, is distributed in 12 provinces, mainly in the provinces of Northeast, Northwest, and Central; the disease is considered to be of moderate magnitude in the country. The trend in case detection stabilized in the 1990s at 450–500 new cases per year; the prevalence decreased from 0.82 per 10,000 population in 1997 (the year that marked achievement of the goal of eliminating leprosy as a public health problem) to 0.22 per 10,000 in 2005. In the latter year the prevalence/detection quotient was 1.5, while in 1997 it was 5.3. Multibacterial forms predominate in persons older than 15 years old, and there was a decreasing number of cases with grade 2 disability at the time of diagnosis. The current strategy, with a national prevalence under 1 per 10,000 population, gives priority to active case search and the estimation of hidden prevalence.

Acute Respiratory Infections

In 1997–2005, between 800,000 and 1 million cases of **influenza-type syndrome** per year were reported to the National Epidemiologic Surveillance System. The epidemic years were 1999, 2003, and 2004, and in those years hospitalizations increased to the overflow point, especially in pediatric hospitals. In 2005, 959,046 cases of influenza-type illnesses were reported, for a rate of 2,644.9 per 100,000 population. That same year, laboratory surveillance of 22,480 samples from patients with acute lower respiratory infection established 2.8% of positive diagnoses for **influenza A** and 0.5% for **influenza B**; in 2,436 samples from patients with influenza-type syndrome detected in the sentinel units, 5.6% of diagnoses were positive for influenza A and 1.1% were positive for influenza B.

HIV/AIDS and Other Sexually Transmitted Infections

Estimates made in 2005 by the Joint United Nations Program on HIV/AIDS (UNAIDS), the World Health Organization (WHO), and the National Program Against Human Retroviruses, AIDS, and Sexually Transmitted Diseases showed that approximately 127,000 (numbers ranging from 115,000 to 134,000) persons were living with HIV/AIDS in Argentina, 60% of whom were unaware of their serologic status. Between 1982, when the first case was recorded in the country, and December 31, 2005, 30,496 cases of AIDS and 32,411 HIV-infected persons were notified to the National Program. The leading characteristics of the epidemic in Argentina are: 1) it increasingly affects women, which increases the risk of vertical transmission, and the highest concentration of cases occurs in sexually active age groups; 2) it essentially affects the economically active age groups in both sexes, that is, individuals 25–34 years old; 3) it is increasingly being transmitted through heterosexual relations (55.6% of cases in 2004), and 4) it affects the poorest and least educated sectors. The incidence of HIV infection shows a rising trend, with values of 1.5 per 100,000 population in 1990, 4.03 in 2000, and 10.01 in 2004. The male/female ratio for AIDS dropped from 6.5:1 in 1990 to 2.4:1 in 2004; for HIV infection it was 1.3 men for every woman in 2004. Fully half of persons living with AIDS are 25–34 years old. Children under 13 years old represented 9.7% of the total recorded cases, with 94.8% of them caused by vertical transmission. AIDS is concentrated in the main urban centers: Greater Buenos Aires, Rosario, Córdoba, and Santa Fe. The mortality rate from AIDS in 2004 was 3.8 per 100,000 population.

In terms of other sexually transmitted infections, 675 cases of congenital **syphilis** were reported to the National Epidemiologic Surveillance System in 2002; in 2003, 742 cases were reported, and in 2004 and 2005, 838 and 583, respectively, for rates of 0.9–1.2 per 1,000 live births. The most seriously affected regions were Northwest and Northeast, especially the latter, where the rates in 2002–2005 were 4.5, 3.7, 2.6, and 2.1 times higher than the overall national rate. Table 5 shows rates of congenital syphilis and other sexually transmitted infections, by region, between 2002 and 2005.

Zoonoses

In 2005, programs were developed to prevent the entry of **avian flu** and **bovine spongiform encephalopathy** into the country; a drill was held with public and private sector institutions to prepare for the possibility. The program for the control of **foot-and-mouth disease** continues to be implemented throughout the national territory, in order to hold on to the "free with vaccination" status. **Animal rabies** remains endemic in the country's north, with cases reported in dogs and bovines in the provinces of Jujuy and Salta. In 2005, 66 cases of animal rabies were reported nationwide (34 in bovines, 16 in dogs and cats, 8 in bats, and 8 in other animals).

In April 2006, an outbreak of **West Nile virus** in horses was declared in the province of Entre Ríos, the first time such an outbreak had been seen in Argentina. Detection and laboratory diagnosis were rapid and the surveillance system was activated. The country has human and laboratory resources for diagnosing infection with this virus.

TABLE 5. Rates[a] of congenital syphilis and other sexually transmitted infections (STIs), by region, Argentina, 2002–2005.

	Congenital syphilis				Other STIs			
	2002	2003	2004	2005	2002	2003	2004	2005
Central	0.5	0.8	1.0	0.8	41.0	39.4	33.7	30.0
Cuyo	0.1	0.1	0.6	0.5	29.3	28.6	41.6	23.0
Northeast	4.5	4.2	3.2	1.7	236.7	313.0	371.9	339.8
Northwest	1.0	0.8	1.3	0.9	287.6	310.8	344.2	274.3
South	0.3	0.4	0.2	0.3	44.5	49.8	59.7	66.1
Total	**1.0**	**1.1**	**1.2**	**0.9**	**86.8**	**95.7**	**102.9**	**88.4**

[a]Rates for congenital syphilis are presented per 1,000 live births; rates for other STIs are presented per 100,000 population.
Source: National Epidemiologic Surveillance System, Ministry of Health.

TABLE 6. Nutritional and metabolic deficiencies (%), by region, Argentina, 2005.

	Argentina	Greater Buenos Aires	Cuyo	Northeast	Northwest	Central	South
Low weight-for-age	3.8	3.3	4.0	5.8	3.9	3.7	2.6
Low height-for-age	4.2	3.7	3.5	4.8	4.0	4.9	3.6
Low weight-for-height	1.2	1.1	2.8	1.2	1.2	1.1	1.0
High weight-for-height	6.6	8.3	5.1	3.0	4.4	7.2	6.3
Anemia in children 6 months to 5 years	15.9	17.9	10.0	22.1	14.0	13.8	15.6
Anemia in children 6 to 23 months	33.2	34.9	23.5	33.2	44.0	30.1	30.9
Overweight, women 19–49 years	24.9	24.8	24.4	20.2	28.1	24.9	26.5
Obesity, women 19–49 years	19.4	18.2	15.9	21.1	20.4	20.5	22.6
Anemia, women 10–49 years	17.1	20.6	14.7	21.8	15.7	12.6	16.2
Cholesterol >170 mg/dl, women 10–19 years	21.5	23.2	30.5	19.4	19.9	34.3	17.0
Cholesterol >200 mg/dl, women 20–49 years	23.4	27.2	12.0	19.8	17.3	28.1	20.4

Source: 2005 National Health and Nutrition Survey.

NONCOMMUNICABLE DISEASES

Metabolic and Nutritional Diseases

According to the Ministry of Health's 2005 National Nutrition and Health Survey, almost half of Argentine women are overweight or obese (Table 6). A study covering four cities in Argentina's central area showed that between 22.4% and 30.8% of persons older than 20 years old were obese, and between 6.5% and 7.7% of them had **diabetes mellitus** (*24*). According to the data from the National Survey of Risk Factors for Noncommunicable Diseases (2005), 15.8% of the uneducated population older than 18 years old said they had hyperglycemia, as opposed to 5.3% of university graduates.

Cardiovascular Diseases

Various blood pressure studies showed wide variability in the prevalence of **hypertension**. In a study conducted in Córdoba in persons 15–85 years old, the prevalence was 29.9%; just 13.0% of hypertensive individuals were being treated and under control (*25*). In another study involving four cities in the country's central area, the prevalence of hypertension in individuals over 20 years old ranged from 27.9% to 43.6%; the prevalence of hyperlipidemia ranged from 24.2% to 36.4%. According to the Ministry of Health's 2005 National Nutrition and Health Survey, approximately one woman in five aged 10–49 years old has high cholesterol.

According to the National Survey of Risk Factors for Noncommunicable Diseases (2005), 56.8% of the uneducated population had had their cholesterol checked at least once and, of those, 44.4% said it was high. The proportions were 79.1%, and 26% among those who had completed university training. Among Argentineans older than 18 years old with no schooling who were interviewed, 49.2% said they did not have high blood pressure, as opposed to 72.7% of university graduates.

Malignant Neoplasms

Between 1997 and 2004, malignant neoplasms were the second leading cause of death, after diseases of the circulatory system, and represented 18%–19% of all deaths. Between 1980 and 2001, the mortality rate from **lung cancer** declined by approximately 1% per year in men. In women, however, rates rose approximately 1.5% per year, except in Cuyo, where the rates remained virtually the same. In terms of **breast cancer**, mortality rates have declined in women under 65 years old since 1991, but they increased 1.6% per year among women older than 74 years old starting in 1980. In the country as a whole, and more so in certain provinces, **cancer of the uterus** is a serious public health problem. Since 1991, a small decrease in mortality from this cancer has been noted, except in the Northwest region, where there was a slight increase of 0.2% a year.

OTHER HEALTH PROBLEMS OR ISSUES

Disasters

The database of the country's disasters in recent years showed that floods prevailed. In areas vulnerable to floods, community leaders were trained in risk management so they could come up with the solutions most appropriate for their natural, economic, social, and political context (*26*). The worst natural disaster in recent years was doubtless the flood in the city of Santa Fe in April 2003, which left more than 30% of that city's population under water, and resulted in 75,036 people being evacuated, 20,000 homes damaged, and 13% of available hospital beds lost.

Violence and Other External Causes

The Ministry of Justice's Victimization Survey, conducted in the autonomous city of Buenos Aires in 2003, showed that 37.5% of persons older than 14 years old said they had been the victim of at least one crime (mostly crimes against property), a lower figure than ones seen in 2000, 2001, and 2002, according to the National Directorate of Crime Policy.

The Injury Surveillance System was put in place in September 2004; by June 2006, 36 sentinel units had been included. Data accumulated up to that date on 27,836 accidents indicate that 81.3% were unintentional, 10.4% were intentional against others, 1.7% were self-inflicted, and the rest, undetermined. Most accidents are concentrated in persons 15–29 years old (34.6%) and in persons 30–44 years old (19.6%); 68.4% are minor, 25.9% are moderate, and 5.7% are serious. Men are the victims in 66.9% of accidents, the male/female ratio is of 2.02:1, and 0.56% of injury events cause death, with a male/female ratio of 2.8:1.

Mental Health and Addictions

There are no updated national epidemiologic data on mental health, except for the results of the disabilities survey. In 2004, 7.8% of the population 16–65 years old had consumed an illegal psychoactive substance at least once, 2.1% had done so in the year before the survey, and 0.8% had done so in the month before the survey. Marijuana and cocaine are the most used substances, in that order.

Oral Health

Based on prior favorable experiences, such as a more than 40% reduction in the DMF (decayed, missing, and filled teeth) index in the province of Santa Fe between 1990 and 2000, the fluoridation of water for human consumption in provinces that require it was reactivated in 2005. It is expected that in 2010, about 50% of the population will be receiving fluoridated water. Moreover, the criteria for conducting an epidemiological survey in all the provincial jurisdictions were standardized.

Hemolytic Uremic Syndrome

The rate of hemolytic uremic syndrome among children under 5 years old was approximately 8.5 per 100,000 children in this age group between 1995 and 2000; since 2001 it has never fallen below 10.4, and it peaked in 2005 (13.9). The mortality rate remained stable in 1995–2005, with an average of 3.3%, a minimum of 2.2% in 1998, and a maximum of 4.8% in 2001. In 2005 the mortality rate was 3.4%. In 2005, 464 cases of hemolytic uremic syndrome were reported, 62% in children under 2 years old. The majority of cases occurred in the warm months (55%). The provinces with the highest hospital-reporting rates were La Pampa (34.4 per 100,000 children under 5 years old) and Neuquén (31.6).

RESPONSE OF THE HEALTH SECTOR

Health Policies and Plans

Since 2002, a Consultative Council has provided a forum for discussion and for forging national-level agreements on health matters with the country's various sectors. The Council ranks include various players connected to the health system, including representatives of community organizations; health providers, financers, and professionals; universities; and well-respected institutions and individuals. The Council also has four standing committees: Human Resources, Costs and Financing, Technology, and Noncommunicable Diseases.

By constitutional mandate, the provinces are responsible for caring for the population's health. The municipalities, especially those with the highest populations and greatest economic resources, also plan and implement health activities. The transfer, in the early 1990s, of a group of hospitals and specialized institutes from the federal Government to the provinces was one of the last stages in the decentralization of the health services. This complex process resulted in varying levels of hospital autonomy, administrative and financial management, human resources policies, and services delivered to the population. In turn, this diversity made it impossible to offer a standard coverage of public health care for all the population. Moreover, geographic location also affects access to public health units.

In the provinces, the performance of essential public health functions is the responsibility of ministries or secretariats of health, with institutional development varying according to the size of the population and the available resources. Health services are delivered through provincial public sector networks and by the private sector. In provinces with higher populations and more economic resources, municipalities administer primary health care services and, in some cases, more complex hospitals, although proportionally there are few municipal health care facilities. In 2006, some provinces were actively devolving primary health care level services to the municipalities. Social security and the private sector have clearly separate functions: the entities responsible for handling financing (social security and health insurers) do not operate their own services as a rule, and instead contract them out to public and private providers throughout the country.

Health Strategies and Programs

During the social and economic upheaval the country lived through in 2001–2005, dialogue channels became consolidated among various players dealing in health at different levels of the State, and this dialogue continued in subsequent years. Finally, at the Council of Federal Health Agencies (COFESA, by its Spanish acronym), one of the leading forums where provinces and the federal Government formulate health policies by consensus, the bases of the 2004–2007 Federal Health Plan were agreed on; the Plan was submitted by Argentina's President in May 2004. The Plan set four avenues for action and embraced the primary health care strategy as the cornerstone for the system's organization. Priority was given to strengthening equality of access to health care and to promoting community participation at all levels. The established targets complemented the country's agreement in connection with the Millennium Development Goals.

FIGURE 2. General scheme and estimated coverage of the health system, Argentina, 2001.

Total population: 37.1 million

PUBLIC SUBSECTOR	SOCIAL SECURITY SUBSECTOR	PRIVATE SUBSECTOR
Population covered by the public health service delivery system **17.8 million (48%)** (Principally under the direct responsibility of the provinces and, in a few cases, the municipalities and the federal Government)	Population covered by publicly funded social welfare activities (social security institutions) **17.5 million (47.2%)** (Principally through private health service providers)	Population covered by health insurance plans **2.8 million (7.5%)** Of this population **1.0 million** also has coverage through social security

Population covered by public health programs under the responsibility of the federal Government and the provincial governments: **37.1 million (100%)**

Source: Adapted from: González García G., Tobar F. *Salud para los argentinos* 2003. Estimates based on the 2001 National Census of Population and Housing (INDEC) and the 2001 Quality of Life Survey (Social Policy Evaluation and Monitoring System, under the Ministry of Social Development and the Environment).

Organization of the Health System

Argentina's health system reflects the federal nature of the country's government, whereby provinces retain the authority to manage and deliver health care within their jurisdiction. The system encompasses three subsectors: public, private, and social security. The latter two are closely connected, given that the institutions responsible for social security contract out many health services to private health service providers of different types and sizes (Figure 2).

In 2006, the health system was characterized by a high level of segmentation and fragmentation, which resulted in poor coordination among subsectors, inequality in financing, inequities in health care quality, and many access barriers for some population groups. In 2003, social security institutions covered approximately 17.5 million people (47.2% of the total population), distributed throughout almost 300 entities of varying sizes and importance. It is estimated that the public subsector covered 17.8 million persons (48%) and private health insurance plans covered 2.8 million persons, of which 1 million also had social security coverage.

Throughout its history, the health system has operated with a degree of inefficiency and inequity. The diverse coverage that is available affects the 24 provincial public systems, approximately 300 national social security institutions, 24 provincial social security institutions, a few dozen health insurance plans, private health insurance plans, and many mutual insurance systems; the National Institute for Social Services for Retired People and Pen-

sioners, known for its Spanish acronym, PAMI, also is affected. In 1993 a "free choice" option became available to workers affiliated with the social security system, as part of a deregulation effort and to improve efficiencies. The fragmentation and lack of coordination of this group of institutions have curtailed the establishment of a unified, efficient, universal health system. Thus, social security is managed by institutions that are vary greatly in terms of the type of population they serve, the coverage they offer, the financial resources per member, operating modalities, and health service networks they contract out to.

The Ministry of Health is responsible for determining the health sector's objectives and policies and for executing the plans, programs, and projects for the area under its jurisdiction, which are developed in accordance with directives from the Executive Branch. The Ministry also oversees the operation of the health services, facilities, and institutions, and conducts the overall planning for the sector in coordination with provincial health authorities. It is also responsible for issuing regulations and procedures to guarantee the quality of health care, as agreed to by consensus with the provinces, and participates in approving the health facility projects that are built by private companies. Through the National Food, Drug, and Health Technology Administration, the Ministry participates in matters related to the development, distribution, and marketing of products directly related to health. The Administration is responsible for implementing and enforcing compliance with legal, scientific, technical, and administrative provisions under its jurisdiction.

The Superintendency of Health Services is the regulatory and controlling agency overseeing those who handle the National Health Insurance (social security) System. Within the Congress, the Senate's Health and Sport Committees and the Chamber of Deputies' Social Action and Public Health Committees are responsible for passing judgment on health and medical-social activities; hygiene; sanitation; preventive medicine and nutrition; hospital subsidies; and societies, corporations, or institutions that carry out health-related activities.

Public Health Services

The 2004–2007 Federal Health Plan assigns priority to primary care and allocates more funds toward promotion and prevention activities. The Plan considers the gradual, systematic, and organized decentralization of these activities and plans for local governments to take on the implementation of this strategy by developing healthy policies, providing information, and modeling conduct.

Various national programs are being implemented in Argentina with the goal of preventing and controlling certain diseases which, because of their importance, require special efforts from the authorities and civil society. The principal programs and their objectives are described below.

The National Program to Combat Human Retrovirus and Sexually Transmitted Infections aims to prevent sexual and perinatal transmission; to prevent transmission through blood, hemoderivatives, and transplants, and during invasive procedures; to prevent the spread of infection among drug users; to reduce the individual, family, and socioeconomic impact of the epidemic; to reinforce analysis of the epidemic's situation and trend; and to consolidate its administrative and management aspects. The program provides antiretroviral drugs to HIV-infected persons.

The National Program for the Control of Tuberculosis is part of the country's health structure, whereby its activities are carried out through the health services. The Program has four levels (central, provincial, intermediate, and local), each with well-defined responsibilities. The central level is at the Ministry of Health, and the responsible entity is the National Institute for Respiratory Diseases Dr. Emilio Coni, which falls under the National Administration of Laboratories and Health Institutes Dr. Carlos G. Malbrán, headquartered in the city of Santa Fe. The provincial level includes the country's 23 provinces and the autonomous city of Buenos Aires. The Program's goals are to reduce morbidity and mortality from tuberculosis, transmission of tuberculous infection, and resistance of *Mycobacterium tuberculosis* to antibiotics. The Program's strategic objectives are to strengthen the reliance of the Directly Observed Treatment, Short Course (DOTS) strategy in all jurisdictions of the country and target efforts in priority departments where the magnitude of the disease is greater.

The National Program for the Control of Chagas' Disease consists of 19 provincial programs; it conducts health promotion and disease prevention activities, as well as diagnosing and treating the disease. The Program does not include any rehabilitation, although it endeavor to improve the hospital network for caring for cardiopathies and transplants. Different parties plan and execute activities, including agents of the national and provincial jurisdictions, health professionals or health promoters, municipal officials, and community leaders, who have the support and supervision of the national commission for vector control.

In 2004–2005, the Ministry of Health launched the National Mass Parasite Eradication Program. Working through the Programa Remediar (a program that distributes medication without charge to vulnerable populations), the Program began an intense campaign that first worked to identify the most problematic foci in the province of Santa Fe and gradually extended the effort to the other affected provinces; mebendazole was distributed to population groups without basic sanitary services.

The Tobacco Control Program channels its work along five key avenues: restrict tobacco advertising, increase the price of cigarettes, launch a strong social-communication campaign, create smoke-free environments, and offer smoking-cessation services.

The Renal Health Program, executed by the Ministry of Health's Special Programs Administration, aims to prevent kidney disease and promote health within the social security system. Along with the Superintendency of Health Services, the Argentine Cardiology Society, and the Argentine Federation of Cardiology, it has developed a program for identifying risk factors and primary prevention of cardiovascular diseases, targeting men 30–49 years old and women 40–59 years old.

The National Program for Healthy Sexuality and Responsible Reproduction was established in 2002 through the enactment of Law No. 25,673. In its early years, the program focused on strengthening provincial programs by providing technical assistance, training, and financing human resources to reinforce existing teams. In 2006, hormonal contraceptives, IUDs, and condoms were distributed for free to 1,925,950 men and women who sought care through the public system. Women covered by social security or heath insurance plans under the Compulsory Medical Program also were ensured coverage.

Problems with basic sanitation remain unresolved. According to the 2001 National Census of Population and Housing, just 47.2% of the households were connected to a sewer system, 24.2% relied on septic tanks and drainage pits, and the remaining 27% relied on wells or had no means of disposal.

By Executive Branch decree, the National Agency for Water and Sanitation Works has been charged with constructing Argentina's major basic sanitation works. In 1993, the State made Aguas Argentinas responsible for managing the drinking water and sewer services for the autonomous city of Buenos Aires and 17 metropolitan area sections (where a third of the country's

Healthy Sexuality and Responsible Procreation

Beginning in 2001, one-third of maternal deaths in Argentina were due to abortions to terminate unwanted pregnancies, one of every seven women giving birth were adolescents, and two-thirds of reported AIDS cases were acquired by having unprotected sex. In addition, the population's most vulnerable sectors—youths, women, and the poorest groups—had serious problems accessing information on responsible procreation. Moreover, it was clear that nearly all maternal deaths could be drastically reduced through prevention efforts and by providing proper care during pregnancy and delivery.

Given these factors, the Government embraced far-reaching decisions that led to effective actions designed to overcome the problems. In October 2002, Law No. 25,673, which created the national healthy sexuality and responsible procreation program, was enacted by broad parliamentary consensus and strong support of nongovernmental organizations and civil society. Early on, the program aimed at strengthening provincial programs by providing technical assistance, as well as training and financing of human resources to bolster existing teams. The program also acquired and then distributed throughout the country contraceptives at a cost of several tens of millions of Argentine pesos.

In 2006, some two million men and women coming to the public health system for care had access to free hormonal contraceptives, IUDs, and condoms. Women enrolled in the social security system and health insurance schemes also were covered through the Compulsory Medical Program. That same year, the National Congress promulgated Law No. 26,130, dealing with surgical contraception, and Law No. 26,150 dealing with comprehensive sexual education; it also ratified the Optional Protocol of the Convention on the Elimination of All Forms of Discrimination against Women (CEDAW), whereby Argentinean women now can bring claims regarding the infringement of their rights to an international and impartial tribunal of experts.

population lives); it produced 3,100,000 m^3 of water per day. In March 2006 the contract was rescinded, and the State assumed responsibility for providing this service. To this end, it made important investments and created Agua y Saneamiento de Argentina, a state-owned enterprise.

A little more than 2,200 municipalities have been given primary responsibility for handling a household waste management service. In some cases, the collection and disposal of household waste is carried out by the municipality itself; in many other instances, the service has been outsourced to private companies. According to official data for 2004, Argentina produces 12,325,000 tons of household waste every year, with an average per capita rate of 0.91 kg/day. The autonomous city of Buenos Aires is among the heavier producers, with average waste generation of 1.52 kg/inhabitant/day; Misiones is among the lowest, with 0.44 kg/inhabitant/day (5).

In 2004, the Government, through its Secretariat for the Environment and Sustainable Development, drew up the National Strategy for the Comprehensive Management of Urban Solid Waste, in order to assess the solid waste situation and come up with appropriate waste treatment and technology for disposing solid waste in an environmentally sound manner. In September 2004, Law 25,916 on management of household solid waste was enacted. As a supplement to the National Strategy for the Com-

prehensive Management of Urban Solid Waste, the National Strategy on Hazardous Household Waste was presented in 2005. The latter strategy aims to address the handling of this waste by promoting its separate collection. In 2005, the Ministry of Health, assisted by the Maternal and Child Health and Nutrition Program, diagnosed waste management in hospitals; it acknowledged that there were major deficiencies, but also identified potential referral centers for managing waste in health facilities through an appropriate action plan implemented in 2006.

Law 20,284 of 1973 established air-quality standards and set levels for issuing contamination alerts, alarms, and emergencies. Regulations for this law were never enacted, rendering the legislation barely operational. Decree 831/93, which promulgates regulations for National Law 24,051 on hazardous waste, establishes guidelines for gaseous emissions and air quality; values have not been updated, however.

Law No. 1,356 on the atmospheric contamination of the autonomous city of Buenos Aires establishes air quality standards and requires ongoing monitoring. Currently, the autonomous city of Buenos Aires monitors and controls fixed and mobile air-pollution sources. The Dock Sud petrochemical plant, which is located extremely close to the city, has approximately 60 smokestacks that release an average of 15 million m^3 an hour of air with various polluting gases. A recent study shows high levels of benzene, toluene, lead, and sulphur dioxide (*27*), with higher concentrations than WHO recommends.

Argentina is party to the Stockholm Convention on Persistent Organic Pollutants and has a National Implementation Plan (NIP) in place, which is executed through the Secretariat for the Environment and Sustainable Development. In 2004, the National Inventory of Dioxins and Furans was published, and emission factors were identified according to activities and sources that generate these toxins. In 2002, Law 25,670, on the Minimum Requirements for the Elimination and Management of Persistent Organic Pollutants, which provides for their total elimination by 2010, was promulgated.

In 2003, the most important clandestine burial site for organochlorate pesticides (mostly hexachlorocyclohexane) known up to then in Argentina was removed in the province of Santiago del Estero. The toxins had been buried in 1990, and 200 metric tons of residues were removed, treated, and disposed of.

There are 21 centers for toxicological information, advice, and assistance in the country, operating under the aegis of the National Program for the Prevention and Control of Poisoning. Since most centers are located in the wealthiest provinces, the least developed provinces must rely on local programs for their poisoning prevention and control activities. The centers provide advisory assistance on pesticide poisoning, as well as on potentially toxic drugs, substances, and chemical products. In 2005, two national multicentric studies were conducted on agrochemicals and domestic pesticides. The Argentine Toxicology Network, which is comprised of scientific associations, governmental entities, and specialized laboratories, operates with the support of the virtual health and environment library.

The National Food Institute authorizes, registers, controls, and oversees food through a food surveillance system. The National Food Safety and Quality Service protects food by monitoring animal and vegetable products produced for internal use and export. In 2005, in coordination with a very active healthy municipalities network, local initiatives focusing on food production and safety began to be developed. These initiatives operate through integrated programs in which the municipalities, the provinces, and the federal Government participate; the private sector and civil society also play an active part. The process has been coupled with a vigorous development of microenterprises.

The National Directorate of Health Emergencies is the agency charged with preventing disasters and mitigating their effect. There are 1,287 health establishments in the provinces that are at highest risk for earthquakes, 8,548 in the flood zones, and 2,220 in the zones most affected by snowfall. There is no single plan for response to natural disasters, because each province develops its own. Approximately 30% of the hospitals have disaster plans. There also are disaster response teams in place at the national and provincial levels, and the National Directorate also has its own stockpiles of essential drugs and supplies for these emergencies. Unpublished data from the survey on disaster prepara-

tion and mitigation by the health sector, which was discussed at the PAHO Regional Meeting of Disaster Coordinators in May 2006, indicate that 42% of the hospitals built in the past five years guarantee that they can continue to operate in case of disasters, and 20% of the hospitals have carried out structural and nonstructural vulnerability studies.

In 2002, the Ministry of Health began working on a General Contingency Plan for Influenza and SARS Pandemics. The influenza surveillance and control activities were organized around five points: a) surveillance of avian flu; b) surveillance through the National Epidemiologic Surveillance System, sentinel units for influenza, and the respiratory virus network; c) vaccines and antivirals; d) public health measures; and e) communication.

The approval in 2005 of the International Health Regulations provides the country with a framework for addressing new challenges in the control of communicable diseases.

Individual Care Services

All the provinces and the autonomous city of Buenos Aires have a wide network of hospital and outpatient services operated by both public and private providers. There are 17,845 health care establishments in the country, and 153,065 hospital beds available at the national level (about evenly split between publicly owned and privately owned). Localized differences notwithstanding, various subsectors and jurisdictions have in recent years been offering new modalities of care: outpatient care, brief hospitalization, day hospital, home care, and others. There are 14,534 outpatient health facilities in the country (*28*).

In the public sector, the auxiliary diagnostic services and blood banks are integrated into the health service systems that operate mainly in the provinces and, sometimes, in the municipalities. In the private sector, these services are also found in the health care facilities, although in some localities there are autonomous diagnostic support units that contract for services with the social security institutions. In 1983, a National Blood Program was instituted by law. The Ministry of Health and the provincial health authorities promote voluntary donation under the framework of the National Blood Plan. In 2005 there were 578 blood collection centers, 333 public and 245 private. That same year, those centers processed 751,412 blood units. The current trend is toward reduction of and improvement in the quality of those centers (in 1999 there were 781 centers) (*29*).

There were 15,916 public sector psychiatric beds in 2002. There are mental health reform initiatives in varying states of implementation in some provinces and in the capital. Law 448/00 (Law on Mental Health for the city of Buenos Aires), which calls for shifting mental health services from the hospital-based system currently in place to a system incorporated into the overall health system, has not yet been implemented, primarily due to corporate reasons. There is an overall trend toward acceptance of psychiatric reforms, and national legislators from various parties are working on draft mental health laws. Clearly, persons with severe mental illness still lack adequate coverage. Recently, several initiatives to promote and defend the human rights of the mentally ill have been initiated, because of their minimal observance in the hospital system, which is mainly institutional.

The work-risk system provides coverage to 5.3 million employed workers (Law 24,557 on Work Risks, 1995). Work-risk insurers are responsible for providing health coverage to workers. To address on-the-job accidents and deaths, the Work-risk Authority launched the Program for the Prevention of On-the-job Accidents and Occupational Illness for workers in small and mid-sized enterprises (SRT Resolution 1/05). This resolution supplemented the 2000 Work Insurance for All Program, which applied to companies with more than 50 employees and has a Center for Information and Advice on Occupational Toxicology that answers questions from all sectors of the community.

Work hygiene and safety conditions were established by Law 19,587 (1972) and its regulatory decree 531/79 and amending decree 1,338/96. This law's comprehensive regulations seek to protect the worker, affording him or her extensive occupational safety conditions. Construction activity, which was regulated by Decree 911/96, was dealt with separately. Law 19,587 is supplemented with the aforementioned Law on Work Risks and its regulatory decree 1,278/00.

Health Promotion

Various initiatives are being implemented in the country (such as "Free Adults with A Healthy Attitude" and "Heart Attack Prevention in Argentina") in association with university and scientific societies that work in the community to prevention risk factors for noncommunicable diseases. One initiative, the Health Surveillance and Disease Control Program, is charged with providing information needed for making decisions related to the structure and operation of the services and the risks that affect the various population groups. Normative and infrastructure elements for improving the surveillance, prevention, and control of the diseases covered by the program were provided to all agents in the health system, and the National Epidemiologic Surveillance System and the Health Analysis and Monitoring Units were developed and implemented. In addition, a national strategy for the control of tobacco use was designed and implemented and a national baseline for the surveillance of risk factors for noncommunicable diseases was established.

The federal Government, the Argentine Society of Pediatrics, the Argentine Toxicology Network, the Government of the autonomous city of Buenos Aires, and the Argentine Association of Physicians for the Environment are among those lobbying for efforts in environmental health, especially since 2003. Within the Ministry of Health's National Directorate for Maternal and Child Health, a coordinating unit for children's environmental health was established, comprised of representatives of the Directorate

for Health Promotion and Protection and the Secretariat for the Environment. These two entities drew up the profile of childhood environmental health and formulated the guidelines for the National Program on Children's Environmental Health. An objective of the Children's Health in Argentina Project is to protect children's health by identifying environmental threats to which children are exposed. The leading results of the project's assessment are expected to be used to develop an ongoing system for the collection, analysis, and dissemination of information on this subject; carrying out of field research; and implementing interventions in the community.

Health Supplies

Argentina's drug industry includes some 250 laboratories funded by domestic and foreign capital. The Ministry of Health's Strategic Health Research Unit indicated that, as of until July 2006, there were approximately 2,057 active principals (and their combinations), with some 20,000 formulations in the market. According to the same source, in 2001 domestic laboratories had more than a 50% share in local sales, and approximately 22% of the country's demand for drugs was being covered with an external drug supply. In 2003, pharmaceutical imports totaled US$ 475,249,000, 6% of which corresponded to immunological and blood products, and 1.7% to vaccines. In 2001, drug exports totaled US$ 266 million. In 2005, the pharmaceutical industry's invoices totaled more than US$ 2,000 million, including taxes. According to INDEC, total per capita expenditures for drugs in 2006 were approximately US$ 63. According to data from the 1997 household survey and the 2003 National Commission for Health Research Programs, drugs account for 46%–52% of average family expenditures on health, with marked differences among the highest (25%–35%) and lowest (65%–73%) income sectors.

Generic drug use (Law 25,649/02), selection of products to be financed with collective resources, and the free provision of essential drugs to outpatients through the Remediar Program were implemented in 2002. This program extended drug coverage to some 15 million people who were totally or partially excluded from the health system. The distribution of kits with 47 different drugs to more than 5,300 primary care centers was put in place. A survey conducted in these centers in 2003 showed that 82% of Remediar Program beneficiaries were below the poverty line and 84% had no health insurance coverage. That same year, more than 70% of prescriptions were for generics.

In addition to its regular control functions, the National Food, Drug, and Health Technology Administration analyzes drugs already on the market through the so-called Horizontal Sampling Plan, which covers 248 medicinal specialties. Beyond the National Drug Surveillance System, which remains in effect, the regulatory agency has launched a technology surveillance program designed to collect, evaluate, oversee, and organize information on medical product defects. Implementation of this program by the companies is required by the "good manufacturing practices" regulations. The regulatory agency also implemented a program to investigate illegitimate drugs to combat the marketing of these drugs. In 1997, illegally marketed products were found in 76.5% of inspected establishments, and in 24.5% of local establishments investigated in 2003.

Human Resources

The number of health and social service workers was estimated at half a million in 2004; 40% worked in the public sector, and most of them (70%) were women. In the city of Buenos Aires, 54% of doctors 30–39 years old were women. The country's population is growing at the rate of 1.6% per year, while the population of physicians is growing at the rate of 3.5% per year. The distribution of human resources in health is irregular, with a high concentration of physicians in large urban centers. The national average is 3.2 physicians per 1,000 inhabitants. Approximately 65% to 70% are specialists, and there is a shortage of general practitioners or family doctors.

There is a shortage of nursing personnel (some 80,000 professionals, including university trained nurses, nursing auxiliaries, and practical nurses). The doctor/nurse ratio, considering only university trained nurses, is 9.5 doctors for each nurse; if we add the auxiliaries and practical nurses, the ratio is still weighted in favor of doctors: 1.5 doctors for each nurse.

Argentina has 25 medical schools, 10 public and 15 private. Public universities are reasonably distributed throughout the country, but private universities are concentrated in the autonomous city of Buenos Aires and in the Greater Buenos Aires Metropolitan Area (Table 7).

A recent study (30) highlighted many issues that surrounded the training and distribution of human resources for health in the country in 2004, such as: a) a decrease in the rate of growth

TABLE 7. Professionals by selected categories, Argentina, 2001.

Career	Number	%
Biochemistry	19,774	6.5
Nursing	12,614	4.2
Pharmacology	21,177	7.0
Speech therapy	7,924	2.6
Kinesiology	11,908	3.9
Medicine	121,076	39.9
Nutrition	4,654	1.5
Obstetrics	3,931	1.3
Dentistry	35,944	11.9
Psychology	46,931	15.4
Veterinary medicine	17,103	5.6
Total	**303,091**	**100.0**

Source: Developed by Mónica C. Abramzón (PAHO/WHO), based on data from INDEC, Encuesta Permanente de Hogares, 2001.

of the availability of health programs of study; b) the greater participation by private institutions in offering programs of study, especially those that require a low investment; c) a slower rate of growth in the demand for medical studies and expansion of other programs of study, notably nutrition and kinesiology; d) a lack of policies that promote and encouragement certain programs of study with the objective of reversing the marked deficit of some professional categories (e.g., nursing); e) the distortion of ratios within the health team, especially the doctor/nurse ratio; f) a need to establish regulatory mechanisms for nurse training and other technical programs, given the dispersion of institutions; g) the marked inequalities in the geographic distribution of all professional categories; and h) the lack of permanent information systems with key variables for the field of human resources in health.

In 2005, a Community Doctors Program was implemented to guide and strengthen training in primary health care and social and community health among human resources working at the primary level of care. The program seeks to expand the coverage and quality of care at the health care centers by strengthening health promotion, disease prevention, and social participation. In September 2006, 7,500 health professionals in the country's 24 territorial jurisdictions were studying at the postgraduate level in social and community health (60% were doctors and the rest were social workers, psychologists, obstetricians, nursing personnel, and others). There are 17 universities in the country that participate in this in-service training program, using similar curricula, methodologies, and instructional materials.

Research and Technological Development in Health

The National Council for Scientific and Technical Research was established by Executive Order No. 1,291 in 1958, in response to an overall sense that there was a need to establish an academic institution that would promote scientific and technological research in the country. The Council includes 116 research institutes, the national research and services laboratories, and 8 regional centers; 3,896 professional researchers, 2,392 research support technicians, and 3,023 grant recipients participate, and there also is an administrative center.

In 2002, Ministerial Resolution No. 170 established, within the Ministry of Health's Office of the Under-secretary for Health Relations and Research, the National Commission for Health Research Programs as a way to provide ongoing advisory assistance for health, clinical, applied, and basic research in the health sciences; give priority to research programs for health surveillance, prevention, and control of prevalent diseases; and promote research on health problems in the country.

The National Administration of Health Laboratories and Institutes cut back its research budget by 600% in six years (using the dollar as the value), and by 30% in 2002–2004. Argentina suffers from a notable fragmentation of the institutions performing scientific and technology activities. Moreover, institutions created with an eminently technological profile, such as the National Agriculture and Livestock Technology Institute, the National Institute of Industrial Technology, the National Atomic Energy Commission, and the National Institute of Space Activities, fall under different ministries or secretariats. Although in practice these institutions also carry out basic research, this compartmentalization reflects the original concept that separated the function of knowledge creation from that of technological development.

In 2003, 15.2% of the research and development projects were in the field of medical sciences (2,552). In 2002 there were 1,976 Argentine publications on MEDLINE, 20% more than in 2000; 43% were in the field of clinical medicine; 29% were in the basic sciences; and 9% dealt with public health and health systems. According to the Network on Science and Technology Indicators, between 1996 and 2003 the percentage of expenditures on research and development in human health remained stable at 13.7%–15.6%, although in absolute terms, since the end of peso-dollar convertibility, expenditures in this field dropped to one-third (from US $165.4 million in 2001 to US$ 55.9 in 2002).

Health Sector Expenditures and Financing

In the 1990s, although resources intended for health sector financing in Argentina were vast, they were being used inefficiently and the amount of spending in the various subsectors was inequitable. Health expenditures as a percentage of GDP were 7.7% in 1997 and 7.3% in 2003. In late 2001, prior to the devaluation of the peso, per capita health expenditures were deemed acceptable in comparison with those of other countries that had nearly universal coverage. In 2000, those expenditures were approximately 651 dollars/inhabitant/year. However, if private spending is left out, the figure is reduced to US$ 383 a year (31). In 2003, this expenditure was reduced to US$ 263 per capita, as a result of the significant devaluation of the currency and the consequent change in the relative-price structure. However, health expenditures by household represented 44%. Argentina lost its position as the country with the highest per capita health expenditure in the Region.

Technical Cooperation and External Financing

In terms of international cooperation associated with Official Development Assistance, Argentina is considered an intermediate developing country. In terms of technical cooperation, the country plays a dual role: on the one hand, it still receives cooperation; on the other, it offers technical cooperation to other countries since 1992. Despite the growth experienced in certain sectors of the country in the 1990s, Argentina still requires international cooperation, especially for poverty reduction, job production and creation, health, education, and research and development, as well as for political and judicial reform. In June

2002 the country again began to receive technical assistance from the United Nations Development Program (UNDP). International cooperation was aligned with the country's priorities, and loans were reallocated to purchase supplies and drugs and to direct care toward vulnerable populations, cooperation modalities that were, in many cases, unprecedented. Even in this context, there were donations in the face of catastrophes, such as the flood that hit Santa Fe in April 2003, when the province received support from various international donors, including the European Union.

International cooperation funds and technical assistance received by Argentina fall into the following categories: multilateral cooperation; bilateral cooperation; cooperation from nongovernmental and international organizations; and decentralized cooperation. Cooperation may be classified by type: financial, which includes loans and donations, with or without national matching funds, and technical assistance, which includes the provision of technicians and consultants by international organizations, as well as other contributions, such as financing for seminars or participation in international meetings. Programs that have emerged from the Iberoamerican Summits, which embody the commitments issued at the meetings of Chiefs of State and Heads of Government, to bolster Iberoamerican cooperation, also should be taken into consideration.

References

1. World Bank. Available at: http://devdata.worldbank.org/external/. Accessed on 28 July 2006.
2. United Nations Development Program. Human Development Report 2005.
3. Universidad Nacional de La Plata, Centro de Estudios Distributivos, Laborales y Sociales. Available at: www.depeco.econo.unlp.edu.ar/cedlas/arg.htm. Accessed on 28 July 2006.
4. Argentina, Presidencia de la Nación. Objetivos de Desarrollo del Milenio. Informe de País 2005.
5. Argentina, Ministerio de Salud, Secretaría de Ambiente y Desarrollo Sustentable; Programa de Naciones Unidas para el Medio Ambiente. Argentina 2006: Indicadores ambientales. Iniciativa latinoamericana y caribeña para el desarrollo sostenible. Indicadores de seguimiento. Buenos Aires; 2006.
6. Argentina, Ministerio de Salud, Secretaría de Ambiente y Desarrollo Sustentable, Unidad de Investigación y Desarrollo Ambiental. Estudio multicéntrico CONAPRIS. Epidemiología del hidroarsenicismo crónico regional endémico (HACRE) en la República Argentina. Asociación Toxicológica Argentina. In press.
7. Argentina, Ministerio de Salud. Atlas de mortalidad de la República Argentina. Buenos Aires: OPS; Universidad Nacional de Lanús; 2005.

8. Argentina, Ministerio de Salud; Pan American Health Organization. Basic indicators. Argentina 2006.

9. Vega AL, Torcida S, Velázquez GA. Análisis de la evolución de la tasa de mortalidad infantil en los departamentos de Argentina. 1994–2003. Revista Salud Colectiva. 2006; 2(3). Available at: http://www.unla.edu.ar/public/saludColectiva Nuevo/publicacion6/index.php.

10. Argentina, Secretaría de Programación para la Prevención de la Drogadicción y la Lucha contra el Narcotráfico; Instituto Nacional de Estadística y Censos. Segundo estudio nacional sobre consumo de sustancias psicoactivas. SEDRONAR; INDEC; 2004.

11. Argentina, Ministerio de Salud, Programa Nacional de Lucha contra los Retrovirus del Humano, SIDA y ETS. Estudio sobre comportamiento e información en relación con el VIH/SIDA e ITS en la población adolescente. 2005.

12. Argentina, Ministerio de Salud. Encuesta Nacional de Factores de Riesgo de Enfermedades No Transmisibles, 2005. MSAL; 2006.

13. Argentina, Superintendencia de Riesgos del Trabajo. Informe estadístico accidentabilidad 2004 y evolución 2000–2004. Publicaciones anuario 2004.

14. Gutiérrez AP, Koehs J, Schamber P, Suárez F. Informe sobre trabajo infantil en la recuperación y reciclaje de residuos. Organización Internacional de Migraciones; UNICEF; 2005.

15. Argentina, Ministerio de Salud, Programa Nacional de Lucha contra los Retrovirus del Humano, SIDA y ETS. Estudio sobre comportamiento e información en relación con el VIH/SIDA e ITS en trabajadoras/es sexuales de Argentina. 2005.

16. Argentina, Instituto Nacional de Estadística y Censos. Encuesta Nacional de Personas con Discapacidad, 2002–2003. Encuesta Complementaria del Censo 2001. INDEC; 2004.

17. Argentina, Ministerio de Economía y Producción, Secretaría de Política Económica; Instituto Nacional de Estadística y Censos. Encuesta Complementaria de Pueblos Indígenas (ECPI). Primeros resultados. 2005.

18. Argentina, Ministerio de Salud, Programa Nacional de Lucha contra los Retrovirus del Humano, SIDA y ETS. Estudio sobre comportamiento e información en relación con el VIH/SIDA e ITS en población aborigen. 2005.

19. Boletín sobre VIH/SIDA en la Argentina. Año X, N° 24; 2005.

20. Gómez JA., Sordo ME, Gentile A. Epidemiologic patterns of diarrheal disease in Argentina: estimation of rotavirus disease burden. Pediatr Infect Dis Journal 2002;21(9).

21. Giordiano MO, Ferreyra LJ, Isa MB, Martinez LC, Yudowsky SI, Nates SV. The epidemiology of acute viral gastroenteritis in hospitalized children in Córdoba City, Argentina: an insight of disease burden. Rev Inst Med Trop S Paulo 2001; 43(4):193–197.

22. Stupka J, Gómez J. Revisión sistemática de los estudios sobre frecuencia de patógenos asociados a diarrea en Argentina. Not published.

23. Lurá MC, Beltramino D, Carrera EF. Prevalencia de helmintosis intestinales en escolares de la ciudad de Santa Fe. Medicina 2002;62(1):29–36.

24. de Sereday MS, Gonzalez C, Giorgini D, De Loredo L, Braquinsky J, Cobenas C, et al. Prevalence of diabetes, obesity, hypertension and hyperlipidemia in the central area of Argentina. Diabetes Metab 2004 Sep;30(4):335–339.

25. Nigro D, Vergottini JC, Kuschnir E, Bendersky M, Campo I, De Roiter HG, et al. Epidemiología de la hipertensión arterial en la ciudad de Córdoba, Argentina. Rev Fed Arg Cardiol 1999; 28:69–75.

26. Herzer H, Celis A, Bartolomé M, Rodríguez C, Caputo G. El manejo de cuenca y su impacto en áreas urbanas: el caso de la llanura pampeana. Argentina. Documentos presentados en el III Congreso Latinoamericano de Manejo de Cuencas Hidrográficas. Arequipa (Perú): INRENA; FAO; 2003.

27. Argentina, Ministerio de Salud, Secretaría de Ambiente y Desarrollo Sustentable; Banco Mundial. Plan de Monitoreo del Aire para el Área del Polo Petroquímico Dock Sud. Estudio o línea de base de concentración de gases contaminantes en atmósfera en el área de Dock Sud. Informe final. 2002.

28. Argentina, Ministerio de Salud; Pan American Health Organization. Basic Indicators. Argentina 2005.

29. Argentina, Ministerio de Salud; Organización Panamericana de la Salud. Informe anual 2005 del Plan Nacional de Sangre.

30. Abramzón MC. Argentina: recursos humanos en salud en 2004. Buenos Aires: Organización Panamericana de la Salud; 2005.

31. González GG, Tobar F. Salud para los argentinos. Buenos Aires: Ediciones ISALUD; 2004.

ARUBA

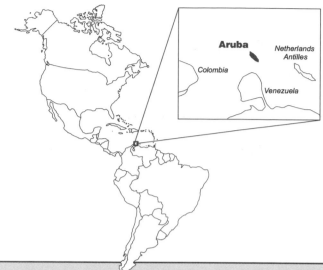

0   10   20   Miles

Aruba

Oranjestad ★

Netherlands
Antilles

Curaçao

Venezuela

The island of Aruba is located at 12°30' North and 70° West and lies about 32 km from the northern coast of Venezuela. It is the smallest and most western island of a group of three Dutch Leeward Islands, the "ABC islands" of Aruba, Bonaire, and Curaçao. Aruba is 31 km long and 8 km wide and encompasses an area of 180 km².

GENERAL CONTEXT AND HEALTH DETERMINANTS

Aruba's capital is Oranjestad, and the island divides geographically into eight districts: Noord/Tanki Leendert, Oranjestad-West, Oranjestad-East, Paradera, Santa Cruz, Savaneta, San Nicolas-North, and San Nicolas-South. The average temperature is 28°C with a cooling northeast tradewind. Rainfall averages about 500 mm a year, with October, November, December, and January accounting for most of it. Aruba lies outside the hurricane belt and at most experiences only fringe effects of nearby heavy tropical storms. While Dutch used to be the sole official language, in 2004 the Parliament of Aruba accepted Papiamento, the native language spoken exclusively on the ABC islands, as an official language. In addition, English and Spanish are compulsory in primary school and are spoken by many Arubians.

Social, Political, and Economic Determinants

Historically, Aruba was part of the Netherlands Antilles, a six-island federation, which also included Bonaire, Curaçao, St. Maarten, Saba, and St. Eustatius. On 1 January 1986, Aruba became a separate entity within the Kingdom of the Netherlands, which now comprises three constituents: Holland, the Netherlands Antilles (five islands), and Aruba. Aruba has its own constitution, based on Western democratic principles. The Queen of the Netherlands appoints the Governor of Aruba, who holds office for an eight-year term and acts as her representative. The Arubian Parliament consists of 21 members elected by universal suffrage; the last elections were held in 2005, resulting in the present Parliament formed by a Social Democratic party (11 seats), a Christian Democratic party (eight seats), and two new parties with one seat each. The Cabinet consists of a maximum of nine ministers and is headed by the Prime Minister. Aruba is responsible for its own administration and policy-making, except for defense, foreign affairs, and the Supreme Court, which are the responsibility of the Kingdom. Despite its separate status, Aruba retains strong economic, cultural, and political ties with Holland and with its "sister" islands.

Estimated real GDP growth for 2005 was 3.2%, a slight contraction of the estimated 2004 growth rate of 3.5%; a further contraction of 2.4% is projected (Table 1). While Aruba has made considerable progress toward alleviating poverty, available data suggest that income inequality is still considerably larger than in countries with comparable income levels.

According to the Centrale Bank van Aruba, at the end of 2005, inflation stood at 3.8%, compared to 2.8% a year earlier. Measured as a 12-month average percentage change, the inflation rate accelerated by nearly 1% to 3.4% in 2005, reflecting mainly price increases for water, electricity, and gasoline following the rise in oil prices on the international market. At the end of 2005, the overall economy continued to show an upward growth trend (Table 2).

The main economic driver is the service sector, in which tourism is the major industry. According to the most recent figures of the Aruba Tourism Authority, the number of stay-over visitors and of their nights spent on the island increased by 2.2% and 2.1%, respectively, during the first 10 months of the year of 2005 compared to 14.5% and 11.9% in the same period of 2004. Most tourists (73%) come from the United States, followed by Venezuela (8.1%) and the Netherlands (5.2%). From 2002 to 2004, the number of stay-over visitors increased from 642,627 to 728,157, that of hotel rooms increased from 6,831 to 7,226, and in 2004 average hotel occupancy rates were 80.7%.

The highest unemployment (28%) experienced over the last three decades was in 1985, when the oil refinery closed down. Accelerated investment in the labor-intensive hotel and construction sectors in the late 1980s and in the first half of the 1990s, coupled with the reopening of the oil refinery, caused enormous pressures on the local labor market: the total number of employed persons rose 43% from 1991 to 2000. Many of the newly created jobs in the economy had to be filled by foreign workers, to the extent that 41% of the working age population in 2000 was non-Arubian. The unemployment rate at the end of September 2005 was 6.2%, which represented a drop of 12.1% (427 persons) to 3,114, compared to a rate of 7.2% in the corresponding period in 2004; most of these were probably structurally unemployed persons, given the mismatch between the needs of employers and the skills and training of the unemployed. Inversely, the number of employed persons rose by 1,967 to 47,350, and most of that increase reflected the greater number of persons employed by the private sector—1,592 more persons thus employed or a 4% in-

TABLE 1. Gross domestic product, Aruba, 2001–2005.

	2001	2002	2003	2004[a]	2005[b]
Nominal GDP (US$ million)	1,942.2	1,954.9	2,056.5	2,182.3	2,326.3
Real GDP (1995 = 100; US$ million)	1,637.7	1,596.0	1,620.6	1,677.7	1,731.4
GDP per capita (nominal in US$)	2,1,140	20,951	21,632	22,346	23,139
Percentage changes					
Nominal GDP	2.2	0.7	5.2	6.1	6.6
Real GDP (1995 = 100)	−0.7	−2.6	1.5	3.5	3.2
GDP per capita (nominal, Aruba florin)	0.7	−0.9	3.2	3.3	3.5

Source: Aruba Central Bank (CBA), Central Bureau of Statistics, International Monetary Fund (IMF).
[a]Preliminary estimates of the CBA.
[b]Preliminary estimates of the CBA and the IMF.

TABLE 2. Inflation, growth, and debt, Aruba, 2002–2005.

	2002	2003	2004	2005
Real GDP (1995 = 100, US$ million)[a]	1,596.0	1,620.6	1,677.7	1,731.4
Inflation, end of period[b]	4.2	2.2	2.8	3.8
Inflation, 12-month average[b]	3.3	3.6	2.5	3.4
Real growth (%)[a]	−2.6	1.5	3.5	3.2
Domestic debt (US$ million)[c]	410	431.2	494.1	516.5[d]
Foreign debt (US$ million)[c]	510.7	413.8	477.5	532.7[d]
Total debt (US$ million)[c]	920.6	845	971.5	1,049.2[d]

[a]Aruba Central Bank, Central Bureau of Statistics, International Monetary Fund.
[b]Aruba Central Bank, Central Bureau of Statistics.
[c]Aruba Central Bank.
[d]End September 2005.

crease to 41,036. The number of public employees also went up by 375 or 6.3% to 6,314. The active portion of the working age population declined slightly to 63.3%.

Demographics, Mortality, and Morbidity

The total population increased from 92,017 in 2001 to 98,829 in 2004 (7.4%), of which 47.7% were males and 52.3% females; most of the increase was attributable to the arrival of immigrants, which ranged from 3,076 in 2002 to 3,906 in 2004. From 2001 to 2004, live births averaged 1,228 and total deaths 482. Between the censuses of 1991 and 2000, the population increased from 66,687 to 90,506, a rise of 35.7%, most of which was likewise caused by immigration. Of the total population in 2000, 66.1% were born on the island and the other 33.9% elsewhere. The density of population increased steadily from 501 inhabitants/km² in 1999 to 549 inhabitants/km² in 2004.

The total fertility rate in 2005 was 1.8. The crude birth rate per 1,000 inhabitants was 14.3 in 2000 and 12.1 in 2004. In 2005 life expectancy at birth was 71.9 years—69.5 years for males, and 74.4 years for females. According to the 2000 census, life ex-

pectancy for males was 70 years and for females 76 years, in each case approximately one year less than life expectancies in 1991 of 71.1 years for males and 77.1 years for females, according to the census of that year (Figure 1). Immigrants concentrated in age groups of high economic activity are an important contribution to the distribution of the population by age. The percentage of persons 65 years of age and older has remained stable: 7% according to the census of 1991 and 7.3% according to that of 2000. Predictions are, however, that a noticeable aging of the population is in the offing, as the mean age of the population has increased from 32.9 to 33.9 years since 1991; notwithstanding, much of the aging is masked by the arrival in recent years of large groups of mostly younger foreign workers.

Between 2000 and 2004, crude death rates for Aruba were consistently around 5 per 1,000 (Table 3). The probabilities of men dying in the 55–70-year age group and of women dying in the 60–70 age group were considerably higher in 2000 than in 1991. In 2004, of a total of 499 deaths defined by cause, 36.3% were attributed to diseases of the circulatory system, 24.7% to malignant neoplasms, 7.8% to external causes, and 6.1% to communicable diseases. Between 2000 and 2004, diseases of the circulatory system and malignant neoplasms consistently occupied first and second place among leading causes of death, while communicable diseases and external causes alternated for third and fourth place.

Among causes of death, mortality from communicable diseases has been under control, but the incidences of diseases of the circulatory system and malignant neoplasms have grown significantly, mainly as a result of unhealthy lifestyles such as poor eating habits and inactivity (Table 4).

More detailed data for causes of death for 2004 show differences between the sexes (Table 5). Diseases of the circulatory system and neoplasms constituted the leading causes of death for both males and females, but external causes of death represented 12.1% of all causes of death for males, while they represented only 2.3% of female deaths. Communicable diseases came in third place for females (8.1%) and in fourth place for males (4.5%).

Conditions originating in the perinatal period account for most of the mortality among children under 1 year of age. For the 1–4-year, 5–9-year, and 15–24-year age groups, external causes are the principal cause of death. Diseases of the circulatory system and malignant neoplasms are the most important causes of death in the 25–64-year age group, followed by external causes; in this age group, men die more often from diseases of the circulatory system and external causes. In the 65 year and older age group, diseases of the circulatory system and malignant neoplasms are the two leading causes of death, while communicable diseases come in third place.

HEALTH OF POPULATION GROUPS

Children under 5 Years Old

The number of infant deaths in the period 2000–2004 ranged from 7 in 2000 to 1 in 2004, and infant mortality rates (IMR) were 5.4, 4.8, 2.4, 2.4, and 0.9 deaths per 1,000 live births. According to the Registry Office, the IMR in 1990 was 4 deaths per 1,000 live births. Over the 15-year period 1990–2004, the IMR fluctuated between 1 and 8 deaths per 1,000 live births, with an average of 4 deaths. Between 2000 and 2004, the most common cause of the 20 registered infant deaths—responsible for 12 deaths or 60% of the total—was related to conditions originating in the perinatal period. Subcategories of these conditions included disorders related to length of gestation and fetal growth, constituting 5 deaths or 25% of all causes of registered infant deaths; followed by congenital malformations, deformations, and chromosomal abnormalities with 3 deaths; fetus and newborn affected by obstetric complications and birth trauma with 2 deaths; and respiratory disorders specific to the perinatal period with 2 deaths. Another important cause of death in infants was external causes with 2 deaths of all registered infant deaths.

In the period 2000–2004, six children 1–4 years old died—three males and three females. The most common cause of death

FIGURE 1. Population distribution, by age and sex, Aruba, 1990 and 2005.

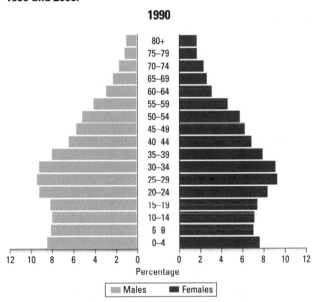

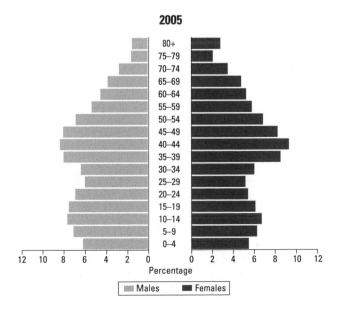

TABLE 3. Crude mortality rates, Aruba, 2000–2004.

Year	Population	Deaths	Number of deaths per 1,000 inhabitants
2000	91,064	531	5.9
2001	92,676	435	4.7
2002	93,945	492	5.2
2003	96,207	501	5.2
2004	98,829	499	5.0

Source: Central Bureau for Statistics and Population, Registry Office.

TABLE 4. Causes of death as a percentage of all deaths, Aruba, 2000–2004.

Causes	2000	2001	2002	2003	2004
Diseases of the circulatory system	34.8	30.3	34.5	35.6	36.3
Malignant neoplasms	22.9	21.7	25.7	27.9	24.7
External causes	6.7	8.7	9.6	8.5	7.8
Communicable diseases	7.3	9.6	7.6	4.7	6.1
Symptoms, signs, and ill-defined conditions	9.2	6.4	5.1	4.3	2.9
Certain conditions originating in the perinatal period	0.4	0.6	0.6	0.2	0.0
All other diseases	18.7	22.6	17.0	18.8	22.2

Source: Department of Public Health, Epidemiology and Research.

TABLE 5. Causes of death, as a percentage of all deaths, by sex, Aruba, 2004.

Causes	Males	Females	Total
Diseases of the circulatory system	36.0	36.7	36.3
Neoplasms	22.5	27.6	24.7
External causes	12.1	2.3	7.8
Communicable diseases	4.5	8.1	6.1
Certain conditions originating in the perinatal period	0.0	0.0	0.0

Source: Department of Public Health, Epidemiology and Research.

in this age group was external causes of injury and poisoning, with three deaths.

Children 5–9 Years Old

Eight children in the 5–9-year age group died in the period 2000–2004. Two deaths occurred due to external causes by injury and poisoning, and two due to congenital malformations, deformations, and chromosomal abnormalities.

Adolescents 10–14 and 15–19 Years Old

In the 10–14-year age group 10 deaths occurred in the period 2000–2004; most (7) were males and five of the male deaths were due to external causes. In the same period, 14 deaths occurred in the 15–19-year age group, of which 11 were males. In this age group, nine died of external causes (eight died in traffic accidents, of which only one death was female).

In 2004 the fertility rate of 15–19-year-old girls was 37 live births per 1,000 adolescent girls—considerably lower than the 2000 rate (51 live births per 1,000) and the 1991 rate (58 live births per 1,000).

Adults 20–59 Years Old and 60 Years and Older

Of deaths occurring in 2004 in the 20–64-year age group, 89 were males (73%) and 33 females (27%). From 2000 to 2004 no maternal mortality was reported. The most common cause of death in 2004 for males in this age group was land transport accidents (10), followed by cardiac arrest (9) and ischemic heart disease (7). The most common cause of death for females in this age group was neoplasms, chiefly carcinoma of the breast (4).

The crude birth rate according to the 2001 census was 13.8 births per 1,000, as compared to the 1991 census rate of 18.5 births per 1,000. Age-specific fertility rates for 2000 were likewise lower than those of 1991. Fertility rates for women in the 20–24-year age group dropped 40% from 1991 to 2000. For women in the 25–29-year and 30–34-year age groups, the decline in fertility was also significant. The total fertility rate decreased from 2.8 children per woman in 1991 to 1.85 children per woman in 2000. From 1991 to 2000, the mean age at which women had their children remained relatively stable at 27 years. According to calculations of the Central Bureau of Statistics, the fertility of Arubian women is currently below replacement level.

The Family Planning Foundation, founded in 1970 to promote responsible parenthood, distributes contraceptives to the general public irrespective of marital status; it is worth noting, however, that from 2000 to 2004 the number of clients dropped from 3,517 to 2,335. In 2004, of those women who used contraception, 60% used oral contraceptives, 25% used injections, 11% used condoms, and 5% used intrauterine devices. All women now have a choice of a general physician, a midwife, or a gynecologist to attend to them during pregnancy, whereas prior to the introduction of the General Health Insurance program—which covers the differences in costs of services for perinatal care—the choices were more limited: women with private health insurance and employed women could always choose which health professional they wanted to attend to their pregnancy, but women with *pour pouvre* cards (cards for people living in poverty) only had access to a midwife.

Of all deaths during 2004 in the 60 years and older age group, 196 were male (52%) and 184 were female (48%). The most common cause of death in males was ischemic heart disease (19), followed by cerebrovascular diseases (17) and diabetes mellitus (13), while the most common cause of death for females was cerebrovascular diseases (20), followed by diabetes mellitus (19) and hypertensive disease (14).

Demand for Foreign Labor Stresses the Health System

The boom in Aruba's hotel and construction industries that began in the 1990s led to a labor shortage that required bringing in foreign workers to fill the gap. By 2000, the number of employed persons had risen by more than 40%, and two in every five persons in the island's working-age population were foreigners. This influx of a younger population of non-Arubians challenges the capacity of the health system to cope with demand: on the one hand, it must cope with injuries and infectious diseases that the younger population faces; on the other, it must address the chronic diseases and disabilities among the ever-aging Arubian population. To address these issues, the Department of Public Health is providing an array of diverse services, as well as contracting and coordinating with nongovernmental agencies to provide additional health care services.

The Family

The 2000 census counted a population of 90,506 persons, 29,264 households, and an average of 3.1 persons per household, as compared to household sizes of 3.5 in 1991 and 4.0 in 1981. Since 1991 the number of individuals living in a small household (1–3 persons) has increased, while the number living in households with more than three persons has decreased. The number of nuclear households—those with a married couple with or without children, father alone with children, or mother alone with children—increased by almost 40% between 1991 and 2000, from 9,800 to 13,693; nevertheless, the percentage of this type of household among all households decreased from 51% to 47%. The relative number of extended households also fell, from 18% to 16%, as did the number of collective households—institutions such as homes for elderly, youths, or the disabled—from 20% in 1991 to 15% in 2000.

Workers

The Occupational Health Center for the public sector, Bedrijf-sgezondheids Dienst, carries out pre-employment health controls and monitoring of sick workers and deals with the prevention and control of occupational risks, workers' health education, and the registry of accidents and occupational diseases. In 2003 the absenteeism index for the public sector was 4.7%, and the average period of absenteeism was 5.5 days. The most frequent causes of morbidity contributing to absenteeism were influenza, digestive disorders, and headaches; injury in the home setting, traffic accidents, and occupational accidents were the largest contributors to accident-related absenteeism.

Persons with Disabilities

According to the 2000 census, 5,034 persons (5.6% of the population) had physical and/or mental disabilities; the most frequent disability was motor impairment (30.3%), followed by visual impairment (20.6%). The prevalence of disabilities was slightly higher among men (5.8%) than women (5.4%). The Foundation for the Mentally Handicapped gives several kinds of services and day care, based in various operating centers: Daycare Bibito Pin for children 2–16 years old; Dununman School for children 8–18 years old who have learning difficulties; Daycare Briyo di Solo for adolescents and adults 16 years old and older; Center Man an Obra, a school that provides craft training and skills; and Home Sjabururi, which offers permanent care for disabled adults. The Foundation Ambiente Felis, which is subsidized by the government and by monthly contributions from clients' parents, provides permanent care for adults with mental impairments. The three most common disabilities among clients at this foundation are Down syndrome, serious mental impairment (low functionality), and double mental and physical disabilities (such as deafness, blindness, and the inability to walk); their most common burdens of disease are: influenza, epilepsy, diabetes, chronic airway infection, and heart problems.

HEALTH CONDITIONS AND PROBLEMS

COMMUNICABLE DISEASES

Vector-borne Diseases

In 2001, 2002, and 2003, 20, 27, and 33 **dengue** cases, respectively, were reported. In 2004 the island experienced a dengue 3 outbreak resulting in 171 cases. At the end of 2005 another dengue epidemic lasted for a period of six months and resulted in 3,880 cases being reported to the Department of Public Health, 42% of which were confirmed in the laboratory; one case of **hemorrhagic dengue fever** was observed; and dengue serotypes 2 and 3 were isolated. All dengue serotypes except for 4 have been observed in Aruba. No other vector-borne diseases have been reported.

TABLE 6. National vaccination program, Aruba.

Vaccination	Age of vaccination
DPTPolio and Hib	3, 4, 5, and 12 months
MMR	14–15 months
DTPolio	5 years
DTPolio and MMR	10–11 years

Source: Youth Health Service, Department of Public Health, Aruba.

Vaccine-Preventable Diseases

As part of the Kingdom of the Netherlands vaccination program (Table 6), all infants and schoolchildren in Aruba are vaccinated for DPTPolio (diphtheria, pertussis, tetanus toxoid, and poliomyelitis), Hib (*Haemophilus influenzae* type b), MMR (measles, mumps, and rubella), and DTPolio (diphtheria, tetanus toxoid, poliomyelitis).

Infectious Intestinal Diseases

Aruba has no history of **cholera**. During 2004, 13 cases of **shigellosis** and 47 cases of **salmonellosis** were registered.

Chronic Communicable Diseases

In 2003 and 2004, 12 and 2 cases of **pulmonary tuberculosis**, respectively, were registered; no cases of other forms of tuberculosis were reported. In the same two years, 19 and 11 cases of **syphilis**, respectively, were registered. No cases of **leprosy** were registered during 2004.

Zoonoses

No cases of **rabies** or other zoonoses were reported from 2001 to 2005.

NONCOMMUNICABLE DISEASES

Nutritional and Metabolic Diseases

According to a 1998 survey of schoolchildren's eating habits and physical activity, 20% of children in the 6–14-year age group did not eat breakfast before going to school, and as they grew older they were less likely to eat something in the morning; about three-quarters of schoolchildren consumed a warm meal every day or almost every day; primary school children were more likely to eat fruits (46%) than vegetables (39%); 45% of children consumed at least one bottle of soft drink per day; more than three-quarters consumed more than two glasses of water per day; and 70% of children carried food and 65% carried a beverage to school, but as they grew older they were less likely to do so.

According to a 2003 survey, 80% of last-born children were still being breast-fed 4 weeks after birth, and 24% of them were being exclusively breast-fed; only 37% were being breast-fed after

17 weeks and 8% exclusively; by 26 weeks 15% were breast-fed and only 3% exclusively. The study suggests that scant practical knowledge of the value of breast-feeding, insufficient trust in breast-feeding capability, and children's refusal to breast-feed are the main reasons that this practice stops.

Overweight is another issue that merits special attention. Anthropometrical measurements from a 2001 survey conducted by the Department of Public Health indicated that only one-quarter of the population had a normal body weight; 16% were mildly overweight; 19.5% were more than mildly overweight, with risk to their health; and 38% were obese (BMI = >30).

The prevalence of **diabetes** is very high. In a 2001 health survey conducted by the Department of Public Health, 5.7% of the population reported that they suffered from diabetes. Concurrent with that survey, a subsample of the participants 20 years of age or older were subjected to medical examination, according to which 13.2% had diabetes and another 9.2% had glucose intolerance. From 2001 to 2004, mortality from diabetes ranged from 25 deaths in 2002 to 37 in 2004.

Cardiovascular Diseases

Diseases of the circulatory system are the leading cause of death. Annual deaths from cardiovascular diseases ranged from 142 deaths in 2001 to 185 in 2004.

Malignant Neoplasms

Malignant neoplasms are the second leading cause of death, accounting for 24.7% of the total 499 deaths in 2004. The most common sites of malignancies leading to death for both sexes combined are the digestive organs and peritoneum, stomach, and colon. In females the leading cause of death is malignant neoplasm of the breast, and in males it is lung cancer.

OTHER PROBLEMS

Oral Health

The Youth Dental Care Service, with two dentists and one hygienist, works closely with the public, especially through kindergartens and elementary schools, to provide information about dental care to parents and children. Preventive dental care service entails weekly flouride wash programs conducted at kindergartens and elementary schools, and curative dental care service involves referral of schoolchildren to the government dentist.

RESPONSE OF THE HEALTH SECTOR

Health Policies and Plans

Health care on the island is founded on general regulations—specifically the Public Health Act that entrusts the Department of

TABLE 7. Laws regulating the functioning of public health care systems and conditions, Aruba.

General regulation
Public Health Act (1989)

Specific regulations
Law on Medical Practice (1996)
Law on Dental Practice (1989)
Law on the Authorization of Pharmacists and Pharmacy Assistants (1960)
Law on Midwives (1999)
Medical Disciplinary Law (1957)
Mental Health Law (1992)
Law on Drug Provision (1969)
Narcotics Law (1960)
Law on Food Safety (1995)
Law on Contagious Diseases (1992)
Law on Quarantine (1992)
Law on Importation of Small Animals (1992)
Law on Pesticides (1961)
Law on Slaughter and Inspection (1996)
Law on Burials (1999)
Law on Death Certificates (1999)
Law on Environmental Protection (1995)
Law on General Health Insurance (AZV; 1992)

Public Health with the organization of health care and the supervision and promotion of health—and specific regulations dealing with discrete public health areas such as health professions, mental health, drug and narcotic supervision, hygiene, and diseases (Table 7).

Organization of the Health System

The Department of Public Health, under the Ministry of Public Health and Environment, is responsible for promotion of public health and administration of the public laboratory. Its services include the youth health care service, youth dental care service, occupational health service, yellow fever and dengue mosquito control service, sanitary and food inspection service, veterinary service, health promotion and education, epidemiology and research, social psychiatric service, and the public laboratory.

The Youth Health Services monitors and assists the growth and development of children, including the conduct of periodic surveillance of the sight, hearing, weight, teeth, and hair of schoolchildren in the first and fifth grades. Children found to have problems are referred to specialists. In addition, for children and youths who have social, emotional, and behavioral problems, three residential institutions operating on the island give temporary care and education to children referred to them by the Department of Social Affairs and the Guardianship Board: Casa Cuna Progreso admits infants and children in the 0–5 age group; Imeldahof takes children and adolescents 6–18

years old; and Cas pa Hubentud handles individuals in the 12–21-year age range.

Public Health Services

The objective of the Epidemiology and Research Unit is to systematically collect, generate, process, and analyze data in order to disseminate relevant health information for policy development, planning, and evaluation. The unit undertakes surveillance implementation; outbreak investigations; data collection necessary to measure needs assessments and to establish health care policies, strategic plans for AIDS, dengue, and nutrition programs, health care research, and health promotion activities; presentations and the production of publications—the Epi-Alert (bulletin on epidemics or outbreaks in Aruba or in the region) and Epi-Info (epidemiological information); provides data to other sections within the Department of Public Health as well as to other governmental and nongovernmental departments; and conducts surveys.

The Social Psychiatric Care Service provides ambulatory services for chronic psychiatric patients, administers drugs and therapy, and offers patients and their families support in their own environment.

The reporting of a number of infectious diseases is mandated by law. Health care providers are required to report diagnosed or suspected cases of those diseases to the Contagious Diseases Service of the Department of Public Health, where public health nurses provide follow-up. The Department of Public Health takes control measures to prevent a possible outbreak.

Aruba has no natural source of fresh drinking water and very little rain. The water and energy company, W.E.B. Aruba N.V., carries out desalination of ocean water to produce drinking water that is of very high quality—quality that is assured by an array of testing measures by both the company and the public health laboratory.

A home nursing organization, the White Yellow Cross, provides care to new mothers and their infants, diabetics, terminal patients, and others in need of care at home. It also offers information and education on health topics such as safety at home, childcare, diabetes, and vaccination.

The sole hospital, Dr. Horacio Oduber Hospital, is administered by a private, nonprofit foundation. Built in 1970 and situated in the northwestern part of the island, it has 305 beds for inpatient care and is well-equipped to provide highly specialized services: internal medicine, surgery, cardiology, urology, gynecology and obstetrics, pediatrics, otorhinolaryngology, ophthalmology, neurology, neurosurgery, orthopedics, dermatology, plastic surgery, and psychiatry. In 2004 the hospital admitted 11,700 and had an occupancy rate of 88.7%; the average length of stay was 8.4 days. In addition, an emergency room operates 24 hours/day; outpatient care facilities provide consultation rooms for most of the specialists; and hemodialysis and auxiliary facilities such as physiotherapy, wound care, and radiology are offered.

Individual Care Services

Over the last few years a new trend has emerged of specialists establishing independent clinics—solo practices and centers of cooperating physicians in the same or related specializations—instead of their using the hospital's outpatient facilities (although many of these independent clinics are concentrated in the area of the hospital). Another trend is the establishment of private clinical laboratories, for which programs need to be set up to assure the quality of the equipment being used and of the tests being done in these laboratories. A private hemodialysis center, the Posada Clinic, mainly provides services to tourists visiting the island, although locals make use of them as well.

Nongovernmental organizations, whose numbers are growing, provide a range of health care services. The challenge for the Department of Public Health is to assure adequate surveillance of all NGO services and to encourage cooperation among them. In addition to the services for children provided by the Department of Public Health, many nongovernmental organizations offer services for children and youth such as shelters for abused and homeless children, recreational opportunities, and job creation. Other NGOs serve the interests of persons with mental, hearing, visual, and physical disabilities. A new nonprofit organization offers halfway houses for chronic psychiatric patients. Several nongovernmental organizations give care to the elderly. Collectively, these organizations manage three elderly homes in Oranjestad, Savaneta, and San Nicolas with a total of 253 beds. In the years to come, the aging of the population and increased life expectancy at birth will pose ever-greater and changing demands on the health system. Meanwhile, shortages in long-term care facilities for the elderly are already a reality: in 2004, 85 persons were on the waiting list to gain admission to a geriatric home.

Human Resources

In 2005, there was approximately one physician in general practice for every 2,900 persons, one surgeon general for every 16,500 persons, one dentist/orthodontist for every 4,000 persons, and one psychiatrist or neurologist/psychiatrist for every 16,500 persons (Table 8).

Research in Health

In addition to its epidemiological data management function, the Epidemiology and Research Unit conducts health research.

Recent activities include surveys on eating habits and physical activity among primary school children; surveys of knowledge, attitudes, beliefs, and practices with respect to HIV/AIDS, nutrition, and exercise among adolescents; a national health survey on the population's general health; studies on the consumption of medical services; and research on lifestyle—eating habits, physical activity, smoking, alcohol consumption, etc.—and preventive behavior.

TABLE 8. Health personnel, Aruba, 2005.

General physicians	**34**
Specialists	**66**
Anesthesiologists	5
Surgeons general	6
Dermatologists	3
Gynecologists	4
Internists	8
Pediatricians	6
Neurosurgeons	2
Neurologists/psychiatrists	3
Psychiatrists	3
Ophthalmologists	3
Orthopedic surgeons	4
Radiologists	4
Traumatologists	2
Otorhinolaryngologists	4
Pathologists	0
Urologist	1
Plastic surgeons	2
Cardiologists	3
Nephrologist	1
Gastroenterologist	1
Oncologist	1
Physicians employed by the Government	**18**
Other physicians	**29**
Other health personnel	
Dentists/orthodontists	25
Pharmacists	21
Veterinarians	9
Midwives	7

Source: Department of Public Health, Aruba.

BAHAMAS

United States
of America

Bahamas

Cuba

Dominican
Republic

Jamaica   Haiti

Grand Bahama

Freeport

0   50   100   Miles

Nassau
★
New
Providence

F a m i l y   I s l a n d s

Cuba

The Commonwealth of the Bahamas is located off the southeast coast of Florida, United States of America, and northeast of Cuba. It consists of approximately 700 islands and cays with a land mass of 13,940 km². Tourism, followed by international banking and investment management, constitute the industries of most importance to the national economy.

GENERAL CONTEXT AND HEALTH DETERMINANTS

The 2000 population and housing census reported a total population of 303,611, a 19% increase over the 1990 population of 255,000. The population density per square mile increased from 47.4 in 1990 to 56.7 in 2000. More than 95% of the population lives on seven of the islands. The two major population centers are the capital of Nassau (210,832 inhabitants), located on the island of New Providence, and Freeport, which is on Grand Bahama (46,994 inhabitants). The remaining populated islands and cays are known as the Family Islands. The country is divided into four regions: Region 1 (New Providence and Grand Bahama); Region 2 (Abaco, Andros, and Eleuthera); Region 3 (Exuma and Long Island); and Region 4 (other Family Islands).

Social, Political, and Economic Determinants

The Commonwealth of the Bahamas gained independence from the United Kingdom in 1973. The country is governed by a parliamentary democracy based on the Westminster model, with a Governor General who represents the monarchy, a bicameral legislature including an elected Parliament, and an independent judiciary. The government is headed by a Prime Minister. There is a local government system on the Family Islands comprised of a number of locally elected district councils and a central council headed by an island administrator who is an established public officer.

The Bahamas Living Conditions Survey (BLCS) was conducted in 2001. This comprehensive household survey ($n = 6,414$) was the first of its kind ever conducted in the country. In shedding light on general living conditions, it indicated that the standard of living varies greatly among nationalities. Native-born Bahamians, who represent 89% of the population, comprise nearly 88% of those in the wealthiest quintile and just over 84% in the poorest quintile. The BLCS poverty assessment uses per capita, household-consumption expenditure as its welfare measurement. It indicates a poverty rate of approximately 9%, with some 5% of households falling below the annual poverty line of US$ 2,863 per person. The poverty line used is an absolute poverty line in that it represents the minimum amount of money necessary to purchase an adequate diet, with allowances for non-food needs. Nearly 76% of the poor live in the densely populated, urban areas of New Providence and Grand Bahama. The country is characterized by extreme regional disparities in population distribution, which mirror large regional disparities in living standards.

The BLCS 2001 showed that nearly 62% of the workforce was engaged in the private sector, 21% in government services, and 17% were self-employed. The BLCS also analyzed the employment status of children 10–14 years old. The results suggest that child labor was not widespread at the time the survey was conducted, with only 2.4% of children being shown as economically active. This group accounted for less than 1% of the total labor force, yet all of its members were from the poorest quintile. Unemployment was highest among youths (12%), the poor (11.6%), and females (5.4%) in quintile 1. Among nationalities, Haitians had the highest unemployment rate (8%), compared to the national average of 4.6%.

The exchange rate with the U.S. dollar has been 1:1 since 1972. In 2005, per capita income was estimated at US$ 17,883. In the period 2000–2002, tourism and tourism-related commerce accounted for more than 50% of GDP and, directly or indirectly, 60% of employment. The Ministry of Tourism reported that 4.6 million people visited the Bahamas in 2003. Of these, 1.6 million were stop-over visitors. In 2005 the Bahamas received more than 5 million total tourist arrivals.

Financial services were responsible for 15% of the GDP. In 2003, the number of banks and trust companies licensed to operate within the Bahamas stood at 284. The vast majority of these were branches, subsidiaries, or affiliates of major banking institutions in North and South America and western Europe. Data from the Office of the Registrar of Insurance Companies indicate that in 2003, there were 163 licensed insurance companies, brokers, and agents. There were 137 companies operating in the domestic sector and 26 operating as external insurers.

In spite of its high per capita GDP, great inequity existed in the distribution of wealth. The majority of wealth was concentrated in the country's main commercial and tourism centers located on a small number of islands. The GNP increased from US$ 15,447 per capita in 1999 to US$ 16,756 in 2002.

The adult literacy rate in 2005 was 95.8% (males 95.0% and females 96.7%). The Bahamian school system comprises 147 government and 42 private/independent schools. The government educational system includes primary, all-age, junior high, secondary (grades 7–9), and senior high (grades 10–12) schools. Various governing bodies control the independent—mainly church-administered—private schools. However, these schools largely function within the framework of the Education Act of 1996, which establishes the regulations under which public schools operate, and many receive annual government subventions. Primary and secondary education is free and universal throughout the country, and school attendance is compulsory for children 5–16 years of age. National school enrollment for children at the preschool level was 85%, but only 51% among the poor, versus 91% among the non-poor. The country faces an ongoing challenge of ensuring an equitable educational system for students throughout the archipelago, including remote islands and cays. The BLCS 2001 found that 68.5% of persons under 25 years of age were most likely to be enrolled in some type of educational institution, whether a day care facility, primary or secondary school, or university. More than 75% of this school-enrolled population was in the 5–16 age group, and 52% were males. Similarly, males accounted for 52% of those not enrolled. Both international and local educational institutions offer services in the country. Most are located on New Providence, while others have opened facilities on some of the larger of the Family Islands.

In the period 2001–2005, crime and violence became major public health concerns. Annual police reports point to serious challenges with narcotics trafficking, particularly as regards cocaine and marijuana, as well as with the growing numbers of small arms and light weapons illegally entering the country and being employed in criminal activities.

The Water and Sewerage Corporation is responsible for the provision of municipal water supply in the Bahamas. Production from municipal and private water systems is systematically monitored and bacteriological and chemical quality analyzed by the Water Quality Control Program of the Department of Environmental Health Services. This data is provided to the supplier and also used to evaluate trends, determine potential supply problems, and make recommendations for improvements. During the 2001–2005 review period, approximately 96.4% of the total population had access to water supply through household connections and other acceptable piped means. The drinking water supply on New Providence and the Family Islands is drawn from underground source facilities. The population not served by piped systems relies on wells or rainwater tanks. In rural areas, despite the availability of clean and safe water, there are unresolved provision difficulties due to operational, resource, and

technical constraints. In 2000, the mean monthly consumption expenditure on water by Bahamian households was 0.8%.

Most residential dwellings had flush toilets, either linked to a public sewerage system (16%) or attached to a cesspit or septic tank (82%). Approximately 4.5% of households used a pit latrine, while 1.1% reported having no toilet facilities attached to their dwelling unit.

The New Providence regional landfill receives in excess of 181,000 tons of solid waste per year. The high waste generation rate in the Bahamas is a result of the country's considerable reliance on imports, which tend to have substantial packaging; the virtual absence of recycling initiatives to reduce paper, plastic, and metal waste components; and the high volume of waste produced by the tourism industry.

The Department of Environmental Health Services monitors the safety of food offered for public consumption through meat inspections at the abattoir, sampling and testing of imported canned goods at ports of entry, and sanitary inspections of food establishments. Outbreaks of conch poisoning, a serious public health problem, have decreased steadily during the last five years due to the implementation of a number of multisectoral approaches, including the introduction in 2004 of mandatory food safety training for all food handlers.

The annual hurricane season in the Bahamas occurs between 1 June and 30 November. The National Emergency Management Agency is responsible for pre-disaster planning and post-disaster response. During the study period, the Bahamas experienced four hurricanes and various other tropical storms that caused extensive flood and wind damage. Hurricane Michelle, which struck northwestern Bahamas in 2001, caused particularly widespread property damage. Several cases of posttraumatic stress syndrome were also reported. In 2004, Hurricanes Jeanne and Frances caused millions of dollars of severe infrastructure damage on Grand Bahama and Abaco. The cost of Hurricane Francis was estimated at 7% of the country's GDP for that year. In 2005 Hurricane Wilma caused severe property damage on Grand Bahama.

Demographics, Mortality, and Morbidity

The population pyramid (Figure 1) shows a transition from a youthful to a less youthful population due to lower fertility and increased life expectancy rates. Sex differentials were more extreme among the elderly than for other age groups; for every 1,000 females, there were only 708 males. As of 2001, life expectancy for females was 76 years compared to 70 for males. The overall male-female ratio in the country was 95:100. The annual population growth rate declined from 2.2% in 1980 to an estimated 1.9% in 2002.

In 2003, 28.4% of the population was under 15 years of age and 5.2% was 65 years of age or older. The age dependency ratio is estimated at 62.1%. Females constituted 50.5% of the popula-

FIGURE 1. Population structure, by age and sex, Bahamas, 1990 and 2005.

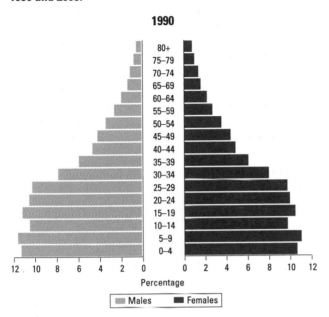

1990

(Percentage — Males, Females)

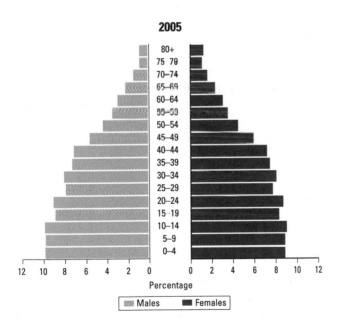

2005

(Percentage — Males, Females)

age) rate decreased from 0.5 per 1,000 children in 1999 to 0.4 in 2003. There were 2 maternal deaths each in 2003 and 2004. The crude birth rate stood at 16 per 1,000 population in 2003. Between 2001 and 2004, the crude death rate increased from 5.4 to 5.7 per 1,000 population, and in 2003 it declined to 5.2 (1,649 deaths). Life expectancy at birth continued to increase steadily, and for the period 1999–2001, it was 73 years (69.9 years for males and 76.4 for females). In 2003, across all ages, the age-specific death rates were higher for males than for females.

In the period 2001–2003, a total of 6,600 deaths occurred. Diseases of the circulatory system accounted for 31.8% of female deaths, compared with 26.2% of male deaths. External causes of injury and poisoning constituted 4% of total female deaths, compared with 11.9% of total male deaths.

Data analysis of the BLCS 2001 reveals an ongoing movement of outlying rural populations to the more developed urban areas. The proportion of the total population living on the Family Islands declined from 16.5% in 1990 to 14.9% in 2000. The census data showed that this declining population trend found on most of the Family Islands resulted largely from migration to either New Providence or Grand Bahama (Region 1) in search of better employment opportunities.

Migrants were for the most part younger persons, with about one-half of both male and female migrants being under 25 years of age. Males comprised 64% of internal migrants. Sustained increased inward migration by the population to Region 1, the influx of immigrants from outside the country, and the booming tourist industry may, over time, produce a concentrated population pattern that could significantly tax the country's health care delivery system.

The large influx of external immigrants presents other challenges to the country's social and economic status, as well. Immigration data shows two distinct migratory patterns: a poorer group in search of employment opportunities and a wealthier middle-aged group arriving in the Bahamas to fill job positions, usually in professional specialties. Poorer migrants have a tendency to increase demand on the country's social services, including government health facilities and schools. Wealthier migrants tend to utilize private facilities (health, education, etc.), even though their consumer habits place additional demands on such public resources as electric utilities and the telephone system.

The country's undocumented immigrants tend to live in substandard housing in overcrowded marginal areas, raising serious environmental health and communicable disease concerns, particularly given the growing population density on New Providence.

Haitians, who represented slightly more than 6% of the population in the 2000 census, accounted for more than 14% of those in the poorest quintile. Within recent immigrant groups (persons who immigrated to the Bahamas within five years prior to the BLCS 2001), nearly 84% of Haitians had a per capita expenditure of less than $8,524. Haitians comprised the single largest immi-

tion. Women of childbearing years in the 15–49 age group comprised 55.3% of the female population and 28% of the total population. Over the 2001–2005 period, the total fertility rate remained more or less constant at approximately 2.3 children per woman. The age-specific fertility rates for the 15–19-year-old and the 20–24-year-old age groups in 2003 were, respectively, 46.1 and 96.5 per 1,000 women.

The infant mortality rate ranged from 12.7 per 1,000 live births in 2001 to 17.3 in 2004; the child mortality (0–5 years of

grant group and accounted for about 33% of recent immigrants. Other immigrant groups included persons from the United Kingdom, the United States, Canada, and other Caribbean islands and territories.

Chronic noncommunicable diseases, influenced by lifestyle choices, accounted for nearly 45% of all deaths in the Bahamas. Taken together, hypertension, diabetes, coronary heart disease, stroke, chronic respiratory diseases, cancers, and injuries dominated the country's morbidity and mortality profile.

HEALTH OF POPULATION GROUPS

Children under 5 Years Old

In the period 1999–2001, the infant mortality rate decreased from 15.8 per 1,000 live births in 1999 to 12.7 per 1,000 live births in 2001. However, the rate rose to 17.2 in 2003 and increased slightly to 17.3 in 2004. The stillbirth rate ranged from 9.5 per 1,000 live births over the period 1999–2001 to 15.4 in 2003. In 2003, registered infant deaths accounted for 3.3% of total deaths. There were 89 infant deaths in 2004. The combined data from the Perinatal Information System showed that the prevalence of low birthweight (less than 2,500 g) ranged from 8.5% in 1999 to 11.2% in 2003.

The BLCS 2001 indicated that approximately 74% of all children 24 months and younger were breast-fed. In the 2002–2004 period, there was no vertical transmission of HIV from mothers on antiretroviral treatment to their babies. According to the National Health Services Strategic Plan 2000–2004, at least 98% of children entering preschool or primary schools were immunized against childhood preventable diseases.

In the period 1999–2000, there were a total of 72 deaths from defined causes among children under age 5. Conditions originating in the perinatal period accounted for 38.9%, followed by congenital malformations with 12.5% of all deaths. There were 7 deaths due to land transport accidents, accounting for 9.7% of deaths in this age group.

In 2003, a total of 10 deaths were recorded in preschool children aged 1–4 years old. This represented a 33% decrease from 2001, when there were 15 deaths. Diseases of the respiratory system were among the leading causes of mortality in children of this age group in 2001 and 2003. Other causes of death included accidental drowning, congenital malformations and chromosomal abnormalities, and pulmonary heart disease. The leading cause of inpatient morbidity during 2001–2003 was acute respiratory infections. Other major causes included injuries and poisonings, intestinal infectious diseases, slow fetal growth, low birthweight, prematurity, and other diseases of the respiratory system. Child abuse in this highly vulnerable 1–4 age group continued to be a cause of concern despite a decrease from 612 to 526 (14%) reported cases from 2002 to 2003. In this period, child neglect and physical abuse were the most commonly reported

types of abuse and accounted for 42% and 32%, respectively, of all cases. Sexual abuse and incest accounted for an additional 23% of reported cases.

The BLCS 2001 results showed that in children 5 years and younger, respiratory illness is a major concern. During the four weeks prior to the survey, among children in this age group, coughs, colds, and runny noses were the most common illnesses (41%), followed by diarrhea (6.6%) and asthma (2.4%). Incidence of diarrhea among children 5 years and younger was 7.8%. The survey also showed that the highest rate of stunting was found among the younger population, with proportions declining as children grew older. Height-for-age z-scores indicated that 15% of children 2–4 years of age were at significant risk for stunting. The overall weight-for-height z-scores (wasting), which reflect current nutritional status, showed that the potential for undernourishment increased as children grew older. Both weight-for-height and height-for-age z-scores showed the highest prevalence of undernutrition on the urbanized islands of Region 1 and the lowest on the less developed Family Islands of Region 4.

Children 5–9 Years and 10–19 Years Old

In 1999–2000, there were 25 deaths in the 5–9-year-old age group and 53 deaths in the 10–19-year-old age group. The leading causes of death in the population 10–19 years of age were homicide, with 13 deaths (26%), and land transport accidents, with 12 deaths (24%).

In 2003, there were 23 deaths among children 5–14 years of age. Leading causes of mortality were primarily external causes such as assault or homicide, drowning and submersion, exposure to smoke and/or fire, and land transport accidents. Together, these comprised 43.5% of all deaths among this age group. In 2001, the mortality profile in this age group showed HIV/AIDS to be the leading cause of death, accounting for 28.6% of all deaths, followed by land transport accidents, with 14.3%.

In 2003, the three leading discharge diagnoses among children in this age group were injuries (13.2%), acute respiratory infections (12.7%), and intestinal infectious diseases (11.5%). Together, these conditions accounted for 37.4% of discharge diagnoses. Injuries and respiratory infections were also among the leading causes of morbidity in children 5–14 years old in 2001 and 2002. There were 8 registered deaths due to HIV/AIDS among this age group during the 1999–2003 period.

Adolescents 15–24 Years Old

During the 2001–2003 period, there were 172 deaths in this age group. External causes, primarily land transport accidents (21.5%) and homicides (18%), accounted for nearly one-half (48.3%) of all deaths. The male-female ratios for land transport accidents and homicides were 5.2:1 and 4.2:1, respectively.

During this same period, there were 412 abortions; 53.9% were due to spontaneous abortions, 29.1% to unspecified abortions, and 10% to ectopic pregnancies. Mental disorders (including alcohol and drug abuse) accounted for 2.5% of primary discharge diagnoses for both males and females. In 2003, there were 9 births among females 10–14 years old, less than half of the 20 births in this same age group in 1994. The birth rates among females 10–14 years and 15–19 years were 0.6 and 23 per 1,000 females, respectively. Findings from the BLCS 2001 showed the prevalence of contraceptive use to be 5.6% in girls 10–19 years.

There were 3 HIV/AIDS registered deaths in the 15–19-year-old age group over the 1999–2003 period. A drug use survey conducted among secondary school students in 2002 showed that alcohol was the most popular drug among students in grades 10 and 12. Among students in grade 10, 3.5% had used tobacco, compared to 1.9% in grade 12. The prevalence of marijuana use increased with age, ranging from 6.7% among students in grade 10 to 7.7% among those in grade 12.

The BLCS 2001 showed that 68% of those between the ages of 16 and 24 had completed high school, while 32% had no academic qualification or credentials (i.e., from high school, vocational school, or another accredited institution). The survey data show that youths from the poorer quintiles exited the educational system earlier and with fewer qualifications than did youths from wealthier quintiles.

Adults 20–64 Years of Age

In the period 1999–2000, there were a total of 1,433 deaths registered in this age group. There were 1,416 deaths due to defined causes and 18 due to ill-defined causes. The five leading causes of mortality in this age group were HIV/AIDS, with 477 deaths (33.7%); assault or homicide, with 95 deaths (6.7%); ischemic heart diseases, with 83 deaths (5.9%); land transport, with 78 deaths (5.5%); and diabetes, with 78 deaths (5.5%). The leading causes of death for men were HIV/AIDS (34%), assault or homicide (9.2%), land transport accidents (7.3%), ischemic heart diseases (6.5%), and cirrhosis and other diseases of the liver (3.3%). The leading causes of death for women were HIV/AIDS (33%), diabetes (5.7%), malignant neoplasm of the breast (4.8%), and ischemic heart diseases (4.2%).

In 2003, the age-specific mortality rate for females aged 25–44 years was 2.6 per 1,000 population, and for males it was 3.7 per 1,000 population. Among women ages 25–44, the three leading causes of death were HIV/AIDS, pulmonary heart disease, and malignant neoplasm of the breast. Together, these accounted for 50% of all deaths in females. Other causes included hypertensive diseases (3%) and cirrhosis and other diseases of the liver (3%).

The combined morbidity data based on hospital discharge diagnoses for 2003 showed that the primary causes of inpatient morbidity in females 25–44 years of age and older were obstetric complications of pregnancy, childbirth, and the puerperium. This cause represented 40.4% of all hospital discharges in 2003. The second and third leading causes were other infectious and parasitic diseases (7.8%) and carcinoma in situ, benign neoplasms, and neoplasms of uncertain or unknown behavior (3.3%). Mental disorders, injuries, and poisonings were also among the five leading causes of morbidity seen at Rand Memorial Hospital in Freeport over the same period.

In terms of morbidity in 2003, the leading public hospital discharge diagnoses among males 25–44 years of age were injuries (28.2%), mental disorders (7%), HIV/AIDS (6.7%), other diseases of the digestive system (6.1%), acute respiratory infections (3.5%), and hypertensive diseases (3.2%).

In 2003, the major causes of morbidity in females ages 45–64 were hypertensive diseases, which represented 8.7% of hospital discharges diagnoses, followed by other diseases of the digestive system (8.1%), injuries and poisonings (6.7%), and carcinoma in situ (6.6%). During the 2001–2002 period, benign neoplasms, hypertensive diseases, diabetes mellitus, and other diseases of the digestive system were also leading causes of morbidity in this age group. The birth control pill was the most popular contraceptive method used among all females (47%), followed by female sterilization (19.7%), which was used primarily by older women. Other methods included injectables (16.1%), condoms (9.1%), and other modern methods (6.5%).

Obesity was most notable in the 31–50-year-old age group (about 35%) and the 51–60-year-old age group (33%), while young adults in the 21–30-year-old age group were predominantly the healthiest in terms of weight.

Older Adults 60 Years Old and Older

The most common causes of inpatient morbidity among persons 65 and older were hypertension, injuries, and poisonings, cerebrovascular diseases (stroke, myocardial infarction), pneumonia, urinary tract infections, diabetes mellitus, and malignancies. Other health conditions affecting this age group included arthritis, cataracts and glaucoma, dementia, depression, and decreased hearing. In 2003, the leading causes of death in adults 65 years of age and older were hypertensive diseases, diabetes mellitus, cerebrovascular diseases, ischemic heart diseases, prostate cancer, urinary tract infections, acute respiratory infections, and malignancies of other areas.

The Family

Female-headed households (FHH) represented a significant portion of all households in the Bahamas, and their poverty rates were double those of male-headed households (MHH). FHHs were found to have more children and had higher economic dependency burdens than MHHs. However, poor female heads of households were better educated than poor male household heads. In poor households, 33% of all youths (ages 19–24) were "unattached," meaning that they neither worked nor were in some type of training in preparation for future employment. Among non-poor households, the unattachment rate for this age group was more than 20%. Nearly 50% of poor children (ages 2–5) were either underweight or overweight.

Housing tenure (ownership, government housing, rental, or rent-free accommodations) as well as housing quality differed markedly between poor and non-poor households. Nationwide, about 70% of households had fewer than two people per bedroom, and 90% had fewer than three people per bedroom. Only 22% of poor households had fewer than two people per bedroom, and 50% had more than three people per bedroom.

Results from the BLCS 2001 showed that individuals from households in higher consumption quintiles had higher levels of health insurance coverage; only 20.1% of those in the poorest quintile had coverage, compared to 76% in the wealthiest quintile. Data from the Ministry of Health in 2003 indicated that higher-income persons were more likely to have comprehensive health insurance packages, while lower-income persons, who purchased lower-priced premiums, faced higher deductibles.

Persons with Disabilities

According to the BLCS 2001, approximately 6% of the sample population ($n = 6,414$) reported having a physical or mental disability. Of those who had a self-reported disability, 68.5% of the disabilities were related to sight, hearing, or speech; 18.2% to limbs; and 13.3% to mental disabilities. A total of 3.7% of children under 5 years of age had a disability, compared to 17.6% of the elderly.

HEALTH CONDITIONS AND PROBLEMS

COMMUNICABLE DISEASES

Vector-borne Diseases

Malaria is not endemic to the Bahamas, although the *Anopheles* mosquito vector is present. Ten imported malaria cases were reported between 2000 and 2003. There were no cases of yellow fever for the 2001–2003 period, although the *Aedes aegypti* vector is present. In 2003, there was a **dengue fever** outbreak resulting in 180 reported cases, presenting predominantly with serotypes 2 and 3; no deaths were registered. Approximately 700 cases of **scabies** were reported annually to the Ministry of Health Surveillance Unit during the 2001–2005 period.

Vaccine-preventable Diseases

In the period 2003–2004, at least 98% of children entering preschool were immunized against **measles, mumps**, and **rubella; diptheria, pertussis**, and **tetanus; polio; hepatitis B**; and *Haemophilus influenzae* **type b**. Since 2000, vaccination

coverage for the first and third doses of all vaccines has exceeded 90%, except for hepatitis B, which was initiated in 2001 as part of the pentavalent vaccine. This vaccine contributed significantly to the Expanded Program on Immunization in the Bahamas.

During the 2001–2005 review period, there were three reported cases of *H. influenzae* meningitis. There was an outbreak of hepatitis A in 2001 in which a total of 46 cases were reported. Only 5 sporadic cases were reported in 2002, 1 case in 2003, and 3 cases in 2004. During the 2002–2003 period, there were 6 reported cases of symptomatic hepatitis B. There were no confirmed cases of polio, diphtheria, measles, or neonatal tetanus. This success is credited to children being routinely vaccinated, immunization campaigns which target adults, and the continuous training of all health care providers.

Figure 2 shows immunization coverage levels by antigen for children under age 2 for the 1995–2004 period.

Intestinal Infectious Diseases

There were three **conch poisoning outbreaks** during the 2001–2003 period. The annual number of reported cases ranged from 122 to 312 during this time as a result of poor food handling by conch vendors; no deaths were registered. Foodborne diseases and **gastroenteritis** continue to pose diagnostic challenges. Between 2001 and 2003, the incidence of reported foodborne diseases ranged from 318.2 to 417.2 per 100,000 population. The number of gastroenteritis cases during the 2001–2004 period ranged from 2,521 to 4,904. Between 2002 and 2003, 564 cases of ciguatera poisoning were reported, and 214 occurred in 2004. Ciguatera poisoning is an important health problem due to the population's high consumption of and frequency of exposure to toxic fishes such as the barracuda. In the 2001–2004 period, reported cases of **salmonellosis** ranged from 4 to 28 cases per year; none, however, were linked to an outbreak.

FIGURE 2. Immunization coverage (%), by antigen, for children under age 2, Bahamas, 1995–2004.

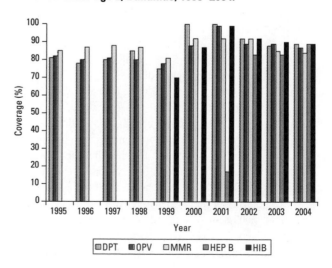

Chronic Communicable Diseases

During the 2001–2004 period, the annual number of reported cases of **tuberculosis** ranged from 44 to 47. Among these cases, the highest proportion occurred in the 25–49-year-old age group. The TB/HIV coinfection rate remained high, standing at 39% in 2002 and 32% in 2003. There were 7 deaths due to coinfection in 2002 and 8 deaths in 2003. Of the reported TB cases, about 7 out of 10 clients were Bahamians, while one in four was Haitian. The male-female ratio for TB infection was 2.1:1 in 2001 and 1.2:1 in 2003.

Acute Respiratory Infections

In 2001–2002, acute respiratory infections were the second leading discharge diagnosis (12.7%) given for children aged 5–14 years. In 2003, there were 388 females and 371 males with hospital discharge diagnoses of acute respiratory infections.

HIV/AIDS and Other Sexually Transmitted Infections

The HIV epidemic in the Bahamas is monitored through seroprevalence surveys conducted among sub-population groups, such as pregnant women attending prenatal clinics, those attending clinics for treatment of sexually transmitted infections (STIs), blood donors, prison inmates, and TB patients. Figure 3 shows prevalence rates for the years 1994–2005 for three of these sub-population groups.

As of December 2005, there was a cumulative total of 10,479 reported cases of HIV infection. The number of new persons testing positive annually for HIV declined by 56.1% from its peak level of 659 in 1994 to 209 in 2003, with the greatest change being noted in the 20–49-year-old age group. The prevalence of HIV in pregnant women declined from 4.2% in 1994 to 2.8% in 2005. Among persons receiving care for STIs, the percentage testing positive for HIV decreased from 7.2% to 5.8% over the 1995–2005 period. Underreporting regarding HIV transmission via injecting drug use remains a challenge.

The prevalence of HIV among blood donors was approximately 0.4% in 2005 and was at its lowest (0.2%) in 2003. Infection rates among the prison population decreased from 3.4% to 2.5% between 2002 and 2004. A decrease in AIDS mortality has occurred for both women and men, with the percentage of registered deaths dropping from 18.4% to 11.8% between 1996 and 2003. The drop is concurrent with improved access to quality health care and ability to diagnose and treat opportunistic infections, as well as the increased affordability and availability of antiretroviral medications.

Zoonoses

There were no reported cases of zoonotic diseases during the 2001–2005 review period.

NONCOMMUNICABLE DISEASES

Metabolic and Nutritional Diseases

In 2005, the Ministry of Health carried out a Chronic Noncommunicable Diseases Prevalence and Risk Factors Survey that found overweight and obesity to be significant risk factors in the population. The overall prevalence of **overweight** and **obesity** was 70.6%; New Providence had the lowest rate (68.7%); on Grand Bahama it was 73.7%, and on the Family Islands 76.9%. Nutritional choices also emerged as a major risk factor, with a significant percentage of those surveyed reporting that they consumed the equivalent of less than one daily serving of fruit (47.1%), vegetables (51.1%), and legumes (80.1%). Current international dietary guidelines encourage five or more servings of fruits and vegetables daily. Of the population 62% reported that they engaged in some sort of moderate or intense physical activity over the course of most days. The remaining 37.5% noted that they engaged in little or no physical activity.

The prevalence of self-reported **diabetes** was 7.0%, while that of clinical diabetes was 9.2%. As with clinical hypertension, males had a lower prevalence (8.6%) of clinical diabetes than females (9.6%).

Cardiovascular Diseases

The 2005 Noncommunicable Diseases Prevalence and Risk Factors Survey showed the prevalence of clinical **hypertension** to be 37.5%, with males experiencing a slightly lower prevalence (37%) than females (38.4%). The prevalence of self-reported **stroke** was 1.1%, self-reported **heart disease** 3.2%, and self-reported asthma 6.1%. On comparison by region, it was found that the prevalence on the Family Islands was consistently higher than the national prevalence, with stroke at 2.5%, heart disease at 7.8%, and asthma at 7.8%.

FIGURE 3. HIV prevalence in pregnant women, blood donors, and STI clients, Bahamas, 1994–2005.

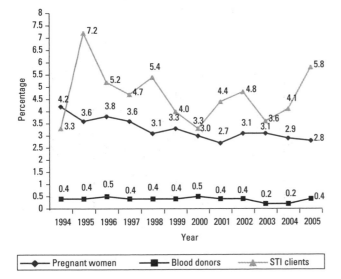

Malignant Neoplasms

National figures showed prostate cancer prevalence among males ages 40–70 years old to be 1% and breast cancer prevalence in women ages 15–74 years old to be 1.3%, while cervical cancer among women in this same age group was 0.8%. Colorectal cancers in men and women ages 50–74 years old were 0.7%.

OTHER HEALTH PROBLEMS OR ISSUES

Oral Health

During the 2001–2005 period, annual school dental screenings provided data on the oral health of children. Twenty-four of the 26 public schools on New Providence were examined during the 2004–2005 school year. Of the 2,566 grade 6 students examined, 82% were caries-free; the decayed, missing, or filled teeth (DMFT) index was 1.54. Over the same period, 2,106 grade 1 students were also examined: 55.6% were caries-free, and the DMFT was 3.48.

RESPONSE OF THE HEALTH SECTOR

Health Policies and Plans

The main objectives of monetary and fiscal policies pursued by national authorities remain the maintenance of macroeconomic stability, improvement of all aspects of economic competitiveness, and stimulation of sustainable development by the private sector in the short and medium terms. A key goal in the Bahamas is diversification of the economy, which is to be accomplished by improving intersectoral linkages between the tourism sector and the rest of the economy and by improving infrastructure on the Family Islands to promote their economic development.

Major health events and developments during the review period include the appointment of a blue ribbon commission in 2002 to study the feasibility of creating a national insurance system; the report was presented to the Cabinet in 2004 and development of an implementation plan was mandated. A cost and financing report was also submitted in late 2005. During 2001–2005, the government increased access to quality health care for persons living with HIV/AIDS by removing cost barriers. Renewed focus was given to ensuring appropriate levels of integration at the policy, programmatic, and service levels, and this approach was successfully applied to maternal and child health, communicable diseases prevention, and oral health. It is now mandatory that medical students complete a rotation with the Ministry of Health's Department of Public Health.

Between 2001 and 2005, the Ministry of Health consulted and collaborated with a variety of agencies on policy initiatives that impact the country's health situation. These culminated in the Workers' Health and Safety Act (2002) and the establishment of the National Emergency Management Agency in 2004.

In the period 2001–2005, several reforms were introduced under the Ministry of Health's leadership. The National Health Services Strategic Plan (NHSSP) 2000–2004 is a comprehensive framework for the advancement of an enhanced, integrated, national health care service delivery system. The plan seeks to foster multisectoral collaboration and participation while strengthening partnerships between the public and private sectors and the population at large. The revised 2003–2004 NHSSP consists of 13 strategic goals; each embodies a main objective, contains key indicators and expected results, and identifies the entities responsible for leading actions. The priority focuses are health promotion and protection, scaling up HIV/AIDS care and treatment, prevention and control of communicable and chronic noncommunicable diseases, environmental protection and sustainability, improved efficiency of health services delivery systems, and enhanced strategic management.

A mid-term review of progress of the original NHSSP 2000–2004 took place in December 2002 in preparation for implementation of the revised plan in 2003, providing an opportunity to make necessary adjustments and emphasize areas of special concern. These concerns included the increasing numbers of deaths due to noncommunicable diseases and teenage deaths attributable to homicides and land transport accidents, the contribution of alcohol and drug abuse to the rising rates of homicides and violent injury, and the growing threat to public health posed by domestic violence. Other areas calling for more focused attention were the status of health legislation, the regulation of professional certification, health financing and infrastructure, and health information systems. In 2001, the National Health Information System acquired databases for mortality and hospital discharges, thereby streamlining data processing and enabling improved health situation analyses.

In the area of occupational health, in addition to the passage in 2002 of the Workers' Health and Safety Act, two other labor statutes were approved that same year. The first entitled women to 12 weeks of maternity leave, and the second provided unpaid paternity leave following the birth of a baby, and/or during the illness of the baby or the baby's mother. Additionally, the Employment Act of 2002 eliminates discrimination in the workplace against those living with HIV.

Results from a 2002 evaluation of essential public health functions indicated that the national health system performed below average in all areas except health promotion and capacity for the development of laws and regulations. Further analysis revealed, at all levels in the health system, an absence of formal evaluation processes and the inefficient and ineffective utilization of established institutional capacity and of management information systems.

Organization of the Health System

The health care organizational model has been centralized and is predominantly curative and disease-based, with all functions (financing, provision of services, and regulation) performed by the Ministry of Health. The health care delivery system consists of public institutions, private-for-profit institutions, and private nonprofit institutions. The government health sector is comprised of four main clusters of services: the Ministry of Health, the Department of Public Health, the Department of Environmental Health Services, and the Public Hospitals Authority. An organizational and management review of the Department of Public Health is currently under way, and within this framework, between 2001 and 2003, a regional health pilot project commenced in southeastern Bahamas to improve the quality of public health services. The Public Hospitals Authority has responsibility for the three government hospitals (Princess Margaret Hospital, Rand Memorial Hospital, and Sandilands Rehabilitation Center) as well as public health services on Grand Bahama.

The Doctors Hospital Health System is the principal provider of private inpatient services through Doctors Hospital located in Nassau, New Providence, which is staffed and equipped for the provision of primary, secondary, and tertiary care. A second private inpatient clinic is the Lyford Cay Hospital. Various nongovernmental organizations, such as the Cancer Society, the Diabetic Association, the Bahamas Heart Association, the Family Life Association, and the AIDS Foundation, provide additional outpatient and community services.

All workers in both the private and public sectors are required by law to participate in the National Insurance Scheme, which provides illness, disability, and death benefits to its contributors, as well as retirement, occupational injury, maternity, and survivorship benefits. Private health insurance also is offered by a number of companies. A small percentage of workers are enrolled in an insurance plan managed by a private insurer on behalf of the Bahamas Public Services Union. At the current time, the group health insurance scheme has proven to be an attractive option for many persons.

Public Health Services

The Department of Public Health holds responsibility for primary health care services on New Providence and the Family Islands. These services are provided through a network of primary health care facilities ranging from level I (complex health centers) to level II (main health centers) and level III (satellite clinics). Home visits by trained public health nurses, which include basic primary care and follow-up, are provided through various of these facilities. The Department is also responsible for supporting the Ministry of Health's public policy development and the management of more than 14 national health programs.

In order to improve program management effectiveness, funding is provided annually in the Department's budget for the following national program areas: maternal and child health services, Expanded Program on Immunization, nutrition services, disease surveillance (general; vector-, water-, and foodborne dis-

eases; STI prevention programs; and tuberculosis control), and training and development (nursing and medical health professionals, allied health professionals, and administrative and other support staff).

In 2003–2004, protocols were put in place for 90% of all diseases that have been identified and targeted for surveillance and control. With regards to tuberculosis, the Directly Observed Treatment, Short Course (DOTS) strategy was being consistently applied on all islands. A specialty clinic for new diabetes cases was established using a team approach to patient management, and treatment and protocols for asthma patients have been developed for implementation at the primary, secondary, and tertiary care levels. To address issues concerning HIV/AIDS and STIs, the prevention of mother-to-child transmission program was expanded, and antiretroviral drugs were introduced as part of the comprehensive treatment program for all patients attending public facilities. During the 2001–2005 review period, the Ministry of Health prepared guidelines for this comprehensive care and treatment strategy, conducted public education programs, and provided US$ 1 million for the purchase of antiretroviral drugs.

In 2001 and 2002 the government received technical support to document key functional and data requirements as part of a long-term strategy to strengthen the public health information system. In December 2003, the Department of Public Health initiated plans for the pilot implementation of an automated, integrated client health records and reporting system (IPHIS). IPHIS supports public health provider interventions, tracking, follow-up, case management, and reporting and has been implemented in four sites on New Providence and Grand Bahama. The IPHIS initiative should improve the quality, collection, and analysis of public health data in the future.

The principal objective of the national laboratory service is to strengthen services to improve case management and disease prevention and control efforts. A National Medical Laboratory Strengthening Committee, with representation from both public and private laboratories, coordinates the national activities of a subregional project being implemented through the Caribbean Epidemiology Center. One component of the project calls for the establishment of a national laboratory information system.

The principal public health laboratories are located at Princess Margaret Hospital on New Providence and Rand Memorial Hospital on Grand Bahama. They provide services in the areas of clinical chemistry, microbiology, immunology, blood banking, surgical pathology, cytology, and hematology. The main laboratory at Princess Margaret Hospital processes an average of 700 tests daily. Laboratory specimens from the Family Islands are transported to the Princess Margaret or Rand laboratories for testing.

During the study period, the government provided a bulk waste collection program and depository sites and implemented a national solid waste education and awareness program. The New Providence Regional Landfill receives in excess of 181,000 tons of solid waste per year.

The Government Strengthens the Health System to Better Respond to Citizens' Needs

The location of the leading commercial and tourism activities drive the population's distribution, as well as inequities in the distribution of wealth, throughout the islands of the Bahamas. Moreover, the health care services are being overloaded as Bahamians migrate from less developed to more economically advantaged islands and as more and more immigrants, mainly Haitians, flow into the country. To better respond to all residents' health care needs, the Ministry of Health is spearheading an effort designed to bolster the health system. At the heart of this endeavor is the 2000–2004 National Health Services Strategic Plan, which envisions an integrated national health care delivery system. The Plan sets forth 13 strategic goals, conferring priority to health promotion and protection, prevention and control of communicable and noncommunicable diseases, environmental protection, efficient delivery systems, and better health services management.

In 2001, the Department of Environmental Health Service's Derelict Vehicle Removal Program disposed of some 7,200 abandoned vehicles taken from vacant properties, roadside garages, and along public thoroughfares on New Providence. The resulting 8,121 tons of compacted metal were then exported to the United States for recycling. In 2002, the program was expanded to address the larger of the Family Islands, and 4,000 additional vehicles were collected, crushed, and exported.

The Department also monitors manufacturers of bottled water to ensure sanitary production conditions and quality control. The Water and Sewerage Corporation evaluated the condition of all municipal sewage treatment systems with the goal of implementing improvements as necessary.

The risk management service within the Public Hospitals Authority was strengthened, and cooperation between health agencies and the National Insurance Board was enhanced. The revised NHSSP 2003–2004 includes efforts to strengthen the Worker's Health and Safety Program and workers' health services, and develop and implement occupational safety training programs.

In 2002, permission was sought from the Cabinet to amend the section pertinent to food handling of the Public Health Act. In November 2003, the Department of Public Health began piloting the new Serve Safe Food training program for food industry workers, and in 2004 a four-hour course became mandatory for all food handlers. Since the training's introduction, 85% of documented food handlers have participated and five persons have been certified as trainers. In 2001–2003, the Public Market and Slaughterhouse Act was reviewed and deemed adequate without further amendment. Poultry regulations were drafted, and a Hazard Analysis and Critical Control Point (HACCP) program based on inspection will be implemented in the poultry and other food industries. Amendments were introduced to the meat importation regulations under the Animal Contagious Diseases Act to protect the Bahamas from the introduction of bovine spongiform encephalitis and foot-and-mouth disease. The Act's amendments focused on the areas of changing technologies, country disease status, and emerging diseases.

In 2001, a group of health centers were designated as hurricane treatment centers and equipped to respond to persons requiring medical care in the immediate aftermath of a hurricane. Ministry of Health, Department of Public Health, and Public Hospitals Authority personnel have been trained in the use of Humanitarian Supply Management System (SUMA) techniques as well as in the medical management of disasters. A disaster preparedness workshop was conducted in August 2002, and a National Disaster Plan was proposed.

The emergence of severe acute respiratory syndrome (SARS) highlighted the need to take proactive measures to counteract emerging communicable diseases that might enter the country through the port system. Reports of West Nile virus on one of the Family Islands strengthened an integrated approach to outbreak investigations. The Ministries of Health and Agriculture remain on high alert in addressing the threat of avian influenza in birds and poultry and pandemic influenza in humans.

Individual Care Services

In 2003, there were five public and private hospitals with a total of 1,068 beds, representing 35 hospital beds per 10,000 population. There were 55 health centers or main clinics; 9 were on New Providence, 5 on Grand Bahama, and 41 on the Family Islands. There were 59 satellite clinics throughout the country and 286 privately owned health care facilities offering primary care and diagnostic services.

In 2001, a state-of-the-art health care center opened to serve south-central New Providence. It is the largest of the country's approximately 115 community health clinics and the only public health facility to offer ophthalmology, laboratory, radiology, and audiology services. The center holds a weekly nutrition clinic for at-risk obese schoolchildren.

Grand Bahama has its own public health services network of clinics and the Rand Memorial Hospital. The clinics make referrals to Rand, which in turn makes referrals to Princess Margaret Hospital in Nassau for those services not available at its own facilities.

A National Mental Health Committee was set up in early 2002. Between 2000 and 2002, a new organizational framework for the creation and implementation of community-based mental health programs and interventions was developed.

In 2003, the National Family Islands Dental Prevention Program was initiated; several dental professionals travel to the Family Islands to provide primary, secondary, and tertiary dental treatment, including dental prosthesis. A National Dental Sealant Program was initiated that same year and incorporated into the National Family Islands Dental Prevention Program.

A Neurodevelopment Clinic was established in 2001 to screen at-risk children between the ages of 6 weeks and 5 years for neurodevelopment disorders. During the 2001–2005 reporting period, the Department of Social Services spearheaded a basic training program for caregivers at the continuing education and extension services of the College of the Bahamas. A revised Parentcraft Education Program was launched in 2003 to prepare expectant couples for the birthing process and teach basic techniques in baby care and breast-feeding.

Health Promotion

The revised NHSSP 2003–2004 identifies health promotion as a strategy leading to the establishment of healthy public policy and healthy individual behaviors. The strategy's expected results include supporting national health programs, strengthening communications strategies, formulating healthy public policies, improving intersectoral collaboration, and capacity-building.

In 2005, the National Health Promotion Three-Year Plan of Action was completed and the Ministry of Health's Health Education Division is now a line item in the Ministry's budget. All staff members of the Division have participated in at least one relevant continuing education health promotion activity. A career path for new and existing posts for the Health Education Division was prepared.

Human Resources

The shortage of nurses in the public sector and the need for recruitment and retention were major issues of concern during the 2001–2005 period. In 2002, the Ministry of Health adopted a three-pronged incentive-based approach: sponsorships and stipends for nursing students were increased, opportunities for continuing education were promoted, and special focus was placed on encouraging high school students to choose nursing as a career. A Nursing Task Force was established which led to the development of a more comprehensive Strategic Plan for Nursing in the Bahamas. During the period 2001–2003, 66 students trained as registered nurses. Training was provided in dialysis

nursing and psychiatric nursing to further meet the growing demand in these specialty areas. Post-graduate medical training has been established in the Bahamas in collaboration with the University of the West Indies in the disciplines of family medicine, obstetrics, gynecology, and internal medicine.

Table 1 shows the total number and ratio per 10,000 population of health professionals by category employed in the Bahamas for the 2002–2003 period.

Health Supplies

The Ministry of Health holds responsibility for the regulation and control of pharmaceutical services. The BLCS 2001 reported that respondents who were outpatients tended to buy their medicines from both public and private facilities. When expenditures at both types of facilities were combined, results showed that, on average, females spent more on medications than males.

Vaccines, needles, and syringes for the public sector are procured by the government through the PAHO Revolving Fund for Vaccine Procurement. The Bahamas National Drug Agency is responsible for the registration of pharmaceutical distributors and the drugs these companies distribute. There is no registration system for individual pharmaceutical drugs. Effective cold chain practices are in place to ensure the viability of vaccines until they are dispatched to health centers and clinics. The national drug formulary consists of approximately 600 pharmaceutical products.

Research and Technological Development in Health

High technology units and equipment were concentrated on New Providence, at both public and private facilities. There were two dialysis units, one located at Princess Margaret Hospital and the other at Rand Memorial Hospital. There were two intensive care units on New Providence and one on Grand Bahama. There were two neonatal intensive care units, both located on New Paradise; one is at Princess Margaret Hospital and the other at Doctors Hospital.

Research activities carried out during the period 2001–2003 included the design of a questionnaire on the health section for the BLCS 2001 and conducting a drug survey of secondary schools in 2002. The Ministry of Health's Family Planning Unit collaborated with the Department of Statistics of the Ministry of Finance to include key questions in the BLCS 2001 reflecting knowledge, attitudes, and practices regarding family planning.

In 2005 the Ministry of Health also completed the Chronic Noncommunicable Diseases Prevalence and Risk Factors Survey.

Health Sector Expenditure and Financing

Health care is financed by the government, private health insurance, users' fees at both public and private facilities, social

TABLE 1. Number and ratio of health personnel, Bahamas, 2002–2003.

Category	Total number	Ratio per 10,000 population
Physicians	523	16.8
Dentists	79	2.5
Hospital administrators	35	1.1
Professional social workers	128	4.0
Nutritionists/dietitians (registered)	15	0.5
Nurses/nurse practitioners	840	26.9
Enrolled nurses/trained clinical nurses	508	16.3
Radiographers	43	1.4
Laboratory technologists/technicians	119	3.8
Pharmacists/dispensers	133	4.2
Pharmacy technicians	7	0.2
Physiotherapists	30	0.9
Occupational therapists	8	1.0
Dental assistants	131	4.0
Public/environmental health inspectors	72	2.0
Statisticians	4	0.1

Source: Annual Report of the Chief Medical Officer.

health insurance (the industrial injury component), and external sources. The total recurrent health expenditure for the 2001–2002 fiscal year was US$ 148,271,603. The 2002–2003 estimated expenditure was US$ 155,261,671. Health expenditure, as a proportion of the total actual recurrent expenditure, was 15% in 2002–2003. In fiscal year 2001–2002, about 69% of the health budget was apportioned to the delivery of health care, with institutions receiving the majority of the share. In the 2003–2004 fiscal year, the distribution of expenditure between the different divisions of the Ministry of Health showed that 65% went to all areas of the Public Hospitals Authority, 18% to the Department of Environmental Health Services, 10% to the Department of Public Health, and 7% to the Ministry of Health headquarters. In 2001, private insurance spent about US$ 102 million, and total per capita out-of-pocket expenditure in 2000 was US$ 309.

Technical Cooperation and External Financing

The agencies providing technical cooperation and direct financing for health projects include PAHO/WHO (the only United Nations agency with a resident representative in the Bahamas), Food and Agriculture Organization, Inter-American Institute for Cooperation on Agriculture, Inter-American Development Bank, Organization of American States, United Nations Development Program, Joint United Nations Program on HIV/AIDS, the European Commission Humanitarian Aid Office, the Clinton Foundation, the Government of Cuba, University of Toronto's Hospital for Sick Children, McGill University, the University of South Florida,

and the U.S. Embassy. In the Caribbean subregion, support was received from CARICOM, the Pan Caribbean Partnership against HIV/AIDS (PANCAP), and the Caribbean Disaster Emergency Response Agency (CDERA).

Bibliography

Commonwealth of the Bahamas, Ministry of Finance, Department of Statistics. Bahamas Living Conditions Survey (BLCS) 2001. Nassau; 2004.

Commonwealth of the Bahamas, Ministry of Finance, Department of Statistics. Report of the 2000 Census of Population and Housing.

Commonwealth of the Bahamas, Ministry of Health. Annual Report of the Chief Medical Officer 2001–2003; April 2005.

Commonwealth of the Bahamas, Ministry of Health. Chronic Noncommunicable Diseases Prevalence and Risk Factors Survey; 2005.

Commonwealth of the Bahamas, Ministry of Health. Communicable Disease Surveillance Manual; August 2005.

Commonwealth of the Bahamas, Ministry of Health, Department of Oral Health. Annual Report 2004.

Commonwealth of the Bahamas, Ministry of Health, Department of Public Health. Communicable Disease Surveillance Report; 2004.

Commonwealth of the Bahamas, Ministry of Health, HIV/AIDS Center; 2006.

Commonwealth of the Bahamas, Ministry of Health. Mid-term Report on the National Health Services Strategic Plan 2000–2004; Revised National Health Services Strategic Plan 2003–2004.

Commonwealth of the Bahamas, Ministry of Health. National Health Services Strategic Plan 2000–2004.

Commonwealth of the Bahamas, Ministry of Health. Secondary school drug prevalence survey; 2002.

Commonwealth of the Bahamas, Office of the Registrar of Insurance Companies. Data; 2003.

Commonwealth of the Bahamas, Public Health Information System. Project charter and implementation strategy, version 1.0; November 2005.

Pan American Health Organization. Country Cooperation Strategy (Draft); 2006.

Pan American Health Organization. Health Services System Profile (Draft); 2006.

Project of the Department of Statistics of the Commonwealth of the Bahamas, the United Nations Population Fund, and the Caribbean Community. CAR/94/PO6. P. 10.

United Nations Development Program and United Nations Population Fund. Draft country program document for the Bahamas 2006–2010; February 2005.

BARBADOS

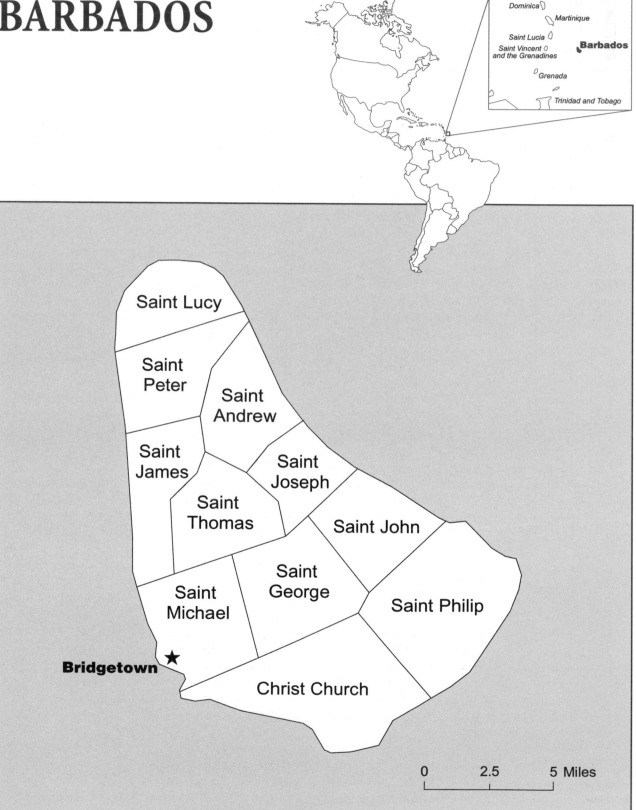

Saint Lucy

Saint Peter

Saint Andrew

Saint James

Saint Joseph

Saint Thomas

Saint John

Saint George

Saint Michael

Saint Philip

Bridgetown

Christ Church

Dominica

Martinique

Saint Lucia

Saint Vincent and the Grenadines

Barbados

Grenada

Trinidad and Tobago

0   2.5   5 Miles

B arbados is the easternmost Caribbean country. The coral island stretches for 34 km and is 23 km wide; its land area is 430 km². The country is mostly flat, with its highest point rising just over 334 m.

GENERAL CONTEXT AND HEALTH DETERMINANTS

The average temperature is 27° Celsius. The annual rainfall is approximately 1,524 mm, with the rainy season falling between June and November. During these six months, there is increased vigilance for hurricanes and attendant disaster planning.

Barbados is divided into 11 parishes. The capital city, Bridgetown, is the most densely populated area. There is a public transportation system and a network of roads, with highways linking the airport, Bridgetown, the seaport, the industrial areas, and the tourist belts on the west and south coasts. Barbados has an international airport, and continues to see significant increases in passenger arrivals and air cargo. In the reporting period, the seaport continued to undergo significant development, which has facilitated the expansion of the cruise ship market.

Barbados has a democratic government with parliamentary elections held every five years. Legislative power is vested in Parliament, which comprises a 28-member elected House of Assembly, a 21-member nominated Senate, and the Governor General, who is the Head of State. The Constitution provides for a Cabinet, comprised of Ministers, that is the principal organ of policy. It is presided by the Prime Minister. The Caribbean Court of Justice has replaced the Privy Council as the final court of appeal in the country.

Social, Political, and Economic Determinants

In 2002–2005, Barbados experienced a sustained annual GDP growth of 3%, low fiscal deficit of 2.5%, net international reserves of six months import cover (in the context of an exchange rate regime which is fixed and stable with a parity of US$ 1/BDS$ 2), and price stability. Unemployment in 2005 dropped to 9.6%.

After recording continuous economic growth between 1995 and 2000, the Barbados economy experienced a downturn in 2001, as a result of a global slowdown from the negative repercussions of the September 11, 2001, attacks in the United States. Tradable goods industries were particularly hard-hit, with tourism output down by almost 6%. The manufacturing and agriculture industries contracted by approximately 8% and 6%, respectively. To mitigate the effects of the global recession, the Government undertook an expansionary fiscal policy, which lim-

ited the extent of the economic fallout, but increased the central government deficit from 1.5% of GDP in 2000 to about 3.6% in 2001 and 6.4% in 2002.

Despite the decline in traded activity, GDP rose by about half of a percent in 2002, principally due to growth of 7.7% in construction and an increase of 6.5% in government services.

The economy strengthened further in 2003, expanding by approximately 1.9%, largely reflecting a turnaround in tourism (up 6.9%) and agriculture not related to the sugar industry (up 2.2%), as well as growth in construction and retail services. In 2004 there were 721,000 cruise arrivals, compared with 559,000 in 2003, for a 29% increase. This continued success in the cruise market was largely due to the increasing number of ships home-porting at Bridgetown Port. Cruise ship calls increased from 442 in 2003 to 539 in 2004. The cruise ship passengers to Barbados during the first quarter of 2004 came primarily from the United States (67%), followed by United Kingdom nationals (13%) and Canadian citizens (11%). During the second quarter of 2004, 72% of cruise ship passengers visiting Barbados came from the United States.

Cruise passenger spending rose by an estimated 35%, from US$ 13.1 million during the first quarter of 2003 to US$ 17.6 million in 2004. Approximately US$ 12.4 million was spent by cruise visitors from the United States and the remaining US$ 2 million by passengers from other countries. In 2005, there were 547,534 stay-over tourists in Barbados, most of them from the United Kingdom (202,764), followed by United States citizens (131,005). New jobs were created as the economy gathered momentum. The rate of inflation in 2005 was 2.4%.

The Government of Barbados is committed to eradicating poverty well before 2015 (Goal 1 of the Millennium Development Goals). An Inter-American Development Bank Poverty Assessment Study undertaken in 1996/1997 calculated the country's poverty line at US$ 2,752, approximately US$ 7.00 per person per day. In 2002, approximately 38% of the poor lived in the largest urban parish of St. Michael and 20% lived in rural parishes. In 2005, there were approximately 35,000 persons living below the poverty line.

The 2004–2005 Barbados Economic and Social Report indicated that labor market conditions had improved, with the annual estimated unemployment rate at 9.8%, compared with the 11.0% figure for 2003. Employment as a percentage of the labor force was 91.3%, as compared with 90.0% in 2003.

The number of unemployed persons totaled 14,300, a fall of 1,700 persons since 2003. Both female and male unemployment declined during 2004, with female unemployment recorded at 7,500 women, compared with 8,900 in 2003. The rate of female unemployment decreased to 10.6%, from 12.6% in 2003. Male unemployment stood at approximately 6,700 males, compared with 7,100 in 2003. The rate of unemployment for males was 9.0%, a reduction compared with the 2003 figure of 9.6%.

The labor force increased by approximately 800 persons from 2003 to 2004, rising from 145,500 persons to 146,300. The labor force comprised 75,000 males and 71,300 females. The employed labor force totaled 132,000 persons, 2,500 persons more than the 129,500 employed in 2003.

During the year, the overall labor participation rate was 69.5% compared with 69.2% in 2003, representing a 0.3 of a percentage point increase. Both male and female participation rates increased by 0.2% to reach 75.3% and 64.2%, respectively.

According to the 2005 UNDP report, Barbados had a literacy rate of 98%, which is attributed to the offer of free public education from pre-primary to university level. In 2001–2005, enrollment in primary education was 100%, and education remained compulsory for ages 5–16 years. Several programs such as school meals provided in primary schools, a textbook loan initiative, subsidized transportation, a uniform grant, secondary schools bursaries (scholarships), and a wide range of grants and scholarships at the tertiary level were available to ensure that all students can actively participate. The performance of girls and women in the educational system has been improving—girls are performing at significantly higher levels than boys in core subjects of English, mathematics, social studies, and integrated sciences. The drop-off rate between primary and secondary schools was lower among females than males.

In 2004, approximately US$ 206.2 million, 17% of the national budget, was allocated to the education and sports sector, an increase of US$ 1.3 million from 2003. More than half of the investment in education and youth supported the continuation of the Education Sector Enhancement Program, which aimed to improve the learning environment by upgrading physical facilities, teaching skills, and teaching tools, including the use of computer technology.

The Government of Barbados continued to emphasize curriculum reform initiatives, the establishment of the National Accreditation Agency, the University College of Barbados, and expansion in access to early childhood education.

With only 170 m³ of available fresh water per capita annually, Barbados is a water scarce country. Nonetheless, the country has universal potable-water coverage, which is piped into 99% of households; 1% of households access their water through standpipes. With 100% access to potable water, Barbados has reached Goal 7, Target 10 of the United Nations Millennium Development Goals. The entire population had access to sewerage and excreta disposal facilities.

Barbados did not experience any natural disasters in the period under review, but the threat of hurricanes has increased in the past four years, and the country has had flooding in low-lying coastal districts. There were no injuries or loss of life due to natural disasters.

Demographics, Mortality, and Morbidity

In 2005, the UN total population estimate was approximately 270,000. National population estimates for the years between 2001 and 2005 vary by no more than 2,000 persons from this estimate, or less than 1%. Figure 1 shows the population structure in five-year age groups for 1990 and 2005, the latter one based on the last census completed in 2000. The figure shows that females accounted for 52% of the total population in 2005 and males, for 48%; the population younger than 15 years old represented 21.5% of the total.

In 2005, the crude birth rate was 11.8 per 1,000 population and the crude death rate, 8.3 per 1,000. That same year, women of childbearing age (15–49 years old) represented 52% of the total female population, with a total fertility rate of 1.5 children per woman. Life expectancy at birth was 72.3 years for men and 78.9 years for women, with an overall life expectancy rate at birth of 75.8 in 2005. The infant mortality rate was 14.3 in 2003. Most of the population lives in Saint Michael, Christ Church, and Saint Philip parishes.

Migration was the major force contributing to variations in population. In 2003, Barbados had one of the largest concentrations of immigrants, with at least 12.3% of the total number of Caribbean migrants in the region. In addition, with the introduction and full implementation of the Caribbean Single Market and Economy, this free movement of labor affected the health care system.

Chronic noncommunicable diseases such as heart disease, cancer, stroke, diabetes, and hypertension continue to be the leading cause of morbidity and mortality among Barbadians. According to information from polyclinics and outpatient clinics, hypertension, diabetes mellitus, and disorders of the circulatory system were conditions commonly seen and treated among older adults (45–65 years old), whereas the impact of road traffic accidents, violence, and HIV/AIDS were more frequently observed among younger adults (20–44-year-olds).

In 2002 there were 2,215 deaths from defined causes, and in 2003 there were 2,436. In those same years, there were only 75 (3.3%) deaths due to ill-defined causes and 71 (2.8%) deaths due to unknown causes. In 2002 there were 2,290 deaths from all causes, of which 1,118 were male and 1,172, female. The largest number of deaths were in persons 65 years old and older (1,680; 932 females and 748 males), followed by deaths in the 5–49-year-old age group (281). The age group 50–64 years old accounted for 272 deaths and the age group under 5 years old accounted for 57 deaths.

FIGURE 1. Population structure, by age and sex, Barbados, 1990 and 2005.

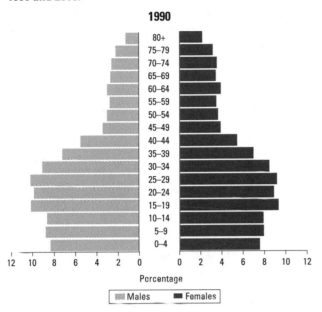

1990

2005

monia (132), malignant neoplasms of the digestive organs except the stomach (114), malignant neoplasm of the prostate (102), septicemia (55), and AIDS (42). In 2003, the leading causes were diseases of pulmonary circulation and other forms of heart diseases (257), diabetes mellitus (246), cerebrovascular diseases (207), ischemic heart diseases (180), hypertensive diseases (159), pneumonia (143), malignant neoplasms of the digestive organs except stomach (115), malignant neoplasm of the prostate (101), septicemia (74), and AIDS (30).

There were 932 deaths in females and 748 in males in 2000. Among persons 15–24 years old, 25 of the deaths were in males and 15 in females. The leading causes of death for males were homicides (5), motor vehicle accidents (3), diseases of pulmonary circulation and other forms of heart disease (3), and accidental drowning and submerging (3). There was one death from AIDS in this age group. The main causes of death among females were diseases of the musculoskeletal system and connective tissue (3), other accidents (2), hypertensive diseases (1), and septicemia (1).

The leading causes of mortality among adults were diseases of pulmonary circulation and other forms of heart disease, which were responsible for 256 deaths, with a rate of 94 deaths per 100,000 population; cerebrovascular diseases, for 207 deaths, with a rate of 76 per 100,000; diabetes mellitus, for 246 deaths, with a rate of 90 per 100,000; hypertensive diseases, for 159 deaths, with a rate of 59 per 100,000; pneumonia, for 143 deaths, with a rate of 53 per 100,000; malignant neoplasms of the digestive organs except stomach, for 115 deaths, with a rate of 42 per 100,000; malignant neoplasm of the prostate, for 101 deaths, with a rate of 37 per 100,000; septicemia, for 74 deaths, with a rate of 27 per 100,000; malignant neoplasm of the breast, for 57 deaths, with a rate of 21 per 100,000; and AIDS, for 30 deaths, with a rate of 11 per 100,000.

HEALTH OF POPULATION GROUPS

Children under 5 Years Old

Infants and children 1–4 years old represented 6.8% of the estimated total population in 2003. That year there were 63 deaths in children under 5 years old; 50 deaths were in infants, of which 32 were neonatal deaths and 18 were postneonatal deaths. The estimated infant mortality rate was 14.3 per 1,000 live births; the corresponding age-specific death rate in children 1–4 years old was less than one death per 1,000 population in 2003.

In 2003, the causes of death in this age group were conditions originating in the perinatal period (37), congenital anomalies (6), pneumonia (3), HIV/AIDS (3), and sudden infant death syndrome (2).

Low-birthweight babies (under 2,500 g) continue to be of concern, with rates fluctuating between 12.8% in 2004 and 13.9% in 2005.

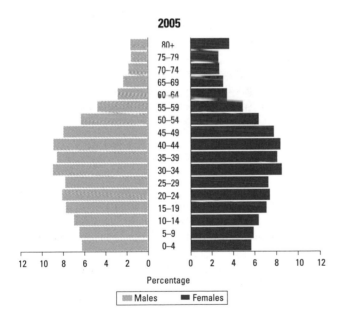

In 2003, there were 2,507 deaths from all causes, distributed virtually evenly in men and women. The largest number of deaths were in persons 65 years old and older (1,822), followed by deaths in the age group 50–64 years old (322) and deaths in persons 5–49 years old (299); there were 53 deaths in children under 5 years old. In 2002, the 10 leading causes of death were diabetes mellitus (221), cerebrovascular diseases (205), diseases of pulmonary circulation and other forms of heart disease (198), hypertensive diseases (162), ischemic heart diseases (150), pneu-

The perinatal mortality rate in 2003 was 14.8 deaths per 1,000 live births, but rates fluctuated over the period. In 2001–2005, the highest rate was in 2001, 22 perinatal deaths per 1,000 live births.

The 2002–2003 Report of the Chief Medical Officer stated that admission to the pediatric ward for malnutrition among children under 5 years old was rare; obesity in children increased, however.

Between 2001 and 2004, immunization coverage was polio, 91%; DPT/HIB, 92%; and MMR, 93%. Children seen in the government clinics are routinely monitored for growth and development.

Children 5–14 Years Old

In 2003, the age group 5–14 years old represented 14.7% of the total population; males represented 7.4% of the population and females, 7.3%. In 2003, there were four deaths in this age group, one due to viral disease, one to leukemia, one due to diseases of the nervous system, and one to malignant neoplasm of unspecified sites. The age-specific death rates were 20 per 100,000 population in 2002 and 10 in 2003.

The number of deliveries among women younger than 15 years old declined from 41 in 2001 to 6 in 2003. The number of terminations of pregnancy halved, decreasing from 8 in 2001 to 4 in 2003.

The 2002 Global Youth Tobacco Survey indicated that tobacco use was initiated at a median age of 11 years among boys and a median age of 13 among girls.

At age 11 years, children are given a booster of diphtheria, tetanus, and polio and the second MMR dose as part of the entry requirement into secondary school. The overall health status of this group is good. There were no deaths in this age group from HIV/AIDS from 2002 to 2003.

Adolescents 15–24 Years Old

In 2003, persons aged 15–24 years old represented 14.7% of the total population; males represented 15.5% and females, 13.9%. There were 34 deaths in this age group in 2002, due to homicide and injury purposely inflicted by other persons (9), motor vehicle accidents (5), diseases of the urinary system (4), and HIV/AIDS (2). In 2003, there were eight deaths in this age group, whose causes were diseases of the musculoskeletal system (3), other accidents (2), diseases of pulmonary circulation and other forms of heart disease (1), accidents caused by fire and flames (1), and homicides and injury purposely inflicted by other persons (1).

In 2003, there were 1,499 deliveries to women 15–24 years, representing 43% of deliveries to women of all ages. In 2003, there were 178 terminations of pregnancy to women 15–24 or 41% of terminations of pregnancy to women of all ages. Statistics from the Maternal and Child Health Services indicated that the number of new acceptors of prenatal services was 1,030 in 2001 and 914 in 2003.

The increasing incidence of violence and illegal drug use is of great concern; young Barbadians are particularly vulnerable in this regard. This group is at risk for violence, deviant behavior, precocious sexuality, mental health disorders, and substance abuse, including coping disorders rooted in depression and psychosocial stress. Marijuana, alcohol, and, to a lesser extent, cocaine were the drugs of choice among this cohort. This increasing drug use has had economic implications for Barbadian society as productive hours are lost by the workforce as a result, as well as the increased health care costs from treating individuals with substance use problems, who sometimes are at an increased risk of acquiring diseases such as HIV/AIDS and other sexually transmitted diseases. The latter consequence could become a serious threat to public health.

There were two persons in this age group who died from HIV/AIDS in 2002; there was one death due to HIV/AIDS in 2003.

A report of the Barbados Risk Factor and Health Promotion Survey conducted in December 2002 suggested that the mean age at which current smokers started to smoke was around 16.5 years. Other studies suggest that smoking may begin at even earlier ages, however. Reports of the 1999 and 2002 Global Youth Tobacco surveys indicated that whereas more than 30% of students may have smoked at some time, only 1% considered themselves to be regular (daily) smokers.

Among the main causes of illness and deaths in this cohort were homicides, motor vehicle accidents, and other accidents. Deaths in this age group fluctuated from 34 in 2002 to 25 in 2003.

Teen pregnancies remained a serious problem. In 2002, births to teenagers were 18% of all births; in 2003 they were 16%. There were 619 teenage deliveries in 2002 and 573 in 2003. Of the total number of abortions in 2002, 16% (514) were in teenage women; they increased to 19% (432) in 2003.

There is an active children's development center, with 2,740 children enrolled in 2004.

Adults 25–64 Years Old

In 2003, adults 25–64 years represented 52% of the total population, with males accounting for 52% and females for 51%. The total fertility ratio in 2005 was 1.5 children per woman 15–44 years old. Data from the Barbados Family Planning Association indicated that in 2003 and 2004 the family planning methods preferred by adults were oral and injectable contraceptives. With the promotion of early registration for prenatal services, women were seen by the 12th week of gestation and regularly thereafter for monitoring maternal health and fetal growth, as well as to prevent medical complications for both mother and baby during pregnancy. There was one maternal death in 2002, two in 2003, and none in 2004 and 2005.

In 2003, there were 84 deaths among 25–44-year-olds. The leading causes of death in this group were diseases of pulmonary circulation and other forms of heart disease (six), pneumonia (six), and homicide and injury purposely inflicted by other persons (five).

In 2003, there were 103 deaths among persons 45–64 years old, and the leading causes were diabetes mellitus (13), other malignant neoplasms (9), malignant neoplasm of the cervix (8), hypertensive diseases (8), and diseases of pulmonary circulation and other forms of heart disease (8).

Morbidity statistics from the primary health care system indicated that in this age group, conditions treated included hypertension, diabetes mellitus, and disorders of the circulatory system. The male clinic of the Barbados Family Planning Association (NGO) reported a rise in new client visits, from 250 in 2003 to 356 in 2004. The total male visits for 2004 rose 60% to 955, from 597 in 2003.

Older Adults 65 Years Old and Older

In 2003, the population 65 years old and older represented 12% of the general population; males accounted for 10% and females for 14%. In 2003, there were 840 deaths among persons 65 years old and older, and the leading causes were diabetes mellitus (131), cerebrovascular diseases (112), diseases of pulmonary circulation and other forms of heart disease (109), and hypertensive diseases (87).

With an increasingly aging population, there were major challenges for the provision of health care and other social services, especially for persons 75 years old and older. About 4% of the elderly live in institutions, with the remainder living at home, either alone or with relatives.

The Family

In Barbados, the average household size is 3.5 persons. More than 80% of households have telephone service and 90% have installed electricity. The Social Welfare Department reported that among family problems seen, the majority related to family maintenance matters, which ranged from 455 cases in 2003 to 1,118 in 2005. In 2003 there were 55 cases of domestic violence, 330 in 2004, and 191 in 2005.

The Department's family services section continued to provide professional service in intervention and management of individual and family problems, and the empowerment of persons in dysfunctional situations.

In 2004, there were 2,465 cases investigated, compared with 851 in 2003. The Fatherhood Initiative Program processed requests from mothers who sought assistance with securing maintenance for their children. The purpose of the program is to protect and preserve the family, provide fathers with the necessary skills to participate meaningfully in their children's development,

and foster better relationships between the parents. There were 1,150 males counseled in 2004 and 1,066 in 2003. In 2005, the Welfare Department continued to offer counseling. In 2004 3,345 children under 16 years old received monetary grants, compared to 3,357 in 2005.

The Child Care Board processed nearly 2000 inquiries, referrals, and complaints concerning 2,300 children in 2005; approximately 900 were new allegations of abuse, affecting almost 1,000 children.

The National Assistance Program responded to material needs of persons by paying utilities and rent; offering emergency food vouchers; providing dentures, spectacles, and hearing aids; and caring for and supporting persons living with HIV/AIDS.

Workers

Statistics from the National Insurance Office, the social security institution and main provider of sickness and injury benefits in Barbados, showed that at the end of 2004 the total claims received was 72,489, a 16.5% decrease from the previous year. Sickness claims account for approximately 70.3% of total claims received, followed by claims for injury on the job. All occupational accidents were reported to and investigated by the Ministry of Labor and Civil Service's Labor Department.

Persons with Disabilities

Statistics from the National Disability Unit showed that the total number of persons with a disability or a major impairment was 13,142 in 2000. Of them, 537 (4%) were under 5 years old, and 4,714 (35%) were 65 years old and older; 2,868 persons with disabilities (21%) were females and 1,846 (14%) were males. Loss of sight was the most common form of disability for both males and females, with a total of 2,446 cases.

The Children's Development Center had a registration close to 3,000 in 2005.

A training program in recreational therapy was conducted to enhance the provision of services at that institution.

HEALTH CONDITIONS AND PROBLEMS

COMMUNICABLE DISEASES

Vector-borne Diseases

In 2004, 566 cases of **dengue fever** were reported, with 2 confirmed deaths. Serotype 3 was the only serotype identified that year. There were 474 cases of dengue fever in 2005.

Malaria is not endemic in Barbados; there were three imported cases of malaria between 2003 and 2005, but no deaths due to the disease.

In 2004, the number of cases of **leptospirosis** increased due in part to unseasonably heavy rainfall: 30 cases and 2 deaths were reported that year, compared to 22 cases and one death in 2003. Most reported cases were among outdoor workers. At the end of 2005, the number of leptospirosis cases was 21.

There were no cases of **yellow fever**, **Chagas' disease**, **schistosomiasis**, or **lymphatic filariasis**.

Vaccine-preventable Diseases

Thanks to a successful Expanded Program of Immunization, in 2001–2005 there continued to be no cases of **polio**, **neonatal tetanus**, **measles**, **rubella**, or **congenital rubella syndrome**. In 2005, vaccination coverage for polio was 91%; for DPT/HIB, 92%; and for MMR, 93%. In 2004, the varicella (chickenpox) vaccine was administered to at-risk staff in the Ministry of Health.

Intestinal Infectious Diseases

There were no reported cases of **cholera** or **helminthiasis** in the period. Cases of **food-borne illnesses** increased from 62 in 2003, to 173 in 2004, and to 226 in 2005. In 2004 there were 40 cases of **campylobacter** reported, compared with 15 in 2003. This was the highest number of reported cases since 2000. In 2004, there were no reported cases of **shigellosis**; five were reported in 2003. The increased use of sanitary facilities for the disposal of fecal waste was associated with the gradual decline of shigellosis.

Chronic Communicable Diseases

During 2004, Queen Elizabeth Hospital reported 20 cases of **tuberculosis**, compared to 13 cases in 2003. Of these, four were HIV co-infections, nine were imported cases, and one was in a 2-year-old child. In 2005 there were 12 reported cases of tuberculosis, 1 of them drug-resistant. The increase in the number of tuberculosis cases is related to HIV-coinfection and an increase in imported cases. The ease of migration and an increased life expectancy of HIV-infected persons due to the Highly Active Antiretroviaral Therapy (HAART) Program will affect the management of tuberculosis. It should be noted, however, that the overall number of tuberculosis cases reported remains low.

At the end of 2005 there were 12 confirmed cases of **leprosy** (Hansen's disease). Of these, two were active cases that had been imported from other Caribbean countries and were being actively treated.

Acute Respiratory Infections

In 2002, there were 132 deaths due to **pneumonia**, of which 85% (112) were in persons 65 years old and older. In 2003 there were 143 deaths from pneumonia, with 60 deaths in persons 65 years old and older. Asthma continued to be a significant cause of morbidity, with more **asthmatic episodes** in all age groups occurring primarily during the rainy season. Asthmatic episodes

treated at the Accident and Emergency Department of Queen Elizabeth Hospital averaged 10,030 cases, of which approximately 3.8% were admitted. In 2003, there were 431 admissions for asthmatic attacks and 406 in 2004.

HIV/AIDS and Other Sexually Transmitted Infections

Information available up to March 2005 shows that there were 34 new HIV cases, compared with the 60 reported for the same period in 2004. Of persons testing positive for HIV, the majority (54%) were 20–44-year-olds, with the highest numbers in persons aged 30–34 years old.

By the end of March 2005, there were 22 new AIDS cases; 35 were reported for the same period in 2004.

There were fewer cases of AIDS reported for both males and females in 2005, but the number of deaths due to AIDS increased, from five by the end of March 2004 to nine by the end of March 2005.

All pregnant women attending prenatal clinics were counseled about and tested for sexually transmitted infections (STIs), including HIV. In 2003, there were 5,360 reported cases of STIs.

NONCOMMUNICABLE DISEASES

Metabolic and Nutritional Diseases

In 2001, there were 25 deaths due to endocrine and metabolic diseases, 24 of which occurred in persons 65 years old and older; in 2003, there were 8 deaths, 7 of which occurred in persons 65 years old and older. There were four cases of protein-calorie **malnutrition** in 2001, one among 35–44-year-olds and three among persons 65 years old and older. There was only one case in 2003, in the age group 45–64 years old. Surveillance of **overnutrition** and **undernutrition** in children under 5 years old is carried out as part of the maternal and child health program.

The 2000 Food Consumption and Anthropometric Survey showed that 30.0% of Barbadian women were obese and 58.0% were overweight; 29.0% of men were overweight and 10.0% were obese. The prevalence of **obesity** increased, mainly due to the adoption of high fat diets and a sedentary lifestyle. Increasing proportions of children are **overweight**, especially among 11–17-year-olds. The prevalence of overweight among preschoolers was estimated to be as high as 3.9% in 2000.

Cardiovascular Diseases

Diseases of pulmonary circulation and other forms of heart disease ranked among the top three of the five leading causes of death, accounting for 256 deaths in 2002 and 198 deaths in 2003. The bottom two of the five leading causes of death were **ischemic heart diseases**, with 150 deaths in 2002 and 180 in 2003, and **hypertensive diseases**, with 162 deaths in 2002 and 150 in 2003.

Hospital discharge statistics for cardiovascular diseases for the years 2000, 2001, and 2002 were 1,092 for 2000, 1,373 for 2001, and 1,763 for 2002.

Malignant Neoplasms

Malignant neoplasm of the prostate remained a concern throughout 2000–2004. In 2000, 63 men were diagnosed with malignant neoplasm of the prostate. In 2000, there were 102 deaths from malignant neoplasm of the prostate, representing 24.2% of all deaths from malignant neoplasms. Other malignant neoplasms included neoplasm of the female breast, with 51 deaths (12.1% of total deaths due to malignant neoplasms); other malignant neoplasms of the digestive organs and peritoneum, with 49 (11.6%); malignant neoplasm of the colon, 46 (10.9%); and malignant neoplasm of the stomach, 32 (7.6%).

In 2004, there were 79 referrals for malignant neoplasm of the breast, 34 for malignant neoplasm of the cervix, and 39 for malignant neoplasm of the prostate; in 2005, the figures were 112, 19, and 41, respectively. The majority of the cases of malignant neoplasms of the breast and of the cervix were among 30–69-year-olds; the majority of cases of malignant neoplasm of the prostate occurred among 50–89-year-olds.

The decrease in cases of malignant neoplasm of the cervix can be attributed to enhanced screening in the public and private sectors. The increase in cases of malignant neoplasm of the prostate points to the need to review and strengthen programs dealing with men's health.

OTHER HEALTH PROBLEMS OR ISSUES

Violence and Other External Causes

The 2004–2005 Barbados Social and Economic Report showed a 3.9% decline in reported crime, following a decline of 17.3% in 2003. The total number of reported crimes was 9,435 in 2004, which represented a drop of 388 cases from the 2003 total. Reported cases of major crimes and of property crimes declined, as a result of the success of policies and programs of the Royal Barbados Police Force. For example, enhanced community-based policing programs have been introduced, including neighborhood watches, setting up of community outposts, and utilizing community profiling. This decline notwithstanding, areas of concern continued to present challenges to the Royal Barbados Police Force, such as the continuing, pervasive use and abuse of illicit drugs, the propensity of resorting to violence to settle disputes, the use of firearms in the commission of certain offenses, and the high number of youth offenders, particularly males.

Mental Health

Most patients in the eight-bed mental health service unit within Queen Elizabeth Hospital were admitted due to a mood disorder; 20% had some kind of a psychotic disorder. In addition, 80% were female and 15%–20% were children or adolescents. The average length of stay was 10 days.

Approximately 1,000 patients were admitted annually to the Psychiatric Hospital, of which 200–250 were first admissions: 60% were male; 70% were admitted involuntarily. In 2004, there were 1,035 admissions to the Psychiatric Hospital. The bed occupancy rate in 2004 was 82%. The number of deaths also decreased, with only 13 persons dying in 2005. The number of outpatient visits were about 13,000 in both 2004 and 2005. Outpatient services were provided in the public sector and by general practitioners in the private sector.

Environmental Pollution

Test results of groundwater and spring water sampled by the Environmental Protection Department in 2001–2005 showed that measurements for dissolved solids, chlorides, electrical conductivity, pH, and nitrates did not exceed WHO standards. The high nitrate values in Barbados' waters, however, seem to indicate that they have been adversely affected by agricultural activities.

Oral Health

Detection of oral health problems and appropriate intervention was provided for all school-age children up to 18 years of age. An emergency service providing extractions was available at no cost for the elderly and children up to age 16 years. Limited oral and maxillofacial services were available at the Queen Elizabeth Hospital.

Between 2001 and 2003 there were 53,567 visits to the dental health clinics within the public primary health care system. Of these, 20,226 (37.8%) were for prophylaxis; 9,426 (17.6%), for extractions; 9,192 (17.25%), for fillings; and 98 (0.18%), for root canals. In that same period, visits to the polyclinics for oral health reasons ranged from 15,000 to 20,000. Dental clinics used improved treatment modalities, including the use of fluoride releasing restorative materials, in all public-sector dental clinics.

RESPONSE OF THE HEALTH SECTOR

Health Policies and Plans

The Government's vision for a healthy people is to empower individuals, communities, and organizations to pursue health and wellness within a health system that guarantees the equitable provision of quality health care. This, in turn, will fully contribute to Barbados' sustained economic, cultural, social, and environmental development. To this end, the National Health Policy rests on the tenet that health care is a fundamental right of every citizen.

The 2002–2012 Barbados Strategic Plan for Health was developed to reform the health system by bringing about greater efficiency, effectiveness, financial sustainability, equity, and social participation in the delivery of quality services. The Plan, which was crafted with input from within and outside the health sector, addresses 10 priority action areas and has broad strategies and measurement indicators.

The Plan represents a shift from a medical model to a more client-focused model of care. It gives greater emphasis to health promotion, disease prevention, and full stakeholder collaboration. Its strategies include programs for vulnerable groups, such as the disabled and persons with alternative lifestyles, who may be reluctant to seek the formal health care system. This new strategic direction requires that there be greater collaboration with nongovernmental organizations, community-based organizations, civil society, and the private sector and encompasses a new regulatory framework with monitoring mechanisms. Thanks to these reforms, there are now new opportunities for the Government to forge new partnerships and strengthen existing alliances with NGOs to provide support, particularly in care, advocacy information, and education. There are approximately 45 health-related NGOs and community-based organizations on record. The Ministry continued to incrementally amend the Health Services Act and regulations to facilitate the implementation of the reform.

Barbados has pockets of poverty, and the Government has embarked on a poverty eradication program since 1999, which has been further strengthened by the formation of the Ministry of Social Transformation.

A national mental health policy to guide the reform on mental health service delivery was approved by the Cabinet in June 2004.

In 2005, the legislature discussed ways to address communicable diseases, food safety, embalming and transportation of human remains, and animal control. Specifically, the Government has introduced legislation to strengthen the control of imported foods. Policies were developed for disease surveillance and institutional hygiene. In 2005, comprehensive solid waste management legislation began to be prepared. That same year, a draft national policy for the country's greening and beautification was prepared, and minimum standards of care for residential facilities for persons with substance abuse disorders were developed and submitted to responsible government authorities so that regulations could be drafted.

The Health Services Act, Cap 44, and its regulations provide for the comprehensive regulation of all public health matters. Through the Act, the Government regulates and monitors new development projects and other commercial and industrial activities, specifically with respect to their impact on drinking water quality, near-shore water quality, solid and liquid waste management, hazardous waste management, and air and noise pollution. The Government also maintains a food inspection program at ports of entry and at local food processors and shops, supermarkets, restaurants, and other businesses to ensure that food offered for human consumption meets minimum standards.

Organization of the Health System

Under Section 12 of the 1969 Health Services Act, the Ministry of Health is responsible for the health of the population of Barbados; it is the executing agency for the delivery of health care. The Ministry provides a steering role, which includes setting the health sector's vision—defining the strategic direction, policies, regulations, norms, and standards. The Chief Medical Officer is the Ministry's technical head.

The Ministry of Health is the major provider of health care services in the public sector. It provides acute, secondary, and tertiary care at the 554-bed Queen Elizabeth Hospital, including medicine, surgery, pediatrics, obstetrics and gynecology, accident and emergency, psychiatry, and oncology. Subspecialty services include cardiovascular surgery, neurosurgery, and orthopedics. A medical aid scheme is also available for persons requiring medical services that are not available on the island. Queen Elizabeth Hospital is also a teaching hospital and is affiliated with the University of the West Indies School of Clinical Medicine and Research. Mental health services are provided at an 8-bed unit within Queen Elizabeth Hospital and at the 627-bed Psychiatric Hospital. The Psychiatric Hospital provides inpatient, outpatient, and outreach services, with additional limited outpatient services offered at the eight polyclinics. In addition, residential services are provided for persons with substance abuse disorders at two privately managed drug rehabilitation centers. The Government has a contractual arrangement with these centers for the provision of care. The Government also operates four long-term care institutions, with a total bed capacity of 706 beds for residential care of elderly persons. Through a contractual agreement with the private sector, the Government is able to provide care for an additional 300 elderly persons.

Services in the private health care sector continue to expand to include in-vitro fertilization, stem-cell therapy, complementary and alternative medicine, cosmetic surgery, and renal dialysis. There are about 50 nursing and senior citizens' homes in the private sector, providing long-term care for persons 65 years old and older.

It is estimated that 20%–25% of the population has private health insurance coverage. Health insurance packages are marketed specifically to credit unions, trade unions, and large organizations.

Environmental health officers and the Environmental Engineering Division are responsible for regulatory functions that safeguard the quality and safety of food, drinking water, air quality, solid and liquid waste management, control of disease vectors, and the management of hazardous waste. In addition, public health nurses collaborate with environmental health officers to maintain surveillance at the air and sea ports for diseases listed in the International Health Regulations, and investigate cases of notifiable diseases.

The safety and effectiveness of drugs and the operations of pharmacies and pharmaceutical manufacturing plants are the responsibility of drug inspectors, who function under the drug control regulations. Three drug inspectors work with the Police Department and the Ministry of Health in issues dealing with narcotics and controlled substances. There is legislation to regulate and monitor the operations of private hospitals and of nursing and senior citizens' homes through a multidisciplinary inspection team that comprises a public health nurse, an environmental health officer, a drug inspector, and a nutritionist. There is a provision to incorporate other professionals as needed.

Public Health Services

Primary health care services are provided through eight polyclinics and two satellite clinics strategically located to allow for easy access by clients. Services include maternal and child health, adolescent health, community mental health, dental health, nutrition, general practice clinics, and environmental health services.

Much effort and many resources are invested in the fight against HIV/AIDS. Thanks to added resources dedicated to this effort, the response of the health care system to HIV/AIDS has radically changed. In addition to implementing best practice models for the treatment and laboratory monitoring of patients living with HIV/AIDS, the Government offered enhanced psychosocial support through the counseling and domiciliary care program. At the end of 2004, US$ 5.6 million was spent on the program, compared with US$ 7.7 million spent in 2003 and US$ 6.9 million spent in 2002.

To reduce the number of TB cases the TB control program has been reviewed and strengthened with the introduction of the Directly Observed Therapy (DOTS) initiatives as well as forging closer links with the HIV/AIDS program.

In 2004, the welfare department provided National Assistance Grants for 180 Persons Living With HIV/AIDS (PLWHA); 183 persons also received in-kind assistance, including food vouchers, furnishings, clothing, and dentures. Total expenditure on these National Assistance Grants was US$ 125,256.

The Barbados Cancer Society launched a breast cancer screening project to promote early detection, and reduce premature deaths due to breast cancer.

During 2004, 320 persons were assessed and referrals made based on these assessments. The Ministry of Health assigned a clinical medical officer from the polyclinics to visit the Children's Development Center to address mental disability rehabilitation.

Medical practitioners are required by law to notify the Ministry of Health of all cases of communicable diseases listed in the health services regulations. The National Epidemiologist leads a team responsible for surveillance of communicable diseases; the team is comprised of environmental health officers and public health nurses who work in collaboration with the public health and private sector laboratories, as well as the Leptospira Laboratory.

The Government of Barbados, cognizant of the importance of environmental sustainability to Barbados' economic and social welfare, remains committed to coordinating sustainable development work programs. To help protect the country's fragile ecology, the Environmental Protection Department periodically monitors groundwater, spring water, and near-shore bathing water.

Active surveillance for the *Anopheles* mosquito was carried out in wetlands as a way to prevent the transmission of malaria. In 2004, US$ 1.35 million was allocated to the vector control program to control vectors associated with the spread of disease. The mosquito control program targeted *Aedes*, *Culex*, and *Anopheles* species of mosquito.

In 2005, the Coastal Zone Management Unit conducted a beach profile to better understand beach dynamics at high-profile locations. That same year, the Unit collaborated with the University of the West Indies in a temperature monitoring project designed to assist in establishing a long-term coastal water temperature profile for Barbados' coasts. In 2005, US$ 2.65 million was spent on the coastal infrastructure program.

The marine pollution control section of the Environmental Protection Department investigated 30 complaints, which comprised oil pollution, foul odors, wastewater and sewerage discharges, and petroleum product discharges. In 2005, a solid waste and hazardous materials management section was added to the environmental protection department. The Solid Waste Unit conducted teacher-training workshops to introduce teachers to various educational tools, including the *Guide to the Integration of Solid Waste Management into the School Curriculum*. Other materials included a brochure series; information on a solid waste website; the game, "Waste Buster"; and an educational storybook, "Timmy Turtle and the Litterbugs."

The Barbados Water Authority provides potable water to households throughout the country. Approximately 99% of dwellings are connected to the supply; the remainder have access to potable water. The water supply strategy involves the use of inland deep-water wells and desalination of brackish water. In 2004, 54 million m^3 of water was consumed. In 2005, nine public and two agricultural supply wells were monitored. In addition, all wells recorded acceptable mean pH values, ranging from 6.97 to 7.46. Groundwater samples were analyzed for 21 water supply parameters. Five parameters which gave the best description of water quality were selected for detailed analysis. The selected parameters were total dissolved solids, chlorides, electrical conductivity, pH, and nitrates. Seven public springs were monitored in 2005; average total concentrations were in compliance with WHO standards.

In 2005, five beaches were added to the sampling regime of the recreational water monitoring program in an effort to determine whether waters are safe for bathing. Weekly samples are taken and analyzed for fecal coliform and enterococci.

The Government is committed to preserving the country's ecosystem by improving sewage disposal along the densely populated south and west coasts and in Bridgetown. The City of

Bridgetown and the country's southwest coastal area are connected to sewerage systems. The primary objective of providing sewerage connections to these areas was to bring the near-shore water to bacteriological standards in line with international standards and to reduce chemical contamination affecting reefs, marine life, and beaches.

The effluent from sewerage treatment plants was monitored for indicators including total nitrogen, total phosphorous, and chemical oxygen demand. Feasibility studies are being undertaken to provide sewerage services on the west coast. In the meantime, however, hotels in this area operate package sewage treatment plants.

The Government gave priority to solid waste management in order to reduce the quantity of refuse in the waste stream and to address concerns with illegal dumping. The Inter-American Development Bank-funded Integrated Solid Waste Management Program included a composting facility and a chemical waste storage facility. Incentives will be provided to stimulate recycling.

The Ministry of Health's Environmental Health Division is responsible for inspecting all food destined for human consumption. In 2003, the Division inspected 24.8 million kg of meat, poultry, and fish (local and imported). Of these, 2.1% were determined to be unfit for human consumption and were condemned. The Port Health Inspection service was responsible for inspecting all food landing at ports of entry for wholesomeness and for taking food samples for bacteriological, chemical, and organoleptic analysis. It also inspected and monitored the handling of food prepared for export on cruise liners and airplanes and the issuing of relevant certificates. The Port Health Officer inspected all food businesses and restaurants and supervised the disposal of condemned food items.

Surveillance of food catering establishments licensed under the Health Services Act—hotels, restaurants, bakeries and shops, supermarkets, food-processing plants, and itinerant food vendors—was kept up. Temporary restaurant permits were approved for vendors operating at street fairs and festivals. Each year, the Ministry of Health provides training courses for food handlers as a strategy to prevent food-borne outbreaks.

The Government operated a school-meals program that provided daily meals at an affordable price for primary school students. The Welfare Board, the Barbados Red Cross Society, church-based organizations, and other NGOs provided food assistance to the needy. In the public sector, the National Assistance Board assigned home helpers to prepare meals for elderly persons living alone. The Ministry of Health facilitated a food bank program for persons living with AIDS stocked by food donations from the public.

Barbados has a national disaster program that seeks to prepare the country in the event of natural or man-made disasters. This program is community focused but each sector is assigned particular duties and responsibilities.

The Ministry's avian influenza plan was developed in 2005 to enhance surveillance at the ports of entry, wetland surveillance to detect illness in all birds including migratory and wild birds, prophylaxis measures for at-risk populations, and appropriate education for the public.

Individual Care Services

Outpatient services are provided in the public and private sectors. Between April 2004 and March 2005 there were some 3,000 surgeries performed at Queen Elizabeth Hospital. There were 105,286 outpatient visits in 2001, 98,171 in 2002, and 96,310 in 2003. Outpatient visits in the Accident and Emergency Department and in the General Outpatient Clinic were 44,048 in 2001 and 47,050 in 2003.

Polyclinics provided a significant share of ambulatory visits in the public sector. In 2005, the polyclinics provided 391,315 primary care clinic attendances, including maternal and child health services, dental services, and general practitioner visits. Since 2000, catheter changes were done in the polyclinics, rather than at Queen Elizabeth Hospital.

According to the 1998 Report on the Barbados Health Sector Rationalization Program, the private sector provided most medical and surgical ambulatory services, by a modest margin. In terms of dental services, however, the private sector was by far the greater provider, because public sector dental care is offered mainly to children under 18 years old and, to a limited extent, to pregnant women and elderly persons.

Children with developmental challenges are assessed at the Children's Development Center, which provides a wide range of services, including speech therapy, ophthalmology, audiology, psychology, psychiatry, and occupational therapy. Long-term institutional care is provided for children with physical and mental disabilities at the St. Andrew's Children's Center.

In 2005, asthma cards were given to all patients with asthma. Protocols for the management of asthma in polyclinics and schools were developed and distributed.

A diabetes protocol was developed and training in the use of this protocol in the primary health care setting and with all staff levels was provided at Queen Elizabeth Hospital.

In an effort to reduce the number of non-emergencies that arrive at Queen Elizabeth Hospital's Accident and Emergency Department and reduce waiting times for medical care, in 1999 the Government instituted a fast-track system at the polyclinic nearest to the hospital. Approximately 70% of patients seen at the polyclinic were walk-ins and 30% were referrals from Queen Elizabeth Hospital's Accident and Emergency Department.

New classes were added to the sign language program in 2004, some of which catered to parents and relatives of children with disabilities; 115 persons graduated in 2004.

In 2004, 67 persons were granted aids to daily living equipment such as canes, shower extensions, wheelchairs, cushions, raised toilet seats, and grab bars. An additional 26 persons with disabilities were placed in occupational activities.

More than 205,492 laboratory requests were conducted at Queen Elizabeth Hospital in 2003. Approximately 81% of all tests are performed at either the hospital's laboratory or at the public health laboratory at Winston Scott Polyclinic. Four private laboratories together account for one-fifth of the country's laboratory testing. Bacteriological testing also is done in collaboration with the Caribbean Epidemiology Center (CAREC). The blood bank that functions under Queen Elizabeth Hospital routinely screens donated blood for HIV infection, hepatitis B, hepatitis C, and syphilis.

There were no reported cases of diseases transmitted through blood transfusions during the period under review. There was no evidence that the six reported cases of acute hepatitis B in 2001 and 2002 had occurred as a result of blood transfusion.

There is a referral system between public sector institutions and private providers of specialized health care services, including ultrasound and mammogram, angioplasty, MRI, renal dialysis, and laboratory work. These services are paid for on a fee-for-service basis.

For more than a decade, an independent living model of care has been in place for older persons, carried out through the local branch of Soroptimist International.

Health Promotion

The Ministry of Health focused on health promotion as an approach to attain and maintain health and wellness. The media took an active role in promoting healthy lifestyles by producing regular features on health and by collaborating with the Government, businesses, and NGOs to promote healthy lifestyles.

As part of the effort to build the personal health skills of Barbadians, health and family life topics were introduced into primary- and secondary-school curricula.

Priority was given to asthma education and training, environmental health, and mental health issues. Community mobilization and organization activities were implemented through a national "Healthy Lifestyle Extravaganza," which included health fairs, smoking cessation drives, and community education activities.

The Child Care Board continued its Child Abuse Awareness Program within primary schools. The program aims at keeping children safe from abuse and equipping them with necessary information that can assist them should they become victims. In 2004, 559 children from 13 primary schools participated.

Human Resources

Barbados continues to face the problem of emigration of health professionals, and this depletion of human resources is putting additional pressures on the delivery of quality care to the population. The health sector continued to experience health human resource shortages, especially in the medical, nursing, physical therapy, occupational therapy, and allied health disciplines. As health professionals have continued to migrate to Europe and North America, the rate of training (especially of nurses) has not kept pace. Between 2002 and 2003, there was a dramatic reduction in registered nurses from 1,422 in 2002 to a mere 648 in 2003. Registered nursing assistants also declined, although not so precipitously, from 363 in 2002 to 307 in 2003.

The Barbados Community College continues to provide training for health professionals such as environmental health officers, medical record clerks, medical laboratory technicians, pharmacists, registered nurses, nursing assistants, and rehabilitation therapy technicians.

In 2004, two staff members of the Convention on the Elimination of All Forms of Discrimination Against Women participated in a workshop for government officials responsible for preparing reports to the Convention.

Health Supplies

The Barbados Drug Service procured essential drugs from a local pharmaceutical manufacturing company and, more extensively, from sources in the United States, Canada, South America, and Europe.

Supplies for medical and other health care purposes are generally supplied for the public sector through a Government central purchasing agency.

The Barbados Drug Service has entered into contract with private participating pharmacies to meet the prescription demands of persons older than 65 years; children under 16 years old; and persons suffering from hypertension, cancer, diabetes, asthma, and epilepsy. In fiscal year 2004/2005 there were more than one million prescriptions submitted by private participating pharmacies through the Special Benefit Service, at a cost to the Government of US$ 11.7 million. This figure represented an 85% increase in prescription volume and a greater than twofold increase in expenditure compared to the figures in fiscal years 1993–1995.

Vaccines for the Expanded Programs on Immunization are purchased through the PAHO's Revolving Fund for Vaccine Procurement. Reagents for laboratory use and for diagnostic procedures are purchased through the main medical laboratory at Queen Elizabeth Hospital for distribution to other laboratories. Automatic and semiautomatic laboratory testing are in use with a new Elecsys Hitachi machine for hormone and cardiac testing.

Research and Technological Development in Health

The Barbados Eye Study ended in 2002. The Barbados Cancer Study, launched in March 2002, examined family connections and risk factors affecting cancers of the prostate and of the breast in the population. The study was a collaborative effort between

Demographic Transition Prompts Health Sector Changes

A declining birth rate and reductions in the incidences of communicable diseases and nutritional deficiencies have resulted in an increasingly older population with a longer life expectancy. To address these new challenges the Government has launched a Strategic Plan for Health that will be in effect through 2012, which provides for more effective health care for the country's aging population. To secure the Plan, the Ministry of Health has undertaken a reform of its health information system.

the State University of New York at Stony Brook (Coordinating Center), the University of the West Indies, the National Human Genome Research Institute, and the Ministry of Health. This comparative epidemiological study was designed to examine environmental and family/genetic risk factors for prostate cancer and breast cancer in Barbados. As a result of the study, a population-based cancer registry was established. Initially the registry only recorded breast and prostate cancer cases, but will eventually be expanded to include other cancers.

Health Sector Expenditures and Financing

The health sector allocation for fiscal year 2005–2006, less emoluments, was US$ 122.4 million, compared to US$ 121.35 million for fiscal year 2004–2005, for an overall increase of 0.7%. The bulk of this expenditure went to hospital services and primary health care. Expenditures for hospital services were estimated at US$ 136.6 million for fiscal year 2005–2006, compared with US$ 70.5 million in 2004–2005.

Expenditures on primary health services were estimated at US$ 27.1 million in fiscal year 2005–2006, an increase of 10.8% from the US$ 24.5 million figure for fiscal year 2004–2005. Further budgetary allocations included those to the pharmaceutical program, which received US$ 17.2 million, or 14.0% of the total budget; to the HIV/AIDS prevention and control program, US$ 4.5 million, or 3.6% of the budget; to direction and policy formulation, US$ 4.4 million, or 3.5%; and to care for the disabled, US$ 650,000, or 0.5% of the budget.

In addition to recurrent funding, the Government allocated US$ 21.5 million for financing various projects within Queen Elizabeth Hospital; an additional US$ 12.5 million loan was allotted to the hospital. Approximately US$ 3.5 million in European Union funds have been earmarked for the development and expansion of the cardiac unit and angiographic suite. The European

Union also will provide US$ 2.75 million for the development of the hospital's information system network.

Technical Cooperation and External Financing

Among the regional and international agencies providing technical cooperation are the Pan American Health Organization (PAHO), Caribbean Regional Drug Testing Laboratory (CRDTL), Caribbean Food and Nutrition Institute (CFNI), Caribbean Epidemiology Center (CAREC), Caribbean Environmental Health Institute (CEHI), the World Bank, the Inter-American Development Bank (IADB), and the European Development Fund. The Ninth European Development Fund program was launched in 2005. This program involves grant funds from the European Union in the amount of US$ 12.5 million, to be executed over a four-year period. The primary objective was to facilitate the development of a comprehensive and integrated strategy that focuses on policies to benefit the poor, including providing fair financing.

Bibliography

Barbados Economic and Social Report 2002–2005.

Barbados, Ministry of Health. Chief Medical Officer's Annual Report 2000–2001.

Barbados, Ministry of Health. Chief Medical Officer's Annual Report 2002–2003.

Barbados, Ministry of Health. National Mental Health Policy for Barbados. 2004.

Barbados, Ministry of Health. Strategic Plan for Health 2002–2012.

Caribbean Commission on Health and Development. Caribbean Commission Report on Health and Development. 2005.

BELIZE

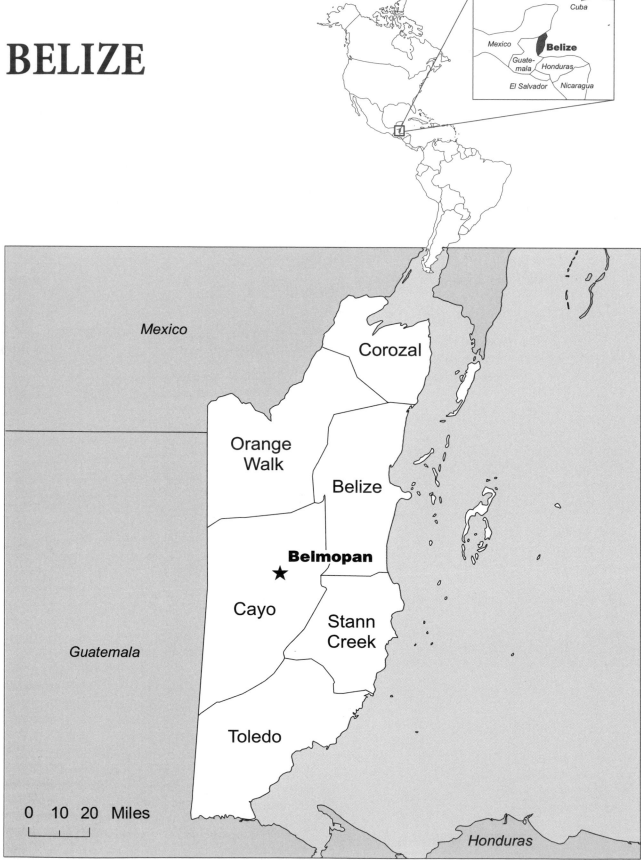

Cuba

Mexico

Belize

Guate-mala

Honduras

El Salvador

Nicaragua

Mexico

Corozal

Orange
Walk

Belize

Belmopan

Cayo

Stann
Creek

Guatemala

Toledo

0 10 20 Miles

Honduras

Belize is located in Central America; it shares a border with Mexico to the north, Guatemala to the west and south, and with the Caribbean Sea to the east. It is 274 km long and 109 km wide. The total land area (mainland and keys) is 22,700 km², with a population density (2005) of approximately 12 inhabitants per km².

GENERAL CONTEXT AND HEALTH DETERMINANTS

In 1970, the government moved the national capital from Belize City to Belmopan, which is located inland, in light of hurricane-related damages to Belize City, which is located at sea level. A former British colony, Belize is the only English-speaking country in Central America. Its culture, politics, and economy are more like those of other English-speaking Caribbean countries; due to its location, however, Spanish is also widely spoken.

Social, Political, and Economic Determinants

Belize is a sovereign state governed by the principles of parliamentary democracy based on the British Westminster system. The titular head of state is Queen Elizabeth II, represented by a Governor-General. A Prime Minister and Cabinet constitute the executive branch of the government, while a 29-member elected House of Representatives and a nine-member appointed Senate form a bicameral legislature, the National Assembly. The Cabinet consists of Ministers and Ministers of State who are appointed by the Governor-General on the advice of the Prime Minister. The country has six administrative districts: Belize, Cayo, Corozal, Orange Walk, Stann Creek, and Toledo. A locally elected town board of seven members administers each urban area. Belize City and Belmopan (Cayo District) have their own nine-member city council. Village councils carry out the village-level administration, with the traditional "alcalde," or mayoral system, incorporated into the structure in the southern part of the country (Toledo District).

In 2005, the mid-year population estimate of Belize was 291,800, comprised of 144,400 (49.5%) females and 147,400 (50.5%) males. The population has more than doubled since 1980, when it was 144,000, while the female-male distribution remains unchanged. In 2005, 50.2% lived in urban areas and 49.8% in rural areas, compared to 49% and 51%, respectively, in 2000. The 2005 mid-year population showed that Belize District continued to maintain the highest proportion of the population (29.8%), while Toledo District maintained the lowest proportion (9.5%). The population density averaged 12 per km² during the years 2001–2005. The population structure, by age and sex, for 1990 and 2005 is presented in Figure 1.

The demographic profile is of a young population. In 2005, 50% of the population was under 15 years of age, while 48% was 20 years and older. The elderly (60 years and older) accounted for 4.2% of the total population. Women of child-bearing age (15–49 years) accounted for 49.2% of the total female population. The dependency ratio was 69.6% in 2005.

Belize has an open economy based primarily on agriculture and services. Agriculture exports, which include sugarcane, citrus and bananas, and marine products, have historically dominated Belize's economy. The country also relies heavily on forestry, fishing, and mining as primary resources. One of the main attractions for foreign investment is the stability of the currency; since 1976, the exchange rate has been pegged to the U.S. dollar (US$ 1.00 = BZ$ 2.00).

In 2000, Belize had an unprecedented GDP real growth of 12.3%, which was associated with growth in revenues from the tourist industry and shrimp exports. Following several natural disasters, a slowing world economy, higher fuel prices, and a programmed reduction in the central government's expenditure, the GDP fell to 4.3% in 2002 and to 3.1% in 2005. However, increases in banana and in farmed shrimp production and exports, coupled with a surge in tourism activity, contributed to the 2003 GDP growth of 9.3%. Data from Belize's Central Statistical Office (CSO) showed that GDP per capita for 2003 was US$ 3,604. Per capita income at constant prices averaged approximately US$ 3,500 over the 2001–2005 period.

The 2002 Living Standard Measurement Survey report used expenditure data for estimating poverty indicators. (The CSO uses a 1990 World Bank definition in defining poverty as "the inability to maintain a minimum standard of living.") In 2003, the overall poverty level in Belize was 33.4%, and estimates indicated that 10.8% of the population was very poor or indigent. The indigent line was defined as the "minimum cost of food requirement necessary for healthy existence" (with the minimum cost being based on CSO's list of basic food items and their unit cost, which in turn was obtained from the February 2002 round of price collection for the Consumer Price Index).

The poverty rates varied by district and were highest in Toledo, where 79% of the population was poor; the lowest rate

FIGURE 1. Population structure, by age and sex, Belize, 1990 and 2005.

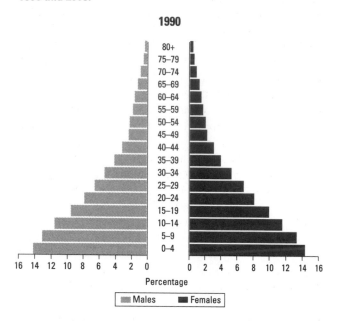

1990

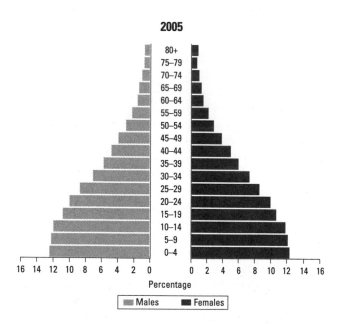

2005

working poor accounted for 29.8% of the labor force. At the household level, 7.5% were very poor and 24.5% were poor. The level of poverty among female-headed households was lower (21.8%) than that of male-headed households (25.5%).

The total adult literacy rate in 2005 was 94.7% (94.8% for females and 94.6% for males). The level of participation in the educational system is expressed in terms of gross and net enrollment rates. The United Nations Children's Fund (UNICEF) estimated that the net enrollment rate for primary school-aged students (number of children 5–12 years enrolled in primary schools expressed as a percentage of all children 5–12 years) was 89.9% for the 2002 school year (91.7% of females and 88.2% of males). The primary school gross enrollment rate (number of children enrolled in primary school expressed as a percentage of all children 5–12 years) was 104.5% in 2002. Between 2000 and 2001, overall enrollment in secondary schools increased by 5%, with a further increase of 6% between 2001 and 2002. Males comprised 49% of overall enrollment and females 51%. At the primary level, Belize District had the highest net (100%) and gross enrollment (112.7%) rates; it also had the highest net enrollment rate at the secondary level.

According to the 2005 Labor Force Survey, women in Belize have just above half the male rate of labor force participation (39.2% female, 76.4% male); just above half the male level of employment (men have 65.8% of available jobs); double the male rate of unemployment (7.2% male, 17.4% female); but more than double the male rate of long-term employment (greater than 12 months) (8.7% female, 3.3% male).

Analysis of health data for the 2001–2005 period indicates that noncommunicable diseases were among the leading causes of morbidity and mortality in Belize. Diseases such as diabetes mellitus and hypertension continued to be the major contributors to mortality and morbidity. During the period 2001–2004, the incidence of reported HIV infections increased 15.6%, but in the period 2004–2005 it decreased 5.0%. The Ministry of Health reported that the average HIV adult prevalence for the 2001–2005 period was 216 per 100,000 population.

Access to safe drinking water continued to improve. In urban areas, coverage increased from 95% in 1990 to 98.8% in 2004 and has remained steady since. In rural areas, coverage increased from 51% in 1990 to 95.4% in 2004. As regards sanitation, limited progress has been made, especially in the rural areas. According to 2002 data from a CSO Poverty Assessment Report, 54.8% of all households had access to improved sanitation (sewer or septic tanks) while 39.7% used pit latrines, 10% of households shared toilet facilities, and 3.5% did not have any toilet facility. Slightly more than 65% of all rural households used pit latrines, compared to approximately 35% of the urban households (except for Belize City). Increased waste generation and inadequate waste management represent a major national problem. It is estimated that Belize produces approximately 112,000 tons of municipal solid waste annually with a per capita generation of approxi-

was in Belize District (24.8%). These two districts also had the highest and lowest percentage of the indigent population, respectively. The poverty rates in Orange Walk and Stann Creek were very similar and only slightly above the national rate. The Cayo and Corozal Districts joined Belize District as the districts with the overall lowest levels of poverty. The level of poverty in households with children 0–13 years of age was 39%, while the corresponding rates in households with youth 14–24 years of age and those 60 years and over were 33.9% and 26.5%, respectively. The

mately 1.32 kg/day. While a national solid waste management plan was developed in 1999, very little progress has been made in implementing it. Collection services in urban centers have improved; however, proper disposal continues to be a major challenge since the country has no proper facilities for solid waste disposal. The situation in rural areas is even more serious, as there are no collection or disposal services.

In the 2001–2005 period, Belize has been directly and indirectly affected by natural events, mainly hurricanes and floods. The last hurricane to hit Belize was Iris, in October 2001. The country, in particular the health sector, has shown a high level of preparedness and response to natural events. However, in view of the increased frequency and intensity of these events, the country remains on high alert and continuously updates its disaster management plans and programs to reduce vulnerability and minimize any catastrophic impact on public health.

Around 75% of the population in Belize is vulnerable to natural disasters, which particularly impact on the poor, with devastation exacerbated by land degradation. Challenges include the need to strengthen national technical and management capacities as part of efforts to minimize the impact of natural and human-made disasters and to address issues related to improper natural resources utilization, including over-exploitation of marine resources and unsustainable land management practices.

In 2003, there were 1,240 cases of domestic violence. The 25–29-year-old age group accounted for the highest number of cases (269), followed by the 20–24-year-old age group (243), the 30–34-year-old age group (237 cases), the 15–19-year-old age group (100), and the 40–44-year-old age group (81). In 2005, there were 969 reported cases of domestic violence. The population segment ages 15–44 comprised 89% and 87% of the cases in 2003 and 2005, respectively.

The 2000 census revealed that the majority of the foreign-born population comes from Central American countries. Guatemalans have remained the single largest group, accounting for 42.5% of the foreign-born population. Approximately 15% of immigrants were under 14 years of age, the majority being in the productive age group.

Demographics, Mortality, and Morbidity

The total fertility rate in 2003 was 3.4 children per woman; it was 3.6 in 2004 and 3.0 in 2005. The infant mortality rate ranged from as high as 21.2 per 1,000 live births in 2000 to as low as 14.3 in 2004. It was 18.4 in 2005. During the 2001–2005 period, the mortality rate in children under 5 due to diarrhea was reduced from 164 per 100,000 children to 23. Life expectancy at birth in 2005 was 71.8 (69.5 for males and 74.2 for females). The crude birth rate in 2005 was 25.7 births per 1,000 population. Teenage pregnancy, as reflected by births to the under-20 population, was 18.5% in 1998 and 17.1% in 2002. The crude mortality rate from 2001 to 2005 was 4.9, 4.8, 4.7, 4.6, and 5.2 deaths per 1,000 pop-

ulation per year, respectively. There were 5 maternal deaths in 2000, 7 in 2002, 3 in 2003, 5 in 2004, and 10 in 2005. In 2005 the estimated underregistration of deaths was 12.8%, while for 2004 it was 6.7%. There were 6,489 deaths during the period 2001–2005, of which 7.8% (504) were from hypertension. Of these, 50.2% (253) occurred among females. Diabetes mellitus ranked among the first 10 leading causes of mortality in the period 2001–2005, accounting for 398 (6.1%). Of these, 228 (57.3%) occurred among females. In 2005, diabetes accounted for 94 (6.9%) deaths. There were 386 (5.9%) deaths from land transport accidents during this same period, with this cause ranking fourth during 2005. Of these deaths, males accounted for 303 (78.5%). There were 372 (5.7%) deaths related to acute respiratory infections between 2001 and 2005. Of these, 199 (53.5%) occurred among males. Acute respiratory infections ranked sixth in 2005. The leading causes of death from defined causes for all ages in Belize in 2005 were diabetes mellitus, ischemic heart diseases, land transport accidents, and HIV/AIDS. For males, the five leading causes of deaths in 2005 were land transport accidents, HIV/AIDS, injuries, ischemic heart diseases, and diabetes mellitus. In 2005, for females, the five leading causes were hypertensive diseases, diabetes mellitus, ischemic heart diseases, cerebrovascular diseases, and acute respiratory infections.

HEALTH OF POPULATION GROUPS

Children under 5 Years Old

In 2001–2005, the leading cause of infant mortality was conditions originating in the perinatal period (62.0%). Of all deaths among neonates due to this disease group, slow fetal growth, fetal malnutrition, and immaturity accounted for 149 deaths (19.0%); hypoxia, birth asphyxia, and other respiratory conditions for 87 deaths (11.1%); other conditions originating in the perinatal period for 35 deaths (4.5%); congenital anomalies for 89 deaths (11.4%); acute respiratory infections for 65 deaths (8.3%); nutritional deficiencies and anemias for 28 deaths (3.6%); and septicemia for 29 deaths (3.7%). Diarrheal diseases and acute respiratory infections were among the leading causes of death in the under-5 population. From 1998 to 2003, cases of diarrhea in children under 5 were reduced from 1,645 to 227. In 2005, the five leading causes of death were slow fetal growth, fetal malnutrition, and immaturity; hypoxia, birth asphyxia, and other respiratory conditions; congenital anomalies; intestinal infectious diseases; and acute respiratory infections.

Between 2001 and 2004, the prevalence of low birthweight (less than 2,500 g) fluctuated from 3.6% to 4.4%; it peaked at 6.9% in 2005.

The highest proportion of deaths in the 1–4 age group was due to external causes of injury for the period 2001–2005. Of these deaths, land transport accidents accounted for 18 (11.5%) and accidental drowning for 13 (8.3%). The second leading cause of death for this age group was communicable diseases, accounting for 44 (43.6%) of all deaths. Of these, acute respiratory infections accounted for 13 (12.9%) of total deaths, and septicemia accounted for 11 (10.9%). In 2005, the five leading causes of death were transport accidents, accidental drowning, acute respiratory infections, septicemia, and intestinal infectious diseases.

In 2005, the main causes of hospitalization among this age group were acute respiratory infections; noninfectious lower respiratory diseases; intestinal infectious diseases; injury, poisoning, and certain other consequences of external causes; and appendicitis, hernia of abdominal cavity, and intestinal obstruction. In 2005, 76.8% of births occurred in public hospitals. In 2001, 90% of mothers breast-fed their babies; 24% breast-fed exclusively for the first three months. Those most likely to have breast-fed were Kekchi Maya women and women who gave birth at home. Of those who did not practice exclusive breast-feeding, most were from urban areas and were younger and better educated. Creole women were the least likely to have practiced exclusive breast-feeding.

Children 5–9 Years Old

The mortality rate for this age group stood at 32 per 100,000 in 2003 and increased to 50 in 2005, with 79 deaths for the 2001–2005 period. External causes accounted for 40.5% of all deaths, transport accidents for 24.1%, and accidental drowning and submersion for 13.9%. Communicable diseases, including acute respiratory infections (12.7%), septicemia (3.8%), and HIV/AIDS (2.5%), together accounted for 19.0% of deaths in this age group. In 2005, the five leading causes of death were accidental drowning and submersion, acute respiratory infection, transport accidents, nutritional deficiency and anemia, and diseases of pulmonary circulation and other forms of heart diseases.

Hospital discharge data for 2001–2005 show that there were 3,151 hospitalizations among this age group. Of these, 574 (23.9 %) were due to injury, poisoning, and certain other consequences of external causes; 297 (12.3%) to appendicitis, hernia of abdominal cavity, and intestinal obstruction; 264 (11.0%) to noninfectious lower respiratory diseases; and 254 (10.6%) to acute respiratory infections.

Adolescents 10–14 and 15–19 Years Old

Those 10–19 years of age accounted for 64 deaths during the period 2001–2005. The mortality rate for adolescents 10–14 years old ranged from 36 per 100,000 population in 2001 to 40 in 2005. External causes of injury were the leading cause of death (40.6%). Most notable were transport accidents, which made up 14.1% of total deaths. Communicable diseases accounted for 12.5% of all deaths, mostly due to respiratory infections. In 2005, the five leading causes of death were accidental drowning and submersion, malignant neoplasms of lymphatic and hemopoietic tissue, transport accidents, acute respiratory infections, and dis-

eases of the nervous system other than meningitis. For the five-year period, adolescents in the 10–14 age group accounted for 2,643 (2.8%) of the 92,813 hospital discharges. Leading causes of hospitalization included injury, poisoning, and certain other consequences of external causes (19.6%); complications due to pregnancy (11.8%); and appendicitis, hernia, and intestinal obstruction (11.2%).

There was an average of 24 live births to mothers under 15 years of age over the same period. There were 1,356 live births to mothers in the 15–19-year age group, representing 18.1% of the total live births.

The mortality rate among adolescents 15–19 years old remained constant at 86 per 100,000 population in both 2002 and 2003. There were 157 deaths in this age group over the five-year period. Of these, 63.1% were due to external causes, of which land transport accidents comprised 21.0%. While males were disproportionately affected by land transport accidents, complications of pregnancy (56.1%) were the leading cause of hospitalization for females.

In 2005, the leading causes of death were land transport accidents, homicide, suicide, other accidents, and diseases of pulmonary circulation and other forms of heart disease. In 2004, the first two causes were the same as 2005; accidents caused by firearm missiles and accidental drowning and submersion were also leading causes in 2004.

During the period 2001–2005, there were 145 (41 males and 104 females) new HIV infections in the age group 10–19 years, which comprised 6.9% of total new HIV infections. Of these, 16 occurred in the 10–14 age group. The early initiation of sexual activity and the prevalence of STIs are public health concerns. Fourteen suicides and self-inflicted injuries were reported in the 10–19-year-old age group during 2001–2005.

Between 2001 and 2005, there were 95 reported domestic violence cases in the age group of under 1 to 14 years of age; of these violent acts, 76.7% were committed against females.

In 2003, studies showed that the prevalence of smoking is very high among school-aged adolescents (13–15 years) and that it is substantially higher among males as compared to females.

Adults 20–59 Years Old

This age group comprised approximately 42.2% of the total population in 2005 and accounted for 35.0% of deaths for that year. In the period 2001–2005, there were 2,147 deaths in this age group, or 33.1% of all deaths (6,489). The leading cause of death for adults was external causes, 762 deaths or 35.5% of all deaths in this age group; 252 of these deaths were due to land transport accidents. In 2003 and 2004, the leading cause of death among those ages 20–59 was land transport accidents, and for 2005 it was injuries. In the 30–39-year-old age group, the leading cause of death in 2004 was land transport accidents, and in 2005 it was HIV/AIDS.

Maternal deaths registered between 2001 and 2005 ranged between 3 and 10 per year. In 2003, 14% of pregnant women accessed prenatal care during their first trimester; 85% obtained prenatal care at some stage of their pregnancy; an estimated 20% who tested their hemoglobin level during pregnancy were found to be anemic; and only 62% took folic acid, iron, and vitamin A supplements before or during pregnancy.

Statistics from the Belize Family Life Association, a nongovernmental family planning services organization, reveal that oral contraceptives remain the method of choice; however, there seems to be a shift to the one-month injection, especially among younger women.

Older Adults 60 Years Old and Older

Belize has a relatively low proportion of older persons (4.2% in 2005); the absolute number of elderly persons is increasing and is projected to double by 2025. Income security in 2000 and 2001 was a key welfare issue; many older persons had only a very small income or none at all.

The mortality rate during 2001–2005 for this age group was 48.3 per 1,000 population. There were 2,780 deaths (42.8% of total deaths), with males making up 56.1% and females 43.9%.

Diseases of the circulatory system accounted for 1,146 (43%) deaths among those 65 years of age and older. In 2005, the five leading causes of death were hypertensive diseases, diabetes mellitus, ischemic heart diseases, cerebrovascular diseases, and pulmonary heart disease and diseases of pulmonary circulation.

The Family

The 2000 population census survey results showed that a higher proportion of persons in rural areas (60%) was married or in a common law union as compared to 52% in urban areas. Toledo District reported the highest proportion (62%) of its population in a union while Belize District reported the lowest (51%).

In 2004, a Rapid Assessment of Orphans and Vulnerable Countries (OVC) conducted by UNICEF indicated that approximately 2,000 children have lost one parent due to AIDS. The report estimated that the number of children affected in Belize is likely to increase to more than 7,000 by 2010. It concluded that some 14,000 children, or more than one in 10 in Belize, are already vulnerable and each adult death from AIDS results in approximately three children left with one or no parent. The OVC assessment also concluded that for every Belizean who has already died, there are nearly three more living with HIV.

The 2000 population census showed that females headed 33% of households. The 2002 CSO Poverty Assessment Report noted that households headed by males are more likely to be poor than households headed by females. Furthermore, the report indicated that households headed by females with a partner are more likely to be poor than a household headed by a female without a part-

ner. Married women comprised 65% of those in a domestic relationship, with the remaining 35% being in a common-law union. The Belize family court system reports that more than half of court orders are for child support and for support of children of unmarried women (paternity suits).

The 2000 census revealed that mean individual income is US$ 414 per month. This represented an increase compared to 1991 (US$ 311). The mean income was higher for males than for females. In urban areas, 1% earned less than US$ 714, compared to 6% in the rural areas. The highest quintile of income—those earning US$ 17,130 and above per annum—was three times as high as the lowest quintile of population, most of whom lived in rural areas. Toledo District reported the highest percentage (23%) that earned less than US$ 694 per annum, while Belize District reported the lowest, less than 1%. Belize District also reported the highest percentage that earned more than US$ 17,130.

Workers

Work-related injuries have increased 70%, from 1,522 cases in 1995 to 2,580 in 2003. The loss of productivity increased from 35,430 days lost in 1995 to more than 70,000 days in 2003, with the construction and agricultural sectors being the most affected. Assessments conducted in the agricultural sector indicate a high incidence of exposure to hazards and of reports of injuries and/or diseases. Underreporting of occupational injuries and diseases, however, contributes to the limited information available and therefore makes it difficult to determine the real magnitude of this problem in the country.

Persons with Disabilities

The 2000 census showed that 5.9% of the national population had a disability, with significantly higher rates of disability found in the populations of Toledo (8.4%) and Cayo (7.5%). The census found that the most prevalent disability was sight loss or impairment (3% of total population), followed by problems of mobility (1.8%), body movement (1.4%), and hearing (1.1%). Cayo District reported the highest prevalence (3%) and Stann Creek District the lowest (0.9%). A disturbing finding was that the cohort under 5 years of age represented 29% of Belize's disabled population. Most of the disabled live in rural areas where services are not available.

Ethnic Groups

A Labor Force Survey conducted in 2004 indicated that Mestizos comprised 48.4%, Creoles 27.0%, Mayan groups (the major two are Mopan and Kekchi) about 10%, Garifunas 5.7%, Mennonites 3.2%, and East Indians 3.0% of Belize's population. Other ethnic groups constituting less than 1% of the population were Chinese (0.9%) and Caucasian (0.7%).

Desirable Tourism Aggravates Undesirable Sanitation Problems

In recent years, increasing revenues from tourism have led to unprecedented real growth in Belize's gross domestic product—to over 12% in 2000 and 9.2% in 2003. Notwithstanding this economic growth and the country's reasonably well-organized social services, tourism is exacerbating sanitation problems that are potentially threatening to the population's health status. The generation of waste is voluminous: an estimated 130,000 tons of municipal solid waste in 2005, and 1.26 kg per person every day. The management of that waste is a national issue and a major challenge for the health sector, as proper facilities to dispose of solid waste do not exist countrywide. A national solid waste management plan, developed some years ago, currently awaits implementation.

HEALTH CONDITIONS AND PROBLEMS

COMMUNICABLE DISEASES

Vector-borne Diseases

The two main vector-borne diseases affecting the country are **malaria** and **dengue**. The principal species causing malaria in Belize is the *Plasmodium vivax* parasite, although *P. falciparum* remains an important and dangerous threat in parts of the country. Malaria cases fluctuated from 1,441 cases in 2000 to 1,066 in 2004 and 1,549 in 2005, of which 653 cases (42%) were from the southern Stann Creek District. Malaria will continue to represent an important public health concern in Belize, especially in rural areas of the southern districts, given that there is an active migrant population that works in the citrus and banana industries, and frequent population movements and substandard housing have provided favorable environmental conditions for mosquito breeding.

Dengue is also endemic in Belize. While the number of cases had been relatively low (under 5 annually), outbreaks were experienced in 2002 (42 cases) and 2005 (652 cases). Of the latter cases, 614 (94%) were from Cayo District. The first confirmed case of dengue hemorrhagic fever (DHF) in Belize occurred in 2005. Serotypes 2, 3, and 4 have been identified in Belize; therefore, the population remains vulnerable to a DHF outbreak.

Recently a few chronic cases of **Chagas' disease** have been reported, and studies reveal the presence of the vector in the western and southern districts.

Vaccine-preventable Diseases

There have been no reported cases of **measles** since 1991 or **poliomyelitis** since 1987. The last case of **neonatal tetanus** was reported from Stann Creek District in 1997, and the last case of **non-neonatal tetanus** was in a 3-year-old from Orange Walk District in 1998. The last case of **congenital rubella syndrome** was reported in 1997. No cases of **diphtheria** or **pertussis** were reported for 2001–2005.

In 2002, two new vaccines, hepatitis B and *Haemophilius influenzae* type b, were introduced into the national infant immunization schedule. The vaccines were constituents of the pentavalent combination vaccine DPT/HepB/Hib. Although rubella elimination activities with vaccination of adults were started in 1997, following introduction of the measles-mumps-rubella (MMR) vaccine the previous year, MMR vaccination of males was carried out in 2004; the effort targeted 66,800 males aged 5 to 35 years and resulted in 96% coverage.

Vaccination coverage of all antigens (diphtheria, BCG, tetanus, pertussis, polio, Hib, hepatitis B, MMR) steadily increased during the 2001–2005 period. During the 2001–2005 period, vaccination coverage for BCG was 96% or higher, and that for 3 doses of polio was 93% or higher in infants. For 2005, vaccination coverage for MMR (children 12–23 months) was 95%; coverage of infants (less than 12 months) for BCG was 96%; and that for third doses of the DPT/HepB/Hib pentavalent combination vaccine and OPV-3 was 96%.

Intestinal Infectious Diseases

Access to safe drinking water (97.2% of the population) contributed significantly to the control of **cholera**. There have been no cases of the disease since 1999. On the other hand, reported cases of **gastroenteritis** ranged from 293 to 3,737 during 2001–2005. The numbers of reported cases of foodborne diseases were as low as 13 in 2001 and as high as 224 in 2005. Improved surveillance contributed to the change in cases reported; nonetheless, these numbers are low.

Acute Respiratory Infections

Acute respiratory infections (ARI) continue to be one of the leading causes of mortality and morbidity in the general population. Information from the Ministry of Health showed that deaths attributable to ARI in the 1–4 age group were 9.4% in 2001 and 8.8% in 2004.

HIV/AIDS and Other Sexually Transmitted Infections

HIV/AIDS constitutes a major public health problem characterized by its increasing feminization, the infection of children, and a growing number of AIDS-related orphans. The highest concentration of infected persons can be found in Belize City

(437 in 2002 and 396 in 2005), with Corozal and Toledo reporting the lowest number of cases—4 in 2002 and 3 in 2005, and 6 in 2002 and 2 in 2005—respectively. A national multisectoral response strategy includes access to antiretroviral drugs for all those in need. However, issues of stigma and discrimination remain obstacles against successful care and treatment.

HIV/AIDS reports from 1986 through 2005 indicated that 3,360 individuals have acquired HIV, 762 have developed AIDS, and there have been 606 registered deaths due to AIDS. Between 2003 and 2005, approximately 185 women tested positive for HIV. The male-female ratio at the end of 2005 was 1.1:1. In 2003, 10 children less than 1 year of age and 12 children 1–4 years of age were newly diagnosed as being HIV-positive. Antiretroviral treatment is provided to 398 patients: 360 are adults (207 males and 153 females), and 38 are children.

In 2005, the mother-to-child transmission rate was 9.5. Underreporting is very likely since clinicians may not indicate AIDS on the death certificate to protect individuals and family from stigma and discrimination. The Prevention of the Mother-to-Child Transmission (PMTCT) Program was implemented within all public health facilities and four private health facilities.

In the general population, new infections with HIV continue to show an upward trend as greater numbers of the population are being tested.

Zoonoses

There have been no **rabies** cases in humans since 1989, and the last canine case was reported in 2000. However, the prevalence of rabies in bovine animals and wildlife, such as vampire bats and foxes, represents an ongoing public health threat.

NONCOMMUNICABLE DISEASES

Metabolic and Nutritional Diseases

In 2005, **obesity** was found in 2.8% of children under 5 years of age who were seen in health clinics. Belize District had the highest percentage (36.4%) and Corozal District the lowest (4.4%). In rural areas, the severity of **malnutrition** was higher for females than for males, while in the urban areas, it was approximately the same.

Cardiovascular Diseases

In 2001, heart diseases ranked second (82 deaths), of which 69 were from **ischemic heart diseases. Cerebrovascular diseases** were another leading cause, with 59 deaths. Cardiovascular diseases accounted for 22.4% of registered deaths in 2001 and for 21.3% of registered deaths in 2005.

Malignant Neoplasms

Hospital discharge data showed 366 and 391 hospitalizations for neoplasms in 2003 and 2005, respectively. In 2005, females accounted for the highest number of cases, of which 183 were benign neoplasms, carcinoma in situ, and neoplasms of uncertain behavior and of unspecified nature. Neoplasms of these same categories in males were 35. In females, there were 28 cases of malignant neoplasms of the uterus (cervix, corpus, and part unspecified). In males, there were 9 cases of malignant neoplasm of the prostate.

In 2001, there were 18 deaths from cervical cancer, 6 in 2002, and 12 in 2003. Cervical cancer statistics from the Ministry of Health showed 14 deaths in 2004 and 10 deaths in 2005. Cervical cancer morbidity data indicate 21 cases in 2004 and 23 in 2005. In 2001, there were 1 and 2 deaths in Stann Creek and Toledo, respectively; however, there were no cervical cancer deaths in Toledo District during the 2002–2004 period. In 2003, malignant neoplasms of the uterus (cervix, corpus, and part unspecified) ranked eighth in the 10 leading causes of death. In 2005, there were 10 deaths from cervical cancer. A 2003 needs assessment report showed that the estimated coverage of cervical cancer screening was 62.7%, with the lowest coverage among illiterate women living in rural areas. The cervical cancer mortality rate in 2005 was 6.9 per 100,000 women.

OTHER HEALTH PROBLEMS OR ISSUES

Mental Health and Addictions

The principal conditions leading to mental health consultations are clinical depression, psychotic disorders, anxiety disorders, substance abuse, and stress-related disorders. In 2005, 12,318 patients were seen at various psychiatric units throughout the country. Psychotic disorders accounted for the highest number of cases seen, affecting 1,904 men and 1,257 females. Child disorders and abuse were 303 and 141, respectively, in 2005.

The Global Youth Survey conducted in Belize in 2003 found that 20% of high school students had used tobacco, 16% had smoked cigarettes, and 9% had used other forms of tobacco. Nearly one-quarter (23.5%) purchased their own cigarettes, and 15.5% reported that they usually smoked at home.

Environmental Pollution

The importation of pesticides in the country increased significantly, from 1.7 million kg in 2001 to about 7 million in 2005. A 2001 study documented 59 severe acute pesticide intoxication cases, including 3 deaths. It was also estimated that about 4,000 acute pesticide intoxication cases occur annually in the country with the majority involving agricultural workers, pesticide handlers, and/or applicators.

A study conducted by the Ministry of Health and PAHO in the Macal River (Cayo District) in 2005 revealed the presence of mercury in several fish species. The average concentrations found were 0.11 µgHg/g and 0.56 µgHg/g in non-predatory and predatory fish, respectively. While these levels are lower than the limits set jointly by the Food and Agriculture Organization and the World Health Organization—0.5 µgHg/g in non-predatory and

1.0 in predatory fish—there are concerns of exposure to mercury due to consumption of fish by residents of rural communities along the river.

Oral Health

Caries prevention strategies for preschool children focus on fluoride prophylaxis applications. Clinics also offer fissure sealants for children, prophylaxis and check-ups, and some limited restorative dentistry.

The Ministry of Health's Dental Health Program is carried out in all six districts with 19 professionals: 9 are dental surgeons and 10 are dental nurses or dental assistants.

RESPONSE OF THE HEALTH SECTOR

Health Policies and Plans

Belize's national health care system is based on the principles of equity, affordability, accessibility, quality, and sustainability through the formation of effective partnerships with other public and private entities to promote attainment by the population of the highest level possible of health and well-being. As part of the Health Sector Reform Project, the Ministry of Health reorganized the country's health services into four health regions: Northern, Central, Western, and Southern. Each has a regional health manager, who, with the support of a management team, is responsible for coordinating the delivery of population-based health services to the communities in the geographical areas under its jurisdiction.

Significant health events and developments occurred in the period 2001–2005. These included the implementation of guidelines for the clinical management of mother-to-child transmission of HIV, the Family Violence Protocol, the Protocol for the Use of Psychotropic Drugs, and the National Policy for Older Persons. A Sexual and Reproductive Health Policy was introduced in 2002, and a comprehensive national plan was developed to make the policy operational.

Other Ministry of Health plans and protocols are in various stages of implementation. These include the Family Plans and Norms, a draft mental health policy, draft Medical Practice Bill, draft General Health Act, draft Policy for Disabled Persons, the National Policy on Health and Family Life Education, the first draft of the Poverty Elimination Strategy and Action Plan, the National Referral System Policy Guidelines and Protocols, the National Plan of Action for Children and Adolescents, National Strategic Plan for HIV and AIDS, and the National Care and Treatment Plan for HIV and AIDS.

Care protocols for victims of domestic violence were developed and implemented by the Ministry of Health for use within public clinics and hospitals and in conjunction with other community social services. The National Action Plan for Gender-based Violence was developed in 2005 to strengthen collaboration among key stakeholders in addressing systematically the issues of gender-based violence and child abuse. The National Action Plan for Children and Adolescents was designed to create greater synergy among key programs addressing childhood and adolescent development issues. The Plan is coordinated by the National Committee for Families and Children and clearly outlines Belize's international commitments and national policies, targets, and strategies as they relate to children and adolescents. At the end of 2003, a process was initiated to review and update all public health-related legislation to create an umbrella act known as the General Health Act.

In the latter part of 2000, the Ministry of Health launched a pilot project of the National Health Insurance Initiative, with the objective of consolidating efforts for the implementation of a national insurance plan to cover health care costs currently being funded by the government through the Ministry of Health and to ensure sustainable universal access to health care by the population.

In 2002 a service agreement between the Social Security Board (SSB) and National Health Insurance Fund (NHIF) was signed that defines the relationship between the two entities, with the latter serving as a sub-unit of the SSB. It instructs the NHIF to purchase services agreed upon by the Ministry of Health, applying certain performance contract principles (productivity, efficiency, and effectiveness indicators linked to targets and bonuses). Service agreements between the NHIF and the four primary care provider (PCP) clinics on Southside Belize City were signed in 2001 and define the NHIF relationship as a service purchaser and the PCPs as service providers. Service level agreements were developed by the Ministry of Health with PAHO technical cooperation in 2003 to define the relationship between the Ministry and health regions. Targets are being set and indicators established to measure progress as part of the health reform principle of shifting emphasis from input to output indicators.

The Ministry of Health applies nominal fees in its hospitals and clinics for imaging and laboratory tests; there are also nominal fees for inpatient services, including deliveries. The National Health Insurance pilot started in August 2001 and did not include any fee for service payments by the consumer, no co-payments were required, and collection rates differed at each institution. Subsequently, co-payments were introduced in Southside Belize City. These fees are less a source of revenue generation than a mechanism to discourage abuse of the system. When the initiative was rolled out in the Southern Health Region, it was felt that a fee structure would be a barrier to access, so no co-payments were required. The NHIF purchases only a primary care package of services; normal inpatient care at public institutions retains a nominal fee structure. The initiative was completely implemented in the Belize District (Southside Belize City) in early 2005 and extended to the Southern Health Region (Stann Creek and Toledo Districts) in June 2006.

Organization of the Health System

The role of the Ministry of Health headquarters is to provide policy advice to the Minister of Health. It holds responsibility for national health planning, public health protection, regulation, research, quality and standards, international and regional collaboration, and monitoring of the overall performance of the national health system. There are two key divisions in the Ministry of Health: the administrative arm, headed by the Chief Executive Officer, and the technical arm, headed by the Director of Health Services. The Director of Health Services is constitutionally responsible for the health of the nation.

The Ministry of Health operates a nationwide network of facilities that includes a total of eight hospitals, one in each district, with the exception of Cayo and Belize Districts, which have two each. Three of the eight hospitals are designated as regional hospitals and provide a wide range of secondary care in addition to routine primary care. Another three hospitals are community hospitals or primary level facilities, which provide a minimum amount of secondary care at the district level. Only the Karl Heusner Memorial Hospital functions as a national referral hospital; it is also the general hospital for Belize District. It provides services for neurology, physiology, ENT (ear, nose, and throat conditions), and orthopedic surgery. Outreach community services include dental health, mental health, and communicable diseases prevention and control. In addition, there is a mental health hospital, a psychiatric unit in Belmopan, and psychiatric units staffed with psychiatric nurses in each of the regional and community hospitals. The psychiatric nurses, as part of a community-based psychiatric program, provide ongoing counseling to survivors of gender-based violence and child abuse, as well as pre- and post-test counseling for HIV. There is a Mental Health Association that serves as an advocate for patients with mental illnesses and their families, while at the same time supporting the Ministry of Health's mental health programs and services. The Mental Health Consumer Association also has been very active, and in 2005 advocated successfully for new psychotropic drugs to be added to the national drug formulary.

Public Health Services

Belize's primary health care strategy ensures equity in health as it relates to accessibility and human resources distribution. The Ministry of Health has an organizational structure that establishes a permanent link between its headquarters, the districts, and communities. Community health workers form the principal link between the formal health system and the community. Village health committees support these workers in identify-

ing community health needs and planning the implementation of corrective measures. In 2003, two of the most significant achievements of the primary health care strategy were the involvement of the lay public in community health projects and intersectorial collaboration. District and village teams were established with community members whose active participation was encouraged in activities developed to enhance the population's general health status. At the national level, a National Primary Health Committee monitors the progress of these efforts and supports the district health committees in the planning and implementation of programs. The Health Sector Reform Project continues to support primary health care initiatives, with the overarching goal of producing a more efficient, sustainable, and equitable national health system which incorporates the participation of communities in the planning, implementation, and monitoring of their own health care systems.

The overall health of the population improved during the reporting period due to the expansion of health services and infrastructure in rural and urban areas. This was evidenced by an increase in life expectancy, improved immunization coverage, a reduction in preventable childhood diseases and the infant mortality rate, a decreased fertility rate, and an aggressive vector control program that was implemented as part of the primary health care strategy. Within this framework, new facilities that include a rehabilitation center for independent living were constructed in 2004. Similarly, in 2005, approximately 12 new psychiatric nurse practitioners were trained to improve the country's response to mental health issues and strengthen its community-based approach.

The national response to gender-based violence has seen dramatic improvements in the areas of detection and treatment since the beginning of the 2001–2005 period. Recognizing the public health challenge, the Ministry of Health's national surveillance system registers cases of gender-based violence and child abuse and analyzes data. In 2003, the surveillance system was evaluated by the U.S. Centers for Disease Control and Prevention, and recommendations for the improvement of its operations were implemented in 2005.

Data from various health situation analyses conducted in 2005 indicate that maternal and infant mortality rates continue to be above acceptable levels. Other trends include a steady increase in noncommunicable diseases (hypertension, diabetes, cardiovascular diseases, and cervical cancer); road traffic injuries and violence; STI/HIV/AIDS, its feminization, and TB coinfection; malaria and dengue cases, including the risk of DHF outbreaks; and occupational injuries. There is also inadequate management of solid waste. In this context, the government's 2000–2006 National Health Plan identifies disease surveillance and strengthened health information systems as national priorities.

In the area of communicable diseases prevention and control, the National Health Plan includes initiatives to decrease the risk and impact of STI/HIV/AIDS; reduce the incidence of tuberculosis, malaria, and dengue; provide sexual and reproductive health services with a life cycle approach and special emphasis on services for pregnant women and children under 5; provide timely and reliable laboratory diagnostic and epidemiological services that are confidential and of high quality for effective patient management, surveillance, and health planning; and provide and disseminate opportune information about priority health events/disease outbreaks. The National Laboratory Services Strategic Plan 2004–2009 seeks to provide quality diagnostic services in compliance with international standards that are timely, confidential, accessible, and affordable to the public.

The Directly Observed Treatment, Short Course (DOTS) strategy continues to be used for the treatment of tuberculosis; public and rural health nurses administer DOTS to patients at public clinics and at the TB Clinic in Belize City; in the rural communities where a public health nurse is not available, family members receive training to administer the medication.

The 2005–2010 Plan of Action for Food and Nutrition Security provides a comprehensive framework to guide the implementation of activities comprising the six programs outlined in the Food and Nutrition Security Policy. These are Information, Education, and Communication on Food Production, Preparation, and Nutrition; Diversified Food Production, Food Processing, Marketing, Storage, and Credit Mobilization; Maternal and Child Care, School Feeding, and Nutrition for the Elderly and the Indigent; Creation of Employment and Income-Generating Opportunities at the Local Level; Food Safety; and Analysis and Reform of National Policies for Food and Nutrition Security.

The Plan's food safety activities include the development of a meat inspection plan; training and monitoring of food handlers in safe food handling techniques and personal hygiene; and the inspection of food establishments. The National Health Plan includes activities to prevent and control waterborne illnesses and to eliminate human rabies. The Ministry of Agriculture, in collaboration with the Ministry of Health, drafted a Plan for the Development of Human Resources in Nutrition. The country's school feeding program was restructured in 2003.

Despite the fact that there are nine dentists and two dental auxiliary nurses spread out across the districts, with the highest concentration in Belize District, most district clinics reported an increase in tooth extraction, particularly among children. Productivity was largely measured based on the numbers of extractions and clinical encounters. Supply and equipment shortages continued to be challenges during the 2001–2005 period.

In 2000, the government instituted a Health Sector Hurricane Management Plan that is updated each year in May. Health managers annually participate in hurricane preparedness meetings. A mass casualty plan was developed in 2004, emergency workers were trained in mass casualty management, and a simulation exercise was carried out in 2004. The Karl Heusner Memorial Hospital is the only public hospital with a mass casualty management plan.

A national response plan to mitigate the emergency effects of a potential Severe Acute Respiratory Syndrome (SARS) pandemic was developed and put into effect at the end of 2003.

Individual Care Services

The national public health system provides universal access for personal and population-based services through a regionalized network of public facilities and programs. This includes the provision of pharmaceuticals and other support services. A system of rural health centers with permanent staff is supplemented by mobile health services, community nursing aides, voluntary collaborators, and traditional birth attendants working throughout rural communities. For 2005, the health care delivery network reported 209,959 outpatient visits (720 visits per 1,000 population), 21,745 hospital discharges (75 per 1,000 population), and 7,457 live births. There were 357 hospital beds (1.2 beds per 1,000 population).

The private health care delivery network is comprised of 54 outpatient facilities or clinics. These are mainly located in Belize City, and some offer specialized services such as dentistry, dermatology, and gastroenterology. In addition, there were five private hospitals, for a total of 79 beds.

In the public sector, the provision of hospital-based care in the four health regions includes inpatient and outpatient care for accident- and emergency-related incidents, as well as services in the areas of pediatrics, obstetrics, gynecology, internal medicine, and surgery. Primary health care needs are addressed through a network of clinics, health centers, and health posts.

The Ministry of Health is responsible for the operations of the Central Medical Laboratory, which serves as a referral and reference center for the four health regions and the public medical laboratories of all districts. Services by the laboratory include bacteriology, serology, cytology, histology, and special chemical and hematological analyses. A Quality Control Program supported by the Caribbean Epidemiology Center (CAREC) is underway. The Belize National Blood Transfusion Services are responsible for the collection, screening, storage, and distribution of blood and blood products. Services depend on voluntary donors.

A community-based approach to addressing mental health illnesses was developed and implemented in 2000. Mental health units have been established in all the districts, and an acute psychiatric unit was constructed in 2001. Mental health services are organized and implemented at three levels of care: outpatient services (crisis intervention and therapeutic services to individuals and families); inpatient services at the Rockview Hospital and Belmopan Hospital; and community services (outreach and ancillary services).

Belize's National Policy for Older Persons was introduced in 2002. The National Council on Aging was established in 2003. There are four institutions that house the elderly: the Sister Cecilia Home and the Raymond Parks Shelter for the Homeless, both in Belize City; the Golden Haven Home in Hattieville; and the Octavia Waight Home in San Ignacio. The Mercy Kitchen and St. Joseph Mercy Clinic in Belize City provide primary health care, home-delivered meals, and visits to the residences of the elderly. The Mercy Kitchen additionally provides socialization activities, spiritual enrichment programs, and laundry facilities for the homeless.

The country's only rehabilitation/treatment center is located at the Karl Heusner Memorial Hospital, where physiotherapy services for adults and children are offered through one trained physiotherapist and one nurse aide.

Health Promotion

Health promotion strategies remain among the national public health priorities, with policies, programs, and plans focusing on domestic violence, road traffic accidents, health education, community participation, and tobacco control. A project was implemented in Toledo District under the auspices of the Institute of Nutrition of Central America and Panama (INCAP) to respond to the nutritional problems identified in that district. Interventions were geared toward the control of malnutrition, micronutrient deficiencies, and other consequences of undernutrition. The major activities included nutrition education, organic vegetable production, food preparation, and fruit and vegetable drying and preservation. In addition to the general health promotion programs organized by the Health Education and Community Participation Bureau (HECOPAB), other aspects of health promotion included, but were not limited to, health and family life education, school health services, and road safety. Extensive efforts were made to engage the media in health promotion initiatives, resulting in a number of award-winning health promotion features. As part of promoting health lifestyles, the Ministry of Education has introduced the Health and Family Life curriculum, and training guides for primary and secondary schools were finalized in 2005. The curriculum, which is now being piloted in 12 schools in the six districts throughout the country, focuses on self- and interpersonal development, managing the environment, nutrition and physical activity, and sexuality and sexual health with an emphasis on STI/HIV/AIDS prevention.

In 2004, 232 children were placed with foster families. In the same year, 2,024 child protection cases were processed (1,330 cases related to child abuse and 694 to other services, such as family support, placement requests, and child custody cases). In 2005, 731 abuse cases were reported for Belize District, of which 242 were related to sexual abuse, 144 to physical abuse, and 70 to child abandonment. The progress made toward achievement of the Millennium Development Goals is the framework used for assessing the social situation of children and adolescents in Belize. In addition, the Convention on the Rights of the Child and the 2002 United Nations' General Assembly Special Session on Children titled "Building a World Fit for Children" continue to be the structure for research and policy analysis concerning the human rights, health, and educational situation of Belizean children.

Human Resources

In 2005, the health staff inventory showed that more than one-half of all health personnel continue to be located in Belize City, where there is the largest number of bed capacity (115) for an estimated population of 87,000. Nationally (public, private, and volunteers), there were 159 specialists, 166 general practitioners, 257 registered nurses, 24 public health inspectors, 27 medical technologists, 21 radiographers, and 248 community nursing aides. A national network of traditional birth attendants is supported and supervised through the maternal and child health program of the Ministry of Health. There are an estimated 70–75 licensed pharmacists, of whom 25 work in the public health system.

Severe human resources shortages have led to the recruitment of health professionals from within and outside of the Caribbean. Many of these professionals, especially medical doctors, are assigned to remote rural areas where human resource shortages are particularly acute. The shortages are compounded by the active recruitment of national health professionals, particularly nurses, by developed countries.

Belize has no national school of medicine. The country depends largely on the utilization of medical training institutions in Cuba. The University of Belize supplies other non-physician health care providers through its Faculty of Nursing and Allied Health Sciences. Training programs include pharmacy, medical technology, and practical nursing; bachelor's degrees in nursing and social work, as well as an associate degree in social work, are also offered. There are approximately 40–90 graduates per year from these programs collectively (2003–2005). In 2005, 16 students graduated from the psychiatric nursing program. Neither the production nor recruitment of health care providers was guided by a human resources plan for health, since none existed for most of the reporting period. In late 2005, measures to address this concern were beginning to be developed.

Between 2001 and 2005, community nurses aides were selected by their communities to receive training by the Ministry of Health in rehydration therapy, including venipuncture for the administration of fluids to severely dehydrated patients who do not have immediate access to health centers and hospitals. Traditional birth attendants received training and were provided with the basic equipment necessary to perform their functions in the community. Health care workers (physicians and nurses) in all six administrative districts were trained to diagnose STIs and

HIV/AIDS based on clinical manifestations. In 2004, 374 parenting workshops were carried out countrywide along with other public awareness activities. Training was provided to health care personnel as well as caregivers in the area of nutrition and HIV/AIDS. Physicians, health educators, nurses, and lay persons were trained in the nutritional management of obesity, diabetes, and hypertension. Special training was provided on simple techniques for the diagnosis of cervical cancer. All of the public health nursing staff was trained in the surveillance of immune-preventable childhood diseases as well as maintenance of the cold chain.

Other study programs designed to fulfill the continuing education needs of health care providers addressed such topics as protecting the human rights of the mentally ill, clinical management of dengue and HIV/AIDS, referral systems, safe motherhood, water and sanitation, proper nutrition, food safety, prevention of geo-helminthes infections, and malaria control.

Health Supplies

Belize has no local pharmaceutical manufacturing capacity even though there are 28 importers in-country. Registration for pharmaceuticals is covered in the draft Pharmacy Act, which currently is pending review and approval. The Act will govern the licensing of professionals, registration of medicines, and the donation policy. A permit is required for the importation of pharmaceuticals into the country. All Belizeans have access to the drugs in the Belize Drug Formulary when using public sector health services. In the period 2001–2005, new psychotropic drugs were included in the national drug formulary. Close to 100 private pharmacies operate in the country.

The antiretroviral and PMTCT programs are parallel systems and separate from the rest of the pharmaceutical management system. Antiretroviral medications are not quantified for, procured, or distributed through the established system for essential medicines or supplies, nor are they dispensed at health facilities. Instead, they are dispensed at voluntary counseling and testing clinics or by psychiatric nurses in hospitals.

A total of US$ 692,669 was used to procure vaccines, needles, and syringes for the period 2001–2005 from the Expanded Program on Immunization.

The total public health budget for 2004–2005 was US$ 9,163,327, of which 44.52% (US$ 4,079,304) was allocated for the procurement of pharmaceuticals.

Research and Technological Development in Health

Several studies were conducted during the review period in order to develop appropriate interventions, including a seroprevalence study among the prison population in 2005, a baseline parasitological survey among schoolchildren that same year, and the Global Youth Tobacco Survey among youths ages 13–15 in 2003. Additionally, a study on consumer practices relating to food safety was carried out in 2003 in collaboration with the Caribbean Food and Nutrition Institute (CFNI) and the University of Belize.

The Belize Virtual Health Library was launched by PAHO/WHO in 2003 and joined the expanding Internet network of libraries containing health sciences information throughout Latin America and the Caribbean. The universal access initiative is targeted to both national and regional users.

Health Sector Expenditures and Financing

Health care is financed by the government, private health insurance, and the private sector. In 2001, the Ministry of Health budget was US$ 20,330,331, which is 8.4% of the total government budget and 2.4% of the GDP. In 2003, it was US$ 23,407,066, which was 8.43% of the government's budget and 2.4% of the GDP. In 2005 the Government of Belize budget increased to 9.1% of the GDP.

In 2005 the Ministry of Health's budget increased to US$ 26,161,413, which was 9.57% of the government's budget and 2.5% of the GDP. Personnel emoluments and medical supplies consume a large share of the budgetary allocation. Procurement of pharmaceuticals and supplies regularly exceeds the annual budgeted cost. Regions are allowed to collect and retain revenues. It has been mandated that the funds be utilized as follows: 5% for staff performance incentives, to be granted at the discretion of regional management teams; 10% for staff development (training, workshops, conferences, and seminars); and 85% for capital investments. As the revenue-generating center for the Central Region, the Karl Heusner Memorial Hospital shares 10% of its revenue obtained from secondary services for the strengthening of primary health care services in the Belize District.

Technical Cooperation and External Financing

Multilateral and bilateral agencies, including UNICEF, PAHO/WHO, and the U.S. Agency for International Development, provided financial support for the process of modernizing and upgrading Belize's public health system. Bi- and tri-national agreements with Guatemala and Mexico also contributed significantly to improvements in the population's health, particularly in the areas of immunization of children under 5 and the prevention and control of rabies, malaria, and dengue fever. In 2004, funds were mobilized from nongovernmental sources for the completion of the National Plan of Action for Children and Adolescents, an 18-month institutional strengthening and capacity-building package for the social sector, development of protocols for the management of cases of children with behavioral problems, publications design and printing, completion of an Addendum Report to the Committee on the Rights of the Child, and consultations for the National Education Summit as part of the Ministry of Education's Action Plan 2005–2010.

Through international agreements with Cuba and Nigeria, health professionals from these countries have provided support in expanding health services coverage to rural areas and introducing specialty services within hospitals.

Technical cooperation activities were carried out with CAREC, CFNI, and INCAP. Other agencies providing technical support included the Inter-American Development Bank, Organization of American States, Inter-American Institute for Cooperation on Agriculture, Regional Inter-governmental Organization for Agricultural Health, United Nations Development Program, UNICEF, United Nations Population Fund, and Joint United Nations Program on HIV/AIDS.

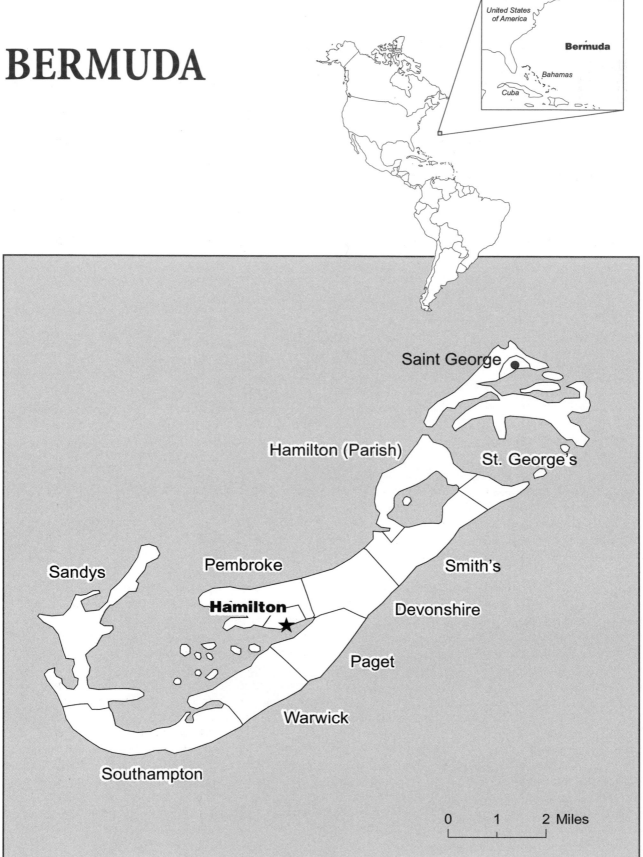

BERMUDA

United States of America

Bermuda

Bahamas

Cuba

Saint George

Hamilton (Parish)

St. George's

Sandys

Pembroke

Smith's

Hamilton

Devonshire

Paget

Warwick

Southampton

0   1   2 Miles

B ermuda, the oldest self-governing British Overseas Territory, is a group of more than 100 small islands in the Atlantic Ocean, the largest seven being linked by bridges. It is located 943 km east of North Carolina, U.S.A. Together, the islands cover an area of approximately 54 km², making them about one-third the size of Washington, D.C., U.S.A. The maximum elevation is Town Hill, at approximately 79 m. The subtropical climate is mild, frost-free, and humid, with temperatures ranging from 65°F to 88°F and an average annual rainfall of 140 cm. Bermuda is famed the world over for its pink-sand beaches and turquoise waters. Hurricanes are the only potential cause of natural disasters, with hurricane season lasting from May to November. Hamilton is the capital city of Bermuda. The Territory has nine parishes: Sandys, Southampton, Warwick, Paget, Pembroke, Devonshire, Hamilton, Saint George's, and Smith's. Pembroke is the most populated parish.

GENERAL CONTEXT AND HEALTH DETERMINANTS

Social, Political, and Economic Determinants

The Bermuda government is based on the Westminster model of parliamentary democracy and consists of a Governor, appointed by and representing the British monarch; a Deputy Governor, appointed by the Governor; a Cabinet; and a Legislature. The Cabinet is responsible to the Legislature, which consists of a Senate and a House of Assembly. Bermuda is divided into 36 constituencies, each represented by one elected member in the House of Assembly. Members sit for a term of five years, unless the House is dissolved earlier. The Senate is composed of 11 members appointed by the Governor. According to Bermuda's Constitution, five members of the Senate are appointed on the recommendation of the head of the executive branch, the Premier, and represent the governing party. In 2005, there were 12 Ministers in the Cabinet. Within the Cabinet, the Minister of Health and Family Services is responsible for health policy, planning, and evaluation and reports to the Cabinet.

Bermuda has one of the highest GDP per capita in the world, estimated in 2004 to be above US$ 65,500. The economy, primarily based on international business and tourism, has enjoyed steady growth in recent years. Approximately one-third of the workforce is employed in wholesale retail trade, one-third in restaurants and hotels, and one-third in community, social, and personal services.

Living standards in Bermuda are high, with good housing and well-developed transportation and communications systems. Roads are of good quality, and the public transportation system includes buses, taxis, and ferries. Private car ownership is high, though limited to one vehicle per household. All of the population has safe drinking water available in the home, as well as hygienic waste disposal.

The country generally showed a balance of payments surplus; the Bermuda dollar is pegged to the U.S. dollar on an equal basis. The consumer price index in 2004 was 127.8 (January 1995 = 100.0). Inflation was estimated at 2.7% per annum in 2000. The tourist industry, which accounts for an estimated 28% of GDP, attracts 84% of its business from North America. Bermuda has very few natural resources. The industrial and agricultural sectors are very small, and almost all consumable goods, including some 80% of foodstuffs, are imported. International business contributes more than 60% of Bermuda's economic output.

The 2000 census determined Bermuda's population to be 62,059, or 6% higher than in the previous (1991) census. While 11% of the population was 65 years of age and older, representing a 25% increase over 1991 figures, 6% was under the age of 5 years, a decrease of 2% from 1991. The racial composition of the population has not changed significantly over the past decade. In 2000, 60% of the population was Black or mixed Black, and 40% was White or of other racial background. Seventy-five percent of the Bermuda-born population was Black, while the foreign-born population was primarily White and other races (79%). The islands have a small but growing Asian community. A significant segment of the population is also of Portuguese heritage, the result of immigration from Portuguese-held islands (particularly the Azores) over the past century. The external immigration community additionally includes several thousand residents engaged in specialized professions, such as accounting, finance, and insurance, principally from the United Kingdom, Canada, and the United States. During the period 2000–2004, more than half of the population belonged to one of three religions: Anglican (28%), Catholic (15%), and African Methodist Episcopalian (12%).

Regarding relative income, poor and near-poor households accounted for 19% and 11%, respectively, of all Bermudian households in 2000, remaining unchanged since the 1991 census; while middle class and upper class households constituted 42% and 27%, respectively, versus 46% and 24% in 1991. Black Bermudian households are overrepresented in low-income households and underrepresented among high-income ones.

Education is free in public schools and compulsory up to the age of 17. In 2005, the literacy rate was 98.5% (98% in males and 99% in females). Many Bermudians study abroad at the tertiary level. The highest enrollment figures were in hotel and business administration (50% of all students) and arts and sciences (35%). Established in 1974, Bermuda College is an internationally recognized community college based in Paget Parish that offers associate degrees, certificates, and diplomas in the applied sciences, liberal arts, business, technology, and hospitality. As the only post-secondary educational institution in Bermuda, the College has developed an extended academic structure linking it to other academic institutions overseas, thus enabling students to easily transfer credits elsewhere to continue their studies.

Economic expansion during the 2000–2004 period occurred primarily in the financial and tourism sectors. In 2004, the total workforce consisted of 38,363 workers. Women made up 50% of this number, and 30% of workers were non-Bermudian. A substantial number of contract personnel worked in the hotel industry and international business sector; by law this group is included in a health insurance scheme that assures equitable access to health care.

As a developed country, Bermuda faces problems associated with declining fertility rates and increasing longevity, such as a shrinking labor force, increasing demand for housing, and a growing elderly population, with consequent health and social needs. Increasing health costs have required the government to find cost-cutting measures while taking into consideration the needs of an increasingly aging population, particularly the elderly poor.

Demographics, Mortality, and Morbidity

The estimated population in 2004 was 63,955, representing a 0.7% increase over 2003 figures. The estimated 2004 male population was 30,821 (48.2%), and the female population was 33,134 (51.8%). Population density was estimated at 1.16 persons per km^2 in 2000. The dependency ratio was estimated at 42 in 2000. In 2004, the crude birth rate was 13.2 per 1,000 population, and the annual population growth rate was 0.7%. Life expectancy in Bermuda in 2000 was 77.7 years (80.4 for women and 74.7 for men); disparities, however, can be observed between the Black and White population segments. Figure 1 presents the population distribution by age and sex for 1990 and 2005.

There were 836 live births recorded in 2004. The birth rate and sex ratio have remained stable over the period under review. Of the total live births recorded in 2004, 445 were male and 391 were female, with a male-female ratio of 1:1.1. There were 287 out-of-wedlock births in 2004, representing 34.3% of the total number of births for that year. Between 2000 and 2004, the cumulative total of live births was 4,168. The percentage of these births to unmarried women over the same period ranged from a low of 34.3% in 2004 to a high of 37.7% in 2001. On average, there were 833 births per year between 2000 and 2004, with approximately 36% occurring out of wedlock; this situation indicated possible financial dependency problems for an estimated 1,500 women on the islands.

The fertility rate was estimated at 1.9 children per woman. Although life expectancy at birth has continued to increase, the difference between the sexes has widened.

There were 25,148 households in 2000, with household size continuing to decrease. In 2000, it was estimated that 36% of households were headed by females.

The number of deaths for the 2000–2004 period totaled 2,156, with an annual range of 404–470 deaths. Stillbirths registered during this period ranged from 0 to 2 per year, with a total of four. An average of 215 males and 216 females died annually during the period.

Of known causes of death for the 2001–2002 period, diseases of the circulatory system accounted for 313 deaths (36.2%), while malignant neoplasms accounted for 246 deaths (28.4%), diabetes mellitus for 48 deaths (5.5%), and influenza and pneumonia for 18 deaths (2.1%). Among males 20–59 years of age, ischemic heart diseases and HIV/AIDS were the two leading causes of death, while among females in this age group, the leading causes were malignant neoplasms of the breast and HIV/AIDS.

According to the Ministry of Health and Family Services, diseases of the circulatory system and malignant neoplasms were the first and second leading causes of death for every year between 1990 and 2003. Between mid-2000 and mid-2004, discharge data from King Edward VII Memorial Hospital (Bermuda's general hospital) showed asthma to be the principal diagnosis, followed by pneumonia and gallbladder calculus. The major health problems, as reflected in mortality data, included cancer, ischemic heart diseases, fatal cerebrovascular disease (stroke), HIV/AIDS, and motor vehicle accidents.

FIGURE 1. Population structure, by age and sex, Bermuda, 1990 and 2005.

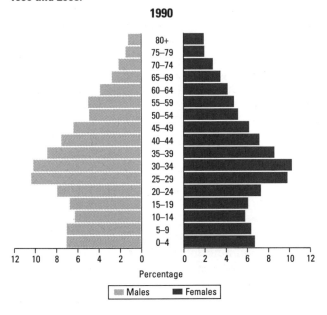

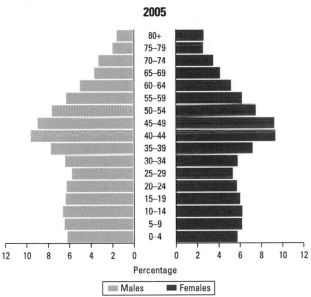

leading cause of hospitalization among children under age 5 and totaled 1,629 cases. During the same period, there were 668 cases of gastroenteritis reported among children in this age group.

Children 5–9 Years Old

There were 559 cases of gastroenteritis in this age group during the 2000–2003 period.

No deaths were registered for this group in 2004.

Adolescents 10–14 and 15–19 Years Old

There were no deaths in either of these two age groups in 2003 and 2004. In the 15–19-year-old age group, there was one death each in 2001 and 2002. Accidents were the leading cause of death among youths 15–19 years of age and one of the major causes of hospital admissions in this age group, along with pregnancy and respiratory diseases.

Obesity is a public health concern in Bermuda. The weight-for-age of approximately 10% of children and adolescents between the ages of 5 and 15 is above the recommended level, and some are obese.

Decreases in the incidence of dental decay have been maintained in the period under review, and oral health in children is generally excellent. This is in large part attributable to a preventive dental care program for infants and children that includes teaching mothers best practices regarding bottle-feeding, as well as the importance of regular teeth-brushing and limiting access to foods high in sugar, and providing free fluoride treatments. The voluntary school-based health program maintained high participation levels during the study period.

Between 2000 and 2004, 12.7% of all deliveries were to teenagers, with 23 deliveries to females under 16 years of age. There were 315 deliveries reported in the 16–19-year-old age group.

Adults 20–59 Years Old

There were 360 deaths among adults in this age group during the 2000–2004 period. Of these, 221 (61.4%) were males; the male-female ratio was 1.6:1. Only 42 (11.6%) of these deaths occurred among those aged 20–34; malignant neoplasms and diseases of the circulatory system were the major causes of mortality.

Accidents were a major cause of hospital admission among adults aged 25–44 years, and diseases of the circulatory and digestive systems and cancers were the leading causes of admission among the population aged 50–64 years old.

Older Adults 60 Years Old and Older

In 2004, the average age of death was 73.6 (79.6 years for females and 67.9 years for males). Those 60 years old and older rep-

HEALTH OF POPULATION GROUPS

Children under 5 Years Old

All births in Bermuda are hospital births. There were nine deaths in the 0–4 age group, five infant deaths, and four stillbirths during the 2001–2004 period. The prevalence of low-birthweight infants (< 2,500 g) was 7% in 2004, an increase from 4.1% in 2000. During the 2000–2003 period, respiratory diseases were the

resent the fastest growing segment of Bermuda's population. Ischemic heart diseases, diabetes, cerebrovascular diseases, and cancer are among the leading causes of mortality in this group.

There were 1,774 deaths between 2000 and 2004, accounting for 82.6% of total deaths. The most common causes of hospitalization among persons aged 65–74 included diseases of the circulatory system, cancer, and diseases of the digestive system. Among those aged 75 years or older, the major causes of hospitalization were diseases of the circulatory and respiratory systems.

The Family

A health and behavioral survey carried out in Bermuda in 2005 showed that 55% of Bermudian adults were married and that the separation and divorce rates were low when compared to other countries in the Caribbean region. Only 9.7% of households were headed by a single parent. The survey examined the population in terms of marital status in 2005 and revealed that 55% were married, 15.8% were separated or divorced, 10% were widowed, and 17% had never married.

Workers

There is no child labor in Bermuda as school attendance is mandatory up to age 17.

The Office of Health and Safety oversees the enforcement of health regulations in the workplace. No-smoking policies are in place in all government offices and virtually all other institutions. There were no industrial site fatalities during the 2000–2004 period.

Persons with Disabilities

In 2000, there were 2,832 individuals (1,265 males and 1,567 females, or 4.5% of the population) with a long-term condition that affected their daily lives. This figure was lower than that of 1991, even though the total population with disabilities remained constant at 5%. Blacks accounted for 60% of all those with disabilities, as opposed to 55% of the total population; Whites, on the other hand, constituted 30% of the population with disabilities, compared to 34% of the total population. The median age in 2000 for this group was 53 years.

HEALTH CONDITIONS AND PROBLEMS

COMMUNICABLE DISEASES

Vector-borne Diseases

In 2005, one imported case of **malaria** was reported and subsequently confirmed. There were also two cases of suspected **dengue** reported and investigated, but not confirmed.

Vaccine-preventable Diseases

The incidence of diseases preventable by immunization is zero or very low, and there were no reported cases of **pertussis**, **rubella**, **tetanus**, **neonatal tetanus**, or **diphtheria** during the 2001–2005 period. Measles has not been reported since 1991, and poliomyelitis has not been reported for more than 25 years. Vaccination coverage against diphtheria, measles, mumps, pertussis, polio, rubella, and tetanus was maintained at levels of over 85% during the 2001–2005 period. The following vaccines are part of the national immunization program: injectable polio, diphtheria, acellular pertussis, tetanus, *Haemophilus influenzae* type b, hepatitis B, pneumococcal disease, measles-mumps-rubella (MMR), varicella, and seasonal influenza. For 2005, the vaccination coverage for MMR was 96%, completion of the third dose for hepatitis B reached 82%, and DTaP/IPV/Hib coverage was 85%.

Chronic Communicable Diseases

There was one case of tuberculosis in 2003, and one imported and confirmed case in 2005.

HIV/AIDS and Other Sexually Transmitted Infections

In 1982, the first case of HIV/AIDS was reported in Bermuda. Since then, the Epidemiology and Surveillance Unit of the Ministry of Health and Family Services has received reports of 555 new HIV infections. Of these, 498 have progressed to AIDS, and 392 persons have died (Figure 2). At the end of 2005, it was estimated that 163 persons were living with HIV/AIDS in Bermuda, with a prevalence of 26 persons per 10,000 population. Males accounted for 75% of all cases, giving an overall male-female ratio of 3:1. Since 1982, less than 3% of all reported HIV infections have been among persons under the age of 20. The 20–29-year-old age group represented 17% of reported HIV infections, while the 30–39- and 40–49-year-old age groups represented 44% and 25%, respectively, thereby yielding a combined total of 69% of all new reported HIV infections. The age group of those 50 years old and older represented 12% of all new reported HIV infections. Eighty-eight percent of reported HIV cases were among those identifying themselves as Black, and 12% were among those identifying themselves as White. From 1982 to 1986, injection drug use was the most commonly reported transmission category among individuals with HIV, accounting for 74% of all HIV cases reported during that time period. While injection drug use continued to be a major route of transmission until 1990, sexual contact has been the most commonly reported transmission category since 1987. Overall, persons exposed through sexual contact account for 62% of all reported HIV cases, with exposure through injection drug use and other routes accounting for 31% and 7%, respectively.

After several years with a consistent declining trend (1989–2002), the number of new HIV infections reported annually stabilized at 11 new cases per year for 2004 and 2005 (Figure 3).

FIGURE 2. HIV/AIDS prevalence and mortality, Bermuda, 1982–2005.

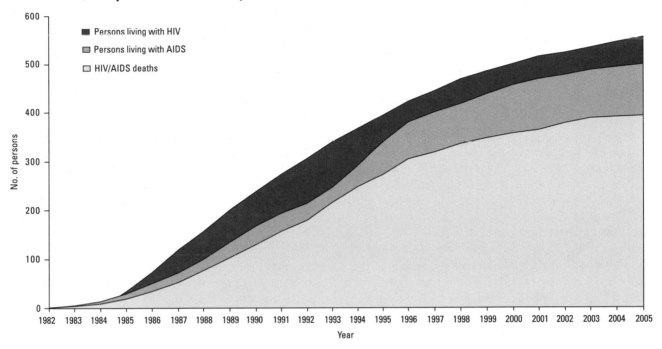

FIGURE 3. Annual reported HIV/AIDS cases and deaths, Bermuda, 1982–2005.

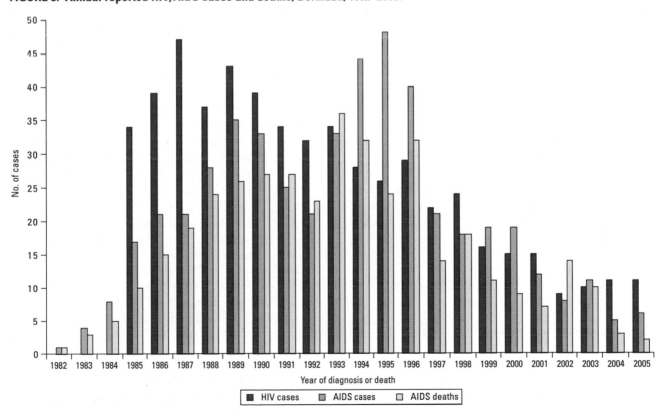

The annual number of cases of sexually transmitted infections during the 2001–2005 period was **chlamydia**, 356; **nonspecific urethritis**, 87; **gonorrhea**, 69; **herpes**, 33; and **syphilis**, 7. During this time, the number of annually reported cases of chlamydia increased by 91%. Reported cases of gonococcal infections and nonspecific urethritis decreased, while the rates of reported syphilis cases increased slightly and the rate of reported herpes cases remained about the same.

Zoonoses

There were no reports of bovine spongiform encephalopathy (mad cow disease), foot-and-mouth disease, or zoonoses, including rabies, during the period under review.

NONCOMMUNICABLE DISEASES

Metabolic and Nutritional Diseases

Obesity is an important risk factor for a number of major health problems in Bermuda, including diabetes. The health and behavior survey conducted in Bermuda in 2005 showed that one in every three adults is obese, one in every two adults is above a healthy body weight, and one in every two adults is also attempting to lose weight.

Cardiovascular Diseases

Cardiovascular diseases are the leading cause of death among females and males and affect the older adult population at much higher rates. For the 2001–2002 period, 162 deaths, or 35.4% of all male deaths, were due to cardiovascular diseases. For the same period, 151 deaths, or 37.0% of all female deaths, were caused by cardiovascular diseases.

Malignant Neoplasms

The number of deaths due to malignant neoplasms is surpassed only by that for cardiovascular diseases. For the 2001–2002 period, malignant neoplasms accounted for 125 deaths, or 27.4% of all male deaths, and 121 deaths, or 29.7% of all female deaths. For males, the malignant neoplasms that caused the most deaths were those of the prostate (24.1%) and trachea, bronchus, and lung (21.6%). For women the most common malignant neoplasms were those of the breast (19.8%) and trachea, bronchus, and lung (12.4%).

OTHER HEALTH PROBLEMS OR ISSUES

Disasters

Hurricane Fabian, a Category Three storm, hit Bermuda in September 2003, causing 5 deaths and extensive infrastructural damage. During the period under review, there were no other natural disasters.

Addictions

Reports from Bermuda's police services and the Epidemiology and Surveillance Unit of the Ministry of Health and Family Services showed that 22 deaths occurred during the 2002–2005 period due to a drug or alcohol overdose. The health and behavior survey conducted in 2005 found that of the adult interviewees who drank alcohol, 67% reported drinking one or more drinks in the past month, and 21% said that they had had less than 1 drink in the past month or that they no longer drink at all. On drinking days, 77% of alcohol consumers said they drank three or more drinks at one time.

The same survey revealed that 12% of the population are abusers of alcohol, 11% of the population is strongly indicated as being abusers of alcohol, and 44% of the adults who were strongly indicated as being abusers of alcohol had moderate to high stress overload scores, compared to 21% of adults with no indication of alcohol abuse having moderate to high stress overload scores.

Binge drinking, which is defined as the consumption of five or more drinks per occasion, was seen in 56% of adults who had consumed alcohol at least once in the past month; 21% of the adults who drank alcohol in the past month binged two or more times. Six percent of adults reported using mood-altering or sleep-enhancing drugs daily, and 11% of adults reported using these drugs several days a week; 69% of this group also had high stress overload scores.

The 2005 survey additionally found that 17% of adults smoked cigarettes, and another 28% reported being exposed to second-hand smoke on a daily basis. According to research conducted by the National Drug Commission (NDC) of the Ministry of Health and Family Services in 2001, 54% of the adult population reported using alcohol during the previous month; 18% used tobacco and 7% marijuana. Reported use of cocaine, crack, and hard drugs, including heroin, was less than 1%.

In 2003, the NDC carried out behavioral studies on middle school and senior high school students. Marijuana use was found to be as low as 1% in middle schools and as high as 21% in senior high schools. Ten percent of those studied reported using marijuana within the previous 30 days; this was 3% less than in 2002. These findings indicate a decline in marijuana use since 1997. Cigarette use also declined from 10% in 2000 to 7% in 2003. Alcohol use stayed more or less stable at 27%.

RESPONSE OF THE HEALTH SECTOR

Health Policies and Plans

Bermuda's health policy emphasizes several key areas, including maternal and child health, health of schoolchildren, community nursing for the elderly, oral health, mental health, and prevention and control of communicable diseases and alcohol and drug abuse. Population groups designated for special attention include mothers and infants, school-age children, and the elderly.

Child health programs and services focus on the following areas: immunizations, periodic growth and development assessments, parental support in the child health and development process, addressing behavioral and nutrition problems, injury prevention, and disease management. Health care services for the 5–9-year-old age group focus on health promotion and prevention activities and screening for early detection of hearing and vision problems and scoliosis.

During the 2001–2005 period, the Bermuda Health Council, a government-appointed entity responsible for regulating, coordinating, and maximizing the effectiveness of the country's health services, focused on the development of an integrated health care delivery system within a general framework that shifted from a disease-focused model to one that incorporates community participation in improving the public health infrastructure. Health education, core public health functions, and professional training were also emphasized.

Legislation governing the formation of the Bermuda Health Council was approved in 2005 mandating the Council to oversee the integration of health services. In 2005, the Medical Practitioners Amendment Act was developed and in 2006 was approved by the Legislature; it calls for periodic registration by this group and continuing medical education training once every two years. Among the Act's provisions is one specifying the responsibility of health professionals to report drug misuse. This Act also revised disciplinary procedures in the medical profession, an activity that is overseen by a subcommittee of the Bermuda Medical Council.

The Tobacco Products (Public Health) Amendment Act was approved by the Legislature in December 2005 and entered into effect on 1 April 2006. The Act bans smoking in enclosed public places and bars, restaurants, hotels, and business vehicles. It also bans cigarette vending machines, limits tobacco advertising, and prohibits the sale of tobacco products to those under age 18. To facilitate transition into the new law, a six-month grace period was allowed for the affected premises, with prosecution for violations beginning in October 2006.

The Nursing Act of 2000 established requirements for nursing categories and continuing education. The rules and regulations needed to implement these changes were modified during the current review period and now allow for nurse practitioners and nurse specialists to be registered.

Under review currently are a pharmacy act and dental practitioners act. The Professions Supplementary to Medicine Amendment Act is being updated to include a code of ethics and improved disciplinary procedures.

Organization of the Health System

The public and private health care systems collaborate closely in the provision of health care. Responsibility for public health care lies with the Ministry of Health and Family Services. The Ministry is mandated to promote and protect the health and well-being of Bermuda's residents and is charged with assuring the provision of health care services, setting standards, and coordinating the health care system. As a Cabinet-level official, the Minister of Health and Family Services reports to this body on all issues related to health policy, planning, and evaluation.

This Ministry is composed of several departments and agencies, including the Department of Health, Department of Child and Family Services, Department of Financial Assistance, and Department of Court Services. Each department is responsible for its own operation, under the authority of the Permanent Secretary, and the direction of the department head or director.

The Ministry is also responsible for Bermuda's two hospitals, the King Edward VII Memorial Hospital (the general hospital) and the Mid-Atlantic Wellness Institute (formerly Saint Brendan's Hospital, the country's psychiatric facility). The King Edward VII Memorial Hospital has 327 beds in private, semiprivate, and public wards. Services are organized into five multidisciplinary programs: continuous care, critical care, maternal and child care, medical care, and surgical care. The culturally diverse nursing and medical staff is recruited locally and worldwide, and provides quality nursing and medical care within the community using up-to-date procedures and technological equipment.

There is a large private health care sector utilizing fee-for-service practices, as well as an increasing number of informal groups and corporations of specialist physicians and allied health professionals; part of their focus is on primary care. Currently, the reimbursement system for physicians is being revised to ensure standardization in the delivery of services.

Bermuda has no universal, publicly funded health insurance system. Health insurance plans are provided through private companies, public agencies, and employers. Public sector workers are insured through the Government Employees Health Insurance Scheme, while several major employers operate their own approved coverage plans for employees. The Bermuda Health Council has a committee that oversees the health insurance plan. This plan has an annual open enrollment period designed to ensure access to hospitalization insurance for all residents of Bermuda. Hospitalization insurance is mandatory for all employed and self-employed persons. Both employers and employees contribute to hospitalization insurance, with employers contributing 50% of the premium costs. Insurance coverage is nearly universal, and some individuals are over-insured. Insurance sold by private companies and public agencies is regulated through the Bermuda Health Council and must include a provision for minimum benefits known as the Standard Hospital Benefit.

A Mutual Reinsurance Fund, also administered by the Bermuda Health Council, covers dialysis, anti-rejection drugs, and hospice care. Hospitalization is provided free of charge to children and the elderly; costs are covered through a government subsidy to the Bermuda Hospitals Board.

Government Deals with Fewer Births, Longer Lives

As its crude birth rate drops and life expectancy rises, Bermuda is transitioning toward an older population—11% of the population is 65 years old and older, while only 6% of the population is under 5 years of age. As a result, the active labor force can be expected to decrease in the years to come, while an aging population will make increasing demands on the health care system. The Government is addressing this situation by providing special attention to the elderly, including free-of-charge hospitalization. The 11 residential care facilities for the elderly include nursing and domiciliary homes that provide care and personal services.

Responsibility for providing public health services rests with the Ministry of Health and Family Services, which is mandated to provide health promotion and disease prevention and control services as well as personal health and dental health care. In its role as a regulatory agency, the Ministry monitors food safety and water and air quality.

The Public Health Service plays a significant role in the provision of personal health services and also administers a number of traditional public health programs, including maternal and child health, school health, immunizations, health promotion and education, communicable diseases control, rehabilitation, and home health care, including health visiting, district nursing, and selected specialized care for conditions such as HIV/AIDS.

Bermuda is divided into three health regions to facilitate the delivery of public health services. In each region, the Ministry of Health and Family Services operates a health center that offers prenatal and child health care, family planning services, immunizations, and other primary care services, as well as dental clinics for children.

Private voluntary agencies provide some specialized services with governmental assistance, such as community-based oncology nursing and personal services for HIV-infected persons, among others.

King Edward VII Memorial Hospital and the Mid-Atlantic Wellness Institute are administered by the Bermuda Hospitals Board, a statutory body appointed by the Minister of Health and Family Services. The Board delegates day-to-day responsibilities for the running of the two facilities to a Chief Executive Officer who is assisted by several senior managers, including a Chief of Staff and a Director of Nursing and Patient Services. Medical staff committees representing the physicians are involved in the administration of the facilities. Both hospitals undergo periodic accreditation reviews by the Canadian Council on Hospital Accreditation. There are no private hospitals in Bermuda.

Public Health Services

As part of its disease prevention and control activities and functions, the Ministry of Health and Family Services provides health analysis and epidemiology services. Routine laboratory tests are conducted within the country; formal arrangements with various overseas laboratories exist for certain types of specialized laboratory testing.

Potable water and sanitary excreta disposal are handled on an individual household basis; hotels and other commercial establishments have their own systems. Since Bermuda has few natural water supplies, water is obtained principally through a roof cistern collection system. Desalinization through a reverse osmosis process and water treatment at the Wellington Water Works supplements hotel and residential water needs. By law, well water is to be utilized only for non-drinking purposes. However, there are some private licensed wells that supplement the tank supply; these are monitored by a team of environmental health inspectors maintained by the Ministry of Health and Family Services.

Sanitary excreta are handled through individual septic tanks, as the islands' limestone formation provides a natural filtering system. Beaches and harbors are monitored to control sewage disposal or dumping into the ocean. Ships hook into a main sewerage line for disposal in the ports at Hamilton and the Royal Navy Dockyard. In the town of St. George's, ship sewage is disposed of in a holding tank. In general, sewage is treated and only then channeled out to sea. Monitoring has been conducted to assure that sewerage is treated prior to disposal into the sea, and although no serious health problems have been reported to date, the process is of ongoing concern and thus warrants permanent vigilance.

The Ministry of Health and Family Services monitors the safety of workers in the areas of pesticide use and those working in the mass burning incinerator; the Ministry also carries out occupational safety assessments for government employees and provides occupational health advice to all government departments.

The Ministry of Health and Family Services also oversees matters relating to food safety and control, including monitoring of food handlers and itinerant food vendors. During the 2001–2005 period, the Ministry initiated continuing health education training for all hotel restaurant personnel, including chefs, in collaboration with Bermuda College.

The Emergency Measures Organization, an entity under the responsibility of the Bermuda Police Commissioner, monitored and instituted preventive measures in preparation for Hurricane Fabian in September 2003 and also offered post-disaster assistance. A preparedness plan for avian and other serious pandemic influenzas has been developed that details operational plans for implementation in the event of an outbreak.

Individual Care Services

Primary health care services, which are generally available on demand, are delivered at government health centers, hospital outpatient clinics, and private physicians' offices. Additional ambulatory care services are provided through specialty clinics and the Emergency Department of King Edward VII Memorial Hospital. A substantial proportion of primary health care is delivered through the private sector. The majority of physicians and dentists are independent, private practitioners. Most other health care providers are employed on a salaried basis by the two hospitals, the Public Health Service, or private physicians.

There are no health maintenance organizations, independent practice associations, or preferred provider organizations in Bermuda. Nor are there provisions for prepaid medical care. There are a small number of multi-specialty group practices and a limited number of partnerships involving specialists. Primary health care physicians, including internists and pediatricians, account for half of all practicing physicians. General practitioners (i.e., family physicians) and other primary health care physicians generally coordinate care and control access to other specialists. Office visits represent the largest portion of physician-patient contact. Almost all physicians have hospital admission privileges.

In addition to its specialty, ambulatory care clinics, King Edward VII Memorial Hospital operates a primary health care clinic for indigent patients. The average length of stay at this facility was 8.2 days during 2003–2004, 7.9 days in 2004–2005, and 8.5 days in 2005–2006. The occupancy rate was 71% in 2003–2004, 69% in 2004–2005, and 73% in 2005–2006. Emergency and outpatient surgery services are only provided at King Edward VII Memorial Hospital. There were over 33,600 patient visits to the Emergency Department in 2005. Between April 2004 and March 2005, surgical procedures were carried out on 2,413 inpatients and on 5,775 outpatients. Other services delivered during this period included 18,710 physiotherapy treatment sessions, 31,584 x-ray examinations, 9,773 cardiac investigations, 9,901 ultrasound scans, 1,397 nuclear medicine investigations, 893 outpatient chemotherapy treatments, 4,851 CAT scans, and 5,112 occupational therapy treatment sessions.

There are no secondary or tertiary care hospitals in Bermuda. However, tertiary care is provided through links with institutions in Canada, the United Kingdom, and the United States.

Bermuda has three special education facilities for children with disabilities and impairments. In addition, a specially equipped housing complex, Summerhaven, is available for adolescents and adults with physical impairments. Students with disabilities are being mainstreamed from special schools into the regular school system, where paraprofessionals are assigned to facilitate the process; a government post has been established to coordinate this activity.

King Edward VII Memorial Hospital provides diagnostic and treatment services for patients with a variety of health conditions. Services include medicine, surgery, obstetrics and gynecology, rehabilitation, and geriatrics. The hospital also provides such specialized services as oncology, renal dialysis, and medical and surgical intensive care.

Mental health services are provided by psychiatrists, psychologists, a psychiatric social worker, mental health welfare officers attached to the Mid-Atlantic Wellness Institute, and the Employee Assistance Program. The Mid-Atlantic Wellness Institute is Bermuda's only psychiatric hospital and provides comprehensive mental health care and treatment. Accredited by the Canadian Council on Health Services Accreditation and recognized by the Royal College of Psychiatry as a training site for psychiatric resident doctors, the Institute covers all areas of psychiatry including acute general adult, adolescent, and child psychiatry; rehabilitation; community care; extended care; and the subspecialties of learning disabilities and substance misuse. Forensic psychiatric services are provided to prison facilities, and consulting services are available to King Edward VII Memorial Hospital and social services agencies. The 120-bed facility, which serves approximately 600 outpatients per year, has undergone a process of de-institutionalization over the past two decades, and today maintains several community group homes as well as a halfway house.

The Board and the government also operate various long-term care facilities. Skilled nursing care facilities include Lefroy House, with 57 beds, and the Extended Care Unit at the King Edward VII Memorial Hospital, with 90 beds. A new residential hospice care facility with 43 beds provides a range of services, including assisted care and skilled nursing care, and it has an Alzheimer's unit. This integration of care facilitates changes in patients' care as their condition alters without the need to transfer them to other facilities. Plans are currently under way to develop a single unit to cover all long-term care for older adults. Agape House, also operated by the Bermuda Hospitals Board and partially subsidized by public funds, provides hospice care for clients with terminal conditions. There are 11 residential care facilities for the elderly, including nursing homes that provide limited nursing care and personal services, as well as domiciliary care homes that provide room and board and limited assistance with personal services. Most of these facilities are partially funded through public monies.

Health Promotion

The Ministry of Health and Family Services' Health Promotion Office develops and coordinates programs that promote healthy lifestyles, environments, and policies and seeks to raise public awareness regarding healthy options, risk reduction, and the availability of professional support and services in the community. It works with a range of partners, both within and outside the Ministry.

One example of interagency collaboration is a comprehensive school health initiative developed jointly by the Ministries of Education and Health and Family Services in cooperation with 12 different government entities. The health-promoting schools initiative operates around a framework of policies, programs, activities, and services designed to enhance students' educational achievement and wellness through 12 different components. It provides practical and strategic opportunities for students, parents and families, educators, health workers, community organizations, and policymakers to interact in a variety of activities that stimulate the creation of healthy behaviors and enhance learning. All of Bermuda's public schools and three private schools are taking part in the initiative. A nutrition policy, food and nutrition handbook, and other health promotion brochures and materials have been distributed to all government schools. Twelve schools have implemented a program to address overweight and obesity issues as part of the health-promoting schools initiative.

Human Resources

In general terms, Bermuda had sufficient human resources to meet its health needs during 2001–2005. During this time, the number of physicians increased, as did the number of visiting specialist physicians. In 2004, there were 161 physicians, or 26 physicians per 10,000 population.

Nurses continue to represent the largest group of health care providers in the country, with a total of 423 in 2004, or 67 per 10,000 population. However, this figure represents a significant reduction from the more than 800 licensed nurses, including registered nurses and psychiatric nurses, who were employed in Bermuda in 1999. Registered nurses accounted for 75% of nurses. Most nurses were hospital-based, and a significant proportion of these were non-Bermudian. There is an ongoing shortage in some nursing specialties.

There were 11 dentists/dental hygienists per 10,000 population in 2004. Seventy dentists/dental hygienists were practicing in Bermuda; most private dentists have independent practices. Specialized forms of dentistry, such as periodontics and orthodontics, are also available. In 2004, there was one optometrist per 10,000 population.

There was a variety of allied health personnel in 2004, including medical laboratory technologists, radiographers, occupational therapists, physiotherapists, 12 nutritionists/dietitians, and speech-language pathologists. There were 44 pharmacists, who provided services ranging from retail pharmacy to clinical pharmacology. Most pharmacists were employed on a salaried

basis. Nurse midwives are registered, but do not provide independent care.

Despite the increase in the number of practicing physicians, shortages persisted in some specialty areas. Physician specialties included general, family practice, internal medicine, anesthesiology, emergency medicine, public health/preventive medicine, pediatrics, psychiatry, general surgery, obstetrics/gynecology, orthopedics, sports medicine, otolaryngology, radiology, cardiology, dermatology, ophthalmology, pathology, geriatrics, and urology.

Bermuda continues to experience difficulties with the retention of nurses and has responded by recruiting from a wider range of countries and by increasing the country's own training capacity.

Even though Bermuda has no medical schools or graduate medical education programs, it nonetheless requires continuing medical education for hospital-based physicians. Refresher courses and a degree program for nurses have been developed at Bermuda College in conjunction with overseas institutions. Training programs for emergency medical technicians have been established by both the Bermuda Fire Service and the Bermuda Hospitals Board.

Health Supplies

There is no local production of pharmaceuticals, drugs, or medical equipment.

Research and Technological Development in Health

In 2004, the Bermuda Hospitals Board formed an Ethics Committee whose objective is to promote greater awareness of moral, ethical, and legal issues at its hospital facilities, endorse medical ethics education, develop an ethics consultation service, and provide guidance to health care professionals when circumstances call upon them to make controversial decisions.

In 2005, a scientific research trial on diabetes was conducted.

Health Sector Expenditures and Financing

In 2004, the Bermudian health system consumed over US$ 376 million, representing 9.05% of GDP, or nearly US$ 6,000 per capita. The largest two sources of funding were private insurers, with over US$ 191 million (51%), followed by the government, with US$ 110 million (29%), which is 15% of the total government expenditure. Household financing, or out-of-pocket expenses paid by Bermuda residents when purchasing health care (such as co-payments on services and products covered by health insurance, or full payments, if not covered by insurance), constituted the third source of financing of Bermuda's health sector, with over US$ 57 million (15%). Finally, the nonprofit sector contributed US$ 12.9 million, or 4% of the total share in 2004. Over the past decade, there has been an increase in the share of private sector financing (from 61% in 1993 to 70% in 2004) and a decrease in the share of public sector financing (from 39% in 1993 to 30% in 2004). Regarding 2004 health expenditure, the Bermuda Hospitals Board represented the largest share, at more than US$ 140 million, or 38% of all expenditure; it was followed by local providers, including care for the elderly, with US$ 107 million (28%); overseas care, with US$ 40 million (11%); and spending on drugs, with US$ 36 million (10%). The latter has experienced the steepest increase over the past five years, rising from 6% in 2000 to 10% in 2004. The Ministry of Health and Family Services accounts for 7% of all expenses, or US$ 26.9 million. Health system costs have outpaced the economy's in the past 15 years: 8.7% and 5.0% per year, respectively, in 1990–2004.

Bermuda's health system delivers high quality levels of care. The distribution of care and financing, however, shows some inequities. The very high life expectancy, extremely low infant and maternal mortality, and excellent record on HIV/AIDS prevention, detection, and treatment are examples of the quality and effectiveness of the country's health care. However, disparities in life expectancy, insurance coverage, and distribution of health financing, in particular affecting low-income, Black, and older adult-headed households, indicate the persistence of pockets of inequity. The Bermuda Health Council has been mandated to address these and other equity-related issues affecting Bermuda's health services and systems.

Technical Cooperation and External Financing

During the 2001–2005 period, the Pan American Health Organization and the Caribbean Epidemiology Center provided technical cooperation in health to Bermuda.

BOLIVIA

0 50 100 Miles

Brazil

Pando

Peru

Beni

La
Paz

La Paz

Cochabamba

Santa Cruz

Oruro

Chuquisaca

Potosí

Tarija

Chile

Paraguay

Argentina

olivia shares borders with Brazil, Paraguay, Argentina, Chile, and Peru. It covers an area of 1,098,581 km², 65% of which is plains, where 26% of the population lives; the Andean valleys occupy 19% of the surface area, with 29% of the population; and 16% is occupied by highlands plateau (the altiplano), with 45% of the population (*1*).

GENERAL CONTEXT AND HEALTH DETERMINANTS

Social, Political, and Economic Determinants

The 2001 census showed that 64% of the total population did not have sufficient income to cover basic needs. According to 2005 projections from the Economic and Social Policy Analysis Unit, the estimated population living in poverty in 2006 would be 5.9 million people (63%) (*2*) and of this group, 2.0 million (35%) would be living in extreme poverty (*3*). This population was concentrated in municipalities of the high Andean valleys and altiplano and was mainly of indigenous descent. The plains area, El Chaco region, and the largest Bolivian cities also have significant levels of poverty, due to migration. In 2002, the estimated Gini index was 0.614 (*4*).

In 2000, the government administration then in office established the Bolivian Poverty Reduction Strategy. This Strategy was implemented following a highly participative national dialogue in which civil society determined areas of intervention where available resources could be applied to reduce the levels of extreme poverty. The objective of the Heavily Indebted Poor Countries (HIPC) initiative—a joint effort of the World Bank and the International Monetary Fund supported by bilateral donors—is to reduce the burden of foreign debt of the world's most heavily indebted poor countries to sustainable levels. Through this Initiative, Bolivia was initially granted a cancellation of external debt equivalent to US$ 1.1 billion; under the HIPC II initiative, US$ 1.5 billion of debt was cancelled, and through the "Beyond HIPC" process, cancellation of more than US$ 2 billion up to 2015 was estimated.

In 2003, the Bolivian Poverty Reduction Strategy was updated for the 2004–2007 period; it proposed broad-based growth favoring the creation of thousands of jobs in micro-, small-, and medium-sized enterprises in order to achieve accelerated social and economic impact (*5*). Part of this effort was also linked to the Millennium Development Goals (MDGs) formulated by the United Nations as a way to reduce global inequities. Bolivia drew up its second revision of the MDGs in 2002 (*6*); this has now become the driving force behind the Poverty Reduction Strategy.

The objective of reducing extreme poverty from 35% to 17.5% by 2015, as set forth in the Strategy, calls for economic growth at a sustained annual rate of 5%–5.5% over the next 15 years (*7*). Gross domestic product increased 0.6% in 1999 and 2.5% in 2003, when the average per capita income was US$ 900, but an income distribution analysis showed that the wealthiest 20% of the population had, on average, income 13 times higher than the poorest 20% segment. The presence of inequalities within poor groups was also noted; thus, in rural areas males had incomes 13 times higher than their female counterparts and, when comparing the data by gender and area of residence, an urban woman was shown to earn seven times more than her rural indigenous peer (Human Development Report, United Nations Development Program).

A change in leadership followed the June 2002 national elections. In February 2003, due to the high fiscal deficit and the Government's efforts to establish tax policies to control it, extensive conflicts arose, along with the demand for a constituent assembly and recovery of ownership of hydrocarbons; these resulted, in October 2003, in the Vice President of the Republic replacing the President through constitutional succession.

The political crisis resulted in several presidential changes between 2004 and December 2005, when a Presidential election was held. In January 2006, a new administration took office; its agenda includes nationalization of Bolivia's petroleum and natural gas reserves, and the development of social policies to reduce the country's cumulative social inequities. Its political plan includes achieving, by 2007, universal public health insurance, giving priority to decreasing undernutrition in children under 5 years old, strengthening the steering role of the Ministry of Health and Sports within the context of the self-governing and decentralization process the country is undergoing, and promoting community participation in health issues.

In 2001, 97% of Bolivian children between the ages of 6 and 13 were enrolled in school. Primary education is mandatory and free up to the eighth grade (*8*). For every 100 boys, there were 94 girls enrolled in primary education and 89 in secondary education. In the population as a whole, the illiteracy rate in men was 6.9%, and in women it was 19.4% (*1*).

Analyzing levels of education and income, it was found that the population's poorest quintile, consisting mainly of indigenous and native people (as opposed to those of European and mestizo origin), had an average of 3.6 years of education (3 years in rural

115

areas and 5.8 years in urban areas). The wealthiest quintile had 5 years of education in rural areas and 10.8 years in urban areas (9).

Various studies have shown that 53% of Bolivian communities are highly vulnerable to food insecurity; 16% of this population, or 7,718 communities, are the most vulnerable, and of these, 78% are extremely poor. By department, 80% of the communities of Chuquisaca and Potosí are highly vulnerable, as are 50% of the communities of Oruro, Cochabamba, and La Paz (10).

In 2004, 41% of the rural population had access to water through household plumbing, as compared to 88% in urban areas; just 5.3% of rural dwellingss had sewer service, as compared to 57.6% in urban areas; 65% of rural households and 91% of urban households had electricity.

The percentage of protected areas in the national territory increased from 1% in 1990 to 16% in 2004. The country has progressively incorporated the principles of sustainable development in national policies and programs as part of its efforts to prevent further loss and degradation of environmental resources.

Demographics, Mortality, and Morbidity

The population grew 8% between 2001 and 2005 (from 8,516,000 to 9,182,000 population). In 2005, 64.4% of the population lived in urban areas and 33.6% in rural areas. According to the 2001 census, 31% of the population identified themselves as being Quechua (i.e., of Incan descent), 25% as Aymara, and 6% as Guaraní or another ethnic minority of the Amazon region; 38% did not identify their ethnic origin.

In the same period, life expectancy at birth increased from 63 years (2001) to 64.9 years (2005). The low increase is due to high infant mortality, 54 per 1,000 live births, principally because of the component of neonatal death. The crude birth rate is 28.5 births per 1,000 population, due to the high fertility rate (3.7 children per woman), women's lack of autonomy in making decisions about and exercising their sexual and reproductive rights, and limited access to reproductive health services. The adjusted gross mortality rate decreased from 1,230.2 per 100,000 population in 2001 to 994.9 in 2005.

In a study conducted in 50 municipalities (of a total of 327 in the country) whose population is at the highest levels of extreme poverty and that included the native monolingual population, it was found that infant mortality is two times higher (48 per 1,000 live births) than in the 138 municipalities in which the poverty situation is less dire.

According to a 2003 study by the United Nations Development Program, the infant mortality rate stood at 78 per 1,000 live births in 2001 and decreased to 54 per 1,000 live births in 2005. But it must be emphasized that the probability of death in a child under 2 years old born to a woman who speaks only Spanish was 75 per 1,000 live births if she lived in the altiplano, 86 if she lived in the Andean valley area, and 92 if she lived in the plains area. In

comparison, the probability of death for a child of an Aymara woman who migrated to the plains was three times higher, or 206 per 1,000 children under 2 years old.

As regards birth rate, the 2003 National Demographic and Health Survey found that on average women had wanted to have 2.5 children and actually had 4.2. This difference was greater in rural areas, where women had wanted 3.2 children and had 6.4, than in urban areas, where women had wanted 2.2 children and actually had 3.3. A woman with an intermediate or higher level of education had, on average, 2.7 children during her childbearing years, whereas a woman with no formal education, generally indigenous or from a rural background, had 7.1 children during her reproductive years. If a woman had no formal education, the average age at which she would give birth to her first child would be 19 years; if she completed secondary education the average age would be 23 years (11).

Women have had little participation in politics and represent only 13% of the country's mayors; moreover, of all members of the bicameral National Congress in 2005, only 18% were female Deputies and 14% were female Senators. Unemployment was higher among women (5.9%) than men (3.9%) in 2003 (12).

The national system of vital statistics had not yet been consolidated in 2005, thereby placing limitations on the analysis of epidemiological data. However, the distribution of mortality in 2005 shows a predominance of cardiovascular diseases (40%), followed by communicable diseases (13%), external causes (12%), malignant neoplasms (8%), certain conditions originating in the perinatal period (5%), and other causes (21%). It should be emphasized, however, that this information may be biased, due to the aforementioned inadequacies in the national health system as of 2005.

Despite the fact that communicable diseases are still an important health problem in Bolivia, noncommunicable diseases are responsible for a much higher proportion of mortality, accounting for more than half of all deaths annually (13). Of these, diseases of the circulatory system are responsible for 40% of deaths, malignant neoplasms for 8%, and external causes (including accidents and other types of violent death) for approximately 12%.

The general mortality rate from all causes was higher in men (1,102 per 100,000 population) than in women (897 per 100,000 population). The mortality rate from diseases of the cardiovascular system was similar in both sexes; from neoplasms it was 1.5 times higher in women than in men; from external causes it was 2.5 times higher in men than in women; and from communicable diseases it was 1.2 times higher in men than in women.

More than half of maternal deaths (53.5%) occurred at home; 22% occurred during pregnancy, 36% during childbirth, and 42% during puerperium. The principal causes were hemorrhage (39% of cases), eclampsia (21%), abortion (10%), and other causes (30%). The coverage of institutional births in 2003 was

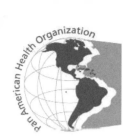

HEALTH IN THE AMERICAS READER'S OPINION SURVEY

Dear PAHO reader:

We greatly appreciate a couple minutes of your time to answer this brief survey. Your responses will help us improve future editions of our publication.

We ask that you respond only if you are an end-user of the book. If you are in charge of the library where the book was sent, we appreciate your passing the survey to a book reader/user and requesting that he/she respond.

1. Country of residence: _____

2. State or province: _____

3. Occupation:

○ Health authority
○ Health and/or related fields professional
○ Health technician and/or related fields
○ Administrator in the health sector
○ Social worker
○ Researcher
○ University professor
○ Student of public health, medicine, or related area
○ Journalist/communicator
○ Librarian
○ Another (specify) :_____

4. Institutional affiliation:

○ Ministry of health
○ Another ministry
○ Local government
○ Health services/ laboratory
○ University
○ Research institute
○ Social security
○ Nongovernmental organization (NGO)/foundation
○ International organization
○ Media (press, radio, TV, news agency)
○ Private sector
○ Self-employed
○ Another: _____

5. How did you obtain this book?

○ Courtesy copy
○ Purchase
○ Through a colleague
○ It arrived at the library/documentation center where I work. (If you marked this option, please pass this survey on to an end-user so that she/he may respond).

6. How do you use or plan to use this publication?

○ Health program/policy development and design
○ In my professional work
○ Staying on top of/up to date on current public health issues
○ Research
○ Education
○ In my university studies
○ To write scientific or journalistic articles

7. Have you previously used the publication?

○ YES   ○ NO

8. Please indicate how useful the following chapters and/or information types were:

	Very useful	Useful	Not useful	Don't know
Vol I: Regional				
An overview of regional health	○	○	○	○
Health in the context of development	○	○	○	○
Health conditions and trends	○	○	○	○
Sustainable development and environmental health	○	○	○	○
Public policies and health systems and services	○	○	○	○
Health and international cooperation	○	○	○	○
Prospects for regional health	○	○	○	○
Vol II: Countries				
Country Chapter	○	○	○	○
Other: Tables, maps, and figures	○	○	○	○
Country highlights	○	○	○	○

9. Additional remarks:

_____
_____
_____
_____

Thank you very much for your time.
Please send your answer to:
DISSEMINATION HIA/B
Postal Service:
PUB/DM
525 23rd St. NW,
Washington DC 20037, USA
Fax: 1-202-338-0869; E-mail: dissemination@paho.org

57%. The probability of maternal death was higher in rural areas, the altiplano, and the high Andean valleys.

HEALTH OF POPULATION GROUPS

Children under 5 Years Old

Vaccination coverage of children aged 12–23 months in 2003 was, on average, 50%. The vaccines whose coverage exceeded 90% were the BCG tuberculosis vaccine, the first dose of DPT (diphtheria, pertussis, and tetanus), and the polio vaccine (11); the lowest coverage occurred mainly with the third doses of DPT and polio vaccine, 49% and 39%, respectively. Just 5.9% of children in this age group had had all their vaccinations, and 4.8% had had none.

In the same year, the prevalence of acute respiratory infections (ARIs) in children under 6 months old was 16.8%, while in children aged 6–11 months old it was 29.8%; 40.6% of children under 6 months of age received care at a health center or post, compared to 36.4% of those aged 6–11 months. The prevalence of diarrhea among children under 5 years of age was 22%, while for those aged 6–23 months, it was 35%, and for the age group under 6 months old, it was 16%. The difference in prevalence between children under 5 living in rural areas and those living in urban areas was minimal (24.1% and 21.1%, respectively). In all three age groups, only 36% received care from a health provider or establishment; 29% received treatment with oral rehydration salts, and 16% were given homemade preparations. During the period 1999–2002, care coverage for cases of diarrhea at health establishments for the poorest population quintile in rural areas remained stable at around 45%, while care coverage for the population's wealthiest quintile stood at approximately 90% in 2002.

Breast-feeding is practiced during the first year of life. In 2003, 93% of children between 10 and 11 months of age were still being breast-fed; however, the rate of exclusive breast-feeding in the first two months of life was 70%, and this percentage decreased to 56% for children between the ages of 2 and 3 months. On average, 54% of children under 6 months old were being exclusively breast-fed; consequently, the introduction of complementary foods began early, occurring among 21% of children during the first two months of life and among 45% of those between the ages of 4 and 5 months of age.

A 2001 study by the Pan American Health Organization concluded that a slow decline in the numbers of neonatal deaths during the review period was related to high prevalences of infectious diseases (32%), of disorders related to prematurity and low birthweight (30%), and of specific respiratory disorders and disorders originating in the perinatal period (22%). Overall infant mortality declined from 67 to 54 per 1,000 live births between 1998 and 2003. For mothers without a formal education, however, the figure was 87 per 1,000 live births; it was 73 in the poorest municipalities; 72 among the poorest population quintile and in the country's poorest department (Potosí); 67 in rural areas; and 61 in the altiplano area (11).

Children 5–9 Years Old

Parasitic intestinal diseases among this age group are a serious public health problem. The prevalence of ascariasis ranged from 5% to 80%, with an average of 40% to 50% in the tropical zones. The prevalence of trichuriasis ranged from 10% to 66%, while the prevalence of uncinariasis is 15%, in contrast to the much lower prevalence found in the Andean regions where there is better access to clean drinking water and sanitation services. In La Paz, the prevalence of oxyuriasis was 29%; in the marginal zones of the city, it was even higher.

Adolescents 10–14 and 15–19 Years Old

The adolescent population accounted for 22.1% of the country's total population in 2004, with 49.3% being female and 50.7% male and 65% residing in urban areas. Economic need forces many adolescents to seek work to help their families. Some 65% work in domestic activities, in which females predominate as household employees. Additional areas in which adolescents work include other types of services to households (26.9%), trade and services (24.1%), and industry (22.9%).

According to the 2003 National Demographic and Health Survey (11), 16% of females ages 15–19 years old had had one pregnancy, and one of every three had had children before the age of 20. The highest percentage of adolescent pregnancies occurred among women without a formal education (47%); by place of residence, the highest percentages of adolescent pregnancies were found among rural women (22%) and among those in the plains area (21%). Of all consultations at public health facilities, 30% were for problems related to complications of pregnancy (including abortion), childbirth, and puerperium.

In the area of family violence, it has been estimated that, in 2003, in the cities of La Paz, Cochabamba, Santa Cruz, and El Alto, 7 of every 10 adolescents suffered psychological violence in the home, manifested by reprimands, yelling, insults, indifference, and prohibition from leaving the house. As regards physical violence, in 2004, the highest number of cases recorded at the national level occurred in La Paz (46%), Potosí (16%), and Cochabamba (12%).

Adults 20–59 Years Old

The total fertility rate dropped from 4 children per woman in 2001 to 3.7 in 2005. Maternal mortality decreased during the same period, from 390 to 230 per 100,000 live births. While 99% of women with a secondary or higher level of education were knowledgeable about modern birth control methods, only 54% of women without a formal education knew about them, and only 7.6% actually used them (*11*).

Older Adults 60 Years Old and Older

In 2005, this age segment represented 7% of Bolivia's population, with a growth rate of 4.4%. According to the Index of Basic Unmet Needs, 63% were living in poverty. Some 46% of this population continued to be economically active, and only 13% of women became inactive due to retirement. The household economic contribution rate for older adults was 33.8% in urban areas and 58.4% in rural areas, with this difference possibly being due to the low coverage by the pension system and the marked poverty in rural areas. Of the population over 60 years old, 47.8% were illiterate; of these, 70% were women. Eighteen percent of Bolivian households were headed by an older adult (*14*). No data are available regarding the situation of this age group among native populations and the rural poor.

The Family

In 2004, slightly more than 90% of the Bolivian population lived in a family environment. Almost 12% of families were headed by a single parent; of these households, 83.7% were headed by women; this phenomenon was due in part to the migration of the male head of household in search of temporary work in other parts of the country. In the cases in which both parents migrate, grandparents or other relatives were often left in charge of the household.

Workers

Sixteen percent of Bolivian workers were insured in 2004; 64% of the urban population performs work associated with the informal sector and, consequently, is excluded from the country's Compulsory Social Security mechanism. Workers in the informal sector reported an average out-of-pocket health expenditure of US$ 20, compared to US$ 25 by their counterparts in the formal sector; this difference is reversed, however, when catastrophic expenses (i.e., those that constitute more than 30% of the household's disposable annual income) are analyzed. Of all households whose out-of-pocket health expenditures exceeded 10%, 61% represented those whose family members performed work in the informal economy, while the remaining 39% held employment in the formal economy.

Many occupational illnesses are misdiagnosed, and the National Health Information System does not keep records of work-related accidents or illnesses, since information collection forms do not include these variables.

Persons with Disabilities

According to information from the Ministry of Health and Sports, 10% of the Bolivian population had some degree of disability. Although there is no clear information regarding the classification of disabilities, in general terms physical disability accounted for 3%, mental disability for 3%, sensory disability for 3.5%, and other types of disability for 0.5%.

Although Bolivia has a law for persons with disabilities, various obstacles hamper an effective response to the problem, including the lack of pertinent health policies, regulations, training programs for health professionals, and new strategies for and approaches to prevention and rehabilitation; moreover, there is a need for coordinated collaboration between social and community actors to find approaches that are feasible within the context of the country's current reality.

Ethnic Groups

According to the 2001 census, there were high rates of infant mortality in the native population. Some 37% of childbirths were attended by a doctor, 18% by another person, and 14.7% by a midwife; 21% were unattended childbirths. In 2005, a study was conducted of institutional birth levels by municipality among native monolingual women. Fewer than 7% of all births in the eight municipalities whose female populations were 80%–89% indigenous took place in a health care facility; among the 12 municipalities in which 70%–79% of the female population was native monolingual, this figure was 10%; in contrast, in the 138 municipalities where the percentage of native monolingual women was 9% or under, 45% of all births occurred in a health establishment (*15*).

Data from the Program for the Improvement of Surveys and the Measurement of Living Conditions show that, between 1999 and 2000, the levels of institutional care during childbirth (approximately 35%) did not increase among pregnant women in the poorest native population quintile in rural areas (*15*).

HEALTH CONDITIONS AND PROBLEMS

COMMUNICABLE DISEASES

Vector-borne Diseases

The information on **malaria** recorded through the National Health Information System for the 2001–2005 period is shown in Table 1. It is worth noting that in 2004, nearly 50% of all malaria cases occurred in the department of Beni, principally in the municipalities of Riberalta (annual parasite incidence [API] 43 per 1,000 population) and Guayaramerín (API 60 per 1,000 population). In 2005, 55% of the cases were recorded in Beni; Beni and Pando have the highest risks of malaria in the country (API 37 and 43 per 1,000 population, respectively).

TABLE 1. Suspected and confirmed malaria cases, Bolivia, 2001–2005.

Year	Suspected cases	Confirmed cases			API[a] per 100,000 population
		Total	Plasmodium vivax	Plasmodium falciparum	
2001	122,926	15,765	14,957	808	5.0
2002	137,509	14,276	13,549	727	4.3
2003	158,299	20,343	19,550	793	6.1
2004	163,307	14,910	14,210	671	4.4
2005	104,300	20,142	19,062[b]	1,031[b]	5.5

[a]API calculated on the basis of the estimated at-risk population in endemic areas.
[b]49 mixed.
Source: National Health Information System.

There were 5 cases of **yellow fever** in 2001, 14 in 2002, 4 in 2003, and 11 in 2004; all of these cases were laboratory-confirmed. In 2005, 73 suspected cases were reported, of which 16 were confirmed (13 in Cochabamba, 2 in Santa Cruz, and 1 in La Paz).

The incidence of **leishmaniasis** was 24 per 100,000 population in 2003 and 37 in 2004. This increase was due to the migration of populations to endemic areas and subsequent modifications to the physical environment. The departments at highest risk were Pando (409 per 100,000 population), Beni (158 per 100,000 population), and La Paz (52 per 100,000 population). Some 2,800 cases were reported in 2004, 48% in La Paz, 20% in Beni, and 9% in Pando.

In 2001, 176 confirmed cases of **dengue** were reported; in 2002, there were 892 suspected cases, of which 278 were confirmed; in 2003, 4,624 suspected cases were reported; in 2004, 7,395 suspected cases were recorded, of which 682 were later laboratory-confirmed; and in 2005, 4,179 suspected cases were reported, with 617 being laboratory-confirmed. Two-thirds (66%) of the national total occurred in the departments of Beni (1,959 cases) and Pando (799 cases); Pando had the highest cumulative risk (1,198 per 100,000 population), followed by Beni (481 per 100,000 population); the figures of both departments were far above the national rate (44 per 100,000 population). In 2004, 48 cases of hemorrhagic dengue fever were recorded, with 6 deaths registered; in 2005, there were 10 confirmed cases of hemorrhagic dengue (7 in Santa Cruz de la Sierra and 3 in Cobija); there were no registered deaths from dengue that year.

The vector for **Chagas' disease**, *Triatoma infestans,* is present in seven of Bolivia's nine departments, which together cover 84% of the country. In 2001, with Inter-American Development Bank funds, household chemical treatment coverage was gradually extended in the endemic area, and in some parts the two cycles were completed and post-spraying entomological evaluations were stepped up. In 2002, due to technical and administrative problems, the original programming targets were not met. In 2003, there was a complete sweep of 670,000 dwellings. In 2004, house-hold spraying was selective, although all positive households were treated. In 2005, guidelines established for stratification were followed, based on the response to earlier control measures.

Up to 2005, the risk of vector transmission following spraying actions was eliminated in 70% of the endemic territory; moreover, there has been a reduction in the risk of disease transmission through increased systematic screening for Chagas of all blood donations to certified blood banks. In 2005, the seroprevalence rates in children under 15 years old (almost 40% of the population) ranged from 10% in urban areas to 40% in rural areas of six endemic departments, which together constitute nearly 50% of the national territory. It has been estimated that some 700,000 children under age 10 live in the endemic area and that of these, some 100,000–140,000 might possibly be infected with *Tripanosoma cruzi.*

Vaccine-preventable Diseases

Since 2000, the number of diseases for which vaccines are available to protect the population under 2 years old has grown from 6 to 11: poliomyelitis; tuberculosis; diphtheria, pertussis, tetanus, hepatitis B, and diseases caused by *Haemophilus influenzae* type b (these five make up the pentavalent vaccine, introduced in 2000); measles, rubella, and mumps (through the triple viral vaccine, also introduced in 2000); and yellow fever. Yellow fever vaccine is also administered to the at-risk adult population, and the vaccine for diphtheria and tetanus is administered to women 15–39 years old. In 2004, coverages of 86% were achieved for BCG tuberculosis vaccine, 84% for the third dose of poliomyelitis vaccine, 84% for the third dose of DPT vaccine, 90% for the triple viral vaccine, and 84% for the third dose of the hepatitis B vaccine in children under 1 year of age.

During the 2001–2005 period, the rate of **acute flaccid paralysis** in children under 15 years old ranged from 1.38 to 1.93 per 100,000 population. For **measles**, the proportion of suspicious cases investigated within 48 hours exceeded 98% during this same period; since 2001 there have been no confirmed cases, and

119

the last follow-up campaign against measles was conducted in 2003. Measles and **rubella** surveillance has been combined since 2004. In 2000–2001, a rubella outbreak occurred affecting 985 individuals; subsequent to the outbreak, the incidence of confirmed rubella has been falling, with 41 cases being detected in 2003, 12 in 2004, and 8 in 2005. Since 2001, an average of 3 cases of **neonatal tetanus** have been reported each year. Case numbers of **yellow fever** have declined due to the implementation of a mass vaccination strategy in the at-risk departments and increased vaccinations in municipalities with high numbers of temporary migrants; thus, during the 2001–2005 period, only 16 confirmed cases of yellow fever were reported. **Pertussis** and **diphtheria** are likewise on the decline, with only 68 cases and 8 cases, respectively, being reported during the entire 2001–2005 period.

Since 2003, Bolivia has joined in the activities carried out every year for Vaccination Week in the Americas. In October 2005, sentinel surveillance of **rotavirus infections** in hospitalized children under 5 years old began, in order to prepare the country for the introduction of this vaccine into the regular vaccination schedule. In December 2005, the Vaccination Law was approved in order to ensure the financial sustainability of the national vaccination program and its ability to procure vaccines. In May 2006, the country joined the Americas-wide effort to eliminate rubella and **congenital rubella syndrome** by carrying out its own national campaign.

Intestinal Infectious Diseases

In children under 5 years old, 541,697 cases of **acute diarrheal diseases** were reported (282.1 per 1,000 population ages 0–4) in 2001; 611,982 cases were reported in 2002 (291.1 per 1,000); and 701,182 cases were recorded in 2003 (269.3 per 1,000). In 2003, 22% of children under age 5 had had an episode of diarrhea in the two weeks prior to the National Demographic and Health Survey conducted that year (*11*). From 2001 to 2003, 80% of all cases of acute diarrhea reported in the country occurred among children under 5 years old (*16*).

No cases of **cholera** were reported during the 2001–2005 period.

Chronic Communicable Diseases

In 2001, the National Tuberculosis Program reported 8,761 new cases of all forms of **tuberculosis**. The incidence rate for all forms was 113 per 100,000 population in 2002, and 80 per 100,000 population for the pulmonary forms with positive bacilloscopy (BK+). In 2003, 7,718 BK+ pulmonary cases were diagnosed (85.5 per 100,000 population), while in 2004 the number of cases decreased to 7,544 (81.8 per 100,000 population). In 2005, of all recorded cases of tuberculosis in all its forms (9,196), 7,527 were BK+ pulmonary (79.8 per 100,000 population). The highest rates for this case finding were in the departments of Pando (113 per 100,000 population) and Santa Cruz (108 per

100,000 population). In 2005, it was found that there is insufficient passive case-finding; there is active case-finding without impact evaluation and without adequate planning vis-à-vis specific human groups or risk areas, and there is no TB/HIV coinfection investigation.

Eighty-five cases of **leprosy** were reported in 2003 (with an incidence rate of 0.07 per 100,000 population) and 76 in 2004, 39 of which were from Santa Cruz. In 2004, the at-risk population was estimated to be 677,280 persons throughout the country. The highest prevalence was recorded in the departments of Santa Cruz (1.34 per 100,000 population) and Pando (0.87 per 100,000 population).

Acute Respiratory Infections

In 2003, approximately 260,000 medical care visits related to ARIs were reported, while the following year the number of visits totaled more than 2 million; of these, half involved children under 5 years of age. By late 2004, 60% of ARI cases involved children under 5 years old. In 2004, 224 medical visits were recorded for every 1,000 persons nationwide. The illness showed a characteristic seasonal pattern, with an increase in the number of cases treated in the autumn and winter, and an average reporting of more than 155 medical visits per 1,000 population in July of each year (*16*).

HIV/AIDS and Other Sexually Transmitted Infections

In 2003, the most affected age groups were the 25–34-year-old group (45%) and the 15–24-year-old group (26%). The most common transmission mode continues to be sexual: 67% heterosexual, 23% homosexual, and 10% bisexual. The male-female ratio is 2.8:1. Half of the 225 persons diagnosed with HIV infection during 2003 already had progressed to the AIDS stage, indicating that early detection remains a serious challenge. Sentinel surveillance detected an HIV prevalence of less than 1% among pregnant women and higher than 5% among populations that engage in high-risk behavior. The country is thus classified as having a concentrated epidemic.

In 2001, the syndromic approach was incorporated in the recording of suspected cases of sexually transmitted infections (STIs), but case recording is very deficient, particularly as regards genital ulcers, a condition characterized by irregular reporting. At the current time, there are no activities aimed at the elimination of congenital syphilis, and syphilis detection during pregnancy and in newborns is not carried out on a regular basis.

According to information from the country's STI/AIDS Surveillance and Referral Centers, which perform monitoring and follow-up activities related to commercial sex work, a decrease in the proportion of individuals with **syphilis** (4.2% to 1.1%) and **gonorrhea** (6.8% to 2.7%) was noted between 2001 and 2004; however, the percentage of cases of **chlamydial infection** has increased: it was almost 13% in 2004, as compared to 7.8% in 2001.

Zoonoses

There were two deaths due to human **rabies** in 2003, six in 2004, and 11 in 2005. With regard to canine attacks of humans, there were 15,182 cases reported in 2004, with children being the most affected group; the majority of the attacks were by stray dogs. Approximately half of the bites (45%) occurred in the department of La Paz, but the risk of attacks was highest in Chuquisaca (286.1 per 100,000 population), followed by La Paz and Cochabamba, with the latter recording 22% of all those injured. In 2005, 14,544 people were bitten (154 injured per 100,000 population), a figure similar to the one for 2004. The high incidence of canine rabies in Bolivia is due to the lack of an operating program overseen by the Ministry of Health and Sports, Departmental Health Services (known as SEDES, for its Spanish acronym), and the municipalities, especially in the nine departmental capitals, that would enable coordination of the various aspects required for effective canine rabies control. In 2004, 408 canines tested positive for rabies, and in 2005, this number increased to 897; of these cases, 54.6% (490) were recorded in the municipality of Santa Cruz and 18.5% (166) in Cochabamba. In the absence of a sustainable national control program, actions to stem the epidemic have been of short duration and limited to mass campaigns which did not achieve the desired results; for example, four mass vaccination campaigns carried out by health authorities and council members in Santa Cruz reached only a 50% coverage rate. Consequently, it is essential for the Ministry of Health and Sports, the SEDES, and the municipalities to have an operating program and the resources necessary to achieve rabies control and eradication in the coming years.

In 2005, the National Service for Livestock Health and Food Safety (or SENASAG, for its Spanish acronym) declared Bolivia free of **foot-and-mouth disease** with vaccination. Based on the fact that no cases of foot-and-mouth disease had been reported for two years and that the World Organization for Animal Health (or IOE, for its acronym in French) had declared the department of Oruro as being free of the disease, SENASAG requested that the Pan American Health Organization provide the support of two experts from the Pan American Foot-and-Mouth Disease Center (PANAFTOSA) for the purpose of training SENASAG veterinarians to conduct national seriologic sampling during 2006. Once the laboratory results are evaluated—and if an absence of viral activity is demonstrated—Bolivia will submit its application to the IOE and request that it be granted status in the category of a country free of foot-and-mouth disease with vaccination.

Between 2001 and 2005, 122 cases of **hantaviral disease** were reported, with 50 of these cases being laboratory-confirmed. Up until 2003, all reported cases had originated in the department of Tarija. In 2004, 10 cases were recorded (0.1 per 1,000 population), 6 originating in the city of Bermejo, department of Tarija, and one originating in Montero, department of Santa Cruz, with a fa-tality rate of 20%. In 2005, 64 suspected cases were reported and 18 were confirmed by laboratory testing.

NONCOMMUNICABLE DISEASES

Metabolic and Nutritional Diseases

Twenty-seven percent of all Bolivian children under 5 years of age suffered from chronic **malnutrition**, the rate being higher for children in rural areas (37%). When analyzing this situation within the context of poverty levels, it was shown that 42% of children under age 5 in the lowest quintile suffered chronic malnutrition, in comparison with only 5% in the highest quintile. Nearly 8% of children in this age group had low weight-for-age. One of every three women of childbearing age exhibited some degree of **anemia**, and one of every two children experienced some degree of anemia, with 25% of all children having mild anemia and 25% having moderate anemia (*11*).

Physical activity levels among Bolivians are generally low, with women being less likely to be physically active than men. Participation in sports decreases with age, and the disparities in activity levels between men and women also tend to increase with age. According to the 2003 National Demographic and Health Survey, 74% of men and 41% of women reported having participated in some type of recreational physical activity during the week prior to the survey (*11*). After the age of 60, more than 83% of women and 60% of men were inactive. Physical activity levels also tend to be lower among the poorest and less educated sectors of the population (*17*).

Malignant Neoplasms

Despite underregistration, available data indicate that cervical cancer is the most frequently reported type of cancer (21%), followed by neoplasms of the digestive system (14%) and those of other female genital organs (11%).

Cervical cancer is one of the leading causes of death among women, particularly those in the 35–64 age group. In 2004, the estimated incidence stood at 151.4 per 100,000 women, while new estimates in 2005 indicated the overall incidence to be 58 per 100,000 women. Higher incidences were recorded in the departments of Oruro and Potosí (60.9 and 93.5 per 100,000 women, respectively).

In some regions, the level of cervical cancer screening is less than 7% among women ages 25–49 years old (*18*). There is a difference between the number of cervical cytology samples taken and the number of samples with results reported. Given the importance of cervical cancer as a public health problem in Bolivia, over the short term the Ministry of Health and Sports plans to address the following areas: the need to develop strategies aimed at empowering women to exercise autonomy in their health care, to improve the recording system, to strengthen the skills of health and laboratory personnel, and to improve the quality of early intervention services and treatment.

OTHER HEALTH PROBLEMS OR ISSUES

Disasters

During 2001–2005, Bolivia was affected by a variety of natural disasters and those caused by humans, including floods, landslides, drought, blizzards, hurricane winds, earthquakes, hailstorms, forest fires, and social conflicts. Of these, floods and social conflicts led to the highest number of deaths (198). Some 150,530 families were affected by disasters, with the presence of poverty further aggravating their fate and the consequences creating a significant setback in terms of the population's overall health and development status.

A flood affecting large segments of the La Paz population occurred in 2003, the aftermath of an intense hailstorm. This event revealed the municipal health system's weak disaster response capacity; in particular, the staff of the emergency and morgue sections of the Hospital de Clínicas soon found themselves overwhelmed with the arrival en masse of the injured and dead.

In 2002, a large-scale forest fire broke out outside the city of Tarija in the Cordillera de Sama. Approximately 2,000 firefighters and other volunteers working to put out the fire suffered burn injuries and conjunctival and respiratory problems. Smoke from other forest fires and the traditional slash-and-burn techniques carried out to prepare land for cultivation also affected local populations and agricultural workers, causing respiratory and eye problems.

Violence and Other External Causes

A 2003 study of six Bolivian municipalities revealed that 55% of married women or women in long-term relationships and of reproductive age had experienced violent acts (physical, sexual, and psychological) committed against them by their intimate partners (19). At the same time, child abuse is a problem of growing concern, affecting as many as one out of every three boys and girls (20).

A series of social conflicts occurring in February and October 2003 and May–June 2005 provoked confrontations among the civilian population, the police, and the army, resulting in more than 80 deaths and 450 injuries; for example, in 2004 there were 3,907 civil disturbances, including marches, strikes, and roadblocks, throughout the country (21). During these incidents, all roads leading into the capital were blocked, which resulted in a shortage of basic foodstuffs and fuel (diesel, gasoline, and gas), and the inability to travel within the city and to access the airport. These events pointed to the vulnerability of the city's infrastructure and, in particular, the weak emergency response capacity of the hospital system.

Estimates by the Ministry of Health and Sports in 2004 indicated that there were 55 traffic accidents every day (2.5 per hour), implying significant social cost and effects on the population's health. In 2004, the mortality rate from accidents was nearly 7 per 100,000 population. In more than 90% of all traffic accidents, there was some human liability and contributory behavior, with failure on the part of the driver to respect traffic regulations, intoxication, and speeding being the most common causes; mechanical failures accounted for only 2.5% of all accidents (16).

Mental Health

A study conducted in La Paz in 2005 found that, at the secondary level of care, there had been consultations due to depressive disorders, disorders related to the use of psychoactive substances, and suicide attempts. In childhood, attention disorders and enuresis were common. The public health care services are experiencing challenges related to adequate training of personnel, availability of guidelines and drugs, case recording and surveillance, and referral services (just 11% of the tertiary-level hospitals nationwide have mental health services or offer specialized care) (21).

Addictions

The 12–18-year-old age group was at highest risk for narcotics use, according to the results of a study conducted by the Directorate for Total Prevention of Drug Dependency and for Mental Health in 2000. In 2004, the prevalence of alcohol use over a month was 43%; it was 61% over a year and 68% over a person's lifetime; it was estimated that 10% of all drinkers were alcoholics; for every ten men with alcohol problems, there were two women with the same problem. This pattern appears to be increasing, as well as initiating at very early ages (22).

Alcohol played a role in the majority of traffic accidents; of the 20,075 accidents occurring in 2004, 10,428 of the drivers were found to be intoxicated (21). Alcohol use and abuse are firmly entrenched in Bolivia and culturally based. The Ministry of Health and Sports and various nongovernmental organizations (NGOs) have made isolated attempts to address this social issue.

In 2004, the prevalence of tobacco use was found to be 25% in a month, 38% in a year, and 48% over a person's lifetime. It was estimated that at least 25% of adults smoked one or more cigarettes a month. About 5% of the population over age 15 were habitual smokers (10 or more cigarettes a day). A 2004 survey of smoking among adolescents ages 13–15 conducted in three Bolivian cities showed that half or more had smoked at some time and that approximately 30% were smokers at the time of the study (23). In general, smoking was more common in males than in females.

Tobacco research has been conducted in Bolivia, and awareness-raising strategies have been prepared for use with members of the National Congress, which facilitated ratification of the Framework Convention on Tobacco Control in 2005. But the implementation of tobacco-related laws, development of tools to promote a reduction in the demand for and availability of tobacco, and the institutionalization of initiatives to promote smoke-free environments are still pending.

Environmental Pollution

A 2004 risk analysis showed that the incidence rates of pesticide poisoning were highest in the departments of Pando, with more than 200 episodes per 100,000 population; Tarija, with 46 episodes per 100,000 population; and La Paz, with 34 per 100,000 population. Contrary to expectations, 63% of the episodes reported occurred in urban areas (*16*).

Oral Health

Data from the College of Dental Surgeons in 2003 showed the index of decayed, missing, and filled teeth (DMFT) in children under age 12 to be 6.7, mainly due to the caries component. The DMFT index for children aged 9 was 6.6, and the prevalence of untreated caries was 84.6% (84% nationally). The DEFT (decayed, extracted, and filled teeth) index in children aged 5–9 was 4.75. There is no oral health care for pregnant women to prevent infection.

RESPONSE OF THE HEALTH SECTOR

Health Policies and Plans

In recent years, Bolivia has promoted important public policies regarding social insurance with the rationale of delivering benefits packages for health recovery and protection, with particular focus on maternal and child health; these insurance schemes were initiated in the mid-1990s with the introduction of the Basic Health Insurance mechanism, and, more recently, with the passage of legislation for a universal maternal and child health insurance system. In the latter case, the goal is to remove economic barriers preventing access to health care, especially in urban and rural centers where health services are available. However, since the country's native, rural, and isolated population segments remain largely excluded from social protection systems, access to this health insurance plan has been much more difficult. A 2005 study by the Economic and Social Policy Analysis Unit showed that 70% of the Bolivian population experiences some form of exclusion from social protection systems for health (*2*).

Following its election in 2005, the current government administration issued a document regarding national health policy focusing on strategies: (1) addressing health issues from the perspective of health determinants, with the goal of eliminating malnutrition in children under 5 years of age, (2) strengthening the national health authority's steering role during the decentralization process, and (3) promoting community participation in health.

Law 1551 on Popular Participation, promulgated in 1994, established the process for the decentralization of funds and responsibility for the administration of educational and health establishments from the State to the municipality level. In 1995, Law 1654 provided for administrative decentralization of some technical and administrative functions from the executive branch to the departmental level.

To further promote policy and administrative decentralization in the country, in July 2006 a nationwide referendum was held addressing further expansion of decentralization activities to the departments. Despite these measures, the poorest municipalities have experienced great difficulties in the local development and implementation of health processes due to their limited operating capacity and ability to mobilize resources.

In 2001, the Ministry of Health and Sports conducted an evaluation of the essential public health functions (*24*), and the best performance was identified in the functions of social participation and empowerment of citizens in health and in the development of policy and planning capacity to support efforts in public health. Average to inferior performance was identified in the functions of research, development, and implementation of innovative public health solutions; promotion of equitable access to necessary health services; ensuring the quality of personal and population-based health services; and human resources development and training. This diagnosis is consistent with the difficulties the Bolivian public health system has experienced in terms of services integration and coverage extension.

The country does not have general public health legislation, although it does have an extensive body of health regulations that require systematization and updating into the corresponding health codes or laws. The Social Security Code (1948), which still governs the tripartite (government, employer, and employee) system of health insurance, and the Health Code (1967), which governs the public and private sectors, have become outdated through the passage of newer legal provisions such as the Law on Community Participation (1994), the Law on Universal Maternal and Child Health Insurance (2003), and other legislation on specific health issues, such as the Law on Safe Blood.

Health Strategies and Programs

Law 2426, effective 1 January 2003, provided for implementation of the Universal Maternal and Child Health Insurance legislation establishing comprehensive health benefits free of cost to all pregnant women from the start of gestation to six months following childbirth and to children from birth to age 5. The maternal and child health care programs, as well as those for nutrition and sexual and reproductive health, were included in the public insurance scheme as packages of established benefits. The benefits are provided at the various levels of the National Health System and the social security system. With the objective of achieving a satisfactory implementation of health sector policies, Ministerial Resolution #0018 dated 15 January 2003 provided that the Extensa Program—whose goal is to increase health coverage in remote rural communities through the use of mobile health teams financed by the World Bank—would coordinate all its activities, whether technical, logistical, or administrative, with pre-existing national health programs and projects under the Ministry of Health and Sports' aegis.

Over the past decade Bolivia has implemented important social policies geared toward the protection of older adults. These include the National Plan for Older Adults, the Bono Solidario, and Old Age Medical Insurance (1998).

Organization of the Health System

The health systems structure is characterized by segmentation, lack of coordination, and inequity. Given this situation, various players have intervened in the provision of health care to the population: the public and private sectors, NGOs, the Church, and traditional medicine practitioners.

The organization of health services is not population-based, nor have the health needs of the population been sufficiently evaluated. Despite recent progress in the decentralization of authority and decision-making to the municipal and departmental levels, vertical programs continue to be established at the central level without sufficiently taking into account important cultural considerations of the target population. This deficiency presents challenges for the identification of viable and effective solutions to the health problems of local populations and thus the provision of appropriate and high-quality care.

The lack of mechanisms to stimulate intersectoral coordination and the fact that the various other players active in the health care arena do not fall under the purview of public health regulations and policies have led to a situation in which the range of activities undertaken by these groups correspond more to institutional priorities and exigencies and do not necessarily contribute to broad, long-term national public health objectives. The fragmentation and lack of coordination in the health care system is one of Bolivia's most insurmountable obstacles to the achievement of universal health services coverage in the near future.

The health insurance system currently covers 26% of Bolivia's population (21% through the National Health Care Fund and 5% through other, smaller funds) (25). It is estimated that 5%–10% of the population utilizes the services of the private sector, and that some 70% of the population is covered by public health sector services. However, due to obstacles limiting access to the public health system, it is estimated that only about one-half of this segment—or some 35%–40% of the population—is able to utilize the services (26). At the same time, it is estimated that half of the population uses traditional medicine techniques, while in rural areas its practice is particularly widespread (1).

Public Health Services

The Ministry of Health and Sports' 2005–2009 National Plan for the Prevention and Control of Noncommunicable Diseases has identified a series of health issues requiring priority attention. These include diabetes mellitus, cardiovascular and rheumatic diseases, and cancer, as well as a group of related risk factors, such as smoking, alcohol abuse, sedentary lifestyles, unhealthy nutritional habits, and overweight. In 2003 and 2004, actions were taken to improve diagnostic strategies; the first national plan for responding to noncommunicable diseases at the primary level of care was developed; and Bolivia joined the CARMEN network, an initiative of the Pan American Health Organization composed of governmental and nongovernmental institutions, academics, and the private sector working together to develop joint activities for noncommunicable disease prevention in the Region of the Americas.

At the same time, improvements in the epidemiological surveillance and control of communicable diseases have been promoted. Prevention and treatment programs still remain largely vertical, and monitoring and evaluation processes either have not been carried out in the majority of the departments or they have been carried out only intermittently. The "epidemiological shield" surveillance strategy has been operationalized and will target malaria, Chagas' disease, tuberculosis, yellow fever, and leishmaniasis. Vector control activities promoted by family and community medicine teams support this effort.

The National Blood Program was officially established in 2002. While the annual rate of donors is very low (less than 20 per 1,000 population), the number of blood donations has increased in recent years. In 2003, 5,498 voluntary donations were received at the departmental-level blood banks, representing 29.4% of the total of 18,317 units obtained, and in 2004, 7,818 voluntary donations were received, representing 34.6% of the 22,581 units obtained. Up until 2004, the country continued to rely to some extent on paid blood donations. Donations are screened for HIV; in 2002, 33,204 serological tests were conducted in 24 blood therapy services in Bolivia, with 30 of these (0.09%) testing positive for HIV.

In 2003, the National System of Health Laboratories was established under the responsibility, control, and technical oversight of the National Health Laboratories Institute.

The quality of water from river sources is poor, largely untreated, and thus not safe for human consumption. Contamination is caused principally by industrial, mining, and agricultural activities utilizing pesticides and fertilizers, and improper domestic use of river water. Populations in the Amazon Basin area are also exposed to heavy metal poisoning, especially mercury, a byproduct of gold-panning activities in streams and riverbeds.

The large number and variety of disasters that occurred in Bolivia over the past five years spurred government officials at the national, departmental, and municipal levels to accord higher priority to disaster prevention and management policies, plans, and activities, resulting in the organization of emergency operation centers in some municipalities and prefectures. In 2003, beginning at the central level, the country began to upgrade its disaster preparedness and response capacity, extending these improvements to the regional level through the development of regulations and training activities. The Ministry of Health and Sports introduced an area specialized in disaster prevention and response, and in recent years, this entity has responded with technical support to several disaster events, working in coordination with the departmental-level SEDES health services. SEDES teams also received training in immediate response techniques, damage assessment and health needs analysis, risk management, the SUMA (Humanitarian Supplies Management) System, the Logistical Support System, and other related tools.

In 2004, the Vice Ministry of Civil Defense, with technical input and support from the health sector, began preparing a manual for the National Emergency Operations Center. The manual, to be used as a tool for the effective management of emergency situations, delineates the functions of disaster preparedness and response personnel and the coordination of efforts with various special committees supporting the Center's work. In 2005, work began on the design of a national health sector plan for emergencies and disasters; it is currently being reviewed by health authorities and key stakeholders.

Individual Care Services

The country's health services are organized into networks that include four levels of operation (national, departmental, municipal, and local or "health establishment") and three levels of care. Health services are concentrated in the urban areas (health posts, centers, and hospitals) and characterized by gaps in access to and quality of care, particularly for vulnerable groups, such as older adults, children who work or live on the street, and those living in extreme poverty. In the marginal urban areas, there are no hospitals or health centers and only a limited number of health posts and trained personnel. In large expanses of rural areas, the scarcity of physicians has led to the assumption by nursing auxiliaries of this responsibility in the provision of health interventions.

In 2004, there were 1.29 physicians and 14 beds per 1,000 population. In that same year, there were 3,021 health care establish-

ments; of these, 77.6% belonged to the public sector, 10.7% to the social security system, 5.5% to NGOs, 3.2% to the Church, and 3% to the private sector. Of this total number of health care establishments, 90% were at the primary care level, 6.6% were at the secondary level, and 3.2% were at the tertiary level (Table 2). The primary-level outpatient establishments in the public system normally include a general physician (or, in the social security system, a family doctor), a nurse, and nursing auxiliaries; this composition, however, may not be strictly adhered to in all establishments due to local circumstances. When health problems require specialized care, the users are required to go to the general hospitals, where outpatient care and hospitalization are provided in four basic specialties: internal medicine, surgery, gynecology and obstetrics, and pediatrics. The users are required to pay for any type of care not included as a benefit in the universal maternal and child health insurance system as an out-of-pocket expense.

Health Promotion

During the 2001–2005 period, there was significant progress in the development of the "healthy municipality" approach. In municipalities such as Chacaltaya and Curahuara de Carangas in the high Andes area, mayors have promoted and incorporated the concept in a variety of local initiatives. In the Chaco lowlands area of eastern Bolivia, the healthy schools and spaces approach has taken root, while in the municipal capital cities, the healthy environments strategy has been adopted.

The Vice Ministry of Sports, under the Ministry of Health and Sports, has launched various interventions to promote physical activity, including the introduction of various programs in the primary school curriculum targeting different age groups, the inclusion of questions regarding the population's physical activity levels in the 2003 National Demographic and Health Survey, and the training of participants in International Challenge Day, a competitive event celebrated in communities around the world to raise awareness regarding the importance of active lifestyles and regular physical exercise.

Promotion of healthy schools, marketplaces, and environments has relied heavily on the active involvement of communities and the support of local government leaders. While these experiences have produced encouraging results, there is a need for

TABLE 2. Health establishments, by institutional type and care level, Bolivia, 2004.

	Primary level	Secondary level	Tertiary level	Total
Public sector	2,210	116	19	2,345
Social security	218	36	70	324
NGO	156	5	4	165
Church	81	16	1	98
Private sector	56	25	8	89
Total	2,721	198	102	3,021

a formal evaluation of their different components in order to build the evidence base and share lessons learned with others in the future. This process will also provide valuable input for the development of healthy public policies and higher visibility on the public health and political agendas, the strengthening of partnerships, expansion of best practices, and improved training and development of human resources.

Human Resources

In 2002, there were 45,189 individuals working in the health field; of these, 35.2% were employed in the public sector, 34.9% in the private sector, 27.5% as part of the social security system, and 2.4% with NGOs devoted to health-related issues. In this group, 24.1% were doctors, 10.5% were nurses, and 22.2% were nursing auxiliaries.

In the public health sector, there were 14,538 workers, of whom 34.8% were professionals, 5.7% were health technicians, 30.6% were auxiliaries, 12% performed administrative tasks, and 16% provided various services. La Paz and Santa Cruz had the highest percentages of public health personnel, 24.6% and 21.2%, respectively, while Oruro and Pando had the lowest proportions, 5.2% and 2.9%, respectively.

In the social security sector, there were 13,138 employees, of whom 41.2% were either physicians or nurses, 3.6% were health technicians, 17.7% were auxiliaries, 22.2% performed administrative tasks, and 15.3% provided various services. Most of these personnel were located in La Paz (38.8%), Santa Cruz (19%), and Cochabamba (12.6%).

In general, most of the medical (43.7%) and nursing (49.9%) personnel were involved in the tertiary level of care, while 56.1% of the nursing auxiliaries performed at the primary level. The social security system had a ratio of 14 doctors, 1.7 dentists, 6 registered nurses, and 11 nursing auxiliaries per 10,000 population; in the public sector, the ratios per 10,000 population were 3.2 doctors, 0.4 dentists, 1.6 registered nurses, and 4.7 nursing auxiliaries (27).

One of the most serious challenges affecting the country's health sector policy is the effective integration of the various types and levels of health care personnel, given the current lack of rationalization and equitable distribution and use of human resources.

Health Supplies

A 2005 study of drug prices revealed that, on average, brand name products are 21 times more expensive than their generic equivalents, and in the case of relatively new drugs, were 65 times more expensive. In comparing the cost of treatment with brand name and generic drugs, a great difference was also noted. For example, treating a respiratory infection cost five times more with brand name drugs (US$ 7, equivalent to 3.8 days of national

minimum salary) than with generic drugs (US$ 1.25, equivalent to 0.72 days of national minimum salary).

In the majority of cases, generic drug prices were lower in the public sector than in the private for-profit sector, yet the limited availability of these drugs in the public sector often required that patients purchase them on the private market, albeit at a higher price.

Research and Technological Development in Health

National science and technology policy is governed by the Ministry of Government (*Ministerio de la Presidencia de la República*). In 2005, the Ministry of Health and Sports promoted the organization of a "Research Board" that called together all the country's public health experts working in the research arena. The board's principal objective was to provide input to the Ministry that would enable it to develop public health research policies and strengthen national regulatory capacity.

In January 2005, the Ministry of Health and Sports issued a resolution for the creation of a virtual public health library on topics of national relevance, and invited various academic institutions, NGOs, and other associations to participate in its development in accordance with the model established by the Latin American and Caribbean Center on Health Sciences Information (BIREME). The methodologies that were adopted facilitated the integration and supplementation of technology and content; a decentralized, yet controlled process for updating of the information modules; secure registration and contents validation processes; and comprehensive sources identification.

An analysis of the scientific and technical works registered in the Latin American and Caribbean Health Sciences Literature (known as LILACS, for its Spanish acronym) and the Pan American Network of Information and Documentation in Sanitary Engineering and Environmental Sciences (or REPIDISCA, for its Spanish acronym) databases showed that, in 2001 and 2002, Bolivia produced an average of 300 publications a year.

Health Sector Expenditures and Financing

Funds allocated for the public sector come from the following sources: the National General Treasury, internal cash generation, foreign credit, and donations; private sector source funds include businesses and institutions, as well as support provided by international cooperation agencies and bilateral support from other countries.

Notwithstanding the above-mentioned sources, much of the sector's funding came from out-of-pocket expenditures. While average estimated out-of-pocket spending was US$ 13 per month in 2002, some households declared annual expenditures on health care that exceeded US$ 5,000. The average out-of-pocket expenditures for individuals living in extreme poverty were US$ 9, US$ 12 for those living in moderate poverty, and US$ 19

Bringing Universal, Comprehensive Maternal and Child Health Care to Underserved Populations

Maternal mortality decreased from 390 per 100,000 live births in 2001 to 230 per 100,000 live births in 2005; infant mortality stood at 78 per 1,000 live births in 2001 and at 54 per 1,000 in 2005, while mortality among children under age 5 also declined during this same period from 77.6 to 65.3 per 1,000 live births. With the goal of sustainably reducing maternal and infant morbidity and mortality, legislation implementing the Universal Maternal and Child Health Insurance initiative was approved in January 2003, providing comprehensive health benefits free of charge for pregnant women from the start of gestation to six months after birth and for children from birth to 5 years of age, including surgical operations, diagnostic tests, and medications. Maternal and child health, nutrition, and sexual and reproductive health programs are included in the insurance initiative as established benefits and are provided obligatorily at all public health and social security system establishments at the primary, secondary, and tertiary care levels and in private for-profit and nonprofit establishments that have joined under special agreements. In 2004, 314 of Bolivia's municipalities were being served through 2,259 care facilities in both rural and urban areas, with the services offered being based on local treatment capacity and available technology.

for those who were not affected by poverty. Out-of-pocket expenditures represented 6% of total household expenditure for families in the middle quintiles of income distribution, while in the wealthiest quintile these expenditures represented only 5.2%.

The social security system recorded the health sector's largest expenditures (35%, equivalent to US$ 151.6 million), despite the fact that the system covers only 27% of the population and actual membership is less than 20%. The public health sector followed with 30%, equivalent to US$ 130 million, and is responsible for financing public insurance programs and national prevention programs. Household out-of-pocket expenditures totaled US$ 123.4 million, and the private sector (NGOs, the Church, and private insurance), with the lowest spending level, reported US$ 32.5 million.

At the global level, 34% of households reported no out-of-pocket health care expenditures, 53% reported spending less than 10%, and 13% reported health care costs of more than 10% of total household expenses. Of these, 63% were urban households and 37% were rural households, indicating a greater income generation capacity among the urban population and, consequently, its greater ability to cover costs.

Technical Cooperation and External Financing

From 2001 to 2003, credits and donations to the Ministry of Health and Sports budget represented 76% of the total budget and 24% came from the National General Treasury. During the 2001–2002 period, financial contributions from external cooperation totaled BO$ 97,097,934 (1 Bolivian boliviano = US$ 0.12), of which 71% represented concessional loans and 29% donations. In 2003, these increased to BO$ 101,857,165, of which 81% were loans and 19% were donations.

The financial resources from donations and the transfer of external credit were allocated mainly to the "nonpersonal services" budget line item, which entails payments for the use, maintenance, and repair of third-party real estate and assets, and includes professional and commercial services. Of the total funds allocated from 2001 to 2003, 53.2% went to nonpersonal services, 21.8% to real assets, 21.6% to materials and supplies, 3% to personal services, and 0.4% to taxes, fees, and royalties.

The total amount disbursed under the heading of cooperation (including donations and loans) between 1998 and 2002 was US$ 3 billion, of which US$ 1 billion corresponded to the social area (health, education, basic sanitation, and rural development). The health sector spent 6% of all funds disbursed by international cooperation (US$ 163 million) in the period under study, thereby becoming the sector with the least relative disbursement within the social area.

Since 1999, Bolivia has had a national policy of cooperation and international relations known as the New Relationship Framework. This policy was proposed during meetings of the Consultative Group on Bolivia sponsored by the World Bank and held in Paris with the goal of "organizing international support for the reduction of poverty levels" (28); under it, Bolivia was able to structure a state policy for governing its international cooperation relations and update it in 2005.

The policy's objective has been to significantly increase the effectiveness of cooperation activities which, combined with the local effort, will be able to more quickly decrease the poverty indexes and consolidate the levels of sustainable growth and development in the 21st century. The various international cooperation partners have developed initiatives and proposals to establish a framework for dialogue with their national counterparts:

- The United Nations Development Assistance Framework, UNDAF (*29*), and the Common Country Assessment, CCA, provide the planning framework for the U.N. system in Bolivia, through which the system's response is organized in order to achieve common development goals. It is also a resource planning tool and establishes methods for the monitoring and evaluation of this cooperation.
- The World Bank, in the context of the Country Development Framework, CDF, has framed a proposal to improve the efficiency of the international community's participation in development activities. The objective of this framework is a results-oriented approach to poverty relief (*30*) through the inclusion of macroeconomic and structural considerations within a comprehensive strategy.
- The Organization for Economic Cooperation and Development, OECD, has proposed, in the document *El Papel de la Cooperación Internacional para el Desarrollo en los Albores del Siglo XXI* (The Role of International Cooperation in Development at the Beginning of the 21st Century), a new strategy for the future based on well-defined roles to be played by the principal bilateral partners for development, taking into consideration comprehensive strategies that include economic, social, and policy elements.

References

1. Bolivia, Instituto Nacional de Estadística. Censo nacional de población y vivienda 2001. La Paz: INE; 2002.
2. Bolivia, Unidad de Análisis de Políticas Económicas y Sociales. Informe económico y social 2005 y Perspectivas. La Paz: UDAPE; 2006. Available at: http://www.udape.gov.bo. Accessed on 9 September 2006.
3. Bolivia, Ministerio de Hacienda. Estrategia de desarrollo nacional (draft). La Paz; 2004.
4. Economic Commission for Latin America and the Caribbean (ECLAC). Social panorama for Latin America 2006. ECLAC; 2006.
5. Bolivia, Unidad de Análisis de Políticas Económicas y Sociales. Revisión de la estrategia boliviana de reducción de la pobreza 2004–2007: oferta estratégica para el diálogo nacional 2003. La Paz: UDAPE; 2003.
6. Bolivia, Instituto Nacional de Estadística; Unidad de Análisis de Políticas Económicas y Sociales; Naciones Unidas. Progreso de los objetivos de desarrollo del milenio. Bolivia 2002. La Paz: INE; UDAPE; 2003.
7. Bolivia, Unidad de Análisis de Políticas Económicas y Sociales. Estrategia boliviana para la reducción de la pobreza 2004–2007: propuesta para la concertación. La Paz: UDAPE; 2003.
8. Bolivia, Ministerio de Educación y Cultura. Sistema de información 2003. La Paz; 2003.
9. Molina GG. Programa de mejoramiento de las encuestas y medición de condiciones de vida 2002. La Paz: UDAPE; 2004.
10. Organización de las Naciones Unidas para la Agricultura y la Alimentación. Políticas de seguridad alimentaria en los países de la Comunidad Andina. Santiago, Chile: FAO; 2005.
11. Bolivia, Instituto Nacional de Estadística. Encuesta nacional de demografía y salud 2003. La Paz: INE; 2004.
12. Bolivia, Ministerio de Salud y Deportes, Prefectura de La Paz. Sistema de salud con enfoque de género, guía para el desarrollo de modelo de intervención. La Paz: MSD; OPS/OMS; 2004.
13. Bolivia, Ministerio de Salud y Deportes, Unidad de Enfermedades No Transmisibles. Prevención y control de enfermedades no transmisibles en la atención primaria de salud: plan nacional 2005–2009. La Paz: OPS/OMS; 2004.
14. Bolivia, Ministerio de Desarrollo Sostenible, Viceministerio de la Niñez, Juventud y Tercera Edad. Programa de atención integral para la promoción del envejecimiento activo y de los derechos de las personas de la tercera edad. La Paz: OPS/OMS; 2005.
15. Calvo A. Equidad en salud, Bolivia. Desigualdad en la población monolingüe nativa, mediciones básicas. Salud Pública Boliviana. 2005; 45(58):25–40.
16. Bolivia, Ministerio de Salud y Deportes, Dirección de Planificación y Cooperación Externa, Sistema Nacional de Información y Vigilancia Epidemiológica. Análisis de situación de salud Bolivia 2004. La Paz; 2006.
17. Bolivia, Ministerio de Salud y Deportes, Viceministerio de Deportes; Instituto Boliviano del Deporte, la Educación Física y la Recreación. Lineamientos para la implementación de políticas de la actividad física. La Paz: OPS/OMS; 2005.
18. Bolivia, Ministerio de Salud y Deportes. Plan nacional de control de cáncer de cuello uterino 2004–2008. La Paz: OPS/OMS; 2004.
19. Bolivia, Ministerio de Salud y Deportes; Universidad Mayor de San Andrés, Facultad de Medicina. Estudio de prevalencia violencia doméstica e intrafamiliar en 6 municipios: Mizque, Viacha, Riberalta, La Paz, Santa Cruz y Cochabamba. La Paz: MSD; UMSA; OPS/OMS; 2003.
20. Bolivia, Ministerio de Salud y Deportes, Dirección General de Salud, Programa Nacional de Género y Salud. Prevención y atención de violencias: plan nacional 2004–2007. La Paz: OPS/OMS; 2004.
21. Bolivia, Instituto Nacional de Estadística. Estadísticas sobre delitos. La Paz: INE; 2004.
22. Bolivia, Ministerio de Salud y Deportes. Salud mental, modelo de abordaje para redes de servicios de salud. La Paz: OPS/OMS; 2005.

23. Bolivia, Ministerio de Salud y Deportes, Servicio Departamental de Salud. Atención primaria de los trastornos de salud mental, guía para servicios públicos de salud. La Paz: MSD/SEDES; 2005.

24. Bolivia, Ministerio de Salud y Deportes. Informe del Ejercicio de medición de las funciones esenciales de salud pública. La Paz: OPS/OMS; 2002.

25. Bolivia, Ministerio de Salud y Deportes; Instituto Nacional de Seguros de Salud. Anuario Estadístico 2002. La Paz: MSP/INASES; 2002.

26. Organización Panamericana de la Salud. Análisis de situación de salud 2003–2004. Washington, DC: OPS/OMS; 2004.

27. Bolivia, Ministerio de Salud y Previsión Social; Universidad Mayor de San Andrés; Instituto de Investigaciones en Salud y Desarrollo. Estudio de mercado de la fuerza laboral del sector salud. La Paz: MSPS; UMSA; IINSAD; OPS/OMS; 2002.

28. Bolivia, Organización Panamericana de la Salud. Alianzas estratégicas para implementar la estrategia de cooperación centrada en el país. Bolivia: versión preliminar. La Paz: OPS/OMS; 2003.

29. Naciones Unidas. La experiencia de la coordinación interagencial en Bolivia: evolución y perspectivas. La Paz: NNUU; 2003.

30. Bolivia, Viceministerio de Inversión Pública y Financiamiento Externo de Bolivia. Nuevo marco de relacionamiento Gobierno Cooperación Internacional. La Paz. Available at: http://www.vipfe.gov.bo/dgfe/nuevomarco/index.html. Accessed on 9 September 2006.

BRAZIL

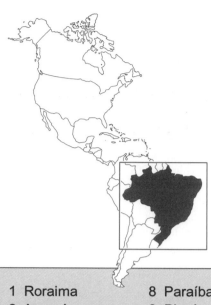

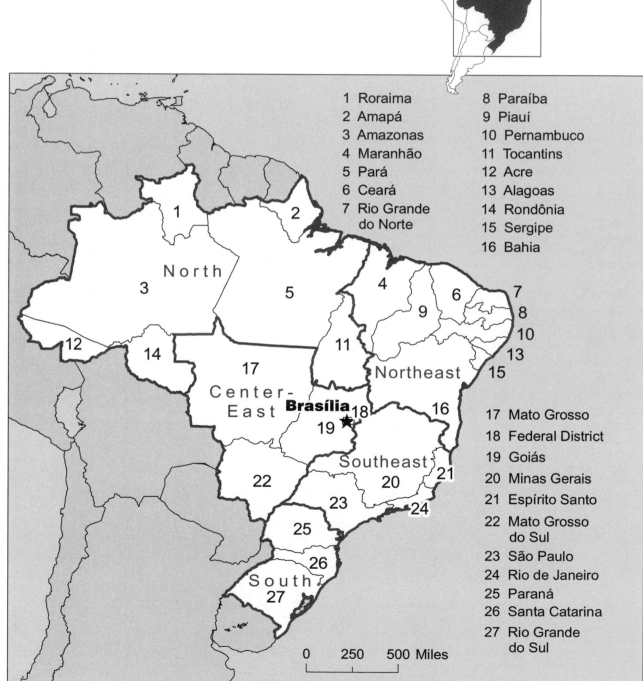

1 Roraima
2 Amapá
3 Amazonas
4 Maranhão
5 Pará
6 Ceará
7 Rio Grande
  do Norte

8 Paraíba
9 Piauí
10 Pernambuco
11 Tocantins
12 Acre
13 Alagoas
14 Rondônia
15 Sergipe
16 Bahia

17 Mato Grosso
18 Federal District
19 Goiás
20 Minas Gerais
21 Espírito Santo
22 Mato Grosso
  do Sul
23 São Paulo
24 Rio de Janeiro
25 Paraná
26 Santa Catarina
27 Rio Grande
  do Sul

North

Brasília

Center-East

Northeast

Southeast

South

0   250   500 Miles

The Federative Republic of Brazil shares borders with all the countries of South America, except Ecuador and Chile. It has a constitutional system of government, with a president as head of state.

GENERAL CONTEXT AND HEALTH DETERMINANTS

The country's political-administrative organization comprises 26 states, 5,561 municipalities, and the Federal District, seat of the federal government. Constitutionally, the Government of Brazil consists of three independent branches: legislative, executive, and judicial. The Federal Constitution of 1988 consolidated the return of democratic government after two decades of military regimes. The country is divided politically and geographically into five regions (North, Northeast, Southeast, South, and Center-West), which share some common physical, human, economic, and cultural features (1).

Social, Political, and Economic Determinants

According to the *Human Development Report 2005* (2), Brazil ranks 63rd in the classification of countries based on the human development index (HDI). Its HDI was 0.71 in 1990, 0.74 in 1995, 0.76 in 2000, and 0.79 in 2003. In 2000, the highest HDI levels were registered in the Federal District (0.84), Santa Catarina (0.82), and São Paulo (0.82), and the lowest were in Maranhão (0.64), Alagoas (0.65), and Piauí (0.66) (3). In 2000, HDI-M (HDI at the municipal level) among the white population was 0.81, while among the black population it was 0.70. If the white population made up a separate nation, that country would rank fourth in the world and would be considered highly developed (HDI of 0.80 or over). The black population, with its medium level of human development (HDI of 0.50–0.79), would rank 10th. Clearly, there is a sizeable gap between whites and blacks. Between 1980 and 1991, the HDI-M of the black population rose relatively more than that of the white population, and the same trend was observed between 1991 and 2000. Over those two decades, the HDI climbed from 0.64 to 0.77 (an increase of 18.8%). The index among the black population rose 24.9% (from 0.56 to 0.70), whereas that of the white population increased 16.5% (from 0.70 to 0.81). Despite this greater growth in the HDI among the black population, however, the difference between the two groups remained significant: in 1980, the HDI-M of the white population was 24.4% higher than that of the black population, and in 2000, it was 16% higher. The difference in human development between these two populations is manifested mainly in income (one of the variables which, together with health and education, are used to compute the HDI). However, as incomes changed little over the two decades—and in fact, they declined between 1980 and 1991—it was the other two factors that contributed the most to the rise in the HDI-M in both groups: education in the case of blacks and longevity in the case of whites. The educational component accounted for 55.5% of the improvement in the HDI-M among the black population between 1980 and 2000, reflecting a decline in illiteracy and an increase in school enrollment; longer life expectancy accounted for 36.3%, and higher income for 8.2%. In the case of the white population, higher life expectancy was the most important factor (51.1%), although education also played an important role (40.6%); higher income accounted for 8.4% of the improvement.

Per capita gross domestic product (GDP) in Brazil was R$ 6,485.64 (6,485.64 Brazilian *reais*) in 2000 and rose to R$ 8,694.47 in 2003. According to data from the Institute of Applied Economic Research (IPEA), the percentage of poor population (monthly income under half the minimum wage) was 33.3% in 2001 and 32.0% in 2004, with major inequalities between the country's various regions and ethnic groups. While per capita GDP in the Northeast region in 2003 was R$ 4,305.86, in the Southeast it was R$ 11,257.54. Similarly, the Northeast and North regions had the largest proportions of poor population in 2004 (55.47% and 43.30%, respectively), while the South and Southeast had the smallest proportions of poor population (17.84% and 20.43%, respectively).

Brazil is committed to achieving the goal of eradicating extreme poverty and hunger. One of the parameters used to measure extreme poverty in the country is the percentage of the population living on less than US$ 1 a day, measured on a purchasing power parity basis (US$ 1 PPP/day) (4). Between 1990 and 2003, extreme poverty decreased by almost half, dropping from 9.9% to 5.7% of the population, a 42.4% reduction. This fall in the rate of extreme poverty is attributed mainly to improvement of the situation in rural areas, where extreme poverty decreased from 24.2% to 13.5% between 1990 and 2003. In contrast, during the same period, the rate in urban areas changed hardly at all, standing at 4.8% in 1990 and 4.2% in 2003. One of the population groups most affected by extreme poverty is that of young people, who encounter difficulties entering the labor market, and when they do find jobs, they generally earn very low wages. In 2003, the unemployment rate among the population aged 16–24 was 19%—almost double the rate for the population as a whole

(10%). The situation is even more serious among young women, for whom the unemployment rate was 24.4%, versus 15% among their male peers.

Opinions regarding inequality in the distribution of income are somewhat divided: according to data from a recent report on Brazil's progress towards the Millennium Development Goals (MDGs) as of 2005 (4), inequality has remained unchanged in the last four years. In 1992, the poorest 20% of the population received scarcely 3% of total income, and in 2003 the figure had gone up by only one percentage point overall, although the size of the change varied with income level. In the poorest parts of the Northeast, the share of the poor rose from 1.5% to 4.4%, while in the Southeast the increase was only from 4.2% in 1992 to 4.5% in 2003. Despite this relative improvement in the situation of the poorest Brazilians, there was virtually no change in the income gap between the poorest and richest segments of the population. In 2003, as in 1992, although there were some regional variations, the richest quintile continued to account for more than half of total income. In the Northeast, for example, the gap between rich and poor decreased, but only because the share of the wealthiest 20% in that region fell from 60.7% in 1992 to 54.6% in 2003. In the Southeast region, on the other hand, the income of the richest quintile increased from 51.8% to 54.1% during the same period. According to the same report, blacks and mulattos are most affected by income inequality. Those two groups make up 68% of the poorest decile, whereas the richest decile is 87% white. Moreover, 32.2% of the poorest members of the population are black. In contrast, another report states that income inequality decreased significantly between 2001 and 2004 (5) and that the proportions of the population living in poverty and extreme poverty must therefore also have diminished substantially. Data from this report indicate that income inequality at the national level fell 4%, with a concurrent decrease in the Gini coefficient from 0.593 to 0.569. This improvement has been attributed to the development of a more effective social protection network, growth in local labor markets, and a reduction in both inequalities associated with education and differences in income by educational level. This study did not address regional differences, which are very marked. It is generally agreed, nevertheless, that there continue to be enormous disparities in income at the national level and that it will take another 20 years or so for income inequality in Brazil to approach the averages found in countries with similar development levels.

One of the most noteworthy changes currently taking place in Brazilian society is the worsening of poverty and social exclusion in metropolitan areas. The rapid exacerbation of social inequalities in the major cities has given rise to the expression "urbanization of poverty" to describe this phenomenon, which has been occurring since the middle of the last decade. The following data highlight the scale of the problem: (1) between 1993 and 2002, unemployment increased in Brazil's large cities in general and in those of the Southeast in particular, where the unemployment rate rose from 9.3% to 13.2%, whereas during the same period the national rate increased from 6.3% to close to 10.0%; (2) employment in the formal sector fell from 55.5% in 1993 to 49.7% in 2002 in metropolitan areas, but increased from 37.5% to 38.4% for the country as a whole; (3) employment opportunities in unskilled jobs (jobs for workers with four to seven years of schooling) also decreased in metropolitan regions; and (4) in 2002, the rate of unemployment among women worsened in metropolitan areas (16.1%) and in the Southeast region, in comparison with the national average (11.7%), as did unemployment among heads of household (6). The growth of urban poverty is not being met with institutional responses that enhance the effectiveness of government policies, and the various levels of government rarely take into account this new geography of social exclusion and the need to address it when making the decisions and coordinating the activities that come under their responsibility (7).

The illiteracy rate among the population over 15 years of age was 11.4% for the country as a whole in 2004, with virtually the same rates among men (11.6%) and women (11.4%). There is considerable difference between the rates in urban areas (8.7%) and rural areas (25.8%), with regional variations ranging from 22.4% in the Northeast (with a high of 29.5% in the state of Alagoas) to 6.3% in the South. In the North, Northeast, and Southeast regions, illiteracy rates were higher among males than among females; in the Southeast and South regions, females had higher rates. The illiteracy rate also varied according to ethnic origin: 7.2% among whites, 16.5% among blacks, and 16.2% among mulattos. The functional illiteracy rate (inability to read, write, and interpret a short, simple text) was 24.4% for the country as a whole, with higher figures among men (25.0%) than among women (23.9%). Functional illiteracy among the rural population was twice as high as among the population living in urban areas (47.5% versus 20.1%). Among the regions, the rate ranged from 37.6% in the Northeast (59.4% for the population residing in rural areas) to 18.1% in the Southeast. Blacks and mulattos showed higher rates of functional illiteracy (32.0% and 31.2%, respectively) than whites (18.1%) (8).

Brazil is close to achieving universal primary education. The challenge now is more one of educational quality than of universality. A significant proportion (19%) of children who finish fourth grade do not perform adequately in reading and mathematics. High rates of enrollment also obscure the fact that more than 700,000 school-age girls still do not attend school because they live in remote rural areas, they are victims of sexual exploitation or child labor, or they suffer from some deficiency. Grade repetition and dropout are common: in 2003, some 2.8 million children left school before the end of the year. Many teachers are not adequately qualified, and their wages are generally extremely low in relation to the importance of the work that they perform (9).

The National Household Sample Survey (PNAD 2004) provided, for the first time, a direct indicator of food security among the Brazilian population, as measured by the Brazilian Food Insecurity Scale (EBIA) (10). Food security is understood to mean that residents of a household have not suffered food shortages, in terms of either quantity or quality, in the three months preceding the interview, and they are confident that they will not face this problem in the near future. At the other end of the scale, severe food insecurity is considered to exist when the residents of a household have gone hungry on at least two days during the three months preceding the interview. Food security was found to exist in 65.2% of the households surveyed, while 34.8% (approximately 72 million people) suffered from food insecurity. The survey's most noteworthy findings were: (1) food security was less frequent among households with at least one member under the age of 18, in comparison with households with no under-18 members; (2) food security rates were lower among household members under the age of 18 and increased with age, with the highest levels being among older adults (aged 65 and over); (3) food insecurity was consistently more common in households headed by women (in both urban and rural areas), and among such households, those that had seven or more members and whose members included children under 18 years of age were more likely to suffer from moderate to severe food insecurity; (4) among households with severe food insecurity, the largest proportion were black or mulatto households; and (5) severe food insecurity was substantially more frequent among households with a per capita income equal to one minimum wage or less.

In summary, Brazil is not a poor country, but it is an extremely inequitable and unequal one, in which a great many people continue to face enormous difficulties in exercising their citizenship. It is a fundamentally urban country, in which the urban poverty rate did not decline to the same extent as the rural poverty rate during the period 1990–2003, and in which labor force growth has outpaced job creation.

Urban violence and environmental degradation both worsened during the 1990s, and those trends continue today. Violence grew in the country's cities and became one of the most important factors in the loss of quality of life among urban populations. It permeates all facets of urban life, with devastating results, and breeds relationships among citizens that are characterized by feelings of insecurity, helplessness, aggressiveness, and self-defense, limiting the exercise of their citizenship and transforming public spaces into unhealthy environments (11).

Since 2003, the National Public Safety Secretariat (SENASP), the agency responsible for the planning, implementation, and monitoring of the national public safety policy, has been working to implement the Unified Public Safety System (SUSP). SENASP views information as the main tool for the work of public safety agencies, and is seeking to build for the first time in the country an information system to support those responsible for planning public safety policies at the national and local levels (12).

Demographics, Mortality, and Morbidity

According to data from the Brazilian Institute of Geography and Statistics, in 2004 the Brazilian population numbered 186 million, and the average population density was 21.9 inhabitants per km^2, with values ranging from a high of 86.1 in the Southeast region to a low of 3.9 in the North. In 2004, 83.0% of the total population lived in urban areas. The sex ratio was 95 males per 100 females, with a higher proportion of men in the North region (101.4). The lowest male-female ratios were found in the metropolitan regions of Recife, Rio de Janeiro, and the Federal District (87.4, 87.9, and 87.6, respectively). The annual geometric population growth rate decreased from 1.9% during the 1980s to 1.6% during the period 1991–2000, with the lowest rates in the Northeast region (1.31%). The crude birth rate in 2004 was 20.6 per 1,000 population. Whites made up 51.4% of the population, mulattos 42.1%, and blacks 5.9%. While blacks constitute the largest proportion of the population in the North, Northeast, and Center-West regions (75.6%, 70.2%, and 56.1%, respectively), whites make up the majority in the South and Southeast (82.8% and 61.2%, respectively).

The total fertility rate has shown a downward trend, dropping from 2.9 children per woman in 1991 to 2.1 in 2004. This decrease has occurred in all regions, both among white women (2.4 in 1991 and 1.8 in 2004) and among blacks (3.5 in 1991 and 2.4 in 2004). The highest total fertility rates are found among white and black women in the North region (2.4 and 3.0 children per woman, respectively). Among women with eight or more years of schooling, the total fertility rate was 1.5 children, while among those with three or more years of schooling it was 3.9. Life expectancy at birth has risen from 67.0 years (1991) to 71.7 years (2004). For men, life expectancy increased from 63.2 years (1991) to 67.9 years (2004), and for women, from 70.9 years (1991) to 75.5 years (2004). Life expectancy at birth varies by sex and subpopulation. For white men, for example, it increased from 58.7 in 1980 to 64.4 in 1991 and to 68.2 in 2000, while for black men, life expectancy rose from 54.1 (1980) to 58.2 (1991) to 63.3 years (2000). Among white women, the corresponding figures were 63.4 years, 71.8 years, and 73.8 years (2000), and among black women, 60.6 years, 65.6 years, and 69.5 years, respectively (13).

The proportion of children under 5 decreased from 13.8% in 1980 to 9.7% in 2004, as Figure 1 shows. During the same period, the proportion of Brazilians aged 60 and over climbed from 5.8% to 7.8% (men) and from 6.4% to 9.2% (women). In 2004, the economically dependent population (under 15 and over 65 years of age) amounted to 35.4% of the total population.

FIGURE 1. Population structure, by age and sex, Brazil, 1980 and 2004.

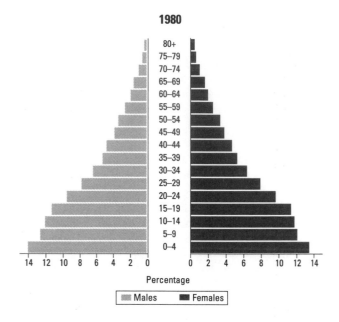

1980

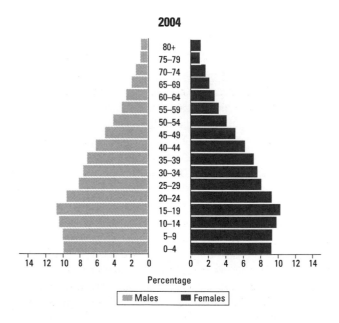

2004

to the largest proportion of residents born in other regions of Brazil (31.4% in 1991 and 31.1% in 2004).

Mortality in Brazil has changed markedly over the years, with a decline in some infectious diseases and a resurgence of others, and with changes in the frequency of some non-infectious diseases and conditions, such as heart disease, diabetes, cancer, and death due to violence. The Mortality Information System (SIM) of the Ministry of Health recorded 1,024,073 deaths nationwide in 2004, of which 126,922 (12.4%) were due to ill-defined causes (Table 1).

Among the deaths from defined causes, cerebrovascular diseases were the leading cause, accounting for 10.1% of deaths, and ischemic heart diseases were the second leading cause (9.7%). These findings reflect the growing concentration of deaths in older age groups, coupled with the improvement of living conditions and the impact of public policies (for example, policies relating to basic sanitation, access to health services, and immunization) on the health of children and the consequent reduction in childhood deaths. Homicide ranks third as a cause of death in the general population and is the foremost threat to the lives of persons aged 10–59. Homicide is the third most frequent cause of death for males, but does not even figure among the first 10 causes for females. Males between the ages of 10 and 19 are six times more likely to be homicide victims than females of the same age. For men aged 20–59, the risk is seven times greater than among women in the same age bracket. Land transport accidents were the fourth cause of male death, but, again, do not figure among the 10 leading causes of female death. Diabetes mellitus was the third most frequent cause of death among women and the ninth among men.

The only communicable diseases among the first 20 causes of death were pneumonia and influenza, which ranked sixth. This may reflect problems with reporting of deaths, since pneumonia may be listed as the immediate cause of death, but there may be other, underlying causes that are not reported.

A comparison of mortality data for 1996 and 2004 reveals an increase in the risk of death from homicide (8.8%), diabetes mellitus (30.5%), and hypertensive diseases (38.0%). The risk of death from perinatal problems has declined 27.3% overall, although during the aforementioned period the risk of death from birth trauma increased 6.5%. The risk of death from land transport accidents fell 13.0%, possibly as a result of the adoption of more rigorous traffic laws in 1997.

During the period 1996–2004, deaths of children under 1 fell by 34%. By cause, the largest reductions were seen in deaths from meningitis (86.3%), human immunodeficiency virus (HIV) infection (69.8%), and intestinal infectious diseases (65.1%). Although mortality in the group aged 10–19 declined 11.0%, the risk of death from homicide increased 26.3%; in the group aged 20–59, the risk increased 6.1%. In the latter age group, the risk of death from alcoholic liver disease and from diabetes mellitus also rose (39.9% and 11.2%, respectively).

The Northeast region continues to experience significant emigration of its population to other regions in the country. In 1991, the proportion of emigrants in relation to natives of the region was 15.1%, and in 2004 the proportion increased to 17.7%. Most of these emigrants move to the Southeast (10.4% of Brazilians born in the Northeast were residing in the Southeast in 1991, and by 2004, it had risen to 12.1%). The Center-West region is home

TABLE 1. Leading causes of death (rate, percentage change, and proportion of total mortality), Brazil, 1996 and 2004.

Cause category	Rate			Proportion of total mortality	
	1996	2004	% change	1996	2004
Total deaths	580.2	571.8	−1.4		
Ill-defined causes	87.5	70.9	−19.0	15.1	12.4
Defined causes	492.7	500.9	1.7		
Cerebrovascular diseases (I60–I69)	51.7	50.8	−1.9	10.5	10.1
Ischemic heart diseases (I20–I25)	47.0	48.5	3.0	9.5	9.7
Acute (I20–I24)	38.5	40.0	3.8	7.8	8.0
Chronic (I25)	8.5	8.5	−0.6	1.7	1.7
Assault (homicide) (X85–Y09)	24.8	27.0	8.8	5.0	5.4
Certain conditions originating in the perinatal period (P00–P96)	23.8	17.3	−27.3	4.8	3.5
Birth trauma and other obstetric causes (P01–P03, P10–P15)	1.4	1.5	6.5	0.3	0.3
Immaturity and related disorders (P05–P07)	2.2	1.8	−19.4	0.4	0.4
Respiratory disorders specific to the perinatal period (P20–P28)	13.9	7.7	−44.6	2.8	1.5
Bacterial sepsis of newborn (P36)	2.6	2.5	−3.4	0.5	0.5
Hemorrhagic and hematological disorders (P50–P61)	0.6	0.5	−29.8	0.1	0.1
Heart failure (I50–I51)	23.5	17.9	−24.0	4.8	3.6
Land transport accidents (V00–V89)	22.5	19.6	−13.0	4.6	3.9
Influenza and pneumonia (J10–J18)	21.7	21.0	−3.2	4.4	4.2
Chronic lower respiratory diseases (J40–47)	20.0	21.5	7.3	4.1	4.3
Diabetes mellitus (E10–E14)	16.8	21.9	30.5	3.4	4.4
Hypertensive diseases (I10–I15)	12.5	17.2	38.0	2.5	3.4

HEALTH OF POPULATION GROUPS

Children under 5 Years Old

This group made up 9% of the population in 2004 and accounted for 6.1% of total mortality. Data from SIM indicate that most of these deaths occurred in the under-1 age group (87%). The Live Births Information System (SINASC) of the Ministry of Health, with an estimated coverage of 90%, recorded 3,026,548 births in 2004. Data for the period 2000–2004 indicate that around 8.0% of liveborn infants had low birthweight. The Southeast region had the highest proportion of low-birthweight babies during the period (9.0%), while the North and Northeast regions had the lowest proportions (6.6% and 7.1%, respectively). Those figures were higher than would be expected under optimum intrauterine growth conditions, although they are lower than the maximum of 10% established as a goal at the global level (14).

Three national studies on breast-feeding, carried out in 1975, 1989 (15), and 1999 (16), found a steady increase in the proportion of children who were still being breast-fed at 6 months of age (69% in 1999). At 12 months of age, however, the situation remained unchanged from 1989 (37%) to 1999 (35%), except in the Center-West region, where the proportion of babies still being breast-fed increased from 17% to 38%. As for exclusive breast-feeding, half of the children studied in 1999 were no longer being exclusively breast-fed at 30 days of age, and deficiencies exacerbated by that cause were observed in those children at 4 months

of age (18%) and at 6 months (8%), with no significant variations among the major regions. Brazil has a National Network of Breast-milk Banks, which in February 2006 included 187 units and 29 storage and distribution facilities; the network is operational in all states of the country (17, 18).

An analysis of the profile of liveborn infants by race or color showed differences in the following characteristics: (1) indigenous and black babies were more likely than white babies to have adolescent mothers; (2) white babies were more likely than indigenous or black babies to have mothers who had received seven or more prenatal checkups, while indigenous and black babies were more likely to have mothers who had not received any prenatal care; (3) white babies were more likely to have been born by cesarean section than black babies; (4) indigenous babies were more likely have been born premature; and (5) black babies were more likely to have been born with low birthweight, but both black and white babies in the Southeast, South, and Center-West regions were more likely to have been born with low birthweight than those in the North and Northeast regions (19).

The infant mortality rate decreased from 33.7 per 1,000 live births in 1996 to 22.5 per 1,000 in 2004. The causes of infant mortality have changed in recent decades, with a decline in deaths from infectious and parasitic diseases. In 1996, intestinal infectious diseases accounted for 8.0% of deaths of children under 1, but by 2004 the proportion had dropped to 4.0%. During the same period, the proportion of infant deaths due to perinatal causes increased from 57.0% to 61.2%. The geographic inequalities are evident from the figures for 2004, when the risk that a child would die before reaching the age of 1 year was 2.23 times greater in the Northeast than in the South (*20*). The states with the highest and lowest rates, respectively, were Alagoas (47.1 per 1,000 live births) and Santa Catarina (13.6).

More infant deaths have tended to occur in the neonatal period as the proportion of avoidable deaths has decreased, thanks to basic health and sanitation interventions. In 2004, 66.5% of infant deaths occurred in the first month of life and 50.9% in the first week; in 1996, these figures were 60% and 47%, respectively. In 2004, the Northeast region had the largest proportion of infant deaths in the post-neonatal period (35.3%).

Among children 1–4 years old, the leading causes of death in 2004 were influenza and pneumonia (13.5%), congenital malformations (8.6%), intestinal infectious diseases (6.5%), land transport accidents (6.3%), and drowning (6.0%). Between 1996 and 2004, the risk of dying from influenza and pneumonia decreased 43.5%; from intestinal infectious diseases, 41.3%; from land transport accidents, 34.6%; and from meningitis, 88.5%. The Northeast region accounted for 56% of deaths from intestinal infectious diseases.

The implementation of several programs and activities since 1996 has helped to bring about a marked decline in infant mortality, among them the Comprehensive Women's Health Program (PAISM), the Comprehensive Child Health Program (PAISC), the strategy of Integrated Management of Childhood Illness (IMCI), the National Immunization Program (PNI), incentives to encourage breast-feeding, and monitoring of child growth and development. In addition, the Family Health Program has experienced substantial growth since 1999, achieving a coverage level of 47.7% of the Brazilian population—83 million people—in August 2006. The program boasts 26,000 teams comprising a doctor, a nurse, and a community health agent. Basic sanitation and poverty reduction programs have also played an important role, as have certain demographic factors, such as the decline in the fertility rate (*21*).

Children 5–9 Years Old

Primary-school-age children made up close to 9.0% of the population and accounted for less than 0.5% of total deaths in 2004. The main causes of death in this group were land transport accidents (18.1%), drowning (9.2%), leukemia (5.9%), influenza and pneumonia (5.5%), and congenital malformations (4.9%). During the period 1996–2004, the risk of dying from influenza and pneumonia fell 26.0%; from land transport accidents, 38.5%; from meningitis, 88.6%; from drowning, 17.8%; and from leukemia, 6.8%.

In 2005, 457,338 children from this age group were admitted to public hospitals (4.0% of total hospital admissions). The leading causes of hospitalization were diseases of the respiratory system (29.2%), especially pneumonia (12.1%) and asthma (8.7%), and communicable diseases (17.9%), especially diarrhea and other intestinal infectious diseases (10.7%).

Adolescents 10–14 and 15–19 Years Old

Adolescents represented about 20.3% of the country's population and accounted for 2.4% of total mortality in 2004, with most of the deaths in this group being male deaths caused by accidents and violence. The death rate among adolescent boys (99.0 per 100,000 population) was far higher than the rate among girls of the same age (34.9 per 100,000 population). The leading causes of death among males in this group were assault (34.2%), land transport accidents (16.9%), drowning (6.3%), events of undetermined intent (4.0%), and intentional self-harm (3.2%). During the period 1996–2004, deaths from assault increased 26.3%, but the risk of dying from the other causes decreased—for example, the risk of death from land transport accidents fell 22.3%; from drowning, 28.2%; from suicide, 8.5%; and from leukemia, 8.0%. The mortality profile of this group differs between males and females. Among males, the first five causes of death are external, while among females the first two causes of death are external, but causes related to pregnancy and childbirth rank third (4.6% of deaths).

Injuries due to accidents and violence accounted for 9.4% of the total of 1,314,408 hospital admissions recorded in this age group in 2005. The leading external causes of hospitalization were falls (41.8%) and transport accidents (15.8%).

In 2004, a total of 661,290 births to adolescent mothers aged 10–19 were reported (21.8% of all births), a slightly lower proportion than in 1998 (24.0%). An estimated 26,726 live births (0.9% of the total) in 2004 were to mothers aged 10–14. The prevalence of low birthweight in this group (13.5%) was higher than the average in the general population (8%).

Adults 20–59 Years Old

Adults constituted 52.7% of the total population and accounted for 32.1% of all deaths registered in 2004 (37.9% of male deaths and 24.2% of female deaths). The mortality rate in the adult male population (501.5 per 100,000 population) was a little over twice the rate in the female population (219.8 per 100,000 population). The leading causes of death were assault (12.7%), land transport accidents (8.4%), ischemic heart diseases (7.7%), cerebrovascular diseases (7.1%), and cirrhosis and other diseases of the liver (4.8%). Between 1996 and 2004, the risk of dying from assault increased 6.1%. At the same time, mortality from other causes decreased, as did the risk of dying from land transport accidents (10.7%), cerebrovascular diseases (16.2%), ischemic heart diseases (3.3%), and HIV disease (38.1%). The risk of dying from external causes for a man 20–59 years of age (rate of 77.0 per 100,000 population) was 10 times higher than the risk for a woman in the same group (5.9 per 100,000 population). The risk of dying from land transport accidents was six times higher for men than for women (rates of 47.1 and 7.8 per 100.000, respectively). Breast cancer (5.5%) and diabetes mellitus (4.6%) figure among the five main causes of death for women.

Maternal mortality in 2004, calculated for nine states that had consistent data, ranged from 44 deaths per 100,000 live births in the Federal District to 84 deaths per 100,000 live births in Mato Grosso do Sul. Although maternal deaths statistics are known to be deficient, it is estimated that the average rate for the country is probably around 76 deaths per 100,000 live births, based on an adjustment factor (1.4) obtained from a 2002 study of mortality among women aged 10–49. In 2004, 61.4% of maternal deaths were due to direct obstetric causes, notably eclampsia and antepartum hemorrhage. Important indirect causes—i.e., preexisting conditions complicating pregnancy—include infectious diseases, diabetes, anemia, and cardiovascular disorders.

In 2005, about 6 million hospitalizations of adults were recorded in public institutions, predominantly of women (67.3% of the total). Most were due to conditions related to pregnancy, childbirth, and the puerperium, which together accounted for 33.1% of all adult hospital admissions and for 49.1% of admissions among women. Excluding that group of causes, the main reasons for hospitalization were diseases of the digestive system (13.8%), circulatory system (12.9%), and genitourinary system (12.0%). External causes accounted for the largest proportion of hospital admissions among men (17.6%), followed by diseases of the digestive system (14.6%). Among women, excluding hospitalizations for pregnancy, childbirth, and the puerperium, diseases of the genitourinary system were the leading cause (18.2%).

In 2004, data on 3 million births showed that 52% of the mothers had seven or more prenatal visits, with the percentages ranging from 22% in Amapá to 69% in Paraná. The proportion of cesarean births was 41.8%. In 2000, support mechanisms were introduced with a view to establishing state systems for hospital referral of women with high-risk pregnancies, and special resources were allocated to humanize care during childbirth and newborn care, as well as to improve access, coverage, and quality of care. Data from the Ministry of Health on the first evaluation of the impact of the activities aimed at humanizing care during childbirth in the 29 principal maternity hospitals showed a reduction of 6.9% of neonatal deaths between 2004 and 2005.

Older Adults 60 Years Old and Older

In 2004, older adults made up 9.0% of the total population and accounted for 58.4% of total mortality. The proportion of adults over 60 years of age in the general population has increased steadily in all regions of the country, with women outnumbering men in this age group. In 1991, 7.8% of all Brazilian women and 6.8% of all Brazilian men fell into this age group; in 2004, the corresponding proportions were 9.2% and 6.8% (22, 23). The aging

of the Brazilian population is the result of the combination of high fertility rates in the past and lower mortality in younger age groups in recent decades. The proportion of people of advanced age within this group has also grown: persons older than 80 made up 0.8% of the population in 1991 and 1.1% in 2004.

The number of deaths among persons over the age of 60 has risen steadily, from 38% of all deaths during the three-year period 1979–1981 to 54% in 1998 and 58.4% in 2004. In the latter year, the proportions ranged from 45.8% in the North region to 63% in the South. The main causes of death were cerebrovascular diseases (13.6%), ischemic heart diseases (12.5%), chronic lower respiratory diseases (6.5%), diabetes mellitus (5.9%), influenza and pneumonia (5.2%), and heart failure (5.0%). During the period 1996–2004, the risk of dying from chronic respiratory diseases increased 3.0%; from diabetes, 28.5%; and from influenza and pneumonia, 14.0%. The risk of dying from cerebrovascular diseases and from ischemic heart diseases, on the other hand, fell 3.0% and 2.2%, respectively. The mortality profiles of males and females in this age group are very similar. Although a high percentage of deaths continue to be attributed to ill-defined causes (14.4%)—a proportion which is higher than the average in Brazil and is growing in the oldest subgroups—this figure represents an improvement in the quality of information on causes of death in comparison to the figure recorded in 1998 (18.0%).

The older adult population accounted for 9.5% of admissions to public hospitals in 2005, the main causes of hospitalization being diseases of the circulatory system (28.9%), respiratory system (17.7%), and digestive system (10.2%). The activities aimed at this segment of the population are governed by the National Policy on the Health of Older Adults, adopted in 1999 (24), which establishes guidelines, general strategies, and program priorities for promoting healthy aging, maintaining and improving the functional capacity of the elderly, preventing specific diseases, treating the sick, and rehabilitating persons with limited functional capacity. One of the major preventive interventions for this group is vaccination against influenza and pneumococcal pneumonia. Influenza immunization for those aged 65 and over was introduced in 1999, and the target population was subsequently expanded to include those aged 60 and over. Vaccination coverage rates reached the goal of 72% in 2000 and 84% in 2005. In 2006, 13.5 million people in this age group were vaccinated—a coverage rate of 85.7%.

Workers

Responsibility for workers' health in Brazil is shared by the health, labor, social welfare, and environmental sectors, each of which has specific functions and spheres of action. In the health sector, various recent federal regulations guide technical and operational activities aimed at improving the coverage and quality of services for workers. Information on occupational diseases and accidents comes primarily from the system of coverage for injuries, disability, or death established under the country's social insurance scheme, which covers only the population working in the formal sector. In 2004, there were 31.4 million workers in the formal sector (17% of the population). The Southeast region had the heaviest concentration of formally employed workers (51.8%), while the Northeast and South regions claimed 17.0% and 17.9%, respectively. During the period 2002–2004, employment in the formal sector increased 9.5%, with the entry of 2.7 million workers into the formal labor market.

An analysis of information on sick leave benefits during 2004 reveals that the most frequent causes of absenteeism among workers were diseases of the musculoskeletal system and connective tissue—which accounted for 30% of all sick leave benefits—external causes (18.0%), diseases of the circulatory system (11.0%), and mental and behavioral disorders (10.8%) (25). Among Brazilian industrial workers a high prevalence of several risk factors for cardiovascular disease was found: arterial hypertension (25.2%), current tobacco use (15.9%), diabetes mellitus (3.2%), elevated total cholesterol (7.9%), obesity (13.4%), and sedentarism (17.2%) (26).

Ethnic Groups

Since 1999, the Ministry of Health has exercised direct responsibility for indigenous health through 34 special indigenous health districts linked to the National Health Foundation (FUNASA). Each district has a health team that provides basic care, with linkages to the formal health care system, under the supervision of local and district indigenous health councils. Villages and communities all over the country are served by indigenous health agents trained in basic health care. These services are linked to formal health care services at the secondary and tertiary levels by means of indigenous health units located in municipal referral centers. To support the indigenous health activities carried out at the community level, FUNASA implemented the Indigenous Health Care Information System (SIASI) in 2000.

In 2003, the Brazilian indigenous population was estimated at 770,000 people, who belong to some 210 groups and speak more than 170 languages. Although they make up only 0.2% of the total population, indigenous peoples are found in all states of the country. Each group has its own forms of social, political, and economic organization and its own way of relating to the environment and utilizing the land. Close to 44% of the indigenous population and 98.7% of indigenous lands are concentrated in the North and Center-West regions. During the period 2000–2004, SIASI recorded 4,584 deaths in the indigenous population, 45% of them among children under 5 years of age. In 2003, SIM recorded 2,116 deaths, 33% among children under 5. The main causes of death were external causes (16.8%), diseases of the circulatory system (16.5%), diseases of the respiratory system (13.9%), and infectious diseases (13.8%).

The indigenous population receives the vaccines provided for under the health system in accordance with the basic immunization schedule for this population. Since 2003, Brazil has been taking part in Vaccination Week in the Americas, a joint initiative of the Ministry of Health and the Pan American Health Organization (PAHO) that resulted in increased vaccination coverage in 2006.

The black population of Brazil, which includes both blacks and mulattos, is the largest of any country outside the African continent. This population has some distinctive genetic features resulting from miscegenation—or mixing of races and cultures—of individuals from various ethnic groups originating from different regions of sub-Saharan Africa (27). In 2004, this population was estimated at 10.7 million blacks and 76.6 million mulattos, and it made up 48.0% of the total national population. Approximately 80% of blacks reside in the Northeast and Southeast regions. Additionally, there are remnants of some 1,000 fugitive slave communities scattered around the country. In 2003, approximately 350,000 deaths of black persons were recorded, some 280,000 of which were of mulattos.

The leading defined causes of death among the black population were diseases of the circulatory system (29.9%), external causes (20.6%), neoplasms (12.4%), and diseases of the respiratory system (9.1%). In that year, the black population was at greater risk than the white population of dying from infectious diseases, endocrine diseases, and complications of pregnancy, childbirth, and the puerperium. The mulatto population had a higher risk of dying from causes related to pregnancy, childbirth, and the puerperium and from external causes than the white population, but a lower risk of dying from neoplasms and from diseases of the circulatory, respiratory, digestive, and genitourinary systems. However, rates of death among mulattos may be underestimated because they are often listed as being of unknown race/color and also because a wide variety of people are classified as mulattos (since in the various regions of Brazil mulattos may be the result of different race/color combinations). The most frequent health problems in the black population—malnutrition, drug use, septic abortion, and violence, among others—are associated with long-standing social inequalities that lead to poverty and reduce access to health services. These inequalities are aggravating factors in diseases such as arterial hypertension, diabetes mellitus, and glucose-6-phosphate dehydrogenase deficiency, which seem to be more prevalent in the black population.

Among the genetically determined diseases that occur in this population, the principal one is sickle cell anemia, the most common monogenic hereditary disease in Brazil (28). It is estimated that between 8,000 and 50,000 persons have the disease and between 2 million and 10 million carry the sickle cell gene, which implies a high degree of underreporting of cases, since only around 4,000 cases have been identified. An estimated 80% of those with sickle cell anemia die by the age of 30, but 85% of these deaths are not accurately registered (29). In 1995, a Government initiative aimed at improving the situation of the black population (*30*) helped mobilize civil society, the scientific community, and health professionals, resulting in the formulation of a program for control of sickle cell anemia and other measures to protect the interests of this population group.

HEALTH CONDITIONS AND PROBLEMS

COMMUNICABLE DISEASES

Vector-borne Diseases

Malaria is endemic throughout the Brazilian Amazon region, which encompasses the whole of the North and parts of the states of Maranhão (Northeast) and Mato Grosso (Center-West). More than 99% of the cases reported in the last 10 years occurred in this area, where the annual average number of positive exams was 530,000. The incidence of malaria surged in this area in 1999, returning to 1970s levels. Some 632,600 new cases were reported—34% more than in 1998—resulting in 21,100 hospitalizations, mainly of adult and adolescent males aged 15–34. The high endemicity of malaria in the Amazon region is related to changes in extractive activities, which lead to internal migration and the establishment of unplanned rural settlements. In 2000, the Ministry of Health launched the Plan for Intensification of Malaria Control Activities in the Amazon Region (PIACM), which facilitated a restructuring of local health services designed to include malaria control in the network of health services, employing a strategy that emphasizes early diagnosis and immediate treatment. By the end of 2002, the number of malaria cases had decreased 45% in comparison to 1999. In 2003, the Ministry of Health introduced the National Malaria Control Program (PNCM) with a view to maintaining the successes achieved under the PIACM through strengthening of the structure of services. Despite all the resources invested, however, the number of cases rose 17.3% (408,795 cases) from 2002 to 2003. The number continued to rise in 2004 (464,231 cases, an increase of 13.6% over 2003) and in 2005 (599,690 cases, 29.2% higher than in the previous year). The increase in malaria cases is due mainly to intensive and unplanned growth of the peripheral areas surrounding the major cities.

No cases of urban **yellow fever** have been reported since 1942. However, since the 1970s there has been a progressive reinfestation of the national territory by the *Aedes aegypti* mosquito, the urban vector of the disease. Sylvatic yellow fever is endemic in some regions, although the number of cases has fallen steadily since 1999 as vaccination coverage rates in the endemic areas have risen. In 1999, 76 cases were reported, and in 2005, three. Over the period 1999–2001, epidemics occurred mainly in the Center-West region. The last outbreak began among simians in the Amazon region and then spread to the savanna region in the Center-West part of the country. The virus continued to spread in a southeasterly direction, with epizootics occurring in 54 municipalities in six states. In 2000, human cases were detected in São Paulo and Bahia, both of which had been free of the disease since the 1950s. In 2001, an outbreak of human cases occurred in the state of Minas Gerais, and there were epizootics in the state of Rio Grande do Sul, in areas that theretofore had not been considered susceptible to yellow fever. In 2003, 64 cases of yellow fever were confirmed, with 22 deaths. Cases were reported in 18 municipalities in the states of Minas Gerais, Rio Grande do Sul, Mato Grosso, Roraima, and Pará. Most of the cases since 1999 have occurred among men (more than 80%) and among farmers and ecotourists. From 1999 to 2003, based on the cases reported to the surveillance system, the case fatality rate was around 40%. Brazil's immunization policy with respect to yellow fever calls for vaccination after 6 months of age for all persons residing in endemic areas, vaccination after 9 months of age for all persons residing in transition zones, and vaccination of all persons traveling to endemic areas.

The mosquito vector of **dengue**, *Aedes aegypti*, is found in all cities of the country, except in the states of Rio Grande do Sul and Santa Catarina. The dengue virus was reintroduced into Brazil in 1981 and 1982. The first clinically documented and laboratory-confirmed epidemic occurred in Boa Vista (Roraima) and was caused by serotypes 1 and 4. Other epidemics have occurred since 1986, affecting Rio de Janeiro and several capital cities in the Northeast region, and dengue has now become endemic in Brazil, with epidemic spikes. The number of cases decreased from 794,000 in 2002 to 118,000 in 2004, but 2005 brought a new increase: 217,000 cases, including 447 cases of dengue hemorrhagic fever, with 43 deaths. Circulation of serotypes DEN1, DEN2, and DEN3 has been detected.

During the 1960s, areas at risk of household transmission of **Chagas' disease** were identified in more than 2,000 municipalities in 18 Brazilian states. *Triatoma infestans* was detected in 711 municipalities in 13 states. The prevalence, based on serological screening, was 4.2% for the country, with values as high as 8.8% in Minas Gerais and Rio Grande do Sul. The Initiative of the Southern Cone Countries for the Elimination of *T. infestans* and Interruption of Transfusional Transmission of American Trypanosomiasis has helped to consolidate the control of this species, which is the main, and virtually the only, vector for household transmission. In 1998, national commissions began carrying out reviews in the states, which were followed by international evaluations in 1999. An intergovernmental meeting held in Rio de Janeiro in 2000 certified the interruption of transmission in six states (Goiás, Mato Grosso, Mato Grosso do Sul, Paraíba, Rio de Janeiro, and São Paulo). In the ensuing years, with the intensification of operations in the other states, transmission was interrupted and certification was obtained in the states of Minas Gerais, Pernambuco, Piauí, and Tocantins. In 2005 and 2006, the international commission evaluations sponsored by PAHO recommended certification of the interruption of transmission for the last three endemic states: Paraná, Rio Grande do Sul, and Bahia. The current challenge is to strengthen epidemiological surveillance, especially in the Amazon region, and to ensure medical care and social services for those who were infected in the past.

Little information is available on the frequency of **lymphatic filariasis** in the country as a whole. The main focus of the disease is in the metropolitan area of Recife, in the state of Pernambuco. A residual focus exists in the state of Alagoas, although no cases were detected there in 2005. Under the National Program for the Elimination of Lymphatic Filariasis (PNEFL), being carried out as part of the WHO-led global effort to eliminate the disease, old foci of the disease are being reassessed, and states not considered to be at risk are being included in surveillance of lymphatic filariasis morbidity.

Transmission of **schistosomiasis** is most intense in the Northeast region and the northern portion of the state of Mato Grosso, but the disease is widely distributed across the country. Analyses by health services of stool samples from the population show a reduction in the prevalence of the infection. In the last 15 years, the percentage of samples testing positive has ranged from 5.5% to 11.6%. Of the slightly more than 4 million tests conducted during the period 2000–2005, the prevalences were 7.1% (2000), 6.4% (2004), and 5.5% (2005). The expansion of water supply and sanitation coverage based on epidemiological criteria, coupled with greater medical care coverage, has helped to reduce the frequency of schistosomiasis cases and deaths.

Visceral leishmaniasis, or kala-azar, has shown an upward trend, with epidemics reported during the 1980s and the 1990s. In 1999 and 2000, a new upsurge in cases occurred (close to 4,000 per year), mainly in the Northeast region. The rise in the prevalence of leishmaniasis in several regions of Brazil in recent years can be explained by changes in the disease's pattern of geographic distribution, which has spread toward the periphery of urban centers as a result of mass migration of the rural population to the cities. At the same time, the process of organizing the health care system, together with better diagnosis and treatment, has resulted in increased detection of cases. In 2004, 3,386 cases were reported.

During the period 1987–2004, reported cases of American **cutaneous leishmaniasis** ranged from 13.5 per 100,000 population to 23.0 per 100,000. In 2004, 28,575 cases were reported. The North and Northeast regions account for the largest number of cases (37% and 33%, respectively, of total reported cases during the period).

The first cases of **hantaviral disease** were detected in 1993 in São Paulo. The South region and the states of São Paulo, Minas Gerais, and Mato Grosso have had the highest incidence of this disease. Up to 2003, a total of 338 cases had been reported in 11 states, with a mean case-fatality rate of 44.5%. In 2004, 159 cases were detected. The Ministry of Health has taken steps to put in place epidemiological surveillance of the disease, develop labora-tory diagnostic capability, disseminate information on appropriate treatment to reduce fatalities, and track the circulation of hantaviruses in wild rodents in Brazil as part of eco-epidemiological surveillance activities.

Vaccine-preventable Diseases

The National Immunization Program, which marked its 31st anniversary in 2005, provides specific vaccines, free of charge, for more than 10 diseases and has achieved high routine immunization coverage among children, adolescents, adults, and the elderly. Program implementation is decentralized, with activities in all municipalities, although procurement of immunobiologicals takes place at the central level.

The hepatitis B vaccine and the bivalent MR (measles-rubella) virus vaccine were introduced gradually into the routine immunization schedule (Table 2) after 1992, and by 2000 they were being administered in all states. The vaccine against *Haemophilus influenzae* type b (Hib) was introduced in 1999, and since 2002 it has been administered routinely as part of a combined tetravalent vaccine (DTP + Hib: diphtheria-tetanus-pertussis and *Haemophilus influenzae* type b). The influenza vaccine was introduced in annual vaccination campaigns for the older population in 1999.

TABLE 2. Basic immunization schedule, children up to 10 years old, Brazil, 2006.

Age	Vaccines	Number of doses
At birth	BCG - ID	single dose
	Hepatitis B vaccine	1st dose
1 month	Hepatitis B vaccine	2nd dose
2 months	Rota (oral human rotavirus vaccine)	1st dose
	OPV (oral polio vaccine)	1st dose
	Tetravalent vaccine (DTP + Hib)	1st dose
	Rota (oral human rotavirus vaccine)	2nd dose
4 months	OPV (oral polio vaccine)	2nd dose
	Tetravalent vaccine (DTP + Hib)	2nd dose
6 months	OPV (oral polio vaccine)	3rd dose
	Tetravalent vaccine (DTP + Hib)	3rd dose
	Hepatitis B vaccine	3rd dose
9 months	Yellow fever vaccine	single dose
12 months	MMR (trivalent measles-mumps-rubella)	single dose
15 months	OPV (oral polio vaccine)	booster
	DTP (trivalent diphtheria-tetanus-pertussis)	1st booster
4–6 years	DTP (trivalent diphtheria-tetanus-pertussis)	2nd booster
	MMR (trivalent measles-mumps-rubella)	booster
6–10 years	BCG - ID	booster
10 years	Yellow fever vaccine	booster

Source: Ministry of Health, National Immunization Program Information System. Available at: http://pni.datasus.gov.br/calendario_vacina_Infantil.asp (in Portuguese only).

Vaccination coverage for the following vaccines among children under 1 year of age (3.2 million children) was over 95% in 2005: BCG (100%); OPV, 3 doses (98%); and tetravalent DPT-Hib, 3 doses (96%). Coverage for the hepatitis B vaccine (3 doses) was 92%. Coverage for the trivalent MMR (measles-mumps-rubella) virus vaccine among children aged 12 months was 100%. Of the 5,564 municipalities in Brazil, 62% had DTP3 and MMR coverage levels of over 95%.

The National Influenza Pandemic Preparedness Committee was established in 2003, and the National Influenza Pandemic Preparedness Plan was drawn up and implemented in November 2005. The various states are developing their local strategies based on the national plan, which is regularly updated. The Butantán Institute is developing a vaccine against the H5N1 influenza virus. The country already has a strategic reserve of the antiviral drug oseltamivir, and other influenza preparedness and response planning activities are being carried out at the health service level.

It was decided in 2005 that the rotavirus vaccine would be introduced into the immunization schedule starting in 2006. Brazil is the first country in the world to incorporate this vaccine into its routine immunization program.

Measles elimination activities began in Brazil in 1992 and in the Region of the Americas as a whole in 1999. In addition to surveillance, the elimination strategy included rapid interruption of viral circulation in the community by means of a single mass vaccination campaign targeting the cohort of children between the ages of 9 months and 14 years. The mass vaccination campaign carried out in 1992 brought the number of measles cases down from 42,934 in 1991 to 2,396 in 1993. The elimination strategy also called for the achievement of routine measles vaccination coverage of at least 95% in order to ensure permanent interruption of viral circulation. To address the inevitable accumulation of measles-susceptible children in each successive birth cohort (the 5% who fail to receive primary immunization), periodic follow-up vaccination campaigns must be carried out among children aged 1–4. The first national follow-up campaign was conducted in 1993. In 1997, there was a serious measles epidemic, with more than 50,000 cases reported initially and 61 deaths. A second nationwide follow-up campaign was carried out in 1997, achieving a national coverage rate of 66%. It was followed by campaigns in 2000 and 2004, with coverage levels of 93%. The number of measles cases decreased from 908 in 1999 to 36 in 2000. Since 2001, the measles vaccine has been administered to children at 12 months of age, with a second dose of trivalent virus vaccine during the preschool years. No indigenous cases of measles have been reported since 2001.

Surveillance of **rubella** was incorporated into Brazil's measles surveillance activities in 1996, and surveillance of congenital rubella syndrome (CRS) was added in 2001. The rubella vaccine was introduced in some Brazilian states in 1992, which changed the age group affected by the disease. In the outbreaks reported during the period 1999–2002, high incidence was observed among women of childbearing age. Since 2002, all states in the country have been using the MMR vaccine in their routine childhood immunization programs, and in 2001, the country adopted a strategy of rapid control of rubella through vaccination of women of childbearing age. The impact was significant: cases of both rubella and congenital rubella syndrome dropped markedly (233 and 4 cases, respectively, in 2005).

Brazil was certified free of **poliomyelitis** in 1994 (the last case was reported in 1989). In addition to routine immunization with the oral polio vaccine (OPV-Sabin), two national mop-up campaigns are conducted each year, with high coverage rates being achieved (95% during both the first and second campaigns of 2005). In 2005, routine vaccination coverage among children under 1 year of age was 98%. Surveillance of acute flaccid paralysis (AFP) is carried out routinely. More than 80% of suspected cases were investigated in a timely manner, but stool samples were obtained promptly from only around 70% of patients with AFP in the last three years. Efforts to develop a National Plan for the Containment of Wild Poliovirus in Laboratories began in 2002, and containment activities were initiated in 2003 with a national survey of 289 high-risk laboratories in 173 institutions. Following the new recommendations of WHO (2005), the country opted to repeat the national survey in order to evaluate all active laboratories in the country.

The incidence of **neonatal tetanus** has fallen steadily for more than a decade: 66 cases in 1999, 34 in 2000, 15 in 2003, 14 in 2004, and 10 in 2005. However, cases are still being reported, mostly in areas where the coverage and quality of basic health care services are low. The Plan for Elimination of Neonatal Tetanus was launched in 1992, with the goal of reducing the incidence of the disease to under 1 per 1,000 live births. In 2000, some of the strategies for epidemiological surveillance in small municipalities were reformulated. Vaccination coverage for Td (tetanus and diphtheria toxoids) among women of childbearing age is below the national goal, and additional efforts are needed to ensure the protection of this population group. In 2005, 74% of the country's municipalities had less than 50% tetanus vaccination coverage among pregnant women. The incidence of other forms of tetanus has remained relatively unchanged in recent years (439 cases reported in 2000 and 420 in 2005). The vast majority of tetanus cases occur in men (81%).

The incidence of **whooping cough** has also remained stable in recent years, with a total of 764 cases in 2000 and 1,328 in 2005. The most serious forms of the disease and the highest number of fatal cases occur in children under 1 year of age. The number of confirmed cases of **diphtheria** fell from 46 in 2000 to 27 in 2005.

A total of 1,358 cases of **meningitis** due to *Haemophilus influenzae* type b (Hib) were reported in 1999, of which 617 (45%) occurred in children under 1 year of age. Following the introduction of the Hib vaccine that year, the number of cases fell to 153 in 2000; children under 1 continued to be the most affected group (accounting for 43% of cases). In 2005, only 108 cases of Hib meningitis were reported.

Epidemiological surveillance of **viral hepatitis** consists of mandatory reporting of confirmed cases of hepatitis B and C. A seroepidemiological study has been under way since 2004 in representative areas of the five regions of the country, with the aim of estimating the frequency of hepatitis A (IgG anti-HAV) among persons aged 5–19 and of hepatitis B (IgG anti-HBc, HBsAg, anti-HBs) and hepatitis C (anti-HCV and HCV RNA) among persons over the age of 9 (age cohorts 10–19 and 20–69).

Chronic Communicable Diseases

Tuberculosis is a high priority public health problem in Brazil affecting mainly the poorest populations at the most productive ages of life. Analysis of a 10-year time series (1993–2004) reveals that the incidence of the disease has remained quite stable, with a slight decline in all forms of tuberculosis. The states of Rio de Janeiro and Amazonas had the highest incidence rates in 2004: 94.5 and 70.6 per 100,000 population, respectively. In 2004, 91,855 cases were reported, with an incidence rate of 45.2 per 100,000 population. Of those cases, 88.1% (80,960) were new cases of tuberculosis in all its forms and, of those, 84.9% (68,744) were pulmonary cases and 62.5% (42,972) were pulmonary cases with positive sputum smears. The estimated prevalence was 50 million infected individuals, with approximately 111,000 new cases and around 6,000 deaths a year. Multidrug-resistant tuberculosis is not a significant problem in Brazil. Tuberculosis occurs as an opportunistic infection in 15.2% of AIDS cases and in around 8.0% of HIV-positive tuberculosis cases. The 2004–2007 Plan of Action established the goal of instituting the strategy of Directly Observed Treatment, Short Course (DOTS) in the 370 high-priority municipalities that account for more than 70% of the country's tuberculosis burden. The DOTS strategy was introduced in 1997 in several pilot areas of the Center-West region, but progress in extending its coverage has been slow. Nevertheless, the population covered by the strategy has grown steadily in recent years, increasing from 3% in 1998 to 52% in 2004. In the high-priority municipalities, DOTS coverage is around 70% of the affected population.

Despite progress in recent years, **leprosy** remains a significant problem, with a prevalence rate of 4.9 cases per 10,000 population in 1998 and 78,000 leprosy patients on record. In the same year, 42,055 new cases were diagnosed (detection rate of 2.6 cases per 10,000 population). In the North and Center-West, the disease remained hyperendemic (more than 4 new cases per 10,000 population), but the Northeast had the highest absolute numbers of current leprosy cases (25,267) and of detection of new cases (14,015). In 2004, Brazil began to calculate point prevalence (proportion of individuals in a population suffering from the disease at a given point in time) rather than registered active cases, which had been calculated up to 2003. In late 2005,

the registered prevalence was 1.48 per 10,000 population (27,313 leprosy patients in treatment), with a detection rate of 2.1 per 10,000 population (38,410 new cases detected). Notwithstanding the reduction in prevalence observed during the period 1985–2005—from 19.0 to 1.48 per 10,000 population—leprosy remains a public health problem, and intensified action is needed to accelerate its elimination.

Acute Respiratory Infections

Acute respiratory infections are among the leading causes of mortality among children under 5 years of age. Although **bacterial pneumonia** is not a reportable disease in Brazil, epidemiological surveillance of this form of pneumonia has been strengthened through the implementation of a system of sentinel surveillance of invasive pneumoccocal disease. According to data from the Hospital Information System of Brazil's Unified Health System (SIH-SUS), from January 2005 to March 2006, pneumonia accounted for approximately 6% of all hospitalizations, 21.5% of them of children under age 5, and 6.5% of persons over the age of 60. Data for 2005 from the pneumococcal infections surveillance network of the Regional Vaccine System (SIREVA) show that in *Streptococcus pneumoniae* samples isolated from children under age 6 with pneumonia, the most frequent circulating serotypes were 14, 1, and 6B. However, these data are not representative of the country as a whole. The proportion of samples of *S. pneumoniae* with intermediate or total resistance to penicillin increased from 10.2% to 27.8% between 1993 and 2004.

HIV/AIDS and Other Sexually Transmitted Infections

In Brazil, AIDS currently affects mainly injection drug users and men who have sex with men. In the early 1980s, recipients of blood transfusions and blood products were also disproportionately affected. In recent years, incidence rates have remained high—19.2 cases per 100,000 population—owing to a steady rise in the number of cases among women. Among men, the proportion of cases due to homo/bisexual HIV transmission has remained stable, while the proportion due to heterosexual transmission has increased and the proportion due to injection drug use has declined steadily and significantly. The mean number of AIDS cases recorded annually ranges from 25,000 to 30,000, depending on the origin and source of the data consulted. The cumulative number of AIDS cases reported since the start of the epidemic is 400,000, and the number of people living with HIV/AIDS is estimated at more than 600,000. AIDS death rates rose until the mid-1990s, leveling off and remaining at around 11,000 per year from 1998 onwards. The policy of universal access to antiretroviral treatment—which combines medications with different modes of action in the regimen known as highly active antiretroviral therapy (HAART)—has led to a substantial decline in mortality. Nevertheless, the continued growth in the proportions of AIDS cases among women and among blacks and

Inequalities Have an Impact on Health

Inequality in Brazil mainly affects the black population (which refers to brown- and black-skinned persons) and indigenous peoples. Blacks account for 68% of the poorest decile, while whites account for 87% in the wealthiest one; also, 32.2% of the very poor are black. The Afro-descendent population is larger than in any other country outside Africa and presents special genetic characteristics owing to the mixture of races and cultures involving people who came from different parts of sub-Saharan Africa. In 2004, there were an estimated 10.7 million brown-skinned Brazilians and 76.6 million blacks, totaling 48.0% of the country's population. The most frequent health problems in the black population—malnutrition, drug use, septic abortion, and violence, among others—are associated with long-standing social inequalities that lead to poverty and reduce access to health services. These inequalities are aggravating factors in diseases such as hypertension, diabetes mellitus, and glucose-6-phosphate dehydrogenase deficiency. In 1995, a Government initiative aimed at improving the situation of the black population helped mobilize civil society, the scientific community, and health professionals, and resulted in the formulation of a program to control sickle cell anemia and other measures to protect the interests of this population group. The Ministry of Health and the Special Secretariat on Policies to Promote Racial Equality are working together to propose and systematize management and assistance strategies for the implementation and monitoring of actions related to the health of the black population in the National Health Plan (PNS), with the aim of promoting racial equality.

mulattos of both sexes between 1998 and 2004 points up the inequity that exists in access to early diagnosis and treatment services among the most socially and economically disadvantaged populations.

NONCOMMUNICABLE DISEASES

Metabolic and Nutritional Diseases

The Periodic Family Budget Survey (POF 2002–2003) conducted by the Brazilian Institute of Geography and Statistics (*31*, *32*) indicated that the prevalence of **underweight** has declined in Brazil (except in the rural North), falling from 6.8% in 1989 to 5.4% during the period 2002–2003 among females and from 3.8% to 2.8% among males. In the same period, the prevalence of **overweight** and **obesity** among males increased from 29.5% to 41.0% and from 5.1% to 8.8%, respectively, while among women overweight decreased slightly, from 40.7% to 39.2%, and obesity remained virtually the same: 12.8% to 12.7%.

During the period 2002–2003, a household survey was conducted in 15 state capitals to identify risk factors in the population aged 15 and over (*33*). Analysis of overweight and of degree of excess weight (body mass index [BMI] $\geq 25 \text{kg/m}^2$) revealed a somewhat higher prevalence in the Southeast, South, and Center-West regions (9.8%, 9.7%, and 8.4%, respectively) than in the North and Northeast regions (7.8% and 6.8%, respectively). Data from the Periodic Family Budget Surveys of 1974, 1989, and 2002–2003 show that the prevalence of obesity is rising in all regions of the country, both in rural and in urban areas, and al-

though the increase is larger among men, women have higher obesity figures. As for physical inactivity, the proportion of individuals classified as insufficiently active was highest in João Pessoa (Paraíba) (54.5%) and lowest in Belém (Pará) (28.2%); no characteristic pattern was observed among the regions. More women than men were found to be physically inactive. The highest rates of physical activity were observed in the group aged 15–24.

Cardiovascular Diseases

Diseases of the circulatory system were the leading cause of death for both sexes (284,685 deaths in 2004, 28% of total mortality). **Cerebrovascular diseases** were the most frequent cause of death in the country (10.1% of total mortality), followed by **ischemic heart diseases** (9.7% of total mortality). Analysis of the period 1990–2003 shows a downward trend in death rates for diseases of the circulatory system. The risk of death from cerebrovascular diseases and ischemic heart diseases has declined in the last 15 years among both sexes in all Brazilian states, except in the states of Pernambuco and Mato Grosso, where the risk is rising significantly.

Malignant Neoplasms

Registered deaths from cancer totaled 134,683 in 2003. The first three causes among women were cancer of the breast (15%); trachea, bronchus, and lung (9%); and cervix uteri (6.8%). Among men, the foremost cause was cancer of the trachea, bronchus, and lung (15%), followed by prostate cancer (12%) and stomach cancer (11%).

The crude mortality rate for cervical cancer in 2003 was 4.7 per 100,000 women. The risk of death during the period 1980–2003 remained stable for women aged 30–59 but increased in a statistically significant manner for women aged 60 and older. Analysis of cervical cancer mortality is limited by the high number of cases of uterine malignancies coded as unspecified (29%, with rates as high as 50% of cases of uterine cancer in some states). The crude mortality rate for breast cancer in 2003 was 10.4 per 100,000 women. The risk of death from this cause in the period 1990–2003 rose significantly in all age groups, except for the group aged 60–69. The South region had the highest rates.

The crude mortality rate for cancer of the trachea, bronchus, and lung in 2003 was 9.3 per 100,000 population. Men have a higher risk of dying of cancer than women everywhere in the country. Among men aged 30–49 years, the risk of death during the period 1990–2003 remained stable at around 4 per 100,000 population; it fell substantially among men aged 50–59, remained the same among those aged 60–69, and rose significantly among those aged 70 and over. Among women, increasing risk was observed in all age groups.

OTHER HEALTH PROBLEMS OR ISSUES

Disasters

According to data from the 2002 Global Environment Outlook (GEO) report for Brazil (*34*), the most common natural disasters during the period 1991–2001 were low water levels (55.1%); dry weather (19.9%); flash floods (20.6%); gradual flooding (1.7%); gales and storms (0.9%); severe gales and extratropical cyclones (0.3%); forest fires (0.4%); and hail, water-logging, and other phenomena (1.0%).

Mental Health and Addictions

A national survey conducted in 2002–2003 to identify the risk factors among the population aged 15 and over (*13*) found that the prevalence of cigarette-smoking was highest in Porto Alegre (Rio Grande do Sul) (25.2%) and lowest in Aracajú (Sergipe) (12.9%). Of the eight cities with the highest prevalence, seven were located in the South and Southeast regions. In all the cities surveyed, the estimates of smoking prevalence were higher among men. These sex differences were statistically significant in all cities of the North, Northeast, and Center-West regions, except for the city of Natal (Rio Grande do Norte). Among young people aged 15–24, the prevalence of tobacco use ranged from 6.8% in Aracajú to 24.1% in Porto Alegre. Among those aged 25 and over, the highest prevalence was found in Porto Alegre (25.6%) and the lowest in Aracajú (15.5%). With regard to alcohol use, the proportion of individuals who reported consuming at least one alcoholic drink in the 30 days preceding the survey ranged from 32.4% in João Pessoa to 58.6% in Florianópolis (Santa Catarina).

Oral Health

In 2003, the Ministry of Health, with the participation of academic institutions and health services, concluded a broad and comprehensive national survey of oral health, which yielded the following findings: there is a high rate of dental caries among persons older than 12; three out of four older adults have no functional teeth; less than 22% of adults and less than 8% of the elderly have healthy gums; and the prevalence of caries was 49% higher in municipalities without fluoridated water. In light of the results of this study, the Ministry of Health launched the "Smiling Brazil" program, which aims to bring about a significant increase in the number of oral health teams within the Family Health Program (PSF) and ensure the addition of fluoride to drinking water in 2,000 municipalities and the construction of specialized oral health care centers. In 2004, there was a 67.3% increase in the number of oral health teams distributed among 2,944 municipalities (*35*).

RESPONSE OF THE HEALTH SECTOR

Health Policies and Plans

The national health policy is based on the Federal Constitution of 1988, which sets out the principles and guidelines for the delivery of health care in Brazil through the country's Unified Health System (SUS). This system, whose operating regulations were established in 1990 (*36*), is guided by the principles of universal and equitable access to services for the promotion, protection, and recovery of health, integrated in a regionalized, multilevel network under the responsibility of the three levels of government (federal, state, and municipal). The private sector plays a complementary role. The SUS operational guidelines call for decentralized management, integrated care, and community participation. Under the Constitution, the activities of the federal government are to be carried out in accordance with multiyear plans (PPAs) approved by the national congress for periods of four years.

The PPA for 2004–2007 establishes the federal government's high-priority initiatives for the four-year period, identifying the following priorities in the area of health: (1) plant and animal health safety; (2) investment in science, technology, and innovation to promote competitive import substitution in strategic areas; (3) sanitation; (4) increased access to low-cost medicines through the Government's *farmácia popular* program; (5) improvement of the quality of care provided through the Unified Health System (QualiSUS project); (6) monitoring, evaluation, and oversight of the health activities and financial resources transferred to states, municipalities, and institutions in the framework of the SUS; (7) formulation of regulations for implementation of Constitutional Amendment 29, which establishes the allocation of resources for the SUS; (8) oral health (through the "Smiling Brazil" program); (9) mental health; (10) women's health; (11) control of leprosy and tuberculosis; (12) organ transplant; (13) professional civil service in the health sector; (14) enhancement of the SUS's capacity to produce blood products, immunobiologicals, and pharmaceuticals; (15) indigenous health; (16) approval of the National Health Plan; (17) decentralization of the SUS to the regional level and improvement of its management; and (18) improvement of the quality of care provided under private health plans.

The SUS was established immediately after the adoption of the Federal Constitution of 1988 with the aim of ensuring universal and equitable access to health care. The system underwent an institutional reorganization pursuant to the regulations adopted in 1990 and the process of decentralization called for under the basic operational guidelines approved by the governing bodies of the system: the Tripartite Interagency Commission (CIT) and the National Health Council (CNS). In 2006, a new instrument of commitment was adopted, the "Pact for Life, Strengthening the SUS and Its Management" (37), the result of a long process of negotiation among stakeholders initiated in 2003. The Pact, approved by the CIT and the CNS in February 2006, establishes a new dynamic in the collective management of the SUS and introduces changes in the way the federal, state, and municipal levels of government interact with one another, including: (1) replacement of the qualification process with voluntary adherence to the Terms of Commitment for Management; (2) regionalization on a basis of solidarity and cooperation as the guiding principle for the process of decentralization; (3) integration of the various methods of federal resource allocation; and (4) harmonization of the various preexisting agreements (Basic Health Care Pact, Surveillance Pact, and other agreements).

To ensure coordination of the activities of the SUS in the three spheres of government administration, there are two negotiating and consensus-building bodies, which meet regularly: at the state level, the Bipartite Interagency Commission, with equal representation of the State Secretariat of Health and the Council of Municipal Secretaries of Health (COSEMS); and at the national level, the Tripartite Interagency Commission, with equal representation of the Ministry of Health and of the National Councils of State and of Municipal Secretaries of Health (CONAS and CONASEMS). The agreements reached by these commissions are formalized at the corresponding level of government. Social participation in the SUS occurs primarily through two formal bodies: health councils and health conferences. The councils are permanent bodies that formulate strategies and monitor the implementation of health policy, including the economic and financial aspects. The conferences are convened every four years, with broad stakeholder participation. They assess progress with regard to the health situation and they propose public policy guidelines for the sector. Government agencies, service providers, health professionals, and users are represented on the councils and at the conferences, the numbers of users and health professionals equaling the number of representatives of the other two

groups combined (38). The 12th National Health Conference, held in December 2003, formulated recommendations on a wide variety of issues relating to the SUS (39).

The health councils are organized on the federal, state, and municipal levels. They were established with the aim of ensuring the existence of functioning state and municipal councils during the process of decentralization, as a condition for the regular and automatic transfer of federal financial resources (40). The National Health Council established guidelines for the organization of the state and municipal health councils (41), and in 1999 it established training guidelines for council members (42), for which purpose it distributed several documents aimed at providing guidance for social participation and representation on the councils, especially at the municipal level. In 2005, national guidelines were approved for the process of continuing education on social oversight of the SUS, which includes training for health council members, initiatives related to continuing education policies and strategies, and health communication and information for the entire population (43).

The Ministry of Health is responsible for leading the process of regionalization of health care networks and ensuring that the public health system has adequate response capacity. To that end, it proposes and approves general guidelines and standards for regionalization, in accordance with the norms and agreements of the Tripartite Interagency Commission currently in effect. The Ministry, through the states and municipalities, is also responsible for providing technical and financial cooperation to the health regions, giving priority to the most vulnerable regions and promoting equity among regions and states.

The regulation of professional practice in the various health occupations is the responsibility of professional boards, which maintain regional delegations with jurisdiction in each state of the country. The boards are autonomous public entities, created by law, which supervise ethical and legal aspects of professional practice in the various health occupations within their respective jurisdictions. The practice of health professions is also subject to federal health oversight regulations.

The Ministry of Health establishes the criteria for regulation, monitoring, and control of the production of all goods and services in the health sector. It regulates all health activities, including those of both ambulatory care facilities and hospitals, at the various levels of the health care system (primary, intermediate, and tertiary) and the access of users to care at those levels. The strategy for regulating supply and demand in the health sector is based on "regulatory complexes," which organize all the activities relating to regulation of access to care (inpatient care, outpatient visits and exams, treatment protocols) in a coordinated and integrated manner, aiming to tailor the supply of health services to actual needs (44).

The Brazilian Hospital Accreditation Program, which has been in existence since 1995 (45), evaluates hospital services based on standards established at the federal level (46). Since 1998, health services provided under private plans have also been subject to regulations, standards, monitoring, and oversight, in accordance with specific legislation (47). The National Supplementary Health Coverage Agency (ANS) monitors trends in the prices of private plans, as well as the activities of private providers and the use of resources; it also authorizes corporate subdivisions, mergers and acquisitions, incorporations, and modifications, and it oversees coordination with consumer protection entities (48).

Since government regulation began, important changes have taken place in the sector which have had an impact on the dynamics of the private health insurance industry and on competitive strategies. A recent study showed a reduction of 17% between 2000 and 2003 in the number of prepaid group practices and of 23% in the number of self-managed company health plans. In the same period, the number of registered insurance companies increased from 4 to 14, and the number of plan administrators grew from 28 to 37 (32%). Production and marketing of health-related goods and services, processes, inputs, and technologies are regulated by the federal, state, and municipal agencies that comprise the National Health Surveillance System. The Ministry of Health coordinates the System through the National Health Surveillance Agency (ANVISA) (49), which is also responsible for health regulation at ports, airports, and borders.

Health inspection activities are being decentralized to the state and municipal governments, which participate in technical analysis of product registration processes. At the central level, the Ministry of Agriculture is responsible for registration and industrial inspection of products of animal origin, drinks, pesticides, and drugs for veterinary use. Agricultural export products are subject to direct inspection by the federal government. The health and agriculture sectors have their own laboratory networks to support food safety activities.

Brazilian environmental policy derives from specific legislation (50) and from the Constitution of 1998, which established the National Environmental System, an advisory and deliberative body (51). The executive agency for the system is the Brazilian Institute for the Environment and Renewable Natural Resources (52).

Health Strategies and Programs

The National Health Plan (PNS) approved in 2004 (53) provides explicit guidelines for the activities of the health system during the period 2004–2007 with regard to: (1) the reorganization of health care with a view to improving quality and increasing access to comprehensive care and strengthening the system's capacity for regulation; (2) health conditions, identifying a variety of actions for prevention and control of the most prevalent diseases, and activities aimed at providing adequate protection for the most vulnerable groups (women and children, adolescents and young people, the elderly, black and indigenous populations, persons with disabilities, workers, the prison popula-

tion), as well as increasing strategic activities (oral health, mental health, healthy eating, communicable diseases control, and environmental surveillance); and (3) health sector management, including improvement of access to and quality of care, sustainability of financing, strengthening of social participation processes and participatory management practices, as well as monitoring, evaluation, and control of health activities and of the use of financial resources by the SUS, and also strengthening of international cooperation. The PNS also calls for the formulation of a National Plan for Investment in Health, aimed at enhancing the response capacity of the health services system and reducing regional inequalities.

Organization of the Health System

The health sector in Brazil comprises a complex network of services encompassing both public and private suppliers and financers. The private sector includes for-profit providers and nonprofit charitable organizations. The private system of health plans and insurance covers 24.5% of Brazilians (54), 44% of the privately covered population being primary beneficiaries of health plans and 56% dependents of primary beneficiaries. Most of the clientele of the private system reside in the cities of the Southeast and South regions. The private system underwent considerable growth during the 1990s, especially in the second half of the decade.

The public health sector, to which access is universal, is the sole provider of health care coverage for 75% of the population, in addition to providing public health services (e.g., epidemiological and health surveillance, control of communicable diseases) for the entire population. Some of the population covered by private health plans also use the services of the SUS, especially for highly complex or costly procedures or treatments (e.g., transplants, HIV/AIDS treatment, pharmaceuticals). SUS health services are delivered through federal, state, and municipal government networks and by private contractors, including both nonprofit and for-profit entities. The SUS includes subsystems at the level of each state (state SUS) and each municipality (municipal SUS). By law, municipalities have primary responsibility for providing health care and services to their respective populations, with technical and financial assistance from the federal government and the states. Nationally, the SUS is managed by the Ministry of Public Health, which has primary responsibility for regulatory and coordination functions and plays a major role in financing of the system. The Ministry retains direct responsibility for some areas, such as health education, research, tertiary care, and delivery of special services, such as indigenous health care. Other parts of the federal government also provide health services directly, notably the system of university hospitals, health care facilities operated by the Ministry of Education, and the armed forces health services. The SUS carries out ongoing functions of coordination, planning, linkage, negotiation, monitoring, control, evaluation, and auditing, which are incumbent on the three levels of government.

Public Health Services

Since the mid-1990s, Brazil has been working to strengthen primary health care (first level of the health system) as a strategy for reducing inequalities in access and encouraging the reorientation of care in the framework of a universal and comprehensive model which before had been excessively focused on hospital care. The principal mechanisms used to expand coverage and reduce interregional inequalities are the basic health care package (*Piso de Atenção Básica*, or PAB) and the Family Health Program (PSF).

The PAB is a strategy for allocating resources to primary care for the implementation of previously defined activities and for the achievement of goals negotiated by means of integrated, consensus-based programming. Municipalities are responsible for providing a set of basic health care services for their respective populations. For that purpose, they receive capitation payments, which are transferred from the Ministry of Health to the Municipal Health Funds, replacing the previous fee-for-service system of resource allocation. The most important of the incentives is associated with the implementation of the Family Health Program, launched in 1994, which incorporates and builds upon a previous initiative focused on the work of community health agents. The program provides comprehensive health care to a particular population in a particular territory, assigning patients to a multi-professional team composed of at least one doctor, one nurse, nursing auxiliaries, and community health agents (one agent per 150 families, or 750 people, maximum). Each health team is responsible for some 1,000 families. The team members are trained at education and training centers located in all regions of the country. The training promotes an intersectoral approach to address the various determinants of health.

In 2005, the PSF was being carried out in 4,837 Brazilian municipalities, with 22,683 family health teams providing care for approximately 73 million people (40% of the population). The teams give priority to areas not covered by the rest of the system, and their coverage therefore varies greatly from one jurisdiction to another. The program also applies differentiated strategies in the poorest areas and the areas with lowest coverage; in particular, rural areas of the Amazon region and municipalities with fewer than 30,000 inhabitants and an HDI of 0.7 or less.

Since 2002, the Ministry of Health, together with PAHO, has been working on the design and application of a model for enhancing the Family Health Program, seeking to incorporate the dimension of quality into the principles that guide the program (targeting of a specific geographic area and population, comprehensive care and continuity, accountability to and linkage with the community, multi-professional teams, and encouragement of social participation) and into its lines of action. The dimensions of structure, process, and results are also incorporated, taking into account relevant contextual factors. To determine the degree of user satisfaction, various mechanisms are used, including surveys and studies, in addition to the information obtained from social participation in the SUS health councils and conferences.

Since 2004, through the "Smiling Brazil" program, resources have been allocated to expand oral health teams and establish oral health care centers. In 2005, 137 such centers were operating in 86 municipalities of 21 states.

Another important specific financial incentive is the provision of essential drugs through tripartite funding mechanisms. The federal government transfers one Brazilian real (R$ 1.00) per capita each year to the subnational levels for the purchase of essential drugs for primary care, and the states and municipalities contribute an equal amount. Municipalities targeted by the Zero Hunger Program receive R$ 2.00. The Zero Hunger Program has several components, one of the most important being the family food subsidy (*Bolsa Família*).

Epidemiological surveillance systems also receive financial incentives for the identification and control of communicable diseases and health surveillance activities. All surveillance and disease prevention and control activities are currently overseen by the Secretariat of Health Surveillance (SVS), an area within the Ministry of Health.

With the process of decentralization, municipalities have taken on a larger role in carrying out health surveillance. States are responsible for coordination and supervision, as well as execution, of supplementary or complementary surveillance activities. Standardization and coordination at the national level remain the responsibility of the federal government (55).

The SVS is responsible for coordinating the activities of the National Epidemiological Surveillance System, the National Environmental Health Surveillance System (which includes surveillance of workplace environments), the National System of Public Health Laboratories (aspects of their work relating to epidemiological and environmental health surveillance), the Epidemiological Information Systems, and the National Immunization Program (PNI). The Secretariat is also responsible for drafting and disseminating health information for use in establishing priorities, monitoring the health situation in the country, and assessing the impact of disease prevention and control activities.

The municipal governments are responsible for basic sanitation activities, but in most communities, sanitation services are actually provided by state sanitation companies. The federal government plays a major role in financing the system, contributing resources from the regular budget and offering lines of credit. The health system also carries out basic sanitation activities in small communities, generally in conjunction with vector control activities undertaken in the framework of endemic disease prevention. The National Health Foundation (FUNASA) carries out sanitation works in communities of up to 30,000 inhabitants in rural and indigenous areas and in urban fringe areas with critically low quality-of-life indicators. Activities aimed at preventing and controlling diseases of public health importance are undertaken in accordance with the guidelines established by the specialized technical divisions of the Ministry of Health in the form of plans and programs to be executed by municipal and state agencies of the SUS.

According to the national MDG monitoring report (56), Brazil continues to show inadequacies and inequalities in relation to housing conditions and services and in the distribution of services. The proportion of the urban population with connections to the general water supply system rose from 88.3% in 1992 to 91.3% in 2002. In rural areas, access to water supply systems remains limited although it has improved, increasing from 12.3% in 1992 to 22.7% in 2002. In many places, the reliability and quality of the water supplied are uncertain, however, owing to periodic interruptions of service or deficiencies in water treatment.

With regard to sanitation, the proportion of the urban population served either by the general sewerage system or by septic tanks grew from 65.9% in 1992 to 75.9% in 2002. Such services are scarcer in the North, Northeast, and Center-West regions. In rural areas, the proportion of population covered by sewerage systems or septic tanks increased from 10.3% in 1992 to 16.0% in 2002. The results of the National Basic Sanitation Survey (PNSB 2000) carried out by the Brazilian Institute of Geography and Statistics (57) reveal a grim reality: more than 70% of the sewage collected not only receives no treatment, but it is released directly into freshwater sources, thus worsening, not improving, environmental conditions.

Data from the same survey (57) also show inadequacies with regard to final disposal of solid waste: 64% of municipalities are still disposing of their solid waste in open-air dumps, seriously undermining the effectiveness of the policies of other sectors, including the health sector. The existence of a large number of potentially contaminated areas is recognized. The extent and complexity of the potential environmental risks associated with this situation include environmental degradation, higher incidence of diseases, loss of biodiversity, and limitations on the use of water and soil—all of which have negative economic and social consequences. In rural areas, the use of agrotoxins has increased 2.5 times over the last four years.

The National Food and Nutrition Policy (PNAN) (58), approved in 1999, seeks to guarantee the quality of foods intended for human consumption and to promote healthy eating habits, as well as to prevent and control nutritional disorders. One of the current government administration's foremost social initiatives is the Zero Hunger Program, created to bolster action aimed at ensuring an adequate diet for the entire population and to help to reduce poverty. The program seeks to combat the causes of hunger through such complementary initiatives as the mobilization of civil society, job creation and income generation, and access to food and emergency assistance programs for the most vulnerable groups. In this context, the *Bolsa Família* program was launched in 2003, and it has since become the cornerstone of current efforts to alleviate hunger and poverty. The program provides cash transfers to the neediest families as a means of ensuring their access to such basic rights as food, health care, education, and social services. The goal of the *Bolsa Família* program for 2006 is to provide monetary assistance to 11.2 million poor families. As part of the Zero Hunger Program, the National Food and Nutrition Security Program carried out activities that include the purchase of goods produced by small farmers, the establishment of low-cost restaurants with affordable prices for the poor, and improvement of public school meal programs. A similar program provides subsidies to families who promise to ensure that their young and adolescent children will not engage in the harmful and dangerous forms of child labor and that they will attend school. The Program for the Eradication of Child Labor (PETI) assists some 980,000 children.

Individual Care Services

Access to health services seems to be assured for the vast majority of the Brazilian population. According to data from the National Household Sample Survey (PNAD 2003), 98% of the respondents who reported having sought health care during the survey period did, in fact, receive care (48). The percentage was slightly lower for the population with income equal to or below the minimum wage (97%) and higher in the population with income equal to 20 times the minimum wage (99.5%). Nevertheless, the 2003 World Health Survey revealed a high degree of user dissatisfaction (57.8%) with the services provided by the country's health systems, including both public and private. Users of private health plans and users of the SUS differed in their assessments, however: 72% of private plan users said they were dissatisfied versus 53.3% of SUS users. The organization of health services is marked by strong involvement of the private sector in the supply of hospital services and diagnostic and treatment support services; at the same time, the public sector is the major supplier of ambulatory services (59).

In 2002, 71% of the facilities in the health system (46,428) were ambulatory care facilities (with no inpatient care provided). Of those facilities, 76% (35,086) belonged to the public system and 73% (33,747) to municipal networks. Less than 15% (1,619) of the private facilities not offering inpatient care were SUS-contracted facilities. The municipal network provides basic health care and most intermediate-level care, and is composed of small health care units (health centers and posts).

In 2002, there were 7,397 hospitals, of which 4,809 were private, and 70% of the latter were providing services to the SUS (60). Approximately 95% of diagnostic and treatment support facilities (e.g., clinical analysis laboratories, radiology clinics) were private, and of those facilities, 35% were providing services to the SUS. The total number of available inpatient beds in 2002 was 471,171, including 146,319 (31%) in public facilities and 324,852 in the private system. However, in addition to beds in public facilities, the SUS covers 83% of those in private facilities, which means that close to 88% of the country's inpatient beds are accredited for use by the universal public system. SUS hospital admissions in 2005 totaled nearly 13 million; the average hospital stay was 5.9 days.

The National Transplant System (SNT) operates in 22 states and comprises 540 health facilities and 1,338 medical teams authorized by the System to perform transplant procedures. The number of transplants performed within the public system has grown steadily: in 2004, the SUS financed 13,000 organ and tissue transplants.

Ambulatory care under the SUS comprises basic care (including health promotion, disease prevention and control, and basic medical care); intermediate-level specialized care (including consultations with specialists); and tertiary care (involving the use of more complex equipment and technologies). The most recent data (48) indicate that in 2003 the number of yearly doctor visits per capita was 2.4 for the country as a whole and 1.8 in rural areas. The North region has the most problems with access to health services, owing to insufficient supply of services and to population dispersion. Oral health care is considered a critical area: 22% of the population aged 5–19 has never had any dental care. In the public system, 63% of the outpatient procedures performed were related to basic care; in the North, this figure was 72%.

The SUS Mobile Emergency Care Service (SAMU/192), established in 2003, is the main component of the National Emergency Care Policy. The Ministry of Health has equipped 94 services of this type, which are currently operating in 647 municipalities.

Human Resources

During the period 1999–2004, the number of registered physicians increased from 237,000 to 292,000; the number of dentists, from 145,000 to 178,000; and the number of nurses, from 72,000 to 98,000 (61). During the same period, the number of doctors per 1,000 population in the country as a whole rose from 1.4 to 1.6, although in 2004 there continued to be significant regional differences: 2.2 in the Southeast, 1.0 in the Northeast, and 0.8 in the North. The number of dentists per 1,000 population during the period ranged from 0.9 to 1.0, and the number of nurses, from 0.4 to 0.5, with similar differences in regional distribution. Of the 730,000 positions existing in high-level occupational categories in 2003, 64% were occupied by doctors, 12.2% by nurses, and 7.8 by dentists. Between 1999 and 2002, the job market for nurses grew more than the job market for doctors (26.7% versus 9.7%). In 2002, the public sector accounted for 45% of all physician jobs and 65% of nursing jobs. The share of the public sector in all health care jobs in 2002 was higher in the North (76%) and Northeast (65%) than in the South (48%). Training for high-level health personnel is provided by public and private institutions, with growing participation by the latter, which include both for-profit and community-philanthropic entities. In 2002, 53 of the 115 training programs in medicine, 81 of the 275 nursing programs, and 52 of the 159 dentistry programs were affiliated with the public sector (62).

Health Supplies

Brazil is one of the largest consumer markets for pharmaceuticals and is highly dependent on imported drugs. A study by the Brazilian Government (63) revealed that the value of the 1,028 most widely used imported drugs on the Brazilian market virtually doubled between 1990 and 2000, rising from US$ 535 million to US$ 1 billion. This expansion of imports is only partially explained through updating of the therapeutic arsenal and the launching of new-generation drugs on the domestic market. Of all drug imports in 1998, 83% had original patents issued prior to 1977, and of these, 47% had been issued before 1962. Imports of finished drugs increased from US$ 212 million to US$ 1.28 billion between 1990 and 2000. The value of drug sales (excluding taxes) on the domestic market was US$ 6.7 million in 2004 (64). Spending on drugs accounts for the largest share of family expenditure on health, amounting to 76% among the lowest-income families. The National Drug Policy (65), approved in 1998, seeks to ensure the safety, efficacy, and quality of drugs, as well as rational use and access for the population to essential products. Its implementation presupposes decentralized management of resources, based on a national list of essential drugs and a set of essential products whose supply is mandatory. The three levels of government share responsibility for financing basic drug assistance: states and municipalities are responsible for procurement and distribution of drugs, while the federal government is responsible for ensuring the availability of strategic products (antiretrovirals, blood products, and special antimicrobials) and high-cost drugs. The National Drug Assistance Policy (PNAF) (66), formulated by the Ministry of Health in conjunction with the National Drug Policy, establishes that drug assistance is to be understood as a public policy guideline for the formulation of sectoral policies. To expand the population's access to drugs, incentives have been offered for the marketing of generic products (67), which cost an average of 40% less than brand-name products. As of 2006, 1,847 generic drugs had been registered, comprising 310 active substances in 91 drug classes produced by 66 laboratories. Of these registered products, 1,449 (79%) are now being manufactured domestically and 398 are imported, with India (51%) and Canada (16%) being the largest suppliers.

With regard to the production of immunobiologicals, public laboratories are primarily responsible for the production of the vaccines and sera used in public programs. Brazil produces vaccines against tuberculosis, measles, diphtheria, tetanus, pertussis, yellow fever, and human and canine rabies, and heterologous sera (snakebite, tetanus, diphtheria, and rabies antisera). Strengthening of public laboratories has been a priority in recent years: between 2002 and 2005, the federal government invested around R$ 200 million for that purpose. The Institute of Immunobiological Technology (Bio-Manguinhos), a unit of the Oswaldo Cruz Foundation (Fiocruz), is the largest supplier of vaccines for the Ministry of Health. In 2002 alone it produced more than 120 million doses—meeting nearly 60% of national public demand for vaccines. Together with other Brazilian public laboratories, Bio-Manguinhos supplies the SUS with immunobiologicals for the National Immunization Program.

Quality control of blood used for transfusions began in 1980, with the offering of incentives for voluntary donation and the establishment of a network of public blood centers. The use of blood and of human tissue, cells, and organs for treatment is regulated and monitored by the National Health Surveillance Agency (ANVISA) (68), which coordinates the National Blood Surveillance System, a nationwide system for gathering and assessing information on adverse or unexpected effects of blood products use. In 2006, the network included 33 coordinating blood centers and more than 2,000 blood therapy services registered with ANVISA. The blood centers work in association with universities and contribute to the training of specialized personnel and to scientific and technological development in this area.

Research and Technological Development in Health

Research and technological development in health are financed jointly by the Ministries of Health, Science and Technology, and Education. In addition, in some states there are foundations that receive state budget funding. The Ministry of Health carries out its activities of coordination, promotion, and development of research and technology through the Secretariat of Science and Technology and Strategic Inputs (SCTIE) and Fiocruz. The Secretariat of Science, Technology, and Innovation, a branch of the Ministry of Health (69), is responsible for setting guidelines and overseeing the assessment of technologies. It also seeks to introduce new products and processes through health decision-makers, providers, and professionals. To that end, in January 2006, the Ministry of Health put in place a procedure for the incorporation of technologies in the SUS. Brazil's investment in research and development as a proportion of GDP rose from 0.8% in 1996 to 1.0% in the period 2001–2003. The number of scientific articles by Brazilian authors published in LILACS increased from 5,916 in 2000 to 7,221 in 2003, and the number of articles in the MEDLINE database more than doubled between 1999 and 2003, increasing from 3,123 to 6,418.

Health Sector Expenditures and Financing

There are three major sources of funding for the Brazilian health system: the Government (through taxes and social security contributions collected by the three spheres of government), companies, and families. As Brazil does not have a system of local

health accounts, no accurate data are available on total expenditure (public and private) on health based on internationally comparable criteria. Nevertheless, the World Health Organization (70) estimates that in 2004 total health spending in Brazil amounted to 7.9% of GDP. Private expenditure accounted for 51.9% of that total, and out-of-pocket spending by families accounted for nearly 64% of private expenditure. Private spending on health includes expenditures by both families and companies, the latter through the provision or purchase of insurance plans or through health plans for their employees and their dependents, such coverage being voluntary, not mandatory. In 1996, 9% of consumer spending by families was devoted to health (37% for drug purchases, 29% for payment of health plans and insurance, and 17% for dental services). Spending by the richest segment of the population represented a significant portion of total health expenditure, while spending by the poorest decile constituted only a very small fraction. According to the Periodic Family Budget Survey, the three wealthiest deciles accounted for 68% of total health spending, while the poorest 30% accounted for just 7% (71). There are also qualitative differences in expenditure by the richest and poorest segments: while drugs constitute the main item of expenditure for the latter, among the highest-income deciles, health plans accounted for an increasing proportion of spending, although in all income deciles spending on drugs accounted for a considerable proportion of total health expenditures. In particular, in the poorest decile, 54% of health spending went to the purchase of drugs and 6% to payment for health plans, while in the wealthiest decile 24% of spending was for drugs and 33% for health plans.

The SUS is financed by public resources from the three levels of government. In 2004, the federal government contributed 50.7% of total funding for the SUS; the states and the Federal District, 26.6%; and the municipal governments, 22.7%. Resources for the federal government come from general taxes and social security contributions. In recent years, spending by the Ministry of Health has represented 9% of the total actual (nonfinancial) expenditure of the federal government. Of the social areas, health accounts for the second highest level of spending, exceeded only by social security. In 1995, the budget of the Ministry of Health was R$ 36.8 billion (in 2003 values). In 2003, R$ 30.8 billion was allocated to the Ministry of Health, close to 50% of which was transferred to states and municipalities for the implementation of health activities and services following consolidation of the process of health system decentralization. In 1995, in contrast, direct expenditures by the Ministry of Health accounted for 72% of its total budget and only 8% was transferred to subnational entities. There are important regional differences in the allocation of public resources for health: in 2002 per capita public spending in the Northeast region was R$ 168.43, while in the Southeast region the amount was R$ 250.56. Federal resources represented 62% of per capita public expenditure in the Northeast region and 49% in the Southeast region. Investment in health by the Ministry of Health in 2004 amounted to around R$ 1.9 billion, 5.1% of its total expenditure: 1.9% in direct investments and 3.2% in resources transferred for investment by states and municipalities.

Technical Cooperation and External Financing

Various programs are being carried out in Brazil with support from bilateral and multilateral cooperation organizations, including the Inter-American Development Bank; the World Bank; PAHO; the United Nations Population Fund; the United Nations Development Program; the United Nations Educational, Scientific, and Cultural Organization; and the European Union. Notable among these initiatives are three projects, one aimed at strengthening basic health care attention (Project for the Expansion and Consolidation of the Family Health Program [PROESF]), another at reorganizing health care for the indigenous population, and the third at enhancing disease surveillance [VIGISUS].

International cooperation stresses public health services and training, especially in the areas of disease management and prevention and control. This cooperation is either national in scope or it targets the states where the health situation is most precarious, particularly those in the Northeast region. The broad thematic areas for cooperation include: (1) reduction of infant and maternal mortality through promotion of women's and children's health and expansion of the Family Health Program; (2) improvement of the quality of health services through physical restructuring, strengthening of management, and training of human resources; and (3) improvement of access to health services and interventions.

Several international foundations are also active in Brazil, providing direct financing for projects or individuals in fields related to the Program of Action of the International Conference on Population and Development (Cairo, 1994) and to the achievement of the MDGs. PAHO technical cooperation in Brazil is based on rights, equity, gender, and life-course approaches (a new approach aimed at promoting neonatal care as part of a continuum of care for mothers, newborns, and children), evidence-based decision-making, and consonance with national policies. Through its communication and knowledge management activities, PAHO promotes integration of various technical areas, thus facilitating technical cooperation with the country.

Brazil also participates in cooperation initiatives in the Southern Hemisphere involving large amounts of financial resources. Several neighboring countries, including Bolivia, Colombia, Guyana, Paraguay, Peru, and Venezuela, are benefiting from control activities targeting endemic diseases such as malaria, schistosomiasis, leishmaniasis, tuberculosis, and leprosy, and from HIV/AIDS prevention activities. The MERCOSUR countries are currently engaged in intensive conversations aimed at establishing common health regulations. In addition, Brazil continues to provide support to the Portuguese-speaking countries of Africa and to East Timor.

References

1. Brasil, Portal do Governo Brasileiro. Available at: www.brasil.gov.br. Accessed on 26 May 2006.
2. Brasil, Programa das Nações Unidas para o Desenvolvimento. Relatório de desenvolvimento humano: Racismo, pobreza e violência; 2005.
3. Brasil, Programa das Nações Unidas para o Desenvolvimento. Atlas do desenvolvimento humano no Brasil 1991–2000; 2003.
4. Brasil, Instituto de Pesquisa Econômica e Aplicada. Objetivos de desenvolvimento de milênio, relatório nacional de acompanhamento; 2005.
5. Brasil, Instituto de Pesquisa Econômica e Aplicada. Sobre a recente queda da desigualdade de renda no Brasil; August 2006.
6. Ramos L, Ferreira V. Geração de empregos e realocação espacial no mercado de trabalho brasileiro: 1992–2002. Rio de Janeiro: IPEA; 2004.
7. Brasil, Instituto de Pesquisa Econômica e Aplicada. O Estado de uma nação: Capitulo III: Pobreza e exclusão social; 2005.
8. Brasil, Instituto Brasileiro de Geografia e Estatística. Síntese de Indicadores Sociais: Serie Estudos e Pesquisas Informação Demográfica e Socioeconômica, número 17; 2005.
9. Nações Unidas no Brasil. Uma leitura das Nações Unidas sobre os desafios e potencias do Brasil. Avaliação conjunta do país, August 2005.
10. Brasil, Instituto Brasileiro de Geografia e Estatística. Pesquisa Nacional por Amostra de Domicílios 2004. Segurança Alimentar; Rio de Janeiro; 2006.
11. Carrión F. De la violencia urbana a la convivencia ciudadana. In: Seguridad ciudadana, ¿espejismo o realidad? Quito: Facultad Latinoamericana de Ciencias Sociales; OPS/OMS; 2002. Pp. 13–19.
12. Brasil, Ministério da Justiça. Relatório descritivo. Perfil das organizações de segurança pública. Volume 1. Perfil das organizações estatais e municipais de segurança pública: corpos de bombeiros, forças armadas (2004), polícia militar (2004), polícia civil (2004), guardas municipais (2003). Brasília; 2006.
13. Brasil, Programa das Nações Unidas para o Desenvolvimento. Atlas Racial Brasileiro, 2005.
14. United Nations Children's Fund. World Declaration on the Survival, Protection, and Development of Children. New York; 1990.
15. Venâncio S, Monteiro C. A tendência da prática da amamentação no Brasil nas décadas de 70 e 80. Revista Brasileira de Epidemiologia. 1999; 1(1).
16. Brasil, Ministério da Saúde. Prevalência de aleitamento materno nas capitais brasileiras e no Distrito Federal. Relatório preliminar. Brasília; 2001.

17. Brasil, Ministério da Saúde; Rede Brasileira de Bancos de Leite Humano. Bancos de Leite Humano em Brasil. Available at: http://www.fiocruz.br/redeblh. Accessed in July 2006.

18. Brasil, Ministério da Saúde; Organização Panamericana da Saúde. Guia alimentar para crianças menores de 2 anos. Brasília; 2005.

19. Brasil, Ministério da Saúde. Saúde Brasil 2005: uma análise da situação da saúde. Brasília; 2005.

20. Brasil, Ministério da Saúde; Organização Panamericana da Saúde. Painel de indicadores do SUS. Año 1, Nº 1; 2006.

21. Costa MCN, Mota ELA, Paim JS, Silva LMV, Teixeira MG, Mendes CMC. Mortalidade infantil no Brasil em períodos recentes de crise econômica. Revista de Saúde Pública. 2003; 37(6): 699–709.

22. Brasil, Instituto Brasileiro de Geografia e Estatística. Pesquisa Nacional por Amostra de Domicílios (PNAD), 1999. Rio de Janeiro; 2000.

23. Brasil, Instituto Brasileiro de Geografia e Estatística. Censo demográfico 1991.

24. Brasil, Ministério da Saúde. Portaria Nº 1.395, 9 December 1999.

25. Brasil, Ministério do Trabalho e Emprego. Anuário Estatístico RAIS. Empregos por setor. Available at: http://anuariorais.caged.com.br/emprego.asp?tab=01&arq=Emprego1#. Accessed in September 2006.

26. Brasil, Serviço Social da Indústria. Perfil epidemiológico de fatores de risco para doenças não transmissíveis nos trabalhadores das indústrias do Brasil, resultados preliminares; 2006.

27. Alves AL, Barbosa RB. A saúde da população negra, realizações e perspectivas. Ministério da Saúde e Ministério da Justiça. Grupo de Trabalho Interministerial para Valorização da População Negra. Brasília; 1998.

28. Universidade de Brasília, Faculdade de Ciências da Saúde, Departamento de Saúde Coletiva. Manual de doenças mais importantes, por razões étnicas, na população brasileira afro-descendente. Mimeo, 102 p. Publicação elaborada sob o patrocínio do Ministério da Saúde. Brasília; June 2000.

29. Alves AL. Grupo de Trabalho Interministerial de Valorização da População Negra. Informe Epidemiológico do SUS, 1998.

30. Brasil, Presidência da República. Decree of 20 November 1995.

31. Brasil, Instituto Brasileiro de Geografia e Estatística. Pesquisa de Orçamentos Familiares (POF) 2002–2003. Análise da Disponibilidade domiciliar e estado nutricional no Brasil. Rio de Janeiro; 2004.

32. Brasil, Instituto Brasileiro de Geografia e Estatística. Pesquisa de Orçamentos Familiares (POF) 2002–2003. Primeiros Resultados. Rio de Janeiro; 2004.

33. Brasil, Ministério da Saúde; Instituto Brasileiro de Geografia e Estatística: Inquérito Domiciliar sobre Comportamentos de Risco e Morbidade Referida de Doenças e Agravos não Transmissíveis em 15 capitais brasileiras e no Distrito Federal 2002–2003; 2004.

34. Brasil, Instituto Brasileiro do Meio Ambiente e dos Recursos Naturais Renováveis. GEO-Brasil 2002. Perspectivas do Meio Ambiente no Brasil. 1ª ed. Brasília: IBAMA; 2002.

35. Brasil, Ministério da Saúde. Projeto Saúde Bucal Brasil. Levantamento das Condições de Saúde Bucal da População Brasileira; 2004.

36. Brasil. Leis Nº 8.080 e Nº 8.142, 19 September 1990 and 28 December 1990, respectively.

37. Brasil. Portaria GM Nº 399, 22 February 2006.

38. Brasil. Leis Orgânicas da Saúde: Nº 8.080 e Nº 8.142, 19 September 1990 and 28 December 1990, respectively.

39. Brasil, Ministério da Saúde, Conselho Nacional de Saúde. 12ª Conferência Nacional de Saúde, Relatório Final; 2003.

40. Brasil, Ministério da Saúde. Norma Operacional Básica do Sistema Único de Saúde (NOBs-SUS 01/93 y 01/96).

41. Brasil, Ministério da Saúde, Conselho Nacional de Saúde. Resolução CNS Nº 333/2003.

42. Brasil, Ministério da Saúde, Conselho Nacional de Saúde. Diretrizes Nacionais para Capacitação de Conselheiros de Saúde. Brasília; 1999.

43. Brasil, Ministério da Saúde, Conselho Nacional de Saúde. Resolução CNS Nº 354/2005.

44. Brasil, Ministério da Saúde, Secretaria de Atenção à Saúde. Departamento Nacional de Auditoria do SUS. Secretaria de gestão do Trabalho e da educação na Saúde. Curso Básico de Regulação, Controle, Avaliação e Auditoria da Atenção à Saúde do SUS: Noções básicas sobre os processos de apoio à gestão no âmbito da atenção à saúde. 1ª ed. Brasília: Série Cadernos da SAS; 2005.

45. Brasil, Ministério da Saúde. Portaria GM/MS Nº 1.107, 14 June 1995.

46. Brasil, Ministério da Saúde, Secretaria de Políticas de Saúde. Manual Brasileiro de Acreditação Hospitalar. 2ª ed. Brasília; 1999.

47. Brasil. Lei Nº 9.656, del 3 de junio de 1998; Medida Provisória N.º 1.665.

48. Brasil, Ministério da Saúde. Agência Nacional de Saúde Suplementar. Available at: www.ans.gov.br. Accessed in September 2006.

49. Brasil. Lei Nº 9.782, de 1999. [Some of its provisions were subsequently altered in October 2000.]

50. Brasil. Lei Nº 6.938, 1981.

51. Brasil, Ministério do Meio Ambiente. Available at: www.planalto.gov.br/paginas_governo/19.htm.

52. Brasil, Ministério do Meio Ambiente, Instituto Brasileiro do Meio Ambiente e dos Recursos Naturais Renováveis. Available at: www.ibama.gov.br.

53. Brasil. Portaria MS/GM Nº 2.607, 10 December 2004. Aprova o Plano Nacional de Saúde—Um Pacto pela Saúde no Brasil; 2004.

54. Brasil, Instituto Brasileiro de Geografia e Estatística. PNAD 2003, Suplemento de Saúde; 2003.

55. Brasil. Portaria Nº 8 de 29 de junho de 2004.

56. Brasil, Instituto de Pesquisa Econômica e Aplicada. Relatório Nacional de Acompanhamento dos ODM; 2005. Available at: http://www.ipea.gov.br/sites/000/2/estudospesq/odm/cap7.pdf. Accessed in July 2006.

57. Brasil, Instituto Brasileiro de Geografia e Estatística. Pesquisa Nacional de Saneamento Básico, PNSB 2000. Available at: www.ibge.gov.br/home/estatistica/populacao/condicao devida/pnsb/pnsb.pdf.

58. Brasil, Ministério da Saúde. Portaria Nº 710, 10 June 1999.

59. Viacava F, Souza-Júnior PR, Szwarcwald CL. Coverage of the Brazilian population 18 years and older by private health plans: an analysis of data from the World Health Survey. Cad Saúde Pública. 2005; 21(Suppl 1):S119–128.

60. Brasil, Instituto Brasileiro de Geografia e Estatística. AMS 2002.

61. Brasil, Ministério da Saúde. Rede Interagencial de Informações para a Saúde. Indicadores e Dados Básicos. Brasil, 2000 a 2005 (IDB 2000 a 2005). Available at: www.datasus. gov.br.

62. Brasil, Ministério da Educação. INEP. Censo Nacional da Educação Superior; 2000.

63. Brasil, Diretrizes de Política Industrial, Tecnológica e de Comércio Exterior; 2003.

64. Brasil, Federação Brasileira da Indústria Farmacêutica, Departamento de Economia; 2006. Available at: http://www.febrafarma.com.br/.

65. Brasil, Ministério da Saúde. Portaria Nº 3.916, 30 October 1998.

66. Brasil, Ministério da Saúde, Conselho Nacional de Saúde. Resolução Nº 338, 6 May 2004.

67. Brasil. Lei Nº 9.787, 1999.

68. Brasil. Lei Nº 10.205, 21 March 2001.

69. Brasil. Portaria Nº 1.418/GM, 24 July 2003.

70. Organización Mundial de la Salud. 2002–2004. Available at: www.who.int/nha/country/BRA.

71. Brasil, Instituto Brasileiro de Geografia e Estatística. Pesquisa de Orçamentos Familiares 1995–1996.

BRITISH
VIRGIN ISLANDS

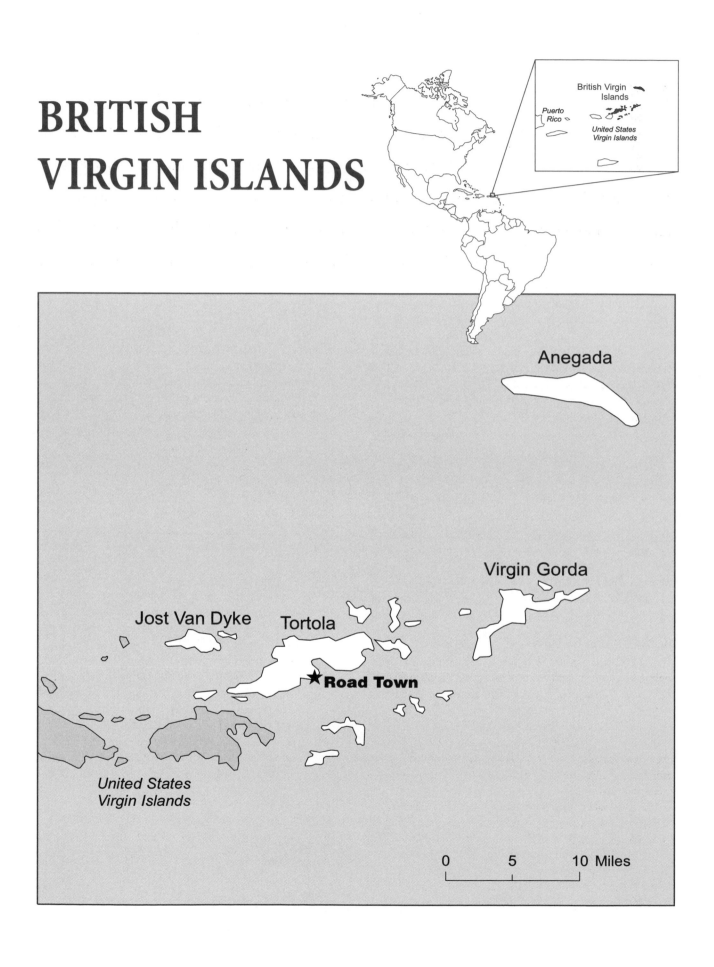

British Virgin
Islands

Puerto
Rico

United States
Virgin Islands

Anegada

Virgin Gorda

Jost Van Dyke

Tortola

★ Road Town

United States
Virgin Islands

| 0 | 5 | 10 Miles |

The British Virgin Islands is a cluster of about 50 islands, cays, and rocks strewn over 3,445 mi^2 in the northeastern corner of the Caribbean Sea, east of Puerto Rico. The British Virgin Islands' total land area is 154 km^2. Of the 15 inhabited islands, the largest are Tortola (56 km^2), where Road Town, the capital, is located; Anegada (39 km^2); Virgin Gorda (22 km^2); and Jost Van Dyke (8 km^2). Topography varies from extremely flat land in Anegada to mountainous and rugged terrain on Tortola, which has the highest point, Mount Sage, rising 543 m above sea level.

GENERAL CONTEXT AND HEALTH DETERMINANTS

The British Virgin Islands is an overseas territory of the United Kingdom with internal self-government. A 13-member Legislative Council is democratically elected. The Queen appoints a Governor to represent her and exercise reserve powers on behalf of the Crown. The Governor, in turn, appoints the Executive Council ministers: a Chief Minister, who is the head of government; an Attorney General (an ex-officio member); and four other government ministers. The Executive Council is chaired by the Governor. The Governor acts on the advice of the Executive Council. Because the territory is so small, there is no need for a local government. District officers with administrative functions have been appointed for Virgin Gorda, Jost Van Dyke, and Anegada.

Social, Political, and Economic Determinants

The British Virgin Islands uses the US$ as currency (one of only three dependent territories of the United Kingdom that do). GDP grew by an average of 9% annually between 1991 and 2001. GDP at current market prices was estimated at US$ 765 million in 2000 and US$ 830 million in 2003. Nominal per capita GDP in 2001 reached US$ 35,954. GDP produced by the financial services sector grew by an average of 23% between 1991 and 2001. Tourism grew by 12% annually over the same period and now accounts for 14% of GDP.

The financial services sector is the major contributor to the economy (38% of GDP), and accounts for more than half of the government's revenue. Since the enactment of the 1984 International Business Ordinance Act and the 1990 International Business Company Act and its subsequent amendments, the financial sector has steadily grown—more than 650,000 companies had been incorporated by the end of 2005. The International Business

Company is the designated venue for initiating international business ventures and is responsible for the expansion of various sectors in the financial services industry, such as the management of insurance, mutual funds, trusteeships, and companies. The Business Companies Act of 2004 (which went into effect in 2005) removed the differential tax obligations that existed between companies conducting business locally and internationally, while providing flexibility and choice in a larger range of corporate products such as restricted, purposed, and segregated portfolio companies. The British Virgin Islands is a major jurisdiction for the incorporation of mutual funds. At the end of 2005 a total of 3,724 mutual funds were registered or recognized. The British Virgin Islands continues to be an extremely conservative banking jurisdiction. At the end of 2005, 8 banks were authorized to conduct business in or from within the territory. In the area of fiduciary services, 117 general trust licenses and 119 restricted trust licenses were issued. The territory also provides ship registration services. At the end of 2005, 2,531 ships had been registered.

Tourism is the next major contributor to the territory's economy. The figure of 2,500 visitors per day set by the cruise ship policy is often exceeded, because multiple, large-capacity cruise ships often dock simultaneously. Government infrastructure projects and commercial and residential developments continue to fuel activity in the construction industry.

The current labor force is around 11,700, 95% of whom are employed. The unemployment rate remained constant at 3.6% in 2001–2005. The unemployment rate for women in 2003 was 3.4%, compared to 3.8% for men. In 2001 there were 15,227 persons older than 15 years of age; of the 13,543 persons employed in this age group, 48% were males and 52% were females. These figures remained constant in 2002. The five leading employers in 2001 were public administration and social security (4,742), followed by hotels and restaurants (2,164), construction (1,071), education (1,382), and wholesale and retail trade (1,050).

The population living in poverty[1] in the British Virgin Islands in 2003 hovered around 22% of the population (16% of households). Indigence is nearly absent.

With few exceptions, the poor in the British Virgin Islands did not exhibit characteristics typically associated with poverty. Housing characteristics and other indicators such as access to water and electricity supply and overall health levels are little different from those of non-poor households. In addition, school enrollment for 5–16-year-olds among the poor neared 100%. Many poor households also owned assets such as vehicles, telephones, washing machines, refrigerators, and stereos, and had access to services such as cable TV at levels comparable to those in non-poor households (for example, 20% of poor families have cell phones and more than one-third have computers). Almost 30% of poor households also owned land that they considered to be developable and which represented a potential source for additional funds.

More than 80% (95% if single elderly households are excluded) of poor households have at least one person working; just under one-half have two or more working members. Unemployment, although higher than among not poor households, was only 11%, but workers from poor households tend to be less skilled. The minimum wage (US$ 4/hour) provides sufficient income for adults working full-time to exceed the poverty line. The elderly living on their own made up virtually all of poor households with no one working. This subgroup had little income generating potential, and depended on the government, their families, or NGO assistance for support.

Single-parent households made up one-fifth of all poor households, although it should be noted that more than 70% of them are not poor. The more serious matters dealing with unstable family relationships are issues such as family and marital problems, domestic and spousal violence, single parenting, and teenage pregnancy or motherhood.

There was little evidence that children were seriously affected by lack of income. Their health was generally good, school enrollment was nearly universal, and there was no evidence of malnutrition. The main problems have to do with children's welfare, particularly when parental relationships break up.

The British Virgin Islands has 26 primary schools, 16 public and the remainder private. School attendance is compulsory up to age 15 years, and the average length of school attendance is 9.4 years; most students complete 12 years of combined primary and secondary education, however. There are four public secondary schools and one private. Adult literacy rates in 1998–2000 were 98.3% for females and 97.8% for males.

The British Virgin Islands currently generates more than 80 tons of solid waste per day during the peak tourist season and less than half that at other times of the year. In 2004, waste generated on Tortola, Jost Van Dyke, Virgin Gorda, and Anegada amounted to approximately 31,964 tons. In 2004, 26,506 tons were delivered to the incinerator plan compound; 5,458 tons were delivered to sister island dumpsites to be used as landfill.

As of this writing, there is no government-run public transportation system; vehicle ownership rates are high, however, and private transportation services are readily available. A fairly extensive network of roads provides access to all settlements. Inter-island transportation is mostly by ferry, although limited air taxi services are available to Virgin Gorda and Anegada.

The major source of potable water is cisterns (each home is required to have one before it can receive planning approval for construction) and wells. Two companies produce reverse-osmosis, desalinated water distributed by Tortola's Water and Sewerage Department in Tortola, which supplies about 75% of the population on that island. The remainder of the population relies on cisterns. Virgin Gorda has its water supplied by two systems, one at North Sound and the other at The Valley. Municipal public water supplies also are available on Anegada and Jost Van Dyke. Bottled water is imported or locally produced by at least five companies that bottle and distribute locally. Several hotels operate their own seawater desalination plants.

Tortola's food establishments continue to increase. In 2000 there were 237 food establishments, increasing to 278 in 2003 and representing a growth of 17.3%. During the first three quarters of 2003, 176 food premises were inspected: 143 were found to be satisfactory. Major problems involved improper food thawing practices, poor maintenance, improper storage of food and utensils, and inadequate screening of buildings to keep away insects and other pests.

Hurricanes and seismic activity pose the greatest threats to the British Virgin Islands, as the territory lies in the expected path of Atlantic hurricanes. No major storms or hurricanes affected the territory during 2001–2005. In November 2002, major flooding affected many low-lying and coastal areas, damaging property and causing minor damage to the road infrastructure. Although no major incidents have occurred since then, the potential for flash flooding in low-lying and coastal areas remains an area of concern, particularly during periods of very heavy and prolonged rainfall. The islands are also prone to disasters caused by humans, such as exposure to hazardous chemicals, explosions, and transportation accidents. Oil spills are considered to be the greatest manmade threat to the British Virgin Islands.

Demographics, Mortality, and Morbidity

The population of the British Virgin Islands is highly concentrated in the working age group (45–64-year-olds); fewer than half of households had children and only 14% contained an eld-

---

[1]The poverty definition is set on the basis of indigence lines (based on minimum food requirements) and poverty lines (minimum food requirements plus an element of non-food expenditure), and is derived according to the Caribbean Development Bank's (CDB) methodology. The indigence line for an adult is US$ 1,700 per annum; the poverty line for an adult is US$ 6,300 per annum.

erly person. In 2002, the estimated population was 20,987, with persons under 15 years old accounting for 24.9%. Persons 15–44 and 45–64 years old comprised 47.6% and 22.4% of the general population, respectively, while those 65 years and older accounted for 5.1% of the population. The total population in 2004 was 21,689—11,152 were men and 10,537 were women.

Population growth was most marked in the age group 45–64 years old, which almost doubled between 1991 and 2004. This is the population group likely to have the highest incidence of early stage noncommunicable disease and most likely to benefit from secondary (and to some extent primary) prevention efforts. The aging of the population can be clearly seen by a comparison of population pyramids from 1991 to 2005 (see Figure 1).

The British Virgin Islands depends heavily on migrant labor and this group influences the distribution of the population. In 2004, immigrants accounted for more than 50% of the population (11,269). Migrant labor contributes to the bulge in the 19–45-year-old group in the territory's population pyramid. Employment by nationality is as follows: nationals, 44%; immigrants from other Caribbean countries, 43%; and other non-nationals, 13%. The Government provides just under 30% of all employment; most of the remainder is provided by private employers, and only 13% of workers are self-employed. Non-nationals dominate the private sector (70% of employed) although they also fill one-third of all government jobs. While they are strongly represented in all occupations, they are more likely to be employed in the less skilled occupations. They especially fill the ranks of employees in hotels, construction, trade, and domestic services (more than 60%).

Life expectancy at birth remained constant at 75.1 years in 2001 and 2002, and at 73.8 years in both 2003 and 2004. In 2001–2004, life expectancy at birth for males was 73.2 in 2001, 76.6 in 2002, 78.9 in 2003, and 69.9 in 2004. For females it was 77.7 for 2001, 75.9 for 2002, 75.9 for 2003, and 78.5 for 2004.

In 2003, the crude birth rate was 12.6 births per 1,000 population, rising to 14.7 births per 1,000 population by 2004. The total number of births increased from 267 in 2003 to 318 in 2004, an increase of 18%. The total fertility rate averaged 1.5 children per woman in 2003, slightly dropping to 1.4 in 2004.

Chronic diseases, their complications, and consequences are the major causes of morbidity and mortality in the territory. Cancers, hypertensive diseases, diabetes, cerebrovascular accidents, and coronary artery disease consistently have been the leading causes of death and hospital admission in the territory. In 2004, 23 patients were admitted to the hospital for diabetes and 15 for hypertension. Use of dialysis increased, with the primary contributing factor to renal failure being diabetes. Diabetic leg ulcers and diabetic foot problems are also a concern. Accidental injuries, including drowning, and mental health disorders are two other major causes of morbidity and mortality in the territory. Diabetes, hypertension, arthritis, and mental disorders were among the significant reasons persons gave for seeking care at the community health clinics in 2001–2004.

FIGURE 1. Population structure, by age and sex, British Virgin Islands, 1991 and 2005.

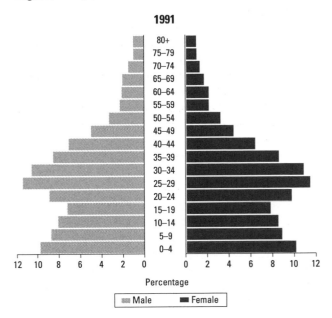

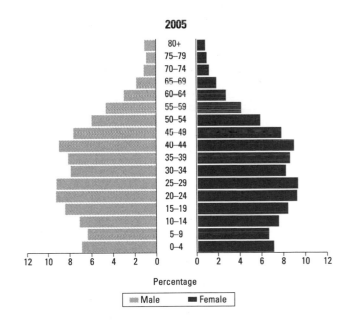

There were 422 deaths in 2001–2004. The number of total annual deaths varied from 101 in 2001 to 120 in 2004, representing crude death rates of 4.9 to 5.3 deaths per 1,000 population for the period. There were no maternal deaths during the reporting period. The five leading causes of death in this period were hypertensive disorders, malignant neoplasms, drowning, coronary artery disease, and pulmonary embolism. In 2003–2005, malignant neoplasms ranked first, followed by hypertensive diseases. Specific causes within the five broad causes included ischemic heart disease, diabetes mellitus, cerebrovascular diseases, and accidental drowning and submersion. In 2003 the leading causes of death in males were malignant neoplasms (17), hypertensive diseases (10), drowning and submersion (6), ischemic heart disease, (6) and alcoholic liver disease (2). The leading causes of death in females in that same year were malignant neoplasms (6), hypertensive disease (11), drowning and submersion (1), alcoholic liver disease (2), and diabetes mellitus (2).

HEALTH OF POPULATION GROUPS

Children under 5 Years Old

In 2001, children in this age group represented 8.5% of the population (20,647); in 2004 they represented 8.1% of the population (21,689). Coverage of the Expanded Program on Immunization (EPI) in 2004 for this age group was as follows: BCG, 100%; polio, 90.97%; DPT, 90.61%; and measles and MMR, 100%. In 2001–2005, the national immunization program's schedule included BCG, DPT, HepB, Hib, OPV, and MMR vaccines. Coverage of this highly successful program reached more than 90% of children with all recommended vaccinations during the first 12 months of life.

In that same period, there were 23 perinatal deaths, 2 neonatal deaths, and 4 infant deaths. The breakdown of annual perinatal deaths during the period was six deaths each in 2001 and 2002, one death in 2003, and five deaths each in 2004 and 2005. Causes of death related to labor and delivery included complications of placenta, cord, and membranes; birth asphyxia; and neonatal aspiration of meconium. Prenatal causes of death in the same period included hypertensive disease during pregnancy, placental abruption, and intrauterine infection, accounting for 7 of the 23 (30%) deaths; conditions originating in the perinatal period accounted for 8 of the 23 (35%) deaths; and genetic and other abnormalities accounted for 8 of the 23 (35%) deaths.

In 2001, of 126 hospital discharges in this age group, the major cause of discharges was elective circumcision (53), followed by asthma (20), neonatal jaundice (11), pneumonias (11), gastroenteritis (9), viral infection (7), and external causes (5).

There were 1,477 live births in 2001–2005. In 2004, there were 316 live births, 22 (7.0%) of which were low-birthweight babies. That same year, there were three stillbirths. In 2005, there were 282 live births and 6 stllbirths; of these, 18 (6.4%) were low-birthweight babies.

Children 5–9 Years Old

In 2001, this age group represented 9.0% of the population. There were no deaths in this age group that year. Of the 58 hospi-

tal discharges in this age group, the leading discharge diagnoses were asthma (18), elective circumcisions (14), fracture of the forearm (6), and gastroenteritis (5).

Adolescents 10–14 Years Old

Adolescents in this age group represented 8.6% of the population in 2001 (20,647). There were no deaths in this age group that year. Of the 43 hospital discharges in this age group, the leading discharge diagnoses were asthma (9), sickle cell disease (8), viral infections (6), elective circumcision (4), appendicitis (4), and bronchopneumonia (4). There were two deliveries to 14-year-old mothers. All children entering high school are given full medical screenings.

Young Adults 15–24 Years Old

This age group represented 14.5% of the population in 2001. There were two deaths in this age group in 2001, one due to pneumonia and the other to external causes. There were 57 hospital discharges in this age group; the leading discharge diagnoses were unspecified abortions (15), viral infections (5), mental and behavioral disorders due to alcohol use (5), appendicitis (5), acute asthma and pneumonia (3), and motor vehicle accidents (3).

Pregnant women attend prenatal clinics up to 32 weeks of pregnancy, after which they are referred to Peebles Hospital, where deliveries are usually performed. A significant number of women go to the United States to deliver their infants, although the figure varies considerably from year to year. There were 25 deliveries in the age group 15–19 years old.

There is an active family planning program that is part of the community health services. Available family planning methods include condoms, oral contraceptives, injectable contraceptives, and intrauterine devices. Diaphragms and contraceptive foams and jellies were phased out by 2006 due a decline in use and increased promotion of condoms. Pap smears are offered as part of the Community Health Services' family health program.

Adults 25–64 Years Old

This age group represented 54.4% of the population in 2001 (20,647). There were 33 deaths in the age group. The leading causes of mortality in 2001 were hypertensive diseases (6), malignant neoplasms (4), drowning and submersion (6), ischemic heart disease (3), external injuries (4), and renal failure (1). There were 325 hospital discharges in this age group in 2001; the leading discharge diagnoses were unspecified abortions (31), deep vein thrombosis (27), malignant neoplasms (24), sickle cell disease (22), and leiomyoma of the uterus (21). There were two AIDS-related deaths in this age group in 2001.

Older Adults 65 Years Old and Older

Adults 65 years and older represented 4.9% of the population in 2001. There were 53 deaths in this age group. The leading causes of mortality were malignant neoplasms, mainly in the prostate, cervix, gastrointestinal tract, and lungs (16); hypertensive disorders (15); ischemic heart disease (3); diabetes (3); cerebrovascular accidents (3); and pneumonia (2). Of the 97 hospital discharges in this age group in 2001, the leading discharge diagnoses were malignant neoplasms (17), congestive heart failure (15), cataracts (12), diabetes (10), and hypertension (22).

The Family

More than half the adult population are immigrants, mainly from other Caribbean countries; one-half of them have been residents of the British Virgin Islands for at least 10 years. One in five households are "mixed," having at least one adult from the territory and one from another country, twice as many household as in 1991. This implies that the integration of non-national residents in households is on the rise. One-third of households are exclusively composed of British Virgin Islands nationals; the rest (46%) are exclusively composed of non-nationals. Household size has remained virtually unchanged, at 2.9 persons per household on average, since 1991. One-half of the British Virgin Islands' households have one or two persons living in them; only 16% have five or more. Mixed households tend to be larger than exclusively British Virgin Islanders or exclusively non-British Virgin Islander households. One in eight households is headed by a single parent; one in seven has an elderly person; and under half include children, half of which have no adult male present.

Persons with Disabilities

According to the Development Planning Unit within the Chief Minister's office, 4.4% of the population of the British Virgin Islands has some form of disability, including mental retardation (4.6%) and reported mental retardation and sight (12.6%), hearing (3.1%), and speech (2.9%) impediments. Slightly more than 59% of the disabled are females, 80% had education levels at or below primary level, and 24% were formally employed.

The Esylen Henley Richard Children Center is the main facility providing care for children with special needs. A volunteer group, the Friends of Esylen Henley Richard, provides funds for meals and helps to arrange medical care. BVI Services is a vocational rehabilitation program established in 1982 to assist disabled adults reincorporate into the society through occupational therapy and training. Social security invalidity benefits are payable to insured persons who have become permanently unable to work or who have received sickness benefits for at least 26 weeks and have been issued a medical certificate attesting that they are likely to remain incapacitated. Benefits are dependent on a minimum number of contributions to the scheme.

HEALTH CONDITIONS AND PROBLEMS

COMMUNICABLE DISEASES

Vector-borne Diseases

Dengue is the vector-borne disease of greatest concern in the territory. There were no cases of dengue or dengue hemorrhagic fever reported to the Ministry of Health in 2004; there was one case of dengue fever in 2005. The house index of *Aedes aegypti* mosquitoes ranged from 1.2 to 3.2 in 2002, compared to 1.7 to 1.8 in 2003. In 2004, the house index for *Aedes aegypti* ranged between 0.77 and 1.5. There were no cases of **malaria** or **yellow fever** in 2001–2005.

Vaccine-preventable Diseases

There were no confirmed cases of **polio, diphtheria, rubella, measles, mumps,** or **neonatal tetanus** between 2001 and 2005. There were also no confirmed cases of *Haemophilus influenzae meningitis* during the period. The territory's Expanded Program of Immunization (EPI) is a component of the Family Health Program. Under the program, children under 1 year old receive BCG, hepatitis B, DPT, Hib, and OPV vaccines. Children 1 year old receive MMR, DPT, and polio vaccines; boosters are given according to the immunization schedule up to 11 years of age.

Acute Respiratory Infections

In 2001–2004, acute respiratory infections represented an important proportion of communicable diseases reported to the Ministry of Health. In 2001, there were 308 cases of acute respiratory illness in children under 5 years old, compared to 179 in 2004. Reported **influenza** cases ranged between 1,283 in 2001 to 120 in 2004. In 2002, one case of **tuberculosis** was confirmed in a person with a history of an extended visit to Guyana. A full course of treatment was completed. In 2004 two cases were confirmed, both of which were among residents who spend only part of the year in the territory. Both completed a full course of treatment. No cases were reported in 2003 or 2005.

HIV/AIDS and Other Sexually Transmitted Infections

The first case of AIDS was reported in the territory in 1985. By the end of 2005, there were 62 reported cases of HIV infection (33 males and 29 females). Of these, 21 males and 14 females have died. In 2005, 27 persons were living with HIV/AIDS and receiving antiretroviral therapy; 9 were cases of HIV infections without AIDS (4 males and 5 females) and 18 were AIDS patients (8 males and 10 females). Of those receiving antiretroviral therapy, ten were receiving care overseas. The predominant mode of transmission was heterosexual contact (43), followed by homosexual contact (5), blood-borne (2), mother-to-child (1), and not reported (11). The age distribution of persons with HIV/AIDS is 25 to 35 years (9), 35 to 65 years (15), and over 65 years (3).

Zoonoses

There were no reported cases of zoonotic diseases in 2001–2005.

NONCOMMUNICABLE DISEASES

Cardiovascular Diseases

In 2001, cardiovascular diseases accounted for 21 of 126 (16.7%) hospital discharges; 12 deaths that year were due to cardiovascular diseases. **Ischemic heart disease** was the leading contributor, with eight deaths, and **hypertensive heart disease** and **cardiomyopathy** accounted for two deaths each. In 2004, 15 of 84 deaths were attributable to cardiovascular disease; the main contributors were ischemic heart disease (8 deaths), cardiomyopathy (4), and hypertensive heart disease (3).

Malignant Neoplasms

In 2001, malignant neoplasms accounted for 41 of 126 (32.5%) hospital discharges. In that same year, 20 of 97 (20.6%) deaths were due to malignant neoplasms. Prostate cancer accounted for 6 of the deaths, followed by cancer of the gastrointestinal tract (3), lung cancer (2), and female genital tract cancer (2). In 2004, 28 of 84 deaths (33.3%) were due to malignant neoplasms, with prostate cancer accounting for 5, followed by gastrointestinal tract cancer (13), breast cancer (3), and cancer of the female genital tract (1).

OTHER HEALTH PROBLEMS OR ISSUES

Mental Health and Addictions

In 2004, there were 69 hospital admissions of psychiatric cases at Peebles Hospital (47 males and 22 females); 102 new psychiatric cases were registered at the Ministry of Health's Mental Health Division. The active patient case load by the end of 2004 was 500. Services provided at the Mental Health Division include psychometric assessment, psychotherapy, and management of the Crisis Intervention Team.

According to results from the 2002 National Secondary School Survey, 97% (960) of the 991 respondents attended public schools; the remainder were enrolled in private schools. There was a greater proportion of female students (55.8%) among those surveyed. The study found that one in every six students (18.3%) had tried cigarettes in their lifetime, one in every 26 (3.9%) had tried them in the 12 months prior to the survey, and only 1.3% had smoked cigarettes in the month before the survey. Alcohol rated highest of any drug category surveyed: six of every 10 students (61.6%) reported having tried alcohol in their lifetime, almost one in three (38.1%) reported having used alcohol in the past year, and about one in five (21%) reported having used alcohol in the month prior to the survey. Marijuana was by far the most frequently used illicit substance (including inhalants). Lifetime use of cocaine and crack cocaine was very low overall (reported by only eight students), and reportedly used exclusively by males. Students also reported very little lifetime use of tranquilizers or stimulants.

Violence and Other External Causes

The number of violent crimes averaged two murders, six attempted murders, and five reported cases of rape per year throughout 2001–2005. In the same period, there were 6,179 road traffic accidents, 14 of them fatal and 975 resulting in injuries.

Oral Health

The Dental Service Unit, which is part of the Community Health Services, monitors fluoridation in primary schools and provides dental health services to the population at large. Between 2001 and 2004 the number of annual extractions ranged from 257 to 303, and the number of restorations ranged from 1,213 to 1,469. In 2004, there were 1,383 tooth fillings and 257 teeth extractions performed, for a 5:1 ratio of teeth filled to teeth extracted. There are two government dentists based on Tortola; they also provide dental services once a week on Virgin Gorda and once a month on Anegada.

RESPONSE OF THE HEALTH SYSTEM

Health Policies and Plans

The Ministry of Health and Social Development is charged with executing the government's national health policy, as established in the Public Health Act, Cap 194. In 2005, with the passage of the British Virgin Islands Health Services Act, the British Virgin Islands Health Services Authority was established. As a result, the role of the Ministry will shift from that of provider of services to that of procurer of services. Following the Ministry's general policy direction, the Health Services' Board answers to the Ministry in regard to the delivery of health services.

In accordance with the 1976 Public Health Act, which provides the statutory framework for protecting and promoting the population's health, government health services are provided free at the point of use to certain groups, including full-time schoolchildren, nursing mothers, the elderly, the mentally ill, the indigent, health workers, firefighters, the police, prisoners, and prison officers. Given the low user fees and a poor fee collection scheme, the health system does not generate revenues, and the Government is forced to heavily subsidize it. In 2006, the Government began to explore the design of a national health insurance scheme to improve the inflow of revenue into the system.

The Government's health priorities, as stated in the 2003–2007 legislative agenda, are: improving health care and social services by insuring access to health services for every citizen on all islands; reaching out to those at risk; improving access to health care by completing the hospital annex, working towards the completion of the new hospital, installing the hospital board, upgrading clinics, and exploring options for training and attracting more local doctors and nurses; and meeting social challenges by exploring a national mobile pension plan, developing a national health insurance plan, and strengthening unemployment benefits.

The legislative framework for environmental management was revised in 2001–2005. The 2000 Derelict Vehicle Ordinance regulates and authorizes the removal of derelict vehicles from roads or public places and sets a schedule of fines for handling the vehicles; the Merchant Shipping Act (2001) was established to control oil pollution; the Slaughterhouses Act (2001) is designed to regulate the establishment and control of Government abattoirs and other slaughterhouses; the 2001 draft Labor Code is designed to allow labor inspectors to act in cases where safety and health are threatened.

The territory's regulatory framework on food safety needs strengthening to include provisions for setting standards, monitoring, and incorporating up-to-date criteria to promote food safety.

Organization of the Health System

The Ministry of Health and Social Development is responsible for providing health and social services, as well as for monitoring and regulating health providers. The Permanent Secretary is responsible for the Ministry's administration and also provides support to the Minister in his policy role. The Director of Health Services is the chief technical adviser on health matters.

The territory has a dynamic and expanding private health sector, encompassing both inpatient and ambulatory care. Private health care facilities include Bougainvillea Clinic, specializing in plastic surgery; four private dental surgeries; seven private medical clinics; and nine private physician offices. It is estimated that about 50% of local medical consultations are in the private sector. Many residents seek care off-island, mainly in the United States Virgin Islands or Puerto Rico, either by choice or because they require specialized care unavailable locally. British Virgin Islands residents also have access to specialist care in the United Kingdom, which is arranged through the International Division of the United Kingdom's Department of Health.

Public Health Services

Public sector primary care services are offered at the British Virgin Islands' 10 health clinics and 2 health posts: Road Town Health Center and seven other clinics on Tortola, two on Virgin Gorda, and one each on Jost Van Dyke and Anegada. The Road Town Health Center serves as a referral point for the district clinics. The clinic in The Valley, on Virgin Gorda, is staffed by two physicians; the clinic at North Sound is staffed by a resident nurse supported by The Valley clinic physicians. The clinic on Jost Van Dyke is staffed by a nurse practitioner, and the clinic on Anegada, by a public health nurse; both clinics are visited regularly by a physician. The clinics on Tortola and Virgin Gorda are adequately staffed and function well; the others are understaffed.

Catchment populations fluctuate, depending on the arrival of tourists and temporary residents such as yacht dwellers, who may seek care through the public health services.

District clinics provide a full range of child health services, including growth and nutritional monitoring, development assessment, treatment of common illnesses, counseling, school health, and screening for anemia, including sickle cell anemia. District clinics also offer another range of services, including maternal and child health clinics, special chronic disease clinics, treatment of common illnesses, nutritional counseling, and school health services. A voluntary screening program for prostate cancer began in 2000 and continues to operate. A Community Health Pharmacy Program was established in 2002—a community health pharmacist is stationed at Road Town Clinic and also provides services to Virgin Gorda and to East End and West End on Tortola.

The Environmental Health Division of the Ministry of Health is responsible for food hygiene; vector control; water quality surveillance; hygiene in institutions; and investigation of complaints such as septic tank problems, rodent infestations, and abandoned vehicles.

The two main instruments that deal with sewage disposal in the territory are the Public Health Ordinance and the Public Health Regulation (Nuisances). Both need to be amended to be able to regulate the use of holding tanks in yachts and the discharge of sewage effluents from ships and yachts. The Water and Sewerage Department is responsible for providing public sewerage services in the British Virgin Islands. A sewerage system currently serves Road Town, with waste being collected and pumped through an outfall located on Tortola. Cane Garden Bay, on Tortola's western end, is also served by two sewerage systems that include a secondary treatment plant. In addition, some hotels have sewage treatment plants that produce water for garden irrigation. Most of the rest of the territory relies on individual septic tanks and soak-away systems. Poor soil percolation has led to sewage disposal problems in the East End/Long Look community on Tortola; a sewage collection and treatment system is being implemented in that area.

The Environmental Health Division administers a water quality surveillance and institutional hygiene program designed to protect residents and tourists from water-borne disease outbreaks and ensure that public institutions adhere to a basic standard of sanitation. The inspection of schools and water supply systems is a major component of the program. In 2003, 105 samples were taken and analyzed; 25 of them were contaminated and subsequently treated with chlorine.

The vector control program targets mosquito-borne diseases in the British Virgin Islands. The outputs outlined were improved quality of work and reduction of the house index from current levels. The goal to reduce the incidence of mosquito-borne diseases was achieved. Other activities included are conducting training sessions for workers, providing workers with protective equipment, and fogging areas with a house index of 2% and above.

The food safety program of the Environmental Health Division conducts regular inspections of food production and distribution outlets. Clinics for food handlers were conducted at Road Town, Virgin Gorda, Jost Van Dyke, and Anegada, which included lectures on the use of "ServSafe" materials and the hazard analysis and critical control point (HAACP) approach. Some of the sessions were held at the larger food establishments.

The Community Nutrition Unit and the Hospital Dietary Unit together provide nutrition and dietetic services. At the community level, the nutrition program is run by a nutritionist based at the Road Town Public Health Clinic and who also provides scheduled services to the clinics at Anegada, Capoon's Bay, East End, Jost Van Dyke, Long Look, and Virgin Gorda. Services include nutrition consultations for persons requiring both normal and therapeutic diet therapy, nutrition surveillance, and nutrition screening among vulnerable groups (e.g., 0–5-year-olds and senior citizens) to aid in program planning and for research. The Unit also is involved in the development and implementation of nutrition education programs to promote healthy lifestyles and nutrition projects to help to assist in the fight to reduce the incidence of noncommunicable chronic diseases.

The Community Nutrition Unit works with public health nurses; school health, health promotion, environmental health, and mental health units; and with the Social Development and Education Department. The Caribbean Food and Nutrition Institute, headquartered in Jamaica, provides invaluable technical cooperation to complement the national nutrition programs.

The Department of Disaster Management's mission is to reduce loss of life and property due to disasters by ensuring that adequate preparedness and mitigation measures are in place and that response and recovery mechanisms are established to offset the impact of natural and technological hazards. A health disaster coordinator post was established in the Ministry of Health and Social Development in 2003 to coordinate health disaster mitigation efforts. The Department operates under the 2003 Disaster Management Act.

Individual Care Services

The British Virgin Islands has one 44-bed public hospital—Peebles Hospital—and one 8-bed private hospital—Bougainvillea Clinic, both located in Road Town. Peebles Hospital offers inpatient specialist services in obstetrics and gynecology, internal medicine, pediatrics, general surgery, ophthalmology, and psychiatry. Eleven medical specialists and nine general practitioners are employed at the hospital. Bougainvillea Clinic offers mainly general medical, primary care, and surgical services.

Peebles Hospital's physical plant is currently undergoing major development. Construction of a 120-bed hospital is scheduled to commence late in 2006. An annex building housing a refurbished accident and emergency department, imaging services, medical diagnostic laboratories, the dialysis unit, and office space was completed in 2006. This annex serves as a transitional facility to relieve cramped services in the current hospital.

In 2001–2005 there were 10,746 admissions at Peebles Hospital, and the average length of stay for all wards was 5.8 days; the bed occupancy rate averaged 52.2%. Hospital admissions in the period ranged from 2,200 in 2001 to 2,131 in 2005 at Peebles Hospital. Bed occupancy rates increased steadily from 61% in 2001 to 63% in 2004. In 2005 occupancy rates were 72%. Total inpatient days also steadily rose, increasing from 9,865 in 2001 to 11,540 in 2005.

There were 23 medical emergency evacuations from the island in 2005, compared with 26 in 2004, with conditions ranging from childbirth to road traffic accidents. Cases that could be dealt with by the nurse were triaged and appropriate care was given at the clinic.

The national blood bank service is located at the Peebles Hospital medical diagnostic laboratory. The laboratory relies on the Caribbean Regional Standards for blood banking.

There were 343 blood donations in 2004, compared to 318 in 2003. All blood for transfusion is screened for HIV, hepatitis B, and syphilis. All donations are collected on a voluntary basis and there is no remuneration for any donation.

Programs aimed at improving the management of both communicable and noncommunicable diseases are available through the Community Health Services and Peebles Hospital. Hypertension and diabetes clinics are conducted on Tortola at Road Town, Iris Smith-Penn (East End), and Capoon's Bay clinics, and on Virgin Gorda at North Sound and Iris O'Neal clinics.

The dialysis unit was upgraded to eight stations in 2005; currently there are 19 persons receiving dialysis. Pathology services and diagnostic radiological services, including x-rays, ultrasound, and mammograms, are also available in the public sector. CAT scans are available in the private sector; patients who require MRIs travel to Puerto Rico or the United States Virgin Islands. Patients requiring tertiary care are referred to Puerto Rico, Jamaica, Barbados, the United States, and the United Kingdom.

The Mental Health Division within the Community Health Services is the lead agency providing mental health services in the British Virgin Islands. The central office is located in Road Town, and it provides outpatient mental health care through its outreach psychiatric services. It receives referrals from a broad cross section of agencies and the general public.

The incorporation of new values and beliefs led to the redefinition of the Mental Health Unit as a coordinated service covering all psychiatric clients, including those with substance abuse

The British Virgin Islands' Migrant Workers

Immigrants seeking work account for more than half of the British Virgin Islands' population; many of them stay on for years, even for decades. The British Virgin Islands relies heavily on this migrant labor force. Non-nationals dominate the ranks of private-sector employment and fill about one-third of Government jobs. They tend to work in less skilled occupations, mostly as employees in hotels, construction, trade, and domestic service. With migrant workers being disproportionately represented among 19–45-year-olds, the health system must address both the problems of the younger migrant population and those of the older British Virgin Islands national population.

problems. The Unit's mission is to provide a comprehensive range of services to assist the people of the British Virgin Islands in achieving their fullest potential and optimal level of mental wellness. The territory's mental health service approach emphasizes treating individuals in their communities, including monitoring and administering medication, providing family counseling, and promoting self-care.

Mental health services are directed by a psychiatrist who also manages the inpatient care of psychiatric patients at Peebles Hospital. The mental health team includes a clinical psychologist, a school psychologist, three mental health officers, and three orderlies.

The mental health team visits the hospital, the prisons, and geriatric homes as required. Mental health officers also travel regularly to outer clinics in Tortola, Virgin Gorda, Jost Van Dyke, and Anegada. Psychiatric patients are admitted to Peebles Hospital Medical Ward. There are only two secured rooms on the medical ward and non-disruptive patients are admitted to the general medical ward.

Health Promotion

In 2003, the Health Education Division was reorganized to become the Health Promotion Unit. It provides leadership and strategic direction for the development, coordination, and integration of health promotion programs aimed at improving the health and quality of life of the people in the British Virgin Islands. The unit delivers programs that focus on promotion of health and wellness, and also emphasizes behavior modification and lifestyle changes, targeting vulnerable groups such as primary and secondary school children and young adults, as well as community groups.

The main objective of the Dental Health Services is to provide optimum lifetime dental health for all British Virgin Islands citizens by providing and maintaining services directed towards limiting and preventing the occurrence, progression, and recurrence of dental disease. Preventive strategies include a school-based program to administer fluoride rinse to children aged 3 to 13 years on a weekly basis. Schoolteachers conduct the program,

and a Dental Division dental hygienist provides periodic monitoring. In 2004, a program was started to provide each kindergarten and primary-school child with a toothbrush each school term; the program was terminated due to lack of funding. Fluoride toothpaste is also made available in the schools. Schoolchildren are regularly checked during the dental hygienist's regular visits to the roughly 20 public and primary schools for dental caries and other dental-oral abnormalities and referred when necessary for treatment. The dental hygienist instructs the children on oral hygiene, home care, diet, nutrition, and brushing techniques, sound dental health, and the development, progression, and prevention of dental caries.

Human Resources

There were 45 physicians practicing in the British Virgin Islands as of December 2005. Of these, 29 work in the public sector and the remainder in the private sector. As of the end of 2005, there were six registered dentists in practice, two in the public sector and four in the private sector. Medical and dental practitioners are registered by the British Virgin Islands Medical and Dental Council.

There are 121 registered nurses employed in the public sector; 24 of them work in Community Health Services and 97 at Peebles Hospital. There is no nursing school in the territory, so nurses are principally trained in other Caribbean islands, the United States Virgin Islands, or the mainland U.S. Nurse recruitment is primarily from other Caribbean countries. In 2004, the Government launched the Health Scholarship Program to recruit young people into the health professions. Under this initiative, special scholarships were offered in medicine, nursing, pharmacy, radiography, and medical technology.

Health Supplies

There is no local production of drugs, vaccines, or medical equipment. The Peebles Hospital Pharmacy is the central purchasing agency for the public health services. Drugs are purchased through the Organization of Eastern Caribbean States

Pharmaceutical Procurement Service Unit. Some drugs that are not included in the Unit's formulary are purchased directly from private suppliers. The Unit's formulary is revised every two years. Narcotics are not available at district clinics. Private sector practitioners make their own arrangements to purchase drugs. A certificate from the Director of Health Services is required to import narcotics into the territory; all other drugs used in the private sector are purchased independently and are not regulated by the Government. The Peebles Hospital Pharmacy supplies pharmaceuticals to the district health centers (primary care units). There are privately owned pharmacies in Tortola and Virgin Gorda. The Medical Act (2000) requires that a registered pharmacist be present at both private and public pharmacies. Standardized treatment protocols for conditions such as asthma, eclampsia, hypertension, and gastroenteritis are available.

Vaccines are purchased through the Pan American Health Organization (PAHO) Revolving Fund. When urgently needed, some vaccines are purchased through a vendor in Barbados. Some vaccines are provided at no cost to private sector practitioners as a way to boost vaccination coverage. A limited number of vaccines are ordered directly by the private sector.

Most of the equipment, including laboratory, x-ray, ultrasound, and dialysis, is located at the public hospital. CT scan and mammography are available in the private sector; there also are three private medical diagnostic laboratories in the private sector. Maintenance employees at Peebles Hospital have received biomedical technology training from the suppliers; service contracts also are maintained with some suppliers.

Health Sector Expenditure and Financing

Public health care currently is financed mainly through the Government's annual budget allocations to the health services, by out of pocket payments, and by insurance reimbursements. The Government is actively investigating the development of a National Health Insurance scheme to increase access and share risk. Private health care is financed by out of pocket payments and private insurance. There is a growing sector of the population that accesses care overseas. This is generally funded by private insurance, out of pocket payments, and Government assistance to those requiring overseas tertiary care. User fees generally raise only 8% of the hospital and primary-care operating costs. In 1997, expenditures on public health services (hospital and primary health services only) were US$ 7.14 million, with hospital services accounting for 65.5%. By 2004, the total figure had increased to US$ 16.89 million, with hospital services accounting for 69%. Total private health expenditure, including out of pocket insurance payments, was estimated to be US$ 10.5 million.

The budget for hospital and primary care services represented 7.8% of the national budget and has ranged from 6.6% to 7.5% between 1999 and 2004. The budget for solid waste management rose from US$ 2.38 million in 1997 to US$ 3.42 million in 2003. Total health expenditure as a percentage of GDP stood at 2.4% in 1999 and rose to 3.1% in 2004. Total per capita spending on health is estimated at US$ 1,050 in 2004, up from US$ 760 in 1999.

Capital investments in health between 2004 and 2005 have included the construction of Peebles Hospital Annex, helipads for emergency medical evacuation, and a new municipal incinerator on Tortola. A compulsory social security scheme covered all paid employees, with employees and employers contributing equally to the premiums; some persons are covered 100% by the government. Self-employed workers are also required to participate in the plan. The social security benefits include maternity, occupational injury, unemployment, old-age pension, sickness, and survivor's benefits, as well as a funeral grant.

Technical Cooperation and External Financing

The Ministry of Health and Social Development currently benefits from technical assistance provided by several regional and international health institutions, including the Pan American Health Organization (PAHO), which provides access to World Health Organization technical resources and manages the revolving fund for purchasing vaccines for the Expanded Program on Immunization. The Caribbean Epidemiology Center (CAREC) provides support in epidemiology and medical laboratory. The Caribbean Health Research Council (CHRC) promotes research on diseases and health issues important to the territory by developing national capacity to conduct essential national health system and services research. The Caribbean Environmental Health Institute (CEHI) provides technical assistance in the field of environmental health. The British Virgin Islands' Medical and Dental Council participates in meetings of the Caribbean Association of Medical Councils (CAMC). CAMC was established by CARICOM to help ensure the quality of doctors practicing in the Caribbean after the University of the West Indies medical schools stopped being accredited by the United Kingdom's General Medical Council. The Caribbean Regional Drug Testing Lab (CRDTL) provides quality testing of pharmaceuticals for the territory. The Organization of Eastern Caribbean States Pharmaceutical Procurement Service (OECS PPS) provides drugs to the territory at considerable cost savings realized by the pool procurement of drugs for nine Eastern Caribbean countries.

Bibliography

British Virgin Islands, Chief Minister's Office, Development Planning Unit. Development Planning Statistics 2000.
British Virgin Islands, Health Services Authority, Community Health Services. Annual Reports 2001–2004.

British Virgin Islands, Ministry of Health and Social Development, Environmental Health Division. Unit Reports 2001–2004.

British Virgin Islands, Ministry of Health and Social Development. Health Services and Systems Profile 2003–2004.

British Virgin Islands, Ministry of Health and Social Development. National Development through Health Improvements: A Multi-Sectoral Partnership. Draft. 2006.

Caribbean Development Bank; Government of the British Virgin Islands. Country Poverty Assessment: The British Virgin Islands, 2003. Halcrow Group Limited; 2003.

Caribbean Epidemiology Centre, Caribbean Drug Information Network (CARIDIN). National Secondary School Survey. The British Virgin Islands 2002. Integrated Risk Behaviour: Drug Consumption and Sexual Behaviour. 2002.

CANADA

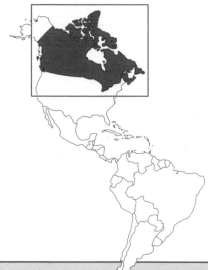

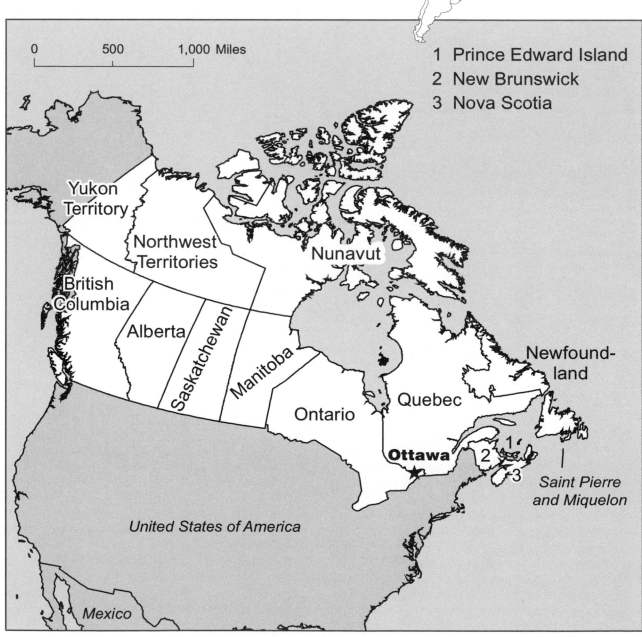

0   500   1,000 Miles

1 Prince Edward Island
2 New Brunswick
3 Nova Scotia

Yukon Territory

Northwest Territories

Nunavut

British Columbia

Alberta

Saskatchewan

Manitoba

Ontario

Quebec

Newfoundland

Ottawa

Saint Pierre and Miquelon

United States of America

Mexico

In the 1990s, Canada's economy underwent rapid and profound changes, largely shaped by the global economy. Growth in the late 1990s was dominated by sectors such as high-tech and auto manufacturing and information and communications technology services. These sectors slowed since 2001, in favor of long-neglected areas such as construction, resources, health, and education.

GENERAL CONTEXT AND HEALTH DETERMINANTS

In 2005, the country's real gross domestic product (GDP) growth was stable at 3%. Owing to the high corporate profits and surpluses, Canada also posted the largest gain in business investment over the last three years. The surge in commodity prices and exports in turn helped push the exchange rate up from US$ 0.65 early in 2003 to US$ 0.86 in late 2005, the most rapid currency shift in the country's history.

The thriving energy and mining sectors helped to drive unemployment to 30-year lows, especially in western Canada. While other regions did not benefit as much, they did fare well in their own right. Quebec's unemployment hit a 30-year low of 8.3%, while Ontario experienced a 1.3% gain in employment, with the unemployment rate being less than a point above its record low of 5.8% set in 2000.

Its sheer size has allowed Canada's economy to weather repeated shocks in recent years, ranging from the stock market decline between 2000 and 2002, to the attacks in the United States on 11 September 2001, to the recent exchange rate and energy price surge. By comparison, much discussed health events such as the SARS epidemic or the mad-cow disease crisis have had little impact on the economy.

Social, Political, and Economic Determinants

In 2002, Canada supported the agreement to achieve the Millennium Development Goals, defined under the Monterrey Consensus. Developing countries assumed primary responsibility for them, while industrialized countries, including Canada, committed themselves to support the former's efforts through aid, trade, and debt relief. Among the most salient indicators reported for Canada by the United Nations are the following: net school enrollment for both sexes increased from 97.0% in 1999 to 99.5% in 2001 (97.0% to 99.7% for girls; 96.9% to 97.3% for boys); the share of women in wage employment in non-agricultural sectors increased from 48.8% in 2001 to 49.4% in 2004; the percent of seats held by women in national parliament has remained steady at 20.6% since 2001; the percentage of children inoculated against measles dropped from 96% in 2001 to 95% in 2004; the percent of married women between the ages of 15 to 49 years using contraception has remained at 75% in the period under review; the proportion of the population using safe drinking water and improved sanitation was 100% in urban settings and 99% in rural ones; the net official development assistance as a percent of the GDP declined from 0.25% in 2004 to 0.24% in 2005.

A focus on health promotion, public health, and population health aims to improve the health of the entire population and to reduce health inequities among population groups (1).

The economic growth in 2001–2004 discussed earlier also has led to several improvements in conditions of low-income families and individuals (see Table 1). Fewer than 8% of families composed of two or more persons had low incomes in 2004, down from under 10% in 1999. Similarly, approximately 36% of single-parent families headed by women had low incomes in 2000, compared to 39% five years earlier. The percentage of children living in low-income families also has consistently fallen since 1996; in 2001, it was at its lowest (12%) since 1980. Table 1 shows the percentage of families below the low-income cutoff, by family type. Since 2001, however, low-income rates for children have remained essentially unchanged (just under 13% in 2004).

The trends in the distribution of household income, on the other hand, have shown a rise in inequality in disposable income. From 1995 to 2004, the average income of families in the highest economic quintile rose by approximately 26%. The rise in income of the families in the lowest economic quintile, however, has been more modest, just under 13%. The dollar gap between these two income groups increased by 30% between 1995 and 2004 (2).

Major health disparities also have been detected. For example, of Canadian men living in cities, those in the highest income quintile live five years longer than do those in the lowest income quintile; the men in the highest income bracket also were about one-quarter less likely to die of heart disease. These health disparities are differentially distributed among specific populations (such as among Aboriginal peoples), by gender, by socioeconomic status, by educational attainment and income, by geo-

TABLE 1. Percent of families below the low-income cutoff, by family type, Canada, 1996, 1998, 2002, and 2002–2004.

Family type	Year					
	1996	1998	2000	2002	2003	2004
Families of two persons or more	12.1	10.1	9.0	8.6	8.5	7.8
Senior families	3.3	3.9	3.1	2.9	2.7	2.1
Non-senior couples without children	8.4	6.7	6.9	7.1	6.6	6.2
Two-parent families with children	10.8	8.5	8.3	6.5	6.7	6.7
Single-parent families headed by females	52.7	42.9	36.3	39.4	38.8	35.6
Single persons	37.3	35.1	32.9	29.5	29.6	29.6

graphic location, and by other markers of disadvantage or inequality of opportunity (3).

Health disparities most affect Aboriginal peoples in the lowest socioeconomic quintile. Because they are more often and more severely sick or injured, people in the lowest income quintile use approximately twice as much health care services as those in the highest income quintile. Approximately 20% of total health care spending may be attributable to income disparities. In contrast, middle-income households utilize 8.1% of health care spending (4).

Women also face a higher incidence of poverty than men, and this social factor leads to an increased risk to health. Single mothers are at particular risk: the great majority are low-income (81% vs. 15% of partnered mothers); more than half experience food insecurity (54% vs. 10%); and 40% experience violence, compared to 7% of partnered mothers (4).

Canadian rural residents are more likely to be living in poorer socioeconomic conditions, to have lower educational attainment, and to exhibit less healthy behaviors. For all age groups up to 64 years, the mortality risks for all causes were higher in rural than urban areas (5).

Canada has been affected by various disasters during the reporting period, including forest fires, a hurricane, and serious winter storms. The frequency of flood disasters also is increasing in the country. Snowmelt accounts for about 40% of all floods in Canada, although they are also caused or compounded by heavy rainfall, ice jams, glacier outbursts, coastal storms, tsunamis, cyclones, and hurricanes.

The most commonly measured outdoor air pollutants in Canada include ground-level ozone, particulate matter, carbon monoxide, sulphur dioxide, and nitrogen oxides. According to 73% of Canadians, air and water pollution are the most significant risks to health.

The Canadian Medical Association estimated that there were 5,800 premature deaths due to air pollution in 2005 in Ontario, and projected that the figure will increase to 10,000 premature deaths by 2026 unless effective steps are taken to reduce smog. In 2005, air pollution in Ontario was estimated to cost in excess of Can$ 1 billion in direct health care costs and lost productivity. In

British Columbia, the Provincial Officer for Health estimated that in 2004, air pollution in the province caused between 140 and 400 premature deaths, 700 to 2,100 hospital stays, and between 900 and 2,750 emergency room visits that year.

The highest human exposure to persistent organic contaminants in Canada tends to be among the northern populations. Aboriginal peoples tend to have greater exposure because they rely on traditional foods that have high levels of contaminants, such as mercury. Research has revealed significantly higher levels of mercury in maternal blood of Inuit women compared to Caucasian, Dene people, or Métis.

Demographics, Mortality, and Morbidity

There are at least four salient factors influencing health care delivery: the aging of the population; differences in health service needs in urban, rural, and remote populations; cultural diversity resulting from high rates of immigration; and Aboriginal health (6).

In 2003, individuals aged 65 years old and older made up 12.8% of the population compared to 7.9% in 1970; this group is projected to represent 20% of the population by 2025. (See Figure 1 for the country's population structure in 1991 and in 2001.)

The total fertility rate declined from 2.3 children per woman in 1970 to approximately 1.5 in 2002, and the birth rate declined from 17.5 births per 1,000 population to 10.7 per 1,000 for the same two years, respectively (6).

According to data from the Department of Agriculture and Agri-Food Canada, in 2001, 79.4% of Canadians lived in urban areas with a population of 10,000 or more, up from 78.5% in 1996; the remainder lived in predominantly rural regions, with the three northern territories and five provinces having more than half of their populations living in predominately rural regions (7). Rural population segments that live far from metropolitan centers present enormous challenges to the delivery of health care in terms of range, quality, and cost of services offered. Canadians in these regions suffer lower health status, while having greater difficulty accessing even basic primary health care services, much less specialized health care services (6).

FIGURE 1. Population structure, by age and sex, Canada, 1991 and 2001.

1991

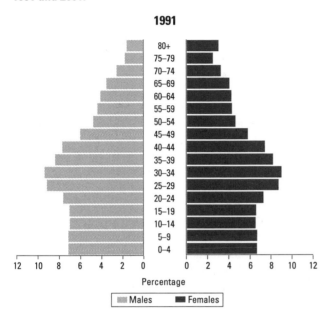

2001

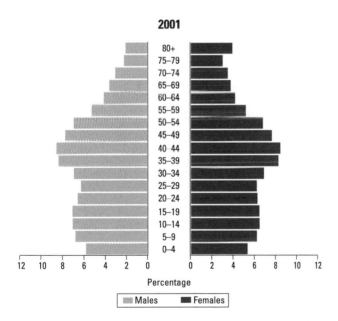

High immigration to Canada after the Second World War also has created a culturally diverse population. Based on the 2001 census, 18.4% of Canadian residents were born outside the country, a majority of whom came from non-English-speaking and non-French-speaking countries. Most recent immigrants come from outside Europe and do not speak English or French as their first language.

Canadians and new immigrants were highly mobile between 2002 and 2004. Most of the provinces and territories had net gains from migration. Relative to its population, Ontario registered the largest net gain with 10.4 new immigrants for every 1,000 population, or 127,300 people in total. British Columbia was second, with a net gain of 10.2, while Alberta was third with 8.3. Nunavut registered the largest net decline relative to its population, losing 5.1 residents per 1,000 population, although the absolute numbers were small.

Among metropolitan census areas, Toronto had the highest net inflow of people, with Vancouver ranking second, followed by Montreal. These three metropolitan areas attracted about three-quarters of the international immigrants. About 65% of the people who moved into Toronto during 2003–2004 came from outside the country, as did 50% of those who moved into Vancouver and 48% of those who moved into Montreal. Without these immigrants, these urban centers would have incurred a net outflow of people during the past several years. With this population concentration in the largest cities, pressure is placed on the health care facilities to provide services in ways that can overcome cultural and linguistic barriers (8).

Canadians reporting some Aboriginal ancestry made up 4.4% of the country's total population in 2001. Almost 50% of Aboriginal[1] Canadians are recognized First Nations people living on or off reservations. A further 26% are non-status Indians, many of whom are concentrated in urban areas; about 30% are Métis living mainly in western Canada, and 5% are Inuit who live in the Arctic regions of Canada (6). Approximately 45% of First Nations peoples are under 20 years old.

Aboriginal health status indicators, such as life expectancy and infant mortality, have been improving over the past 20 years. Aboriginal peoples do suffer disproportionately from chronic diseases and conditions such as diabetes, hypertension, heart disease, tuberculosis, HIV infection, and fetal alcohol syndrome, however. In addition, according to 2004 information from the Canadian Institute for Health Information, the death rate due to injuries and poisoning is four time higher for First Nations people and Inuits than for the overall Canadian population.

Life expectancy for Aboriginal women is 5.2 years less than the national average; Aboriginal men can expect to live 7.4 fewer years than the national average. And although they represent only 2% of Canada's total population, First Nations persons have 7.2% of the national HIV/AIDS cases. The incidence of diabetes also is three to five times higher than the national average, and suicide among young Aboriginals between the ages of 10 and 19 years is 4.3 times higher than for the rest of the country; among the Inuit it is 11 times higher for all ages.

As a result, Aboriginal Canadians account for higher use, and higher cost, of health care services than other Canadians. The

---

[1]Most of the information provided relates to First Nations and Inuit populations, which fall under Health Canada's jurisdiction. The overall Aboriginal population in Canada, unless specified in the text, is not included in the data contained in this publication.

broader social determinants of health, including relative poverty and marginalization, are significant factors that lead to the poorer health outcomes of Aboriginal Canadians relative to other Canadians, and to a consequent greater use of public health care services (6).

In 2004, the crude birth rate edged downward to a record low—despite a second straight increase in the number of live births. The crude birth rate was 10.7 live births per 1,000 population in 2003 and 10.5 in 2004. Rates appear to have stabilized, with the crude birth rate hovering around 10.5 to 10.7 since the start of the new millennium.

The number of births increased in 5 of 13 jurisdictions: Alberta, Nova Scotia, Ontario, Quebec, and Yukon. Labrador and Newfoundland had the largest relative decrease in births (–3.0%), similar to its annual average decline of 2.8% in the number of births throughout the 1990s.

Trends in province-to-province migration, as well as in inflows of international migrants, have a major impact on the number of births in the provinces. In Labrador and Newfoundland, for example, a contributing reason for the decline in births is outmigration to other provinces, especially among men and women aged 20 to 29 years, which has not been offset by immigration from outside the country or from other provinces.

Studies show that immigrants have higher fertility rates compared with Canadian-born women, but they decline to levels of Canadian-born women by the second generation.

Mothers are getting older in Canada. In 2004, women aged 24 years and younger made up 20.6% of all women giving birth that year—one-half of the 40.7% figure seen in 1979. The bulk of the births now occur among women aged 25 to 34, with this age group accounting for 62.1% of all births in 2004, compared with 54.7% in 1979. In 2004, the average age of women giving birth in Canada was 29.7 years.

In addition, the percentage of all births to older mothers—women aged 35 years and older—was almost four times that of a generation earlier. These older mothers accounted for 17.2% of all births in 2004, nearly four times the percent from a quarter century earlier of 4.6%. Migration also is driving the trend towards older motherhood. The average age of mothers who gave birth in the province or territory in which they themselves were born was 29.0 years in 2004, compared with 30.1 years for Canadian migrants and 31.1 for international immigrants. Immigrating women and men may be delaying marriage and childbirth while settling in a new area and re-establishing social networks.

According to data from the Organization for Economic Cooperation and Development, the country's total fertility rate in 2004 was unchanged from the 2003 rate of 1.53 children per woman. The record-low total fertility rate for Canada was set in 2000, at 1.49 children per woman.

Canadian women also are increasingly likely to be having their first child in their thirties. According to information from Statis-

tics Canada, more than one-third (34.7%) of births to Canadian women in their thirties in 2004 were first births.

In 2003, combined life expectancy at birth for both men and women reached a record high—79.9 years. That same year, life expectancy at birth for women was 82.4 years and for men it reached a high of 77.4.

The widest gap between male and female life expectancy in the last quarter century was in 1979, with a 7.4 years difference. From 1979 to 2003, the gap narrowed, as life expectancy for men improved by 6.0 years, while life expectancy for women improved only by 3.6 years. Life expectancy in 2003 for both sexes combined was highest in the provinces of British Columbia and Ontario.

The number of deaths has been on an upward trend for several years, the result of a growing and an aging population. Between 2002 and 2003, the figure rose by 1.2%. In those same years, Canada's population grew by 1.0%. The number of deaths rose in every province and territory, except in Prince Edward Island, Quebec, and the Yukon, where the number of deaths declined.

Life expectancy also improved for Canadian seniors. In 2003, life expectancy for those 65 years old improved for both men and women—on average, men that age could expect to live an additional 17.4 years, while women that age could expect to live an additional 20.8 years. In 2002, the comparable figures were 17.2 years for men and 20.6 for women. The gap between the two sexes remained the same, at 3.4 years.

As can be seen in the following section, improvements in infant mortality are a clear indication of the excellent state of health care in the country. As also will be seen, however, infant mortality rates vary considerably within Canada's borders.

HEALTH OF POPULATION GROUPS

Children Under 5 Years Old

The infant mortality rate declined from 5.4 infant deaths per 1,000 live births in 2002 to 5.3 in 2003. This decrease was due to a reduction in the number of deaths among infants aged 7 to 364 days, which fell by 4.0% in 2003 to 668, compared with 696 in 2002, while the mortality rate declined from 2.1 deaths per 1,000 births to 2.0.

The mortality rates for infants under 1 day old and for infants aged 1 to 6 days old remained unchanged at 2.5 and 0.7 deaths per 1,000 births, respectively. The male infant mortality rate was 5.7 deaths per 1,000 male births in 2003, while the rate for females was 4.8.

Infant mortality rates are substantially higher in northern areas and in regions with large Aboriginal populations. Nunavut, Canada's newest Arctic province, had the highest rate of infant mortality, averaging 14.9 deaths per 1,000 live births between 1999 and 2003. British Columbia was lowest, with an average of

4.08 infant deaths in the same period. This reflects the relatively low income and difficulty in accessing health resources in northern regions. Urban centers generally experience a lower incidence of infant mortality than rural areas.

The leading causes of death for infants in 2003 were congenital anomalies, sudden infant death syndrome, and low birthweight and its associated complications. Congenital anomalies caused a significant proportion (46%) of infant morbidity and mortality, as well as fetal mortality. With the advent of preventive measures such as food fortification with folic acid, promotion of the use of multivitamins containing folic acid in the periconceptional period, pre-pregnancy immunization against rubella, and interventions to reduce alcohol and drug use during pregnancy have greatly improved perinatal and infant health.

First Nations infants are more likely to be born pre-term, yet have heavier birthweights than non-First Nations infants. This is the case in the country's rural and urban areas. In addition, in 2003, infant mortality rates were more than twice as high among First Nations than in non-First Nations people. Post-neonatal mortality rates were 3.6 times as high.

According to the Canadian Hospital Injury Reporting and Prevention Program, in 2002 25,796 children aged 1 to 4 years old were treated for injuries. The most common cause of injury was activity-related (43% of all treatment and hospitalization); 67% of these injuries occurred at home.

Data from the National Longitudinal Survey of Children and Youth, as reported by parents, show that in 1994/1995, 42% of children aged 6 months to 5 years were in some form of childcare. Over the subsequent six-year period, the childcare rate increased steadily to more than one-half of children (53%) by 2000/2001.

Children 5–9 Years Old

Children aged 5 to 9 years make up 5.8% of Canada's population; 963,000 are male and 919,300 are female.

The leading causes of death for school-aged children are injury and cancer. Injuries accounted for almost half the reported morbidities of this group. Motor-vehicle fatalities dropped sharply, with 79 children aged 5–14 dying in vehicle accidents in 2004, down from 120 in 2000. Incidence rates of childhood cancers have remained stable over the past 18 years, with leukemia (3.8 new cases per 100,000 children per year), brain tumors (2.9 per 100,000), and lymphoma (1.4 per 100,000) being the most commonly diagnosed cancers in the age group.

According to police reports, children and youth are victims of sexual assaults to a disproportionate degree. Although they represent only 21% of the population, 6 out of every 10 sexual assaults reported to police involve a child or youth. Children in this age group also were victims in 21% of all physical assaults and 17% of all other crimes involving violence or the threat of violence reported to police in 2003.

Food allergies are an important health problem that affects children predominantly, with up to 8% of Canadian children suffering from food allergies.

Adolescents 10–14 and 15–19 Years Old

While the majority of Canadian adolescents considered themselves to be in "very good" or "excellent" health in 2000/2001, nearly one in three 12–17-year-olds rated their health as no better than "good," according to a 2003 Government study.

Adolescents who considered their health to be poor, fair, or good were more likely to smoke, drink, or be obese. They also were less likely to live in high-income households. The study also found that the lower the adult educational level in the adolescent's household, the worse his or her self-rated health was likely to be.

Boys' self-perceived health tends to be better than that of girls. According to data from the 2000/2001 Canadian Community Health Survey, girls' perceptions of their health become less favorable in mid-to-late adolescence. At ages 12 to 14 years, 73% of both boys and girls reported excellent or very good health. But by ages 15 to 17 years, while the percentage of boys reporting very good or excellent health remained about the same, the percentage of girls reporting so dropped to 66%.

The prevalence of smoking in Canada has reportedly declined among both men and women across all age groups, but the sharpest decrease was among young people aged 12 to 17 years, among whom it fell from 14% in 2000/2001 to 10% in 2003, and to 8% in 2005. The youth smoking rate has declined primarily because of the decreasing numbers of young people who initiate smoking. In 2000/2001, 73% of youth reported that they had never smoked cigarettes. By 2005, the proportion had hit 82%. As a result, there may be further declines in smoking rates among older age groups as today's youth move into adulthood.

An estimated 12% of boys and 13% of girls reported having had sexual intercourse by ages 14 to 15 years. In 2003, over one-quarter (28%) of 15–17-year-olds reported having had sexual intercourse at least once in their lives. By ages 20 to 24, the percent was 80%. About 3 in 10 young people who had sex with multiple partners in the past year had not used a condom the last time they had intercourse. (Sex without a condom was reportedly even more common at older ages—nearly 44% of sexually active 20- to 24-year-olds reported sex without a condom, compared with 33% of those aged 18 to 19 years, and 22% of those aged 15 to 17 years.)

According to data from the Canadian Community Health Survey, 4% of 15–24-year-olds who reportedly had had sex at least once also reported having been diagnosed with a sexually transmitted infection. The true figure is likely higher than that reported, possibly because of a lack of symptoms or awareness. Early age at first intercourse also increased the risk. Those who reportedly had had sexual intercourse by age 13 were more than twice as likely to report a sexually transmitted infection than were those who had waited until they were older to have sexual intercourse.

At ages 12 or 13 years, 26% of boys and 31% of girls reported that they had tried smoking cigarettes. Over the previous two years, more than one-quarter of this group reported that they had had intercourse.

Marijuana use was most prevalent among young people, and its use peaked in the late teens. Close to 4 out of every 10 teens aged 18 to 19 years reported having used marijuana or hashish in the past year. The proportion among 15–17-year-olds was about 3 in 10.

Adults 20–64 Years Old

This group represents the largest proportion of Canada's population, and its mortality and disease patterns vary extensively.

Canadian adults have much higher suicide rates than younger groups. An average of 282 suicides were counted in 2002 for ages 20–34, while an average of 438 were counted for 35–54-year-olds.

In 2004, nearly one-quarter (23%) of adult Canadians were obese. An additional 36% (8.6 million people) were overweight. These people tended to spend their leisure time in sedentary pursuits and ate vegetables and fruit infrequently. Obese adults were at increased risk of high blood pressure, diabetes, and heart disease. Rates of overweight and obesity vary by income, but the relationship is different when the data are disaggregated by sex. According to 2004 information from the Canadian Institute for Health Information drawn from the report "Improving the Health of Canadians," the likelihood of being overweight or obese increases with income among men: 61% of men with annual incomes of Can$ 80,000 or more were overweight or obese, compared with 49% of men who earned Can$ 15,000 or less. The opposite trend is true for women, however, where only 34% of women with incomes of Can$ 80,000 or more were overweight or obese, compared with 43% in the lowest income category.

Men and women also differ in health-related habits. Women were more likely than men to consider overall health, weight, and specific diseases when choosing the food they consumed. In a 2004 Health Canada study, 80% of women were concerned about maintaining or improving health through food choice, compared with 63% of men. While 59% of women considered their weight when selecting foods, just 41% of men did so. And about 48% of women considered the relationship between food and heart disease, compared with only 38% of men.

Individuals aged 45 to 64 are generally in better health than were those in the same age group two decades ago, according to data from the 1998/1999 National Population Health Survey and the 1978/1979 Canada Health Survey.

During the past 20 years, the prevalence of arthritis or rheumatism, high blood pressure, heart disease, and bronchitis or emphysema has decreased in this age group. These trends suggest that efforts in disease prevention and health promotion, along with improvements in the treatment of disease, have contributed to improved health in this group.

Adults living in rural Canada were slightly more likely than those in urban areas to have difficulty finding a regular medical doctor in 2003, according to data from the Canadian Community Health Survey. About 5.5% of individuals in rural areas had difficulty, compared with 4.5% in urban areas. Of the 1.2 million people who reported that they were unable to find a doctor in 2003, 273,000 lived in rural areas and 965,000 lived in urban areas.

Older Adults

In 2005, 74% of seniors assessed their health as good, very good, or excellent, compared to 70% who did five years earlier. Better-educated seniors were more likely to have fewer health problems than have less educated seniors.

However, Canada's roughly four million seniors aged 65 or older, which represent 13% of the total population, are heavy users of the nation's health care system. Seniors account for one-third of all hospitalizations and more than one-half of all hospital days. According to the 2003 Canadian Community Health Survey, 88% of seniors reported consulting a general practitioner or a family doctor at least once during the year before the survey, compared with 76% of people aged 12 to 64 years. Moreover, 92% of seniors reported having taken at least one type of medication in the previous month, 14% reported having been hospitalized in the past year, and 15% reported having received home care.

The Family

Child poverty rates are dependent on parental poverty rates and tend to rise and fall as economic conditions deteriorate or improve. Low-income families live on incomes substantially below the average. In 1991, the average income of low-income couples with children under 18 years old was Can$ 18,800, 32% of the Can$ 58,761 average income for all couples with children under 18 years. In 1996, the average income of low-income couples with children was Can$ 19,915—31% of the Can$ 63,981 average income for all couples with children.

Although the percent of working-age, single-parent families living in poverty has declined, the growth in the percent and number of single-parent families in the population has offset gains in poverty reduction. In 1975, 8.7% of children under age 7 years lived in single-parent families; by 1992, nearly one million children under 7 (14.7%) lived in single-parent families.

The federal government's decision to extend parental leave to 35 weeks from 10 weeks (for those eligible to receive it from employment insurance) has had a marked impact on the family. In 2001, employed mothers were able to increase maternity benefits to 10 months, up from 6 months in the year 2000. Fathers are becoming increasingly involved: the use of paternity leave jumped from 3% to 10% of working males between 2000 and 2001.

The Canadian family portrait taken by the census at the outset of the 21st century shows a continuation of many of the changes in families over the last 20 years. The proportion of "traditional" families—a mother, a father, and children—continues to decline, while families with no children at home are on the increase.

In 2001, married or common-law couples with children aged 24 years and younger living at home represented only 44% of all families in Canada. In 1991, they accounted for 49% of all families, and in 1981 they represented more than one-half (55%).

Behind this shift in living arrangements are diverse factors, such as lower fertility rates, with increasing proportions of couples who delay having children or who are childless. In addition, life expectancy is increasing, with the result that couples have more of their lives to spend together as "empty-nesters" after their children have grown up and left home.

For the first time, the 2001 census provided data on same-sex partnerships. A total of 34,200 same-sex, common-law couples were counted in Canada in 2001, representing 0.5% of all couples. There were slightly more male same-sex, common-law couples than female; census data counted about 19,000 male same-sex couples, 55% of the total. More female same-sex couples have children living with them. About 15% of the 15,200 female same-sex couples had children living with them compared to only 3% of male same-sex couples.

Workers

About one-quarter of workers reported high levels of general stress in their daily lives. For men and women, average job strain levels were significantly lower in 2002 than in 1994/1995. In 2002, 19% of men were classified as having high strain jobs, down from 23%. The decline for women was even larger, from 35% to 27%.

According to the 2002 Canadian Community Health Survey, just over one million adults aged 18 or older had experienced a major depressive episode in the year before the survey. For workers of both sexes, high stress on and off the job was associated with depression. Men in high-strain jobs were 2.5 times more likely than their counterparts in low-strain jobs to have experienced depression. When various sources of stress were considered simultaneously, along with other possible influences, high job strain was associated with depression for men, but not for women.

Persons with Disabilities

In 2005, 30% of Canadians aged 12 years and older reported limitations in participation and activity, while in 2000–2001, 22% reported such limitations. Women were slightly more likely than men to report limitations in physical activity—31% of women reported limitations, compared to 28% of men. Each successively older age group reports a higher percentage of their group as having impairments, from a low of 17% among 12–14-year-olds to a high of 63% for persons aged 75 years and older.

Of persons with disabilities, 44% are not included in the labor market, compared to 19% of persons without disabilities. The disabled also are more likely to have lower employment incomes. According to the Survey of Labor and Income Dynamics data for 2004, the average employment income for persons with disabilities was Can$ 31,700 compared to Can$ 36,100 for non-disabled persons.

Indigenous Peoples

In general, there are gaps between the social, economic, and environmental conditions of Aboriginal peoples and of other Canadians, which have a effect on health. In Nunavut, the average lifespan for women is 12 years less than the average for Canadian women; the gap for males is 8 years. Infant mortality rates among First Nations on reserve and Inuit are twice to three times higher than the Canadian rate.

In 2000, life expectancy at birth for the Registered Indian population was estimated at 68.9 years for males and 76.6 years for females. This reflects differences of 8.1 years and 5.5 years, respectively, from the 2001 Canadian population's life expectancies. In 2005, life expectancy was 5.2 years less for Aboriginal women and 7.4 years less for Aboriginal men than the national average.

Except for male prostate cancer, cancer mortality rates among First Nations peoples are lower than those for the overall Canadian population. Acute myocardial infarction rates among First Nations are about 20% higher than the overall Canadian rate, and stroke rates among First Nations are almost twice as high as the comparable overall Canadian figure.

Between 1981 and 2000, infant mortality rates declined 64% for First Nations peoples living in rural areas, and declined 47% for those in urban areas. Most of the excess infant mortality among First Nations people was due to higher post-neonatal mortality, particularly from deaths due to preventable causes, such as sudden infant death syndrome, infection, and external causes. This suggests a need for improved socioeconomic and living conditions.

In September 2000, Canada's First Ministers established early childhood development as a new federal/provincial/territorial social priority, recognizing the importance of children's early years in shaping long-term outcomes. It includes promotion of healthy pregnancy, birth, and infancy; improved family support; improved early child development, learning, and care; and improved community support.

The maternal and child health program framework for First Nations has been developed in collaboration with the Assembly of First Nations to improve health outcomes for pregnant women and families with infants and young children who live on reserves. The comprehensive program services include: home visits by nurses and experienced mothers in the community during pregnancy, postpartum, and early childhood; links to services for children and families with special needs; and exploration of opportunities to return safe birthing closer to communities.

Some 15% of new HIV infections and AIDS cases occur in Aboriginal peoples. Compared to the general Canadian population, heart disease is 1.5 times higher among First Nations peoples than in the general population; type 2 diabetes is 3 to 5 times higher, with even higher rates among the Inuit; and tuberculosis infection rates are 8 to 10 times higher. In 2005, First Nations peoples, while constituting only 2% of Canada's population, had 7.2% of the national HIV/AIDS cases.

Health Canada's First Nations and Inuit Health Branch (FNIHB) is actively engaged in addressing the HIV/AIDS epidemic among on-reserve First Nations people and in Inuit communities across Canada. FNIHB supports communities in developing the knowledge, skills, and tools they need to prevent HIV transmission and to facilitate care and support for those infected and affected by HIV/AIDS.

The 2000 reported rate of genital chlamydia was very high among First Nations peoples, at 1,071.5 cases per 100,000 population. This is about six times higher than the Canadian rate (178.9 per 100,000 population in 2001). First Nations females suffer much higher rates of chlamydia infection than do males. At a rate of 6,572.2 cases per 100,000 population, females aged 15 to 24 years accounted for 53.5% of all First Nations cases where age and sex were recorded.

HEALTH CONDITIONS AND PROBLEMS

COMMUNICABLE DISEASES

Vector-borne Diseases

Vector-borne diseases formerly regarded as exclusively tropical are finding their way to Canada. The incidence of imported **malaria** has increased steadily since the early 1990s. Malaria remains an important concern for travelers returning from tropical regions, and this disease accounts for illness and deaths among them. There appears to be a cyclical pattern of imported malaria, with notable peaks occurring every four to five years (1986/1987, 1991/1992, and 1996/1997). During the last peak, in 1997, there were 1,029 malaria cases reported in Canada; a 65% decrease was seen the following year with only 368 cases reported. In 2000, fewer than 400 malaria cases were reported.

Vaccine-preventable Diseases

Since Canada implemented its routine vaccination programs, the country has experienced a significant reduction in all diseases preventable by immunization. **Polio** was officially elimi-

nated in Canada in 1994, and since the implementation of routine two-dose measles, mumps, and rubella (MMR) schedules in 1996–1997, the occurrence of **measles** and **rubella** cases has been limited to sporadic importations with infrequent outbreaks. In 2005, a historic low of only six measles cases were reported in Canada, with at least four of these imported. That same year, an outbreak of 309 rubella cases occurred in a small Canadian community that was philosophically opposed to immunization.

During 2003–2004, fewer than 30 cases of **mumps** were reported annually, the lowest incidence ever recorded in Canada. Two mumps outbreaks (of 13 and 22 confirmed cases, respectively) involving adolescents and young adults occurred in 2005.

Childhood immunization rates remain high in Canada. In 2004 approximately 94% of children had received a single dose of the MMR vaccine by age 2 years and 78% of children had received their second dose by 7 years of age. Furthermore, an estimated 94% of children had received at least three doses of vaccines against diphtheria, pertussis, tetanus, polio and *Haemophilus influenzae* type b by their second birthday.

Since the adoption of a Canadian National Immunization Strategy in February 2003, childhood pneumococcal conjugate vaccine and adolescent acellular pertussis programs were implemented in all 13 provinces and territories, along with childhood meningococcal conjugate C and varicella vaccine programs. An oral rotavirus vaccine was approved for use in Canada in August 2006.

Intestinal Infectious Diseases

An estimated 11 million cases of foodborne illness occur each year in Canada, although most go unreported. Of these, 2% to 3% result in chronic health problems. In 2004, **campylobacteriosis** was the most commonly notified enteric infection, with 9,345 reported cases and an incidence rate of 30.2 per 100,000 population; followed by **salmonellosis**, with 4,953 cases and a rate of 16.0 per 100,000; and **verotoxigenic** *E. coli*, with 1,038 cases and a rate of 3.4. The incidence rates of all three diseases have decreased from 1998 levels. Health Canada is leading a number of initiatives to lower the rates of foodborne illness, including mandatory safe handling labels for raw ground meat and ground poultry.

Chronic Communicable Diseases

In 2002, 1,634 cases of new active and relapsed **tuberculosis** (TB) were reported. The highest rate, 93.4 per 100,000, was reported from Nunavut. Individuals between the ages of 25 and 34 years were the largest group represented, accounting for 19% of the total reported caseload of TB. Of the 1,702 cases diagnosed in 2001, 84% were fully cured after completing medical treatment. Approximately 65% of these cases occurred in foreign-born persons. The spread of drug-resistant TB strains throughout the world also represents a threat for Canada. In 2001, 1% of TB infections were drug-resistant. However, in Toronto the rate of drug resistance tends to be much higher, at 14%.

Not all groups of Canadians are equally at risk. Canadian-born Aboriginal peoples have a much higher than average infection rate of 24.3 per 100,000 population, whereas Canadian-born non-Aboriginals have a rate of 1.1. Moreover, 2001 marked the first time that the proportion of cases among Canadian-born Aboriginals surpassed the proportion among Canadian-born non-Aboriginals (18% and 16%, respectively). In Nunavut, 97% of TB cases occurred in the Aboriginal population, where the infection rate was 47.5 per 100,000 population.

A TB elimination strategy was introduced in 1992. National responsibilities include policy-making, care, treatment and surveillance. Activities such as case management, drug supply, maintenance of a TB registry, outbreak management, and community health education are centralized at the regional level, and implemented through primary health services at the community level.

Acute Respiratory Infections

Acute respiratory infections under routine laboratory surveillance in Canada include **influenza, respiratory syncytial virus (RSV), adenovirus**, and **parainfluenza virus**. Influenza and RSV account for the highest proportion of positive laboratory tests reported each year. Influenza positive tests account for 6% to 13% of the total respiratory virus tests conducted each season, with up to 30% positive for influenza at the peak of the season. RSV accounts for approximately 7% to 12% of positive laboratory tests for respiratory viruses in Canada, while adenovirus and parainfluenza virus account for approximately 1% to 4% of positive tests reported.

It is estimated that between 10% and 25% of the population develops influenza every year. Rates of influenza infection are highest among children, but rates of serious illness and death are highest among older persons (older than 65 years) and persons with medical conditions. It is estimated that, on average, 4,000 Canadians, mostly seniors, die every year from influenza, and many others may die from other serious complications of influenza. An average 20,000 Canadians are hospitalized each year from complications attributable to influenza.

About 10 to 11 million doses of influenza vaccine are distributed in the country each year during the influenza season. According to findings from the 1996–1997 National Population Health Survey and the 2000–2001 Canadian Community Health Survey, the proportion of the Canadian population aged 20 and older who reported having received an influenza vaccination in the year prior to the survey nearly doubled, from approximately 15% in 1996–1997 to almost 30% in 2000–2001; it has remained relatively stable since. The population groups with the highest proportion of persons immunized were seniors and people with chronic conditions, two of the groups targeted for influenza vaccination.

In 2003, a previously unknown respiratory infection—severe acute respiratory syndrome (SARS)—emerged in China. Between March and June 2003, a total of 438 SARS cases were reported in Canada. The first Canadian cases were identified in March 2003 in persons who had traveled to Hong Kong and returned to Canada. Since the end of the outbreak, with the last case reported in mid-June 2003, no SARS cases have been reported.

HIV/AIDS and Other Sexually Transmitted Infections

At the end of 2005, an estimated 58,000 people were living with HIV (including AIDS cases), a 16% increase from the estimate for 2002. In 2005, approximately 27% of people with HIV were unaware of their infection. At the end of 2005, an estimated 51% of all prevalent reported HIV infections were attributed to men having sex with men, 27% to heterosexual sex, 17% to illicit injection drug use, and 4% to both risk factors of men having sex with men and illicit injection drug use; the remaining 1% was due to other exposures. As of 2005, approximately 21,000 people have died of AIDS in Canada.

Women accounted for one-quarter (25.4%) of all positive HIV test results in 2005. Although the number of HIV-exposed infants has increased for each birth year, the proportion of HIV-infected infants has decreased dramatically—from 39% in 1994 to just 4% in 2005—because pregnant women have been receiving antiretroviral therapy. Advances in treatments available for persons living with AIDS have significantly increased their life expectancy.

Among adult AIDS cases reported with a known exposure category, the proportion accounted for by men having sex with men fell from above 75% in the years prior to 1994 to 38% in 2005. Conversely, the heterosexual exposure category increased from 10% to 38% over the same period.

In December 1999, it was estimated that 11,194 HIV-infected persons were also infected with **hepatitis C** virus. An estimated 250,000 people in Canada are infected with hepatitis C, with approximately 3,300 new cases diagnosed annually. Of those infected, it is estimated that 90,000 of them are unaware of their infection. Recent outbreaks of **lymphogranuloma venereum** among men having sex with men have been associated with co-infections of HIV, hepatitis C, and other sexually transmitted infections.

There has been a rise in sexually transmitted infections in Canada since the late 1990s. **Chlamydia** accounted for a total of approximately 63,000 infections in 2004 and is most commonly diagnosed in young women aged 15–24 years and young men aged 20–29. **Gonococcal infections** are the second most commonly diagnosed sexually transmitted infection, with young males between the ages of 20 and 29 accounting for two-thirds of the reported cases in 2004.

The most dramatic increases in sexually transmitted infection rates since 1997 have been in infectious **syphilis**, which have been associated with outbreaks primarily among 30–39-year-old men having sex with men.

Zoonoses

There has been only one case of a variant of **Creutzfeldt-Jakob disease** (mad cow disease) in Canada, which was reported in 2002. The patient had spent some years in the United Kingdom and was likely exposed to contaminated beef while in that country.

NONCOMMUNICABLE DISEASES

Metabolic and Nutritional Diseases

In Canada, the national prevalence of breast-feeding is 85%, but there are marked differences in breast-feeding prevalence by age, income, marital status, and place of residence. Women older than 29 years of age who have higher education and income levels have consistently higher prevalence rates of breast-feeding, and immigrant mothers are more likely to breast-feed than non-immigrants. Initiation rates increase from east to west across the country, from 53% in Atlantic Canada to a high of 87% in British Columbia.

Obesity rates among children and adults have increased substantially during the past 25 years, according to the results of a 2004 national survey, which directly measured the height and weight of respondents. The percent of obese and **overweight** boys and girls have increased similarly, but trends differ for various age groups. The percent of children 2 to 5 years of age who were overweight or obese remained virtually unchanged from 1978 to 2004. In contrast, the percent of overweight adolescents aged 12 to 17 years more than doubled, from 14% to 29%, while the prevalence rate of obesity for this age group tripled, rising from 3% to 9%. For children aged 6 to 11 years and adolescents aged 12 to 17 years, the likelihood of being overweight or obese tends to rise with the amount of time spent in sedentary activities such as watching TV and playing video games. This surge in obesity among adolescents is of particular concern, because overweight or obese conditions in adolescence often persist into adulthood. The prevalence rates of overweight and obesity among youth varied across the country, with the highest prevalence rates being in the Atlantic provinces.

The likelihood of becoming obese is related to diet and exercise. Canadians whose leisure time is sedentary are much more likely to develop overweight and obesity. In 2004, 27% of sedentary men were obese, compared to just 19% of active men. Among women, obesity rates do not fluctuate between active and sedentary lifestyles.

Conversely, almost 15% of Canadians, or an estimated 3.7 million people, were considered to be living in food-insecure households at some point during 2000/2001. Women who were single parents were at especially high risk. One-third of female single parents reported food insecurity, almost double the figure for male single parents. In contrast, just 9% of people who were partners in a couple without children reported food insecurity.

The rate was also notably high among Aboriginal peoples living off-reserve. About 31% reported some food insecurity, more than double the rate for non-Aboriginal peoples.

Diabetes continues to be a significant health problem in Canada. It is estimated that more than two million Canadians have diabetes, and of these, one-third are undiagnosed. Nine out of ten people with diabetes have type 2 diabetes. Seniors represent almost 48% of the total number of people with the disease, and this number is expected to rise as Canada's population continues to age.

Among persons 20 years of age and older, approximately 1,054,100 persons, or 4.8% of this age group, currently have been diagnosed with diabetes; as many as one-third of all diabetes cases go undiagnosed.

Cardiovascular Diseases

In 2003, cardiovascular disease accounted for 74,255 Canadian deaths. That same year, 32% of all male deaths in the country were due to heart diseases, diseases of the blood vessels, and stroke. For women, the toll was even higher—34% of all female deaths in 2003 were due to cardiovascular diseases.

In 2002, 54% of all cardiovascular deaths were due to **coronary artery disease**, 21% were due to **stroke**, 16% were due to other forms of heart disease and the remaining 9% were due to vascular problems such as **high blood pressure** and **hardening of the arteries**.

In Canada, 80% of the population has at least one modifiable risk factor for cardiovascular diseases; nearly one-third has two modifiable risk factors, and another 11% have three or more modifiable risk factors. The prevalence of some risk factors, such as overweight among men, diabetes, and high blood pressure, is increasing. Individuals who are socioeconomically disadvantaged show higher prevalence rates of the major risk factors. However, data show some narrowing of the risk factor gap between the high and low socioeconomic population groups.

Malignant Neoplasms

An estimated 153,100 new cases of cancer and 70,400 deaths from cancer have been estimated to occur in Canada in 2006. The most frequently diagnosed cancers will continue to be **breast cancer** for women and **prostate cancer** for men. The leading cause of cancer death for both sexes continues to be **lung cancer**.

For men, the rate for lung cancer declined from 81 lung cancer deaths per 100,000 men in 1988 to 64 in 2000. The rate for women climbed, however, rising from 27 lung cancer deaths per 100,000 women in 1988 to 34 in 2000; this reflects trends in smoking.

Though prostate cancer is more frequently diagnosed, lung cancer remains more lethal for men. In 2001, 9,925 men died from lung cancer, whereas only 3,825 died from prostate cancer. In fact, 9% of all male deaths and 29% of all male cancer deaths were caused by lung cancer. By contrast, prostate cancer was responsible for 3% of all male deaths and 11% of all male cancer deaths.

For women, the incidence of cancer has risen slightly since the mid-1980s, while the death rate has remained essentially unchanged. The incidence rate of breast cancer has also risen. One in nine Canadian women will develop breast cancer in her lifetime.

Breast cancer death rates have been declining since 1986, and more rapidly since 1990. This reflects improved screening programs and more effective treatments. As of 2000, the death rate for lung cancer had climbed to 34 deaths per 100,000 women, whereas for breast cancer it had dropped to 25 deaths per 100,000 women.

Tobacco use is the cause of almost 30% of all fatal cancers and a major cause of lung cancer, one of the most preventable cancers. Poor diet—one with a high proportion of dietary fat—causes about 20% of fatal cancers.

OTHER HEALTH PROBLEMS OR ISSUES

Disasters

In the past five years, Canadians have been affected by several natural disasters, including forest fires in Western Canada, Hurricane Juan hitting the Maritime Provinces in 2003, and the severe winter storms that affected Nova Scotia and Prince Edward Island in 2004. People aged 60 and over have the highest death rates of any age group during disasters.

The 2001–2002 drought in British Columbia, the Prairies, Ontario, Quebec, and Nova Scotia was the most expensive in history, with preliminary estimates of Can$ 5 billion in damages. The Canadian Wheat Board estimated that the 2002 drought resulted in production losses for grains and oilseeds of nearly Can$ 2.8 billion. In 2003, Hurricane Juan caused over Can$ 100 million in damages in the Maritime Provinces.

Violence in Children and Youths

According to data from police reports, in 2003 the risk of violent victimization of children and youth is highest for older children. The reported rate of victimization for both male and female children was under 500 victimizations per 100,000 children under 8 years of age. By age 14 years, rates were four times as high, at 2,000 victimizations per 100,000 children for both male and female youth.

One-fifth of all violent crimes reported in 2003 were committed against children and youth aged 17 and under. The risk of violent victimization of children and youth increases with age, and the profile of perpetrators of violent crimes against children and youth also changes as children get older. A family member, most often a parent, committed the majority of physical and sexual assaults against children under the age of 6. In contrast, older youth aged 14 to 17 years were more likely to be assaulted by a peer or a stranger. More than half of teenage victims between 14 and 17 years were physically assaulted by a close friend, acquaintance, or coworker; over one-fifth were physically assaulted by a stranger; while 16% were physically assaulted by a family member.

Of the 15,000 sexual assaults reported to 122 police services, 61% of the victims were aged 17 years and under. About four-fifths of the victims 17 years and under were girls and more than two-thirds of these females were between 11 and 17 years old.

Mental Health

Data show that 20% of individuals in the country will experience a mental illness in their lifetime. Approximately 8% of adults will experience major depression at some time in their lives, and about 1% will experience bipolar disorder. Schizophrenia affects 1% of the Canadian population. Anxiety disorders affect 5% of the household population, causing mild to severe impairment.

In 2002, 1 of every 10 persons aged 15 years old and older (about 2.7 million people) reported symptoms consistent with a mood anxiety disorder, or alcohol or illicit drug dependence. Major depression was reported in 6.3% of women and 5.3% of men. Anxiety disorder is the second-most common mental disorder, with 4.8% of men and 5.9% of women reporting symptoms.

Suicide rates differ between men and women and between young and old. Men are more likely to commit suicide than women, but women are more likely than men to be hospitalized for suicidal ideation. In 2001, there were 3.5 suicides among men for every suicide among women. For men, the risk of suicide was greatest between the ages of 40 and 44 years. For women, the risk peaked at ages 45 to 49 years. People in their forties accounted for almost one in four suicides.

Suicide accounts for 24% of all deaths among 15–24-year-olds and 16% among 25–44-year-olds. Suicide is one of the leading causes of death in both men and women from adolescence to middle age.

Addictions

In 2004, 79% of Canadians aged 15 or older reported consuming alcohol, although most drank in moderation. Of those reporting consumption of alcohol, 44% reported drinking weekly. Drinking rates peaked among youth aged 18–24 years, with about 90% of that group consuming alcohol during 2004. Of drinkers, 6% reported heavy drinking (for men, five or more alcoholic drinks on a single occasion and four or more for women) at least once a week.

The proportion of women drinkers identified as high-risk is 9%, compared to 25% of men. More than 30% of those under 25 years of age were high-risk drinkers. Less than 5% of seniors 65 years of age and older were in the high-risk drinking category.

Beer consumption, which makes up about 80% of all alcoholic beverages consumed, rose to 80.3 liters per person over 15 years of age in 2005. At the same time, the consumption of wine has continued to increase over the last ten years reaching 13.9 liters in 2005. Spirit consumption, at 7.5 liters, remained fairly stable from a year earlier.

In 1989, 6.5% of the population reported using marijuana and 7.4% did in 1994; by 2002, the proportion had reached 12%. Nearly half (47%) of those who had used marijuana in the previous year had done so less than once a month. About 10% of those using marijuana in the previous year reported they used it on a weekly basis, and another 10% said they used it daily. Men were more likely than women to have tried marijuana at least once. Lifetime use of marijuana was highest among young adults aged 18 to 24 years.

Overall, 2.4% of people aged 15 years or older reported to have used cocaine, crack, ecstasy, LSD, amphetamines, or heroin in the past year. This figure is up from 1.6% in 1994. An estimated 321,000 people (1.3% of the population) had used cocaine or crack, making it the most commonly used of these drugs.

Oral Health

In the population 15 years old and older, 66% of women and 61% of men reported having made a visit to a dentist in 2003. The highest rate of dental visits was reported by people 15 to 24 years old, 35 to 44 years old, and 45 to 54 years old; 69% of each age group had visited the dentist in 2003. However, the frequency dropped sharply, to 46%, among people aged 65 and over. Dental insurance was an important factor influencing dental visits. In 2003, 74% of people who had benefits to help cover all or part of their dental expenses had consulted a dentist in the past year, compared to 48% of the non-insured. Income was also an important factor, as only 36% of the non-insured and 57% of the insured individuals from low-income households had a dental consultation in the previous year. Low-income Canadians were the least likely to have dental insurance, or to have visited a dentist during the past year. Among Canadians in the low-income group, only 44% visited a dentist in the previous year. By contrast, 77% of high-income Canadians had reported a visit to a dentist in the previous year. Education and geographic location were also factors in people accessing dental care. Of those who had not completed high school, only 47% reported visiting a dentist, while 71% of college/university graduates did. In rural areas, 56% of residents reported consulting a dentist in the past year, compared to 65% of urban residents.

Health Canada endorses the fluoridation of drinking water to prevent tooth decay, but does not participate in the decision to fluoridate water supplies, because this falls under the jurisdiction of provincial and territorial governments. In collaboration with their municipalities, the provinces and territories decide whether or not to fluoridate and the amount of fluoride to be added;

42.6% of the Canadian population has fluoridated drinking water and 57.4% does not have fluoridated drinking water.

RESPONSE OF THE HEALTH SECTOR

Health Policies and Plans

Canada's health care system reflects the underlying right to access health care. It provides first-dollar, universal coverage for hospital and physician services (i.e., no user fees are payable by any patient, rich or poor, for medically necessary hospital and physician services). It is predominately funded by taxes, but the delivery of services is largely private. In accordance with the constitutional division of powers between the two levels of government, the federal government provides funding through transfer payments to the provinces and territories to help pay for health care services, but the provinces and territories actually are responsible for managing and delivering the services.

The Canada Health Act is the country's federal health care legislation. It sets out the criteria that provinces and territories must meet in order to receive the full federal cash transfer under the Canada Health Transfer. The five principles embodied in the Act are public administration, comprehensiveness, universality, portability, and accessibility.

The responsibility for Aboriginal health services is shared by the federal, provincial, and territorial governments and by Aboriginal organizations. Through its First Nations and Inuit Health Branch, Health Canada is responsible for community health programs on First Nations reserves and on Inuit land claim areas, administering the non-insured health benefits program and the funding and management of public health and health promotion initiatives for these groups.

The mandate of the First Nations and Inuit Health Branch is to provide targeted disease prevention and health promotion programs for all Aboriginal peoples; to ensure the availability of, or access to, health services for First Nations and Inuit communities; to assist First Nations and Inuit communities to address barriers to health and disease threats, and to attain health levels comparable to other Canadians living in similar locations; and to build strong partnerships with First Nations and Inuit to improve the health system. Other Aboriginal populations in Canada are provided access to health services by provincial and territorial governments.

Responsibility for public health also is shared with the federal Public Health Agency of Canada which was created in 2004 following the 2003 SARS outbreak. The Agency works closely with other federal departments and agencies, provinces, and territories, and collaborates with various stakeholders, including those in the private sector, the not-for-profit sector, and health professionals such as family physicians. Initiatives promote health, prevent and control infectious and chronic diseases, support public health research and surveillance activities, and protect the public from the consequences of health emergencies (1, 6). Through its activities and in partnership with the public health community, the Agency not only improves health and quality of life, but also can relieve some of the pressure on the health care system, helping to contain costs and shorten patient wait times.

Canadians are in the midst of the second phase of health reforms marked by an increase in public health expenditures and measures to ensure the fiscal sustainability of public health care. Data from the Canadian Institute for Health Information show that there has been a dramatic increase in the use of advanced medical diagnostic imaging, such as CT scans and magnetic resonance imaging, and that this spike has created a demand that has outstripped the available supply of equipment, medical radiation technologists, sonographers, and diagnostic radiation and nuclear medicine physicians who operate, maintain, and use such technology. This, in turn, has had a negative impact on the speed of treatment (6).

To cope with these and other pressures on the system, the Prime Minister, provincial premiers, and territorial leaders met in 2003 and agreed to an Accord on Health Care Renewal. The Accord constitutes a renewed commitment by governments to a sustainable public health care system in Canada and to the values that underlie it. An action plan was developed whereby First Ministers agreed to provide first-dollar coverage for a basket of services for short-term and acute home care, including acute community mental health and end-of-life care. They also agreed that by 2011, 50% of the Canadian population would have access to a primary health care provider.

Subsequently, a 2004 Health Accord built upon the previous agreements by addressing home care, catastrophic drug coverage, and pharmaceutical management. The Ministers agreed that no citizen should suffer undue financial hardship for needed drug therapy.

The Ten Year Plan to Strengthen Health Care, articulated in September 2004, committed First Ministers to reduce wait times in priority areas such as cancer, heart, diagnostic imaging, joint replacements, and sight restoration by March 31, 2007. They also agreed to an ongoing focus on primary health care reform, human resources in health, and home care in post-acute, mental health, and end-of-life circumstances. They further agreed to establish a best practices network to share information and find solutions to barriers inhibiting progress in primary health care reform. With the exception of Quebec, both levels of government created a ministerial task force to work on a national pharmaceutical strategy.

The 2003 and 2004 federal budgets supported this action plan by increasing federal investments in health care. The federal government also increased its funding to territorial governments and Aboriginal organizations in order to facilitate reform and improve access, including medical transportation infrastructure for remote northern communities.

In June 2001, the Government of Canada established a Secretariat on Palliative and End-of-Life Care to act as a focal point and facilitator of collaborative action on these issues. Community working groups also were created to address issues in the areas of best practices and quality care, education, public information and awareness, research, and surveillance. Through the Canadian Strategy on Palliative and End-of-Life Care, Health Canada has supported initiatives such as curriculum development for providers, standards for accreditation, and networks of researchers.

In 2004, the Government of Canada also introduced the Employment Insurance Compassionate Care Benefit, which provides a maximum of six weeks of employment insurance to assist families caring for a dying loved one. Furthermore, in 2004, First Ministers agreed to provide first-dollar coverage for home palliative care services, including case management, nursing, palliative care medications, and personal care.

Canada has a highly decentralized health system with a mix of public and private health delivery. The national regulatory authority rests in the Federal Government. The provinces have primary jurisdiction over the administration and delivery of public health care services, but "delegate" actual delivery to health organizations, as well as to physicians working on fee-for-service schedules or mixed remuneration arrangements, the terms of which are negotiated with the provincial governments. Health facilities and organizations, from the hospital to the regional health authority, are accredited on a voluntary basis through the Canadian Council on Health Services Accreditation. Most health care providers, including physicians, nurses, dentists, optometrists, chiropractors, and psychologists are organized as self-governing professions under provincial framework legislation (6, p.61).

Health Canada's Biologics and Genetic Therapies Directorate is the federal authority that regulates biological drugs (products derived from living sources) and radiopharmaceuticals for human use.

Nutrition labeling regulations became mandatory for most prepackaged foods on December 12, 2005.

The management of persistent organic contaminants is performed through a variety of tools, including legislative, regulatory, and policy instruments, guidelines, and codes of practice.

The use of pesticides for the protection of food crops is approved and registered by the federal government's Pest Management Regulatory Agency, once its use is shown to be affordable, efficacious, and having acceptable levels of environmental and human health risks. The Regulatory Agency's role as the Canadian regulatory body for pest control products contributes to the protection of food crops from an economic and social point of view.

Public Health Services

As the final report of the 2002 Romanow Commission on the Future of Health Care in Canada states, "there is almost universal agreement that primary health care offers tremendous potential benefits to Canadians and to the health care system .... No other initiative holds as much potential for improving health and sustaining our health care system."

Approximately 80% of contacts with the Canadian health care system occur through the primary health care sector, which makes it critical to have integration and coordination within the system to ensure both comprehensive care and continuity of care. The key feature of primary health care renewal is, therefore, a shift from the current practice of single family physicians to a model that has greater coordination and collaboration among a range of health care providers who, collectively, provide comprehensive services to their clients.

Telephone advice lines, tele-health services, and electronic medical/health records are being introduced. These technologies help to improve access, support information-sharing, and improve the quality of care. In remote communities, tele-health services have been instrumental in providing quicker access to care, by allowing Canadians to access more services right in their community, resulting in better care and in cost savings for users and for the system itself.

All provincial and territorial ministries of health devote resources to communicable disease control in their jurisdictions. But because communicable diseases spread extremely rapidly and easily across geographical boundaries, the federal government often has been called upon to play a larger role in this effort. The 2003 SARS outbreak and the ensuing Naylor Report were the catalysts for a policy change, whereby the federal government expanded its national infectious disease control and prevention infrastructure along the lines of the Centers for Disease Control and Prevention in the United States (6).

In addition, as a result of a national consensus conference in 2005 on the goals and objectives for six vaccine preventable diseases, four new vaccine programs (against meningococcal disease, pneumococcal disease, varicella, and acellular pertussis) are under way in almost all provinces and territories.

Screening programs for early detection of cancer also are operating at the provincial and territorial levels. With funding from Health Canada, the Canada Breast Cancer Screening Initiative, which focuses both on public education and program development, has been operational since 1990.

The 2004 Canadian Community Health Survey incorporated nutrition-related indicators, thus filling a critical 35-year gap in national food consumption data.

As part of Canada's environmental health surveillance, levels of environmental chemicals in humans are monitored through the Northern Contaminants Program; environmental radiation is monitored; children's environmental health and air health indicators have been developed; drinking water advisory systems are applied to track enteric diseases from water- and food-borne sources; and, beginning in 2007, the Canadian Health Measures Survey will include a substantial bio-monitoring component.

The Canadian Hospitals Injury Reporting and Prevention Program is a surveillance program based in emergency departments in 10 children's and 4 general hospitals that is operated by Canada's Public Health Agency. The program tracks the number of people visiting associated emergency departments for treatment of injuries, as well as the location and cause of the injury.

Canada's National Microbiology Laboratory is responsible for identifying, controlling, and preventing infectious diseases. The laboratory's activities include reference microbiology, support to epidemiology programs, surveillance, emergency response, applied and discovery research, and management of intellectual assets to improve public health in Canada and internationally.

The Office of Laboratory Security, within the Public Health Agency of Canada, is the country's national authority for biosafety. Its mission is to ensure effective, evidence-based biosafety interventions on a national scope through regulatory control, surveillance, applied research, and timely dissemination of information related to needs, priorities, and strategies. The Office was designated as a WHO Collaborating Center on Biosafety Technology and Consultive Services in 1983, and provides guidelines and safety programs for microbiology laboratories worldwide including consultative services in biocontainment technology and biosafety, biosafety training, the dissemination of information, the provision of a biosafety resource center, surveillance, and applied biosafety research programs.

The Public Health Bureau manages programs to protect the health of people traveling within Canada and to ensure safe drinking water for federal employees. Under the Traveling Public Program, Health Canada provides three types of services: inspections and audits, investigations of disease outbreaks, and surveillance of gastrointestinal diseases.

Inspections also are conducted to verify the safety of food, water, and other environmental health conditions on board cruise ships, passenger ferries, passenger trains, and their ancillary services. Unannounced inspections are conducted on cruise ships traveling within Canadian waters once per year during cruise ship season.

Under the International Health Regulations, international cargo vessels are required to obtain a de-ratification exemption certificate every six months declaring the ship free of rats or evidence of rats. A certificate is issued upon completion of a full inspection of the ship by a Health Canada inspector.

Approximately 78% of Canadians are served by central water distribution systems. An estimated 6.8 million Canadians rely on private water supplies, primarily groundwater wells. Approximately 74% of Canadians living mostly in urban areas are serviced by municipal sewer systems, and three-quarters of them receive high-level treatment. Some surveys indicate that between 20% and 40% of wells, particularly in rural areas, may be contaminated by nitrates or bacteria. All the data on drinking water quality for public systems are collected and categorized differently across the provinces and territories.

The federal/provincial/territorial Committee on Health and Environment has been created to strengthen a multi-level government surveillance of waterborne contamination; it published guidance documents on safe drinking water in both 2002 and 2004.

Through the Infrastructure Canada Program, the Government of Canada has committed additional funds over five years (2003–2007) to upgrade, maintain, and monitor drinking water and wastewater systems on First Nations reserves and to promote green municipality initiatives.

Canada promotes an environmentally sound, science-based system for monitoring waste shipments. Canada's guidance manual for sustainable communities promotes the use of waste as a resource, and encourages reduction, reuse, and recycling to reduce waste. Canadian federal, provincial, territorial, and municipal governments and businesses evaluate, develop, and implement new waste management programs and policies.

Canada has banned leaded gasoline in automobiles and over the past decade has passed several regulations controlling the formulation of various fuels. Sulphur regulations have been in place in the country since January 2005.

Internationally, Canada ratified a Heavy Metals Protocol under the United Nations Economic Commission for Europe's Convention on Long Range Trans-boundary Air Pollution, thus committing itself to enhance regional cooperation for reducing transboundary air pollution.

The National First Nations Environmental Contaminants Program was launched in 1999 as a collaborative research program between the Assembly of First Nations and Health Canada. The objective of the Program is to help First Nations assess the extent of exposure to environmental contaminants and the potential for associated risk to the health and well-being of First Nations in Canada.

Canada bans the use of pesticides with high levels of 2,3,7,8-tetrachlorodibenzodioxin (TCDD) levels, and is monitoring the amount of polychlorinated biphenyls (PCBs) in food, air, and water to reduce health risk. Guidelines have also been developed to minimize the release of dioxins and furans from municipal solid waste and hazardous waste incinerators.

As a way to eliminate children's exposure to lead, Canada has put in place the Lead Risk Reduction Strategy for Consumer Products. Ingestion of lead in house dust is currently the major source of intake of lead on children.

The Canadian Center for Occupational Health and Safety is a federal government agency that supports the elimination of all work-related illnesses and injuries in the country. The Center provides Canadians with unbiased, relevant information and advice that supports responsible decision-making and promotes safe and healthy working environments. It disseminates a vast scope of occupational health and safety information for the public and for health and safety professionals.

The Government of Canada, through the Public Health Agency's Center for Emergency Preparedness and Response works with multiple partners to ensure that Canada is prepared to respond to the public health risks posed by all disasters, natural or caused by humans, such as infectious disease outbreaks, hurricanes, floods, earthquakes, and criminal or terrorist acts such as explosions and the release of toxins. The Center's approach includes the provision of preparedness training exercises, security for laboratories that handle dangerous human pathogens, and the maintenance and expansion of national stockpiles of emergency supplies across the country.

The maintenance and improvement of quarantine services at Canada's major international airports is a priority, as was the passage of a revised Quarantine Act, which was approved by Parliament on May 12, 2005. This Act provided new powers and modern tools to quarantine services.

In collaboration with the provinces, Emergency Response Assistance Plan teams are deployed across the country. The teams are comprised of various professionals prepared to respond to transportation issues involving infectious substances that pose high individual and community risk.[2] In 2005, the newly renovated laboratory rated for containment Level 3[3] became operational and now serves as a biological threat response lab for the National Capital Region.

Individual Care Services

Canadians benefit from a strong and healthy federal public service, which is achieved through the Public Service Health Program and the Employee Assistance Services. The Program includes health evaluations; communicable diseases; workplace investigations; office ergonomics; and health education, promotion and training.

Health Canada's First Nations and Inuit Home and Community Care Program in 1999 began to allow individuals with chronic or acute illnesses and the elderly to receive care in their own home delivered primarily by First Nations and Inuit community members. The program's guiding principles include a respect for First Nation and Inuit approaches to healing and wellness and for community-focused planning.

In addition, the Canada Prenatal Nutrition Program—First Nations and Inuit Component assists pregnant women, including those living in poverty; pregnant teens; and women living in isolation or with poor access to services. Activities include food and vitamin supplementation, breast-feeding support, one-on-one nutrition counseling, counseling on lifestyle issues, food-preparation training, transportation, childcare, and referral to other services.

Health Promotion

Both the federal government and the provinces and territories run several health promotion and education programs dealing

---

[2] WHO Risk 4 Group.
[3] Capable of handling indigenous or exotic agents which may cause serious or potentially lethal disease as a result of exposure by the inhalation route (applicable to clinical, diagnostic, teaching, research, or production facilities).

with alcohol and drug abuse, family violence, fetal alcohol syndrome, food and nutrition, mental health, physical activity, safety and injury, and sexuality, including AIDS prevention. Health Canada also has spearheaded a comprehensive e-health information website that provides reliable information for all Canadians on how to stay healthy and prevent illness (6, p. 90).

As Health Canada works to improve the health status of First Nations and Inuit peoples, one of its priorities is to develop and implement a National Aboriginal Youth Suicide Prevention Strategy. The Strategy aims to increase resiliency and protective factors, and reduce risk factors associated with Aboriginal youth suicide.

In 2005, the Government announced a major new investment in health promotion and chronic disease prevention for the coming five-year period and beyond, the Pan Canadian Healthy Living Strategy. Approved by Canada's federal, provincial, and territorial ministers of health, the Strategy aims to improve overall health outcomes and to reduce health disparities, with an initial emphasis on healthy eating and physical activity and their relationship to healthy weight.

In addition, the Public Health Agency directs its health promotion activities through community grants and contribution programs delivered both nationally and regionally. Examples include the Community Action Program for Children, the Canadian Diabetes Strategy, and the AIDS Community Action Program.

The Family Violence Initiative brings together 14 federal departments as partners and takes a coordinated approach to promoting public awareness of the risk factors of family violence and the need for public involvement in responding to it.

In 2005, the Ministers of Education and of Health formed an intergovernmental partnership and developed an action plan to address a variety of health, social, and learning-related problems of school-aged children and youth.

Canada's Drug Strategy, spearheaded by the Health Canada's Office of Demand Reduction, is a federally coordinated intersectoral initiative to reduce the harm associated with the abuse of narcotics and other controlled substances, alcohol, and prescription drugs. The Strategy focuses on youth and includes education, prevention, and health promotion initiatives, as well as enhanced enforcement measures. It also provides best practices to front-line health and social services providers in the areas of prevention, treatment, and rehabilitation.

The Canadian Center on Substance Abuse manages the national program, Health, Education and Enforcement in Partnership. In 2004, a program implementation team comprised of provincial coordinators was created to share information and foster intersectoral networks for the development of strategies addressing substance abuse.

The Federal HIV/AIDS Initiative (2005) is a partnership of the Public Health Agency of Canada, Health Canada, the Canadian Institutes of Health Research, and Correctional Services Canada. Working closely with all stakeholders, the initiative supports research and programs benefiting persons living with AIDS.

Health Canada recognizes that maintaining good oral health is an important part of good overall health. To emphasize this link, Health Canada created the Office of the Chief Dental Officer in October 2004. The Office is charged with improving the oral health status of Canadians and increasing awareness about the prevention of oral diseases.

Human Resources

In 2004, there were 315,139 regulated nurses employed in their discipline—78.2% were registered nurses, 20.1% were licensed practical nurses, and 1.6% were are registered psychiatric nurses. Canada's nursing workforce is still predominantly female. In 2004, 5.4% of registered nurses were male, compared to 6.9% of licensed practical nurses, and 22.7% of registered psychiatric nurses.

Data from the Canadian Institute for Health Information showed that there were 69,519 physicians, including interns and residents, working in Canada in 2005; 51% were family physicians and 49% were specialists. The growth in the number of physicians has kept pace with the growth of the population.

Canada's physician workforce is increasingly female: the number of female physicians increased by 14%, rising from 16,945 in 2000 to 19,365 in 2004, whereas male physicians increased only 0.6% in the same time period. Most physicians are concentrated in urban areas, and there tend to be acute shortages in rural and isolated areas, where nurses continue to play a primary role in delivering health services.

Health Canada, working through the Pan-Canadian Health Human Resources Strategy, is collaborating with provinces, territories, and stakeholders to strengthen health human resources planning, to promote and put in place inter-professional education among health care professionals, and to develop and implement recruitment and retention strategies to ensure a better supply of health care professionals over the longer term.

Complementing that effort is the Aboriginal Health Human Resources Initiative, which addresses issues about human resources in health in Aboriginal and remote communities by seeking to increase the number and improve the skills of health providers in those communities.

Health Supplies

Health Canada's Biologics and Genetic Therapies Directorate is the Canadian federal authority that regulates biological drugs (products derived from living sources) and radiopharmaceuticals for human use.

The Common Drug Review was established in 2002 to provide a single process for reviewing new pharmaceuticals and provid-

Boosting Health among First Nations and Inuits in Canada

The Government of Canada, through Health Canada, is actively working to close health gaps between the country's indigenous peoples and the rest of the Canadian population. For example, despite significant gains in health, infant mortality rates among First Nations and Inuits still are from two to three times higher than the rates for non-Aboriginal persons. In an effort to narrow health inequities, Health Canada's First Nation and Inuit Branch seeks to ensure that these communities have adequate access to health services. In building strong partnerships with First Nations and Inuit communities, the Branch more effectively combats disease threats and helps bring down barriers to health.

ing recommendations concerning formularies to all provinces and territories, with the exception of Quebec (6, p.69).

Research and Technological Development in Health

The Canadian Institutes of Health Research is the Government of Canada's agency for health research. It coordinates research through a unique, interdisciplinary structure made up of 13 "virtual" institutes, which are networks of researchers brought together to focus on important health problems. Each institute embraces research that ranges from fundamental biomedical and clinical research, to research on health systems, health services, the health of populations, societal and cultural dimensions of health, and environmental influences on health. Priority health research themes include Aboriginal peoples' health, aging, cancer research, health services and policy research, human development, child and youth health, nutrition, metabolism, and diabetes.

In 2004, Canada Health Infoway launched a strategy targeting investments in a series of tele-health applications in Aboriginal, official language, minority, northern, rural and remote communities. To date, there have been few systematic studies of the impact of tele-health applications (6).

Health Sector Expenditures and Financing

In 1975, total Canadian health care costs represented 7% of the Gross Domestic Product. By 2005,[4] Canada's total health care expenditures as a percentage of GDP grew to an estimated 10.4% (or Can$ 4,411 per person). According to the Canadian Institute for Health Information, public health expenditures in 2005 accounted for seven out of every 10 Canadian dollars spent on health care. The remaining three of every ten Canadian dollars came from private sources and covered the costs of supplementary services such as drugs, dental care and vision care.

How health care dollars are spent has changed significantly over the last three decades. On average, the share of total health expenditures paid to hospitals and physicians declined, while

spending on prescription drugs greatly increased. Still, expenditures for hospitals and physicians take up 43% of the amount that is directed to health care.

In 1975, a much larger share went to hospitals (45%) than in 2005 (30%). Payments to physicians in 1975 (15%) accounted for the second largest share of expenditures; this declined to the third largest area of spending (13%) by 2005. In contrast, drug therapies, particularly those prescribed by physicians, accounted for 9% of total health expenditure in 1975. This had nearly doubled by 2005, and at almost 18% had become the second largest share of total health expenditure. The share of publicly funded health expenditure stood at 69.6% in 2005, on par with its 2002 level. These shares are the lowest on record since 1975.

Growth in total health expenditures varied greatly across provinces in 2005. At 11.3%, Alberta recorded the fastest pace of expenditure growth. At the low end, Prince Edward Island, Newfoundland, and Labrador recorded growth rates below 5%.

Per capita health spending by province was generally similar. Per capita health expenditure ranged from a low of Can$ 3,878 in Quebec to a high of Can$ 4,820 in Alberta in 2005. Most of the remaining provinces recorded per capita health spending within plus or minus Can$ 300 of the national average. The three territories have significantly higher per capita expenditures (with Nunavut being much higher than Canada's average). These elevated costs per capita are a result of the remoteness of the Canadian territories and lower population density, which lead to important transportation costs.

In 2005, hospitals and drugs accounted for Can$ 67.2 billion, or nearly half of total health expenditures. Meanwhile, expenditures on health professionals (physicians and other health professionals) represented almost one-quarter of health spending.

Technical Cooperation and External Financing

The Government of Canada is participating in large-scale, multi-donor programs based on developing-country priorities that use local institutions and systems for their implementation. This reinforces the capacity of well-governed developing coun-

[4]Data for 2004 and 2005 are forecasts.

tries that have assumed primary responsibility for achieving the Millennium Development Goals, and it also helps coordinate and focus aid.

Canada considers the Pan American Health Organization (PAHO), Regional Office of the World Health Organization, as a strategic partner in efforts to improve the health status of the people of the Americas. This is reflected in the degree of support that the Canadian International Development Agency provides to address key health issues such as communicable diseases, immunization, HIV/AIDS, pandemic preparedness, and disaster management, as well as health human resources and institutional capacity-building in Latin America and the Caribbean.

Canada does not use PAHO's Biennial Program Funds for work within Canada. Instead, these funds are used in partnership with Latin American and Caribbean countries and with PAHO itself to mobilize Canadian health experts for specific health needs as identified by the countries. Approximately 20 projects a year are supported in a two-way partnership that serves to reinforce the guiding spirit of Pan Americanism.

Internationally, Canada is addressing the "10/90 research gap" through the Global Health Research Initiative. The Initiative constitutes a partnership among four leading Canadian health organizations, each with a different comparative strength: the Canadian Institutes of Health Research, the Canadian International Development Agency, Health Canada, and the International Development Research Centre. This collaborative approach serves as a framework for activities aimed at shaping and responding to the global health research agenda, influencing policy and policy coherence relating to global health research and facilitating information sharing among partner agencies.

The International Development Research Council, through its Globalization, Growth, and Poverty Initiative, also supports policy reforms in developing countries aimed at promoting inclusive, equitable growth and poverty reduction, as well as appropriate international integration strategies by generating necessary evidence and policy analysis.

In addition, Canada has been acting as Secretariat to the Global Health Security Initiative, in which 180 countries have been participating since 2001. The Secretariat's tasks include preparing and disseminating a vaccine procurement protocol and developing coursework in containment and isolation for smallpox and other contagious diseases.

Canada also is one of several country partners to the WHO's Commission on Social Determinants of Health, and is providing funds to support three of nine knowledge network hubs on early child development, globalization and health, and health systems in South Africa. Canada has also taken a leading role with WHO in identifying chronic disease prevention and control initiatives by helping establish a Framework Agreement for Cooperation on Chronic Diseases in 2005. It is anticipated that a partnership with PAHO and the countries of the Americas will continue to expand in this area over the coming years.

The country also is committed to building capacity in water management internationally. For example, Health Canada participates in the WHO-organized international network on small community water supplies. This project is designed to address problems associated with providing safe water to remote communities in developed and developing countries, as a means to progress towards the Millennium Development Goals, specifically those related to water and sanitation.

Since 2002, when it hosted the hemisphere-wide Health and Environment Ministers' Meeting (HEMA), Canada has been supporting a health and environment agenda, including developing a broader policy framework for building bridges between health and environment. The HEMA Task Force, comprised of ten senior government representatives from the health and environment sectors of the five American subregions, has since advanced measures throughout the Region to prevent and mitigate environmental threats to human health at the national and regional levels. The subsequent Declaration and Cooperative Agenda calls for building strategic alliances that underscore connections among the health, environment, education, and labor sectors in particular; developing public policies on sustainable development that endeavor to alleviate poverty and inequality; and protecting the environment and public health within the framework of human rights.

References

1. Public Health Agency of Canada, Treasury Board of Canada, Secretariat. 2005–2006 Performance Report (DPR-Part III Estimates). Available at: www.tbs-sct.gc.ca/dpr-rmr/0506/PHAC-ASPC/PHAC-ASPC_e.asp.

2. Statistics Canada. Income in Canada 2004. (Statistics Canada Catalogue Number 75-202-XIE). Ottawa, Ontario: Statistics Canada; 2006.

3. Federal/Provincial/Territorial Advisory Committee on Population Health and Health Security, Health Disparities Task Group. Reducing Health Disparities—Roles of the Health Sector: Discussion Paper. December 2004.

4. Yalnizyan A. Getting Better Health Care: Lessons from (and for) Canada. Canadian Centre for Policy Alternatives; 2006.

5. DesMeules M, Pong R. How Healthy Are Rural Canadians? An Assessment of Their Health Status and Health Determinants. Ottawa: Canadian Institute for Health Information; 2006.

6. Marchildon GP. Health Systems in Transition: Canada. Volume 7, Number 3. Copenhagen: WHO Regional Office for Europe on behalf of the European Observatory on Health Systems and Policies; 2005.

7. Canada, Department of Agriculture and Agri-Food Canada. 2002.

8. Statistics Canada. 2001 Census Analysis Series. A profile of the Canadian population: where we live. Catalogue Number 96F0030XIE.

CAYMAN ISLANDS

Cuba

Mexico

Cayman Islands

Jamaica

Honduras

Nicaragua

Cayman Brac

Little Cayman

Grand Cayman

George Town

0   25   50 Miles

The Cayman Islands, a British overseas territory, comprises the islands of Grand Cayman, Cayman Brac, and Little Cayman. The territory spans approximately 250 km^2 in the western Caribbean Sea, about 240 km south of Cuba and 290 km west of Jamaica. Grand Cayman is by far the most populous and largest island, with an area of 197 km^2.

GENERAL CONTEXT AND HEALTH DETERMINANTS

The two "sister islands" of Cayman Brac and Little Cayman are located about 145 km east of Grand Cayman and have areas of 36 km^2 and 26 km^2, respectively. The capital, George Town, is located on Grand Cayman. All the islands are generally low-lying, with the exception of a massive limestone bluff that rises on Cayman Brac.

Social, Political, and Economic Determinants

The Governor, who represents the Queen of the United Kingdom, heads the territorial government and presides over the Executive Council, which includes three official members and Ministers elected by the Legislative Assembly; Ministers delegate policy implementation and administrative matters to Permanent Secretaries. The Parliament has 15 seats, two of which are held by women.

The Cayman Islands are politically stable and economically strong. With an average income of around $42,000, Caymanians enjoy the highest standard of living in the Caribbean. The islands print their own currency, the Cayman Islands Dollar (KYD), which is pegged to the U.S. dollar at a fixed rate of 1 KYD = 1.227 USD.

The GDP growth rate in 2002 was 5.3% and an estimated 1.7% in 2005. Economic growth is mainly fueled by the finance and tourism sectors, as the islands can receive as many as 10,000 visitors a day.

At year-end 2005, the population was estimated to be 52,466 (residents only, including those with work permits) compared to 40,200 in 2000. Of the total population, 50.2% is male and 49.8% female. The vast majority of the population resides on Grand Cayman, with a population of over 50,000. Cayman Brac is the second most populated with about 2,000 residents, followed by Little Cayman with around 200 permanent residents. The sharp increase in total population over the past five years is attributed to the rapid increase in the number of foreign work-permit holders and their dependents; although this influx has served to fill the gap left by a shortage of local workers, it has burdened the territory's services, including health care. The population growth rate for 2005 stood at 2.6%, an increase compared to the 2.1%

rate for 2001. In 2005, life expectancy at birth was 80.0 years (77.3 years for males and 82.6 years for females) and represented an increase over the 2002 figure of 79.2 years (76.4 years for males and 81.6 years for females). The crude birth rate in 2005 was 12.9 births per 1,000 population, compared with 13.5 births per 1,000 population in 2002.

The population comprises a mix of more than 100 nationalities. About half the population is of Caymanian descent; some 60% is of mixed race; and, of the remaining 40%, about half is Caucasian and half of African descent. The inhabitants are almost exclusively Christian, and the largest denominations are Presbyterian and Anglican.

With regard to some of the leading determinants of health, the adult literacy rate in 2005 was estimated at 99%, and schooling is free and compulsory for all children between the ages of 5 and 16; health care is provided free of charge to all schoolchildren, and all persons in Cayman have equal access to health care; approximately 95% of the population has access to safe piped water, and the remaining 5% have access to safe water provided by tanker trucks; public sewerage covers approximately 10% of the population, with the remaining 90% served by onsite wastewater treatment plants such as septic tanks, aerobic wastewater treatment plants, and cesspool onsite wastewater treatment plants.

Demographics, Mortality, and Morbidity

A comparison of the population distribution between 1990 and 2005 shows an aging population (see Figure 1). In 2005, the population under 20 years of age comprised 3% less of the total population than in 1990, and the population in the 60 years and older age group comprised 3% more of the total population than in 1990.

All deaths in the Cayman Islands, whether of Caymanians or of work-permit holders, are registered. Deaths of residents average approximately 120 per year, and the annual crude death rate held steady from 2002 to 2005, fluctuating between 5.2 and 4.8 deaths per 1,000 population (mortality data of tourists are analyzed separately). The leading causes of death can be seen in Table 1. Ischemic heart disease, cerebrovascular diseases, and neoplasms are the three leading causes of death and account for 30.4% of all deaths. Patterns for causes of death in males and females differ: disaggregating leading causes of mortality by gender shows that malignant neoplasms of the trachea/bronchus/lungs and the prostate are leading causes of death for males, and acute respiratory infections (influenza and pneumonia) along with malignant neoplasms of the breast are the leading causes of death for females. During the period 1994–2000, 90 deaths occurred due to external causes, which represents an annual average of 13 deaths (11% of total deaths). Leading external causes of death are road traffic accidents at 30 deaths (33.3%), accidental drowning at 20 (22.2%), homicides at 16 (17.8%), suicide at 5 (5.6%), undetermined intent at 4 (4.4%), house fire at 3 (3.3%), and all other accidents at 12 deaths (13.3%). The male-to-female ratio for external causes of death was 4 to 1, with a male-to-female ratio of 15 to 1 for homicides. It is worth noting that the territory is particularly vulnerable to hurricanes, and that in September 2004 Hurricane Ivan caused two deaths and an estimated US$ 10 million in damages to the territory's infrastructure.

HEALTH OF POPULATION GROUPS

Children under 6 Years Old

During the period 2002–2005, a total of 20 infants died, five of them in 2005. For the four-year period, the infant mortality rate was 7.9 deaths per 1,000 live births, the neonatal mortality rate was 5.1 deaths per 1,000 live births, the postneonatal death rate was 2.8 deaths per 1,000 live births, and the perinatal mortality rate was 13.9 per 1,000 births. The main causes of death were extreme prematurity, congenital abnormality, dysfunction of a diseased brain, and neonatal asphyxia. The proportion of newborns weighing less than 2,500 g at birth was 7% in 2005.

In the period 2002–2005, 22 deaths occurred in children under 5 years of age. Of total hospital discharges in 2002, 409 (10%) were of patients in the under 6 year age group. The five leading final diagnoses on discharge from the hospital in the under 6 year age group were diseases of the respiratory system

TABLE 1. Leading causes of mortality, numbers, and percentage of total deaths, Cayman Islands, 1998–2000.

Causes of death	No.	% of total deaths
Ischemic heart disease	68	18.1
Cerebrovascular diseases	24	6.4
Malignant neoplasms of trachea/bronchus/lung	22	5.9
Influenza and pneumonia	21	5.6
Diabetes	17	4.5
Malignant neoplasms of prostate	14	3.7
Heart failure and complications	13	3.5
Hypertensive disease	12	3.2
Land transport accidents	10	2.7

FIGURE 1. Population distribution (%), by age and sex, Cayman Islands, 1990 and 2005.

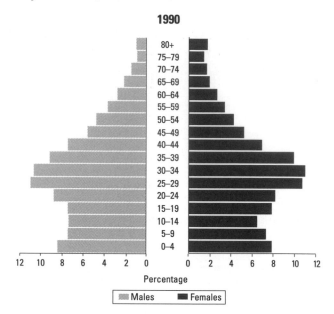

1990

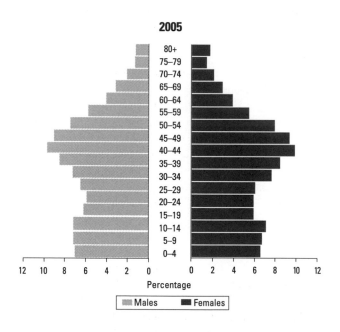

2005

(34% of all final diagnoses for this age group); symptoms, signs, and abnormal clinical and laboratory findings (15%); intestinal infectious diseases (14%); diseases of the digestive system (12%); and injury, poisoning, and other external causes (7%). Of all discharges from the hospital in 2002, children under 6 years of age accounted for 35% of all asthma cases and 69% of all cases of respiratory conditions due to chemicals, gases, fumes, and vapors (including reactive airway dysfunction syndrome).

Chronic Diseases and Sickle Cell Anemia

Ischemic heart disease, cerebrovascular diseases, and malignant neoplasms took the greatest toll in the Cayman Islands between 1998 and 2000—they were the three leading causes of death, accounting for 30% of all deaths. Sickle cell anemia follows closely. To help ease the burden from these diseases, the Government has stepped-up screening and follow-up for those affected with this disease.

Children 6–10 Years Old

In 2002 in the 6–10-year age group, 174 children were discharged from the hospital, comprising 4.3% of total discharges. Leading final diagnoses for 6–10-year-olds discharged from the hospital included diseases of the respiratory system (27%); diseases of the digestive system (20%); injury, poisoning, and other external causes (16%); symptoms, signs, and abnormal clinical and laboratory findings (9%); and certain infectious and parasitic diseases (6%).

Immunization coverage of school-age children in 2005 for measles, mumps, and rubella (MMR) and diphtheria, tetanus, and pertussis (DTaP) or tetanus and diphtheria (TD) was 98%.

Adolescents 11–14 and 15–19 Years Old

In 2002 there were 94 hospital admissions in the 11–14-year age group. The five leading causes of admission to the hospital of this group were injury, poisoning, and other external causes (24%); diseases of the digestive system (23%); diseases of the respiratory system (14%); diseases of the genitourinary system (7%); and symptoms, signs, and abnormal clinical and laboratory findings (6%).

In 2002, 67 adolescents 15–19 years of age were admitted to the hospital. Admissions of this group comprised complications of pregnancy, normal delivery, and cesarean sections (25.4%); injury, poisoning, and other external causes, with a 2:1 male-to-female ratio (20.9%); symptoms, signs, and abnormal clinical and laboratory findings (10.4%); disorders of the digestive system (7.5%); diseases of the respiratory system (7.5%); and mental disorders, of which all were females under 18 years (6.0%), including three cases of depressive episodes and one adjustment disorder. Of all births between 1995 and 2004, 2.4% were to women under 18 years, but the yearly percentage steadily declined from 4.1% in 1995 to 1.6% in 2004; during that 10-year period, only three pregnancies occurred in the <15-year age group—one each in 1996, 1997, and 1998 and none since 1999. To assist youth in making responsible decisions, the Life Skills program in schools offers family life education sessions. All adolescents graduating high school in 2005 were fully protected against tetanus.

Adults 20–64 Years Old and 65 Years and Older

In 2002 patients in the 15–64-year age group accounted for 2,009 hospital discharges (49% of all discharges). Excluding 550 discharges for hospitalizations due to pregnancy, childbirth, and the puerperium (27%), 1,459 discharges were due to illness. The leading discharge diagnoses of persons in this age group were injury, poisoning, and other external causes at 251 (17%); diseases of the digestive system at 221 (15%); diseases of the genitourinary system at 167 (11%); diseases of the circulatory system at 147 (10%); and mental and behavior disorders at 100 (7%).

The proportion of women attended by trained personnel during pregnancy fluctuated very little from 2002 to 2005, when it stood at 98.6%. The proportion of women attending clinic during the first trimester of pregnancy increased from 45% in 2002 to 62% in 2005. In 2002 the cesarean section rate at the Cayman Islands Hospital was 8.2%. In 2004 the total fertility rate was 1.9 children per woman. Over the last 10 years only one maternal death occurred, in 2005.

According to the Health Services Authority (HSA), in 2002 there were 588 hospital discharges for those 65 years of age and older—46% of which were male and 54% female (14.4% of total discharges). The leading causes of 543 hospital discharges defined by cause in this age group were diseases of the circulatory system with 151 discharged patients (27.8%); diseases of the respiratory system with 78 (14.4%); diseases of the digestive system with 64 (11.8%); endocrine, nutritional, and metabolic disorders with 38 (7.0%); diseases of the genitourinary system with 35 (6.4%); injuries and other consequences of external causes with 33 (6.1%); diseases of the musculoskeletal system and connective tissue with 24 (4.4%); diseases of the eye with 16 (2.9%); and malignant neoplasms with 15 (2.8%). Half of the patients were admitted once; the remainder were admitted more than once, usually for the same condition.

The Family

Females 15–49 years of age comprised 62% of the total female population. The number of households increased from 8,115 in the 1989 census to 14,908 in the 1999 census, representing an average annual increase of 679 households. Single-parent households—those without a spouse or common law partner—increased from 951 to 1,425 in the same 10-year period, but as a percentage of total households dropped slightly from 11.7% to 9.6%. In 1999, the proportion of single-parent households with 1 or 2 children out of all such households increased to 83.5%, as compared to 78.6% in 1989, while the proportion of single-parent households with 4 or more children decreased from 10% in 1989 to 5.8% in 1999.

Workers

Child labor does not exist in the Cayman Islands, as compulsory schooling precludes employment of children under 16 years of age. Prostitution is illegal, but in certain areas there is an illicit commercial sex trade; an HIV/AIDS strategic plan makes provision for educating and counseling those who work in that high-risk trade.

HEALTH CONDITIONS AND PROBLEMS

COMMUNICABLE DISEASES

Vector-borne Diseases

Three cases of **malaria** were reported in 2004, and one in 2005. One case of **dengue** fever was reported in 2004, and none in 2005.

Vaccine-preventable Diseases

During the period 2001–2005, no cases of **diphtheria, neonatal tetanus, pertussis, rubella**, or *Haemophilus influenzae* **type b** were reported. The last reported case of **polio** was in 1957, and of **measles** in 1991. The national immunization program includes the following vaccines: injectable polio, diphtheria, acellular pertussis, tetanus, *Haemophilus influenzae* type b, hepatitis B, MMR, varicella, and seasonal influenza; the varicella and pentavalent combination (DTaP/IPV/Hib) vaccines were introduced into the national schedule in 2000. Vaccination coverage of antigens administered from 2001 to 2005 ranged from 87% to 92%. In 2004, 92% of children had received the three-dose primary series of DPT, Hib, and polio vaccines; 87% had received the first dose of the MMR vaccine; 92% had received BCG; 77% had received three doses of the hepatitis B vaccine; and 81% had received the varicella vaccine. After the ravages of Hurricane Ivan in 2004, public health staff offered tetanus boosters to anyone who had not had a booster in the previous five years—about 15,000 doses, for a coverage of 40%; 85 cases were reported in 2004, and 33 in the first six months of 2005.

Infectious Intestinal Diseases

Food-borne illnesses and **gastroenteritis** continue to pose significant health problems. Flooding and limited water supplies due to Hurricane Ivan increased the incidence of gastroenteritis on the islands: 1,399 cases were reported to the Public Health Department in 2004. Cholera, typhoid, and hepatitis A are not endemic.

Chronic Communicable Diseases

The reported incidence of **tuberculosis** is very low, ranging from 0–4 new cases per annum and with one case reported in 2004. No case of tuberculosis has been reported in children for the past 20 years.

Acute Respiratory Infections

In 2004, 310 cases of **influenza** were reported. Of all hospital admissions 9% were due to diseases of the respiratory system; excluding asthma and respiratory neoplasms, 51% of admissions for all other respiratory diseases were due to acute respiratory infections. In 2004, 20 cases of asthma were admitted, 35% of which were children under 5 years of age.

HIV/AIDS and Sexually Transmitted Infections

From 1985, with the first reported case of AIDS, to mid-year 2005, 68 residents tested positive for HIV, including one new case in 2004. By mid-year 2005, 36 cases of AIDS had been reported, of which 25 (69%) had died. By September 2005, 34 persons were reported to have tested positive and were living with HIV/AIDS; 29.7% of those were between 25 and 39 years of age. An estimated 70% of HIV infection was transmitted via heterosexual contact; the next most common mode of transmission was by homosexual contact; and a small percentage was due to perinatal transmission and drug use. Illegal residents and foreigners seeking employment within the country are not included in these statistics—an important consideration given the impact that foreigners seeking employment have on the islands' HIV services. It is mandatory for those seeking work permits to be tested for HIV, and those individuals represent the largest category of people accessing HIV testing services. Mandatory testing also exists for antenatal clinic attendees, prisoners, prisoners' contact officers, and returning expatriates. The guidelines and procedures are in place for two prenatal screenings of women, and HIV-positive mothers are given AZT to prevent transmission of the infection to their infants. Between 2001 and 2005, 575 pregnant women were tested for HIV, and none of them tested positive. Two cases of mother-to-child transmission of HIV occurred between 1989 and 2005. In September 2005, 23 persons were receiving antiretroviral drugs.

Illicit intravenous drug abuse is not a problem in the Cayman Islands. No cases of HIV transmission through transfusion of blood and blood products or needle stick injuries have been reported.

NONCOMMUNICABLE DISEASES

Metabolic and Nutritional Diseases

Consistent with the recommendation of WHO, breast-feeding is encouraged as the best, and preferably exclusive, source of feeding for infants from birth to 6 months; moreover, all island hospitals observe the Code of Marketing of Breast Milk Substitutes. The Cayman Islands Hospital complies with many criteria of the WHO/UNICEF Baby-Friendly Hospital Initiative and is working towards certification as a "baby-friendly hospital." A 2005 study revealed that 94% of mothers started breast-feeding, 76% continued to breast-feed when their infants were six weeks of age, but that as children grew older and mothers returned to work the proportion breast-feeding dropped to 60% at four months and 35% at six months.

The rate of newborns at **low-birthweight** (< 2500 g) has held steady at 7%.

In 2001, the Health Services Authority Nutrition Services, with the assistance of the Caribbean Food and Nutrition Institute, conducted a survey on local young child feeding practices. Based in part on that survey and a follow-up workshop, a young child feeding policy was developed in 2003. Body mass index (BMI) assessments were conducted in 2003–2004 of children 10–13 and 3–5 years of age. The assessments found that 24.6% of schoolchildren aged 10–13 years were overweight and 14.7% were at risk of being overweight (compared to 20.9% overweight and 16.3% at risk in 1997–1998); that is, 39.3% of children 10–13 years were already observed to have a serious health risk factor. The assessments further showed that, of children 3–5 years old, 14.1% were overweight and 13.1% were at risk for overweight—indications of an early onset of abnormal weight gain.

Pregnant women and preschoolers are routinely provided with vitamin supplements.

Cardiovascular Diseases

In the period 1998–2000, **ischemic heart disease** was the leading cause of death, accounting for 68 deaths or 18.1% of all deaths defined by cause.

Malignant Neoplasms

The number of cases of malignant neoplasms reported annually from 2001 to 2005 ranged from 33 to 49, with an annual average of 41. In the period 1998–2000, malignant neoplasms of the trachea/bronchus/lung were the third leading cause of mortality, accounting for 22 deaths; malignant neoplasms of the prostate were the sixth leading cause, accounting for 14 deaths; among females, seven deaths occurred due to malignant neoplasms of the breast.

OTHER HEALTH PROBLEMS OR ISSUES

Disasters

As mentioned above, the territory is prone to hurricanes, and in September 2004 Hurricane Ivan proved particularly destructive. HAS opened district medical shelters to house special-needs patients and nearby residents and deployed physicians, nurses, and other health care workers, as well as ambulances, to those shelters. Cayman Islands Hospital provided shelter, food, and potable water to almost 1,100 persons for a week, greatly depleting hospital resources. Some 80% of the health care workers had moderate-to-major damage to their houses.

Mental Health and Addictions

In 2002, 131 hospital discharges for mental and behavior disorders were related to: psychoactive substance use (42 discharges or 32.1%); mood affective disorders (likewise 42 or 32.1%); schizophrenia and delusional disorders (24 or 18.3%); neurotic, stress-related, and somatoform disorders (12 or 9.2%); and other disorders such as adult personality, physiological development and emotional disorder, and organic, including symptomatic, mental disorders (5 or 3.8%).

A drug and alcohol survey of 985 households, carried out in 2000, found that alcohol and tobacco are by far the most commonly used substances, with 61.2% and 46.6% of respondents reporting having ever used these substances, respectively, over their lifetimes. Men were significantly more likely to have consumed alcohol over the previous 12 months (68.5%) than were women (44.8%). The highest percentage of heavy drinking (an average of four or more drinks in one drinking session) was found among 20–29-year-olds (41.7%). Smoking among men over the past 12 months exceeded that among women, and the 20–29-year-olds were the most likely to smoke. The percentage of persons using marijuana over the past 12 months was small (3.5%), as was the use of other illicit or nonmedical drugs; marijuana use is most prevalent among persons under 30 years old and, more specifically, in the 15–19 age group. About 30% of the population was using at least one form of prescription drug at the time of the survey. Half of respondents using a cough syrup or painkiller containing codeine (15% of the adult population) did so without the advice of a physician or used more than the physician advised; barbiturates were used by 5% of the population, and about one-fifth reported at least some use without a prescription.

RESPONSE OF THE HEALTH SECTOR

Health Policies, Plans, Strategies, and Programs

The Health Services Authority initiated development of a five-year strategic plan, the six key components of which are: design of an efficient organizational structure for HAS; implementation of steps to ensure the financial viability of HAS; implementation of measures to ensure that health care delivery meets or exceeds internationally accepted standards; creation of an environment in which patients and families are encouraged to participate actively in achieving wellness; improvement in external communication to gain public confidence and support to achieve the mission and objectives of HAS; and establishment of an environment that ensures internal communication, fosters job satisfaction, and encourages staff commitment to improve productivity and customer service.

Among initiatives in health legislation and regulation, the national breast-feeding policy was updated in 2001 to include provisions of the new WHO standard of exclusive breast-feeding. Although the Convention of the Elimination of Discrimination Against Women (CEDAW) was ratified by the United Kingdom, it has not yet been extended to the Cayman Islands. No legislation deals with family planning and reproduction. With regard to sexual rights, the legal age of consent is 16 for both males and females. Abortion is prohibited, the only exception permitted by law being when abortion is necessary to preserve the life of the mother. The Health Insurance Law makes it mandatory for everyone to have health insurance coverage, thereby ensuring that it is extended to children. Various sections of the Health Services Law dealing with health service fees ensure the right of children to basic health care services and state that a Caymanian and spouse do not have to pay fees for antenatal or contraceptive services, including those of clinics, devices, and drugs provided at health care facilities.

The Health Practice Commission has responsibility for the inspection and certification of health care facilities and the registration and licensing of health professionals through the health practice councils. It was set up under the Health Practice Law (2002), which defines "health care facilities" as premises where a registered practitioner provides health services: clinical examination, nursing care, dental care, provision of blood and blood products, diagnostic procedures, provision of medical and surgical services, and provision of pharmaceuticals, advice, or counseling. The Commission also advises the Director of Planning on applications for development of health care facilities and the Minister of Health Services on policy relating to health practice, including determining the types of health professions that should be permitted to work on the islands; and it provides guidance to the Health Practice Councils and monitors their performance. Health professionals are regulated by the Health Practice Councils, the Medical and Dental Council, the Nursing and Midwifery Council, the Pharmacy Council, and the Council for Professions Allied with Medicine (e.g., chiropractors, mental health counselors, opticians, optometrists, and radiographers).

Organization of the Health System

The Ministry of Health and Human Services oversees and regulates health care services. Health care is provided by both the Health Services Authority, a Crown corporation, and the private sector. Cayman Islands Hospital is located in the capital of George Town, and health centers, which provide all primary care services, are located in various districts; full-time nurses are present at all health centers, and the frequency of physicians' visits varies depending on a community's size. Given the islands' small population and area, the management of health services is centralized, but senior managers have decision-making authority in accordance with general policies and guidelines.

The privately owned and operated Chrissie Tomlinson Memorial Hospital is open to all visitors and residents. The hospital includes an outpatient department, two major operating rooms, a maternity ward, an intensive care unit, and a pharmacy; it offers the following services: urgent care, computerized axial tomography scanning, radiology, ultrasound, mammography, magnetic resonance imaging, nuclear scanning, laboratory, physiotherapy, endoscopy, physical therapy, occupational therapy, and ambulatory surgery. In addition, several dental practices are available, including a new private dental clinic, Cayman Dental Services, in George Town with resident dental surgeon/specialists on call 24 hours/day.

The Health Insurance Commission (HIC) monitors the performance of the health insurance industry and serves five major functions: advising the minister responsible for health insurance on any matter relating to health insurance; requiring every health care facility and registered health practitioner to file with the HIC annually and whenever they change their fees for services provided; investigating and settling disputed claims to health benefits and answering questions about the provision of health insurance; providing advice to the Governor-in-Cabinet on premium rates charged by health insurers; and managing the segregated insurance fund, including the collection of monies on behalf of the government from premiums charged by approved insurers to cover medical costs for indigent persons. CINICO is a government-owned insurance company formed to provide health insurance coverage to civil servants (employees and pensioners) and other residents who have had difficulty obtaining coverage through their employer or from the private insurance market. According to HIC, in 2006 59% of the population was covered by private insurance, 24% was covered by CINICO, and 17% was not covered.

PUBLIC HEALTH SERVICES

The Health Services Authority is governed by a 15-member Board of Directors that sets broad policies for the Authority; its day-to-day operations are managed by a Chief Executive Officer and a team of senior managers.

Prominent among health promotion activities is Breast-feeding Awareness Week, observed every year in August. A breast-feeding support group is actively involved in weekly breast-feeding clinics at the Women's Health Center, in school education programs, in a young parents program, and in workplaces for mothers who are returning to work. Instruction on healthy eating during pregnancy and lactation and on infant feeding (from birth to 1 year) is offered free of charge through prenatal education classes.

The Department of Environmental Health works closely with the Public Health Department to conduct field investigations of food-borne illnesses and similar suspected or confirmed disease outbreaks. Both departments also offer health awareness training to barbers, beauty parlor operators, cosmetologists, and those doing tattooing and body piercing; training focuses on specific diseases, such as skin infections and blood-borne pathogens, general health, and sanitation.

An active surveillance system is in place for collecting notifiable disease data; a nurse epidemiologist visits the hospital several times a week to identify any communicable disease occurrences. An epidemiological team set up in 2000 and comprised of representatives from the Environmental Health and the Public Health departments and the Cayman Islands Hospital Laboratory, which serves as the territory's public health laboratory, regularly assesses the epidemiological situation; staff from the Veterinary Department, the Mosquito Research and Control Unit, and other physicians are consulted as the need arises. In addition, a new information system has been set up to render health care delivery more efficient and patient centered, while enabling sound financial management through adequate capturing of charges and relevant statistical information.

The Water Authority, a statutory body of the Government, is charged with providing and implementing the Cayman Islands' water and sewage infrastructure and protecting its water resources. In Grand Cayman, the authority supplies water to the district of George Town and eastward into the village of East End. A private company holds a government franchise to provide piped water supplies to the West Bay Beach area and the district of West Bay. The Water Authority operates a small piped water supply system in Cayman Brac to serve a few customers. Potable water is provided via water tankers to customers not on the piped system. A private operation has been granted a government franchise to provide piped water to a very limited area of Little Cayman Island. Water quality is monitored internally by the companies and externally by the Department of Environmental Health.

In addition, the Water Authority operates a sewerage system that provides services to the tourist hotel areas of Grand Cayman. All other sewage treatment and disposal is through septic tanks with deep-well injection or soak-away fields. Septic tank collection services are available through private companies, and the waste is treated at the Authority's wastewater treatment plant. Adequate excreta disposal facilities cover 99.5% of the population.

Residential solid waste is collected twice a week in Grand Cayman and three times a week in Cayman Brac and Little Cayman. Commercial collection is carried out at least on a weekly basis, with restaurants having daily collections. All three islands have sanitary, government-managed landfills—the only legal disposal

sites in the territory. According to a 2005 PAHO report on the regional evaluation of municipal solid waste management in Latin America and the Caribbean, 57.7 tons of solid waste is generated by the Cayman population daily. Such a quantity of waste emphasizes the importance of proper disposal techniques, without which the risk of leptospirosis, hantavirus, and other rodent-borne diseases, as well as water and air pollution, multiplies.

The Environmental Health Laboratory is equipped to analyze and monitor food quality, and a program to monitor ready-to-eat foods is in place at selected food establishments. Based on a financial evaluation, the Social Services Department provides financial assistance to obtain food to those who are economically deprived.

Individual Care Services

The Health Services Authority provides patient care through the Cayman Islands Hospital and Faith Hospital on Cayman Brac. The 125-bed Cayman Islands Hospital is the principal health care facility, with accident and emergency services, a wide range of medical and surgical services, a critical care unit, and pharmacy and laboratory services (including a forensic unit). Faith Hospital, an 18-bed facility, serves the residents of Cayman Brac and Little Cayman and provides primary, basic secondary, and emergency care; it also has an inpatient unit, an operating theater, a maternity unit, an accident and emergency department, outpatient clinics, and a public health department. In Little Cayman, clinics are conducted throughout the week by a registered nurse and are complemented by a weekly physician visit. The resident nurse also makes home visits and, together with a paramedic, provides pre-hospital care service including 24-hour emergency care and transport service for the residents in Cayman Brac. Primary health care is offered at four district health centers in Grand Cayman and at another in Little Cayman. Dental and eye care services are offered at the health service complex in Grand Cayman.

Radiological and laboratory facilities are available in all public and private hospitals. There is a central blood bank in Grand Cayman and a collecting center at Faith Hospital, which performs the immuno-hematology testing for units collected at their site, while all spectrum-analyzer screens are performed at the Cayman Island Health Services Pathology Laboratory. Procedures are in place for the collection of autologous and therapeutic units. All units collected are screened for HIV, hepatitis B, hepatitis C, and syphilis. The donor pool is small and does not support the production of random platelets, making it necessary to import platelets when requested. Blood is also imported in emergency cases. Donations ranged from 710 in 2001 to 864 in 2005.

The primary objective of the school health program is to promote health and wellness and to facilitate health education for all levels of students. School health services are made available to all students regardless of race, gender, or nationality. Schools are required to conduct health screening, including vision and hearing, problem identification, and immunization; all public schools have a resident or visiting school nurse to offer those services, and private schools are also offered health checks and the updating of immunizations.

The Health Services Authority provides a comprehensive newborn screening program at both the Cayman Islands Hospital and Faith Hospital that covers over 50 inherited disorders, identifies infants at risk, and establishes early diagnosis and treatment. Pregnant women are offered testing for sickle cell disorder as well as for other disorders if their family history so indicates; they also receive genetic counseling and follow-up recommendations regarding tests for partners, other children, and the like. A school health coordinator, public health nurse, and genetics coordinator are on a multidisciplinary committee of an early intervention program that focuses on children 0–5 years of age who are at risk, are developmentally delayed, or have specific disorders. If a child is suspected of having a genetic disorder, the physician can order genetic tests and the parents can receive pre-test counseling. The Lighthouse School has approximately 60 children with special needs, including cerebral palsy, autism, Down syndrome, and various learning disabilities. A school nurse from the Public Health Department visits the school twice weekly to provide immunization coverage and to attend to chronic and acute problems. A general practitioner and a genetic coordinator perform annual physical examinations on the students, making referrals as needed to specialists. The Public Health Department offers a monthly pediatric genetics clinic for persons with known disorders as well as for those with suspected disorders who need evaluation and testing. As part of genetic counseling, pedigrees are drawn on persons with known genetic traits or disorders. Public awareness talks aim to make adolescents aware of certain disorders with an historically high incidence due to the isolation, and consequential consanguinity, of the Cayman Islands population over several hundred years; the incidence of disorders has decreased greatly as the islands have become a multinational community.

A no-tolerance approach to domestic violence prevails throughout the territory, which has a number of agencies that fight domestic violence: the Royal Cayman Islands Police Service, which has a family support unit that is responsible for the investigation of cases; the women's resource center, which educates and informs the public on issues relevant to women and the family; and the Cayman Islands Crisis Center, established to provide a safe home for the victims of domestic violence—mainly women and children. Annual reports of the Royal Cayman Islands Police Service for 2000 and 2002 indicate an increase in domestic violence cases from 917 to 1,517; some of that increase is real, while some of it may be due to improved reporting procedures.

The Mental Health Department provides comprehensive psychiatric and psychological services to adults, children, and geri-atric patients. Outpatient clinic services, with two psychologists, see adults, children, and adolescents in all the districts and sister islands, with daily outpatient clinics and emergency coverage 24 hours/day in George Town; disorders treated include schizophrenia, depression, anxiety disorders, dual diagnosis disorders, and developmental disorders with behavioral features. Monthly clinic services are offered to prisons and consultations are provided to the police. An eight-bed acute psychiatric inpatient unit, staffed with psychiatric nurses and an occupational therapist, provides day hospital services. Two community nurses provide community outreach, follow-up, and treatment for chronic patients. In addition, detoxification services in conjunction with substance abuse services are offered. Schools are supported by psychologists who offer educational testing and therapy interventions.

Health Supplies

As no drugs or other medical supplies are manufactured locally, all drugs, reagents, syringes, needles, and equipment are imported; any such supplies that have been approved in the United States or the United Kingdom are automatically approved for use in the Islands (any other drugs or medical equipment must be approved by the Health Practitioners' Board). Vaccines are procured through the Revolving Fund operated by the Pan American Health Organization. The Health Services Formulary includes all essential drugs.

Human Resources

In 2004 the following health workers were registered: 74 doctors, half of whom worked in private practice; 18 dentists, two-thirds of whom worked in private practice; 226 nurses, one-sixth of whom were in private practice; and 236 other health care workers.

Health Sector Expenditures and Financing

The budget of the Health Services Authority increased steadily from US$ 46.8 million in 2000 to US$ 54.9 million in fiscal year 2003–2004, US$ 62.1 million in 2004–2005, US$ 71.9 million in 2005–2006, and US$ 72.3 million in 2006–2007. The steep increase in 2005–2006, the year following Hurricane Ivan, relates to subsequent reconstruction efforts. On average, the health budget represents 12.5% of the Government's budget (the range in recent years has been from 11.4% to 14.5%). Data on private sector financing are not available.

PAHO, CAREC, and CFNI provide training through fellowships and workshops—support that amounts to US$ 25,000/year. The Cayman Islands receives no external funding for health care delivery.

CHILE

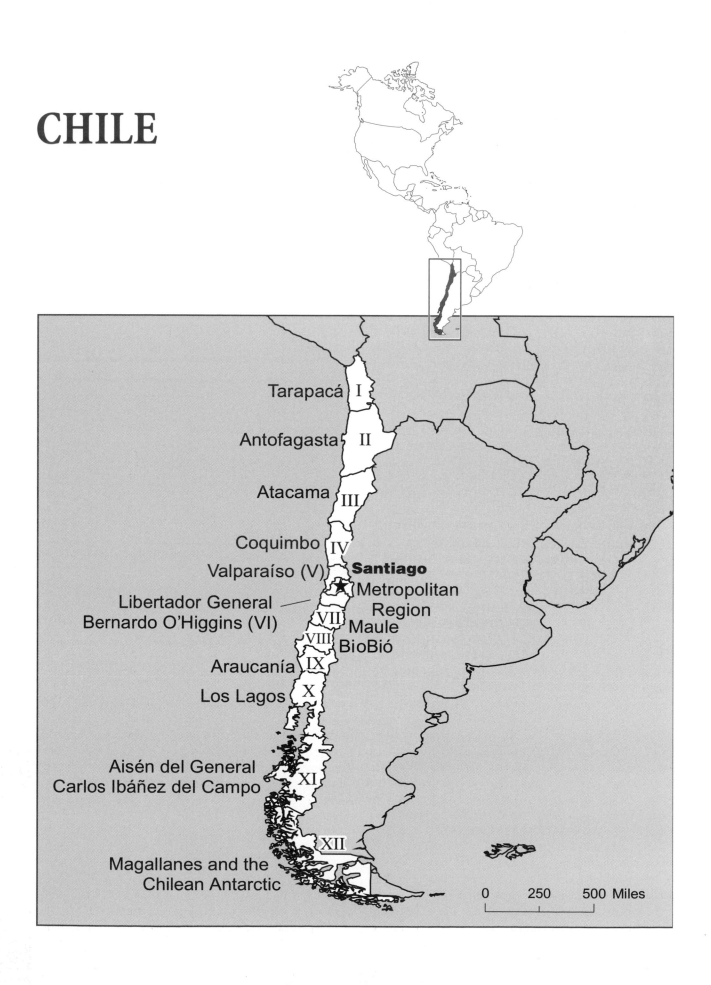

Tarapacá I

Antofagasta II

Atacama III

Coquimbo IV

Valparaíso (V)

Libertador General —
Bernardo O'Higgins (VI)

Santiago
Metropolitan
Region

VII

Maule

VIII

BioBió

Araucanía IX

Los Lagos X

Aisén del General
Carlos Ibáñez del Campo

XI

XII

Magallanes and the
Chilean Antarctic

0   250   500 Miles

C hile is situated in the extreme southwest of South America, bordering Peru, Bolivia, and Argentina. Continental Chile has a length of 4,329 km and an average width of 177 km. Its continental and insular surface area is 756.626 km^2, and its Antarctic territory covers 1,250,000 km^2.

GENERAL CONTEXT AND HEALTH DETERMINANTS

The country is divided into 13 political-administrative regions: Tarapacá (I); Antofagasta (II); Atacama (III); Coquimbo (IV); Valparaíso (V); the Santiago metropolitan region (RM); Libertador General Bernardo O'Higgins (VI); Maule (VII); BioBió (VIII); Araucanía (IX); Los Lagos (X), Aisén del General Carlos Ibáñez del Campo (XI), and Magallanes and the Chilean Antarctic (XII).

Social, Political, and Economic Determinants

Chile's economy has continued to experience solid growth, with a GDP of 6.1% in 2004. The inflation rate decreased from 4.5% in December 2000 to 2.4% in December 2004. Unemployment figures, however, have only marginally improved since 2000. According to Chile's Central Bank, the country's unemployment rate was 8.8% in 2004. The natural resource sectors that have been specifically associated with the economic upturn include mining, forestry, and agriculture.

Environmental protection concerns have been mounting on critical issues such as air quality in the Santiago metropolitan region and in areas surrounding copper smelting facilities located in the northern part of the country. Chile has progressively strengthened its environmental policies based on a model of multi-sector environmental coordination.

The adult population is very concerned about environmental and social problems, as evidenced by the fact that environmental pollution and sanitation rank second and problems associated with alcohol and drug addiction rank third among perceived problems. According to a national survey on socioeconomic conditions (CASEN 2003), potable water coverage nears 100% in urban areas and exceeds 90% in more densely populated rural areas; 96.1% of households have electricity coverage; and only 2.7% of households lack access to excreta disposal systems in urban areas, while this figure increases to 3.5% in rural areas (1). By 1994, nearly 100% of the urban population had regular residential trash collection service. Some urban sanitary landfills were closed as they reached the end of their useful life. As municipalities have outsourced their trash collection services, prob-

lems have emerged, because there are only a few companies controlling the market.

The Ministry of Planning and Coordination, using the CASEN survey, assesses the country's poverty levels and the coverage, distribution, and impact of social protection programs. In Chile, people are considered "poor" if their income falls under a minimum necessary to meet basic needs; persons are considered indigent when they cannot satisfy their nutritional needs. Between 2000 and 2003, absolute poverty—or the sum of non-indigent poor plus the indigent population—decreased by 1.8%, for a rate of 18.8% at the end of 2003. This stands in sharp contrast to the 38.6% rate seen in 1990. Rural poverty and indigence are always greater than in urban areas. In 2003, the income of the wealthiest 20% of Chileans was 14.3 times higher than that of the poorest 20%. Upon factoring in all government financial and non-financial subsidies, the figure falls to 7.6%. In 2003, 31.6% of the country's indigenous population in rural areas lived below the poverty line; 27% of indigenous peoples in urban areas lived below the poverty line.

In 2002, there were 11,226,309 persons 15 years old and older, of whom 5,877,149 made up the workforce, accounting for a 27.2% increase with respect to 1992 census data. The number of females in the workforce increased by 7.5%, while the number of males decreased by 1.5% over the same period.

Since 2000, job creation activity has been more vigorous, and there has been a moderate but sustained decrease in unemployment. Women, young people, and low-skilled workers face significant obstacles to their insertion into the job market, as well as greater job instability. Women in the workforce are subject to employment discrimination by different sectors and in their wages, with most female job opportunities being limited to the services sector. Managerial jobs are largely occupied by men and the average hourly salary received by women is 20% less than that of their male counterparts. Since 1994, the percentage of young people in the job market has been declining, while unemployment rates have remained high. From a geographical standpoint, the highest employment rates during 2002 occurred in the Santiago metropolitan region (43%), and in regions VIII (11%) and V (10%).

During 1992–2002, the housing stock increased (30.6%), with the largest rise (34.2%) occurring in urban areas, as compared to 13% in rural areas. The stock of permanently occupied housing increased by 31.6%, while temporary housing decreased by 48.2%, which indicates that the population has better access to more stable housing arrangements (2).

In 2002, the literacy rate among the population over age 10 was 98.5%, nearly evenly distributed by sex throughout the country (2). Upon comparing data from the previous census (1992), a slight improvement was observed (1.2%), with increases in the levels of preschool (children under age 5 years old), basic, and higher education. Preschool education coverage has increased, and 1 of every 3 children currently has access to this type of education. Chileans attend school an average of 10.2 years, ranging from 8.7 years in region VII to 11 years in the Santiago metropolitan region. The literacy rate is lower among indigenous groups, especially among women, 10.4% of whom can neither read nor write, according to the CASEN 2003 survey (3).

Civic engagement among the adult population is low—55% of adults 15 years old and older do not belong to any organization. Local citizen action groups have the highest membership and participation, followed by religious and sporting groups. Moreover, only 57% of adults claim to have social networks that offer emotional and material support.

Demographics, Mortality, and Morbidity

According to 2002 census data (2), Chile has a population of 15,116,435; 7,447,695 are male and 7,668,740, female. In terms of the total population, persons under 15 years of age account for 25.7%, and those aged 60 years and older, for 11.4%. Population density is 20.4 inhabitants per km^2 and the average age is 30.04 years. Between 1992 and 2002, Chile's annual population growth rate was 1.2% (0.6 percentage points lower than the growth experienced over the previous decade). Rural dwellers account for 13.4% of the country's population; the urban population (86.6%) is concentrated in the Santiago metropolitan region and in regions VIII (12%), V (10%), and X (7%). According to the 2002 census, 4.6% of the population reported belonging to one of eight indigenous groups recognized by the country's Indigenous Law: 87.3% belong to the Mapuche community and 7% to the Aymará. The number of resident aliens in the country was reported to be 184,064, or 1.2% of the total population; 77.1% are immigrants from other countries of the Americas, including Argentina, Peru, and Bolivia.

The country's birth rate has steadily declined, and was estimated at 15.5 births per 1,000 population in 2003 (3). Infant mortality has followed a similar trend, and was 7.8 per 1,000 live births in 2003, as illustrated in Figures 1 and 2. In addition, life expectancy at birth in 2005–2010 was estimated at 78.5 years.

Mortality indicators come from the National Statistics Institute's (INE) vital statistics registries and cause-of-death codes of the International Classification of Diseases, 10th revision (ICD-10) (Ministry of Health). The most recent published fig-

ures (2003) (3) reveal sound quality indicators: 98.9% of deaths are medically certified, and only 2.8% are coded as ill-defined (R00–R99). In 2003, there were 83,672 deaths, for a crude general mortality rate of 5.25 per 1,000 population. Age-adjusted mortality for the standard world population is 5.0 per 1,000 population. By and large, a downward trend in the age-adjusted mortality rates was observed between 2000 and 2003 (5.17 and 5.0 per 1,000 population, respectively). Differences by sex remained constant in these years for all age groups, with excess male mortality of 1.2%. Figure 3 shows the leading causes of death per 100,000 population by broad groups of causes.

In 2000–2003, maternal mortality decreased from 1.9 per 10,000 live births (49 deaths) to 1.4 (35 deaths), which was attributable to a decrease in maternal mortality due to abortion from 0.5 per 10,000 live births (13 deaths) to 0.3 (7 deaths). Fetal mortality in 2003 was 5.7 per 1,000 live births; it has experienced a sustained increase since 1999 (rate of 4.1 per 1,000 live births). There were 909 late fetal deaths (rate of 3.9 per 1,000 live births) in 2003, which represents a sizable reduction in comparison to the figures from 1998 (rate of 4.3 per 1,000), taking into account that these rates had remained stable from 1978 through 1988, and from 1988 through 1998.

Between 1983 and 2003, the total fertility rate decreased from 2.5 children per woman to 1.9. In 1983, the fertility rate was highest among 20–24-year-olds (137.6 per 1,000 women), whereas it was highest among 25–29-year-olds (100.6 per 1,000 women) in 2003. The desired fertility rate is 2.76 children, which is not much different from actual fertility data captured by the 2002 census. Among the population with low socioeconomic status, the rate approaches 3.2 children per woman (2003), which indicates that this group will bear more children than the desired rate due to a lack of access to family planning information and programs.

The 2003 National Health Survey (ENS 2003) reveals elevated rates of morbidity from adult chronic diseases, which account for most of the disease and mortality burden. Mortality from cardiovascular disease, diabetes, and cancers combined accounts for 58% of deaths in the country (4). The 2000 National Quality of Life and Health Survey (ECV 2000) showed that the general population was well satisfied with their health (greater than 5 on a scale from 1 to 7); women and population groups with low socioeconomic status were less satisfied, however (5).

HEALTH OF POPULATION GROUPS

Children under 5 Years Old

There were 1,935 deaths in children under the age of 1 year in 2003, accounting for 2.3% of total deaths and an infant mortality rate of 7.8 per 1,000 live births. The decrease in infant mortality has been mainly due to reductions in late infant mortality. In 2003, neonatal mortality accounted for 64% (4.9 per 1,000 live births) of

FIGURE 1. Birth, mortality, and natural growth rates, Chile, 1983–2003.

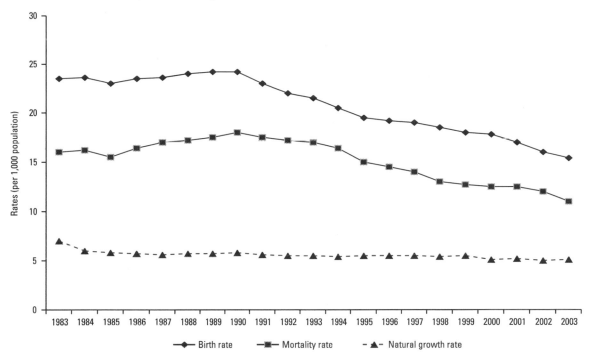

Source: Instituto Nacional de Estadísticas, INE (2003). Anuario de Estadísticas Vitales 2003.

FIGURE 2. Infant mortality rates, Chile, 1983–2003.

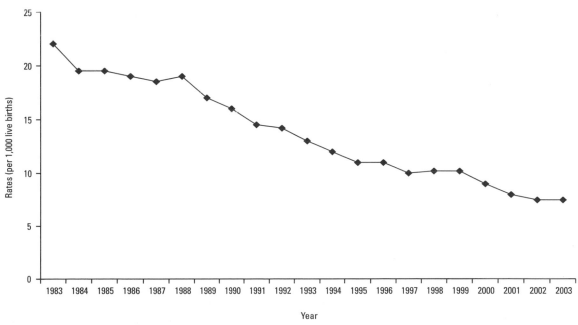

Source: Instituto Nacional de Estadísticas, INE (2003). Anuario de Estadísticas Vitales 2003.

FIGURE 3. Adjusted mortality rate,[a] by broad groups of causes and by sex, Chile, 2000–2003.

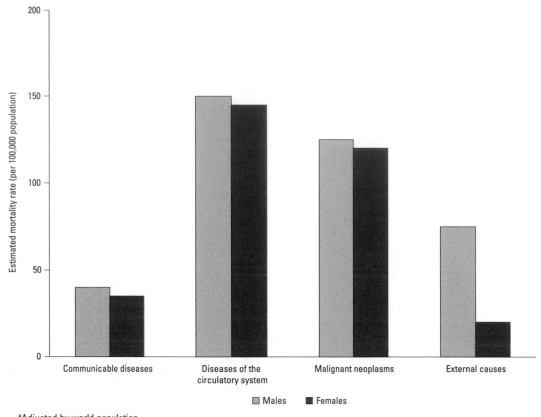

[a]Adjusted by world population.
Source: Ministerio de Salud, Departamento de Estadísticas e Información en Salud.

infant deaths and 75% (723 deaths) of these occurred during the first week of life. Studies on infant mortality in the country's regions reveal fluctuations ranging from 9.6 per 1,000 live births in the Aisén del General Carlos Ibáñez del Campo region to 7.1 in the Atacama and Santiago metropolitan regions. The leading specific causes of death among children under 1 year old are: extreme prematurity, congenital heart defects, pneumonia, sudden infant death syndrome, and central nervous system defects, which together account for 48% of all deaths in this age group.

Approximately 5.2% of newborns weigh less than 2,000 g and 16.5% have low birthweight (between 2,500 and 2,999 g). These figures have remained relatively stable in recent years. Very-low-birthweight infants (less than 1,500 g), while representing only 0.9% of all births, nevertheless account for one-third of infant mortality. The survival rate for this group is 69%, ranging between 8% of newborns weighing 500–599 g and 90% of those weighing 1,250–1,499 g. With respect to hospital discharges for this group, most were due to certain conditions originating during the perinatal period (36.8%), followed by diseases of the respiratory system (31.4%), infectious and parasitic diseases (7.4%), and congenital birth anomalies, deformities, and chromosomal abnormalities (5.4%).

In 1990, a national program was launched to reduce mortality from acute respiratory infections (ARIs) among children under 1 year old. The program reduced the mortality rate from 23.9 per 1,000 live births in that year to 3.4 per 1,000 by 2003. Pneumonia in children under 1 year old accounts for 90% of total deaths from acute respiratory infections (ARIs), and remains the leading cause of preventable childhood mortality. Bronchiolitis obliterans syndrome is the leading cause of hospitalization, accounting for 23% to 25% of all pediatric morbidity medical consultations in Santiago, and affecting one-quarter of all children under 1 year old. With regard to congenital anomalies, Chile gives priority to two conditions: central-nervous-system and cardiovascular anomalies. Data from maternity wards of the Santiago metropolitan region show a decrease on the order of 40% in the incidence of neural tube closure defects. Chile's program of flour fortification with folic acid, implemented in 2000, is credited with this accomplishment. Cleft palate represents another significant problem, with an estimated incidence of 1.8 per 1,000 live births. In 1992–2004, the country's mass phenylketonuria and hypothyroidism screening program performed 1,780,457 tests (100% coverage), identifying 644 children carrying congenital hypothyroidism (incidence of

1 per 2,764 newborns) and 114 carriers of classic phenylke-tonuria (incidence of 1/15,618 newborns).

According to data compiled by the Ministry of Health's nutritional evaluation and surveillance system, the prevalence of malnutrition among children under the age of 6 years has been declining over the past ten years and remains stable to date. Moreover, between 1990 and 2003, an increase was observed in overweight and obesity, while figures on overweight remained stable in 2004 and 2005, at 15% and 7.4% respectively.

It is estimated that at least 16% of children younger than 2 years are afflicted with delayed psychomotor development. Although child abuse is underreported, it is estimated that half of children under age 6 years have been subjected to severe mistreatment. The United Nations Children's Fund estimates that 74% of Chilean children are exposed to or have experienced violent situations within their families (6).

Children 5–9 Years Old

The age group 5–9 years old accounted for only 0.3% of deaths in 2003 and, consequently, had the lowest mortality rate, at 0.17 per 1,000 population. Boys accounted for 59% of such deaths. Reported deaths in 2003 were due primarily to external causes (35.2%); malignant tumors (17.6%); and congenital anomalies (10.8%). Among specific external causes, traffic accidents were responsible for 45.5% of deaths. With respect to deaths related to malignant neoplasms, different types of leukemia were responsible for 45.5%. In terms of hospital discharges for this age group, most were attributable to diseases of the respiratory system (26.3%), followed by diseases of the digestive system (14.2%); infectious and parasitic diseases (7.4%); diseases of the genitourinary system (7.0%); malignant neoplasms (5.5%); and congenital anomalies, deformations, and chromosomal abnormalities (5.1%). Among patients discharged for respiratory system diseases, 23% were pneumonia related; among digestive diseases, 55% were for appendix-related conditions; and among infectious and parasitic diseases, 53% were for diarrheal diseases.

A study of schoolchildren conducted by the Ministry of Health's National Organization for Student Aid and Scholarships found that 5.9% of the sample studied was hyperactive in the home environment, 4.2% at school, and 1.2% in both. With the aid of tools designed to detect mental health problems in elementary schoolchildren through teacher-parent observation, such as the Teacher Observation of Classroom Behavior-Revised (TOCA-R) and the Pediatric Symptom Checklist (PSC), the checklist was administered to the aforementioned sample and showed that 11.9% of the girls and 17.1% of the boys were at risk for developing mental health problems. The study revealed that in 30% of cases, the father does not live in the home with the child; 54.2% of families do not participate in social activities; 17.2% of families have a child required to be absent from school frequently; and 9.4% have a family member receiving treatment for some form of mental illness (7).

Adolescents 10–14 and 15–19 Years Old

The mortality rate among adolescents 10–19 years old is 0.33 per 1,000 population. Mortality in this group (934 deaths) accounts for 1.1% of total deaths. The leading causes of death per 100,000 population by broad groups of causes are: external causes (17.2), malignant neoplasms (4.5), and diseases of the nervous system (3.1). Most hospital discharges in this group were due to diseases of the digestive system (13.1%), followed by diseases of the respiratory system (7.3%), diseases of the genitourinary system (5.1%), and malignant neoplasms (4.4%). In 2003, there were 34,832 live births to women under 20 years old. The women in this age group accounted for 14.9% of total live births, representing a significant decrease with respect to the 16.2% figure reported in 2001. Between 1993 and 2003, the specific fertility rate among adolescent females decreased from 63.9 children per 1,000 adolescents to 54.7. The number of pregnant adolescents accounted for in the National Health Services System (SNSS) remained stable between 2002 (21.1%) and 2004 (21.7%). The country's 2003 national youth survey revealed that 33.1% of adolescents 15–18 years old had been sexually active; 6% of women 15–17 years old had already borne children; 80.4% of women 15–20 years old who had given birth were not currently studying; and 31.6% of persons 15–29 years old had initiated sexual relations at age 15 or younger (8).

According to the 2003 Global Youth Tobacco Survey, schoolchildren have very high smoking rates, especially young women (9). According to the National Drug Control Council, drug abuse prevalence rates among adolescents from the highest-income families double those of young people from the lowest-income families (9), which is consistent with the difference in the consumption pattern of adults observed in the National Health Survey (2003). The prevalence of illegal drug use among adolescents 12–18 years old decreased from 8.6% in 2000 to 6.5% in 2004. In contrast, persons 19–25 years old continued to have high rates of drug use between 2000 (16.3%) and 2004 (16%). Use of all types of illegal drugs by women increased. In 2004, the Tarapacá and Santiago metropolitan regions had the highest drug use rates among the general population. The 2003 National Child Labor Survey revealed a 7.1% prevalence rate of "unacceptable work" among adolescents 15–17 years old, defined as work that prevents young people from studying or that requires them to work at night, outdoors, or involves excessive working hours.

Adults 20–64 Years Old

In 2003, there were 7,273 deaths among 20–44-year-olds, accounting for 8.7% of total deaths and a mortality rate of 1.2 per 1,000 population. The leading causes of death per 100,000 population by broad groups of causes are: external causes (51.9), malignant neoplasms (20.3%), diseases of the circulatory system (12.2), and diseases of the digestive system (9.1). The leading reasons for hospital discharge in this age group were diseases of the digestive system (9.5%), followed by diseases of the genitourinary system (6.9%) and malignant neoplasms (5.1%). The mortality rate in the age group 45–59 years old was 4.6 per 1,000 population, with 11,288 deaths, which accounted for 13.5% of total deaths. In 2003, the distribution of mortality by broad groups of causes in this age group was malignant neoplasms (146.6 per 100,000 population), diseases of the circulatory system (105.1), diseases of the digestive system (63.3), and external causes (62.2). The leading causes for hospital discharges in this age group were diseases of the digestive system (18.2%), malignant neoplasms (15.0%), diseases of the genitourinary system (11.7%), diseases of the circulatory system (10.9%), and diseases of the respiratory system (5.2%).

The mortality rate for the age group 60–64 years old was 11.6 per 1,000 population, which accounted for 7.4% of total deaths (6,177 deaths). Deaths by broad groups of causes in this age group were due to malignant neoplasms (397.8 per 100,000 population), diseases of the circulatory system (302.9), diseases of the digestive system (149.2), external causes (71.6), and endocrine diseases (66.7). With respect to hospital discharges for this age group, the leading causes were diseases of the digestive system (17.7%), diseases of the circulatory system (15.8%), malignant neoplasms (13.8%), diseases of the genitourinary system (10.5%), and diseases of the respiratory system (8.1%). The 2003 National Health Survey revealed that Chile was at an advanced stage in its epidemiological transition, highlighting elevated prevalence rates of smoking, of non-traumatic musculoskeletal symptoms, depressive symptoms in the previous year, and high rates of hypertension (Table 1).

The population with low levels of education is at greater risk for most chronic health problems, with the exception of smoking, which poses a greater risk to the more educated among the population. Chilean women have a higher prevalence for conditions that affect quality of life: tooth loss, musculoskeletal symptoms, obesity, impaired vision, and depressive symptoms. Chilean men, on the other hand, have an increased prevalence for determinants associated with cardiovascular risks, which is consistent with their higher mortality rates from this cause. The rural population has significantly higher rates of cognitive decline and tooth loss, which suggests some degree of disparity in access to basic education and health services. The urban population has significantly higher rates of depressive symptoms. There is a high degree of disparity by region in the prevalence of chronic health problems. Some 83% of adults suffering from multimorbidity (patients with two or more chronic diseases) are younger than 65 years old and 46% have less than eight years of formal schooling.

Among men and women 15 years old and older, 47.5% use some type of contraceptive to postpone pregnancy (either person or his/her partner): 16.7% use the intrauterine device or "IUD," 15.6% use oral contraceptives, and 4.6% use condoms; 7.6% of Chilean women have been voluntarily sterilized. There are some differences by age. The age group 20–44 years old prefers oral

contraceptives (26.3%) and the IUD (25.8%), and to a much lesser degree, condoms (5.7%). In contrast, among persons 15–19 years old, 10.1% use condoms, 9.4% use oral contraceptives, and far fewer use the IUD (3.2%).

Older Adults 65 Years Old and Older

The mortality rate for the age group 65–79 years old was 28.7 per 1,000 population, with 28,247 deaths, accounting for 33.8% of total deaths. The leading causes of death in this age group are diseases of the circulatory system (916.3 per 100,000 population), malignant neoplasms (866.4), diseases of the respiratory system (243.2), and diseases of the digestive system (238.0). With respect to hospital discharges for this age group, the leading causes were diseases of the circulatory system (18.6%), diseases of the digestive system (14.5%), diseases of the respiratory system (12.7%), malignant neoplasms (12.4%), and diseases of the genitourinary system (9.9%).

In 2003, the population 80 years old and older had a mortality rate of 116.8 per 1,000 population, accounting for 27,172 deaths or 32.5% of total deaths in 2003. The distribution of deaths per 100,000 population is as follows: diseases of the circulatory system (4,178.0); tumors (2,056.8); and diseases of the respiratory system (1,723.3). With respect to hospital discharges for this age group, the leading causes were diseases of the respiratory system (22.5%); diseases of the circulatory system (20.0%); diseases of the digestive system (10.6%); diseases of the genitourinary system (7.3%); and tumors (7.3%).

Chronic health problems are more prevalent among adults older than 60 years old, with the exception of depressive symptoms and smoking, which are lower in this group than in the general population older than 17 years old (4). Some degree of hearing loss affects 66.6% of men and 49.2% of women 60 years old and older. According to 2006 estimates based on the 2003 National Health Survey, 33% of older adults may need hearing aids. The prevalence of impaired long-distance visual acuity (with correction) is 34.5% for men and 44.2% for women aged 60 and older; 41.8% of men and 61.8% of women in this age group experienced tooth loss. Cognitive decline (confirmed by the Mini Mental State Examination and the Pfeffer questionnaire to detect senile dementia) was 8.5% for the population aged 60 and older. The prevalence of impaired visual acuity, tooth loss, and cognitive decline is higher among women, especially in rural areas. Some 7.8% of older adults have difficulty walking on flat surfaces. The prevalence of prostate-specific antigen levels higher than 4 ng/ml was 13.6% in males aged 60 and older.

The Family

Between 1990 and 2003, approximately 720,000 women entered the job market, and account for 38% of the workforce. Some 60% of working women are in their childbearing years (under

TABLE 1. Prevalence of certain chronic health conditions, rates per 100 adults, Chile, 2003.

Health condition	Men	Women	Total
Arterial hypertension (SBP ≥140 or DBP ≥90 mmHg)	36.7	30.8	33.7
Dyslipidemias			
Total elevated cholesterol (>200 mg/dl)	35.1	35.6	35.4
Low HDL (<40 mg/dl)	48.4	30.6	39.3
Nutritional status			
Normal	36.6	36.9	36.9
Underweight (IMC <18.5)	0.6	1.1	0.8
Overweight (IMC 25 < 30)	43.2	32.7	37.8
Obesity (IMC >30)	19.4	27.0	23.2
Morbid obesity (IMC >40)	0.2	2.3	1.3
Diabetes	6.1	6.5	6.3
Smoking (current smoker)	48.0	37.0	42.0
Metabolic syndrome	23.0	22.3	22.6
High global cardiovascular risk (ATPIII)	64.2	46.2	54.9
Symptoms of angina and high cardiovascular risk	11.7	13.8	12.8
Sedentary lifestyle	87.9	90.8	89.4
Musculoskeletal symptoms			
Symptoms over last 7 days, pain ≥ 4 (scale of 1–10)	26.1	42.2	34.3
Inability to work and disability among those with symptoms	2.4[a]	5.1[a]	4.0[a]
Depressive symptoms (within the last year)	10.4	24.3	17.5
Renal function			
Elevated creatininemia (age-and-sex adjusted)	6.1	7.3	6.7
Diminished clearance 30–80 ml (body-surface adjusted)	19.4	22.4	21.0
Low clearance 30 ml	0.14	0.21	0.18
Chronic respiratory symptoms	22.2	21.3	21.7
Oral health problems			
Tooth loss in maxilla (0 teeth present in maxilla)	9.1	17.2	13.3
Tooth loss in both maxilla (0 teeth present in mouth)	3.2	7.7	5.5
Prevalence of dental caries	68.6	63.3	66.0
Vision (best eye, with correction, Snellen, normal 0.4–1)			
Loss of visual acuity (0.1–0.3)	7.9	14.2	11.2
Blindness (<0.1)	1.9	3.2	2.6
Hearing loss			
"Whisper" and "tic toc" test findings	18.9	16.3	17.6
Gastric reflux (pyrosis or regurgitation of food)	26.5	33.1	29.9
Cognitive degeneration in older adults			
Cognitive decline + disability (MMSE < 13 + Pfeffer ≥6)	8.3	8.6	8.5
Anemia (hemoglobin ≤12 mg%)	[b]	5.1	[b]
Elevated prostate-specific antigen > 4 ng/ml	3.8	[c]	[c]

Source: Ministerio de Salud, Encuesta Nacional de Salud 2003.
[a]Symptomatic patients only.
[b]Women only.
[c]Men only.

age 40). The percentage of female heads of household increased from 25% in 1992 to 32% in 2002, as did the percentage of families where both spouses work (from 27% in 1990 to 39% in 2000). Extended families account for only about 10% of families. Traditional patterns in the division of household labor persist, causing women to become overburdened. On average, women typically work 41.5 hours per week, whereas men work 44.5. More than 30,000 children and adolescents living in female-headed households work to supplement the family's income. Of them, 2,000 are between 5 and 8 years old. Approximately 42,000 girls and teenaged females are responsible for caring for their siblings or offspring at the expense of their own development.

Among the country's health objectives slated for 2000–2010 is the need to implement a comprehensive program for the prevention and treatment of domestic violence, to include a component for the evaluating and monitoring of child abuse. To date, survey data indicate that more than 50% of women in depression treatment programs exhibit signs of domestic violence. Given the estimated magnitude of this problem and the fact that it is currently underreported, a component to identify cases of domestic violence, child abuse, and sexual abuse was added to the data intake system at the primary health care level between 2002 and 2003. In 2004, domestic violence programs were implemented at 30 "communes" (*comunas*), which provided care to approximately 4,500 women for these problems. As a result, domestic violence care roughly doubled in 2005 compared with 2004.

Workers

In 2004, there were at least 297 fatal accidents in the workplace, or 10.3 accident fatalities per 100,000 workers. Accidents en route to the workplace accounted for 28% of this figure. While this trend has been declining since 2000, when there were 14.12 accident fatalities per 100,000 workers, the distribution of fatal accidents by site of accident has remained the same. The rate of workplace accidents remained relatively stable between 2000 and 2004, ranging from 8.66% to 8.24%. The incidence rate for occupational diseases reported in 2004 was 0.15%, as compared to 0.10% in 2000. In 2004, an average of one workday per worker was lost due to workplace accidents, and .03 of a day per worker for occupational diseases. In 2004, there were 240,000 workplace accidents in companies enrolled in employers' mutual insurance plans (Law No. 16,744).

Poisonings involving workplace pesticides are classified as workplace accidents. Since reporting became mandatory in 2004, the number of reported poisonings has doubled. There were 461 cases of workplace poisonings in 2005, or 63 per 100,000 workers. In 2005, the regions with the highest rates of workplace poisonings were the Santiago metropolitan region (148 cases per 100,000 population), region V (101 cases), and region VI (92 cases). These cases included many workers from the agricultural, hunting, and fishing sectors of the economy. Men were most affected (53%), averaging 33 years of age. Twenty-five cases of workplace poisoning were reported involving persons younger than 18 years old.

One of Chile's health goals is to reduce morbidity and mortality associated with workplace conditions. Consequently, the country has developed an ongoing monitoring system to ensure that 100% of workplace accidents involving a fatality are investigated within 48 hours of the event. Coverage of inspection visits has been stepped up, from 8% in 2005 to 15% in 2006, with a view to preventing risks and ensuring adequate oversight of companies whose activities are considered high risk. Occupational health and safety teams and peer committees have received training to enhance their investigations into such accidents. Steps have also been taken to improve funding and the allocation of financial resources for the program.

Persons with Disabilities

Conducted in 2004, Chile's first national survey on disability (*10*) revealed that 12.9% of the population, or 2,068,072 persons, are living with some degree of disability. Adults are four times more likely to have disabilities than children, while disabilities among older adults are 14 times more likely than among children. One of every two persons living with a disability had not completed basic education, and only one in three persons of working age with disabilities had a paying job. Of people with disabilities, 6% reported no access to rehabilitation services. One of every 40, or 403,842 persons, had a severe disability. There were 34.6% of households that had at least one member with a disability. Women account for 58% of persons with disabilities. The highest prevalence is observed among the age group 30–64 years old (51%). The most prevalent disabilities are physical (31.3%), followed by visual (19%). Some 10% of disabled persons have multiple disabilities. Chronic diseases are the leading cause of reported disabilities.

Ethnic Groups

The country's first sociodemographic and epidemiological study of indigenous groups was conducted in 1997 (*11*), revealing disparities between these groups and the rest of the country. For example, indigenous peoples had excessive infant mortality rates (more than 40 points higher than the national average in the case of the Atacameño population); lower life expectancy at birth (10 years less for the Aymará); a low Swaroop index, which is roughly equivalent to that of the country at the start of the 1980s; a pattern in the causes of death indicative of the situation prior to the epidemiological transition (Aymará); and worse health conditions among indigenous peoples living in cities than those of indigenous peoples living in rural areas. Subsequent studies have shown that the incidence of death from bronchial pneumonia among Mapuche children under 5 years old is higher than among children of non-Mapuche ancestry (*12*). Likewise, the incidence of tuberculosis is higher in areas with large concentrations of indigenous peoples. This is especially true of the Aymará, which, according to the Arica Health Service, have a tuberculosis mortality rate twice the national average. Studies show that both Mapuche children and adults tend to have short stature, and this difference is partly explained by their poverty and social vulnerability. The Araucanía (region IX), with its high concentration of Mapuche, has higher mortality from gallbladder cancer, as well as a high prevalence of colelitiasis and poor access to colonoscopy screening.

HEALTH CONDITIONS AND PROBLEMS

COMMUNICABLE DISEASES

All information in this section comes from the Ministry of Health's Epidemiology Department (*13*).

Vector-borne Diseases

In 2000, the **dengue** vector, *Aedes aegypti*, was detected on Easter Island, with household infestation indices on the order of 70%. In response, a vector control campaign was launched and a

AUGE Plan: Basic Health Guarantees

The centerpiece of health care reform in Chile is the law that establishes the Plan for Universal Access with Explicit Guarantees (AUGE Plan, established by Law 19,966, known as the General System of Health Care Guarantees) and a law that strengthens the health authority and generates the conditions whereby hospitals can be managed with greater flexibility (Law 19,937 pertaining to the Health Authority and Network of Autonomous Hospitals). The AUGE Plan specifies four basic guarantees for a group of health problems: access, timeliness, quality, and financial protection. The AUGE Plan began to be implemented in the public sector in August 2002, with guarantees provided for three health problems. In 2003, two additional health problems were included, and by 2006, the 40 diseases that most affect family health and spending were being covered under the plan. The AUGE Plan implementation foresees including all 56 leading health problems by 2008. Guaranteed benefits include medications and medical inputs required to treat diseases. Benefits will be provided only at medical centers, hospitals, and clinics that comply with the Ministry of Health quality standards. Persons seeking care are ensured that they will receive treatment within an established time frame; if they do not, they can bring a complaint to the Office of the Health Superintendent.

dengue fever surveillance system put in place. In March 2002, the first case of indigenous dengue fever was confirmed on Easter Island, the index case of an epidemic outbreak that continued until mid-May. It affected 17% of the population, but did not result in any deaths. DEN-1 was the circulating serotype, which is phylogenetically identical to the strain that surfaced in Polynesia at the end of the previous year. No new outbreaks have been detected since. Continental Chile has remained free of the dengue vector.

In 1999, Chile achieved interruption of *Trypanosoma cruzi* transmission. The country's area of endemic **Chagas' disease** extends from regions I through IV, and includes the Santiago metropolitan region. Since 1992, the mortality rate for Chagas' disease (0.3 per 100,000 population) has stabilized at an average of 52 deaths annually. In 2001, the number of deaths jumped to 68 (0.44 per 100,000 population), but has been trending downward in the years since; 80% of these deaths are due to Chagas-related heart disease and the remainder to other visceral manifestations. Since 1996, the notification of infected blood donors has increased, for an annual average rate of 0.4 per 100,000 population (2003).

No cases of **yellow fever**, **plague**, or **schistosomiasis** have been reported in the country. Since 1945, there have been no reported cases of **indigenous malaria**. However, *Anopheles* foci are present in areas of the Yuta Valley (Arica) and Quebrada de Tarapacá (Iquique); region I has remained free of *Plasmodium* infection.

Vaccine-preventable Diseases

Information in this section comes from the Ministry of Health's Expanded Program on Immunizations (*14*).

Vaccination coverage of infants younger than 12 months old with BCG, Hib, three doses of OPV, and three doses of DPT is over 95%, as is coverage with measles, mumps, and rubella triple vaccine at age 1 year old.

With regard to **poliomyelitis**, since 1975 the country has been free of wild poliovirus circulation. In 2001, coverage with three doses of DPT/Hib vaccine was 96.6% and coverage with oral polio vaccine was 96.1%; in 2004, it was 95.1%. In 2005, reported cases of flaccid paralysis were 2.2 per 100,000 children younger than 15 years old, a figure similar to that in the 1990s.

Since the beginning of the 1990s, **diphtheria** evolved from being endemic to having sporadic cases, with the last case occurring in 1996. From 2002 to 2005, seven suspected cases of diphtheria were detected through surveillance activities, all of which were ruled out. Coverage with three doses of DPT in 2004 (*15*) was 93.1%.

Since 2004, there have been no confirmed cases of **measles**. Between 2001 and 2005, periodic vaccination campaigns of children under 5 years old were carried out to ensure that the country would hold on to the goal of eradication. In 2003, a case of imported measles was confirmed in a 33-year-old Chilean returning from Japan, in which the H1 virus was isolated. Vaccination coverage of 1-year-old children has remained over 90% for the last five years, reaching an all-time high of 94.4% in 2004.

Between 1996 and 2000, the rates of **pertussis** increased. This situation stabilized by 2001, reverting to a low endemic level (6.6 per 100,000 population in 2004), although the last weeks of 2005 witnessed an increase with respect to the previous 5-year period, for an annual rate of 7.7 per 100,000. In 2005, rates among adolescents and adults up to the age of 44 years increased with respect to previous years. The lethality rate for pertussis is approximately 0.2% to 0.4% (5–11 annual deaths). In 2003, the disease resulted in 11 deaths, 10 of which were diagnosed as "unspecified pertussis."

Tetanus cases have been sporadic, at between 7 and 10 cases annually over the past 11 years, and with incidence rates ranging between 0.04 and 0.12. In 2005, nine cases were reported for a rate of 0.06 per 100,000 population. No cases of **neonatal tetanus** have been reported since 1996. In Chile, children between 18 months and 4 years of age receive two DPT booster doses; the diphtheria toxoid vaccine is administered during second grade.

In 2005, there were 1,607 cases of **mumps** reported, for an incidence rate of 9.96 per 100,000 population.

Due to an upsurge in the number of **rubella** cases in 1997, more than 70% of which affected persons between 10 and 28 years old, a rubella immunization campaign was carried out in August 1999. The campaign targeted females 10–29 years old, with a view to preventing congenital rubella syndrome (CRS), and achieved 99% coverage. As a result, the rate decreased from 31 per 100,000 population in 1998 to 11 per 100,000 in 1999, and there was a drop in the incidence rate to only 1.9 in 2002 (94% decrease). Most cases of rubella (68%) occurred in children under 5 years old. In 2003, there were 128 confirmed cases, for a rate of 0.8 per 100,000 population, which represented a 58% decrease with respect to 2002, and a 97% decrease as compared to the year when rubella was at epidemic levels (1998). In 2004, a number of isolated cases were confirmed. In 2005, the first postimmunization campaign outbreak occurred at a military installation in region V, where 46 young men were infected. As of June 2005, there have been no other confirmed rubella cases in the country. In September 1999, a CRS surveillance system was launched. Between 1999 and 2000, 18 CRS cases were detected, 14 of which presented birth defects at the time of the examination. From 2001 to 2005, there were no new confirmed CRS cases.

In 1996, surveillance of invasive infections associated with *Haemophilus influenzae* **type b** (Hib) was launched, targeting children between the ages of 2 months and 5 years. That same year, a program of free vaccination against the disease was implemented, following which reported cases decreased from 10.6 per 100,000 children under 5 years old in 1996, leveling off at approximately 2.0 per 100,000 over the last five-year period. In 2005, 19 cases of Hib infection were confirmed among the targeted age group, 58% of which affected males. The age range was 2 months to 3 years of age, with a median age of 1 year.

Influenza epidemics occur every three to four years. In 2004, the number of cases more than doubled compared with the figure for the same period in 2003 (5,143 cases), which qualified the outbreak as an epidemic. The cumulative rate in 2005 was 633 cases per 100,000 population, which was down from the figure seen for the same date in 2004. Rate increases were observed for all age groups between 2003 and 2004. Moreover, the difference between those two years was significantly less among the population 65 years old and older (37%), which may be attributable to vaccination efforts that targeted this age group. Over the past decade, variations in the mortality rate from influenza have been observed every three years, associated with outbreaks. In 2001, 82% of deaths attributable to this cause (56 deaths; rate of 0.4 per 100,000 population) occurred in people 65 years old and older (4.1 per 100,000 population). In 2002 and 2003, a drop in mortality from this cause was observed (16 and 19 deaths, respectively), including in persons 65 years old and older (2003 rate of

1.6 per 100,000 population). In 2001 (year in which influenza was epidemic), a higher mortality rate from pneumonia was observed among people 65 years old and older, which subsequently decreased. In 2005, vaccination coverage for influenza was 94.6% for chronically ill adults 65 years old and older, 93.7% for pregnant women, and 95.1% for health workers.

Intestinal Infectious Diseases

Typhoid fever and **paratyphoid fever** are endemic diseases that tend to be seasonal in nature (March, October, and November). These diseases have been at low endemic levels since 1984. They occur as localized outbreaks in schools or daycare centers and are linked to the consumption of bacteria-contaminated food and water. Incidence rates for 2004 and 2005 were similar (4 per 100,000 population), with 488 cases reported in 2005. The groups at greatest risk are males and females 5–19 years old; the regions at greatest risk are II, X, VIII, and VI.

Hepatitis A is a disease of intermediate endemicity with epidemic outbreaks every four to five years, mainly in institutions. The most recent epidemic cycle began in 2002 (2001 in some regions) and remained within expected levels during 2004. In 2005, there was a 62.4% drop in cases as compared to the previous year, and cases were 57% lower than expected for a nonepidemic year, for a cumulative incidence rate of 14.4 per 100,000 population. Weekly incidence rates for 2005, which were on the order of 0.3 cases per 100,000 population, remained lower than those observed in 2003 and 2004. The age group 5–14 years old accounts for 40% of the cases. Moreover, a significant increase in the disease has been observed among adolescents and young adults 15–24 years old, affecting more men than women. The disease is distributed throughout the country. The Tarapacá region has the highest incidence rate, at 81 per 100,000 population, followed by the Antofagasta and Coquimbo regions.

Since 1998, there have been no new cases of **cholera**. Deaths of children under 5 years old associated with diarrheal diseases have dropped significantly, from 3.8 per 100,000 children in 1990 to 0.6 in 2003. Due to the cholera epidemic, epidemiological surveillance of **acute diarrheal diseases** was stepped up and mandatory reporting of all diarrheal diseases with dehydration was instituted. Since 2003, data on morbidity and its causes have been available from a network of sentinel centers. During 2005, a total of 8,672 cases of diarrhea in children under 5 years old were reported, for a rate of 9 per 1,000 children. Diarrhea in this age group occurs seasonally, typically in summer (weeks 1 through 16). Infants under 1 year old are most at risk for developing diarrhea, for a rate of 89 per 1,000 children. Rates for most regions range between 6 per 1,000 children under 5 years old to 9 per 1,000. In 2004, surveillance of **rotavirus infection** began at 13 selected diarrheal sentinel centers, following the detection of rotavirus in December 2005 in 14.8% of samples analyzed. The Coquimbo region had the highest percentage of positive samples (21%), whereas the Antofagasta region had the lowest (8.3%).

The virus affects men (14%) and women (13%) in similar proportions, and the highest number of samples are in children under 12 months old (32%).

Chronic Communicable Diseases

Morbidity from **tuberculosis** was similar in 2001 and 2004 (18.4 per 100,000 population). During those years, activities of the national program of tuberculosis prevention and control have been ongoing: bacilloscopy to evaluate suspected cases and monitor treatment, cultures for diagnosing and monitoring the disease, and implementation of the Direct Observed Therapy Short Course (DOTS) strategy for all forms of tuberculosis in the country. In 2004, these activities paved the way for 11 million Chileans to enter the elimination phase of the disease (rate lower than 20 per 100,000 population).

HIV/AIDS and Other Sexually Transmitted Infections

Since the first AIDS case was reported in 1984 up to 31 December 2004, a total of 13,728 cases had been reported in the country, 6,509 of which have been classified as symptomatic AIDS and the remaining 7,219 as HIV positive, asymptomatic individuals. The cumulative HIV/AIDS incidence rate is 98.1 per 100,000 population. The national incidence rate of reported HIV/AIDS cases in 2004 was 7.18 per 100,000 population (12 in men and 2.44 in women). The majority of cumulative cases affect men (85.2% of cases). The male-to-female ratio for 1999–2003 was approximately 5:1, and the cumulative rate for 1984–2004 was 5.7. Most affected are persons 15–49 years old, who account for 90% of cases. The highest cumulative incidence rates for 1984–2004 by region are the Santiago metropolitan region (152.2 cases per 100,000 population), Tarapacá (137.1), and Valparaíso (129.6). The main form of transmission is sexual contact (86.1%), 56.4% through homosexual or bisexual relations. The first AIDS deaths in Chile occurred in 1984. To date there have been 4,644 deaths: 4,086 men (88%) and 558 women (12%). The accumulated mortality rate for 1984–2003 was 33.4 deaths per 100,000 population. Since 1998, AIDS mortality has been unstable but increasing, reaching its highest point in 2001 (3.5 per 100,000 population). The 2003 rate (last official year) was 2.7 AIDS deaths per 100,000 population. In 2003, the rate for men was 4.5 per 100,000 population and for women, 0.8. The age group 25–44 years old accounts for 68% of deaths. Between 1993 and 1997, AZT was the treatment of choice, but beginning in 1998, combination therapy with antiretroviral drugs began to be used. Beginning then and up to 2005, vertical transmission of the disease was reduced from 30% to 1.8%.

Mandatory notification is required for both **syphilis** and **gonorrhea**. The syphilis incidence rate was 23.9 per 100,000 population in 2000 and 17.4 (2,831 cases) in 2005, although underreporting of the disease is probable. Women accounted for the majority of reported cases in 2005 (52.9%). In 2005, 276 cases were reported in pregnant women and 44 cases of congenital syphilis also were reported, which remained within the median for the period 2000–2005. In 2005, the highest rates were observed in the Aisén del General Carlos Ibáñez del Campo and Antofagasta regions, which had rates four and two times the national average, respectively. The gonorrhea incidence rate was 16.1 per 100,000 in 2000 and 10.7 in 2005 (1,739 cases), with men accounting for 77.2% of reported cases. The most reported cases occurred in the Tarapacá region, which were in excess of seven times the national rate, followed by the Los Lagos and Aisén del General Carlos Ibáñez del Campo regions, with more than three times the national rate.

Hepatitis B surveillance is universal, with daily case-by-case and clinical laboratory notification. The 2003 National Health Survey found the prevalence rate of hepatitis B surface antigen carriers to be 0.1% among the population older than 17 years old. Currently, high-risk groups—health workers and chronic hemodialysis patients—are vaccinated. Discussions are under way concerning the possibility of including this vaccine as part of the childhood immunization schedule.

According to the 2003 National Health Survey, 15% of sexually active women are carriers of the **human papillomavirus** (a self-administered vaginal test kit had been distributed to test for the virus). The highest prevalence is seen in women younger than 35 years old (over 23%).

Zoonoses

Hydatidosis is endemic in Chile, especially in rural areas where sheep are raised. Mortality from hydatidosis has remained stable over time, and is the second leading cause of death from parasitic infections after Chagas' disease, with 30 to 40 deaths seen each year. The hydatidosis mortality rate was 0.2 per 100,000 population in 2003, and remained unchanged between 2001 and 2002. Reported cases of hydatidosis have held steady since 1989, at approximately 2–2.5 per 100,000 population. In 2005, 345 cases were reported, or 2.14 per 100,000 population. Despite the high figure and the fact that notification of the disease is mandatory there is significant underreporting, as evidenced in hospital discharge records. Accordingly, 1,220 patients were discharged due to hydatidosis in 2003, but only 337 cases were reported that year. Consequently, hydatidosis was the leading cause of hospitalization due to parasitic diseases that year. Hospital admissions vary greatly by region, with the highest rates observed in the country's rural areas. The Aisén del General Carlos Ibáñez del Campo region (XI) had the highest hospitalization rate, with 41 discharges per 100,000 population, followed by region IX with 38 discharges.

Anthrax outbreaks occur sporadically in Chile. During 2004, there was an increase in outbreaks compared with previous years (incidence rate of 0.07 per 100,000 population); but no cases were reported in 2005. There are also sporadic outbreaks of **brucellosis**. Nine cases were reported in 2005, originating in region X and the Santiago metropolitan region, but no brucellosis deaths were reported. **Trichinosis** emerges in sporadic outbreaks among family groups, with incidence rates that range between 0.7 and 0.2 per 100,000 population. There are between 0 and 2 deaths from trichinosis each year. During 2005, 55 cases were reported, for an incidence rate of 0.4 per 100,000 population. All outbreaks were attributable to unlicensed slaughter facilities.

NONCOMMUNICABLE DISEASES

Metabolic and Nutritional Diseases

Nutritional diseases due to insufficient caloric intake have declined dramatically, while nutritional problems associated with overeating have been on the rise. In 2003, some 5.6% of newborns weighed less than 2,500 g and 1% weighed less than 1,500 g. In 2004, the prevalence of underweight pregnant women as a percentage of all those monitored in the public health care system was only 12.2%, whereas obesity prevalence reached 32.2%. This figure remained unchanged in 2000–2004, although it was higher than its 1994 level of 26.4%. Malnutrition rates among children under 6 years old who are monitored at the primary health care level have decreased, while the prevalence of obesity in the group has increased, although obesity figures have been stabilizing in the reporting period. The prevalence of underweight (BMI < 18.5) in adults is 0.3%, while the prevalence of obesity is 23.2% (19.6% in men and 29.3% in women). More than 60% of the population is either overweight of obese, and 1.3% is morbidly obese (BMI ≥ 40). The highest rates of obesity in adults were observed in women of low socioeconomic status. Obesity among people with less than eight years of schooling is 33.4%. Approximately 29.5% of adults have central or visceral obesity (increasing waist circumference), which jumps to 44.3% among the population with a low level of education. Obesity rates are highest among the lower socioeconomic strata and in the country's deep south (Magallanes region).

The estimated prevalence of **diabetes** among males 60 years old and older is 22.7%; it is 18.6% for females in this age group. The prevalence of diabetes is significantly higher among the population with less than eight years of schooling. Age-adjusted mortality rates for diabetes are increasing. In 2003, diabetes claimed the lives of 3,278 persons, for a rate of 20.6 deaths per 100,000 population.

Among the general population, nonpregnant women older than 17 years old have a 5.1% prevalence of anemia (< 12 g/dl). Exclusive breast-feeding through the fifth month after childbirth in the population accessing the primary health care level in the public services increased from 16% in 1993 to 39.5% in 2000; it was 43.1% in 2002.

Cardiovascular Diseases

Mortality from **ischemic diseases** declined from 53.8 per 100,00 population to 50.9 in 1998–2003. Over the same period, mortality from **cerebrovascular diseases** held steady at 50.1 per 100,000 population. According to estimates, a decrease in age-adjusted mortality from ischemic and cerebrovascular diseases is expected, as is an increase in mortality from hypertension. The rate of hospital discharges owing to ischemic heart disease is 127.9 per 100,000 population and that due to cerebrovascular diseases is 124.7 per 100,000 population.

Hypertension rates among the adult population are high (33.7% of screening tests are positive), especially among young men. The real prevalence of hypertension is estimated at approximately 26% (after diagnostic confirmation). According to the 2003 National Health Survey, hypertension detection, treatment, and control rates are 59.8%, 36.3%, and 11.8%, respectively, and rates are higher among women. Some 12.8% of adults who complain of effort-related chest pain also have more than two cardiovascular risk factors, diabetes, or a preexisting cardiovascular disease. The prevalence of **high total cholesterol** (> 200 mg%) or low HDL cholesterol (< 40 mg%) is 63% among adults older than 17 years old. The most prevalent type of dyslipidemia is low HDL (39.3%). Metabolic syndrome affects 28% of adults (ATPIII).

More than half of adults have two or more of the five risk factors for cardiovascular disease: smoking, age, positive family history for the disease, HDL < 40 mg/dl, and hypertension. Some 6.6% of adults older than 17 years old are at extreme risk for developing cardiovascular disease based on an evaluation of risk factors (smoking, sex, age, systolic pressure, HDL, and total cholesterol). Consequently, according to the Framingham study probability (without considering diabetes), this group's risk for developing a coronary heart disease event over a 10-year period is greater than 20%. Based on the ATPIII classification, which considers risk factors such as diabetes or equivalent cardiovascular conditions, 13% of the population would be at extreme risk. With regard to the determinants of cardiovascular risk, 89.4% of the general population has sedentary lifestyles, increasing to 95.4% among the population with less than eight years of schooling. In the age group 24–44 years old, 29% smoke, are either overweight or obese, and lead sedentary lifestyles simultaneously.

Malignant Neoplasms

Malignant neoplasms are responsible for 23% of total annual deaths and are the second leading cause of death, following diseases of the circulatory system. In 2003, malignant neoplasms claimed the lives of 20,123 Chileans of both sexes, for a rate of 123.7 per 100,000 population. According to estimates, each year malignant neoplasms are responsible for 96,000 hospital discharges and there are 30,000 new cases diagnosed. In 2003, there were 3,115 deaths from malignant neoplasms of the stomach (19.6 per 100,000 population) and 2,016 from malignant neoplasms of the lung (12.7 per 100,000 population). Among men, the leading sites for cancer deaths are the stomach (26.1 per 100,000 population), prostate (18.7 per 100,000 population), and lungs (16.6 per 100,000 population). Among women, the leading sites for cancer are the gallbladder (17.6 per 100,000 population), breast (13.3 per 100,000 population), and stomach (13.1 per 100,000 population).

In the 16 years since the national pediatric cancer program has been in operation, it has proven its effectiveness in improving survival rates and reducing the lethality of most pediatric cancers. In 2000–2002, mortality decreased 26.4%. Acute leukemias have declined by 35.5% and lymphatic leukemias, by 44.1%. Hodgkin's disease has declined by 70.5%, and cohorts treated since 1999 have a 73.2% complete remission rate, a 5-year survival rate of 87%, and a total survival rate of 98%. Malignant neoplasms of the central nervous system in children account for 17% of pediatric cancers in the public health sector, and a reporting system has been in place since 1997.

Age-adjusted mortality for cancer of the cervix between 1999 and 2003 was reduced by 40%. Rates among the early detection program's target group (people over age 25) decreased from 17 per 100,000 population in 1999 to 14.4 per 100,000 in 2003.

The prevalence of prostate-specific antigen at levels above 4 ng/ml is 3.8% in men over 35 years old. Since 2000, coverage of the palliative care program has increased, which treated 13,900 patients in 2004.

Musculoskeletal Conditions

In 2003, the prevalence of musculoskeletal symptoms of nontraumatic origin was 34.3% among the population over 17 years old. Prevalence rates are significantly higher among the elderly, women, and groups of low socioeconomic status. The most prevalent complaint site is the knees, followed by the lumbar region, ankles, and hands. Of the population with musculoskeletal symptoms, 64% retains normal functionality; only 4.2% has a disability or handicap. Most cases follow a chronic course, and only a small percentage has received a specific medical diagnosis. The estimated prevalence of rheumatoid arthritis is approximately 1%. No other demographic studies carried out in the last 5-year period have provided statistical data on the prevalence of specific causes. Musculoskeletal diseases represent an important co-morbidity of chronic adult diseases; according to 2003 estimates, approximately 7% of adults over the age of 17 years presented co-morbidities of dyslipidemia, hypertension, and chronic musculoskeletal symptoms.

OTHER DISEASES AND HEALTH PROBLEMS

Disasters

Chile suffered 19 natural disasters in 2000–2005. Earthquakes caused 11 deaths, 182 injuries, and affected the lives of another 27,463. Although the country is located in a high-risk zone for earthquakes (more than 10 million inhabitants exposed), it has an average vulnerability of 1 to 10 deaths per 1 million population exposed. Extreme temperatures have affected 25,000 persons during the period. Floods claimed the lives of 47 Chileans

and affected 40,886, per year, on average; 221,842 persons were affected between May and June 2002. The floods of June 2000 and of May–June 2002 are among the 10 disasters that affected the most people between 1996 and 2005.

Violence and Other External Causes

Since 1995, accidents have ranked as either the third or the fourth leading cause of death. In 2003, 9% of deaths were due to this cause, for a mortality rate of 46.5 per 100,000 population, which represents a 7.7% decline with respect to 1999. The average excess mortality for men is 4.3 times that of women, although excess mortality is observed in all age groups, in all parts of the country, and for all the different types of accidents, with the exception of falls. The regions with the lowest and highest rates are Atacama and Aisén del General Carlos Ibáñez del Campo, respectively. The Santiago metropolitan region has rates lower than the national average and rates seem to be decreasing. Mortality from trauma and poisonings primarily affects adults 20 years old and older. During 2003, 31% of external deaths among men were due to traffic accidents and 23.5%, to self-inflicted injuries. Among women, 29% were due to traffic accidents and 21%, to falls. In 2003, trauma events, poisonings, and other external causes accounted for 10% of hospital discharges and were the fourth leading cause of hospitalization, representing the leading cause of hospitalization for men, with 17% of cases (102,718 discharges), and the sixth leading cause for women, with 6% of cases (54,652 discharges).

Mental Health

Although awareness about the significance of mental health problems has been on the rise since the 1990s, no specific studies have explored the situation in detail over the last 5-year period. The prevalence of **depressive disorders** among the population ranged between 13% and 17% during the reporting period. In 2004, a national program to diagnose and treat depression served 103,166 patients at the primary health care level and 7,500 patients at the specialized level. The annual incidence of **schizophrenia** among the population older than 15 years old is 12 per 100,000 population. Between 2000 and 2003, the age-adjusted suicide rate increased from 9.7 to 10.4 per 100,000 population. Depression is a significant problem; however, the combination of anxiety and consumption disorders (including alcohol abuse) carried more relative weight in studies conducted in the 1990s.

Addictions

Consistent with the findings of the 2003 National Health Survey and 2000 National Quality of Life and Health Survey, the National Drug Control Council (CONACE) affirms that **smoking** prevalence rates in 2000–2004 stabilized, at 42% (*16*). However, as is the case in the school-aged population, more and more women are taking up smoking, especially those of childbearing age (19–34 years old). In 2004, 55% of women 19–25 years old were smokers.

Due to its link to mortality from cirrhosis, accidents, and violence, **alcohol consumption** is an extremely important if often dismissed topic. According to the above-mentioned National Quality of Life and Health Survey, 15% of adults were problem drinkers in 2002, with the highest prevalence among men, the rural population, and persons with a low level of education. Alcohol consumption among the general population exceeds 50% at all income levels, according to statements of respondents about their alcohol consumption in the 30 days before the survey (2004). Alcohol consumption rises with family income; however, the most significant problems and cases of alcohol-related dependency are seen among the population at the lowest levels of income. Household surveys conducted by CONACE since 1994 show a sustained increase in illegal drug use through 2000 (in annual consumption rates, as well as in consumption in the last year and the last month before the survey). This trend stabilized in 2000–2004.

Oral Health

During the reporting period, there have been no national-level epidemiological studies to provide a comprehensive assessment of the country's oral health situation. In a partial study to determine the effectiveness of eight years (1996–2004) of water fluoridation in the Santiago metropolitan region, which targeted the population between the ages of 6 and 8 years and 12-year-olds, it was observed that the number of permanent teeth damaged by caries in children 6–8 years old decreased 49.6% (decayed, missing, and filled teeth index, or DMFT, decreased from 1.17 teeth to 0.59 teeth). In children 12 years old, this indicator dropped by 16.9% (DMFT 3.13 teeth to DMFT 2.60 teeth) (*17*). The 2003 National Health Survey revealed that 66% of adults older than 17 years old had dental caries and that 13.3% had lost one or both molars. In adults, the prevalence of total tooth loss is 5.5%, which increases to 33.4% among adults over 65 years old, and is highest among women, the rural population, and people with less than eight years of schooling. Tooth loss prevalence rates are lowest in the country's northern portion and highest in the south, which is consistent with the natural fluoride content in water. According to estimates, coverage of the population with fluoridated water was 70.5% in 2004.

Meningococcal Disease

Since 2001, the disease began to decline toward low endemicity (rates of 2.7 and lower), until reaching an incidence of 1.5 per 100,000 population in 2005 (235 cases). The greatest risk of infection, which is slightly higher for men, is found in the Santiago metropolitan region. Mortality has remained stable, with rates between 0.2 per 100,000 population and 0.3, decreasing to 0.1 over the last two years. The lethality rate, which reached 11.2% in 1990, dropped to 5.5% in 2005. During 2005, a change was ob-

served, as meningitides decreased by 34% and meningococcemias increased by 45%. Children under 5 years old accounted for half of all cases. Of the 121 confirmed cases in 2005, 84% were serogroup B strains; 6%, C strains; and 9% ,Y and W-135 strains.

Hantavirus Cardiopulmonary Syndrome

The etiological agent identified in Chile is the Andes virus, whose only confirmed reservoir to date is *Oligoryzomys longicaudatus*. Since the first sporadic cases were detected in 1995, the disease has become endemic, with seasonal outbreaks (70% between November and April) focalized in several areas of the country. From 1995 through December 2005, there were 461 confirmed cases of hantavirus cardiopulmonary syndrome (HCPS). The highest incidence occurred in 2001, but has stabilized subsequently. In 2005, incidence reached 0.42 per 100,000 population. The HCPS lethality rate declined from 60% in 1997 to 31% in 2005 (20 deaths). Its lethality rate is higher among women (37%) than men (27%). The mortality rate has remained stable during the past three years, ranging between 0.11 and 0.13 deaths per 100,000 population. During 2005, there were 67 confirmed cases of HCPS and 7 mild cases (without respiratory failure), which was higher than expected. HCPS cases are observed from the Valparaíso to the Aisén del General Carlos Ibáñez del Campo regions. The greatest risk of infection, however, is found in the latter region, where the incidence rate has reached 3 per 100,000 population. Moreover, the greatest number of cases was observed in region VIII (20 cases). The reservoir of the Andes virus is widely distributed, and the virus has been found in rodents from regions IV to XI.

RESPONSE OF THE HEALTH SECTOR

Health Policies and Plans

Current health sector reforms were officially set in motion by a set of draft laws that the former Administration (2000–2006) submitted to the Parliament in 2002. At the core of the reforms are two laws: Law No. 19,966, known as the General System of Health Care Guarantees, which established the Universal Access Plan with Explicit Guarantees, or "AUGE" Plan, and Law No. 19,937 on Health Authority and Network of Autonomous Hospitals, which strengthens the health authority and establishes conditions for greater flexibility in managing hospitals. The proposal for reforms also considered two draft laws, one to modify private health insurance providers (ISAPREs) and another to finance such changes.

The AUGE Plan specifies the following four basic guarantees for 56 health problems (see Box 1 for a list): access, timeliness, quality, and financial protection. Law No. 19,937, which entered into force on 1 January 2005, split the former Under Secretariat of Health into two under secretariats: the Under Secretariat of Public Health and the Under Secretariat of Health Care Networks. It also reorganized the former ISAPREs Oversight Office into the Office of the Health Superintendent, which is responsible for overseeing ISAPREs, the National Health Fund (FONASA), and public and private health care providers. Execution of the AUGE Plan began gradually and is expected to be finalized for all health problems covered under the plan by 2008.

The health policy framework and plans slated for the current Administration's term (2006–2010) call for completing the implementation and strengthening of the aforementioned reforms. Specifically, this includes increasing the number of covered health problems under the AUGE Plan from 56 to 80 by 2010; strengthening institutional reforms aimed at separating out the delivery of health care services from oversight functions, as well as the implementation of the system of autonomous hospital network; strengthening the family-oriented focus of primary care; enhancing private health care by introducing more competition into the ISAPRE market and streamlining its health plans; and laying the foundations for an elder care policy (18). Looking forward to 2010, the health objectives are reducing disparities in health, addressing the new challenges associated with the aging of the population and the society's changing demographics, and providing quality health care according to the population's needs and expectations.

Chile's health care system is governed by regulations issued by the Ministry of Health, whose programs determine coverage levels, the frequency of contact between users and care providers, and the responsibilities inherent at each level of care in the health system. These regulations constitute mandatory frameworks for care at public and private health establishments, in agreement with the public sector, and represent a frame of reference for the organization of private-sector health care establishments.

Before the changes introduced by Law No. 19,937 (Health Authority Law), the public and private sectors were regulated by health service bureaus, working through the offices of medical and paramedical professionals located in their respective territorial jurisdictions. Beginning 1 January 2005, this responsibility and the technical offices themselves were transferred to the Ministry of Health's Regional Secretariats (SEREMIs) in each region, thereby strengthening them.

Organization of the Health System

The Ministry of Health is the lead agency in the sector. It formulates and establishes health policies and issues general standards and plans, as well as supervising, monitoring, and evaluating compliance with them. The Health Services, the National

BOX 1. Health problems covered under Chile's AUGE Plan.

1. Delivery care with analgesia
2. All childhood cancers
3. Cervicouterine cancer
4. Breast cancer
5. Leukemia (adults)
6. Lymphoma (adults)
7. Testicular cancer
8. Prostate cancer
9. Stomach cancer
10. Gallbladder and bile duct cancer
11. Terminal cancers (palliative care)
12. Ischemic disease (myocardial infarction)
13. Behavioral disorders
14. Congenital heart disease (operable)
15. Neural tube defects
16. Cleft lip/palate
17. Chronic renal insufficiency
18. HIV/AIDS
19. Cataracts
20. Major burns
21. Polytrauma patients with or without medullary lesion
22. Hernia of the nucleus pulposus
23. SNC tumors and cysts
24. Aneurisms
25. Diabetic retinopathy
26. Refractive errors
27. Tooth loss in older adults
28. Surgery requiring prosthesis
29. Hypoacusis
30. Benign hypertrophy of the prostate
31. Pneumonias in older adults
32. Orthotics for older adults (canes, wheelchairs, others)
33. Hemophilia
34. Cystic fibrosis
35. Scoliosis
36. Depression
37. Alcohol/drug dependency
38. Psychosis (severe psychiatric disorders)
39. Bronchial asthma
40. Chronic obstructive pulmonary disease (COPD)
41. Arterial hypertension
42. Encephalitic vascular accident
43. Diabetes mellitus, types I and II
44. Prematurity
45. Retinopathy of prematurity
46. Difficult breathing of newborn
47. Accidents requiring CPU care
48. Rheumatoid arthritis
49. Degenerative osteoarthritis
50. Epilepsy (program to improve management in children)
51. Eye trauma
52. Detached retina
53. Strabismus (children under 9 years)
54. Acute respiratory infections (children under 15 years old)
55. Comprehensive oral health
56. Dental emergencies

Source: Ministry of Health.

Health Fund (FONASA), ISAPRE's Office of the Health Superintendent, the Public Health Institute (ISP), and the Central Supply Clearinghouse (CENABAST) report to the Ministry. According to the most recent legislative changes to the health reforms, Law No. 19,937 delegates responsibility for managing the health care network to the 29 health service bureaus, having transferred health authority functions to the Ministry of Health's Regional Secretariats in each of the 13 regions of the country. The Public Health Institute is responsible for regulating drugs and medical inputs.

In Chile health services are a mixed system in terms of financing, health insurance, and service delivery. By law, all workers are required to pay 7% of their monthly wages into public (FONASA) or private (ISAPREs) health insurance. In addition to contributions from its members, FONASA receives transfers from the Government's Department of the Treasury to cover indigents and to carry out public health programs. The private insurance sector is represented by the ISAPREs, private health insurers that administer the obligatory contributions from wage earners; their members can pay additional premiums to improve their insurance-plan coverage. The ISAPREs and FONASA are both overseen by the Office of the Health Superintendent. Implementation of the AUGE Plan has consolidated this authority. There are also employers' mutual insurance plans that specifically administer insurance for on-the-job accidents and occupational diseases and whose financing is under the responsibility of the employers. Although FONASA and the Office of the Health Superintendent are autonomous, they are subject to oversight by the Ministry of Health, which bears responsibility for sector policy. The Public Health Institute controls drugs and medical inputs and acts as the national reference laboratory. CENABAST procures products for the public sector.

The delivery of services also is mixed. The vast majority of primary care facilities are administered by the municipalities; hospitals fall under the responsibility of the Health Services. Law No. 19,937 provides for a network of autonomous hospitals, which permits greater flexibility in the management of the country's 56 highly complex hospitals. In 2005, autonomy authorization was granted to five hospitals; by 2009, all 56 of the country's highly complex hospitals will be granted this authorization. In addition, there are a series of clinics, centers, laboratories, and pharmacies that are managed by private individuals or companies. There are only a few not-for-profit nongovernmental organizations, and their work is limited to some rural health centers and hospitals operated by religious organizations.

FONASA covers 68.3% of the population and the ISAPREs 17.6%. The remaining 14.1% is covered by other private plans (such as the armed forces plan) or has no insurance at all (19).

ISAPREs can be restricted or open. In restricted institutions, membership is limited to individuals working in a given company or sector of the economy, such as large public copper mining companies. Open institutions allow anyone to become a member. Most ISAPREs (15 nationwide) work through private providers, but may also enter into agreements with public health institutions for some services (e.g., hospitalization in private wings of certain hospitals, emergency care, and care in intensive care units). Some ISAPREs have their own networks to provide care for their subscribers, a trend that has been increasing as the AUGE Plan has been progressively implemented. The insurance contract is negotiated individually between the ISAPRE insurer and the contributor, who is required to make a co-payment, the amount of which varies considerably. ISAPREs may not offer health insurance plans with fewer benefits than FONASA offers, however. The guaranteed financial protection specified under the AUGE Plan sets the maximum co-payment amounts for FONASA and ISAPRE beneficiaries (guaranteed financial protection) for the list of covered health conditions.

Public health services must meet all demands for emergency services. Moreover, the public health programs (such as immunization and tuberculosis control) target the entire population, without discrimination. Peak coverage under ISAPREs was reached in 1995, with coverage of 26.3%. Since 1997, there has been a migration of subscribers from ISAPREs to FONASA, which is attributed to the effects of the Asian financial crisis at the end of the 1990s, to improved public health services, and to the recent implementation of the AUGE Plan (20).

FONASA is responsible for supervision and control of public health sector financing. As is true for all public sector institutions, the Office of the Controller General has ultimate control over its management.

Public Health Services

The Ministry of Health's basic programs (targeted to children, women, adults, and oral health) and their respective subprograms have been designed to take a comprehensive approach, including promotion, prevention, treatment, and rehabilitation. The Ministry of Health has established specific prevention programs, including immunization, food supplements, control of respiratory diseases, prevention of traffic accidents, control of the toxic algal bloom known as "Red Tide," and eradication of Chagas' disease. By December 2004, coverage of the cervical cancer screening program (Pap smears in women aged 25–64 years) was 68%, and 67% for the group at greatest risk (ages 35–64). Coverage of the breast cancer prevention program reached 54% in 2003. These two screening programs will be further enhanced when cervical and breast cancer are added to the health conditions covered under the AUGE Plan.

The Public Health Institute carries out epidemiological surveillance in cooperation with the Ministry of Health's Epidemiology Department. Through the National Control Department, the Public Health Institute monitors the national system for the control of pharmaceutical products, food, cosmetics, pesticides for public health and domestic use, and medical articles. The Institute also acts as the national reference center and is the body that certifies clinical laboratories and blood banks nationwide. Thus, the Institute provides support for ministerial programs designed to control communicable diseases and monitor the quality of pesticides, clinical laboratories, and blood banks. Vital statistics (birth and death certificates) are the most reliable element in the information system. Their coverage is approximately 99%. The system for surveillance of communicable diseases is universal.

With regard to the prevention and control of air pollution, the health sector is responsible for overseeing the elimination or control of all environmental factors, elements, or agents that can harm the health, safety, and well-being of Chileans. There are programs in basic sanitation, air pollution, hazardous chemicals, hazardous waste and liquid industrial waste, food hygiene, vectors of health importance, zoonoses, microbial and parasitic diseases, environmental impact assessment, occupational health, public places, and environmental emergencies. Health reforms transferred control of the environmental departments under the Health Services to the Ministry of Health's Regional Secretariats (SEREMIs) in each region, as was the Environmental Health Service in the Santiago metropolitan region. Consequently, the SEREMIs are now responsible for prevention, control, inspection, and oversight activities in the environmental sphere. Environmental testing is conducted by 20 laboratories that operate in coordination with the Public Health Institute, which acts as the national reference laboratory in microbiology, food science, environmental pollution, and occupational health.

Program guidelines on environmental quality are geared toward controlling the population's health risks due to airborne pollutants. The health authority develops air quality surveillance programs by monitoring compliance with current air quality standards and performs ongoing inspections of airborne pollutants released in emissions of high- and medium-complexity facilities, according to the risks associated with such emissions. Regular diagnosis involves an inventory of fixed sources and fuels used by fixed sources and estimates of emissions from fixed sources, monitoring stations, contaminants measured, measurements on specific dates of the year, and the population affected. The National Environment Commission (CONAMA), under the Ministry of the Interior, is an intersectoral agency and the country's steering authority on environmental matters. The Regional Environmental Commissions (COREMA) are the lead agencies in each region.

Food safety and control systems are based on the Health Code. Food Health Regulations, which establish specifications for food products for human consumption in Chile, went into effect in 1996. Originally, departments of environmental programs that fell under the responsibility of the Health Services were responsible for inspections and overseeing compliance with the legislation. Beginning 1 January 2005, these duties were assumed by each region's SEREMI.

Chile has a national supplementary food program, whose beneficiaries are children under 6 years old and pregnant women. Food is delivered through primary care facilities. Milk, grains, and rice are provided in amounts tied to the nutritional condition of the beneficiaries. Recently, additional supplementary food programs were created for premature infants and children suffering from phenylketonuria. There is also a supplementary food program for schoolchildren operated by the National School Assistance and Grants Board, which provides breakfast and lunch in schools, based on the socioeconomic classification of the children and their families. In recent years, a supplementary food program has been established for older adults. The country also operates wheat flour fortification and salt iodization programs.

New regulations governing food safety are designed to provide basic health standards for the health, safety, and nutritional value of food, as well as dietary guidelines. There also is a nationwide control and hygiene program and coordination, which is supported by the national network of food science. In terms of food safety and control activities pursuant to the Health Code, 60,000 food samples are analyzed each year. The samples are subjected to microbiological tests (75%), chemical-bromatological tests (20%), and parasitological tests (5%).

In light of the 2002 outbreak of avian influenza in Chile, measures have been stepped up to prevent this and other pathologies of interest in animal health from being introduced into the country. Currently the Agricultural and Livestock Services carry out control and surveillance activities on birds, pigs, and horses, but no new outbreaks of avian influenza have been detected in the country since 2002.

Individual Care Services

The public health care network is composed of outpatient and hospital facilities offering services of different complexity. They include 196 hospitals, 60 of which are high-complexity hospitals (23 type-1 and 37 type-2). There are 99 rural (type-4) hospitals. Additionally, 14 private hospitals also are part of the network, providing services to persons covered by public insurance plans under a delegation agreement. The public outpatient network includes 594 primary health care centers: 258 general clinics located in urban areas and 151 rural clinics; 115 primary health care clinics attached to hospitals; and 70 family health centers. The country also operates 40 outpatient mental health centers; 5 health referral centers, which offer services in four core medical specialties (internal medicine, pediatrics, surgery, and gynecology/obstetrics); and 5 diagnostic and treatment centers or high-complexity outpatient facilities. The outpatient network also includes 1,165 rural health posts.

The National Health Services System performed 38,089,674 medical consultations and checkups in 2004, or 3.6 consultations per FONASA beneficiary. This represents an increase of 7.5% since 1999. Of this total, 93.7% were consultations and 6.3%, checkups. Between 2000 and 2005, primary health care medical consultations increased 27%; major surgeries, 17%; emergency care visits, 22%; and hospital discharges remained stable. With regard to oral health, 14,773,772 consultations were reported in 2004, of which 3,770,032 (25.6%) were for preventive treatment and 7,835,598 (53.2%) were for dental repair; the remainder involved specialized care and emergency consultations. In 2005, 54,859,829 laboratory tests and 4,989,970 imaging studies were performed, which represent 2.2 and 0.2 tests per medical consultation, respectively. The Office of the Health Superintendent reported that 12,162,032 medical consultations, 13,844,703 laboratory tests, 3,002,066 imaging studies, and 315,777 surgical procedures were performed in the private sector in 2005, which represent 4.5 medical consultations and 5.1 laboratory tests per ISAPRE beneficiary.

The number of hospital beds in the public sector was 28,135 in 2005, or 2.6 beds per 1,000 FONASA beneficiaries; this represents a reduction of more than 10% in comparison to the 1990s, but the figure has stabilized over the last five years. The private sector has about 11,000 beds distributed among 223 hospitals, clinics, and maternity facilities.

In 2003, there were 1,599,280 discharges from the country's hospitals, of which 1,155,787 were public beneficiaries (72.3%); 252,879, ISAPREs beneficiaries; and the remainder other types of beneficiaries (especially workplace accident victims and schoolchildren). The bed occupancy rate in the public sector in 2003 was 76%, with an average length of stay of 6.1 days. The five most frequent causes of hospitalization were complications of pregnancy, childbirth, or the puerperium (20%); diseases of the digestive system (12%); diseases of the respiratory system (11%); injuries and poisonings (10%); and diseases of the genitourinary system (8%).

Emergency care is provided by hospital emergency services in hospitals and by emergency primary care services. The main private hospitals and clinics also offer emergency care. A prehospital emergency care system has been in place since the closing years of the 1990s; it includes rescue ambulances of different complexity and response capabilities, and a dispatching center. The system operates in the three most heavily populated regions (metropolitan Santiago, Valparaíso, and Bío-Bío); work is under way to extend it to the rest of the country.

Auxiliary diagnostic and therapeutic services are offered by the public and private sectors. In the public sector, services are located in hospitals and serve demand generated in ambulatory services, as well as in hospitals. They are complemented with a few community laboratories in urban "communes" in the major cities. In the private sector, auxiliary diagnostic and therapeutic services are offered by units in private hospitals or clinics or through establishments that offer these services exclusively. Blood banks are primarily linked to public hospitals and to the largest private hospitals. In an effort to improve quality and safety by adopting international quality standards in the processing of blood and blood products, the number of blood banks has been reduced from 120 to 70. The objective is to limit pro-

duction nationwide to only four major blood and tissue banks. Another focus of blood-bank policy has been to promote volunteer donations, which helped increase volunteer blood donations from 2% in 2002 to 8% in 2005. The public health system receives about 180,000 blood donations annually.

Dental care is provided by public and private providers. In the public sector, the oral health program gives priority to comprehensive care for children and pregnant women and offers emergency services for the rest of the population. Treatment is provided through primary health care clinics, with some hospitals providing specialized services. The Ministry of Health's program for children has stepped up its preventive approach by including comprehensive oral health among the 56 health problems covered in the AUGE Plan. This effort is complemented by the operation of dental clinics in municipal schools, which are subsidized by the Ministry of Education through the National School Assistance and Grants Board. Some ISAPREs are beginning to institutionalize private dental care in provider networks, although coverage is still low. Treatment has been complemented by public health actions, such as fluoridation of drinking water.

Mental health is the area with the greatest mismatch between supply and demand in both the public and private sectors. In the public sector, long-term specialized hospital care is only provided in three establishments. Acute care is provided in those same establishments, as well as by psychiatric services in some general hospitals. In recent years, under the national plan for psychiatric care and mental health, the establishment of shelters to deinstitutionalize some patients and encourage their reentry into society has been promoted. The public system also provides outpatient care at community mental health centers in some urban "communes," which are administered by the respective municipalities and include 40 establishments nationwide. The ISAPREs offer only minimal coverage for psychiatric care in their health plans. The conditions covered under the AUGE Plan include depression, alcohol and chemical dependency, and psychoses, which are expected to improve the supply of mental health services and reduce disparities in access among different groups of the population.

Reproductive health services are provided by the network of public and private suppliers. The Ministry's program includes family planning and contraceptive distribution (hormonal, intrauterine devices, diaphragms), which are provided free of cost at primary health care establishments. Normal pregnancies are monitored at primary health care facilities and high-risk cases are referred to hospitals. Both the public and private sectors have centers that offer infertility treatment, but coverage remains low. Emergency birth control has only recently been added to the services offered at public health establishments.

Geriatric services are scarce in the public and private sectors. Public care is offered through the general services provided by primary-level facilities and general hospitals. There is only one specialized center (the Geriatric Institute in the Santiago metropolitan region), which has limited capacity. The private sector has residences for older adults that offer care.

Cancer treatment is provided in some specialized public and private facilities, which offer surgery, chemotherapy, and radiotherapy. The National Cancer Institute and three other regional centers that are somewhat less developed are operated by the public sector. The Ministry has established national chemotherapy programs for certain types of childhood and adult cancers. The private sector has centers that offer radiation therapy, and some have entered into an agreement whereby they provide treatment for public insurance beneficiaries. Childhood cancers, cervical cancer, breast cancer, leukemia and lymphoma (adults), testicular cancer, prostate cancer, stomach cancer, gallbladder and biliary tract cancers, and terminal cancers (palliative care) are included under the AUGE Plan's covered health problems.

Rehabilitation services are provided in public and private establishments, although coverage is low in both. In the public sector, there are some national reference centers for adults in the Northern Metropolitan Santiago Health Service and centers for children in the Eastern Metropolitan Santiago Health Service. Some establishments in other regions also offer rehabilitation services, such as the regional hospital in Concepción. In the private sector, the most important services are provided by a nonprofit foundation, the Children's Rehabilitation Institute, which has centers in the Santiago metropolitan region and other parts of the country. The National Disability Fund was created in 1994 as an agency of the Ministry of Planning and Coordination; it conducted the first national survey on disabilities in 2005.

Health Promotion

The broad objectives of the 1997 National Health Plan are to promote healthy lifestyles and a healthy environment, increase individual and community understanding and capacity for self-care, and bolster the State's regulatory function with respect to health determinants. The National Council for Health Promotion (Vida Chile) was established as an intersectoral agency composed of 24 national institutions; it is responsible for advising ministries and regional and local governments, supporting implementation of community plans, and recommending public health policies. To achieve these objectives it relies on strategies that include programs for healthy communities, health-promoting schools, the "Health for People" program, healthy workplaces, and the CARMEN project. In 2001, there were 305 community health promotion plans; the strategy of health-promoting schools has been introduced in 2,435 educational institutions and 32 schools have been accredited by the health sector as health-promoting schools. Chile's Government is signatory to the agreements issued at the Fifth Global Conference on Health Promotion (Mexico, 2000). In 2002, the country's health promotion plan evaluated, revealing positive results among the group exposed to health promotion plans, as compared to similar target populations that had no such exposure.

Health Supplies

Chile's pharmaceuticals market is characterized by the circulation of significant amounts of generic drugs, a large presence of national laboratories, and operation of the Ministry of Health's Central Supply Clearinghouse. There are no price controls on drugs. In 2002, generic drugs accounted for 39.3% of units sold; trademark generics, 38.5%; and brand-name products, 22.1% (21). In terms of sales, generic drugs account for only 7.7% of the market, trademark generics for 49%, and brand-name drugs for 43.3%. This large share of the market held by generic drugs has reduced the average price of drugs, to US$ 3.03 in 2002. The leading laboratory was Laboratorio Chile (27% of the market). In terms of the total number of patent applications filed with the Ministry of Economy between October 1991 and April 2002, 19% were for pharmaceutical patents. With respect to patents granted, 43% originated in the United States and 24% in Europe. There are some 1,500 community pharmacies in the country, of which 37% are owned by three franchises (Salco-Brand, Ahumada, and Cruz Verde) that control 90% of the market (22). This oligopoly leads to a problem in the vertical integration between the production and sale of a number of pharmaceutical products. In addition, 35 of the country's "communes" with more than 10,000 inhabitants do not have a community pharmacy.

The objective of the national drug policy is to ensure that the entire population has access to an adequate supply of the drugs included on the country's essential drugs list. Furthermore, it seeks to guarantee drug efficacy, quality, and safety; affordable prices for drugs; and a rational use of drugs, with a view to obtaining the maximum benefits while controlling costs. The annual average cost per beneficiary in the public sector is US$ 8.00 (23). Pharmaceutical sales dropped from US$ 567 million to US$ 501 million between 1999 and 2002; nevertheless, the number of units sold held steady at about 168 million. In 2002, the price per unit of generic, trademark generic, and brand-name pharmaceuticals was US$ 0.59, US$ 3.86, and US$ 5.96, respectively. There is a 6.5 times difference in the spending of the highest income quintile and the lowest. Moreover, the highest-income quintile accounts for half of all drug purchases, while the lowest-income quintile accounts for only 7.3% (20). In the public sector, the Ministry of Health's Central Supply Clearinghouse consolidates and facilitates procurement for facilities that want to use its services. It also functions as the official distributor of the products included in national public health programs, such as vaccines and tuberculosis drugs. Private pharmacies, where most drug units in the country are sold, are required to have a pharmacist on board. A pharmacist must also be on the premises in public hospitals, but not private clinics.

In 2003, the Public Health Institute suspended its production of immunobiologicals (DPT, diphtheria toxoid, typhoid, rabies, and tetanus vaccines) to instead concentrate on improving its regulatory, supervisory, and control functions as an agency of the national health authority. Reagents and immunobiologicals produced by private sector companies must be authorized by the Public Health Institute before they can be sold on the national market.

During the 1990s, some US$ 260 million was invested in the public network for construction works and medical equipping, most of which was used to build or rebuild 13 hospitals. Another 53 hospitals and 13 clinics or specialty facilities were renovated, at a cost of US$ 180 million and US$ 105 million, respectively. Regional studies carried out by the public health network during the late 1990s inventoried equipment valued at US$ 571 million, of which US$ 523 million was medical and industrial equipment, and the remaining US$ 48 million vehicles. Investments associated with implementation of the AUGE Plan included US$ 24.6 million in 2005, US$ 22.3 million in 2006, as well as an additional US$ 66.3 million for the construction of 31 new clinics.

Human Resources

According to recent studies (22), the country has 25,542 practicing physicians, of whom 2,276 were trained abroad and directly accredited by the Ministry of Foreign Relations, while 963 are immigrants who have had their medical degrees reaccredited in Chile. Of them, 14,306, or 56%, are physicians certified in specialized areas of medicine. According to the College of Physicians, the country currently has 20,146 physicians (membership in the College of Physicians is not mandatory). The physician-population ratio increased from 1:921 in 1998 to 1:612 in 2004. With respect to public (FONASA) beneficiaries, there are 8.45 physicians per 10,000 population, and their distribution by region ranges from 6 to 16 physicians per 10,000 beneficiaries. Of all licensed physicians, only 42.3% are employed by the National Health Services System. Most physicians working in the public sector are medical specialists (61%). Of them, 13% are employed by the municipalities. The 12 faculties of medicine (9 public and 3 private) graduate about 600 new doctors a year. According to estimates, the country has 18,000 nurses, but only 8,000 work in the public sector. In 2004, there were roughly 60,000 professionals, technicians, and health assistants in the public sector, and one nurse for every three physicians. In that year, the public health sector employed 90,000 people, which indicates that administrative and service staff accounted for one-third of the total. Despite an increase of approximately 5,000 physicians and 1,000 nurses between 1990 and 2000, there are glaring shortages of certain professionals, such as nurses and ophthalmologists.

Professional degrees may be granted only by universities, which are regulated by the Ministry of Education. The legal framework does not make it mandatory to obtain certification in a medical specialty after obtaining a degree in general medicine. Certification of a specialty (or subspecialty) is granted by universities after a period of formal training. For physicians who have not followed a formal course taught by a university, there is an al-ternative mechanism for certification of medical specialists through a national certification board; universities and specialist scientific societies sit on the board.

According to the changes mandated by the health reforms (Law No. 19,937), the Ministry, in conjunction with the Ministry of Education, is charged with establishing a certification system for individual providers in medical specialties and subspecialties. The Office of the Health Superintendent is charged with certification oversight for all public and private health care providers, including individuals. Accordingly, the Office of the Health Superintendent is required to compile a national list of certified individual providers and another one of certifying entities.

Research and Technological Development in Health

The Government, through the National Science and Technology Council, provides incentives for health research, which is geared more toward basic sciences and clinical areas than to public health. To promote essential research on the country's priority health problems, the Ministry of Health has developed a national research policy directed to health policies and has established the Research and Technology Commission, whose members are drawn from the faculties of medical and public health schools and departments in the country's main universities; it also has created the National Health Research Fund. Since 1994, the Fund has hosted an annual competition for public health research projects. The competition attracts some 600 project submissions each year, from which about 30 are selected. The maximum amount of funding per project is about US$ 40,000.

In the last few years, scientific information has begun to be presented electronically to facilitate access by different users. Progress has been made in establishing a virtual health library, whose consultative committee is composed of representatives of the Ministry of Health, the library of the University of Chile's Faculty of Medicine and Public Health School, the National Science and Technology Research Council, the National Library of Congress, and the Society of Editors of Scientific Journals.

The Health Technology Assessment Unit began operations in 1997; this agency of the Ministry of Health became the Chilean Health Technology Assessment Agency a year later. The Agency maintains institutional ties to the International Network of Agencies for Health Technology Assessment and the International Society for Technology Assessment in Health Care. At present, the focus of the Agency's work includes drafting assessment reports which examine and summarize scientific evidence to assist authorities and other users in decision-making; preparing methodology guidelines which scrutinize topics associated with the compilation, analysis, and application of scientific information in the health field, and for hospital quality management applications; and disseminating controlled clinical trials at the national level.

Health Sector Expenditures and Financing

According to national health statistics compiled by FONASA (23), average per capita spending in 2003 for the FONASA beneficiary population was US$ 177; for the ISAPRE beneficiary population, the figure was US$ 332. The public sector is financed from Government contributions, quotas, and co-payments by members of FONASA and the ISAPREs. In 2003, Government contributions accounted for 27.2% of total funding for the health sector; FONASA contributions, for 17.4%; mandatory ISAPREs contributions, for 15.8%; and voluntary contributions, for 6.7%. Out-of-pocket spending represented 26.3%, half of which was co-payments for medications. In 2003, direct contributions by municipalities were estimated to average US$ 6 per capita. With respect to public sector funding, Government contributions accounted for 51%, quotas for 34.9%, operating income for 6.4%, and user co-payments for 7.3%.

External Technical Cooperation and Financing

In 2000–2004, external technical cooperation was received for projects on quality of life, transfusion medicine, mental health, and HIV/AIDS. Technical cooperation in the amount of US$ 13 million was received to develop the first phase of a project aimed at expanding the response to HIV/AIDS (2003–2005), and US$ 24.6 million for the second phase (2006–2008). In 2002, the Inter-American Development Bank (IDB) processed a US$ 45 million loan for a two-phase indigenous health promotion project based on a multisector approach, the first of which was concluded in 2006. The total financial cooperation from PAHO was approximately US$ 2.15 million for 2004–2005, and roughly the same for 2006–2007.

References

1. Chile, Ministerio de Planificación y Coordinación. Encuesta de Caracterización Socioeconómica Nacional; 2003.
2. Chile, Instituto Nacional de Estadísticas. Censo de Población; 2002.
3. Chile, Ministerio de Salud, Departamento de Estadísticas e Información en Salud; 2003.
4. Chile, Ministerio de Salud. Encuesta Nacional de Salud; 2003.
5. Chile, Ministerio de Salud e Instituto Nacional de Estadísticas. Encuesta Nacional de Calidad de Vida y Salud; 2000.
6. Fondo de las Naciones Unidas para la Infancia-Chile. Informe Anual de Actividades 2005. Santiago de Chile: UNICEF; 2006.
7. Chile, Ministerio de Educación, Junta Nacional de Auxilio Escolar y Becas; 2006.
8. Chile, Ministerio de Planificación y Coordinación, Instituto Nacional de la Juventud. IV Encuesta Nacional de la Juventud; 2003.
9. Chile, Ministerio de Salud, Departamento de Epidemiología. Encuesta Mundial de Tabaquismo en Jóvenes; 2003.
10. Chile, Ministerio de Planificación y Coordinación, Fondo Nacional de la Discapacidad. Encuesta Nacional de Discapacidad; 2004.
11. Toledo V. Situación de salud de los pueblos indígenas de Chile. Organización Panamericana de la Salud; Ministerio de Salud; 1997.
12. Oyarce A, Bustos P. Características socioculturales de la mortalidad por neumonía en niños mapuches, 1996–2003 [Unpublished document]. 2004.
13. Chile, Ministerio de Salud, Departamento de Epidemiología, División de Planificación Sanitaria.
14. Chile, Ministerio de Salud, Programa Ampliado de Inmunizaciones.
15. Chile, Organización Panamericana de la Salud. Informe del Programa Ampliado de Inmunizaciones presentado en la Reunión de la OPS de Programas PAI; 2005.
16. Chile, Ministerio del Interior, Comisión Nacional para el Control de Estupefacientes; 2005.
17. Chile, Ministerio de Salud, Departamento de Salud Oral.
18. Programa de Gobierno Michelle Bachelet. "Estoy contigo." Santiago de Chile; octubre 2005.
19. Chile, Ministerio de Salud, Fondo Nacional de Salud; 2003.
20. Inostroza M, Muñoz A, Sánchez M. Migración de afiliados en el sistema ISAPRE. Rev Chil Salud Pública 2005; 9(3): 177–181.
21. Chile, Ministerio de Salud. Política Nacional de Medicamentos en la Reforma de Salud. Resolución exenta N° 515. Santiago de Chile; 2004.
22. Román O, Acuña M, Señoret M. Disponibilidad de médicos en Chile al año 2004. Rev Méd Chile 2006; 134(8): 1057–1064.
23. Chile, Ministerio de Salud, Fondo Nacional de Salud. Cuentas de Salud de Chile; 2005.

COLOMBIA

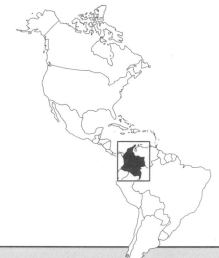

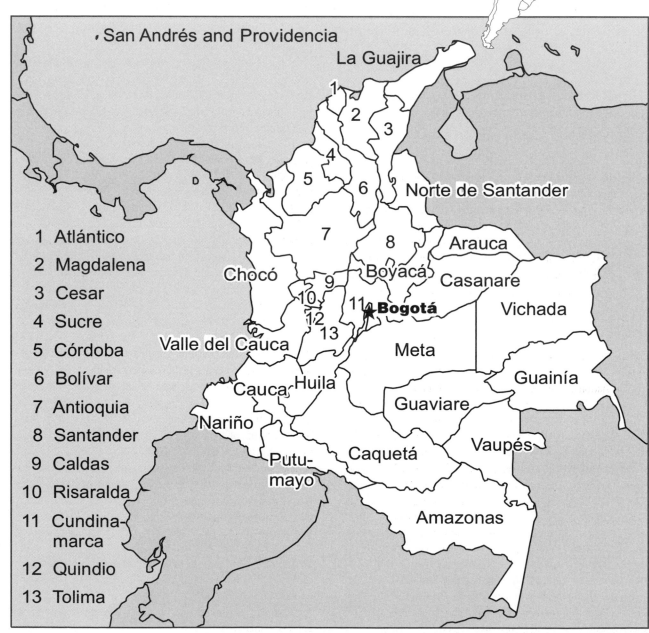

San Andrés and Providencia

La Guajira

Norte de Santander

Arauca

Boyacá

Casanare

Bogotá

Vichada

Choco

Valle del Cauca

Meta

Guainía

Cauca

Huila

Guaviare

Nariño

Vaupés

Putu-
mayo

Caquetá

Amazonas

1 Atlántico
2 Magdalena
3 Cesar
4 Sucre
5 Córdoba
6 Bolívar
7 Antioquia
8 Santander
9 Caldas
10 Risaralda
11 Cundina-
   marca
12 Quindio
13 Tolima

Colombia has a land area of 1,141,910 km^2 with a topographic profile defined by three branchings of the Andes mountain range. It has 1,098 municipalities, which are divided into 32 departments, 4 districts (the Capital District of Bogotá, Barranquilla, Cartagena, and Santa Marta), and the San Andrés and Providencia Archipelago. A 2005 population census registered 41,242,948 inhabitants (1). Bogotá, with 6,776,009 people, is the most populated city and, together with Barranquilla, Cali, and Medellín, accounts for 29.5% of the country's inhabitants. The population is predominantly urban (72% live in administrative centers) (2), and the population density stands at 36.2 inhabitants per km^2 (1).

GENERAL CONTEXT AND HEALTH DETERMINANTS

Social, Political, and Economic Determinants

Colombia is currently overcoming the economic crisis that characterized the end of the 1990s and beginning of the new century. In recent years, the country has shown clear signs of growth in its gross domestic product (GDP); in 1999, the GDP stood at –4.3% and by 2005 it had risen to 5.1% (3). Between 2002 and 2005, poverty decreased from 57% to 49% for the population segment living below the poverty line and from 20.7% to 14.7% for the population segment living below the indigence line (4). The Human Development Index rose slightly over 7% between 1991 and 2003 (from 0.728 to 0.781), putting Colombia in 77th place among 177 countries (5). Still, the inequality in income distribution has become more obvious: the GDP per capita in 2004 was estimated at US$ 2,004.80, according to purchasing power parity (6). The national Gini coefficient increased from 0.544 in 1996 to 0.563 in 2003. Inequality between rural and urban areas continues to persist: in urban settings, indexes come close to those of countries classified as highly developed, whereas they fall to mid-level ranges for rural areas. Inequality among departments is also seen to range from one extreme to the other: Chocó is the least developed region, whereas the Capital District of Bogotá is the most developed. The departments of Chocó (with its large population of African origin) and Cauca and Nariño (with significant indigenous populations) have shown the least human development over the last 14 years (5). The leading strategies in the fight against poverty highlight the importance of providing opportunities to the poor to secure housing and land, an adequate education, and access to credit, as well as of strengthening the Social Protection System, which aims to reduce the population's vulnerability in the areas of health, labor and labor-related risks, and pensions (7).

Another important aspect of current Colombian reality is the internal armed conflict that has afflicted the country for four decades. After the failure of the negotiation strategy of past governments—which had its salient expression in the "distention zone" assigned by President Andrés Pastrana's government (1998–2002) to the Revolutionary Armed Forces of Colombia (FARC)—the current government of President Álvaro Uribe Vélez has carried out a "democratic security" policy based on armed confrontation of the insurgents (Plan Colombia and Plan Patriota). This strategy has brought about a withdrawal of guerrilla groups and stepped-up road travel security, resulting in an 82% decrease in the number of massacres, a 68% reduction in the number of terrorist acts, and an 81.9% decline in the number of kidnappings between 2000 and 2005. As a result, there is a significant difference in today's security situation as compared to that of 2002, when the first term of the Uribe administration began (8). In 2004, the demobilization of the paramilitary United Self-Defense Forces of Colombia (AUC) began; by mid-2006, the demobilization was nearly complete with the withdrawal of about 30,000 troops who began a "reinsertion" process in accordance with the provisions of the Justice and Peace Law approved by the Colombian Congress in 2005.

The most important political topic has been the reelection on the first round of voting of President Uribe for the 2006–2010 period, made possible through constitutional reforms passed in 2005 allowing incumbents to seek a second term. The coalition of parties supporting Uribe also obtained a clear majority in both the Senate and House of Representatives.

Over the past two years, the Government has incorporated the Millennium Development Goals (MDGs) into its political agenda and assigned MDGs oversight to the National Planning Department, which coordinates the activities of various governmental entities—including the Ministries of National Education; Social

Protection; Foreign Affairs; the Environment, Housing, and Territorial Development; and the National Administrative Department of Statistics—with those of various United Nations cooperation agencies. As a result of this initiative, in March of 2005 the CONPES 91 document was issued defining the targets set and strategies to be used to achieve each of the eight MDGs, as well as the budget allocations that will support this process. The MDGs are considered to be the foundation for the Uribe administration's social policies, and the General Health and Social Security System (SGSSS) will play a leading role in helping to secure gains in the social development arena. With the aim of upgrading the SGSSS coverage and quality, two legislative reform initiatives have been brought before Congress, seeking to promote the inclusion of currently uninsured low income population sectors; improve efficiency in the provision of public services, including health; and increase capacity-building and accountability at the regional (territorial) levels.

Between 2001 and 2005, unemployment and underemployment decreased from 17% to 13.2% and from 31.7% to 28.2%, respectively (9). In 2003, the illiteracy rate was 7.6% for the population over age 15; in rural areas this rate was more than double (15.4%). Of the children who entered primary school in 1995, only 33% are expected to complete the 10th grade (10). The probabilities for entering the educational system and remaining in it are lowest for the poor population and residents of remote rural areas. In 2000, the average number of years of schooling for the population over age 15 was 7.3 (with similar figures for both men and women) (6). The quality of basic education is deficient, particularly in rural areas. Slightly over one-third of schoolteachers hold no formal diploma (11). Since 1991, the country has been undergoing an educational reform process initiated by the enactment of a new Constitution, which made education compulsory between the ages of 5 and 15 including, as a minimum, one year of preschool and nine of the 11 years of basic education. According to the 2005 National Survey on Health and Nutrition, 59.4% of the population belonging to the poorest socioeconomic level reported not having adequate access to sufficient, safe, and nutritious foods, in contrast to 16.4% of the population at higher economic levels.

In spite of women's wide participation in society as a whole, their inclusion in the political sphere continues to be disproportionately low in comparison with men. A provision in the 1991 Constitution allowing for the popular election of departmental governors has had minimal impact on this gender disparity: only seven women have served as governors since the reform was introduced. For the 2004–2007 period, of Colombia's 1,098 municipalities, only 9 had achieved equal numbers of female and male political representation; in 73 municipalities, women held 30%–49% of local government positions, and in 184 municipalities, women occupied only 1%–9% of these positions. At the national level, 12 women currently are serving in the Senate (12%) and 17 in the House of Representatives (10.2%).

Demographics, Mortality, and Morbidity

Like other countries of the Region of the Americas, Colombia is undergoing demographic changes typical of societies in transition. Its population is aging, and life expectancy at birth is continuing an upward trend, increasing from 72.17 during the 2000–2005 period to a projected 73.23 for the 2005–2010 period (76.67 for women and 70.34 for men). The crude birth rate decreased from 22.31 per 1,000 population during the 2000–2005 period to a projected 20.57 for the 2005–2010 period (6, 12). Demographic data show a decrease in the proportion of the population aged 15–35 years as a result of migration and violence and an increase in the proportion of the population older than age 60 (Figure 1). External migration has affected the overall national population structure. In recent years, it is estimated that 10% of the Colombian population has left the country, a phenomenon which on the one hand has led to a weakening of social structures to protect adolescents and youth and, on the other hand, has had a positive economic impact (it is estimated that remittances from Colombian emigrants accounted for 3.9% of the GDP in 2003) (13).

Internal migration is determined to a great extent by the circumstances of displacement. The violence spawned by illegally armed groups, common delinquency, and narcotics trafficking has created a generalized feeling of insecurity in the country. This, in turn, has impacted on overall health conditions and access to health services and has led to a sizable migration of Colombians to bordering countries, whether motivated by strong

FIGURE 1. Population structure, by age and sex, Colombia, 2005.

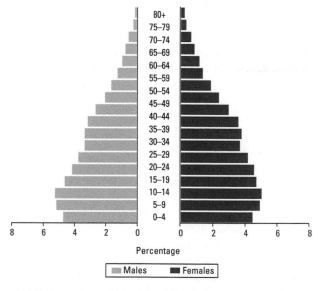

Source: Departamento Administrativo Nacional de Estadísticas, preliminary data, 2005 census.

TABLE 1. Leading causes of death, Colombia, 1990.

	Number of deaths
Assaults (homicides)	24,033
Ischemic heart disease	15,853
Cerebrovascular diseases	9,459
Heart failure	6,052
Pneumonia	5,198
Hypertensive disease	4,794
Diseases of the respiratory system	4,748
Motor transport accidents	4,410
Malignant neoplasms of the stomach	3,605
Other accidents, including late effects	3,570

Source: Departamento Administrativo Nacional de Estadísticas, Vital Statistics Group.

TABLE 2. Leading causes of death, Colombia, 2003.

	Number of deaths
Assaults (homicides)	25,612
Ischemic heart disease	23,532
Cerebrovascular diseases	13,949
Chronic diseases of the respiratory system	10,090
Diabetes mellitus	7,576
Motor transport accidents	6,447
Hypertensive disease	5,576
Pneumonia	5,374
Malignant neoplasms of the stomach	4,406
Malignant neoplasms of the trachea, bronchus, and lung	3,324

Source: Departamento Administrativo Nacional de Estadísticas, Vital Statistics Group.

family ties or economic reasons. According to the United Nations High Commissioner for Refugees, approximately 36,000 Colombians requested asylum in Ecuador between 2001 and 2005, an issue of permanent discussion at all bilateral meetings dealing with health agreements and related topics. The effects of forced displacement on the civilian population reached a crisis point in 2002, when nearly 900 of the country's 1,098 municipalities reported being affected by forced migration to and/or from their territories. In 2003, the Government reported a 48% decrease in the registry of the displaced population as compared to the previous year, a trend which continued in 2004 and 2005. During the past decade, the total number of the displaced population has reached 1,796,508. The departments recording the most intense forced emigration are Antioquia, Bolívar, Cesar, Chocó, Magdalena, and Putumayo. The departments receiving the highest numbers of displaced persons are Antioquia, Bogotá, Bolívar, Magdalena, Sucre, and Valle del Cauca.

The indigenous population represents less than 2% of the national total (785,000 persons); some 500,000 individuals of African descent reside in communities along the Pacific coast; the *raizales* (native islanders of San Andrés and Providencia) number around 25,000 and those of Gypsy descent fewer than 2,000. Half of Colombia's 81 indigenous groups number fewer than 1,000 persons each, and 22 of these groups have fewer than 500 members each. Generally speaking, these ethnic minorities are characterized by high poverty rates and markedly inadequate basic sanitation services; they also experience higher degrees of marginalization, violence, and health problems than other population groups.

Between 1990 and 2003, assaults (homicides), ischemic heart diseases, and cerebrovascular diseases retained their positions as the first, second, and third leading causes of mortality, respectively (Tables 1 and 2).

From 1998 to 2002, no changes were observed in the structure of mortality by broad groups of causes. In 2002, diseases of the circulatory system were in first place (117.7 per 100,000 population), followed by external causes (110.7), neoplasms (67.3), and communicable diseases (28.6). The first three groups of causes increased in frequency in relation to 1998 (circulatory, 105.1; external, 105.1; and neoplasms, 62.1), while there was a decrease in the frequency of communicable diseases (30.0). These rates varied among regions, with Vaupés maintaining its high profile as regards infectious diseases (2.46 times the national rate), exter-

221

FIGURE 2. Infant mortality, Colombia, 1975–2005.

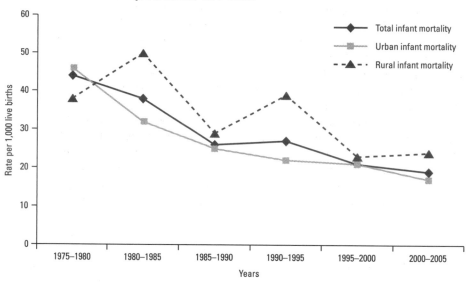

Source: Profamilia: Encuesta de Demografía y Salud, 1980–2005.

nal causes predominating in Caquetá (2.39 times the national rate), Tolima showing high rates of diseases of the circulatory system (1.51 times the national rate), and Risaralda presenting a high frequency of tumor-associated causes (1.34 times the national rate) (*6*). In relation to age and gender, communicable diseases appeared among the first five causes of death only in the male and female population under age 5. Above that age, both sexes showed a progressive increase in causes associated with transport accidents, homicides, intentional self-harm, malignant neoplasms, and diseases of the circulatory system. In the population aged 45 and older, diabetes mellitus replaced external causes as one of the leading five causes of death (*6*). Under-registration of deaths was estimated at 17.5%.

HEALTH OF POPULATION GROUPS

Children under 5 Years Old

In 2005, this age group represented 10.3% of the total population (*1*). Data from the 2005 National Demographic and Health Survey reveal that, during the 2000–2005 period, the infant mortality rate was 19 per 1,000 live births (17 per 1,000 in urban areas and 24 per 1,000 in rural areas) (Figure 2). Departments with the highest infant mortality rate in 2005 were Chocó and Cauca (54 per 1,000 each) and La Guajira (33 per 1,000), while the lowest rates were recorded in Atlántico (14 per 1,000) and Santander (19 per 1,000) (*14*). The infant mortality rate among women without formal schooling was 43 per 1,000 live births, compared to 14 per 1,000 live births for women with higher levels of educa-

tion. The neonatal mortality rate fell from 23 per 1,000 live births in 1980–1985 to 12 per 1,000 live births in 2005, a 48% decrease. Postneonatal mortality fell from 18 to 6 per 1,000 live births during this same period, representing a 66% reduction. Mortality during the first five years of life diminished by 60% during 1980–1985, falling from 51 to 22 per 1,000 live births.

The 2005 National Survey on Health and Nutrition found that 6% of newborns had low birthweight. In Colombia, no statistics are kept on late fetal mortality, thus preventing calculation of perinatal mortality (according to the National Administrative Department of Statistics, early neonatal mortality was 8 per 1,000 live births in 2002). The principal cause of neonatal death was hypoxia, which accounted for 60% of all deaths, followed by obstetrical trauma and prematurity. The following leading causes of death were reported for children under age 1: respiratory illnesses specific to the perinatal period (396 for females and 306 for males per 100,000 population, respectively); congenital malformations and chromosomal abnormalities (246 and 230, respectively); other disorders originating in the perinatal period (116 and 90, respectively); and acute respiratory infections (101 and 84, respectively). Among boys and girls 1–4 years of age, the major causes of mortality were acute respiratory infections (8.5 and 8.2 per 100,000 population, respectively), nutritional deficiencies and anemias (6.1 and 8.2, respectively), accidental drowning and submersion (8.4 and 4.6, respectively), and intestinal infectious diseases (6.0 and 6.1, respectively). Exclusive breast-feeding rose from an average of 0.5 months to an average of 2.2 months between 2000 and 2005. Prevalence of exclusive maternal lactation at six months was 47%, and mean duration of lactation was 14.9 months (*15*).

Children 5–9 Years Old

This age group represented 10.8% of the population, according to data recorded by the National Administrative Department of Statistics for 2002. During that year, 1,449 deaths were registered in this group, for a rate of 30.6 per 100,000 population (60% males and 40% females); this represented a slight increase over 2000, when there were 1,443 deaths (16). Leading causes of mortality were motor vehicle accidents, followed by acute respiratory infections and diseases of the blood (malignant neoplasms of lymphoid, hematopoietic, and related tissue). In this age group, 13% of children showed growth retardation and 5% presented low-weight-for-height proportions. Data from the 2005 National Survey on Health and Nutrition showed that growth retardation is most frequent among boys in rural areas (15).

Adolescents 10–14 and 15–19 Years Old

According to the National Administrative Department of Statistics, the 10–14-year-old age group made up 10.3% of the total population. For that same year, 1,694 deaths were registered (a rate of 35.8 per 100,000 population ages 10–14 years old); 71% of the deaths occurred among males and 29% among females. The majority of deaths were due to external causes, including homicides and transport accidents (17).

The 15–19-year-old age group represented 9.4% of the total population, according to 2002 National Administrative Department of Statistics data. Deaths registered that year numbered 6,738 (156.5 per 100,000 population), a 28% decrease from 2000 figures. Of these, 67% were violent deaths, the majority caused by firearms; for each female mortality, there were six male mortalities. The specific fertility rate among adolescents aged 15–19 was 90 per 1,000 population in 2005 (18). The proportion of adolescent pregnancies rose from 19% to 21% between 2000 and 2005. The number of adolescents aged 15–19 who have had one or more pregnancies has nearly doubled over the past 15 years, increasing from 10% in 1990 to 19.7% in 2005. In a 2002 survey conducted among displaced populations, it was found that 30% of females aged 13–19 had been pregnant at some time, 23% had given birth, and 7% were pregnant with their first child at the time of the interview (19). The adolescent fertility rate was found to be higher than the national average among marginalized populations, with two out of every three females already having given birth by age 19.

Adults 20–59 Years Old

This age group made up 52.2% of the total population in 2002, according to the National Administrative Department of Statistics. The total fertility rate for the 2002–2005 period was 2.4 children per woman (14), representing a decrease since the 1960s, when the rate was 7 children per woman. In urban areas, the fertility rate was 2.1 children, and in rural zones it was 3.4. From 2000 to 2005, the interval between births increased from 37 to 42 months. The median age at first childbirth was 22, and the median age for women's first sexual experience was 18.3 years. In 2005, women without formal schooling had an average of 4.5 children, and women with higher education had 1.4 children. The rate of contraceptive use among women without formal education was 67%, and in women with secondary-level education it was 79%.

According to the National Administrative Department of Statistics, maternal mortality in 2002 was estimated at 84.6 per 100,000 live births, a decrease from 2000, when it stood at 104.9 per 100,000 live births (Figure 3). There were significant differences by region, area of origin, age groups, levels of schooling, and individual circumstances, such as displacement. The maternal mortality rate varied from 315.7 per 100,000 live births in Chocó to 35 per 100,000 live births in Risaralda; 90% of these deaths were due to preventable causes, such as pregnancy-induced hypertension, postpartum hemorrhage, and abortion (7). Of the total deaths, 84% occurred in health institutions and 88% had received medical care (7). It is estimated that one of three pregnancies ends in abortion and that almost 60% of the abortions seen at governmental institutions have been induced (20). In 2006, the Constitutional Court decriminalized abortion whenever the mother's or the fetus' life is at risk, or in cases of rape.

Older Adults 60 Years Old and Older

In 2003, this age group represented 7.6% of the total population, according to the National Administrative Department of Statistics. Morbidity from nutritional diseases was the second most important cause and, as in the case of the population under age 10, these provoked a higher frequency of deaths due to anemia and nutritional deficiencies (42%). In this age group, the leading causes of death are cardio- and cerebrovascular diseases, diabetes, gastrointestinal diseases, obesity, cancer, and osteoporosis (21). During 2005, financial subsidies were received by 173,822 older adults and 41,123 more benefited from supplementary nutrition through the Juan Luis Londoño de la Cuesta Program (22).

The Family

In Colombia, nuclear families are the most common family type (53.4%), followed by extended families (33.6%). Persons living alone make up 7.7% of total households, and blended families make up 5.4% (23). Household size diminished from 4.1 children in 1998 to 2.6 in 2002, but families living in poverty have an average of 4.7 children. Despite the predominance of male-headed households, the proportion of those headed by females is increasing: in 1995, according to the National Administrative Department of Statistics, 24% of households were headed by females, and in 2000 this figure rose to 28%.

FIGURE 3. Maternal mortality rates, Colombia, 1990–2002.

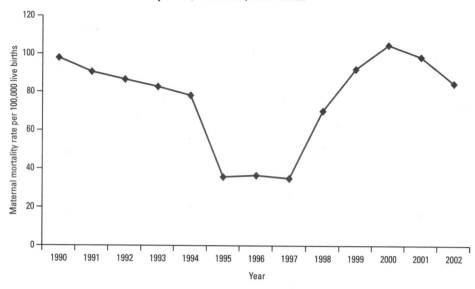

Source: Departamento Administrativo Nacional de Estadísticas, Vital Statistics Group.

The national rate for reported incidences of domestic violence was 184 per 100,000 population. National Demographic and Health Survey data for 2005 showed that psychological violence affecting women rose from 46% in 1995 to 50% in 2000. Physical abuse by male partners fell from 41% in 2000 to 39% in 2005. In the same year, about one-fifth of abused women visited a health center to seek information; there are no data that allow comparison with 2000. Between 2001 and 2003, the rate of working children (5–17 years old) decreased from 12.8% to 10.4%. In rural zones, the rate was twice as high (16.1%) as in urban areas (8%) (*24*).

Workers

The rate of occupational illnesses reported in 2004 was 1.4 cases per 10,000 workers. These were most numerous in the departments of Antioquia, Cundinamarca, and Valle del Cauca, especially in the manufacturing sector. The three leading causes of illness were carpal tunnel syndrome (20%), neurosensory hypoacusia (19%), and lumbosacral spine disorders (18%) (*25*).

The mortality rate registered for 2003 reached 18.29 per 100,000 unionized workers, with an increasing trend in the fishing industry and decreasing trend in the other industries. According to reports issued by private-sector occupational risk management organizations, 96% of workplace accidents were caused by circumstances related to social violence, principally in such economic subsectors as private security, law enforcement, and transport; 3% were caused by traffic accidents, and 1% were due to professional reasons.

Persons with Disabilities

Preliminary data from the 2005 census reveal that there was a 6.4% prevalence of permanent impairments in the population (6.6% in men and 6.2% in women). Among this group, 71.2% reported having one impairment, 14.5% reported having two, 5.7% reported having three, and 8.7% reported having four or more permanent impairments. The principal impairments were related to eyesight (43.2% despite the use of eyeglasses or contact lenses), the ability to move or walk (29%), hearing (17.3% in spite of wearing special equipment), talking (12.8%), and understanding and learning (11.9%) (*26*).

The Colombian Insurer's System of Union Information disclosed that in the 2000–2003 period, 255 cases of disability were recorded in the country's five leading economic activities. The number of cases decreased in the community services sector and increased in the manufacturing industry. The most common causes of disability were trauma-related (83%).

Ethnic Groups

In the jungle and plains areas, parasitic and infectious diseases and nutritional deficiencies prevail, whereas in the Andean region periodontal diseases predominate. The Sierra Nevada de Santa Marta region on the Caribbean coast is home to various indigenous groups, including the Arhuacos, Kankuamo, Kogis, Wiwa, and Yupka, where the predominant health concerns are acute diarrheal diseases, acute respiratory infections, malnutrition, and nutritional deficiencies, as well as tuberculosis, periodontal diseases, and skin disorders. The health situation is better among the

FIGURE 4. Malaria cases by *Plasmodium* species, Colombia, 1993–2005.

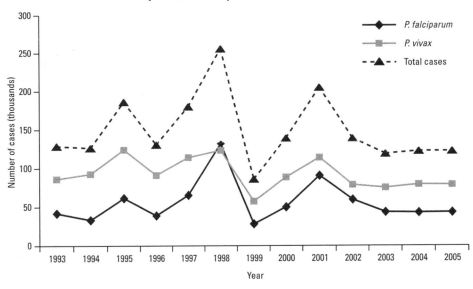

Source: Ministerio de la Protección Social, Grupo ETV.

Gypsy population, even though cardiovascular and respiratory diseases are present among this group. In the Pacific region, where a large part of the Afro-Colombian population lives, the prevalent diseases are tuberculosis, acute diarrheal diseases, acute respiratory infections, malnutrition, malaria, typhoid fever, yellow fever, cancer, and HIV/AIDS. Factors influencing health problems among ethnic groups are loss of ancestral lands, natural resources destruction, and environmental deterioration; social and cultural changes associated with increased contact and interaction with the external environment; gradual abandonment of traditional medicine; difficulties in accessing health services and scarcity of these services in ethnic territories; and poverty and social and geographical marginalization, along with other cultural barriers (*27*).

Displaced Populations

More than half of all households in this group are headed by women, illiteracy is three times higher than the national average, living conditions and access to public services are more precarious, and overcrowding is a serious problem. Infectious diseases are treated with the greatest frequency, especially acute respiratory infections and acute diarrheal diseases, which primarily affect children under 5 years old. In infants under 1 year old, the prevalence of acute respiratory infections was 37.5%, compared to 21.8% among the general population. Frequency of acute diarrheal diseases was 81% among displaced populations and 64% in host populations. Thirty-five percent of adolescent women are mothers (twice the national rate). Insurance coverage among the

displaced population was 24%, compared to 34% among the host population (*28*). With regard to mental health, the sequelae to experiences of violence represent an additional burden for displaced populations already faced with instability and uncertainty. A survey to establish the prevalence of mental disorders in 13 neighborhoods in the cities of Sincelejo and Sucre found a prevalence of 27.6% (*29*).

HEALTH CONDITIONS AND PROBLEMS

COMMUNICABLE DISEASES

Vector-borne Diseases

Over the past three decades, **malaria** morbidity has shown an increasing trend, with an annual average of 142,297 cases recorded between 2001 and 2005; in 60% of the cases *Plasmodium vivax* was the etiological agent, in 38% it was *P. falciparum*, and 2% of the cases were mixed infections (Figure 4). In 2005, the annual parasite index (API) was 14.5 per 1,000 population. The region encompassing Alto Sinú, Bajo Cauca, and Urabá had the highest API that year (26 per 1,000 population). Around 60% of all malaria cases were concentrated in 27 municipalities of the departments of Antioquia, Córdoba, and Nariño. Males aged 15–44 were the most affected population group. Mortality from malaria also follows an ascending trend in the country, with an annual average of 130–150 deaths; under-registration, however, is considered to be close to 70% (*30*). Due to the growing problem of resistance to amodiaquine and sulfapyrimethamine used to treat uncomplicated *P. falciparum* malaria, artemisimin-based combination treatments were introduced in 2006.

In 2004, 24,460 cases of **dengue** (54 per 100,000 population) were reported; 2,261 of them (10 per 100,000 population) were dengue hemorrhagic fever, with 23 deaths. In 2005, there were 43,257 reported cases (187 per 100,000 population); 4,322 were dengue hemorrhagic fever (17 per 100,000 population), with 48 deaths. In recent years, circulation of all four dengue virus serotypes has been confirmed. In 2005, the population age groups most affected were those 45–84 years old (48%) and 5–14 years old (26%) (*31*).

There are jungle **yellow fever** infection foci, mainly in the Amazon, Catatumbo, and Orinoco river basin areas and the foothills of the Sierra Nevada de Santa Marta. Over the last five years, 179 cases have been reported, with a 47% case fatality rate. In 2003, there was an epidemic with 102 cases, which in particular affected the Norte de Santander department. Most cases appeared in male agricultural workers 15–44 years old (*32*).

There were 15,000 cases of **leishmaniasis** reported in 2004 and 22,000 in 2005; 99% of the cases were cutaneous leishmaniasis. Almost 80% of the cases occurred among the 15–44-year-old population segment, with male farmers being the most affected group. In 2005, approximately 75% of the cutaneous and mucocutaneous cases were clustered in the departments of Antioquia, Caquetá, Guaviare, Meta, Nariño, Santander, and Tolima. Confirmed cases of visceral leishmaniasis were largely concentrated in the departments of Bolívar, Córdoba, Sucre, and Tolima (*33*).

A 1999 national study on seroprevalence and risk factors for **Chagas' disease** reported an infection prevalence of 35 per 1,000 in children under 15, especially in the eastern part of the country. In detailed studies of morbidity in the adult population, between 19.4% and 47% tested positive for this disease, and between 25% and 47.8% showed electrocardiographic alterations. An annual average of two to five cases of acute Chagas' disease have been sporadically reported (*34*).

Vaccine-preventable Diseases

The eradication of **poliomyelitis** in 1991, the elimination of **measles** in 2002, and the elimination of **neonatal tetanus** and **diphtheria** as public health problems, as well as the current initiative to eliminate rubella and congenital rubella syndrome by 2010, place Colombia among the first Latin American countries to reach these regionwide goals. From August 2005 to June 2006, 17,697,717 persons between the ages of 14 and 39 years (96.9% of the goal) were vaccinated against measles and rubella. Achievements included interruption of the circulating rubella virus and no reported cases of newborns with congenital rubella syndrome. In 2005, there were 139 reported cases of **whooping cough**, 2,366 clinical cases of **mumps**, 84 cases of **rubella** (53 were laboratory-confirmed cases), 5 cases of **congenital rubella syndrome** (all were reported prior to National Vaccination Day against measles and rubella), and 19 cases of *Haemophilus influenzae*

type b **meningitis**. In 2005, the seasonal flu vaccine was given to adults over age 65 in geriatric residences and hospitals, and children aged 6–18 months with respiratory illnesses. Altogether, 423,648 vaccine doses were administered.

Intestinal Infectious Diseases

Based on sentinel surveillance of **acute diarrheal diseases** carried out by the National Health Institute, Colombia's national reference laboratory, data obtained from the processing of 1,335 samples in 2003 showed that 17.5% were positive for the following microorganisms: *Rotavirus* (7%), *Giardia duodenalis* (6%), *Cryptosporidium sp.* (3%), *Shigella sp.* (0.8%), and *Salmonella sp.* (0.7%). Corroboration of test results between the National Health Institute and sentinel posts ranged from 66% to 100% (*35*). No **cholera** cases were detected.

Chronic Communicable Diseases

Incidence rates for all forms of **tuberculosis** were 26.2 per 100,000 population in 2001, 26 in 2002, 28.5 in 2003, 24.8 in 2004, and 22.5 in 2005. The Amazon and Orinoco river basin areas were those most affected; 53% of the departments are classified as very high-risk (incidence above the third quartile) or high-risk (incidence above the national median). The most affected group was persons 25–34 years old. Based on partial information regarding the cohort receiving treatment in 2003, the cure rate was 72%; the treatment completion rate, 9%; treatment abandonment rate, 8%; death rate, 5%; transfer rate, 5%; and treatment failure rate, 1%. Coverage for the Directly Observed Therapy, Short Course (DOTS) strategy was 35% in 2004. The average percentage of deaths due to tuberculosis between 1991 and 2000 was 0.7%. Among HIV/AIDS patients, tuberculosis deaths averaged 10.8% during the 1997–2001 period (*36*).

Leprosy prevalence has diminished from 9,604 cases under treatment in 1990 (3.0 per 10,000 population) to 1,716 cases (0.3 per 10,000 population) in 2004. Leprosy incidence also showed a downward trend, from 2.90 per 100,000 population in 1990 to 1.31 per 100,000 population in 2004. In 2004, only two departments showed prevalence rates above the elimination goal of 1 per 10,000 population: Amazonas (1.4) and Arauca (1.1). The highest proportion of cases occurred in men (66%); the median age was 46 years, and individuals aged 15–44 years were the most affected population segment (*37*).

Acute Respiratory Infections

In 1990, the mortality rate for acute respiratory infections in children under 5 years old was 48.5 per 100,000, whereas in 2002 it was 34.7. Potential years of life lost (PYLL) per 100,000 children under age 5 amounted to 3,225 in 1990, but by 2002 PYLL had fallen to 1,803. The risk factors related to mortality from acute respiratory infections include the absence or low percentage of breast-feeding, low birthweight, premature birth, secondhand smoking, use of domestic fuels such as firewood and kero-

FIGURE 5. Trends in HIV/AIDS, by sex, Colombia, 1985–2004.

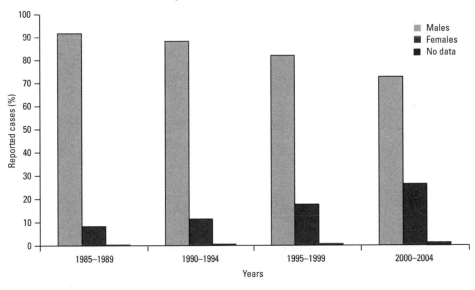

Source: ONUSIDA: Infección por VIH en Colombia. Estado del Arte 2000–2005.

sene, and other predisposing factors, such as overcrowding and seasonal climatic changes (*38*). As regards surveillance of respiratory illnesses, distribution by etiologic agent in 2005 was 33% for **respiratory syncytial virus**, 31% for **parainfluenza virus**, and 15% for **influenza A virus** (*39*).

HIV/AIDS and Other Sexually Transmitted Infections

After HIV emerged in Colombia in 1984, its prevalence grew to 0.6% in 2003 (*40*). In 2005, an estimated 171,504 persons aged 15–49 were living with HIV, with an estimated prevalence of 0.7% (*41*). Between 1983 and 2005, a total of 40,809 cases of HIV/AIDS were reported to the Public Health Surveillance System (*42*). In 53.7% of these cases, transmission was heterosexual; in 27.1%, it was homosexual; in 15.1%, bisexual; in 2.9%, perinatal; in 0.6%, through blood transfusion; and in 0.4%, by other means. Analysis of reported cases by gender reveals a feminization of the epidemic: during the 1985–1989 period, 8.2% of cases were among females, whereas during the 2000–2004 period, this figure reached 26.6% (Figure 5). The male-female ratio changed from 9.4 in 1990 to 2.3 in 2005. According to data from the Ministry of Social Protection's National Observatory for HIV/AIDS Management, there were 13,195 deaths from AIDS during the 1995–2002 period (*43*). Currently, 78.5% of all HIV patients belonging to the General Health and Social Security System (SGSSS) are receiving antiretroviral treatment (*44*). The incidence for congenital **syphilis** is on the rise, from 0.75 per 1,000 live births in 2000 to 1.25 per live births in 2005. Data from the National Health Institute indicate that gestational syphilis increased from 0.89 per 1,000 pregnant women in 2003 to 2.51 in 2005.

Zoonoses

The country has been designated free of **foot-and-mouth disease** with and without vaccination in 60.8% of cattle (*45*). In 2001, there were six outbreaks of type O foot-and-mouth disease, and eight in 2002; type A virus was detected in a 2000 outbreak (*45*).

Reports of the presence of the neurologic syndrome associated with **Venezuelan equine encephalitis** increased between 1979 and 2000, with peaks reported in 1995 (88 foci) and 1998 (214 foci). Confirmed cases in humans showed virus activity from 2000 to 2005, when a total of 75 cases were reported (*46*).

Since March 2000, no cases of human **rabies** of canine origin have been reported. In 2005, three cases of human rabies caused by wild-type viruses were reported. Foci of wild rabies virus strains reported between 1982 and 2002 affected 31 of the country's 32 departments, with a median of 21 and an average of 46 foci per department. High-risk areas include the northern parts of the departments of Antioquia, Chocó, Norte de Santander, and Santander; the entire expanse of the departments of Arauca, Cesar, Córdoba, and Sucre; as well as the south-central section of the department of La Guajira (*47*).

NONCOMMUNICABLE DISEASES

Metabolic and Nutritional Diseases

The 2005 National Survey on Health and Nutrition indicated that chronic malnutrition in children under 5 had diminished slightly that year (13.5%) as compared to 2000 (12%), at which time 10% showed moderate malnutrition and 2% severe malnutrition, with children 1–2 years old being the most affected. Acute malnutrition was observed in 1% of children under 5 years of age. The prevalence of anemia in children under 5 increased from 18% in 1977 to 23% in 1995, and to 33.2% in 2005. In the 5–9-year-old age group, 13% showed stunting and 5% showed low weight for height. During 2005, the Atlantic region had the highest malnutrition rates, thus supplanting the Pacific region, where these rates have traditionally been among the highest. Among women, 40% were overweight and 6% had low body mass indexes. Low weight for gestational age was twice as common among pregnant women under age 15 (47%) as among those of average age (21%).

Cardiovascular Diseases

In 2002, diseases of the circulatory system as a broad group of causes were the leading cause of mortality in the general population, representing 27.3% of all deaths. In 1995–1998, they had accounted for 26%–30% of all deaths. Data from the National Administrative Department of Statistics revealed that in 2002 the most frequent causes of death were ischemic heart diseases (52.3 per 100,000 population), cerebrovascular diseases (31.1 per 100,000 population), and hypertensive diseases (12.7 per 100,000 population). The highest mortality rates by diseases of the circulatory system were recorded in the departments of Tolima (178.7), Caldas (158.6), and Santander (155.6). The National Survey on Health and Nutrition identified overweight and obesity as associated risk factors in 33% of males and 31.1% of females in the 18–64-year-old age group. The proportion of the population complying with the minimum recommended levels of physical activity was 26% among the 13–17-year-old age group and 42.6% among the 18–64-year-old age group.

Malignant Neoplasms

Mortality from this cause increased in frequency between 1998 (62.7 per 100,000 population) and 2002 (67.3 per 100,000 population), when it was the third leading cause of death. In 2002, stomach cancer was the first cause of death from neoplasms for both genders (9.7 per 100,000 population), followed by cancer of the trachea, bronchus, and lung (7.2 per 100,000 population), and leukemias and lymphomas (6.2 per 100,000 population). Cancer of the prostate is the second leading cause of death from neoplasms among men (4.7 per 100,000), while in women, it is uterine cancer (5.03 per 100,000), followed by breast cancer (3.9 per 100,000). The departments with the highest mortality rates from neoplasms in 2002 were Risaralda (90.6 per 100,000 population), Antioquia (90.4), and Quindio (88.5).

OTHER HEALTH PROBLEMS OR ISSUES

Disasters

Colombia is most commonly affected by hydrometeorological phenomena, especially floods, and secondly by geological phe-

nomena. Almost 80% of the population lives in areas threatened to some degree by earthquakes. Since 2001, there has been a steady increase in the number of persons seriously affected or killed by disasters, and this can be associated not only with the growing number of natural phenomena and the persistent concentration of the population in high-risk areas, but also with inadequate measures for disaster prevention, preparation, and mitigation as regards the various sectors involved. Between 2002 and 2005, there were 1,343,282 persons affected by natural disasters, which produced 487 deaths. During the same period, there were 371 deaths caused by manmade disasters related, above all, to transport accidents (48). In 2005, there was a monthly case average of 24 deaths and 68 wounded caused by accidents with antipersonnel landmines (49).

Violence and Other External Causes

The mortality rate from homicides and harm intentionally inflicted by another person was 72.6 per 100,000 population; 16.1 from transport accidents; 10.7 from accidents, excluding transport; and 5.5 from intentional self-harm and suicides. There are no data disaggregated by gender. According to the Institute of Legal Medicine and Forensic Sciences, in 2004 there were 203,438 cases of nonfatal wounds from external causes and, compared to 2003, there was an increase in sexually related and accidental injuries (1.6%). There has been a proportional reduction in common interpersonal violence (42.5%) and an increase in sexual crimes (8.8%); nonfatal injuries from domestic violence amounted to 29.4%.

Mortality caused by violent, illegally armed groups decreased from 28.2% in 2003 to 15.1% in 2004. Departments achieving the greatest reductions in homicide rates were Arauca, Antioquia, Caldas, Caquetá, and Norte de Santander; a majority of the country's departments (21) fell below the national rate (50). In several regions, the presence of antipersonnel landmines posed a serious risk of death or mutilation. Within the context of internal conflict, during the 1995–2003 period, the following violations against medical and public health activities were reported: 684 cases (68%) against life and safety, 146 cases (15%) against the health infrastructure, 160 cases (16%) against health activities, and 12 cases (1%) of misrepresentation or deception (51). The number of violations against medical targets increased from 468 during the 1995–1998 period to 1,006 during the 1995–2003 period (51).

Mental Health and Addictions

Two out of five persons (40.1%) experience at least one mental disorder during their lives, with anxiety disorder being the most prevalent form (19.3%). In men, the most frequent disorder is alcohol abuse (13.2%) and in women, major depression (14.9%). The prevalence of lifetime substances abuse (of all types) was higher in men; following alcohol abuse as leading disorders are alcohol dependence (4.7%), nicotine dependence (2.9%), and drug abuse (2.1%). Lifelong prevalence for suicidal ideation was

A System to Protect Vulnerable Populations

In a national effort toward securing the social inclusion of persons who have experienced inequities in the areas of health care, employment, and pensions, Colombia has established the Social Protection System, a body of public policies designed to manage risks, reduce vulnerability, and improve the quality of life of all Colombians, with particular focus on the country's least privileged social groups. In 2002, the Ministry of Health and the Ministry of Labor and Social Security were merged into a single Ministry of Social Protection, which oversees all aspects of the Social Protection System, including policy formulation, adoption, direction, coordination, implementation, follow-up, and monitoring. The documents CONPES 91 and Visión Colombia 2019 and the National Development Plan for 2006–2010 have made a strong commitment to protect universally recognized human rights, reduce existing gaps between the country's social groups and geographic regions, and move toward achievement of the Millennium Development Goals. One of the greatest challenges to this effort is the persistence of violence perpetrated by illegally armed groups, which has led to the displacement of nearly 2 million persons over the last decade. The heightened vulnerability and precarious living conditions limit this group's ability to access health services and protect its health, thus constituting a grave humanitarian concern.

12.3%. Median age for the appearance of affective disorders in a major depression episode was 24 years (52).

Environmental Pollution

Events involving pesticides poisoning are seldom reported to the Public Health Surveillance System, but it can be assumed that there is considerable underreporting due to the fact that the surveillance system was extended to the national level only in 2005. That year, 5,590 poisonings due to chemical substances were reported; of these, 76% (4,251 cases) were due to pesticides. Pesticide sales in 2002 amounted to 20,081,231 kilograms: 75.4% were in fungicides, 13.9% in herbicides, 4.4% in insecticides, 1.5% in fumigants, 1.4% in biologicals, and 3.3% others.

RESPONSE OF THE HEALTH SECTOR

Health Policies and Plans

Law #789 of 2002 defined Colombia's Social Protection System as the body of public policies designed to reduce vulnerability and improve the quality of life of Colombians, especially the least protected, in order to help this group obtain as a minimum the rights to health, a pension, and work (53). As a consequence of this principle, Law #790 of 2002 called for the creation of the Ministry of Social Protection—the product of the fusion of the Ministry of Health with the Ministry of Labor and Social Security. The primary objectives of the Ministry are to formulate, adopt, direct, coordinate, execute, follow up, and oversee the Social Protection System. This system functionally integrates the aggregate of public, private, and mixed institutions as well as the norms, procedures, and public and private resources allocated to prevent, alleviate, and overcome the risks that threaten the population's quality of life. It also encompasses the national system of family

welfare and social services, and the System of Comprehensive Social Security (made up of the General System of Pensions, the SGSSS, and the General System of Occupational Risks) (54).

Framed within Colombia's National Development Plan for 2002–2006 is a component on the protection of human rights and humanitarian international rights, which includes a provision for the design and implementation of a model to follow up, evaluate, and monitor public policies affecting human rights. The component refers not only to policies related to civil and political rights, but also those encompassing the economic, social, cultural, environmental, and collective realms (55). The Public Defender's Office (Defensoría del Pueblo) is the agency of the Colombian Government responsible for protecting, defending, and promoting human rights, democratic principles, popular participation, and pluralism.

Over the past decade, the health sector in Colombia has instituted many reforms; among the most important are political and administrative decentralization and reform of the social security system. Law #715, enacted in 2001, defined competencies and resources at the various levels of the educational and health sectors. Decentralization in the health sector defined health authority and areas of competency at the departmental, district, and municipality levels. Nevertheless, the evolution of the decentralization process in Colombia has been largely influenced by the country's heterogeneity in terms of development levels and economic and technical capacity. On the other hand, the state of transition in which the health sector currently finds itself has allowed remnants of the previous National Health System model to coexist alongside the newer SGSSS in a market of regulated competition.

Evaluations of the performance of Essential Public Health Functions (EPHF) were conducted in Colombia at the national level and in the Capital District of Bogotá in 2002, and in the departments of Antioquia, Caldas, and Valle del Cauca in 2003. The departmental evaluations facilitated the formulation of plans for strengthening public health at this level. Currently, the structure of the EPHF performance evaluation tool is being adapted in order to undertake this exercise at the municipal level. Results of the national-level evaluation showed performance to be below satisfactory in most functions, except for EPHF11 (reduction of the impact of emergencies and disasters on health), which was judged to be of optimum standards. Performance was deemed to be poor as regards EPHF3 (health promotion), EPHF4 (social participation and empowerment of citizens in health), and EPHF10 (research, development, and implementation of innovative public health solutions).

The Colombian health system has a series of statutes and regulations regarding basic issues such as insurance, services delivery, generation/preparation and utilization of financial and human resources, benefit plans, public health, epidemiological surveillance, inspection, and control. The most important are Law #100 of 1993 (creation of the SGSSS); Law #715 of 2001 (competencies and resources) and its regulatory norms; Decree #1011 of 2006 (Obligatory System of Quality Control); and Resolutions #1943, #1045, and #1046 of 2006. During the last decade, domestic violence has gained visibility in Colombia and it is now considered a punishable offense. Law #248 of 1996 is intended to prevent, punish, and eradicate violence against women. Other laws (#294 of 1996, #360 of 1997, and #575 of 2000) penalize violent behavior in the home, including spousal sexual violence and offenses against sexual freedom and human dignity, and confer special protective rights for the victims of these crimes.

Legislative initiatives approved by the National Congress may originate in this body, the executive branch, the Ministry of Social Protection, or other entities involved in issues related to the health sector and its functioning. The Ministry of Social Protection holds responsibility for regulatory activities; when a regulation affects SGSSS members, however, it must be presented before the National Health and Social Security Council (CNSSS). Otherwise, the Ministry of Social Protection holds autonomy in this area.

Health Strategies and Programs

The Ministry of Social Protection, through the National Development Plan, established national goals and strategies to be carried out during the current government administration; as part of this process the Ministry periodically sends directives to the subnational counterparts and respective health personnel on matters of public health interest that require obligatory compliance, such as early detection interventions, specific health protection measures, and other areas provided for within benefit plans. The various mechanisms comprising the health system seek to ensure principles of equity, quality, efficiency, and, particularly, the financial sustainability of interventions, while social participation is enabled by the regulatory mechanisms that oversee social guidance.

Organization of the Health System

The SGSSS comprises the System of Comprehensive Social Security, which, at the same time, is part of the Social Protection System. The new SGSSS was created through Law #100 of 1993. It seeks to guarantee economic and health care assistance to those whose labor situation or financial capability allows for participation in the System, provide complementary social services as specified by the law, and increase coverage until the entire population has access to the system (56). With the new SGSSS, a fundamental change in insurance came about, affecting in particular the model of health care and services delivery.

The SGSSS is a compound organization uniting the contributory and subsidized regimes, both of whose functions will require integration and national coordination and financial solidity. This model also encompasses a regime for transitory affiliates made up of the population's most disadvantaged sectors without the capacity to pay and who are not participants in the regimes previously mentioned. In addition, there are special regimes not covered by the stipulations expressed in Law #100 of 1993, such as the Colombian Petroleum Company, the teaching profession and public universities, the National Congress, and military and police forces.

The SGSSS specifies the compulsory affiliation of all salaried workers and population groups with the capacity to pay, all of whom join the contributory regime through the payment of premiums. Coverage with social security protection extends to all family members of the affiliated individual. Those without sufficient capacity to pay the compulsory premiums receive total or partial subsidies from the SGSSS in order to ensure their affiliation. Access to this latter regime is gained by beneficiaries of government subsidies who are identified through a socioeconomic survey known as the SISBEN and ultimately selected for inclusion by the corresponding territorial entity.

The System has three social security mechanisms: capitation payment units to balance the contributory regime's resources and ensure access under equal terms to premium-paying affiliates and beneficiaries with different income levels; the Solidarity and Guarantee Fund (FOSYGA), whose resources support access for the population in need of subsidization; and availability of current national income for those having access to the subsidized regime.

The SGSSS is integrated by organisms in charge of supervision, surveillance, and oversight; administration and financing; and health services provision, within a model of regulated services delivery and coverage. The CNSSS acts in the area of supervision and oversight, representing the SGSSS's principal stakeholders and managers under the leadership of the Ministry of Social Protection. It functions as the FOSYGA's administrative council, and its main tasks are to oversee the Mandatory Health Plan and its essential medicines component, to establish premium amounts and value for the UPC with their respective differentials, and to regulate the co-payment and moderating fee regime structure. The National Health Superintendency is an entity attached to the Ministry of Social Protection whose functions include inspection, surveillance, and supervision, as well as financial and budgetary oversight of the participating entities and the establishment of mechanisms to evaluate the quality of services delivery. The Ministry of Social Protection has expertise in epidemiological surveillance, directs the SGSSS, presides over the CNSSS, determines overall health sector policy and general policies of the Social Protection System, and provides technical guidance and assistance to decision-makers.

The departmental and municipal health authorities are representatives of the national government at their respective local levels. The departments and municipalities rely on a Territorial Council of Health and Social Security, whose duties at these two levels are similar to those of the CNSSS at the national level.

Health-promoting entities (EPS) form the basic nucleus of the SGSSS and are responsible for subscribing and registering SGSSS participants and collecting their premiums, as delegated by the FOSYGA. The principal function of the EPS is to organize and to guarantee, directly or indirectly, the delivery of Mandatory Health Plan services to subscribers. Special administrators are in charge of managing insurance to the most vulnerable and disadvantaged members of the subsidized regime as part of the duties the Government delegates to the heads of municipalities.

The institutions that deliver health services include hospitals, medical offices, primary health care centers, laboratories, and all other health services establishments and professionals that together or individually offer their services through the EPS. These facilities and individuals may or may not have a dependency relationship with the EPS, but in all cases they are technically and financially independent. The network of public hospitals operating under the former National Health System has been decentralized and transformed into what are known as Social Enterprises of the State, with the purpose of facilitating the country's supply of health services and at the same time ensuring the hospitals' financial sustainability in a competitive services market.

In 2004, 32.8% of the population subscribed to the contributory regime and 34.3% to the subsidized regime; 3.9% were affiliated to special regimes, and 28.9% were not insured within the system (12). Access to SGSSS services is not necessarily guaranteed as a consequence of insurance coverage. Given the existing barriers to access, subscribers often have had to resort to tutelage action as a tool to obtain compliance with benefit plan provisions, and national authorities have had to examine and follow up strictly on these cases to prevent violation of citizens' rights. The population not insured by the SGSSS basically belongs to socioeconomic levels 3 and 4 as determined by the SISBEN survey used to identify potential beneficiaries, but who have not yet been able to enter the system; young adults 18–24 years old who have not yet initiated education beyond the secondary level, but are of legal age and cannot be subscribed by their parents if they do not certify their student status; the un-

employed not surveyed by the SISBEN; and any other individuals remaining outside the system.

Inclusion and participation of indigenous populations in the SGSSS is a governmental priority. The creation of EPS organizations has been advocated, to be constituted by indigenous town councils or traditional authorities, or both, in order to facilitate adaptation of the health system's institutions and services to local ethnic and cultural values, needs, and expectations (57, 58). Law #691 of September 2001 regulates the participation of ethnic groups in the SGSSS.

Public Health Services

Among the strategies to improve access to health services and increase the response capacity of health care providers in Colombia, the national policy on health services delivery focuses on the identification, systematization, dissemination, and support of innovative strategies in the fields of primary health care, family health, and community health. Within this framework, since 2004 the decentralized levels of the health system—districts, departments, and municipalities—have developed and implemented care and management models incorporating the primary health care strategy. For example, a program in Bogotá seeks to guarantee the universal right to health and other primary health care principles throughout the Capital District jurisdiction by promoting the health and well-being of families and communities, with particular focus on the poorest and most vulnerable population segments. In the departments of Antioquia, Cesar, Santander, and Valle del Cauca, models of family and community health based on primary health care concepts have already been developed as well as public policies for their implementation at the municipality level.

Within the decentralization structure, there are no vertical programs for disease prevention and control and activities in this realm form part of the individual health services (Mandatory Health Plan) offered by the SGSSS. The Basic Health Care Plan is the instrument used in the community health sphere, and the Ministry of Social Protection periodically issues directives indicating the priorities, strategies, and goals to be achieved at local levels.

Law #715 (2001) established that municipality-level governments are responsible for health situation analysis and maintenance of the public health surveillance system in their respective jurisdictions. The National Administrative Department of Statistics is in charge of planning, gathering, processing, analyzing, and disseminating the country's official statistics, including vital statistics and demographic data. The Government is responsible for the Comprehensive Social Protection Information System. At the current time, the most developed departments and municipalities regularly collect and publish their respective basic health indicators. The Public Health Surveillance System actively reports throughout the country on communicable disease occurrences and other events due to a common origin or preventable cause. Models and protocols are being introduced for other types of surveillance in the areas of noncommunicable diseases, mortality, the environment, promotion and early detection activities, and medications. Also in progress are designs for a new information system and a model of territorial surveillance management.

The National Network of Public Health Laboratories has as its mission the diagnosis of communicable diseases of public health importance and the detection of risk factors; its structure is aligned with the ongoing decentralization trend. In 2006, the Network was reorganized in accordance with Decree #2323, which also identified strategic activities in the areas of public health surveillance, quality control, services delivery, and research. There are 33 public health laboratories situated in the departmental capitals; these depend technically and administratively upon departmental-level public health authorities. Public health laboratories are financed by the Basic Health Care Plan and by investments of the department's own resources. Territorial entities are free to contract the services of private laboratories. There is a combined total of 6,042 public and private laboratories with diverse specialties in the country; the great majority of these are clinical in nature.

Over the past decade, the coverage levels and quality of public household water and sanitation services have improved; in large urban areas, there are a variety of public, private, and public-private enterprises working in these areas, while in rural areas, community-based entities usually provide water and sanitation services. Thus, between 1993 and 2003, urban water supply coverage increased from 94.6% to 97.4%, and sanitation services coverage rose from 81.8% to 90.2%. In rural areas, current water supply coverage reaches 66%, which represents a 12% increase over the last 10 years, even though water quality remains deficient. Basic sanitation coverage in rural areas is 57.9% (7).

The national production of solid wastes is estimated at 27,300 tons/day, of which 22,800 tons come from urban areas. Solid waste disposal coverage is 95% (59). Of the country's 1,098 municipalities, 350 dispose of their wastes in sanitary landfills and 565 in open air garbage dumps. Hospital wastes amount to 8,500 tons/year, and 40% of this amount involves infectious residues. In 2002, regulations were established requiring municipalities to develop comprehensive management plans for the disposal of solid wastes.

Most emissions of particles smaller than 10 μm, nitrogen oxides, and carbon monoxide are produced by mobile sources (85% by gasoline used in transportation), whereas total suspended particles and sulfur oxides are produced by stationary sources (65% from carbon). Air pollution is mostly produced by land transportation means (86%). Social costs triggered by air pollution have been estimated at Col$ 1.5 billion a year. Diseases such as cancer, asthma, chronic bronchitis, and respiratory disorders are associated with pollution (60).

The Ministry of the Environment, Housing, and Territorial Development has advanced in the consolidation of a national inventory of persistent organic pollutants (POP); an evaluation of the regulatory framework, institutional capacity, and infrastructure available in the country for POP management; information dissemination and raising community awareness; and strengthening national capacity for the management of POP-affected sites. Through the National Inventory of Dioxins and Furans, the principal POP-generating sources were identified and quantified: uncontrolled combustion, 55.1%; incineration, 15.7%; energy and heat transformation, 8.9%; and metals production, 6%. A national inventory of biphenyl polychlorates is now being carried out (61).

Use of the following fungicidal pesticides based on mercury components has been prohibited in the country: leptophos (phosvel) 2,4,5-T, 2.4.5-TP, DBCP, EDB, DDT, chlordimeform, dinoseb, captafol, aldrin, heptachlor, dieldrin, mirex, dicofol, endosulfan, lindane, and camphechlor (toxaphene). Additionally, some restrictions have been established regarding the use of paraquat, parathion, methyl parathion, and methyl bromide.

Surveillance of foodborne diseases in humans is directed by the National Institute of Health, and the inspection, surveillance, and control of food products is directed by the National Institute for Medications and Food Surveillance (INVIMA). In 2005, there were 7,941 cases of foodborne diseases reported, a 30.4% increase over 2004 (6,090 cases). The 15–44-year-old age group was the most affected, with 42% of cases (62). The Colombian Agricultural Institute monitors the incidence of more than 50 pests and 13 endemic and exotic animal and plant diseases. Since there are no official control programs directly related to risk factors of biological or chemical origin, the country lacks baseline information on the presence of pathogenic microorganisms and chemical contaminants in various types of foods (63).

Both bovine brucellosis and bovine tuberculosis are present in Colombia, but the country is free of bovine spongiform encephalopathy, with certification subject to demonstration. Poultry farming is free of highly pathogenic avian influenza, Newcastle disease, and Salmonella. Endemic diseases in the country include classical swine fever, shrimp white spot virus, Venezuelan equine encephalitis, and equine infectious anemia (63). In September of 2005, the presence of low-pathogenic avian influenza virus H9N2 was detected on poultry production farms in the Fresno municipality of Tolima; this focus was controlled, and the virus was not detected in any other parts of the country.

During the 1996–2005 period, the Nutrition and Food Plan was implemented as part of national government policy. Under the coordination of the Colombian Institute of Family Welfare, activities were carried out in the following areas: food security projects covering the entire life cycle, with particular focus on indigenous families; consumer protection through food safety and quality control initiatives; prevention and control of micronutrient deficiencies; prevention and treatment of infectious and parasitic diseases; promotion, protection, and support of breastfeeding; promotion of healthy nutrition and lifestyles; and research and human resources training in diet and nutrition.

The Ministry of Social Protection has institutionalized the Group on Emergencies and Disasters; 72.2% of departments and districts now include staffing in this area. Ongoing training of health sector personnel in disaster preparedness, mitigation, and response has been implemented as a strategy to overcome weaknesses detected at the subnational levels, particularly as regards interinstitutional coordination and development of a comprehensive emergency response approach. Regulatory frameworks and processes have been adopted for the structural reinforcement and refitting of existing health facilities and for the construction of new health establishments that will ensure their compliance with safety structural standards for earthquake resistance. There is a need for better development of the Regulating Centers for Urgent Care and Emergencies, and for mechanisms to ensure adequate coordination among the Centers for Emergency Operations and local and regional health authorities with disaster prevention and response committees.

In September 2005, the Ministry of Social Protection allocated Col$ 12 billion (approximately US$ 5 million) to the development of a plan for the prevention and mitigation of the impact of an influenza pandemic (64). The plan's principal components include emergency preparedness, public health surveillance, research and case management, community disease prevention and control, preservation of basic services, and evaluation.

Individual Care Services

According to the National Register of Health Care Providers, in September 2006 there were 58,010 health care sites and 51,095 health care providers in the country. Of the latter, 82.7% were independently employed health professionals and 16.6% were affiliated to public or private institutions. There were 872 public hospitals functioning as Social Enterprises of the State. Among the country's registered health services, 68% pertain to outpatient consultations; 13.8% to support services, diagnosis, and complementary therapy; 6.2% to external care; 2.5% to surgical services; 3.8% to hospital service; 1.5% to urgent care; and 1.2% to special transportation. There were 54,475 beds registered in the country (58).

In the SGSSS there are 20,332 services that comply with basic established quality requirements. These include radiology and diagnostic imaging, clinical laboratory testing, gastrointestinal endoscopy, cytopathology, cardiovascular diagnosis, transfusion and other blood services, renal dialysis, fibrobronchoscopy, urology/lithotripsy, clinical oncology, radiation therapy, and pharmaceutical services. The blood bank network consist of 110 banks; as Colombia's national reference laboratory, the National Health Institute coordinates the network's functioning and quality control system and offers training and technical advice in support of the promotion of voluntary blood donation. All banks in the network, whether public or private, must comply with SGSSS quality standards. INVIMA oversees inspection and surveillance of the blood banks. There are 11 units of blood per 1,000 population, whereas the standard is 50 per 1,000 population; availability and distribution are not equitable, with remote rural areas at a particular disadvantage. Blood donation, especially voluntary, increased from 41.7% in 2003 to 55% in 2005. The network guarantees 99.9% screening for internationally recommended infection markers (HIV, HBsAg, HCV, syphilis, and Chagas' disease).

Health Promotion

Territorial entities, EPS, and subsidized regime insurers hold responsibility for evaluating, conducting follow-up, assisting, advising, and overseeing the public health promotion activities that form part of the Mandatory Health Plans of both the contributory and subsidized regimes of the SGSSS. The objective of the Basic Health Care Plan is to promote community health and the prevention of disease; all territorial divisions and public administrative levels are expected to participate in this effort, with the municipality level holding responsibility for the provision of basic social services and promotion of the community's participation in these activities.

Health promotion at the national level accords priority to the development and implementation of public policies, strategies, and activities geared to the achievement of health-promoting schools and housing. Health promotion efforts in Bogotá focus principally on improving heath conditions and protecting human rights among residents of disadvantaged communities. In the cities of Bucaramanga, Cali, and Manizales, the initiatives developed have been based on the reduction of risk factors for noncommunicable diseases utilizing the CARMEN strategy. Three Collaborating Centers of the World Health Organization work at the national level in health promotion efforts: the Institute for Research and Development in the Prevention of Violence and Promotion of Social Coexistence, the Center for Development and Evaluation of Public Health Policies and Technology, and the Institute for the Promotion of Health and Sexual and Reproductive Health.

The country now has a very active National Network for Healthy Housing and is developing guidelines for the incorporation of the healthy housing concept in housing projects for vulnerable populations. In educational programs held for community leaders between May of 2003 and the end of 2005, 1,350 facilitators and 4,527 community agents received training. In addition, 28,500 families were visited through healthy housing initiatives carried out in 15 departments. The Network is led by the Ministry of the Environment, Housing, and Territorial Development, and includes as participants the Ministry of Social Protection, the National Learning Service, the Presidential Agency for Social Action and International Cooperation, the academic community, and various nongovernmental organizations.

The environmental component has been strengthened in schools through the development of a toolbox for risk control and support of water quality surveillance through projects such as "Youth, Science, Health, and the Environment," which provides support to teachers, children, and youth with the goal of reinforcing the important linkages between human health and the physical environment.

Colombia is implementing a program designed to prevent violence and reduce crime through "crime observatories" in the country's southwest that involves various activities at the municipality, subregional, and departmental levels. In addition, the establishment of mandatory insurance for traffic accidents backed by the SGSSS has contributed significant resources to road safety programs and strengthened the country's emergency health services network (65).

The National Occupational Health Committee drafted the National Plan for Occupational Health 2003–2007 as a framework and management tool for the General System of Occupational Risks (SGRP). Components in the Plan include promotion of health and safety in the workplace; creating a culture of self-care and occupational risks prevention; establishment of SGRP entities, institutions, and offices; promotion of technical, technological, and scientific advancement; recognition of workers' rights to health benefits; ensuring SGRP economic viability; and extension of SGRP coverage. In November of 2004, the working age population (≥12 years old in urban areas and ≥10 in rural areas) was 33,548,030. Of this number, 4,836,939 workers were affiliated with the SGRP.

Health Supplies

INVIMA is the agency that regulates, inspects, oversees, and controls medications, foods and health supplies, blood banks, tissues, and organs. There has been a National Pharmaceutical Policy since December 2003. The Ministry of Social Protection determines policies, establishes norms, and oversees the pharmaceutical system. Regulations of the drug production and importation registry incorporate Good Manufacturing Practices requirements. According to the pharmaceutical industry's Annual Manufacturing Survey, gross production of medications fell by 2% in 2004 as compared to 2001. In December 2004, the pharmaceutical market amounted to US$ 1.1 million; the market for finished products has expanded to 10.8% imported and 8.8% exported, compared to 2001. Domestic production—both in national and foreign-owned laboratories—has fallen; in 1995 it supplied 90.6% of internal market needs and in 2004, only 74.3%. The relationship between importation of finished products and apparent consumption rose from 7% in 1994 to 27% in 2004 (66). Shortcomings in the SGSSS as regards the availability and timely provision of medications to its participants have been observed: in 2000, 39.8% of SGSSS participants reported being unable to receive needed medications (67), and in 2005, only 51.6% reported being able to access medications on the same day as prescribed;

the remainder experienced difficulties requiring them to purchase these medications elsewhere. Various studies have shown how severely this issue affects expenditures within the context of the family basket of basic goods and services, particularly as regards the country's poorest population segments (68).

In 2004, regulations were established for the surveillance of diagnostic reagents used in vitro for the examination of specimens of human origin. INVIMA holds responsibility for the inspection, surveillance, and oversight of these activities, as well as the work of a special committee in charge of evaluations of diagnostic tests.

In 2005, through regulation of health registry regimes, marketing authorization, and health surveillance, regulations were set for medical devices for human use (production, processing, packaging, packing, storage, sale, use, importation, exportation, marketing, and maintenance). A program was also implemented for the post-marketing surveillance of medical devices (including equipment). In 2004, regulations were established for conducting surveys of hospital infrastructure at the first level of the public health services network (69). Information was gathered in 2006 for the purpose of establishing policies regarding structure and technology.

Human Resources

In 2005, it was estimated that 278,685 persons were employed in the health sector (659.5 direct service workers per 100,000 population); 70.6% were women and 29.4% were men. The average age among women was 38.6 and among men, 40.9. Auxiliary personnel made up 53.3% of all workers; another 41.9% were professional personnel, and 4.8% were technical personnel. During the 2001–2005 period, the number of general care physicians grew from 29,460 to 33,682 (7.3 per 10,000 population). In 2005, there were an estimated 27,034 registered nurses (5.9 per 10,000), 28,373 odontologists (6.1 per 10,000), 17,643 bacteriologists (3.8 per 10,000), 116,204 nursing auxiliaries (25.2 per 10,000), and 5,544 nutritionist-dietitians (1.2 per 10,000).

Information on the nature of contractual relationships in the health services field was available for only 53.7% of the total workforce; of these, 17.3% hold private work contracts; 14.3% hold career service appointments; 7.3% are permanent staff; 5.6% hold temporary short-term appointments; 2.5% work on a freelance basis; and 6.7% work in some other kind of labor arrangement. Estimates based on the perspective of supply and demand of health professionals and auxiliaries for 2000–2005 show a shortage of 6,316 general care physicians and 17,312 nutritionist-dietitians; on the other hand, there is a surplus of bacteriologists (4,787), odontologists (4,374), and nursing auxiliaries (34,780) (70). At the beginning of 2006, there were 909 academic health training programs (34.8% undergraduate and 65.2% postgraduate), concentrated mainly in universities (70.5%) and university-affiliated institutions (26.4%) (71).

Research and Technological Development in Health

The national science and technology policy seeks to strengthen the capacity of the Francisco José de Caldas Colombian Institute for the Development of Science and Technology (known as Colciencias). The nation's general budget includes a specific category for research and a regulation stating that 7% of the income derived from national lottery proceeds must be reserved for allocation to research activities. Between 2002 and 2004, US$ 11,200,000 were devoted to this pursuit: 38% went to basic biomedical research, 37% to clinical investigation, and 25% to epidemiological and public health studies; of the funds allocated to these three types of research, 47% focused on research related to communicable diseases, 46% was invested in studies of noncommunicable diseases, and only 2% was devoted to research on issues relating to violence and injuries from external causes.

During the 1992–2001 period, 168 articles were published in international indexed journals, 68 articles in international nonindexed journals, 71 articles in catalogued national journals, and 123 in non-catalogued national journals. The number of research teams has increased from 73 (1990–1999) to 194 (2000–2004), and the number of researchers holding a doctorate degree has grown from 157 to 373 during the same period. Seventy-five percent of the groups recognized by Colciencias are based in the cities of Bogotá, Bucaramanga, Cali, or Medellín, which together account for 25% of the country's population. The national agenda of health research priorities is currently being retooled to focus on the country's most salient health problems and the development of inter- and multidisciplinary approaches to them (72). There is an information system (Observatory of Science and Technology), and Colciencias has developed the Red Scienti, a virtual network for use in the health research area. Norms have been prepared to guide research work involving human subjects that focus on ethical aspects and also address scientific, technical, and administrative issues.

At the current time, Colombia does not have a policy regarding health technologies development. However, aside from the norms for regulating medical devices and diagnostic laboratory reagents, there are updated guidelines for the regulation, evaluation, and importation of biomedical technologies. A Committee on Medications and Technology Evaluation advises the CNSSS on the definition and updating of the list of medications, procedures, and technology pertaining to the Mandatory Health Plan.

The National Network of Medical Libraries includes university medical libraries and research centers, with the National Institute of Health Library serving as the chief repository of the country's most important research works in the public health field. Development of the Virtual Library on Health began in 1998 and now includes contributions from 45 affiliated institutions. In 2005, with assistance from the Latin American and Caribbean Center on Health Sciences Information (BIREME) and 20 affiliated institutions, the Ministry of Social Protection launched the Virtual Library for Public Health Surveillance. Other virtual libraries on a variety of health topics—such as psychology and children, adolescents, and youth—are currently in the development stages. In 2006, the SciELO (Scientific Electronic Library Online) Colombia project was launched. Managed by the National University of Colombia and based on the model originally created by BIREME, SciELO Colombia features more than 600 full-text articles published in peer-reviewed journals in the health and biomedical disciplines.

Health Sector Expenditures and Financing

Total expenditures on health in relation to the gross national product varied from 9.7% in 1997 to 8.1% in 2002. Per capita expenditures ranged from US$ 255 in 1997 to US$ 149 in 2002. The heaviest burden is borne by families (approximately 30%), especially through payment of SGSSS premiums (13%) and out-of-pocket expenses (9.5%); businesses provide approximately 25%, largely through employers' contributions; the general national budget contributes 21.8%, with one of the largest expenditure items (14%) being resource transfers to territorial-level health entities; in fourth place are resources from the system's agents, represented by their own resources (non-operational income) and by financing of accounting losses (20.5%); and finally, resource expenditures at the departmental and municipality levels (3.8%). A breakdown of average health sector expenditures during the 1993–2002 period shows that 74.6% corresponded to health care costs, 16% to administrative costs (personnel and general expenses), 7.9% to miscellaneous expenditures, and 1.5% to investment costs, including physical infrastructure and equipment, research, and training.

Technical Cooperation and External Financing

During 2005, the Ministry of Social Protection signed 10 cooperation agreements for the strengthening of health activities in Colombia with the following international partners: the Government of Japan, Japan International Cooperation Agency, Hipólito Unanue Agreement, Andean Development Corporation, Organization of Ibero-American States, World Bank, Inter-American Development Bank, International Organization for Migration, Spanish Agency for International Cooperation, and Andrés Bello Agreement. The two Japanese entities provided financial support and the other eight organizations technical support for a variety of health objectives, including strengthening of health systems and the public hospitals network, improving sexual and reproductive health, and health sector reform and financing. In addition, bilateral cooperation agreements were signed with various institutions and governments, among them the International Cooperation and Assistance Fund and the Governments of Brazil, Canada, Ecuador, El Salvador, Jamaica, Mexico, Panama, Peru, and Venezuela.

References

1. Colombia, Departamento Administrativo Nacional de Estadísticas. Boletín Censo General 2005. Bogotá; 2006. Available at: http://www.dane.gov.co/files/censo2005/boletin.pdf. Accessed on 27 July 2006.

2. Colombia, Departamento Administrativo Nacional de Estadísticas, Dirección de Censos y Demografía. Proyecciones de población. Estimaciones de población con base al censo de 1993.

3. Grupo Aval. Indicadores económicos. Producto Interno Bruto (PIB) Histórico. Available at: http://www.grupoaval.com/oc4j/portales/jsp/gaviframes.jsp. Accessed on 27 July 2006.

4. Montenegro S. Estimaciones de pobreza e indigencia en Colombia 2005. Departamento Nacional de Planeación; 2005. Available at: http://www.dnp.gov.co/archivos/documentos/GCRP_Presentaciones/Presentación_cifras_pobreza_2005.pdf. Accessed on 27 July 2006.

5. Naciones Unidas, Comisión Económica para América Latina y el Caribe; Colombia, Departamento Nacional de Planeación, Programa Nacional de Desarrollo Humano; Agencia Colombiana de Cooperación Internacional; Federación Colombiana de Municipios; Cooperación Técnica Alemana. Las regiones colombianas frente a los objetivos del milenio. Bogotá: NNUU; 2005. Pp. 15–16.

6. Colombia, Ministerio de la Protección Social; Organización Panamericana de la Salud. Situación de salud en Colombia. Indicadores básicos 2005. Bogotá; 2006.

7. Colombia, Departamento Nacional de Planeación. Metas y estrategias de Colombia para el logro de los objetivos de desarrollo del milenio–2015. (Documento CONPES Social 91). Bogotá; 2005. Available at: http://www.dnp.gov.co/paginas_detalle.aspx?idp=811. Accessed on 27 July 2006.

8. Colombia, Departamento Nacional de Planeación, Dirección de Justicia y Seguridad. Cifras de violencia. Primer semestre 2005. 2006. Available at: http://www.dnp.gov.co/paginas_detalle.aspx?idp=562. Accessed on 27 July 2006.

9. Colombia, Departamento Administrativo Nacional de Estadísticas. Encuesta Nacional de Hogares 2001–2006; 2006. Available at: http://www.dane.gov.co/files/investigaciones/empleo/ech/ech_TNal_juni06.xls. Accessed on 27 July 2006.

10. Sarmiento A, Tovar LP, Alam C. Cited in: Colombia, Departamento Nacional de Planeación y Sistema de Naciones Unidas en Colombia. Hacia una Colombia equitativa e incluyente. Informe de Colombia sobre los Objetivos de Desarrollo del Milenio 2005. Bogotá: DNP/PNDH; PNUD; CEPAL; 2006. P. 65.

11. Programa de Promoción de la Reforma Educativa en América Latina y el Caribe; Fundación Corona; Corpoeducación. Cited in: Colombia, Departamento Nacional de Planeación y Sistema de Naciones Unidas en Colombia. Hacia una Colombia equitativa e incluyente. Informe de Colombia sobre los Objetivos de Desarrollo del Milenio 2005. Bogotá: DNP/PNDH; PNUD; CEPAL; 2006. P. 65.

12. Colombia, Ministerio de la Protección Social; Organización Panamericana de la Salud. Situación de salud en Colombia. Indicadores básicos 2004; Bogotá; 2005. P. 3.

13. Garzón A. El entorno de las remesas en Colombia: protagonistas y marco legal. In: Seminario Migración internacional, el impacto y las tendencias de las remesas en Colombia, Organización Internacional para las Migraciones, 2004 nov 10–11. Bogotá, 2005. P. 61–64. 2006. Available at: http://www.oim.org.co/anexos/documentos/publicaciones/libro90.pdf. Accessed on 8 August 2006.

14. Asociación Probienestar de la Familia Colombiana; Instituto Colombiano de Bienestar Familiar; Agencia de Estados Unidos para el Desarrollo Internacional. Mortalidad y situación de la mujer. Chapter 9. 2005. Pp. 189. In: Encuesta Nacional de Demografía y Salud. Salud Sexual y Reproductiva en Colombia.

15. Instituto Colombiano de Bienestar Familiar. Lactancia y estado nutricional. In: Encuesta Nacional de la Situación Nutricional en Colombia (ENSIN) 2005. 2005. Pp. 247–277.

16. Colombia, Departamento Administrativo Nacional de Estadísticas. Información estadística. Defunciones por grupo de edad y por sexo según causas agrupadas en la lista 6/67 de la OPS (CIE-10). 2003.

17. Colombia, Ministerio de Salud; Organización Panamericana de la Salud. Situación de salud en Colombia. Indicadores básicos 2002.

18. Asociación Probienestar de la Familia Colombiana; Instituto Colombiano de Bienestar Familiar; Agencia de Estados Unidos para el Desarrollo Internacional. Fecundidad. Pp. 95–108. In: Salud Sexual y Reproductiva en Colombia. Encuesta Nacional de Demografía y Salud 2000.

19. Asociación Probienestar de la Familia Colombiana. Salud sexual y reproductiva en zonas marginales: situación de las mujeres desplazadas la encuesta de salud sexual y reproductiva entre mujeres desplazadas. 2002. Available at: http://www.disaster-info.net/desplazados/informes/profamilia/saludsexual1.htm. Accessed on 12 June 2006.

20. Zamudio L, Rubiano N, Wartenberg L. La incidencia del aborto inducido en Colombia. Bogotá: Centro de Investigaciones sobre Dinámica Social, Universidad Externado de Colombia; 1994.

21. Colombia, Consejo Nacional de Política Económica y Social, Departamento Nacional de Planeación. Lineamientos para la operación del programa nacional de alimentación para el adulto mayor "Juan Luis Londoño de la Cuesta" y la selección y priorización de sus beneficiarios 2004. (Documento CONPES Social 86). 2004.

22. Colombia, Departamento Nacional de Planeación. Revolución educativa: metas y avances. In: Reactivación social. Siete herramientas de equidad. Resultados 2005. 2005. Available at: www.dnp.gov.co/archivos/documentos/DEPP_Seguimiento_

Resultados/Informe_7_Herramientas_ Equidad. pdf. Accessed on 27 July 2006.

23. Instituto Colombiano de Bienestar Familiar y Profamilia Colombia. Encuesta Nacional de Demografía y Salud–2005. Capítulo 3, Características generales de los hogares y de la población. Bogotá: ICDS; 2005:40–41.

24. Colombia, Departamento Administrativo Nacional de Estadísticas. Sistema de información sobre trabajo infantil en Colombia. Módulo de trabajo infantil en ECH 2003. Available at: http://suamox03.dane.gov.co:7778/pls/tic/home. Accessed on 27 July 2003.

25. Colombia, Ministerio de la Protección Social; Servicio Nacional de Aprendizaje (SENA). Diagnóstico actual y prospectivo de la salud ocupacional y los riesgos profesionales en Colombia con enfoques de entorno. Bogotá: Imprenta Nacional de Colombia; 2005.

26. Colombia, Departamento Administrativo Nacional de Estadísticas. Boletín Censo General 2005 Discapacidad–Colombia. 2006. Available at: http://www.dane.gov.co/files/censo2005/boletin2.pdf. Accessed on 27 July 2006.

27. Colombia, Ministerio de la Protección Social; Organización Panamericana de la Salud. Insumos para la conceptualización y discusión de una política de protección social en salud para los grupos étnicos, 2004.

28. Organización Panamericana de la Salud-Colombia. Comparación de la situación de salud entre población en situación de desplazamiento y receptora en seis ciudades. Serie Salud y Desplazamiento en Colombia. 2002–2003.

29. Médicos sin Fronteras. Vivir con miedo: el ciclo de la violencia en Colombia. 2006. Available at: http://www.msf.org/source/countries/americas/colombia/2006/report/Vivir_Con_Miedo.pdf. Accessed on 18 July 2006.

30. Colombia, Ministerio de la Protección Social. Situación de malaria en Colombia. Bogotá: Ministerio de la Protección Social; 2005.

31. Colombia, Ministerio de la Protección Social, Instituto Nacional de Salud. Enfermedades Transmitidas por Vectores (ETV). Dengue. Inf Quinc Epidemia Nac 2006; 11(3):33–44.

32. Colombia, Ministerio de la Protección Social, Instituto Nacional de Salud. Informe situación fiebre amarilla. Bogotá: Ministerio de la Protección Social; 2006.

33. Colombia, Ministerio de la Protección Social. Instituto Nacional de Salud. Informe situación epidemiológica de la leishmaniasis. Bogotá: Ministerio de la Protección Social; 2006.

34. Colombia, Ministerio de la Protección Social. Situación de la enfermedad de Chagas en Colombia. Bogotá: Ministerio de la Protección Social; 2004.

35. Agudelo CI, Duque S, Arévalo A, Flores AC, Peláez D, Izquierdo VF, et al. Vigilancia centinela de la etiología de la enfermedad diarreica aguda (EDA) en seis municipios de Colombia, 2003. Informe preliminar. Rev Infectio 2004; 8:93.

36. Colombia, Ministerio de la Protección Social. Situación de la tuberculosis en Colombia. Informe 2004.

37. Colombia, Ministerio de la Protección Social. Situación de la lepra en Colombia. Informe 2004.

38. Colombia, Ministerio de la Protección Social. Análisis de la situación de salud en Colombia 1990–2002. Documento preliminar. (Unpublished).

39. Colombia, Instituto Nacional de Salud, Laboratorio de Virus Respiratorios, Grupo de Virología. Vigilancia de influenza y otros virus respiratorios. Actualización Semana epidemiológica N° 52 de 2005. Available at: http://www.ins.gov.co/pdf_investiga/influenza_y_otros_virus_resp_10.pdf. Accessed on 18 July 2006.

40. Prieto F, Osorio A, De Neira M, Grupo de Vigilancia Centinela de VIH. Prevalencia de VIH en población general de Colombia 2003: VI Estudio Nacional Centinela de VIH 2003–2004. Primera fase. Informe Quincenal Epidemiológico Nacional 2004; 9:362–75.

41. Luque R. Situación de la epidemia en Colombia. Presentación del Día Mundial de Lucha contra el SIDA, Videoconferencia nacional, Servicio Nacional de Aprendizaje, diciembre 2005.

42. Colombia, Instituto Nacional de Salud, Sistema Nacional de Vigilancia en Salud Pública. Informe hasta el 31 de diciembre de 2005.

43. Colombia, Ministerio de la Protección Social, Observatorio Nacional de la Gestión en VIH/SIDA. Informe de mortalidad por SIDA Colombia 1995–2002. (Unpublished).

44. Programa Conjunto de las Naciones Unidas sobre el VIH/SIDA; Colombia, Ministerio de la Protección Social. Infección por VIH/SIDA en Colombia. Estado del arte 2000–2005. 2006.

45. Correa R. La erradicación de la fiebre aftosa, un compromiso de todos. Revista Ica-Informa 2005; 32(2):8–9.

46. Mesa F, Cardenas J, Villamil L. Las encefalitis equinas en la salud pública. Primera edición. Bogotá: Leoprint Editores; 2005.

47. Brito E, Palacios H, Yunda H, Martínez J, Reyes L. Rabia de origen silvestre en Colombia. Construcción de un modelo espacial para determinar áreas de riesgo en Colombia. Instituto Colombiano Agropecuario; 2005. Available at: http://www.ica.gov.co/pecuaria/modelo_espacial_abia.pdf. Accessed on 18 July 2006.

48. Center for Research on the Epidemiology of Disasters. Emergency Disasters Data Base (EM-DAT). [Electronic database]. 2006. Available at: http://www.em-dat.net/disasters/list.php. Accessed on 18 July 2006.

49. Colombia, Presidencia de la República, Oficina de Comunicaciones. Balance de minas antipersonales; 2006. Available at: http://www.presidencia.gov.co/resultados/2006/minas_6.pdf. Accessed on 12 June 2006.

50. Colombia, Instituto Nacional de Medicina Legal y Ciencias Forenses, Centro de Referencia sobre Violencia. Forensis

2004. Datos para la vida, boletín de violencia en Colombia. Bogotá; 2005.

51. Colombia, Ministerio de la Protección Social; Organización Panamericana de la Salud. Infracciones a la misión médica en el conflicto armado colombiano (1995–2003). Informe de consultoría. 2003.

52. Colombia, Ministerio de la Protección Social. Estudio Nacional de Salud Mental, Colombia 2003. 2005.

53. Colombia. Ley 789 de 2002 por la cual se dictan normas para apoyar el empleo y ampliar la protección social y se modifican algunos artículos del Código Sustantivo de Trabajo. Diario Oficial. 27 December 2002. N° 45.046. Capítulo I.

54. Colombia. Decreto 205 de 2003 por el cual se determinan los objetivos, la estructura orgánica y las funciones del Ministerio de la Protección Social y se dictan otras disposiciones. Diario Oficial N° 45.086. Artículo I.

55. Colombia. Ley 812 de 2003. Plan Nacional de Desarrollo 2003–2006. Hacia un Estado Comunitario. Capitulo II. Artículo 5.

56. Colombia, Ministerio de la Protección Social, Programa Nacional de Salud 2002–2006.

57. Colombia. Decreto 330 de 2001 por el cual se expiden normas para la constitución y funcionamiento de entidades promotoras de salud, conformadas por cabildos y/o autoridades tradicionales indígenas.

58. Colombia, Ministerio de la Protección Social. Base de datos del Registro Especial de Prestadores de Salud, según información reportada por las entidades departamentales y distritales de salud, 2005.

59. Organización Panamericana de la Salud/Organización Mundial de la Salud, Superintendencia de Servicios Públicos. Manejo de residuos sólidos en Colombia. 2002.

60. Colombia, Consejo Nacional de Política Económica y Social, Departamento Nacional de Planeación. Lineamientos para la formulación de la política de prevención y control de la contaminación del aire 2005. (Documento CONPES 3344). 2005.

61. Colombia, Ministerio de Ambiente, Vivienda y Desarrollo Territorial, Dirección de Desarrollo Sectorial Sostenible. Boletín informativo enero–febrero 2006. Convenio de Donación GEF TF 051529. Proyecto de asistencia preparatoria a Colombia para el cumplimiento de los compromisos adquiridos en el marco de la Convención de Estocolmo para Contaminantes Orgánicos Persistentes (COP). Bogotá; 2006.

62. Colombia, Instituto Nacional de Salud. Enfermedades transmitidas por alimentos, 2005. Available at: http://www.

invima.gov.co/version1/noticias/informeETAano2005.doc. Accessed on 24 May 2006.

63. Colombia, Consejo Nacional de Política Económica y Social, Departamento Nacional de Planeación. Política nacional de sanidad agropecuaria e inocuidad de alimentos para el sistema de medidas sanitarias y fitosanitarias 2005. (Documento CONPES 3375). 2005.

64. Colombia, Ministerio de la Protección Social. Plan de prevención y mitigación de una pandemia de influenza; 2005. Available at: http://www.invima.gov.co/version1/BVSalud/lainfluenzaencolombia.PDF. Accessed on 24 July 2006.

65. Federación de Aseguradores Colombianos. Cámara Técnica Seguro Obligatorio de Accidentes de Tránsito (SOAT). 2006. Available at: http://www.fasecolda.com/int/CT_SOAT.php. Accessed on 28 July 2006.

66. Colombia, Ministerio de la Protección Social. Estudio de la Política de Precios de Medicamentos en Colombia. Bogotá; 2005.

67. Colombia, Defensoría del Pueblo. Primera Encuesta Nacional de Calidad en Salud Percibida por los Usuarios, Colombia, 2000.

68. Colombia, Defensoría del Pueblo. Evaluación de los servicios de salud que brindan las Empresas Promotoras de Salud, Colombia, 2005.

69. Colombia. Resolución 0293 de 2004 por la cual se reglamentan los procedimientos para la elaboración del catastro físico hospitalario de las instituciones prestadoras de servicios de salud de primer nivel de atención del sector público.

70. Colombia, Ministerio de Salud. Desafíos para los recursos humanos en el Sistema General de Seguridad Social en Salud. Memorias del foro videoconferencias, octubre 2002.

71. Colombia, Ministerio de la Protección Social, Observatorio de Recursos Humanos, Sistema Nacional de Información de la Educación Superior. Base de datos. 2006. Available at: http://snies.mineducacion.gov.co:8080/pls/iesprogramas/m_programas.programa_acreditado_lista?p_tipo=2. Accessed on 28 July 2006.

72. Instituto Colombiano para el Desarrollo de la Ciencia; Universidad Nacional de Colombia. Foro Mundial para la Investigación en Salud. Construcción de una agenda de priorización de investigación en salud. Memorias primera reunión. Versión 1.0. Bogotá; 2005.

COSTA RICA

Nicaragua

Guana-caste

Alajuela

Heredia

San José

★

Cartago

San José

Limón

Puntarenas

Panama

0   50   100 Miles

C osta Rica has a land area of 51,100 km^2. The country is divided into seven administrative provinces and 81 cantons. The estimated population in 2004 was 4,248,508 inhabitants. Of this number, 49.7% lived in urban areas and 50.8% were male.

GENERAL CONTEXT AND HEALTH DETERMINANTS

Social, Political, and Economic Determinants

The country's macroeconomic performance over the period 2000–2005 was moderately satisfactory. Using national production as a point of reference, measured in terms of gross domestic product (GDP), the economy grew by 6.5% in 2003, but slowed to 4.1% in 2004 and 2005, which was below the 4.6% growth rate achieved over the previous decade. External demand for the country's agricultural and manufactured goods and services, rising sales in the electronics and high-technology sectors, and the growing national tourism market have played a significant role in the country's economic growth.

From a fiscal standpoint, the country has taken steps to curb tax evasion in its efforts to improve public finances and invest in social development policies. However, the central government's final consumption expenditures have stalled due to the country's austere fiscal policy. As a result, social spending has been lower, accounting for between 15.0% and 15.9% of GDP during the period 2000–2005. Inflation, as measured by changes in the Consumer Price Index (CPI), has remained near or above 10% during recent years, increasing from 10.1% in 2001 to 14.1% in 2005, which is also the highest rate observed within the last ten years.

Costa Rica has a democratic tradition and the country holds presidential elections every four years. In recent years, the country's lack of responsible political leadership, weak institutional systems of public expenditure management, and declining quality of governance have fueled citizen discontent with the country's political leadership. This fact has been evidenced in widespread voter abstention, which was 34.8% during the last elections in February 2006. The National Liberation Party (PLN), which will govern the country during the period 2006–2010, did not win a majority in the National Assembly. Consequently, negotiations, alliance-building, and concerted political action with the other parties will be necessary if treaties, legislation, and other legal instruments are to be approved. It was precisely the outgoing legislature's inability to compromise that slowed down the approval of a number of laws, among them a draft bill for a new general health law, which, although endorsed by the Legislative Assembly's Social Affairs Committee, has yet to be approved by the full Assembly. The incoming administration, which took office in May 2006, is seeking to create new sources of jobs and reduce poverty levels as means to reactivate the economy, and is pursuing two courses of immediate action: promoting the Free Trade Agreement in the Legislative Assembly and fiscal reform.

Costa Rica's ranking in the United Nations Development Program Human Development Index slipped from 41st in 2001 to 47th in 2005, effectively downgrading the country from the high human development to medium human development category. This measure of socioeconomic development is based on a series of indicators, especially the poverty level, which has been approximately 20% over the last decade. In 2000, the urban poverty rate was 17.1% as compared to 25.4% in rural areas.

With respect to income distribution in Costa Rica, since 2000 the poorest income decile has witnessed a greater percentage improvement in income than the highest, although in absolute terms, the purchasing power of the country's most poor continues to be negligible. Moreover, the income gap between the poorest and wealthiest deciles, which was a difference of 36.6% in 2001, decreased by seven percentage points to 29.6 in 2004. Consequently, the inequity gap in the distribution of income continues to be quite wide. Open employment increased from 5.2% in 2000 to 6.6% in 2005 (5.0% among men and 9.6% among women).

With a view to fulfilling the Millennium Development Goals (MDGs), ambitious targets have been set for reducing poverty, child mortality, and maternal mortality. In the case of the poverty rate, which was 21.7% in 2004, the established goal is to reduce it to half its 1990 level of 18% or by 9%. However, current trends suggest that a 9.0% reduction is unlikely to be achieved by 2015. In terms of the infant mortality rate, which was 9.2 per 1,000 births in 2004, the goal of a two-thirds reduction of the country's 1990 level (14.4 per 1,000 live births) or 4.8 per 1,000 live births would be impossible to reach by 2015. Infant mortality in 34 of the country's cantons surpasses the national rate, two exceed 20 per 1,000 live births, and 16 have rates equal to or greater than 15 per 1,000 live births. In 2004, national measles vaccination coverage of children under 1 year was 87.4%, while only four of the country's seven provinces had coverage levels above 95%.

Using a Lorenz curve to compare the distribution of infant mortality in 2005 with the period 1995–1999, a more pronounced curve is observed due primarily to a larger gap between the national rate and those of the Huetar Atlántica, Puntarenas, and Chorotega regions (Figure 1).

FIGURE 1. Distribution of infant mortality, by province, Costa Rica, 2005.

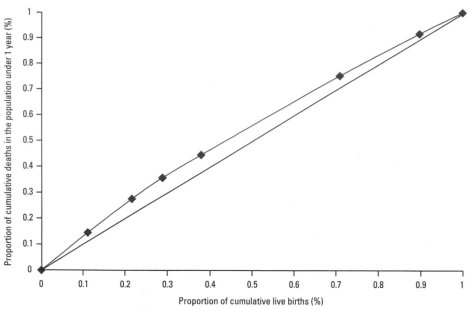

Source: Pan American Health Organization. Basic indicators 2005.

In 2004 the maternal mortality rate was 3.0 per 10,000 live births. Costa Rica has committed to the Millennium Development Goal of reducing maternal mortality by three-quarters between 1990 and 2015. The maternal mortality rate between 1990 and 2004 and the trend for 2015 can be seen in Figure 2.

With respect to malaria, the country's annual parasitic index (API) was 0.3 per 1,000 population in 2004, and 32.8% of the population was at risk for infection. Consequently, reducing malaria by 2015 is completely feasible. Only the province of Limón has an API above the national level (1.88 per 1,000 population). With respect to tuberculosis, whose incidence rate was 16.7 per 100,000 population in 2004, its reduction is also fully feasible by 2015. However, 25 cantons had incidence rates higher than the national average, 10 of which had rates as much as twice or even three times the national average.

Since the 1990s, there have been significant advances in access to education, including expanded participation in preschool education, which increased 28.3% between 1990 and 2004. The primary school net enrollment rate has remained stable at around 99.0% in recent years, dipping slightly to 98.5% in 2004. The increase in secondary education coverage has been less substantial: from 55.3% in 2000 to 63.8% in 2004. Considerable progress has been made in educational coverage. The current challenges in this regard focus on substantially improving educational performance and reducing dropout rates.

The social development index (SDI) is an indicator elaborated by the country's Ministry of National Planning and Economic Policy. The index is based on a combination of seven indicators:

educational infrastructure; special education programs; infant mortality; the burden of childhood mortality; growth delay; residential electricity consumption; and births to single mothers. This index is used to stratify the population into five large groups and serves as the basis for mapping the distribution of poverty in the country. Most cantons in group one (more developed) are located in the San José metropolitan area of central Costa Rica. Conversely, a significant part of the 17 cantons in group five (less developed) are located in border areas (Brunca and Chorotega regions). Of the total population, 15% lives in group one; 32% in group two; 21% in group three; 18% in group four; and 14% in group five. Fifteen cantons have SDIs below the national average of 46.9%.

With regard to environmental quality, it bears mentioning that 25% of the country is under some category of protected area management. In global terms, this is a high percentage, inasmuch as only 14 countries worldwide have more than 23% of their territory under a system of protected area management. Nevertheless, some shortcomings have been observed in regard to urban planning, highway infrastructure, pollution control, and comprehensive water resource management, which, together with hydrometeorological conditions and the increased population density, determine the country's vulnerability to drought and floods, and point to the need to resume efforts to step up protection of the country's water sources.

In 1991 and 2002, access to water for human consumption was 92% and 97%, respectively, and access to sanitary sewer or septic tank systems was 76% and 94%, respectively. Considering this as-

FIGURE 2. Maternal mortality rate, 1990–2003 and projected trend, Costa Rica, 1991ª–2015.

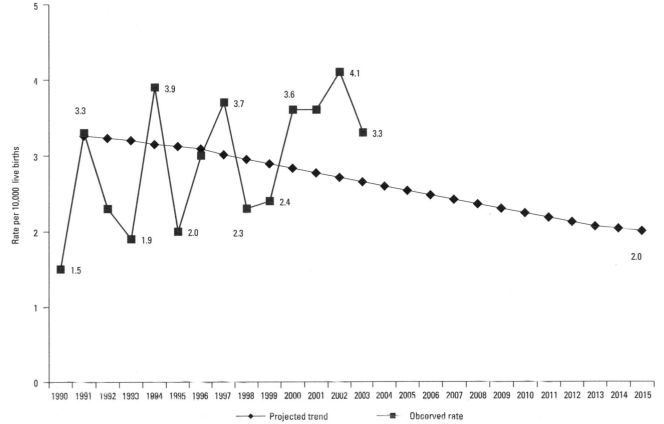

ª1991 is considered baseline year.

pect of environmental sustainability, and based on indicators adopted for monitoring progress on MDG Target 10, the country is making good headway toward achieving the MDGs. However, in contrast to the aforementioned national averages, 62% of households in areas of indigenous population do not have in-house access to potable water. Of these, 10% have an on-premises connection to a water supply; 3.2% an off-premises connection; and 42% have no water pipes. According to estimates, 21% of households have septic tanks and 65% latrines.

Demographics, Mortality, and Morbidity

In 2004, the population density was 83.14 persons per km[2]. The country has experienced profound demographic changes over the last 40 years and is currently in a stage of advanced demographic transition, characterized by low mortality and fertility. The population growth rate continues to be relatively high, but will trend downward with the relative aging of the population. Despite the considerable demographic changes that have taken place in the country, population growth will continue to

figure prominently in the new challenges associated with the demographic transition.

The population pyramid has changed dramatically over the last several decades, bulging at the center (Figure 3). These changes are attributable to the marked decrease in mortality and fertility. Over the past 10 years it has become evident that the country's population has entered a pattern of relative aging that will continue into the coming years.

Mortality (1970: 6.8 per 1,000 population; 2004: 3.6 per 1,000) has not declined at the same pace as fertility and the birth rate, but has been stabilizing since 1985 (1994: 13,313 deaths; 2004: 15,949 deaths).

Another characteristic of this demographic transition is the sustained decrease in fertility and the birth rate, which has been so pronounced that despite the country's larger population and greater number of women of childbearing age in absolute terms, the number of births has actually decreased (1985: 84,337 children; 2004: 72,247 children) to the point that women are currently having only two children. This means that the fertility rate is lower than the population replacement level. Finally, the

FIGURE 3. Population structure, by age and sex, Costa Rica, 1970 and 2000.

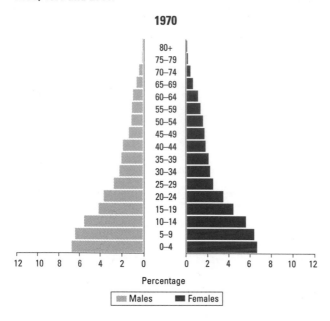

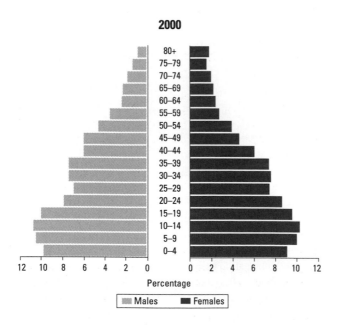

population. Of the total indigenous population, 51.5% were male and 48.5% female, and 79.0% resided in primarily rural areas (INEC 2001). This population is concentrated in the Talamanca and Southern Pacific regions, especially in the border area with Panama. Although indigenous people live in all provinces of the country, more than three-quarters (77.4%) reside in the provinces of Limón (39.2%), Puntarenas (23.5%), and San José (14.4%). The indigenous population is comprised of eight peoples—the Bribris, the Borucas or Bruncas, Cabecars, Chorotegas, Guayamis, Huetars, Malekus, and Teribes, which are distributed among 24 indigenous territories.

With respect to immigration, according to the tenth annual State of the Nation Report, Nicaraguans continue to constitute by far the absolute majority of immigrants in the country. According to the latest census, Nicaraguans accounted for 76.0% of all foreigners in the country and their percentage of the total population increased from 1.9% to 5.9% during that period. There are also significant numbers of immigrants from Panama, the United States, El Salvador, and Colombia; however, only immigration from Colombia and Nicaragua has increased. According to the 2000 census, 10% of all households include persons of Nicaraguan origin. Due to the effects of international immigration, no substantial changes in the makeup of the Costa Rican population by sex or age are expected during the next 25 years. However, depending on the future course of immigration, the natural growth rate of the population may increase anywhere from 24% to 45%.

With respect to the seven broad groups of causes of death in the period 1970–2004, diseases of the circulatory system were the leading cause of death among both men and women. The cumulative rate for these diseases in males ranged between 13.4 in 1970 and 11.0 in 2004. In 2000–2004, the next two principal causes of mortality were other diseases and tumors. Table 1 lists the mortality rates by cause and 5-year period between 1970 and 2004.

An analysis of mortality by cause in the period 1995–2001, with adjusted rates per 100,000 population, indicates that diseases of the circulatory system had been declining since 1997, but trending upward beginning in 2001; the same trend has also been observed with respect to tumors. External causes and diseases of the digestive system have followed a stable trend.

With respect to the relative distribution of hospital discharges by cause in 1990, 1995, and 2005, most cases were associated with pregnancy, delivery, and the puerperium, at 35.9%, 34.2%, and 31.7%. Table 2 provides the distribution of hospital discharges by groups of causes in 1990, 1995, and 2005.

With respect to the risk of emergencies and disasters, the geographic areas of the country most exposed to floods continue to be the Atlantic and Pacific basins, a fact attributable to social disparities. The earthquake-prone regions of the country are located in the provinces of Cartago, Alajuela, and Limón. Other threats have emerged as a consequence of man's exploitation of natural resources, including deforestation, environmental pollution, and

process of demographic transition shows that the most direct effects of the aging of the population will be an increase in the dependency ratio of people over age 65. The dependency ratio is currently 55%; however, the demographic dividend will bring the ratio down to approximately 44% in little more than ten years, after which it will rise again.

According to the Ninth National Population Census (2000), which was the country's first to consider information on ethnic groups, indigenous groups accounted for 1.7% of the national

TABLE 1. Cumulative mortality rates, by cause and 5-year period, Costa Rica, 1970–2004.

	1970–1974 Cumulative rate (%)	1975–1979 Cumulative rate (%)	1980–1984 Cumulative rate (%)	1985–1989 Cumulative rate (%)	1990–1994 Cumulative rate (%)	1995–1999 Cumulative rate (%)	2000–2004 Cumulative rate (%)
Males							
Communicable diseases	4.67	2.45	1.90	1.62	1.83	1.90	1.95
Conditions originating in the perinatal period	0.32	0.24	0.23	0.19	0.15	0.14	0.12
Tumors	6.14	6.39	6.66	6.84	6.76	6.75	6.80
Diseases of the circulatory system	13.44	11.05	11.15	10.80	11.28	11.04	11.00
External causes (injuries and poisonings)	2.24	2.52	1.98	1.95	2.14	2.16	2.14
Other diseases	3.86	4.47	5.06	5.97	5.89	7.25	7.32
Ill-defined signs, symptoms, and morbidity	2.42	1.51	0.87	0.29	0.39	0.26	0.26
Females							
Communicable diseases	4.35	1.95	1.57	1.27	1.26	1.35	1.37
Conditions originating in the perinatal period	0.22	0.18	0.16	0.14	0.11	0.10	0.14
Tumors	5.01	4.70	4.52	4.85	4.42	4.35	4.51
Diseases of the circulatory system	12.38	9.81	9.57	8.85	8.66	8.30	8.28
External causes (injuries and poisonings)	0.66	0.86	0.81	0.85	0.87	0.82	0.80
Other diseases	3.89	4.72	4.58	5.35	4.97	5.60	5.55
Ill-defined signs, symptoms, and morbidity	2.01	1.28	0.64	0.21	0.23	0.14	0.14

Source: Costa Rica, Instituto Nacional de Estadística y Censos y Ministerio de Salud.

TABLE 2. Relative distribution of hospital discharges, by cause, Costa Rica, 1990, 1995, and 2005.

Cause	1990	1995	2005
Health measures	4.2	4.3	5.2
Infectious and parasitic diseases	4.1	3.7	2.8
Tumors	4.1	4.8	4.8
Nutritional support for endocrine conditions	2.2	2.2	0.5
Blood	0.6	0.6	1.8
Mental disorders	2.6	2.0	2.0
Nervous system	3.0	3.3	1.5
Diseases of the eye and adnexa	…	…	2.7
Diseases of the ear or mastoids	…	…	0.5
Circulatory system	5.0	5.0	5.5
Respiratory system	6.2	6.6	7.1
Digestive system	7.6	8.6	9.5
Genitourinary system	6.9	6.7	6.8
Skin and tissue	1.5	1.4	1.4
Musculoskeletal system	2.7	2.6	2.8
Pregnancy, delivery, and the puerperium	35.9	34.2	31.8
Congenital anomalies	1.5	1.8	1.6
Perinatal conditions	3.5	3.5	3.6
Injuries and poisonings	7.2	7.1	6.6
Ill-defined signs, symptoms, and morbidity	1.2	1.1	1.3

Source: Costa Rica, Departamento de Información Estadística de los Servicios de Salud. Caja Costarricense de Seguro Social (CCSS).

the alteration of hydrographic basins. Extensive flooding occurs each year from May through July in the Sixaola region along the country's border with Panama, and from September through October in the Guanacaste region bordering Nicaragua.

HEALTH OF POPULATION GROUPS

Children under 5 Years Old

In the period 1990–2004, the infant mortality rate decreased from 14.4 to 9.2 per 1,000 live births, which is the lowest rate of the previous ten years. According to data of the National Statistics and Census Institute (INEC), the country's neonatal mortality rate decreased from 8.78 in 1990 to 6.73 in 2004, while postneonatal mortality dropped from 6.1 in 1990 to 2.5 in 2004. The highest rates are found in the provinces of Guanacaste (11.2), Puntarenas (9.9), and Limón (9.4), which are also the country's least developed in socioeconomic terms. In 2004, the primary causes of infant mortality by broad groups of causes were certain conditions originating in the perinatal period (49.0%), followed by congenital anomalies (31.0%); respiratory diseases (8.1%); infectious and parasitic diseases (2.1%); and others (9.8%). This pattern has remained steady in recent years. In the period 1990–2004, the relative weight of neonatal mortality in infant mortality increased from 69% to 73% by the last year of the period. Forty percent of infant deaths are preventable.

The 1–4 years age group accounts for 9.6% of the population. In 2002, the mortality rate was 4.8 per 10,000 population. That year, accidents and violence were the leading cause of death (1.7 per 10,000), followed by diseases of the respiratory system; congenital anomalies; tumors; infectious and parasitic diseases; and diseases of the nervous system. In 2002, this group accounted for 4.9% of emergency visits and 5.0% of outpatient consultations. With respect to the causes of morbidity, acute respiratory infections accounted for 35.7% and injuries from external causes for 10.7%. Mortality was greater among boys than girls, at 5.5 and 4.1 per 10,000, respectively.

Children 5–9 Years Old

Children in the 5–9 years age group account for 11.7% of the population. In 2002, the mortality rate for this group was 2.0 per 10,000. The leading causes of death were external causes, tumors, diseases of the nervous system, and infectious and parasitic diseases. That same year, this age group accounted for 10% of emergency consultations, the leading cause of which were respiratory diseases (51.6%), followed by external causes (12.6%) and infectious and parasitic diseases (11%).

Adolescents 10–14 and 15–19 Years Old

In 2002, the 10–14 years age group accounted for 10.6% of the country's total population, and the 15–19 years age group for 10.5%. The leading causes of death among these groups were external causes—10.9 and 29.9 per 100,000 among the 10–14 and 15–19 years age groups, respectively—followed by tumors (4.6 and 8.5 per 100,000) and diseases of the nervous system (3.0 and 5.4 per 100,000). Mortality was greater among males of both groups. The 10–14 years age group accounted for 6.7% of emergency consultations and 4.9% of outpatient consultations at the health services, and the 15–19 years age group for 8.4% of emergency consultations and 6.1% of outpatient consultations. Respiratory infections and external causes were the most common reasons for consultations among both sexes, in addition to pregnancy care visits for women. According to the second report on the status of the rights of childhood and adolescence in Costa Rica (UNICEF, 2002), adolescent girls and young women under 19 years old accounted for slightly more than 20% of births (14,860 births). Eighty percent of this group was unmarried. Moreover, infant mortality among the group was 15 per 1,000 live births, and 25% of these deaths were due to obstetric causes.

Adults 20–59 Years Old

In 2002, the 20–59 years age group accounted for approximately 51% of the total population. The mortality rate was 11.5 per 10,000 population among the 20–44 years age group, and 50.0 per 10,000 among the 45–64 years age group. With respect to the former group, the leading causes of death were external causes, followed by tumors in men, and cardiovascular diseases in women; and in the latter group, external causes followed by cardiovascular diseases in men, and tumors followed by cardiovascular diseases in women.

Young adults aged 20–44 years accounted for 36.6% of emergency services provided, 35.0% of outpatient consultations, and 45.0% of hospital discharges. The most frequent reasons for the demand of all these services were injuries in men and conditions related to reproduction in women. Adults aged 45–59 years benefited from 9.8% of emergency services provided, 14% of consultations, and 8.5% of hospital services. The most frequent reasons

for the demand of these services were diseases of the respiratory tract, diseases of the musculoskeletal system, and injuries.

With respect to reproductive health, fertility levels have fallen in recent decades. The leading causes of maternal death are labor and delivery-related complications, hypertensive disorders of pregnancy, hemorrhages, and infections. Prenatal care administered by qualified health professionals reached 92% and delivery care, 98%. According to estimates, 98% of deliveries are attended in hospitals and 2% in the home or in ambulances. More than 90% of pregnant women had prenatal care, and deliveries by cesarean section increased from 14.1% in 1983 to 22.0% in 2004.

Older Adults 60 Years Old and Older

In 2002, older adults accounted for 7.5% of the country's total population, 90% of which had social security coverage and 36% retirement pensions. According to estimates, 28% live in poverty and one-third of men in this group are still economically active; 10% live alone; and only 1% resides in nursing homes. The leading causes of mortality for this group are cardiovascular diseases (40%), neoplasms (20%–25%), and other conditions (20%–25%), which include chronic respiratory diseases, diabetes, and the default category "senility." Cancer rates are higher among men, while other chronic conditions, especially diabetes, affect women more. Together, these three large groups account for nearly 90% of mortality among older adults. With regard to morbidity, the main causes are hypertension, diabetes mellitus, neurotic disorders, and gastrointestinal and respiratory infections.

The Family

The number of single-parent households headed by women has increased. In 2002, women headed 22.2% of the country's households and also accounted for 32.1% of all poor households, more of which were located in urban (38.6%) rather than rural (26.0%) areas. Trends by sex and marital status of female and male heads of household indicate that the former tend to be single, living in consensual unions, separated, divorced, or widowed. In 2001, the Legislative Assembly approved the Law on Responsible Paternity, which has significantly reduced the percentage of births registered without a recognized father—from 29.3% in 2001 to 8.1% in 2002.

Workers

The annual per worker incapacity rate remained steady over the period 2000–2004. Accordingly, each year 800 of every 1,000 workers are affected by some form of incapacity that causes them to miss work. The area of the country with the highest average of sick leave days per worker is the Brunca region (7.2 days), which is only surpassed by the country's decentralized hospitals (average of 13.41 sick leave days), followed by the

Huetar Norte (6.83 days) and Chorotega (6.83 days) regions. In the San José metropolitan area, an average of only 3.87 sick leave days are provided. The national incapacity rate is 6.84 days of sick leave.

The four most frequent causes of incapacity by annual number of sick leave days are upper respiratory tract infections (100,000 days), back pain (60,000 days), infectious intestinal diseases (45,000 days), and behavioral disorders (35,000 days). Consequently, measures aimed at improving the workplace environment could help to prevent missed days of work.

Agriculture is Costa Rica's second most important industry, employing on the order of 240,000 people. According to estimates, about 3% of agricultural workers become poisoned each year or approximately 7,500 poisoning cases. However, only 600 to 1,000 such cases are reported annually, which points to underreporting of between 82% and 97%. Women account for some 8% of the agricultural workforce, and, due to a combination of biological and other factors, they are more vulnerable to pesticide exposure than men. The rate of occupational poisonings is 2.5 times greater among men, at an average age fluctuating around 31 years. The lethality rate due to occupational poisonings is the lowest for all types of poisonings.

Persons with Disabilities

Data of the INEC's 2000 National Census of Population and Housing revealed that 5.4% of the total population suffers from some form of disability; 52% are men and 48% women. The disabled account for 5% of the urban population and 6% of the rural population. In some rural cantons such as Corredores, Parrita, Osa, and Montes de Oro in the province of Puntarenas, the disability rate surpasses the national average by at least 1.5%. The central part of the country has the highest concentration of the disabled, estimated at 184,452 persons, followed by the Chorotega region (32,586 persons), the Huetar Atlántica region (29,012), the Brunca region (26,109), the Pacific Central region (20,299), and the Huetar Norte region (18,901). Blindness is the most common disability among both men (32,784) and women (29,772), followed by deafness, paralysis, and mental retardation.

Immigrants

According to the most recent census data (2000), there were 226,374 Nicaraguans residing permanently in Costa Rica (nearly 6% of the total population), 50.9% of whom were female and 49.1% male. Approximately half of this population was between 20 and 39 years of age. This figure does not include the population of short-term cyclical migrants from Nicaragua or those not captured by the census for lack of a fixed address.

The distribution and settlement patterns of the Nicaraguan migrant population are irregular and vary by region, but in geographic terms, tend to be concentrated in the central, Atlantic coast, and northern parts of the country, which are home to industries that attract migrant labor (export agriculture, agroindustry, and services). In Costa Rica, 295,456 persons live in "binational" households, of which 36.9% were born in Costa Rica and 62.6% in Nicaragua.

HEALTH CONDITIONS AND PROBLEMS

COMMUNICABLE DISEASES

Vector-borne Diseases

Since reemerging in 1993, **dengue** has become a serious public health problem in Costa Rica. The highest incidence of cases occurred in 1994, 1997, 2003, and 2005 (rate of 55–89 per 10,000 population in this period). It is estimated that 95.7% of the population is at risk of dengue, especially people residing in areas of dengue transmission and high indices of *Aedes aegypti* infestation. In 2005, a total of 37,798 cases were reported. The regions with the highest incidence (81.1%) were Pacific Central (421.3 per 10,000 population), Huetar Atlántica (264.2), Chorotega (172.5), and North Central (67.7). Fifty-two cases of dengue hemorrhagic fever and two deaths were reported for a 3.8% lethality rate. Dengue outbreaks are ordinarily seasonal, with cases increasing at the start of the rainy season. In recent years, however, the seasonal nature of the disease has blurred, resulting in transmission practically throughout the year. Circulation of three serotypes—dengue 1, dengue 2, and dengue 3—has been identified, thus increasing risks for the reemergence of dengue hemorrhagic fever. Over the period 1995–2005, a total of 329 cases of dengue hemorrhagic fever and eight deaths were reported. Upon comparing the cases reported by month during the last three years, increases were observed beginning in May 2003 and 2004, and in April 2005, which peaked in July 2003 and in August 2005. Entomological surveys carried out in the period 2004–2005 revealed infestation indices that fluctuated between 0 and 23.2 cases; some areas were found to have higher Breteau indexes than infestation indices, which points to the presence of more than one breeding foci per household. *Aedes aegypti* larval sites are classified into the following categories: unusable water receptacles (60.6%) such as used tires (which also accounted for the highest percentage of positive larvae tests in this category at 22.7%); cans and scrap metal (33.5%); special man-made receptacles (38.6%); receptacles in use (38.3%), including barrels and containers used to store water for household use (which accounted for the highest percentage of positive larvae tests in this category at 72.8%); and food and water troughs (13.0%).

A sustained increase in **malaria** cases was observed halfway through the period 2001–2005. The number of reported cases jumped from 718 in 2003 to 3,541 in 2005, which represents a 393.2% increase. The annual parasite incidence (API) increased from 1.05 in 2001 to 2.25 in 2005. The highest percentage of cases during this five-year period was reported in the Huetar Atlántica Health Region, located in the northeastern part of the country along the border with Panama, accounting for 66.2% in 2001 and 95.2% in 2005. The 15–49 years age group continues to be most affected, accounting for 62.7% cases in 2001 and 72.0% in 2005. The percentage of males affected fluctuated between 60.6% in 2001 and 62.67% in 2005. No malaria deaths were reported during the five-year period. Of malaria cases reported during the five-year period, 99.7% were caused by *Plasmodium vivax*, which is sensitive to chloroquine. All eight reported cases of *P. falciparum* malaria in 2004 and 2005 (five in 2004 and three in 2005) were imported: five from Nicaragua; two from Africa; and one from the Dominican Republic. Given Costa Rica's geographic, climatic, and land-use conditions, nearly 70% of the country is considered a malaria zone, or favorable for developing the most significant transmission vector, *Anopheles albimanus*. These factors, as well as migratory flows to and within agricultural production zones, and the socioeconomic conditions of the population residing in these places carry significant weight in terms of malaria control.

The country's **filariasis bancrofti** problem is limited to the city of Puerto Limón, located in the Huetar Atlántica region. According to the results of epidemiological (1974–1983) and antigenemia (2002–2003) studies, there is a low probability that the sources of infection needed to maintain active transmission exist. Antigenemia screenings of 3,044 schoolchildren from all neighborhoods of Puerto Limón were negative; 70% of carriers had less than 6 microfilaria per 20 microliters of blood, and residual morbidity occurred only among older adults. *Culex quinquefasciatus* was identified as the primary vector. Inasmuch as lymphatic filariasis has been declared eliminated in Puerto Limón, the pertinent certification process is currently under way.

Vaccine-preventable Diseases

The Expanded Program on Immunization currently includes vaccination against measles, rubella, mumps, diphtheria, tetanus, pertussis, poliomyelitis, hepatitis B, *Haemophilus influenzae* type b, tuberculosis (meningeal and miliary), and against complications due to seasonal influenza (flu) viruses (the latter for groups at risk). In 2004, surveillance of influenza viruses was launched at four sentinel centers—the National Children's Hospital, the National Geriatric Hospital, Hospital Max Peralta, and Clínica de Pavas—in order to strengthen testing aimed at identifying a flu vaccine more consistent with the strains circulating in the country. No confirmed **measles** cases have been reported (the last outbreak occurred in 1999), although one sporadic case was reported in 2005. Beginning in 2001, a program was launched to control **rubella** and eliminate **congenital rubella syndrome** (CRS), which included the vaccination of the population aged 15–39 of both sexes in a campaign that achieved 98% coverage. The program was supplemented with postpartum vaccination of the cohort of pregnant women. **Hepatitis B** is a

disease whose incidence is highest among the 15–44 years age group; however, in recent years it has been rising among the 10–14 years age group. The *Haemophilus influenzae* type b (Hib) vaccine was introduced into the country's basic immunization schedule in March 1998. The most marked decrease in **meningitis** cases has occurred since 1998, when efforts began to achieve national vaccination coverage. No cases of **neonatal tetanus** have been reported in the country since 1988, with the exception of one reported and confirmed case in 2002. As a result, measures were taken to strengthen coverage levels among the adult population and pregnant women at risk. Tetanus cases among adults continue to occur sporadically, with between one and three cases reported annually. No cases of **diphtheria** have been observed in the country since 1976, after introduction of the vaccine against diphtheria and tetanus (DT) into the national immunization schedule six years earlier.

Throughout the last decade and into the present day, the Expanded Program on Immunization has maintained coverage levels of 80% and higher for all antigens. Coverage for tracer vaccines in the official schedule, BCG (bacillus Calmette-Guerin), OPV3 (Sabin oral poliovirus vaccine), and DPT3 (diphtheria-pertussis-tetanus triple vaccine) increased over the period 1998–2002.

Intestinal Infectious Diseases

Acute diarrheal disease rates have been rising over the past years, from 2,917 per 100,000 population in 1992 to 3,939 in 2001 (35% increase). However, hospital discharges attributable to these diseases have been decreasing, from 8,151 in 1990 to 4,821 in 2000 (40.8% decrease). This decrease has been observed in all age groups except older adults over the age of 80 and children aged 5–9 years, whose rates have increased. Mortality from diarrheal diseases has tended to remain stable, with the exception of increases observed in 1994, 1995, and 1996. Their lethality has been declining over the past years, from 0.12% in 1994 to 0.06% in 2001. However, upon a review of the information it bears mentioning that significant underreporting of cases in some areas of the country has hindered the ability to monitor the monthly trends of these diseases; nevertheless, an increase in reported cases has been observed in March and June. Incidence and mortality rates for these diseases are highest among children under the age of 5 years and adults over age 65. Males in the former group are most often affected, whereas those of the latter are least affected. Traditionally, the provinces Puntarenas, Guanacaste, and Alajuela have always had the highest mortality rates.

Chronic Communciable Diseases

Costa Rica is among the countries of the world with the lowest prevalence of **tuberculosis**, with a reported incidence of 17.35 per 100,000 population over the last four years. Pulmonary tuberculosis is the most commonly diagnosed form of the disease, accounting for 85% of total cases. People over the age of 25 are most affected, and men account for more cases than women.

Moreover, the immigrant population accounts for 10% of total cases. Although underreporting of tuberculosis deaths has been a problem, mortality from the disease has been declining since 1999 at an average rate of 2.3 per 100,000 population.

BCG vaccination coverage in recent years has exceeded 90%, and there have been no reported cases of **tubercular meningitis**. Although cases of multi-drug resistant tuberculosis have been reported, this type of tuberculosis is not viewed as a significant problem in Costa Rica. From the operational standpoint, there have been improvements in the screening of patients for respiratory symptoms and an increase in the number of diagnostic bacilloscopies, but this figure is still lower than expected, with 3% culture-positive tests among patients with respiratory symptoms. In this regard, efforts to increase the number and quality of bacilloscopies will help provide a clearer picture of the epidemiological situation.

Coverage with the Directly Observed Treatment, Short-course or DOTS strategy was 100%; in 2001 the cohort of new bacilliferous cases in DOTS areas achieved a 58.2% cure rate and a 25.3% treatment completion rate, resulting in an 83.2% treatment success rate, a 5.6% death rate, and a 10.1% dropout rate. In non-DOTS areas, there was a 34.2% cure rate and 27.9% treatment completion rate, resulting in a success rate of only 62.1%, a 14.6% death rate, and a 22% dropout rate. The most new cases were observed in the health regions covering the Huetar Atlántica, Pacific Central, South Central, and North-Central regions.

In 2002, active surveillance of **leprosy** cases was launched in conjunction with dermatology consultations at national and regional hospitals. Surveillance activities since that time recaptured and identified a total of 114 cases of leprosy during the period 1998–2003, for a prevalence of 0.28 cases per 10,000 population. The province of Puntarenas had the most cases and highest prevalence (0.7 per 10,000 population). Over recent years, some 15 to 20 new cases have been detected annually.

Acute Respiratory Infections

Acute respiratory infections (ARIs) require mandatory notification and are the most common reason for outpatient consultations in the country. ARIs were on the rise through 1999, but began to trend downward in 2000, and remained steady through 2004 (rate of 20,000–25,000 per 100,000 population). Most affected are children under 10 years of age, especially children under 1 year of age, whose hospitalization rates range between 26.7 and 32.8 per 1,000; followed by the age group 1–4 years old with hospitalization rates between 1.65 and 2.41 per 1,000; and finally the 5–9 years age group with rates between 0.36 and 0.79 per 1,000. Children under 5 years of age accounted for between 80% and 90% of hospital discharges for ARIs. The other significantly affected age group is the population over the age of 50, whose hospitalization rates fluctuate between 0.30 and 0.56 per 1,000. However, mortality is higher among this last group than children under the age of 10. The seasonal distribution of reported cases over the last four years points to higher incidence during the months of March, April, and June.

HIV/AIDS and Other Sexually Transmitted Infections

AIDS cases were on a rising trend from 1983 through 1998, which was the year treatment with antiretroviral drugs was introduced. A total of 2,742 cases were reported through 2004. The classification of AIDS cases by mode of infection shows that 84.2% of cases were contracted through sexual contact (43.7% homosexual, 24.9% heterosexual, and 15.6% bisexual), 3.9% exposure to tainted blood (hemophilia 2.1%, transfusions 0.9%, and intravenous drug use 0.9%), 1.2% perinatal transmission, and in 6.8% of cases the mode of infection is unknown. The HIV/AIDS mortality rate has increased steadily since the onset of the epidemic, peaking in 1997 at 4.8 deaths per 100,000 population. That same year, however, a decrease—although not steady—was observed, and in recent years the rate appears to have stabilized at about 3.5 deaths per 100,000 population. The male population has been most affected by the disease. The male-female ratio has been declining: from 12:1 in 1998 to 7:1 in 2001, and down again to 5.4:1 in 2005. In terms of mortality by sex, there has been a slight decrease observed in female mortality. With respect to mortality by age groups, an increase has been observed in the 25–39 years age group.

In regard to other sexually transmitted infections, the highest cumulative incidence rates for **syphilis** were among infants under 1 year of age (105.2 per 100,000 population), followed by the 15–54 years age group (24.0). The rate by sex indicates that for every 1.17 cases of female infection there is one male case. In contrast to all other forms of syphilis, congenital syphilis followed a rising trend in 1996, 1998, and 2004. In 2005, the 15–44 years age group had the highest cumulative incidence rate for **gonorrhea** (37.5 per 100,000 population).

Zoonoses

According to the list of diseases of compulsory notification, the zoonotic disease with the highest cumulative incidence is **leptospirosis**. Studies of the epidemiological trend of leptospirosis during the period 1996–2005 reveal that this disease has become a reemerging zoonosis, which has been trending upward since 1999 due to improved active case finding through fever monitoring activities. Consequently, efforts are needed to strengthen research with a view to establishing cut-off points for each serovar strain and identifying those with the widest circulation in the country. The case distribution by provinces shows that Puntarenas (2.4 per 10,000 population) and Limón (1.1) had the highest incidence, whereas the most affected cantons were Corredores (1.0 per 1,000 population), Golfito (0.7), Talamanca (0.3), and Matina (0.2). The distribution by sex reveals that the male population is disproportionately affected, with a male-female ratio of 4:1. With respect to distribution by age groups, the youngest and oldest of the population had the least incidence, while the highest incidence was found among people employed in agro-industry; residents of flood-prone or marginal areas, or both; and the economically active population.

Costa Rica has had no cases of **canine rabies** since 1987. In 2002, two cases of human rabies were reported involving a rabies virus circulated among vampire bats. The infection was transmitted by a rabid cat in a rural area with a history of bovine rabies. The country's rabies epidemiological surveillance has been strengthened through the coordination of activities with the Ministry of Agriculture and Livestock. **Cysticercosis** is not a disease of compulsory notification and, consequently, no data is available on its incidence. However, upon reviewing the causes of death for communicable diseases, two cysticercosis deaths were discovered in 1995, in addition to four more in 2000. Accordingly, additional investigation is needed to determine whether incidence of the disease is in fact increasing.

NONCOMMUNICABLE DISEASES

Metabolic and Nutritional Diseases

Inasmuch as the most recent national nutrition survey was conducted in 1996, and the latest height census of first grade schoolchildren in 1997, the country has no recent data on the anthropometric situation of the nutritionally vulnerable groups: preschool children; schoolchildren; adolescents; and women of reproductive age. However, a national study of schoolchildren aged 7–15 years was carried out in 2002, which included measurement of body mass index (BMI). The study revealed that 6.2% of the children were underweight, 73.2% normal weight, 12.7% overweight, and 7.9% obese. In 2000, a nutritional assessment carried out in the rural sentinel community of Nicoya, Guanacaste, found that—according to serum ferritin testing—30.4% of preschool children had deficient iron reserves, and 12.1% of women of reproductive age had deficient serum folate levels. The assessment also revealed deficient vitamin A serum levels in 9.9% of preschoolers and in 11.1% of schoolchildren, as well as marginal vitamin A deficiency in 41.1% and 47.7%, respectively.

A 2001 national survey of apparent consumption of foodstuffs in the home revealed that nutritional adequacy rises with family income up to values exceeding 100% adequacy among the higher income households. Food consumption in the home and at the national level is satisfactory; however, differences are observed by degree of urbanization and disparities by income decile, both in urban and rural areas.

The **diabetes** mortality rate has been increasing and gaining momentum in recent years for a rate of 19.3 per 100,000 population in 2004. Data from a 2004 survey conducted in the San José metropolitan area indicate a diabetes prevalence of 7.9% and that 1.9% of those affected are unaware they have the disease. Prevalence is higher among men (8.3%) than women (7.6%) and increases after 40 years of age. Data from the same survey show that

the percentage of persons with a BMI over 25 is 58.9% (males 62% and females 55.9%). It is estimated that 41.2% of the population fails to get 30 minutes of exercise a day at least five times a week.

Cardiovascular Diseases

Diseases of the circulatory system have been the country's leading cause of death since 1970. The mortality rate for this group has been declining since 2002, and the levels for men have been persistently higher. In 2004, the rate was 112 per 100,000 population among men and 103 per 100,000 among women. The mortality rate for **hypertensive diseases** has been increasing and was 13.2 per 100,000 in 2004, without notable differences between the sexes. Data from a 2004 survey conducted in the San José metropolitan area show a hypertension prevalence of 25.2 per 100 population, which increases with age. Mortality from **ischemic heart disease** has been decreasing since 2001 (rate of 50.6 per 100,000 population in 2004, affecting men disproportionately), as well as **cerebrovascular diseases** (rate of 22.1 per 100,000 in 2004, affecting women disproportionately).

Malignant Neoplasms

Malignant tumors are the third leading cause of death. Each year 7,500 new cancer cases are diagnosed, resulting in more than 3,500 deaths. The country's tumor registry, which has been in place since 1980, shows that incidence rates have increased by approximately 40% since the early 1990s, although the mortality rate has not changed significantly in recent years (Figure 4).

The incidence of **breast cancer** reveals a 45% increase in its age-adjusted rates over the period between 1990 (rate of 25.96 per 100,000 population) and 2000 (37.88). Mortality has decreased in recent years from an adjusted rate of 12.09 per 100,000 population in 1990 down to 11.27 in 2003. It is most concentrated in the urban areas of the country's central valley.

The incidence of **cervical cancer** was highest in 2000, with an adjusted rate of 46.94 per 100,000 population. The incidence rates of *in situ* and invasive cancers were 30.90 and 18.17 per 100,000 population, respectively. The adjusted incidence rate of *in situ* cancer increased from 22.62 in 1990 to 30.90 per 100,000 population in 2000, while the corresponding incidence of invasive cancer decreased from 17.48 to 16.80 per 100,000 population, which is attributable to effective screening. During the same period, the adjusted mortality rate decreased from 9.95 to 5.6 per 100,000 population. Its distribution is rural and in the coastal regions of the country.

Costa Rica figures among the ten countries of the world with the highest **stomach cancer** incidence and mortality rates. From 1990 to 2000, there were no notable variations in the incidence rate; however, adjusted mortality decreased from 25.73 to 16.59 per 100,000 population. In 2000, a total of 815 cases were diagnosed, 399 of which corresponded to males. The eastern portions of the central valley and southern Costa Rica have the most cases.

FIGURE 4. Annual incidence and mortality for tumors, both sexes, Costa Rica, 1990–2001.

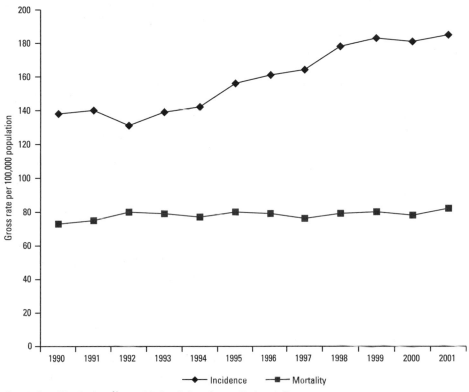

Source: Costa Rica, Instituto Nacional de Estadística y Censos, Registro de Tumores.

The adjusted incidence rate of **prostate cancer** has nearly tripled in the last years from 17.86 per 100,000 population in 1990 to 45.10 in 2000. Likewise, the adjusted mortality rate has been increasing over the same period from 10.29 per 100,000 population to 15.89.

OTHER HEALTH PROBLEMS OR ISSUES

Disasters

Due to the country's geographic location, it is exposed to a variety of threats from natural phenomena and hydrometeorological changes which, together with the vulnerability of the exposed populations residing in the Atlantic coastal areas, shortcomings in terms of implementing appropriate environmental management policies, and the nature of the country's hydrographic basins, have resulted in recurrent flooding. In the period 1998–2005, economic losses sustained by the health sector reached US$ 23 million or the equivalent of 2.7% of total losses from this cause. Given past experiences and the concentration of the population within the areas of the country at risk, the threats posed by volcanic eruptions and earthquakes must always be weighed. Moreover, the risks associated with technological development must also be

considered, which increase at a faster pace than the oversight and control activities of the responsible authorities.

Violence and Other External Causes

In 2004, there were 52,352 traffic accidents that resulted in 587 deaths (13.8 per 100,000 population), which accounted for a 5.6% decrease from the previous year. According to 2005 data of the Highway Safety Board, males accounted for the majority of highway fatalities at the scene of the accident (88.5%). That same year, driver deaths accounted for 23.4% of mortality from traffic accidents and pedestrian deaths for 23.2%. In 2005, there were 7.2% more serious injuries than the previous year. The causes of traffic accidents in 2005 were speeding (29.8%), pedestrian neglect (16.8%), and alcohol (15.3%).

With respect to social violence, the rate of violent deaths (homicides, suicides, and all types of accidents) showed significant increases. Programs of domestic violence assistance offering a variety of institutional services, which include health services, have been growing steadily in recent years. The number of requests for protective orders filed with the court system increased by more than 55% between 1998 and 2002. Violence against women is a serious and growing problem in the country: 58% of women suffered at least one incident of physical or sexual violence, or both, most often at the hands of the men in their lives. The majority of rapes of women (81.9% of cases) over the age of 16 were committed by a male family member or partner; 84.3% of domestic violence occurs in the home. Between 2000 and 2005, there were 152 homicides of women in situations of domestic violence and extramarital sexual violence, or an average of 25.3 women slain each year.

Of the 331 children treated for acts of violence at the National Children's Hospital in 2002, 53.5% were victims of sexual abuse and 25.5% victims of physical assaults. Of the 7,621 individual instances of care provided in 2005 to children under 18 years of age by Costa Rica's child welfare authority (PANI), 49.5% were for physical abuse, 23.3% sexual abuse within the home, 10.6% sexual abuse outside the home, and 16.7% emotional abuse.

Mental Health and Addictions

According to records of the Costa Rican Social Security Fund (CCSS) for 2002, the leading reasons for psychiatric consultations among the population over the age of 10 years were anxiety, depressive, and neurotic disorders. The prevalence of depression in the country is estimated at 7.2%. Twice as many women are treated for depressive disorders than men. The most recent CCSS survey (2001) found that the leading reason for consultations by both sexes was anxiety, followed by alcoholism and depression. Psychoses were the leading cause of discharge from psychiatric hospitals, including schizophrenia. As a percentage, male patients have consistently accounted for more hospital discharges than female patients.

The suicide mortality rate in recent years was as follows: 6.2 per 100,000 population in 1995; 6.3 in 2000; 4.7 in 2001; and 6.7 in 2005. Males accounted for 88.2% of these deaths, and women 11.8%. In 2004, the province of Guanacaste had the highest suicide rate at 7.5 per 100,000 population, followed by Heredia and San José at 7.1, Alajuela at 6.9, and Cartago at 6.7. With respect to homicides, 86% of victims were male and 14% female, for a male-female ratio of 6:1.

Environmental Pollution

According to the 2005 report of the Office of the Controller General of the Republic, over the last ten years there has been increasing use of imported, extremely toxic and hazardous pesticides (WHO classes Ia and Ib), which are likely carcinogenic (classes A and B, according to the U.S. EPA's Environmental Protection Agenda). The report also points out policy, regulatory, and inter-agency cooperation shortcomings, with a view to monitoring and curbing the use of these substances, guaranteeing their quality, and reducing the associated health and environmental risks. Pesticide poisonings continue to pose a significant public health threat in areas of intensive agricultural activity. Costa Rica is among the countries of the world with the highest per capita pesticide use, at 2 kg per person per year.

Oral Health

The most recent national nutrition survey was conducted in 1996. That survey provided information on improvements in oral health among preschoolers and schoolchildren since the previous such survey in 1992. The DMFT (decayed, missing, and filled teeth) index in the preschool population surveyed in 1996 was 3.8, with differences according to area of residence: San José metropolitan area, 3.0; all other urban areas, 2.7; and rural areas, 4.0. Among the school-age population the DMFT prevalence was 49.9%.

RESPONSE OF THE HEALTH SECTOR

Health Policies and Plans

Costa Rica defines its health policies every four years with each administration through participatory negotiations coordinated by the Ministry of Health. The National Health Policy 2002–2006 was developed on the basis of specialized studies, including health sector analysis, performance measurement of the essential public health functions (EPHFs), and evaluations of the steering role in health. The results of these studies were then used to define four core policy areas: strengthening and consolidation of the health sector; the design of health policies based on equity, universality, access, and quality; health promotion; and environmental health and disaster preparedness. These policy areas stem from the Concerted Health Agenda, which sets out the following ten health sector commitments: 1) to strengthen interventions for maintaining or building on achievements in the areas of infant and maternal mortality, communicable diseases, and nutritional deficiencies; 2) to promote the building of a culture of health based on health promotion and the fostering of healthy lifestyles; 3) to prevent and treat noncommunicable diseases and their risk factors; 4) to promote and treat mental health in a comprehensive manner, with an emphasis on social violence; 5) to improve the equity, access, quality, and ethical nature of services, emphasizing the first level of care; 6) to improve environmental health, emphasizing basic sanitation and the comprehensive management of water resources; 7) to promote actions aimed at reducing vulnerability to disasters; 8) to strengthen the institutional framework and performance of the health sector; 9) to ensure that investment, expenditures, and financing are consistent with the values and principles that govern the sector's policies and priorities; and 10) to strengthen the National Health Surveillance System. The Concerted Health Agenda is the framework that guides the work of the sector at the national level. Likewise, each of the country's nine health regions has its own agenda that defines a framework for health action at the regional level.

Health has constitutional status and is considered a basic human right. The health system is based on the principle of universality and the entire population is entitled to the public ser-

Citizen Participation in Health

According to the National Registry of Health Promotion Organizations prepared in 2005 by the Costa Rican Social Security Fund (CCSS), the country has 3,500 active health organizations. Of this number, 143 are health boards, 681 health committees, and the remainder are patients' associations, volunteer groups, and other community-based organizations. The country also has a significant number of social networks working in the areas of domestic violence and HIV/AIDS. Over the past 10 years, the Costa Rican health sector has carried out a number of activities designed to promote increased civil society participation, particularly: community participation in the Health Insurance Regulations; the creation of health boards through the CCSS Hospital Deconcentration Law of 1998 (Law No. 7852); the opening of branch offices of the Health Services Comptroller in 95% of the country's hospitals; the preparation of a 2005 manual for health committees; and the development of strategic plans for social participation in some health regions.

vices the CCSS provides. The country has authorities both inside and outside the health sector to oversee and safeguard the citizens' exercise of this right. First among these are the IV Constitutional Court, responsible for safeguarding the exercise of constitutional rights, including the right to health; and an ombudsman's office called the "People's Defender" [Defensoría de los Habitantes], which exercises oversight on the timeliness and quality of health care. The Ministry of Health, acting through the Office of the Health Services Auditor General [Auditoría General de Servicios de Salud], which was created by law in 2002, promotes the rights and duties of health system users, both public and private. Moreover, the CCSS system includes an Office of the Health Services Comptroller within its health establishments. This office receives and processes user complaints in conjunction with health councils, which are made up of civil society representatives. The functions of the health councils include managerial oversight of health establishments and the use of budgetary resources.

Over the period 2001–2005, the deconcentration of authority and public health services from the Ministry of Health continued, as well as the deconcentration of CCSS assistance and health care services for individuals. The CSSS Hospital Deconcentration Law of 1998 accords legal autonomy to health establishments to administrate human and financial resources through management commitments, which are signed each year with the central level of the CCSS. With regard to public health, the Ministry of Health has decentralized authority for health surveillance activities based on the "Regulations Governing the Organization and Operation of the National Health Surveillance System," which establish the rules for notifying events of compulsory reporting to inter-agency health surveillance committees at the central, regional, and local levels. Moreover, the Ministry has decentralized health regulatory functions such as the accreditation of health and environmental health establishments. Technical cooperation activities have supported decentralization efforts aimed at training public employees to improve institutional capacity with re-

spect to specific oversight tasks, such as measuring performance of the EPHFs and management functions, and to measure social exclusion in health by geographic areas, ethnic groups, age, and other categories of analysis. In 2001, the health sector conducted a national study to measure the performance of the EPHFs, which was subsequently conducted in each of the nine health regions between 2003 and 2004. Corrective plans for improving the performance of specific EPHFs have yet to be developed, including essential research for implementing innovative solutions in public health, human resources development, and public health training.

According to the 2001 report on measuring the performance of the essential public health functions in Costa Rica: "Social protection in health, which is measured in terms of the population covered with health insurance provided by the Costa Rican Social Security Fund, has experienced some ups and downs over the last 5-year period. Between 2000 and 2004, the uninsured population fluctuated between 12.1% and 14.7%, and this is related to the insurance coverage levels of the economically active population, state insurance coverage, insured family members, and insured retirees."

The increase and expansion of social protection in health is the result of the different insurance mechanisms the CCSS has implemented over the years: mandatory insurance for salaried employees; voluntary, out-of-pocket insurance coverage for self-employed workers; special agreements with trade associations, such as taxi drivers and agricultural workers; agreements with different categories of retired workers; and state insurance coverage of the poor, indigent, and prison populations funded by the national treasury. Between 1975 and 1985, the population covered by these mechanisms increased from 60% to 80%. However, over the subsequent two decades—from 1985 to 2004—public insurance coverage increased by only 7%, or from 81% to 88%.

The expansion of public health insurance coverage under the CCSS is facing problems of financial sustainability. All citizens are entitled to CCSS services, but audits of the CCSS' collection system reveal problems of contribution evasion and delinquent payments. As a result, revenues entering the system tend to be less than the benefits paid out by a difference of approximately 0.2% of GDP. This situation reduces the institution's capacity to invest in equipment and supplies and hire new staff, which ultimately leads to long patient waiting lists for treatment, substandard quality care, and limitations on coverage. Moreover, this situation has given rise to some unpopular measures, such as requiring the CCSS workforce (approximately 40,000) to pay the full mandatory social insurance contribution for salaried workers (5.5% of annual income), when for many years they were only required to pay half that amount. Other measures taken to improve institutional management at the CCSS include: reducing the billing payment term (from 30 days in 2002 to 18 in 2005); payroll automation; expanding collection centers and payment systems for providers and workers; decreasing the annual provider delinquency rate (from 13.5% in 2002 to 8.5% in 2005); creation of mechanisms to capture information on new salaried workers and independent contractors; development of regulations for the incorporation of independent contractors and individuals under the voluntary insurance system; the national program for incorporating independent contractors; filing of court actions; and orders to prevent businesses from closing down when they fail to disclose information. Whether or not these measures can actually increase social protection in health and improve the quality of CCSS services can only be determined over the medium term.

Finally, the country also has other social protection mechanisms in place, such as the occupational hazard insurance fund and a mandatory driver's insurance fund. The first covers salaried workers and has provided coverage to 71% of the economically active population in recent years. The latter finances medical care and hospital services for people injured in traffic accidents, both passengers and pedestrians.

The regulation of public health and health care services are steering functions of the health sector. Consequently, the Ministry of Health is responsible for their coordination and establishes national policies which are applicable at all levels of the health system. The Ministry regulates the following three areas: health services, basic health supplies, and the environment.

The Bureau of Health Services [Dirección de Servicios de Salud] is responsible for the regulation of health services. Its regulatory activities are divided into three areas of focus, each of which includes appropriate methodologies and instruments: accreditation of health establishments; hospital accreditation; and comprehensive assessment of the primary care level. The Bureau publishes annual reports with the results of evaluations of public and private health establishments, and advancements made in comprehensive care at the primary care level.

With regard to the regulation of health supplies, the Bureau of Registration and Control defines the guidelines and procedures for the approval and registration of drugs, foodstuffs and products for human consumption, and technical equipment offered on the national market. Currently these activities are still regulated at the central level.

With regard to environmental regulation, the Bureau of Environmental Health is responsible for defining guidelines and procedures at the regional and local levels for construction, waste management, and water quality.

Health Strategies and Programs

The Concerted Health Agenda, as set out in the National Health Policy, defines the strategies of action and institutions responsible for ensuring compliance with the ten health sector commitments. Commitment 2 is concerned with the building of a culture of health based on social participation; commitment 5 with improving the equity, access, quality, and ethical nature of health care services; and commitment 9 with exercising prudence in the financing, expenditure, and investment in health. This agenda forms the technical and political cornerstone for the development of national health programs, which are promoted at the leadership levels of the Ministry of Health. Leadership in the health sector is the main government strategy for promoting the equity, quality, and coverage of health care services, and for ensuring these objectives are met. However, this leadership role has been weakened due to limitations of the Ministry of Health, such as insufficient resources and institutional capacity, although efforts to correct these problems are under way and the situation is gradually improving. Leadership of the health sector in Costa Rica is based on a series of general and specific laws and executive orders such as the General Law on Health, the Ministry of Health Act, the Public Administration Act, and executive orders regarding the organization and functions of the national health system. Upon taking office in May 2006, among the first actions of the incoming administration was the issuance of an executive order to regulate the internal operations of the Executive Branch, which established the Ministry of Health as the country's leading health authority and incorporated the health boards under the Executive Branch, which are comprised of the Minister of Health and the administrative officers of the decentralized institutions. Follow-up will be needed to decipher if these measures successfully strengthen the leadership role in health.

Organization of the Health System

The Costa Rican health system is defined as the set of health institutions, programs, and establishments whose mission is to safeguard the health of the individual, the family, and community which, by definition, also includes citizens, local governments, and intersectoral action. The Ministry of Health oversees the performance of the essential public health functions and exercises the steering role in the health sector. The CCSS is the sole public insurer of comprehensive health care services for the population; the National Insurance Institute (INS) administers mandatory insurance funds that offer protection against occupational risks and traffic accidents. The INS also offers voluntary insurance plans for health care (INS-Salud) and accident liability coverage, through private health care providers and its own facilities. The Costa Rican Institute of Water and Sewerage Systems (AyA) regulates the supply of water for human consumption and wastewater management. The Costa Rican Institute for Research and Education in Health and Nutrition (INCIENSA) performs the functions of a national public health reference laboratory. The Costa Rican Institute on Alcoholism and Drug Dependency (IAFA) administers programs for the prevention and care of addictions. The Costa Rican Cancer Institute (ICCC) was created to develop human resources, promote research, and coordinate the national cancer program. The University of Costa Rica and municipal governments were incorporated into the health sector by a 1989 executive order. The Ministry of Health is part of the Executive Branch, whereas the CCSS, INS, and AyA are all autonomous agencies governed by a board of directors. Each of these autonomous agencies was created through specific laws which provide them with their own resources.

As part of the reform of the health sector during the period 2002–2006, the Ministry of National Planning and Economic Policy approved the structural reorganization of the Ministry of Health with a view to continue efforts to modernize and strengthen its steering role. This reorganization included the creation of several new units to enhance the performance of specific steering functions in health that were performing below expectations, such as expenditures and financing, research and technological development, and public health insurance.

The health sector reform effectively transferred responsibility for service delivery and financing—which were formerly exercised under the leadership role of the Ministry of Health—from the Ministry to the CCSS, where they are administered in accordance with local legislation. However, the Ministry is still responsible for assistance programs such as the program to educate and feed poor children under 7 years of age and the vector control program, the latter of which is currently under study by authorities at the nine health regions to determine whether or not it should be transferred to other agencies.

The Health Sector Council decides the major issues involving the health system. Its members are the incumbent authorities of each of the aforementioned institutions. However, the Council meets sporadically at best, due to a lack of political will on the part of its members. Despite this limitation, the Council has proven useful with respect to coordinating sectoral actions, including national vaccination campaigns and emergency and disaster relief in areas of the country prone to these events, and, more recently, has developed a National Pandemic Influenza Plan.

Public Health Services

Primary care is the responsibility of Basic Comprehensive Health Care Teams (EBAIS). Each team is comprised of a general physician, an auxiliary nurse, and a primary health care technician. Costa Rica has 893 EBAIS teams, each of which administers care to approximately 4,000 people. National EBAIS coverage is on the order of 90%, which means additional EBAIS teams are still needed to ensure full coverage of the population.

Each health area is supported by a certain number of EBAIS teams. Some teams are not CCSS employees, but workers of cooperative organizations and programs whose services are funded by the CCSS under previously negotiated management commitments. In addition to providing health care to the population in their assigned areas, EBAIS teams also perform field work in health promotion and disease prevention, which is not fully successful due to a lack of community work. Since 2005, all the health areas have signed annual management commitments. During the negotiation phase, prior to signing the commitment and budget approval, each health area is required to submit a situational analysis of the area under its control. This analysis includes the plans and proposed levels of coverage to be carried out over the course of the year.

Health care services for the population are based on a primary care strategy and provided through health promotion and disease prevention programs. These includes programs in the areas of nutrition, early stimulation techniques, immunization, vector control, food fortification, basic sanitation, water supply, solid waste disposal, recreation and sports, and social communication in health. Different agencies of the health sector are responsible for administering these programs. However, the Ministry of Health is responsible for sectoral coordination and supervision of such programs. Social networks, organized community groups, volunteer community health agents, nongovernmental organizations, and local governments are also involved in the planning, implementation, and evaluation of these programs, although their role is limited.

During the period 2005–2006, the Bureau of Health Surveillance was reorganized and the new Health Situation Analysis Unit was created to supplement the Bureau's existing Epidemiological Surveillance and Health Statistics units. This brought about a change in the distribution of work within the Bureau and among its units. In addition, the Bureau of Health Surveillance was assigned responsibility for issues related to pharmacovigilance, the indigenous populations, and migrants. The Ministry of Health coordinated two health sector analyses for the periods 1998–2002 and 2002–2006, which served as a basis for formulating national health policies and the Concerted Health Agenda 2002–2006. During this process, the Bureau of Health Surveillance played a pivotal role in terms of identifying the limitations of information: a lack of organized, up-to-date, and uniform intersectoral and inter-agency databases; deficient mapping for data management; and specific situations lacking sufficient risk analysis. The primary deficiencies observed in the data included underreporting in the notification system for various health situations, improper completion of death certificates, and improper completion of event notification reports. The public health laboratory network is operated by the Costa Rican Institute of Research and Education in Health (INCIENSA), which comprises 85 laboratories and a national reference center. This center is in the last stages of a reorganization which will result in a national network of reference centers and may eventually include a national health institute.

Water pollution, improper management of solid waste, and air pollution are persistent problems in urban areas of the country. The highest levels of pollutants are traditionally observed in the Grande de Tárcoles River Basin of the central valley, which is the most populated area of the country. Moreover, the waters from the basin flow into and pollute the Gulf of Nicoya.

Only 25% of the population is covered with sewage disposal via sanitary sewerage lines and only an estimated 2.4% is covered by functioning sewer systems and wastewater treatment plants. Seventy percent of wastewater is released untreated into the Virillas and Reventazón rivers. Approximately 70% of the population has septic tanks, but many are improperly designed and/or installed without the benefit of instructions on their use and maintenance, and, hence, pose the risk of contaminating aquifers. In spite of progress made in terms of sanitary landfills, only 42% of municipalities use them appropriately. More controls are needed to ensure compliance with existing standards, as well as new regulations governing the use of hazardous compounds. Volatile organic compounds have been detected in wells and increasing nitrate levels are being discovered in wells and springs of the San José metropolitan area, posing a very significant threat to the aquifers of the northeastern part of the central valley.

According to 2005 water access and quality data of the Costa Rican Institute of Water and Sewerage Systems (AyA), there are 2,206 aqueducts that supply 93.4% of the population's water; another 4% either have easy access to water or are supplied by developers or other collective organizations. AyA supplies 46% of the population with 176 aqueducts; the municipalities 18% with 243 aqueducts; the Heredia Public Utility Company (ESPH) 4.7% with 13 aqueducts; and rural associations and committees 24.7% with 1,774 aqueducts. Approximately 18% of the population is supplied with non-potable water. In terms of the population served by systems operated by the AyA, the ESHP, the municipalities, and rural organizations, 1%, 0%, 30%, and 35%, respectively, are supplied with non-potable water. Although disinfected water is distributed by all water systems serving areas with more than 50,000 inhabitants, disinfected water is only distributed by 35% and 10% of systems serving areas with 500–2,500 inhabitants and less than 500 inhabitants, respectively.

In order to close the current gaps in access to sanitary sewerage systems with sufficient treatment of wastewater in the San José metropolitan area, AyA has projects under way that include the rehabilitation and expansion of collection sewers and sewer networks, and the construction of wastewater and sludge treatment plants with sanitary disposal of waste. The first phase of the project will provide 65% coverage (1 million inhabitants), and has financing of US$ 230 million. The second phase will provide 85% coverage (1.6 million inhabitants).

Sanitary landfill permits are issued by the Ministry of Health, in coordination with the Ministry of the Environment's Technical Secretariat for the Environment (SETENA), which is supported with advisory services from the Municipal Development Authority (IFAM). The Office of the Controller General of the Republic reviews the budgets of municipal landfill service providers in each canton, either directly or through contract operators. There has been no comprehensive management of landfills, and with only a few but promising exceptions, no waste reduction, reuse, or recycling initiatives either. The amount of refuse generated per capita in the greater San José metropolitan area has doubled over the last 20 years.

With regard to the prevention and control of air pollution, a study of 100,000 emissions samples from gasoline-operated vehicles subjected to technical review showed that traffic emissions from this source have been successfully reduced by 47%. However, this is of little consequence considering the rapidly growing number of motor vehicles and percentage of used vehicles on the road. Over the period 1994–2004 vehicle traffic increased by an average of 8.3% and fiscal policies favor the entry and continued use of used vehicles. High fuel costs have encouraged the use of diesel-powered vehicles whose emissions contain greater levels of particulate matter and sulfurous oxides than gas engines. With regard to the Ministry of Health's "Clean Air" project, the health costs of air pollution in the greater San José metropolitan area are estimated to be US$ 280 million. The study indicates that 78% of the population in the San José metropolitan area is exposed to PM-10 particulate levels in excess of 60 $\mu g/m^3$.

The Food and Nutritional Safety (SAN) strategy has been deployed in marginal municipalities since 2000, with a view to enhancing the comprehensive development of low-income families through support in the form of projects designed to boost food production and income. By 2005, 19 priority cantons had SAN councils with operating plans and a portfolio of food production projects, administered by local organizations and institutions. At the national level, the SAN strategy is managed by the ministries of Health, Agriculture and Livestock, Economy, and Commerce, in conjunction with the Food and Nutrition Policy Secretariat (SEPAN). The country also has a national food policy and an intersectoral food and nutrition plan.

With respect to disaster preparedness, the Ministry of Health's Risk Management and Ionizing Radiation Control Unit was created through Ministerial Decision No. 129 of 2005, which exercises health sector leadership in this area. In 2005, the CCSS Emergency Command Center was established and a fire engineering unit was added, with a view to strengthening teamwork and organization among the different institutions of the health sector. Among the Ministry of Health's main challenges are the development of a comprehensive health plan for disasters and the strengthening of management at the regional and local levels. Currently, several isolated efforts and shortcomings have been identified toward the implementation of coherent and sustainable strategies for disaster alleviation and prevention aimed at the hospital level. The loss of a wing of the Calderón Guardia Hospital complex due to a fire should serve as a "wakeup call" in terms of the need for establishing a hospital safety plan, managed as a core element of design, standards, and implementation, in order to ensure that the hospital network can adequately respond to such events.

Costa Rica has continued to bolster its response capacity to new diseases (emerging and reemerging), and specifically the threat of pandemic influenza. These efforts have included an expansion of intensive surveillance at 12 sentinel sites located throughout the country, with emphasis on border areas and ports. The country has carried out annual vaccination campaigns against seasonal influenza in which an estimated 250,000 doses of flu vaccines were given to risk groups, created the National Influenza Commission, and work is under way on a National Pandemic Influenza Plan.

Individual Care Services

The CCSS is responsible for public health care services for individuals. The CCSS organizes and operates these services according to two types of criteria. In the case of the first, the complexity of infrastructure, equipment, and costs are organized and operated as a network of layered services at the primary, secondary, and tertiary levels of care. The second is based on the seriousness of the condition to be treated, according to which services are organized as either outpatient or hospital services. Both criteria complement each other, but their differences prove useful in terms of allocating resources and organizing the flow of patients through referral and counterreferral mechanisms, as well as for operating a model of comprehensive care. It bears mentioning that the model of care determines the extent of the services to be provided to the population in the tri-level care network. Moreover, the current care model was the result of the reorganization carried out as part of the health sector reform. Services are grouped into five program care categories—children, adolescents, women, adults, and older adults—each of which includes a predetermined portfolio of services.

As mentioned previously, the service model and network are oriented to the primary level of care, under the supervision of the Basic Comprehensive Health Care Teams (EBAIS), which operate out of small establishments located among the population. EBAIS teams are assigned to health areas, and each health area has a central clinic that includes resources such as x-ray equip-

ment and a laboratory to aid in the diagnosis and treatment of patients. The central clinics are staffed with a multidisciplinary health team to support the work of the EBAIS teams. In areas of the country with insufficient CCSS infrastructure, these services are provided by external public (University of Costa Rica, since 1999), private (Costa Rican Medical Services Association or ASEMECO, since 2002), or self-managed cooperative (Pavas, Tibás, and Santa Ana, since 1989) providers. The CCSS contracts with these external providers though special agreements under a per-capita cost arrangement. In turn, these providers offer the same services and insurance coverage as the CCSS and cover 10% of the country's population. The country's 104 health areas—which include those operated by the CCSS and external contractors—negotiate their operating budgets each year with the central level of the CCSS, after submitting a situational analysis of the population under their control, which includes the plans and proposed levels of coverage to be carried out over the course of the year. Each team receives its budget by means of a management commitment. At the end of the contract year, the teams' results are evaluated and form the basis for the next year's budget negotiations. Evaluations of these management commitments reveal differences in the form of disparities, both in terms of the coverage and quality of health care services by age groups and health regions. To cite examples, this has been observed in programs of cervicouterine cancer screening through the Papanicolaou or Pap test, and in the vaccination coverage of children under 5 years of age. In general, Pap test coverage is low in comparison to vaccination coverage, and the Huetar Atlántica and Brunca regions have the lowest coverage levels of all regions.

The secondary level of care offers specialized outpatient consultations, hospitalization, and medical-surgical treatment in the core areas of internal medicine, pediatrics, gynecology-obstetrics, and surgery, through a network of ten health centers, 13 peripheral hospitals, and seven regional hospitals. The tertiary level provides high-tech medical and surgical services in three national general hospitals (México, San Juan de Díos, and Calderón Guardia hospitals) and five specialized hospitals (women's, children's, geriatric, psychiatric, and rehabilitation). Due to insufficient investment in hospital infrastructure during the 1980s and 1990s, the supply of some services such as radiation therapy, ophthalmology, and pathology was gradually eclipsed by demand. As a result, there have been long waiting lists for care and user complaints. To alleviate these problems, the sector contracted with private hospitals and providers to close the gap in the demand for these services. However, this measure has proven to be insufficient considering that by early 2005, the number of patients on the waiting list had grown to 14,000. Moreover on a variety of occasions, the quality of contracted care services, the transparency of contracting mechanisms, and the prices agreed for private services have been called into question by civil society, the Office of the People's Defender, and state agencies, such as the Office of the Controller General of the Republic.

In short, access to the care system should be through the primary level of care. However, in the event of medical or surgical emergencies, patients may go to any hospital or clinic offering these services in the nine health regions. Where the seriousness of a condition so warrants, patients are referred from the primary level to a unit of the secondary level of care or to third-level hospitals. Once patients receive care in the hospital network, they are counterreferred to the primary level of care for control and follow-up by EBAIS teams. Shortcomings in the referral and counterreferral system have resulted in long waiting lists for treatment, and this is especially true for oncology procedures, some surgeries, and specialized studies. Comprehensive care provided in the CCSS system is supplemented with other services such as the Ophthalmology Clinic, the Center for Pain and Palliative Care, the Center for the Early Detection and Treatment of Gastric Cancer, the Laboratory of Human Molecular Genetics ("Responsible Paternity"), the National Cytology Laboratory, and the National Blood Bank, among others.

Health Promotion

According to the National Registry of Health Promotion Organizations created by the CCSS in 2005, the country has 3,500 active health organizations. Of this number, 143 are health boards, 681 health committees, and the remainder patients' associations, volunteer groups, and other community-based organizations. The country also has a significant number of social networks working in the areas of domestic violence and HIV/AIDS.

Over the past ten years, the Costa Rican health sector has carried out a number of activities designed to promote increased civil society participation. These include: community participation in the Health Insurance Regulations; the creation of health boards through the CSSS Hospital Deconcentration Law of 1998 (Law No. 7852); the opening of branch offices of the Health Services Comptroller in 95% of the country's hospitals; the preparation of a 2005 manual for health committees; the development of strategic plans for social participation in some health regions; Law No. 8239 regarding user rights and duties of public and private health services; implementation of initiatives such as the Healthy and Ecological Cantons Network; the Network of Health-Promoting Schools; the Healthy Dwellings Network; the Ecological Blue Flag program; and canton food security boards.

Moreover, the nationwide performance measurement studies of the essential functions of public health (EPHFs) conducted by the Ministry of Health in 2001 and in 2004–2005, revealed some strengths in function 4, "health participation," such as the existence of formal citizen participation processes at the national and local levels, and information strategies for users on their health rights. However, they also revealed weaknesses with respect to the lack of strategies, actions, or processes to foster participation, as well as in the monitoring and evaluation of actions.

The foregoing involve some challenges, such as drafting institutional guidelines for carrying out and monitoring local strategic planning, based on an intersectoral approach, and establishing institutional and inter-institutional mechanisms (CCSS-Ministry of Health) for conducting and coordinating ongoing social participation in health, in coordination with the existing social network. It is important to note that social participation and citizenship in health have been gaining momentum on the agendas of political and technical levels as a key mechanism of accountability and the social production of health.

Human Resources

The 2001 document on the evaluation of the essential public health functions as well as other studies underscore the problems of maintaining up-to-date information on the situation of the country's human resources in health. In this regard, the country's 2002 health sector analysis points out that one problem with human resources information is the "scattered, fragmented, and 'non-interrelated' nature of the available information," and that it is therefore "crucial to strengthen all human resources information systems of the sector's institutions," arguing that doing so would "generate new data for use in strategic planning of human resources development," and would also facilitate "the development of institutional capacity for human resources management." Moreover, the National Health Policy 2002–2006 defines as strategies for developing human resources policies "the development of human resources information systems for each health sector employer that would likewise be integrated into a sector-wide human resources system," and the "development of an information system that would integrate educational centers in health with those of the sector's employers."

Information on the country's health professionals is available from the databases of the 2000 census, health sector employers, professional associations, and educational institutions. Based on data from the 2000 census, the ratio of physicians, nurses, and dentists per 10,000 population is 13.6, 8.9, and 3.8, respectively. According to 2005 data provided by the country's professional associations, these ratios were 20.0 physicians per 10,000 population (8,500), 15.3 for nurses (6,537), and 6.5 for dentists (2,800).

With regard to human resources, disparities are observed both in the distribution of these resources—and consequently, there is no specific information on the needs of heath sector employers—and in their management (hiring, salaries, incentives, and access to the human resources decision-making bodies). In terms of employment, the health reforms and structural adjustments carried out in the country over the period 1986–2004 have led to a decrease in the number of health professionals employed by the Ministry of Health. In contrast, the staff of the CCSS has nearly doubled in the last 15 years, reflecting the health system's commitment to providing the population with health services. The number of health science educational institutions has grown over the past 15 years. By 2005, the country had 17 schools of psychology, eight of medicine, eight of nursing, five of dentistry, five of pharmacy, three of nutrition, two of social work, two of veterinary science, and one of microbiology. In addition to the fragmented nature of information on human resources in health, other problems have been identified, such as educational curricula that lack adequate emphasis on the primary level of care; the persistence of a biological rather than holistic approach to care that promotes the development of biologically driven human resource competencies, instead of those that respond to the needs of the country's social profile; as well as a lack of definition governing the required skills of each category of health professionals. To address the problems identified in human resources for health, the Technical Commission for the Development of Human Resources in Health was created through Presidential Decree No. 32209-5 of 2005, which incorporated the University of Costa Rica into the sector.

Health Supplies

Costa Rica does not have a policy in place to regulate the cost of drugs. Consequently, prices are determined by supply and demand. The health system is permitted access to drugs through the social security system, although such access is a slow process. Policies have been enacted to improve access in the private sector, which has resulted in greater competition and a liberalization of the pharmaceuticals market. The current drug registration and control policy has developed in a satisfactory manner and is responsive to the needs of the population. However, a more aggressive strategy of pharmacovigilance is needed. The country does not have a national institutional policy regarding biomedical supplies and equipment. The Ministry of Health is currently working to develop regulations to govern the importation, control, and registry of biomedical equipment and supplies.

Research and Technological Development in Health

In 2004, the Ministry of Health initiated a process to strengthen research and technological development in health. One outcome of this process was the creation of the Bureau of Research and Technological Development in Health (2005), with a view to leading, monitoring, and strengthening initiatives to create the knowledge base among the different groups involved in the research, promotion, and evaluation of technology, in order to satisfy priority needs in the health field, in compliance with its steering role in the public and private sectors. Accordingly, the Ministry of Health defines the National Agenda of Health Research by preparing, reviewing, and updating standards and procedures; developing techniques and instruments for health re-

search; exercising the leading role in scientific and technological research in health, in coordination with the pertinent social actors; establishing research networks in specialized areas to facilitate the sharing of information, services, opportunities, and contacts; developing and maintaining an information system on technological research and innovations in health, which makes it possible to monitor developments and update the work of the sector in this area; and establishing networks of scientific ethics committees, accredited by the National Council on Health Research, which are governed by processes of standardization and accreditation, with systems to control, monitor, and evaluate compliance with the principles of ethical and scientific research mandated by national legislation, among other functions. The National Agenda of Research and Technological Development in Health 2005–2010 was approved in 2005, and a registry was compiled of the research projects carried out in this field during the period 2000–2005.

Health Sector Expenditures and Financing

In 2000, the country's expenditures on health were 5.2% of GNP. Over the last three years, this figure has remained relatively unchanged at 5.7% of GDP. While no specific data is available detailing the private sector health expenditure, it is thought to be increasing and estimated at approximately 2.5% of GDP. The 2000 per capita expenditure in health was US$ 209, which increased to US$ 234 in 2004; nevertheless, the impact of inflation must be factored in with a view to evaluating the change in purchasing power. Health sector spending as a percentage of domestic production increased from 4.0% in 2000 to 4.5% in 2005.

With regard to public health expenditures, in 2004 the CCSS accounted for approximately 82.7% of health sector expenditures, which is slightly higher than the 80.3% registered in 2000. This is the result of policies designed to expand services, acquire more equipment, and build new facilities at the different levels of care. Expenditures of the Ministry of Health also increased from 6.1% in 2000 to 7.1% in 2004. The percentage of health sector expenditures attributable to the Costa Rican Institute of Water and Sewerage Systems decreased from 8.2% in 2000 to 7.3% in 2004. Health sector expenditures of the Costa Rican Cancer Institute accounted for 0.1% of GDP in 2004.

Upon analyzing CCSS expenditures by level of care, spending for outpatient care services increased from 32% in 2001 to 35% in 2005. In contrast, spending for hospital services decreased from 50.6% in 2001 to 46.2% in 2005, which is in keeping with policies designed to strengthen the primary level of care. It bears mentioning that institutional expenditures for research and development accounted for 1.5% of total sector expenditures in 2005.

As a result of the country's epidemiological transition and decisions of the IV Constitutional Court ordering the CCSS to purchase additional health supplies, CCSS institutional expenditures

TABLE 3. External cooperation, non-reimbursable and reimbursable, Costa Rica, 2002–2004.

Type of cooperation	2002 Total[a]	%	2003 Total[a]	%	2004 Total[a]	%	2002–2004 Total[a]	%
Non-reimbursable	41.1	4.9	89.3	10.7	62.8	7.6	193.2	23.2
Reimbursable	148.3	17.8	487.4	58.6	3.2	0.4	638.9	76.8
Total[a]	189.4	22.7	576.7	69.3	66	8	832.1	100

[a]In US$ millions.

Source: Costa Rica, Universidad para la Cooperación Internacional; Ministerio de Planificación Nacional y Política Económica, 2006.

TABLE 4. Approved international cooperation, by year and type, Costa Rica, 2002–2004.

Year	Bilateral cooperation (in US$ millions)	Multilateral cooperation (in US$ millions)	Total (in US$ millions)
2002	25.3	164.0	189.3
2003	115.7	461.1	576.8
2004	52.1	13.9	66.0
Total	193.1	639.0	832.1
%	23.2	76.8	100.0

Source: Costa Rica, Universidad para la Cooperación Internacional; Ministerio de Planificación Nacional y Política Económica, 2006.

TABLE 5. Approved international cooperation, by sector, Costa Rica, 2002–2004.

Cooperation by sector	Amount (in US$ millions)	%
Environment, energy, and telecommunications	378.9	45.5
Economy and finance	103.8	12.5
Foreign trade	87.2	10.5
Public works and transport	79.2	9.5
Local development	28.7	3.4
Health	27.3	3.3
Agriculture and fisheries	25.2	3.0
Housing and urban development	23.9	2.9
Tourism	15.3	1.8
Science and technology	12.5	1.5
Education	11.6	1.4
Others (culture, security)	38.5	4.6
Total	832.1	100.0

Source: Costa Rica, Universidad para la Cooperación Internacional; Ministerio de Planificación Nacional y Política Económica, 2006.

for drugs have increased in recent years, rising from 7.5% of total health sector expenditures in 2001 to 8.6% in 2005.

With respect to sector financing, workers' social security premiums accounted for approximately 83% of total income in 2001, which decreased to 79% in 2004. In 2004, the total income of the CCSS accounted for 4.5% of GDP, whereas its total expenditures accounted for 4.7%, which underscores the financial weakness of public health insurance.

Technical Cooperation and External Financing

Between 2002 and 2004, external technical cooperation amounted to US$ 832.1 million (Table 3). Of this amount, only 23.2% was for non-reimbursable technical cooperation. The percentage of external resources was highest in 2003, for a total of US$ 576.7 million (69.3% of the total during this period).

Bilateral technical cooperation for Costa Rica in the period 2002–2004 was 23.2% (US$ 193.2 million), while loans from multilateral organizations accounted for 76.8% (US$ 638.9 million). During this period, international cooperation for the health sector was US$ 27.3 million, which accounted for 3.3% of total technical cooperation and ranked sixth among favored sectors (Tables 4 and 5).

The available information does not facilitate the breakdown of health sector data by origin of funding or type of cooperation. The multilateral and bilateral sources of technical cooperation to the sector include the Japan International Cooperation Agency, the Japan Bank for International Cooperation, the World Bank, the

Inter-American Development Bank, the Organization of American States, the Pan American Health Organization/World Health Organization, the Government of South Korea, the Government of the Netherlands, the European Union, the Regional Coordinating Committee of Potable Water and Sanitation Institutions of Central America, Panama, and the Dominican Republic, the Norwegian Agency for Development and Cooperation, the Central American Bank for Economic Integration, and the International Regional Committee for Plant and Animal Health. The primary work areas of projects financed by these cooperation agencies are: strengthening and modernization of the health sector; strengthening of the steering role of the Ministry of Health; strengthening of the country's response to HIV/AIDS; air quality improvement; control of environmental pollution; creation, expansion, and/or maintenance of hospital infrastructure and equipment; incorporation of the bio-psychosocial model in the National Rehabilitation Center (CENARE); accreditation of academic fields and teacher training; strengthening of the first level of care; improving gastric cancer early detection and care; access to potable water in urban centers; and the rehabilitation of health infrastructure in rural communities. In addition, training of health sector personnel with technical cooperation assistance facilitates new knowledge for applications in specialized health areas and the management of social projects. Based on the trend observed since the 1990s, Costa Rica is increasingly receiving less preference for technical cooperation than other countries of Central America.

Bibliography

Alfaro A, Pizarro D, Navas L, Kivers G, Penniecook T, Pérez E. La organización y efectividad de una unidad especial de atención de dengue del área de salud de Limón, Costa Rica, 1999. Memorias de la Academia Nacional de Ciencias (Costa Rica). 2001;7(El Dengue):11–21.

Caja Costarricense de Seguro Social. Egresos hospitalarios, 1990, 1995 y 2000.

Castañeda A, Gómez X, Montiel H. Desarrollo y salud de los pueblos indígenas en Costa Rica, 2003.

Costa Rica, Ministerio de Salud; Caja Costarricense de Seguro Social; Instituto Costarricense de Investigación y Enseñanza en Nutrición y Salud. Informe de país: Costa Rica. Reunión del Grupo Técnico Asesor (TAG), noviembre 2002.

Costa Rica, Ministerio de Salud. Informe de vigilancia de la salud. Foro Nacional de Salud: Hacia la construcción colectiva de la salud. Costa Rica, 1998.

Costa Rica, Ministerio de Salud. Medición del desempeño de las funciones esenciales de salud pública en Costa Rica. San José; 2001.

Costa Rica, Ministerio de Salud. Medición del desempeño de las funciones esenciales de salud pública en el nivel regional en Costa Rica 2004–2005. San José; 2005.

Costa Rica, Ministerio de Salud; Organización Panamericana de la Salud. Análisis sectorial de salud Costa Rica, 2002 y 2006.

Costa Rica, Ministerio de Salud; Organización Panamericana de la Salud. Situación de salud en Costa Rica. Indicadores básicos 2005. Washington, DC: OPS; 2005.

Costa Rica, Ministerio de Salud. Política Nacional de Salud 2002–2006. San José: Ministerio de Salud; marzo 2003.

Fondo de las Naciones Unidas para la Infancia. Estado de los derechos de la niñez y la adolescencia en Costa Rica. Primera edición. San José: UNICEF; 2002.

Mendieta A, Holst B, Montiel H. La discapacidad en Costa Rica: situación actual y perspectivas, febrero 2004.

Montiel H. Desigualdades de salud en Costa Rica: una aproximación geográfico-poblacional, 2004.

Morales A, Acuña G, Gómez X, Montiel H. Migración y salud en Costa Rica: elementos para su análisis, julio 2003.

Morice A, Carvajal X, León M, Machado V, Badilla X, Reef S, et al. Accelerated rubella control and CRS prevention strengthens measles eradication: the Costa Rican experience. J Infect Dis. 2003; 187:S158–63.

Morice A, Navas L, Carranza M. Impacto de la vacunación contra *Haemophilus influenza b* en Costa Rica. Documento técnico.

Sánchez V. Estudio descriptivo del dengue en la Gran Puntarenas, cantón central de Puntarenas 1993–2000. [Tesis de grado]. Costa Rica, 2001. Documento inédito.

Soto-Vásquez ML, Rivera E, Faingenzicht I. Impact of *Haemophilus influenzae* type b (Hib) conjugate vaccine in decreasing the incidence of Hib bacterial meningitis in Costa Rica. Presentado en el Congreso de Pediatría.

Trejos SM. Factores de riesgo materno para sífilis congénita: un estudio de casos y controles en Costa Rica, 1995–1997. Memorias del VII Congreso Nacional de Salud Pública, septiembre 2000.

Villalobos de Chacón, I. Epidemiología del dengue en Venezuela. Memorias de la Academia Nacional de Ciencia, Vol. 7; 2001.

CUBA

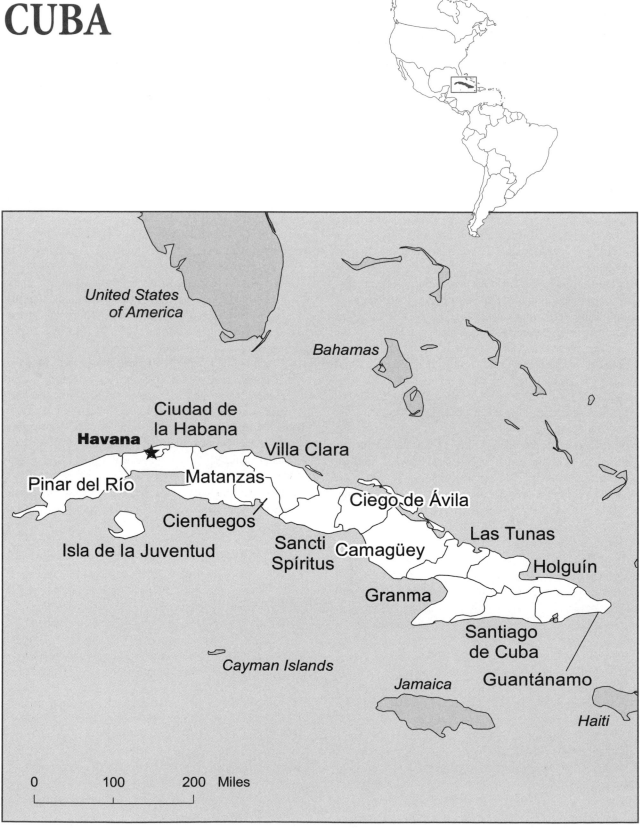

United States
of America

Bahamas

Ciudad de
la Habana

Havana

Villa Clara

Pinar del Río

Matanzas

Ciego de Ávila

Cienfuegos

Las Tunas

Isla de la Juventud

Sancti
Spíritus

Camagüey

Holguín

Granma

Santiago
de Cuba

Cayman Islands

Guantánamo

Jamaica

Haiti

0   100   200   Miles

The Republic of Cuba is an archipelago consisting of two major islands—Isla de Cuba and Isla de la Juventud—and some 1,600 islets and keys. It covers a total area of 110,860 km² and lies at the entrance to the Gulf of Mexico, in the Caribbean Sea. It is divided into 14 provinces and the special municipality of Isla de la Juventud.

GENERAL CONTEXT AND HEALTH DETERMINANTS

Social, Political, and Economic Determinants

Cuba's economic reform process is a different, unique experience for Latin America, geared to protecting the country's social progress and advancing its economic and social development based on the efficient and effective use of available resources. Despite financial hardships, it has managed to sustain its social achievements. Utilization of an applied fee system in the health, education, culture, and sports sectors has helped improve computations of value added by these services in GDP. The country's GDP grew at an average annual rate of 5.1% during the 2000–2005 period. Growth in GDP per capita averaged 5% a year, with very little change in the population dynamics. More than 60% of current budgeted expenditures were earmarked specifically for health, education, social security, and social welfare activities. Cuba has faced a number of adversities such as hurricanes and droughts; the stepping up of the blockade, with a cumulative commercial and financial cost of over US$ 82 billion; and an increase in the average price of oil from US$ 25.90 a barrel in 2001 to US$ 56.50 in 2005. The U.S. Government embargo has affected the national health care system by creating shortages of drugs, equipment, and other supplies.

The agricultural sector has been hard hit by adverse climatic factors. The drought and the 8 devastating hurricanes directly or indirectly affecting the island over the 2001–2005 period resulted in losses totaling US$ 7.8 billion. Key economic activities such as exports; social, personal, and community services; construction; and freight shipping have recovered in the last few years.

The revival of the tourism industry brought 2.3 million tourists to Cuba in 2005, a 35.3% increase over 2000. Its foreign exchange earnings from tourism rose over the course of this same period.

Socioeconomic reforms have turned around unemployment rates in the last few years, bringing unemployment down from 5.4% in 2000 to 1.9% by 2005. The average monthly wage in government and semi-public agencies and enterprises nationwide was 328 pesos in 2005, up 40% from 2000. The Government has managed to control liquidity at levels considered appropriate in light of the country's current economic situation. The budget deficit as a share of GDP has been held at acceptable levels. The State budget covered the implementation of budgeted activities throughout this period.

The country's limited access to external financing contributed to the slow growth of the economy. Despite this constraint, important payment obligations were met, enabling the country to gradually reduce its external debt and take on new loans, stepping up investment and trade. There are still unmet demands in the areas of new home construction and housing repairs, passenger transportation, and supplies of certain types of foods and clothing.

Demographics, Mortality, and Morbidity

The low rate of population growth over the past few years is attributable to trends and changes in the dynamics of population movement (fertility, mortality, and migration), which are closely correlated with socioeconomic development. As of 30 June 2005, the country's total population was estimated at 11,257,105, with 75.8% living in urban areas. The decline in the number of births over the last 15 years steepened in 2004 and 2005. The crude birth rate fell from 12.4 to 10.7 births per 1,000 population between 2001 and 2005. During that same period, the average annual rate of population growth fell from 2.0 to 0.2 per 1,000 population and the general fertility rate decreased from 45.7 to 39.9 births per 1,000 women aged 15 to 49. The plotting of age-specific fertility rates for 2005 by five-year age groups forms a curve with a plateau-shaped top. A comparison of this curve with the curve for 1990 shows fertility rates for younger age groups on the decline and fertility rates for older age groups on the rise (Figure 1).

The size of the population aged 60 and older has been steadily growing as a result of low mortality rates and improvements in life expectancy. The over 60 age group made up 15.4% of the total population in 2005 (Figure 2).

The crude death rate was 7.5 deaths per 1,000 population in 2005, and the risk of death, according to the age-standardized mortality rate, was 4.8 per 1,000 population, or 4% lower than in 2001. Mortality rates were higher in the central and western regions of the country, with the Havana City province showing the highest rate, at 9.0 per 1,000 population, followed by Villa Clara (8.6), with both figures being above the national average. The sex-specific mortality rate was slightly higher for males (54.1%)

FIGURE 1. Fertility rate, by mother's age, Cuba, 1990 and 2005.

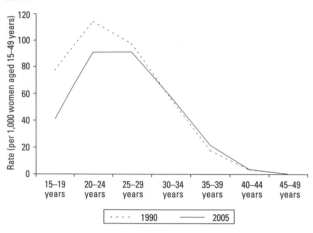

than for females. Life expectancy for the 2001–2003 period was 77.0 (75.13 for males and 78.97 for females).

The country has attained three of the Millennium Development Goals, namely Goal 2 ("ensure that all boys and girls complete a full course of primary schooling"); Goal 3 ("eliminate gender disparity in primary and secondary education, preferably by 2005, and at all levels by 2015"); and Goal 4 ("reduce by two-thirds the mortality rate among children under 5").

Infectious diseases accounted for 1.1% of all deaths in 2005. Diseases of the circulatory system were the top cause of death, with a rate of 306 deaths per 100,000 population in 2005 (Table 1). Age-adjusted rates for all causes of death, with the exception of neoplasms, decreased between 2001 and 2005. The 5–14-year-old

FIGURE 2. Population distribution, by age and sex, Cuba, 2005.

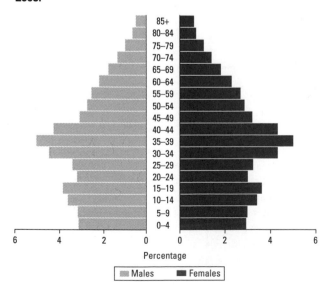

age group had the lowest age-specific mortality rate, and the population aged 65 and older had the highest rate.

The leading causes of death in Cuba are chronic noncommunicable diseases, which accounted for more than 90% of deaths between 2001 and 2005. These diseases and, to a lesser extent, violent deaths (accidents in particular) have emerged as new development problems with a growing impact, requiring new approaches to their prevention and control.

Heart disease, malignant neoplasms, and cerebrovascular diseases are the top three causes of death across all age groups and, together, account for more than half of all deaths (58.9%) (Table 2). The risk of death from malignant neoplasms increased by 12.4% between 2001 and 2005, while mortality rates for accidents; diseases of the arteries, arterioles, and capillaries; and intentional self-harm declined. A look at age-adjusted mortality rates for the leading causes of death shows an across-the-board decline in rates for all causes of death with the exception of malignant neoplasms, diabetes mellitus, and cirrhosis (Figure 3). Causes of death were coded according to the WHO International Statistical Classification of Diseases and Related Health Problems, 10th Revision (ICD-10).

Sex-specific mortality rates for all causes of death except cerebrovascular diseases (0.9) and diabetes mellitus (0.5) were higher for males than for females. Malignant neoplasms, heart disease, and accidents accounted for the largest number of years of potential life lost in 2005, with 16.6, 11.2, and 7.1 years, respectively, per 1,000 population aged 1–74 (Figure 4).

HEALTH OF POPULATION GROUPS

Children under 5 Years Old

There has been a steady decline in infant mortality, which stood at 6.2 per 1,000 live births in 2005, accounting for 0.9% of all deaths across all age groups. The neonatal mortality rate decreased from 3.9 per 1,000 live births in 2001 to 3.4 in 2005, with no change in the postneonatal mortality rate during this period. Regional disparities in infant mortality rates are narrowing. Together, the five leading causes of death in children under 1 year of age in 2005 accounted for 76.5% of all deaths in this age group. The highest risk of death was associated with certain conditions originating in the perinatal period, with a rate of 2.5 per 1,000 live births, followed by congenital malformations (1.6 per 1,000 live births), influenza and pneumonia (0.3), sepsis (0.2), and heart disease (0.2). The share of children with low birthweight dropped from 5.9% to 5.4% between 2001 and 2005.

The mortality rate for all causes of death among children ages 1–4 was 0.4 per 1,000. The top five causes of death in this age group were accidents, congenital malformations, malignant neoplasms, influenza and pneumonia, and bacterial meningitis (Table 3).

Deaths of children under the age of 5 accounted for 1.1% of all deaths in 2005, with a mortality rate of 8.0 deaths per 1,000 live births. The survival rate for children in this age group was 99.2%.

TABLE 1. Mortality by broad groups of causes (rate per 100,000 population), by age, Cuba, 2001 and 2005.

Broad group of causes	Age groups										Total			
	0–4		5–14		15–39		40–64		65 and older		Crude rate		Ajusted rate	
	2001	2005	2001	2005	2001	2005	2001	2005	2001	2005	2001	2005	2001	2005
Diseases of the circulatory system (I00–I99)	4.0	4.4	1.1	1.0	11.1	9.9	204.7	178.5	2,381.3	2,267.6	295.6	306.0	203.9	188.2
Neoplasms (C00–D48)	6.5	4.5	5.5	4.8	16.1	15.2	189.6	178.4	959.4	1,022.7	153.6	172.7	114.8	116.4
External causes (V01–Y98)	14.5	11.9	11.4	10.0	47.4	40.2	58.2	50.5	274.1	253.6	65.2	61.0	52.0	45.4
Communicable diseases (A00–B99, G00–G03, J00–J22)	18.6	26.1	1.8	1.6	6.5	5.5	32.3	28.7	576.9	560.9	70.0	73.9	46.7	44.4
Certain conditions originating in the perinatal period (P00–P96)	54.1	44.0	0.3	0.2	—	0.1	0.1	0.0	—	—	3.6	2.8	4.1	3.3
Other causes (A00–Y89)	51.6	49.7	5.1	5.6	19.8	18.7	112.0	103.9	774.6	864.5	119.1	137.1	87.9	91.0
Total	149.3	140.6	25.2	23.2	100.8	89.6	596.9	540.0	4,966.3	4,969.4	707.0	753.5	509.5	488.7

Note: Age-adjusted rate, standard population derived from the 1981 census.

TABLE 2. Leading causes of death (rate per 100,000 population) all age groups, Cuba, 2001 and 2005.

Causes	2001	2005
Heart diseases (I05–I52)	185.5	197.4
Malignant neoplasms (C00–C97)	149.8	168.4
Cerebrovascular diseases (I60–I69)	71.9	78.1
Influenza and pneumonia (J09–J18)	61.6	64.4
Accidents (V01–X59, Y85–Y86)	42.8	39.5
Diseases of arteries, arterioles, and capillaries (I70–I79)	36.3	28.6
Chronic lower respiratory diseases (J40–J47)	25.0	26.7
Diabetes mellitus (E10–E14)	13.9	17.6
Intentional self-harm (X60–X84, Y87.0)	14.7	12.2
Cirrhosis and other chronic liver diseases (K70, K73, K74, K76, K76.1)	8.7	10.2

Note: Causes of death were coded according to the International Statistical Classification of Diseases and Related Health Problems, 10th Revision (ICD-10).

Source: Sistema de Información Estadístico de Defunciones y Defunciones Perinatales.

FIGURE 3. Age-adjusted mortality rates for leading causes of death, Cuba, 2001 and 2005.

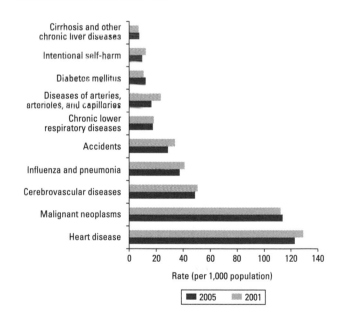

Children 5–9 Years Old

The mortality rate for this age group in 2005 was 0.2 deaths per 1,000 population (0.3 for males and 0.1 for females). That year, together, the three leading causes of death, namely accidents (with a rate of 7.3 per 100,000 population), malignant neoplasms (5.4), and congenital malformations (0.7), accounted for 64.4% of all deaths of school-age children. The main communicable diseases affecting this population group were acute respiratory infections and acute diarrheal diseases.

Adolescents 10–19 Years Old

Adolescent health is an integral part of all health programs and interventions. In 2005, this age group accounted for roughly 15% of the total population and 73.8% of all adolescents lived in urban areas, with no major differences between the sexes or different age subgroups. The fertility rate for the adolescent population decreased from 48.3 to 41.1 per 1,000 females between 2001 and 2005. Adolescent deaths accounted for less than 1% of all

FIGURE 4. Years of potential life lost among the population aged 1–74, by leading causes, Cuba, 2005.

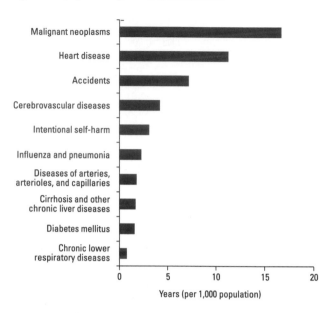

Years (per 1,000 population)

TABLE 4. Leading causes of death (number of deaths and rate per 100,000 population) among adolescents aged 10–19 years, Cuba, 2001 and 2005.

Causes	2001		2005	
Accidents (V01–X59, Y85–Y86)	241	15.0	212	12.9
Malignant neoplasms (C00–C97)	90	5.6	71	4.3
Intentional self-harm (X60–X84, Y87.0)	65	4.0	52	3.2
Assault (X85–Y09, Y87.1)	43	2.7	47	2.9
Congenital malformations, deformations, and chromosomal abnormalities (Q00–Q99)	31	1.9	34	2.1

Note: Causes of death coded according to the WHO International Statistical Classification of Diseases and Related Health Problems, 10th Revision (ICD-10).

Source: Sistema de Información Estadístico de Defunciones y Defunciones perinatales.

deaths in 2005. Accidents were the leading cause of death, followed by malignant neoplasms, intentional self-harm, assaults, and congenital malformations (Table 4).

Adults 20–59 Years Old

The size of the adult population was estimated at 6,495,506 as of 30 June 2005 (57.7% of the total population), of which 3,243,164 were women. Deaths among members of this age group accounted for 18.8% of all deaths in 2005. The mortality rate for all causes of death was 2.4 per 1,000 population (3.0 for

TABLE 3. Leading causes of death (number of deaths and rate per 10,000 population) among children aged 1–4 years, Cuba, 2001 and 2005.

Causes	2001		2005	
Accidents (V01–X59, Y85–Y86)	60	1.0	49	0.9
Congenital malformations, deformations, and chromosomal abnormalities (Q00–Q99)	45	0.8	38	0.7
Malignant neoplasms (C00–C97)	40	0.7	24	0.4
Influenza and pneumonia (J09–J18)	20	0.3	20	0.4
Bacterial meningitis (G00–G03)	—	0.1	10	0.2

Note: Causes of death were coded according to the WHO International Statistical Classification of Diseases and Related Health Problems, 10th Revision (ICD-10).

Source: Sistema de Información Estadístico de Defunciones y Defunciones Perinatales.

males and 1.9 for females). The five leading causes of death were malignant neoplasms (70.3 per 100,000 population), heart disease (45.4), accidents (22.6), cerebrovascular diseases (15.6), and intentional self-harm (12.3). The most common communicable diseases affecting this age group were acute respiratory infections and acute diarrheal diseases.

Women's and children's health, under the Maternal and Child Health Program, are a high public health priority. The average number of prenatal visits was 15 per birth, with 92.8% of first visits taking place prior to the 14th week of pregnancy. Nearly all women (99.9%) gave birth in health facilities, and most births were to women between the ages of 25 and 29, with a rate of 91.1 births per 1,000 women in this age group for 2005. Women completing their pre-university (upper secondary) education accounted for a larger share of births. The direct maternal mortality rate for 2005 was 37.3 per 100,000 live births.

Older Adults 60 Years Old and Older

Deaths of older adults have been on the rise in the last few years. The share of deaths involving adults aged 60 and older increased from 76.8% in 2001 to 79.2% in 2005 (52.3% males and 47.7% females). The five leading causes of death, in descending order, were heart disease (with a rate of 1,105.7 per 100,000 population in 2005); malignant neoplasms (820.3); cerebrovascular diseases (446.4); influenza and pneumonia (385.6); and diseases of the arteries, arterioles, and capillaries (176.1). The risk of dying from one of these causes decreased between 2001 and 2005, except in the case of malignant neoplasms, in which the risk rose by 4%. There was a pattern of higher male mortality associated with all causes of death except for cerebrovascular diseases, from which women ran a slightly higher risk of dying.

The Family

The family structure is diverse and complex, with multigenerational living arrangements and an increase in the number of reconstituted families with children from previous unions and of female-headed households. There have been changes in the family's traditional canons of formation, stability, and partner relationships associated with factors such as age, skin color, nationality, and religious and ideological affiliation, as well as in union formation and in decisions on divorce and parenthood. These have affected certain intra- and intergenerational relationship patterns in various ways. The economic crisis beginning in the 1990s, the deterioration in physical living and working conditions, the complex typology of family models, family survival strategies, the migration problem, changes in family relationship patterns, shifts in ethical and moral values in times of crisis, and the multiple roles the family is called upon to play simultaneously in response to social demands are all part of the challenges affecting the Cuban family.

A 2005 survey of 294 families in selected municipalities around the country found 51% of those interviewed in a family transition process, without their family traits posing any health risks. Of the households surveyed, 43% had family traits with a low or moderate and, in some cases, high criticality level, and 6% had major family health issues.

Workers

A total of 13,584 workplaces were subject to government health inspections in 2005. To prevent occupational diseases, workers exposed to occupational safety and health risks from lead, mercury, organophosphate and carbamate pesticides, silica sand, noise, and *Leptospira* are closely monitored through Watson-Schwartz tests of urine coproporphyrin III levels, urine mercury tests, checks of blood cholinesterase levels, chest X-rays, hearing tests, and other mechanisms. Workers exposed to *Leptospira* are immunized to prevent infection and, in general, proper personal safeguards are taken.

Occupational accidents have been on the decline over the past five years, and mortality rates from this cause have been steadily decreasing. There were 26.5% fewer work-related accidents in 2005 compared with 2000, as illustrated in Figure 5. The agricultural sector and the sugar, electric power, and construction industries accounted for the largest numbers of occupational accidents.

As part of the surveillance system for workers exposed to specific risks, 43 specialized consultations were made in 2005 involving 18,116 workers at high-risk for or with a presumptive diagnosis of an occupational disease. There were 310 diagnoses of occupational diseases, among which the most common diagnoses were chronic nodular laryngitis in primary and secondary school teachers, dermatosis caused by petroleum products, hypoacusia among workers in the metallurgical and mechanical industries, and chemical poisoning.

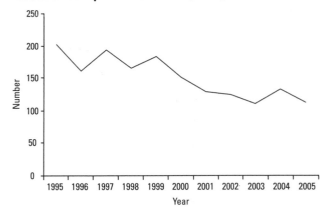

FIGURE 5. Occupational accidents, Cuba, 1995–2005.

Persons with Disabilities

The Government develops policies and carries out programs with nationwide coverage designed to promote equity and equal opportunities for persons with disabilities, particularly in the areas of health, education, sports, culture, employment, and social security. The National Health System has established an extensive network of comprehensive rehabilitation services, which includes all polyclinics and other primary health care units, hospitals, and highly specialized facilities. It also has a human resources training and development program in this area.

There is a special educational subsystem for children and adolescents with all types of disabilities, with 427 schools. Sports and physical fitness are an integral part of human development projects for persons with disabilities and, at the same time, afford recreational opportunities.

The Employment Program for Persons with Disabilities begun in 1995 promotes social mainstreaming and job placement for this population group, with the emphasis on functioning in a normal work environment. Sheltered employment is considered only in the cases of individuals with severe disabilities. Initially, the program focused on finding jobs for the blind and visually impaired, the deaf and hard of hearing, and persons with physical-motor impairments, but has gradually expanded to include persons with intellectual disabilities. As of the end of 2005, there were 28,650 persons with disabilities performing some type of work.

There is an extensive social services network for persons with disabilities requiring economic or social assistance (care, self-care, or other types of services) geared to improving their quality of life.

HEALTH CONDITIONS AND PROBLEMS

COMMUNICABLE DISEASES

Vector-borne Diseases

The increase in *Aedes aegypti* infestation levels since 1997 accelerated in early 2001, triggering a **dengue** outbreak in five of the country's provinces, with 50% of the country-wide infestation concentrated in Havana City. The high household indices (0.9) in the capital contributed to the disease's transmission from a single imported case in the Playa district. By the end of 2001, dengue transmission had been brought under control in most parts of the city, but was still on the rise in other affected provinces. In 2001, senior government officials instituted an intensive strategy aimed at controlling the *A. aegypti* mosquito and breaking the chain of transmission with the participation of most government agencies, as well as the general public. When the campaign began, there were 3,143 dwellings testing positive for *A. aegypti* around the city, with a household index of 0.6. The infestation index was brought down to 0.09 in 42 days and to 0.01 in 77 days, which is equivalent to one positive household per 10,000. The last case developed symptoms on 22 February, and the chain of transmission was broken a month later. The epidemic produced 12,889 cases and three fatalities.

The increase in travelers from areas with endemic diseases previously unknown in Cuba is heightening current risk factors. There were reports of 17 imported cases of dengue between 2004 and 2005, but no reports of any indigenous cases. There were three outbreaks in 2005, with 216 cases in Havana City and Camagüey linked to travelers from dengue-endemic countries. All the outbreaks were brought under control. There is strict border surveillance in the face of the current dengue situation in the Americas. Thus far, efforts to prevent the disease from becoming endemic have been successful.

The last indigenous case of **malaria** was reported in 1967 and the country received its certification of malaria eradication in October 1973. There were 145 reported cases during the 2001–2005 period, 144 of which were imported and one introduced in Guantánamo province. The main vector was *Plasmodium falciparum*.

Vaccine-preventable Diseases

The National Immunization Program protects the public against 13 diseases and has successfully eliminated **polio** (in 1962), **diphtheria** (in 1979), **measles** (in 1993), **whooping cough** (in 1994), **rubella** (in 1995), and **neonatal tetanus** (in 1972). There were no reported cases of **tetanus** anywhere in the country in 2004 or 2005. Morbidity rates for meningoencephalitis caused by *Haemophilus influenzae* **type b** remain low. There were only two reported cases in 2005 (33 fewer than in 2000), due mainly to the inclusion of the Cuban-manufactured *H. influenzae* type b (Hib) vaccine in the official vaccination schedule in 1999.

The impact of the **meningococcus B and C** and **hepatitis B** vaccines is reflected in the continued decline in morbidity rates for these diseases. There were only 25 reported cases of meningoencephalitis associated with meningococcus B and 47 cases of hepatitis B in 2005, compared with 56 cases of meningoencephalitis from meningococcus B and 451 cases of hepatitis B in 2000. The world's first synthetic *H. influenzae* type b vaccine was introduced in Cuba in 2004, and the tetravalent DPT+HB vaccine was introduced in the first quarter of 2005. Both vaccines have

been incorporated into the official vaccination schedule for children under 2 years of age.

A strategy for the elimination of hepatitis B was initiated in 1992 based on the universal vaccination of newborns, vaccination of an under-20 cohort that was completed in 2000, and vaccination of risk groups. There is a perinatal hepatitis B prevention program in place with provisions for the screening of pregnant women for hepatitis B surface antigen (HBsAg) and separate vaccinations of infants born to HBsAg-positive women. By 2005, the incidence of acute hepatitis b had been reduced by 97.9% compared with figures for 1992. There have been no reported cases of acute hepatitis B in children under the age of 5 since 2000.

Intestinal Infectious Diseases

The mortality rate for intestinal infectious diseases fell from 6.4 to 2.9 per 100,000 population (54.7%) between 1995 and 2005. Health care visits for **acute diarrheal diseases** went from 93.0 per 1,000 population in 1995 to 77.8 in 2005. Surveillance for intestinal parasitosis is based on cross-sectional coproparasitological studies of children ages 1–4 attending day-care centers (*círculos infantiles*) in May and October of each year. These examinations are monitored by the nurse and physician attached to the center or by the family physician's office associated with the facility in question. A single sample test is taken from all asymptomatic children enrolled in these centers, who make up 14.7% of the total child population in this age group. In the last five years, the highest positivity rates were associated with protozoal infections (12.4% of all samples tested in 2004).

Chronic Communicable Diseases

Tuberculosis is considered a low-prevalence disease in Cuba. Its incidence has been declining by 3% to 5% annually since 2000, with figures of under 10 per 100,000 population. The incidence rate for tuberculosis in 2005 was 6.5 per 100,000, with the population aged 60 and older being the group most affected. The incidence of tuberculosis in the population under age 15 years is down to below 1 per 100,000 population. There have been no reported cases of tuberculous meningoencephalitis in children under the age of 4 since 1997.

Coinfection with tuberculosis and HIV is under control and accounts for only approximately 3% of all new cases. Thus, in 2005, only 27 HIV/AIDS patients contracted tuberculosis in the course of the disease. There are virtually no reported cases of multidrug resistant tuberculosis (0.3%), and the study of drug-resistant strains among new cases treated at the national reference laboratory for tuberculosis is closely monitored.

Leprosy was eliminated as a national public health problem in 1993, when its prevalence was brought down to 0.79 per 10,000 population. The prevalence rate in 2005 was 0.2. The disease has been successfully eliminated from all provinces. The number of new cases has leveled off in the last few years, putting the incidence rate in 2005 at 1.8 per 100,000 population. The incidence of leprosy among the population under 15 years of age was 0.4

per 100,000 in 2005, accounting for 3.8% of all new cases. In the last few years, the country has been working to strengthen the technical diagnostic capabilities of health personnel and step up surveillance in population groups exposed to the disease.

Acute Respiratory Infections

Most acute respiratory infections are mild and self-limiting, but constitute a national health problem in the sense that they are responsible for large numbers of health care visits each year (4,731,614 in 2005). The main circulating causative agent is the influenza A virus (H3N2) and, to a lesser extent, H1N1 and B viruses. The most severe complications from these types of infections are reported in adults aged 65 and older and in immunosuppressed individuals. The highest mortality rates for influenza and pneumonia are associated with the population aged 65 and older and, within this population, the over-80 age group. Since 1997, all of the population residing full-time or part-time in facilities for older adults and attending senior day-care centers have received seasonal flu shots every year. New risk groups are given the vaccine every year, which was administered to everyone over the age of 85 and to workers on poultry farms during the last two flu seasons (2004–2005).

HIV/AIDS and Other Sexually Transmitted Infections

As of the end of 2005, there were 6,967 reported HIV-seropositive cases nationwide; of these 2,806 had developed into AIDS, with 1,338 fatalities. The HIV/AIDS epidemic has been growing slowly. The number of reported AIDS cases has decreased, and the mortality rate has stabilized. As a result, the total number of persons infected with HIV/AIDS nationwide is leveling off but, apparently, not diminishing. The estimated prevalence rate in the population aged 15–49 is still under 0.1%. The prevalence rate in the 15–24-year-old population dropped from 0.07% in 2001 to 0.05% in 2005. Moreover, 99.4% of all persons diagnosed with HIV and AIDS were infected through sexual contact. There are very few cases of infection through mother-to-child transmission (0.3%) and by blood and blood products (0.3%). Males account for 80% of all reported cases, and the highest risk group (86%) was that of homosexual males. There are over 1.5 million voluntary HIV tests administered each year to members of different population groups. Screening of the blood supply since 1986 and the development of programs promoting voluntary blood donations have virtually eliminated HIV transmission through blood transfusions. Access to prenatal care and prevention programs for mother-to-child HIV transmission (including separate mother and child therapies, elective cesarean sections, and artificial breast-feeding, with clinical and laboratory monitoring of affected infants for the first 18 months following birth) have helped minimize transmission through this mode, keeping the total number of such cases down to 25 in a 20-year-long epidemic. Over 3 million pregnant women have been tested for HIV.

Syphilis and **gonorrhea** cases declined during the 2001–2005 period, while cases of infection by the human papillomavirus

were on the rise. There were no reported cases of late or congenital syphilis. Congenital syphilis has not been a public health problem since 1998, with an incidence rate of 16.9 per 10,000 population in 2005 (down 79.4% from 2000). The incidence of reported cases of gonorrhea in 2005 was 63.6 per 10,000 population, reflecting a 62.6% reduction in the risk of contracting the disease compared with figures for 2000.

Zoonoses

Human **rabies** reemerged in 1988, transmitted by a non-hematophagous bat. There were nine reported cases as of 2005, eight attributable to nonhematophagous bats and one to a wild cat. Most cases of animal rabies have involved dogs, cats, mongooses, and cattle, and the disease has also been diagnosed in nine other animal species, albeit on a smaller scale. Canine rabies is confined to a few suburban and rural areas and is nearly always associated with mongoose attacks, its main mode of transmission in land animals. Nonhematophagous bats are the species of major epidemiological importance in the transmission of human rabies.

There was a sharp surge in human **leptospirosis** in the first half of the 1990s to rates of over 10 per 10,000 population, with a pattern of both endemic and epidemic behavior, followed by a slow decline in morbidity and mortality rates. Figures for 2001–2005 were consistently under 5 per 10,000 population. Most cases of the disease still involve males and subjects between 15 and 44 years of age. The availability of a Cuban vaccine against leptospirosis and of doxycycline prophylaxis have enabled the country to institute an intervention strategy in high-risk areas for contracting the disease. The vaccine has been administered to more than three million people exposed to the infection since 1996. Other zoonoses of medical importance such as **brucellosis, toxoplasmosis**, and **fascioliasis** are associated with low morbidity rates, which is not the case for **teniasis**, which still carries a moderate morbidity rate.

NONCOMMUNICABLE DISEASES

Metabolic and Nutritional Diseases

According to data for 2004, 1.9% of children under 5 years of age had low weight-for-height (more than 2 SDs below the median) and 4% showed signs of some degree of **stunting** based on U.S. National Center for Health Statistics standards. **Iron deficiency** is one of Cuba's most serious micronutrient deficiency problems, primarily affecting children under age 2, women of child-bearing age, and pregnant women, in that order. A 2005 survey conducted in five provinces among children between the ages of 6 months and 4 years put the prevalence of **anemia** (hemoglobin < 110 g/L) at 32.5%. Most cases were mild. The prevalence rate in pregnant women in the third trimester of pregnancy was 24%. There are drug supplementation strategies promoting the use of iron salt tablets targeted at pregnant women, women of child-bearing age, and children up to 5 years of age. Wheat flour is fortified with iron and folic acid and distributed in government-subsidized rations of 80 g of bread per person per day (providing approximately 26% of the daily recommended dose of iron). Pureed fruits for children under the age of 3 are fortified with iron lactate, and evaporated milk for children under age 1 is fortified with protected iron. According to studies of serum retinol levels, **vitamin A deficiency** in preschool- and school-age children is not a public health problem.

Median urinary iodine excretion in school-age children was 246 µg/L in 2005. Over 90% of all salt consumed by Cuban households is iodized. The International Council for Control of Iodine Deficiency Disorders determined that the country was in a position to achieve the sustained elimination of **iodine deficiency** disorders.

Obesity is an increasingly serious problem in all population groups and is on the rise. The Second National Survey of Risk Factors and Noncommunicable Disorders in the Cuban Population, based on a representative sample of 22,851 subjects and concluded in 2001, found 29.7% of males and 31.5% of females to be overweight (with a body mass index [BMI] of 25–29.9) and 7.9% of males and 15.4% of females suffering from obesity (BMI > 30). Looking at body fat distribution patterns, the study found that approximately 25% of the population had an upper-body pattern of obesity, indicating a risk of obesity-related chronic diseases. The share of obese children under 5 years of age was 13%.

Prevalence rates for **diabetes mellitus** have risen in the last five years. As of the end of 2004, there were 342,371 patients (30.5 per 1,000 population) participating in an organized, ongoing, aggressive evaluation and treatment process utilizing an epidemiological and social clinical approach, an increase of 4.1% over the previous year. There was a steady decline in the risk of dying from this cause between 1998 and 2002, followed by a rise in mortality in 2003 and 2004, to 16.5 per 100,000 population.

Cardiovascular Diseases

Heart disease has been the leading cause of death for more than 40 years and the second leading source of years of potential life lost. The decline in mortality levels for this cause during the late 1990s into the beginning of the next decade was followed by a rise in mortality in 2004 and 2005, by which time the death rate stood at 197.4 per 100,000 population (a jump of 5.4% from 2004 and 6.4% from 2001) (Figure 6). Males had a higher risk of dying from heart disease than females, and the most deaths (86.5% of the total) involved adults aged 60 and older. The leading cause of death in 2005 was **ischemic cardiopathy,** which was responsible for 72.1% of all deaths from heart disease. Acute myocardial infarctions accounted for 45.3% of all deaths from ischemic cardiopathy, with an in-hospital case fatality rate of 17.6% in 2005.

There has been major progress in the detection of **hypertension** since 1999 thanks to active case investigation by family physicians and nurses, boosting the prevalence rate in patients under treatment to 194.6 per 1,000 population in 2005.

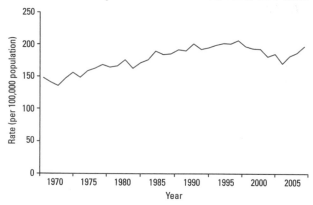

FIGURE 6. Mortality due to heart disease, Cuba, 1970–2005.

Cerebrovascular diseases are the third leading cause of death across all age groups, accounting for 10.2% of all deaths. They are the sixth leading cause of death in the population aged 25–34 and rank ninth among the leading causes of death in the 15-24-year-old age group. Age is the main nonmodifiable risk factor, and arterial hypertension is the leading modifiable risk factor. Cerebrovascular diseases are the third leading cause of death in women aged 35 and older and the seventh leading cause in the female population aged 15–24. The gender mortality gap began to reverse itself in 1992, with recent data indicating more deaths among females than among males. There is a shift in the pattern of these diseases toward younger age groups. Hemorrhagic forms of cerebrovascular disease are the leading cause of death among older adults. Crude death rates are consistently higher for females (21.9 per 100,000 population) than for males (11.0), due primarily to the higher morbidity prevalence in women (38.8 per 1,000) compared with men (22.2 per 1,000).

Malignant Neoplasms

Malignant neoplasms are the second leading cause of death and the number one cause of years of potential life lost. The crude death rate rose from 149.8 per 100,000 population to 168.4 (Figure 7) between 2001 and 2005. Male rates were higher than female rates, and roughly 75.2% of all deaths involved older adults aged 60 and older. Cancer incidence rates were 271.7 per 100,000 population for males and 253.4 for females. According to data for 2002, cancer of the lungs, skin, prostate, larynx, and colon accounted for approximately 63% of the incidence of cancer in males, while the leading cancer sites in females were the breast, skin, cervix, lungs, and colon. The highest mortality rates for malignant neoplasms in 2005 were associated with neoplasms of the trachea, bronchus, and lung (23.5%); prostate (11.8%); and colon (8.9%) in men and neoplasms of the breast in women, which accounted for 6.3% of all deaths. Over the last 10 years, deaths from lung cancer rose by less than 1% a year in males and 2.3% a year in females.

There were 2,478 deaths from cervical-uterine cancer between 2000 and 2005. As part of the National Early Detection Program

FIGURE 7. Mortality due to malignant neoplasms, Cuba, 1970–2005.

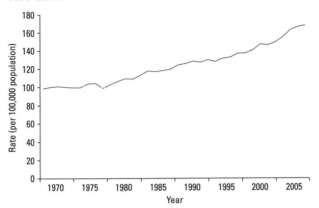

for this form of cancer, 682,232 women aged 25 and above were examined in 2005, for an examination rate of 179.0 per 1,000 women in this age group, with 82% of cancer cases detected in clinical stage 0. The mortality rate for 2005 was 7.3 per 100,000 women, down 69.6% from 2000.

OTHER HEALTH PROBLEMS OR ISSUES

Disasters

In 2005, the country was hit by tropical storm Arlene; Hurricanes Dennis, Katrina, Rita, and Wilma; and heavy rains in its central and eastern regions. Interventions by civil defense personnel significantly reduced the numbers of injured and dead from these disasters. Part of this success was attributable to the training of civil defense workers and the public-at-large, timely shipments of essential supplies and equipment for disease prevention, and the rapid deployment of health personnel, drugs, generators, food supplies, and health transport vehicles to areas facing possible isolation.

The national disaster response plan focuses on taking the necessary steps to ensure that there is no interruption in service in local facilities, as well as heightening other protective measures, particularly as regards evacuations of at-risk populations. The National Health System and Civil Defense System are integrated under current legislation and, as such, carry out coordinated efforts. Cuba also provides neutral aid and support to disaster-stricken countries as a form of international cooperation.

External Causes

The rate of accidental deaths decreased from 44.3 per 100,000 in 2000 to 39.1 in 2004. The rate of incidents of intentional self-harm dropped from 16.5 per 100,000 population to 13.3. Accidental falls as a result of the aging of the Cuban population pose the highest risk. The mortality rate for accidental falls was 15.6 per 100,000 population in 2004, with traffic accidents involving

motor vehicles ranking second, at a rate of 10.0 per 100,000 population. The risk of death from an accident is higher among males than females, with a male-female ratio of 1.5. The pattern is similar for intentional self-harm, with a male-female ratio of 3.1.

Mental Health

The suicidal behavior prevention and control program systematically conducts risk assessments based on epidemiological stratification in all parts of the country. The death rate from suicide dropped from 14.7 per 100,000 population in 2001 to 12.2 in 2005. The strengthening of community-based services for the treatment of patients suffering from schizophrenia has resulted in their successful social and occupational rehabilitation. The number of beds in long-term care units in psychiatric hospitals has been cut back. There is a new strategy for the treatment of alcohol dependency and related problems based on screening tests for the detection of alcohol use disorders.

Environmental Pollution

Exposure to chemicals is monitored under the National Occupational Safety and Health Program, which includes systematic surveillance of working conditions, environmental and biological monitoring, and specialized health care and training for exposed workers, with special emphasis on the productive sectors in general and agriculture in particular. Under the program, all workers exposed to chemicals are given preventive checkups. Timely job removals account for 70% of occupational safety measures, removing workers from exposure to harm and, thereby, preventing them from becoming ill. This measure has helped reduce the number of workers harmed by chemicals. There have been no reported deaths from occupational exposure to these health hazards.

The use of biopesticides for pest control purposes has reduced occupational exposure to farm chemicals. On-site working conditions are evaluated and special measures are taken to limit exposure risk. There is a National Pesticide Registry whose main functions include the performance of chemical, biological, and environmental pesticide assessments prior to authorizing their use in Cuba, the publication of an annual list of authorized pesticides in the *Gaceta Oficial*, and the revocation of pesticide licenses in the event of the establishment of any adverse health or environmental effects, in line with standards proposed by the Pan American Health Organization/World Health Organization (PAHO/WHO). The program monitors exposure to heavy metals and other chemical compounds and determines any necessary measures based on indicators established under current regulations. As of 2005, there were more than 23 instruments dealing with the handling, transport, storage, preparation, use, assessment, and inspection of farm chemicals, industrial chemicals, and hazardous wastes and corresponding safety and health measures, bans, violations, classification schemes, safety requirements, and occupational illnesses, among others, including laws, resolutions, and regulations.

Oral Health

Oral health is a key component of the national health system. According to data for 2005, 55% of 5- and 6-year-olds experienced adequate oral health. The decayed, missing, and filled teeth index at 12 years of age was 1.62%, and 76% of 18-year-olds still had all their teeth. There is an ongoing nationwide preventive oral health program. In 2005, 14,682,226 fluoride rinses were administered to children between 5 and 14 years of age, and 1,337,471 fluoride varnish treatments were administered to children under the age of 12. The rate of oral cancer (including cancer of the lips, oral cavity, and pharynx) stood at 5.2 per 100,000 population in 2005 and is the ninth leading cause of death from malignant neoplasms, by cancer site. The risk of dying from oral cancer in 2005 was 7.7 in males and 2.6 in females.

RESPONSE OF THE HEALTH SECTOR

Health Policies and Plans

The country is committed to achieving a sustained improvement in the health status of its population, as well as in the quality and efficiency of health services and the level of satisfaction of patients, family members, and workers, while providing free aid and assistance to patients from a number of other countries in the Region of the Americas and on other continents. In 2003, it began remodeling, expanding, and installing high-quality medical equipment in 52 of its largest, most advanced, most sophisticated hospitals and in 129 polyclinics representing over 20% and 25%, respectively, of all such facilities nationwide. New health care services were established for the treatment of patients with serious conditions, chronic illnesses, and other common problems in locations more accessible to the general public. In addition, 121 intensive therapy units and 452 rehabilitation units were created to guarantee adequate access to these essential services for residents of all 169 municipalities. These stepped-up investments in technology were paralleled by specialized training activities for professionals and technicians, as needed.

Legislation has been in place since 1983 setting out the underlying principles governing social relations in the area of public health to help ensure health promotion, disease prevention, health restoration, patient social rehabilitation, and social welfare. Progress in health legislation paved the way for the establishment of basic requirements and procedures for the registration of tobacco products with the Ministry of Public Health and the delineation of the functions of the Public Health Protection and Regulation Agency, the regulation of cross-border movements of samples of biological material, and the banning of imports and exports of products with potential human health effects. There are two compendiums of major current domestic legal texts in this area entitled *Legalidad y Sida en Cuba* (Legality and AIDS in Cuba) and *Aspectos Legales sobre Maternidad y Paternidad Responsables* (Legal Considerations for Responsible Parenthood).

Health Strategies and Programs

Health sector strategies are grounded in basic Cuban tenets of public health; namely, the social and governmental nature of medicine, free access to health care, a preventive health approach, the effective use of scientific and technical progress, community participation, and international cooperation. These strategies are designed to achieve equity in health and to strengthen the health system, improving management efficiency and the quality of public health care through active community participation. At the same time, they establish a system of differential care, giving priority to risk groups or life-threatening illnesses or illnesses affecting people's quality of life, delivered under different National Health System programs, such as maternal and child care and older adult health care programs and control programs for communicable and chronic noncommunicable diseases. In addition, new programs are being carried out for the delivery of specialized care at the primary health care level to improve its effectiveness and accessibility to the public.

There have been major changes in primary health care in the past few years, such as the shifting of specialized services previously delivered at the secondary and tertiary levels to the primary health care level, requiring a major investment in physical and financial resources and human resources training. The structure of Cuban society allows for the involvement of all segments of the population in resolving health problems in different regions of the country. The three cornerstones of social participation in the solution of health problems are the country's political/administrative structure, with the National Assembly of People's Power as an organ of government; the influence and timeliness of different approaches and strategies devised by the Ministry of Public Health; and the development and growth in the number of national and international nongovernmental organizations (NGOs) working in the health sector.

Organization of the Health System

The Ministry of Public Health is in charge of administering State and government health policy. The Public Health Protection and Regulation Agency establishes and enforces regulations governing pharmaceutical and diagnostic products, medical equipment, food products, cosmetics, and chemicals with potentially hazardous health effects through the State Drug Quality Control Center, the State Quality Control Center for Medical Equipment, the Food and Cosmetics Registration Department, and the Center for Pharmacoepidemiological Development. The Public Health Protection and Regulation Agency's External Health Service Monitoring Subdivision regulates good practices and oversees the accreditation and certification of different health organizations. Other components of the regulatory system include marketing regulations and permits, clinical trials, good practice compliance inspections for research, manufacturing, quality control, distribution, importing and exporting, and the licensing of corresponding

Health Policies for Older Adults

Low mortality rates and improvements in life expectancy have led to a steady increase in the size of the population 60 years old and older. In 2005, the age group older than 60 years old represented 15.4% of the total population. The Comprehensive Senior Health Care Program is charged with providing a full range of health care services for older adults and meeting their growing health needs through community-based care, institutional care, and hospital care. Community-based care includes disease prevention, health promotion, health care, and rehabilitation services delivered by the National Public Health System in conjunction with other interested agencies and organizations, the family, the community, and older adults themselves, all searching for local solutions to problems. To this end, there are interdisciplinary geriatric teams and counseling and recreational groups that provide older adults with an opportunity to socialize and prepare them to deal with day-to-day problems and to embrace healthy lifestyles. Senior day-care centers are community-based facilities run by a social worker working closely with the interdisciplinary geriatric teams, helping to improve the quality of life for older adults through physical exercise, meal-delivery programs to homes and institutions, telephone counseling hotlines, and assisted-living housing.

facilities, lot releases for selected products, import permits, and post-marketing inspections, including the monitoring of adverse drug reactions and studies of drug usage. The National Pharmacy Division is responsible for health inspections of narcotic drugs and psychotropic substances and inspections of pharmacy procedures. Public Health and Epidemiology Centers are in charge of general health inspections.

Public Health Services

The need to strengthen epidemiological surveillance and analysis systems at all levels of the national health structure, along with active case-finding systems and response capabilities to identify short-term changes and implement different intervention options in a speedy, timely, and efficient manner, became apparent in the early 1990s. The Ministry of Public Health established central-level Health Trend and Analysis Units in all provinces and municipalities to consolidate the information generated by the surveillance system. These units are viewed as an intelligent data analysis and decision-making system, capitalizing on a combination of theoretical and practical knowledge in the area of epidemiology and other public health areas, technological features associated with developments in information technology, and the possibilities afforded by the use of information to gain new insights into current health conditions and make prospective evaluations as the basis for decision-making. They conduct analyses of health situations and trends and studies of forecasting and epidemiological stratification, and have facilitated the establishment of more than 30 surveillance subsystems in the areas of maternal and child health, older adult health, and communicable, noncommunicable, and emerging diseases, among others. There

is also an epidemiological and entomological surveillance system for the monitoring of exotic and vector-borne diseases of medical importance and the implementation of control and elimination measures, tied to a surveillance system for febrile syndromes.

The nation has sufficient water resources to meet household, agricultural, and industrial needs. Groundwater resources account for 72% of the water supply, with the remainder furnished by surface water resources. A total of 2,737 communities had water supply systems in 2005 delivering 1,544.4 hm^3 of water, 100.8 hm^3 less than in 2004 due to water shortages at source points as a result of the drought, as well as to power failures and breakdowns in pumping equipment. Water quality indicators for 2005 were satisfactory, with a wastewater treatment rate of 97.9%, a continuous chlorination rate of 99.1%, and a bacteriological water potability index of 95.6% for water distribution systems.

Most urban households have hook-ups to sewerage systems or septic tanks, whereas latrines are common in rural areas. A total of 562 communities are equipped with sewer systems, which carried 571.1 hm^3 of sewage in 2005, of which 37% was treated.

Spending in the water supply and sewerage sector rose faster than expected in 2005, with 86.4% of all such spending going to the water supply and sewerage program, with a large share allocated to water treatment plants producing drinking water for public consumption.

A study of the country's solid waste sector was conducted in 1997 with assistance from PAHO/WHO, leading to the formulation of a work strategy and development program for that sector. Eight years of institution-building in this sector have borne fruit, with the emphasis on human resources development. The State has been investing in technology for the satisfaction of residential solid waste collection and final disposal needs, while continuing to use other waste collection and transportation alternatives such as animal traction wherever possible. It is continually expanding manual sanitary landfills as the definitive solution for final waste disposal in villages and towns with up to 20,000 inhabitants. Even with existing problems, solid waste services are improving. The hospital waste management, collection, and final disposal program remains in place.

The country has a national surveillance program for food contaminants which samples products posing a high epidemiological risk twice a month, monthly, and yearly for manufacturing and storage facilities and distribution and consumption centers. Technological development processes in certain industries have played an important role in the operation of the surveillance system and the institution of the HACCP (Hazard Analysis and Critical Control Points) approach. The system has 52 health surveillance laboratories for the sampling of food products. The sound, effective use of these laboratories has helped cut costs by 30%. Program design was based on an analysis of performance data for the previous 10-year period and major problems presented by food-borne diseases, as well as an evaluation of hygienic conditions in food centers and findings from sampling processes conducted by other agencies.

Compliance with good manufacturing and handling practices throughout the food chain was considered an important factor. Analysis quality was assured by the laboratory, with the Nutrition and Food Hygiene Institute serving as the reference center for establishing major problems or conducting investigations of interest to the Ministry of Public Health.

With respect to emerging and reemerging diseases, necessary measures have been taken to ensure the stepping up of epizootiological and epidemiological surveillance for avian flu. Health personnel have received training to increase their knowledge regarding response to the threat of a future global flu pandemic. The threat posed by the West Nile virus prompted the formulation of multisectoral, integrated surveillance, prevention, and control strategies for the timely identification of infected birds and the implementation of measures to prevent the appearance of the disease in humans and animals. In response to worldwide flu surveillance efforts in 2002, and in the face of the appearance of SARS (severe acute respiratory syndrome), a national multidisciplinary group developed an emergency plan as a basis for the mounting of training, diagnostic, and surveillance activities which prevented the disease's introduction in Cuba.

Individual Care Services

The hospital network consists of 248 hospitals providing preventive, curative, and rehabilitative services to the entire population. The country has worked arduously to improve quality in each of these facilities, strengthen hospital regulations, and develop hospital epidemiology departments as basic approaches to modernizing medical technology through the use of innovative,

sophisticated equipment ensuring high standards of quality, efficiency, and patient safety. All procedures have been computerized to improve performance efficiency, and there is systematic human resources training.

The integration of primary and hospital care has been crucial to the work of secondary level facilities and has had positive outcomes, both with respect to patient care and to teaching and research, addressing basic health problems in each local area.

Emergency services, urgent care, and critical care come under the Integrated Emergency Medical System forming a chain of survival with six links, in which the first link is on-site early detection and the last link is intensive care for critically ill or injured patients.

Polyclinics at the primary health care level are equipped with urgent care units. In 2004, a preliminary needs assessment encompassing remote areas or areas at large distances from high resolution-capacity hospitals prompted the establishment of municipal intensive care units (*áreas intensivas municipales*, or AIMs) in 121 municipalities around the country staffed with trained physicians and nursing personnel providing round-the-clock service in an endeavor to improve public access to emergency or urgent care services. As of the end of 2005, AIMs had treated a total of 51,978 patients, with a general survival rate of 97.6%. The survival rate for the top 10 illnesses and health problems treated by these units was 98.2%.

AIMs administered thrombolysis to 498 patients in 2004 and to 602 patients in 2005, or to 41.3% and 52.3%, respectively, of all thrombosis victims treated by such units. Mobile emergency services were restructured in 2005, with 121 municipalities equipped with new ambulances and all actively employed ambulance drivers receiving comprehensive paramedic training.

Over 70,000 patients aged 15 years and older were admitted to hospital-based intensive therapy units in 2005.

The National Health System includes 470 clinical laboratories installed in polyclinics (primary care facilities) and another 248 in secondary-level facilities with a level of sophistication capable of meeting current nationwide physician and patient demand. Specialized institutes and national health units around the country (at the tertiary level) have been equipped with 40 chemical analyzers capable of performing 300 tests an hour, 25 blood gas analyzers with ion-selective electrodes, and more than 25 hematology units capable of performing 32 determinations on 60 patients an hour.

Imaging departments in general and clinical-surgical hospitals and national health units and institutes have been equipped with high-tech equipment such as 64-slice CT scanners, nuclear MRI equipment, and three-dimensional echocardiograms.

The National Blood and Transfusion Medicine Program, with its Hematology and Immunology Institute, includes 27 provincial blood banks, 35 municipal blood banks, 121 permanent blood collection centers, 162 transfusion units, and a blood processing plant. There were 524,351 voluntary blood donations made in

2005. All donated blood is screened for syphilis, HIV-1 and HIV-2, hepatitis B surface antigen (HBsAg), and anti-HCV antibodies. The latter three diagnoses are made using a locally produced ultramicroanalysis system. In 2005, testing procedures were instituted for the detection of HCV-RNA in plasma pools used in the manufacturing of hematology products. The prevalence of hepatitis B and C in blood donors was 0.7% in 2005.

There were 17,943,732 patient visits to the country's network of 1,338 oral health services in 2005. Such services are available at 165 dental clinics, polyclinics, hospitals, and other public primary and secondary care facilities. In addition, tertiary multidisciplinary services are provided by clinical-surgical hospitals and the Network for Facial and Buccomaxillary-Facial Prostheses. A comprehensive general oral health care model has been developed for use at the primary health care level by specialists in comprehensive general oral health care and dental technicians working with family physicians and nurses. The introduction of new technology such as laser and implant technology has gone hand in hand with the promotion of different forms of natural and traditional medicine such as acupuncture, homeopathy, and herbal medicine. The country strengthened its oral health councils, dental health care for healthy children and adolescents ages 0–18, and JUVEDENTI, an oral/dental health promotion strategy in which dental health professionals spend time working in special adolescent dental services geared specifically to the requirements and needs of the 12–18-year-old population group. The goal is to provide preventive, curative, and rehabilitative services at the primary care level and, where secondary level care is required, through consults. The fluoride prevention and early oral cancer detection program has been stepped up. Clinical practice guides have been developed, and oral health services have been reorganized in line with changes in population dynamics; in particular, the aging of the Cuban population.

Family planning and reproductive risk management services have been strengthened and new facility-based services are being developed in response to established needs, with a strategic approach for the prevention of preconception reproductive risks and the expansion and stabilization of the preconception and prenatal care system (care beginning six months prior to a potential planned, wanted pregnancy) designed to reduce high-risk pregnancies and lower pregnancy risks. The main cornerstones of the growing family planning services network at the primary care level are community-based physicians and nurses and provider groups in polyclinics in 432 health districts, supported, in turn, by secondary and tertiary level facilities. There is universal access to these services based on an informed decision freely made by the woman or couple in question. Nationwide contraception coverage with modern methods of contraception, primarily third-generation IUDs, is 77.1%. All indirect indicators measuring the effectiveness of the family planning strategy are positive. Health care services for women in the 40–59 age group are delivered at the primary care level by a multidisciplinary team based on medical-social diagnoses, including diagnoses of hidden morbidity, as well as couple, family, or work-related problems. Chronic health problems are treated at the appropriate level of care.

The country now has a National Cardiology and Cardiovascular Surgery Network which keeps records of all surgical procedures performed nationwide and delivers necessary care for the treatment and follow-up of conditions related to this specialty. A total of 14,632 patients, including 3,992 with acute myocardial infarctions, have been admitted to health care facilities through this network, which includes all hospitals nationwide and primary health care units and is successfully used in municipal intensive care units; more than 2,376 pacemakers have been implanted.

The Hemodynamics and Interventional Cardiology Section has performed 5,008 diagnostic procedures and 1,354 major surgeries with a medium to high level of sophistication, including highly complex repairs of congenital malformations and heart transplants, with patient longevity exceeding 10 years.

The tissue and organ transplant program is making satisfactory progress. Data for 2005 shows 138 kidney transplants, 17 liver transplants, 2 heart transplants, 2 lung transplants, 8 bone marrow transplants, 197 corneal transplants, and more than 500 bone grafts.

The nephrology program provides hemodialysis treatment to approximately 1,944 patients and has a total of 458 dialyzers and 50 water treatment plants, with a patient-dialyzer index of 4.3 and a mortality rate under 30% a year.

The national cancer program has state-of-the-art radiation therapy, cobalt therapy, brachytherapy, and superficial radiation therapy technology, localization equipment/simulators, a planning system, immobilization equipment, and computer equipment capable of meeting current needs. Cuban health services use a broad spectrum of cytostatics and have strengthened diagnostic procedures.

The Comprehensive Senior Health Care Program is in charge of providing comprehensive health care services for older adults and meeting their growing health needs through community-based, facility-based, and hospital-based care. Community-based care includes disease prevention, health promotion, medical care, and rehabilitation services delivered by the National Public Health System in conjunction with other interested agencies and organizations and the active involvement of the family, community, and patient in seeking local solutions to problems. To this end, there are interdisciplinary geriatric teams (436 as of 2005) and counseling and recreational groups (1,435) giving older adults a chance to socialize and preparing them to cope with day-to-day problems and embrace healthy lifestyles. There are also intersectoral social programs targeted specifically at older adults living alone or with no family support network in which the Ministry of Labor and Social Security and the Ministry of Public Health both play leading roles, designed to meet the economic and psychosocial needs of this segment of the population.

Senior day-care centers (*casas de abuelos*), community-based facilities run by a social worker working closely with interdisciplinary geriatric teams, and senior community centers (*círculos de abuelos*) helping to improve the quality of life for seniors through physical exercise, home-delivered and congregate meals programs, counseling services, telephone hotlines, and sheltered housing are examples of achievements in the area of older adult health care. In 2005, there were 201 senior day-care centers with 5,562 registered older adults (representing 0.3% of this population group) and 14,701 senior community centers (with an enrollment figure representing 43.1% of the older adult population). Facility-based care is delivered through the country's network of hospitals and institutions for the elderly. As of 2005, there were 143 homes for the elderly with a total of 11,764 beds and 350 physicians devoted to geriatric care (267 specialists). Other health personnel involved in caring for this segment of the population are also being given training to improve the standard of care. Older adult health care policies are designed to keep this population group engaged in the national development process, effectively protect its health, and provide a positive environment.

The Cuban Constitution and Family Code establish family rights and obligations with respect to health, parenthood and matrimony, the mutual responsibilities of parents and children, and the right to free access to curative and preventive health services. Comprehensive Family Health Care Program services are delivered at the primary health care level by the family physician's office health care team, supported by various specialists attached to the basic provider group and polyclinic for that area. The core health care team delivers family health promotion and disease prevention services and curative and recuperative care and conducts educational activities during home visits, at the physician's office, and through community counseling groups for parents, adolescents, and the elderly. Family data is systematically recorded by the family physician's office in Family Health Histories which, in addition to information on family members, also include data on the makeup of the family unit, its living conditions, functioning, major problems, and action plan, with one year of follow-up. The nationwide coverage of the comprehensive family health care program, the existence of high-level multidisciplinary teams in charge of program implementation, human resources training programs which integrate family health components, and the country's current political-administrative structure based on a regionalization model promoting intersectoral participation in family services all help bolster family health care.

The workers' health subsystem is part of the National Health System and, as such, is governed by the same principles of free health care, accessibility, universality, and community participation. All programs and services are planned and monitored from central Ministry of Public Health headquarters; by the Occupational Health Group attached to the National Environmental Health Unit, working closely with local offices; the Ministry of Labor and Social Security; and the unions. Environmental monitoring activities come under the jurisdiction of the Ministry of Public Health's Health and Epidemiology Division, with provincial and municipal offices conducting state health inspections. Primary health care services are delivered by specialists in comprehensive general medicine based at community physicians' offices, workplaces, and educational institutions dispensing free preventive, medical, and rehabilitative care to the public-at-large, including occupational health care for the working population. Specialized care is available at hospitals around the country from highly skilled personnel, including physicians specializing in occupational health, and at the National Occupational Health Institute.

A Government Group was formed in 1983 at the national government level to coordinate and head up a multisectoral effort to control the AIDS epidemic. Among the entities involved are the Ministry of Education, the Federation of Cuban Women, the Ministry of Tourism, the population living with HIV/AIDS, the Ministry of Culture, the Ministry of Trade, and the Ministry of Labor and Social Security. International agencies and organizations have been helping to implement the control plan through specific projects designed to strengthen interventions in furtherance of strategic objectives. Counseling services were expanded in 2004 and 2005, which helped improve the coverage of programs targeted at high-risk groups. The peer education method is being used at the national level in schools and communities and within the HIV-positive population. A network of AIDS prevention and control centers was set up in different provinces and municipalities to increase HIV/AIDS awareness among youth. The National Health System ensures access by HIV-positive individuals to all levels of care, with guaranteed access to antiretroviral therapy and treatment for opportunistic diseases. As of the end of 2005, 2,098 individuals were receiving antiretroviral therapy.

Health Promotion

The health promotion strategy is geared to reinforcing the notion that health interventions are not the sole responsibility of the health sector. The National Health System encourages community participation in problem-solving and engages and trains different social stakeholders to identify needed programs. These programs are underpinned and endorsed by government proposals, as part of a cross-sector, interdisciplinary approach designed to improve the quality of life for the general public. There are undergraduate and graduate-level course offerings in health promotion and health education including scientific disciplines designed to help ensure excellence in all health services. School programs geared to encouraging younger generations to embrace healthy lifestyles have helped the Cuban population develop a comprehensive general culture of personal and public health protection. The health-promoting schools model has triggered a national movement, with all educational establishments aspiring to qualify as health-promoting schools, with all ensuing benefits. There are great expectations for a number of national projects with predominantly educational and behavioral components, such as programs for the prevention and control of tobacco addiction and cancer, sexual and reproductive health education, nutrition and oral health programs, and programs for the prevention and control of sexually transmitted infections and HIV/AIDS. The social communication media and other national structures are actively involved in the mapping out and attainment of individual, family, and community counseling goals promoting healthy lifestyles and self-care.

Provincial Health Promotion and Education Centers, municipal government structures, and people's councils, as the embodiment of community participation in problem-solving processes, help tailor programs to the features and capabilities of each region and ensure the efficient and effective use of available resources for the development of a health culture designed to promote the population's general welfare.

Human Resources

The National Health System has 70,594 physicians (62.7 per 10,000 population), including 33,769 family physicians providing health care coverage for 99.4% of the population. It also has 10,554 oral health specialists (9.4 per 10,000 population), 110,483 high-level technicians (25,022 with degrees in nursing), and 158,726 mid-level technicians (64,440 nursing technicians).

Since 1959, 87,690 physicians, 12,937 oral health specialists, 29,983 registered nurses, and 501 specialists in health technology have graduated from national study programs. The first 1,610 ELAM-CARIBE project physicians graduated in 2005. New training models in the areas of nursing and health technology helped add 15,142 basic technicians to the country's health services. There are polyclinic-based programs of study at the primary health care level in the fields of general medicine, oral health, nursing, health psychology, and health technology in all 169 municipalities as part of the "universalization" of education. To date, 2,242 National Health System units have been transformed into university centers. The first year of the program of study in general medicine was initially offered in 2004 at 75 university polyclinics in 42 municipalities around the country and immediately expanded to 113 polyclinics in 68 municipalities the following year. A six-task research project referred to as the University Polyclinic Project was designed as an evaluation tool for this process. Emerging training programs for nurses were started up in eight provinces, open to candidates at the 9th, 10th, and 11th grade levels, using health facilities as simulators.

The performance of interns (sixth year medical students) in their various rotations has been excellent.

Human resources training programs in the health sector include students from more than 80 countries. Training programs for the so-called "New Latin American Physician" have been started up in the provinces of Havana City (Cojímar), Cienfuegos, and Holguín.

The establishment of eight distance master's degree programs has made it possible for vast numbers of health professionals, not only from Cuba, but also from Venezuela and 13 other Integrated Health Program countries, to work toward graduate degrees. There are a total of 60 health science specialties (51 medical specialties, 5 oral health specialties, 3 nursing specialties, and 1 health psychology specialty). Training in basic biomedical science, public health and epidemiology, and biostatistics specialties is available to all health professionals. A total of 66,051 health professionals were trained as specialists over the period between 1962 and 2005. Graduates of the Latin American School of Medicine (ELAM) were given an opportunity to do their graduate work in the comprehensive general medicine specialty and, later, complete a second specialty. Thus far, 13,449 students in 14 different specialties have graduated from the *Haciendo Futuro* (Shaping the Future) program for the training of specialists to meet basic staffing needs for the operation of Integrated Diagnostic Centers in Venezuela and fill human resources shortages in Cuban health services. Right now, there are 574 Cubans holding doctoral degrees in the health sciences, with work already underway on a degree-training strategy to turn out another 25,000 doctoral recipients in the next few years.

A total of 700,000 health workers in all occupational categories graduated from the In-Service Training Program between December of 2002 and the end of 2005.

Health Supplies

There are ample supplies of locally manufactured drugs, including immunobiologicals and in vitro diagnostic products (diagnostics), and drug regulation activities are being constantly stepped up. Cuba has domestic regulations governing good manufacturing and quality control practices for these products in line with WHO norms, as well as for biologicals, radiopharmaceuticals, cytostatics, metered-dose inhalers, clinical laboratories, blood banks, and human clinical research. The State Drug Quality Control Center certifies compliance with these standards. There are health licensing systems in effect for all establishments manufacturing, distributing, importing, and exporting pharmaceutical and diagnostic products, under which corresponding licenses are issued based on inspections for compliance with recommended practices in each case and are subject to revocation based on post-marketing surveillance data.

The country participates in the WHO Certification Scheme on the Quality of Pharmaceutical Products Moving in International Commerce and requires and issues all corresponding certifications for marketing permits.

The regulatory process with respect to medical equipment begins with the manufacturer's registration and includes product evaluation and registration. This has led to better quality imports and has helped boost demand for domestic products as part of the major technological retrofitting effort by the National Health

System. Manufacturer compliance is monitored by means of audits and other procedures. There are ongoing quality programs, and the adoption at the country level of ISO 13485:2003 (an international system standard for medical devices) is currently under consideration.

Research and Technological Development in Health

The Health Science and Technology System consists of 32 science and technological innovation entities, 21 of which are recorded in the Ministry of Science, Technology, and Environment Registry as accredited research centers and institutes, four as scientific-technological service centers, and seven as scientific-technological development units. Health research is conducted by medical education centers at the higher education level (4 medical universities; 21 schools of medicine, 4 schools of dentistry, 4 nursing schools, and 4 schools of health technology; the National School of Public Health; the Latin American School of Medicine; 35 medical affiliates; 169 municipal university centers; and 273 university centers, including 113 university polyclinics in 68 municipalities). There are 11 "branch" scientific/technical programs at the country level. As of the end of 2005, there were 48 national, 580 branch, 216 provincial, and 1,448 health facility-based research and development and technological innovation projects. Each hospital and municipality has a scientific council in charge of approving projects prior to their submission to the appropriate authority.

The National Health System includes 574 scientific doctoral recipients, 1,413 registered researchers, and 11,502 medical professors. The average age of researchers is 39.

The country has 12 PAHO/WHO Collaborating Centers for health and housing, research and education on human reproduction, occupational health, nutrition and food safety, integrated diabetes care, viral diseases, dengue research and control, reference and research on tuberculosis and mycobacteria, medical malacology and biological vector and host control, child growth and development, development of the virtual health library, and development of genetic approaches to health promotion. It encourages health technology evaluation and impact assessments of new National Health System programs and services.

The Virtual Health Library and the Cuban scientific and technical information network known as Infomed are recognized throughout the Region of the Americas and around the world for their intensive and creative use of information and communication technology. The emphasis on the social use of these resources and on the development of local information flows helping to bring scientific knowledge to bear on the health sector is pivotal. The use of scientific and technical data has become an integral part of continuing professional education and training activities nationwide. All health districts have Virtual Health Library servers, and more and more training activities at all levels are being conducted via the Virtual University. Infomed is the product of a joint effort by health institutions and health workers and is constantly expanding in line with the growing numbers of virtual communities of practice and knowledge established on Infomed Web sites. This process is still in the developmental stage, but is slowly crystallizing. A scientific article recently published in the *Journal of Medical Internet Research* refers to Infomed as "a model of interest for integrating health care information, research, education, and services delivery."

Health Sector Expenditures and Financing

Total national public health spending in 2005 was up 24.2% from the previous year, or by over 507.2 million pesos, outstripping the average annual growth rate, which had been 9.6% up until 2000. A breakdown of expenditures showed wage costs up by 452.8 million pesos, accounting for 65.0% of total spending, along with spending on drugs and related supplies, which consumed 308.0 million pesos (4.0% more than the previous year). The 3,193,300,000 peso appropriation for this important sector in 2006, topping the 2005 appropriation by 23.0%, was designed to help continue to strengthen health care services in search of excellence. Personnel costs amounted to 255.6 million pesos, or 64.4% of total spending, with a 2,007,700,000 peso wage bill. The approved budget for drugs and related supplies came to 347.0 million pesos. Of the total budget, 1,309,200,000 pesos (41.0%) were allocated to primary health care, 85.5 million pesos (2.6%) to scientific and technological development, and 1,660,500,000 pesos (52.0%) to hospital care. The remainder, which came to 138.0 million pesos (4.4%), was allocated to items such as administration and other system support centers.

Technical Cooperation and External Financing

Cuba has continued strengthening its international relations in the area of health cooperation, particularly as regards aid and assistance to other countries (Table 5). A number of new cooperation plans and programs were implemented over the five-year period 2001–2005, such as *Barrio Adentro* (Inside the Barrio) in Venezuela and *Operación Milagro* (Operation Miracle), designed to cure visual impairments in the Cuban population, as well as in Venezuelan patients and those from other Latin American and

TABLE 5. Number of aid workers sent abroad, by year, Cuba, 2001–2005.

Year	Number of aid workers
2001	4,317
2002	6,190
2003	17,033
2004	26,014
2005	31,243
Total	84,797

TABLE 6. Breakdown of external funding for National Health Services, Cuba, 2005.

Agency	Commitment (US$)
PAHO/WHO	771,000.00
UNFPA	308,000.00
UNICEF	826,922.00
UNDP/UNAIDS	20,000.00
UNDP/Government of Japan	284,837.00
UNDP/AIDS	2,879,081.81
WFP	258,000.00
Grants	21,963,943.00
Total	27,311,783.81

Caribbean nations. As of December 2005, a total of 172,306 operations had been performed on patients from several Latin American countries as part of the *Operación Milagro* project. The Henry Reeve Brigade was formed in 2005 in the wake of Hurricane Katrina's devastation of New Orleans, Louisiana, U.S.A., to provide emergency medical assistance following natural disasters and combat disease outbreaks, as an expression of solidarity by the Cuban people. The country has also continued to send medical teams on missions under the Integrated Health Program and other cooperation programs. Cuba has helped train health personnel at the Latin American School of Medicine, whose stu-

dent body currently includes youths from Africa, Latin America, the Middle East, and the United States.

Cuban physicians dispensing health care in other countries also serve as instructors, training local physicians to ensure continuity of care.

In addition to its technical cooperation resources, as indicated in Table 6, funding and grants from international organizations and NGOs came to a total of more than US$ 27 million, which facilitated the implementation of numerous projects.

Bibliography

Cuba, Oficina Nacional de Estadísticas. Anuario Estadístico. La Habana: ONE; 2005.

Cuba, Ministerio de Ciencia, Tecnología y Medio Ambiente. Informe Anual. La Habana: CITMA; 2005.

Cuba, Ministerio de Economía y Planificación. Informe Anual. La Habana: MEP; 2005.

Cuba, Ministerio de Salud Pública. Informe de Programas; 2005.

Cuba, Instituto Nacional de Recursos Hidráulicos. Plan Nacional de Acción, 2005.

World Health Organization. International Statistical Classification of Diseases and Related Health Problems (ICD-10). Geneva: WHO; 2003.

DOMINICA

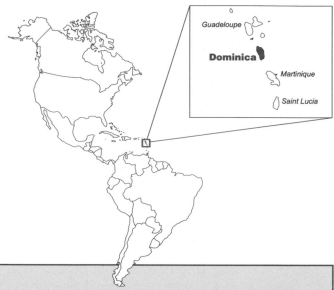

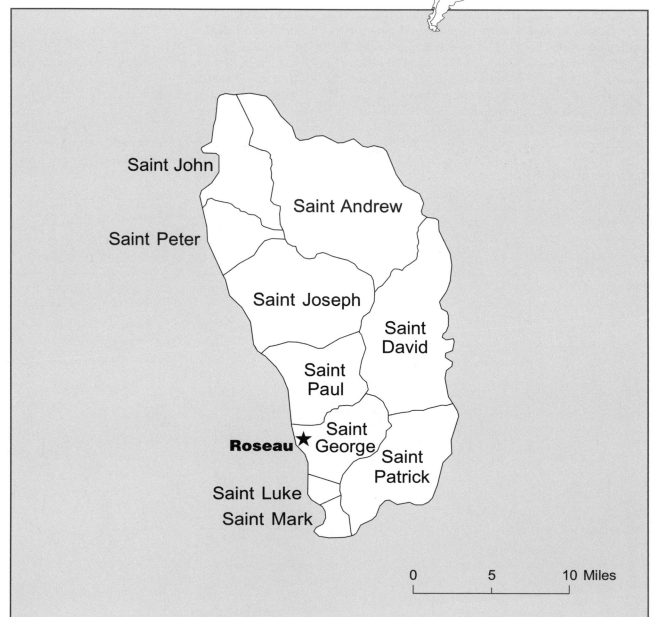

The Commonwealth of Dominica is the northernmost and largest (790 km^2) of the Eastern Caribbean's Windward Islands. It lies between the French islands of Guadeloupe to the north and Martinique to the south. Dominica's climate is humid, tropical, and marine, characterized by little seasonal variation between wet and dry seasons.

GENERAL CONTEXT AND HEALTH DETERMINANTS

The country's pronounced high rainfall during the wet season contributes to its lush vegetation. The island's topography is rugged: it has steep, luxuriant rain-forest mountains; deep, river-incised valleys; and tree-covered hills that produce and sustain pristine rivers, perennial streams, and tumbling mountain waterfalls. The country has great diversity of flora and fauna. Dominica's relatively undisturbed and rugged landscape, extensive forest, and pristine fresh- and seawater ecology have made the country a much-sought tourist destination for nature lovers and environmental adventure seekers. Visitors mainly come from elsewhere in the Caribbean, the United States of America, and Europe. Arrivals increased by 54.2% between 1993 and 2004, reaching 80,087 in 2004. Cruise liners brought 383,614 passengers in 2004.

Dominica attained political independence from England in 1978, retaining a political organization based on the British Parliament, multi-party democracy. The official language is English, but most of the population speaks a patois "kweyol," a blend of African and French linguistic structures.

Dominica is subdivided into ten parishes—Saint Andrew, Saint David, Saint George, Saint John, Saint Joseph, Saint Luke, Saint Mark, Saint Patrick, Saint Paul, and Saint Peter. The capital, Roseau, is located in Saint George.

Social, Political, and Economic Determinants

Dominica's economy has traditionally been based on agriculture. Agriculture—especially banana cultivation—represented 20.0% of the Gross Domestic Product in 1997 and 17.7% in 2003. Recent global and regional events have contributed to a decline in agriculture, particularly in banana cultivation. Dominica pursues a free-market and liberal economy.

During 2004, the economy grew an estimated 3.57%, compared to 0.1% growth in 2003. As a way to address ongoing economic difficulties, the Government strengthened its fiscal policy and generated additional external financial support. Once fiscal efforts took effect, the Government embarked on a more comprehensive reform program to foster growth and move towards debt sustainability, keeping debts from growing further as an essential condition for economic stability.

The Government cut salaries by 5% as a short-term measure designed to reduce employment, which it subsequently intends to follow with a more comprehensive public service reform.

These measures notwithstanding, inflation (as measured by the Annual Consumer Price Index) rose by 2.5% in 2004, compared to 1.4% in 2003. Cost increases were recorded in fuel and electricity (7.5%), housing and utilities (4.7%), educational expenses (3.5%), and food (2.8%).

In 2001–2005, the dominant sector in the country's economy was government services, followed by tourism, construction, manufacturing, and agriculture. Tourism contributed 10%–12% of the Gross Domestic Product (GDP) and more than 30% of foreign exchange earnings—three times the earnings from banana cultivation. Nominal per capita GDP (at factor cost) in 2001 was around US$ 3,100 (US$ 2.72 = EC$ 1). The Government's finances deteriorated sharply in the period, giving rise to a precarious fiscal situation (1).

In 2003, GDP was about US$ 257.6 million, the same as it was in 1998. Government services; agriculture, fishing, and forestry; wholesale and retail trade; bank and insurance; and transport contributed about 22%, 18%, 13%, 11%, and 8% of GDP in 2003, respectively.

Household poverty in Dominica was 29% in 2002, which means that about 7,000 households were assessed as poor in the country. Approximately 11% of households—about 2,500—were considered indigent. Persons living in these households had average annual per capita expenditures under US$ 740 and could not meet their basic food needs. Households which adequately met their basic food needs but were unable to meet all their non-food needs (average per capita expenditure at least US$ 740 but less than US$ 1,251) were classified as poor and represented 18% of all households, or 4,400 households.

Dominica's poverty is largely income poverty, mainly triggered by the rapid decline in revenue from banana cultivation that affected all sectors of the economy. However, the fact that the poverty head count (39%) is higher than the level of extreme poverty (15%) suggests that the majority of Dominicans can meet their basic needs. The poverty gap, which measures the extent to which the income of poor households falls below the poverty line, is 10.2%. Therefore, 4,300 households, on average, have expenditures below the poverty line (2). The Carib population is one of the poorest in Dominica, with prevalence rates of poverty and indigence well above the average for the country as a whole.

Dominica's Country Poverty Assessment revealed that one factor that contributed to the level of poverty and loss of well-being, especially among the indigent, is the abandonment of the elderly to fend for themselves, a situation often exacerbated by sickness and disability. While conditions for the indigent are substandard, attitudes among the relatively poor are very optimistic. Many strongly decry the idea that they are poor, which shows a clear lack of correlation between income poverty and well-being for this group.

According to the country's 2002 Social Protection Review—designed to establish the characteristics, scope, and causes of poverty and identify ways to reduce it—the gender gap in the workforce was particularly high among the poor—49% of poor women were unemployed, compared to 33% of poor men. The unemployment rate decreased for both sexes between the 1997 and 1999 Labor Force Survey periods and the 2001 Population and Housing Census. Men's participation in the labor force was higher for all age groups throughout this same period. The participation rate for both sexes decreased over the years, with women's rates decreasing more sharply. The construction and agriculture sectors were largely dominated by males.

In the reporting period, there was serious overcrowding in the prison, and inadequate diets for persons with hypertension and diabetes, potential communicable disease transmission (such as HIV/AIDS and tuberculosis), inadequate human waste disposal, and inadequate bedding also were problems of concern there.

Dominica achieved universal primary and secondary education in 2005, and the country has already attained the Millennium Development Goal target of having equal access to all levels of education for boys and girls.

In 1998–2004, the net primary-school enrollment for boys was higher than for girls (83% and 79%, respectively). In 2002, three tertiary institutions merged into Dominica State College. More women than men took advantage of tertiary-education opportunities, which, over time, has led to a significant growth in the number of women in senior management positions in both the private and public sectors. More men sought vocational training, and more male students were granted Government scholarships.

In 2001, 4.5% of households did not have access to safe drinking water, down from 7.5% in 1991.

In 2004, the Dominica Water and Sewerage Company, Ltd. (DOWASCO), which manages the country's public water supply systems, operated 43 individual water supply systems that provided drinking water to 100% of urban areas and approximately 95% of rural areas; the remaining 5% of the rural population is served either by private systems or by other means such as springs, rivers, or rainwater catchments.

Per capita water consumption in 2004 was estimated at 40 to 60 gallons per person per day. DOWASCO managed approximately 13,285 service connections and 549 standpipes; 78.30% of the total service connections were metered. Approximately 60% of the population has access to all Solid Waste Management Corporation solid waste storage, collection, and disposal services; the remaining 40% use composting, reuse, burning, and burying. A small percentage of households still practice open dumping. Littering is a major problem island-wide, affecting the lower reaches of rivers and costal zones.

Before 1980, some 60% of households had access to a solid waste collection system. Coverage increased to about 70% in 1991 and to approximately 84% by 2001. The increased coverage of water and excreta disposal facilities resulted in a decrease in helminthiasis and typhoid among the population.

In 2005, 213 restaurants and 229 food establishments seating fewer than five patrons (snackettes) were registered with the Environmental Health Department—70.9% and 66.4%, respectively, achieved satisfactory (70% and above) test scores on the restaurant inspection form.

Dominica is under constant threat of floods, and hurricanes are common in the late summer months. In 2003, there was a major landslide in the south of the country that claimed the lives of two utility workers working in the area. In late 2004, Dominica was hit by an earthquake measuring 6.0 on the Richter scale that caused US$ 33 million in damages, particularly in the country's north. Portsmouth Hospital sustained significant damage. Three months later, aftershocks measuring 4.7 and 5.4 on the Richter scale continued to cause stress among residents.

Demographics, Mortality, and Morbidity

According to the 2001 Population Census, the country's population was 69,625. End-of-year population estimates for 2003, however, put the figure at 70,340, comprising mainly African descendents, with a small population (4.0%) of indigenous Kalinago (or Carib) people, the last surviving tribe of the first Caribbean people, and one of the poorest population groups in the country. The 2001 Population and Housing Census recorded a noninstitutional population of 14,539 for the city of Roseau.

In estimates provided by the U.S. Bureau of the Census, the population 0–20 years old made up a smaller percentage of the total population in 2005 (36%) than in 1991 (45%). The biggest difference in the distribution of the total population between 1991 and 2005 was in the age group 20–60 years of age, which accounted for 46% in 1991 and 54% in 2005. In the age group 60 years old and older little difference is seen: 1991, 11%; 2005, 10%. Differences by sex across age groups were small, with the largest being in the group 60 years of age and older in 2005—males, 9% and females, 12%; in 1991 the proportions in this age group were males 10% and females 13%. Over the last decade, the population has shifted toward the middle of the age-sex pyramid, where an increased impact from chronic diseases is expected. (See Figure 1.) Population density decreased slightly by 2.1% from 95 per km^2 to 93 per km^2.

Life expectancy at birth in 2005 was 74.7 years (71.7 for males and 77.7 for females). A decade ago, in 1990–1995, life expectancy was estimated at 67.8 years (males, 63.5, and females, 69.8). The total fertility rate remained the same between 1991 and 2001 at 3.0 children per woman. The average childbearing age was 27.2 years in 1991 and 27.8 years in 2001. There were 2 maternal deaths between 2000 and 2003, both due to complications of pregnancy. On average, there were 1,137 live births per year in the same period. The crude birth rate averaged 16.1 per 1,000 persons in the same period. The crude death rate averaged 7.7 per 1,000 population; 2,172 deaths were reported.

In 1991–2001, 8,866 persons emigrated from Dominica, continuing the ongoing decline in the population. The most popular destinations for Dominicans were other Caribbean countries and the United States. Outmigration surges in Dominica following hurricanes, as skilled workers lose their jobs and seek better employment conditions elsewhere. On the other hand, outmigration in 2003–2005 slowed, with only 23 persons moving to other countries in 2003. Reduced population outflow and an increase in the birth rate continued to stimulate population growth (3).

In 2003, the ten leading causes of death (and the number of deaths) were malignant neoplasms (123), hypertensive diseases (86), heart diseases (71), diabetes mellitus (31), cerebrovascular diseases (26), diseases of the respiratory system other than acute respiratory disease (20), acute respiratory infection (16), conditions originating in the perinatal period (14), other diseases of the digestive system (13), and diseases of the nervous system except meningitis (12).

In 2002, there were 39,728 visits to district medical officers or to family nurse practitioners. In general, females made twice as many visits (67.7%) as males (32.3%). The largest discrepancy is found in the age group 30–64 years of age, in which the number of visits by females is threefold that by males.

Most children 0–5 years old (88.8%) had normal nutritional status in 2001; 9.4% of children in this age group were obese. In 1990–2000, 30% of the adult population was overweight (body mass index [BMI] between 25 and 30); 17.9% was obese (BMI over 30). The main causes of morbidity and mortality were influenced by such lifestyle practices as inadequate physical activity, poor diet, and poor management of life events, including driving practices. The toll from motor vehicle accidents and violence and injuries increased in Dominica.

HEALTH OF POPULATION GROUPS

Children under 5 Years Old

According to the 2001 census, children 0–4 years old represented 8.9% of the population—4.5% male and 4.4% female.

During 2001–2005, 7,010 births were recorded. The crude birth rate in 2001 was 17.2 per 1,000 population; in 2004 it was 15.1 per 1,000. The infant mortality rate in 2001 was 19.8 per

FIGURE 1. Population structure, by age and sex, Dominica, 1991 and 2005.

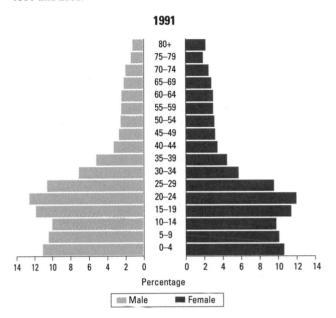

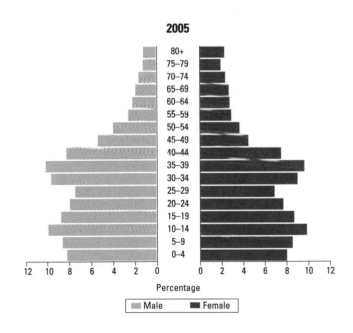

1,000 live births; in 20003, 18.9; and in 2004, 13.1. The neonatal mortality rate was 14 per 1,000 live births in 2001 and 10.3 per 1,000 in 2004. The perinatal mortality rate ranged from 26.8 per 1,000 births in 2001 to 28.8 per 1,000 in 2004; 70 perinatal deaths were recorded during the period. The major causes of death in this age group were respiratory distress syndrome of the newborn (19) and fetal malnutrition (33). Deaths in children under

1 year old ranged from 21 in 2000 (11 males, 10 females) to 14 in 2004. The death rate among children under 5 years old was 4.3 per 1,000 in 2001 and 2.8 per 1,000 in 2004.

The prevalence of low birthweight was 8.2% in 2002, compared to 9.8% in 2004. Immunization coverage for the EPI diseases is over 99%. A few parents refused vaccination on religious grounds.

The breast-feeding initiation rate is 98.7%, and 33.9% of women breast-feed exclusively up to six months; 74% of babies are being introduced to the family cooking pot at six months.

In 2004, 10% of the population was identified as being obese.

According to the National AIDS Program, there were no infants born to HIV-positive mothers between 2003 and 2004. In 2005, there was a 20% increase in the acceptance of HIV testing by pregnant women, which led to the identification of three HIV-positive infants; they are awaiting final testing to determine their status.

Children 5–9 Years Old

Two deaths were recorded in this age group in 2003. Two children in this age group were orphaned by AIDS during the period.

Adolescents 10–14 and 15–19 Years Old

According to the 2001 census, the age group 10–14 years old represents 10% of the population, 4.9% male and 5% female; the 15–19-year-old age group represented 9.6% of the population, with equal distribution of the sexes.

The birth rate for mothers under 20 years of age remained constant, ranging from 43 per 1,000 in 2001 to 44 per 1,000 in 2005. There are no special adolescent health services within the government health system. Condoms were the only contraceptive method available at government health facilities. The fertility rate for adolescents 15–19 years old was 140 births per 1,000 adolescent girls in 2001.

There were 37 deaths in this age group during 2000–2004, with the highest number (11) occurring in 2002. The main causes of death were motor vehicle accidents (6), malignant neoplasms (unspecified) (6), diseases of the circulatory system (6), assault homicides (3), suicide (1), and maternal deaths (1). Data collected from the Global Youth Tobacco Survey (GYTS) in 2004 revealed that 34.4% of secondary- and primary-school students smoked (39.4% of boys and 26.4% of girls).

In 2000, the percentage of students who had ever smoked was 33%–41%; in 2004 it was 25%–38%. According to the data, about 27% of the students surveyed in 2000 and 2004 had started smoking before age 10 years. Current tobacco use and age at initiation remained constant for both survey years. Data for 2004 revealed that there was a 20% susceptibility to smoke among female respondents.

Almost 60% of the students were exposed to tobacco smoke in public places, and there was an increase in the number of students who indicated that one or more of their parents smoked.

Adults 20–59 Years Old

In 2003, there were 32,518 persons 20–59 years old, representing 47.6% of the total population—the highest percentage of any age group: 16,018 females and 16,500 males. That same year, females in this age group comprised 22.8% of the total population, while males accounted for 24.9%.

The total fertility rate in 2001 was 2.5 children per woman and the mean age at childbearing was 27.8 years.

According to the 2004 report of the Dominica Planned Parenthood, the most commonly dispensed contraceptives were condoms, oral contraceptives, and injectible contraceptives. Pap smear screening at this facility declined from 605 clients in 2000 to 363 in 2004.

The sharp decline in the use of spermicides, which do not protect against acquiring HIV/AIDS, might be related to an increased awareness about how to prevent HIV/AIDS.

New acceptors of contraceptives increased 7%, rising from 244 in 2003 to 261 in 2004, and the number of visits for contraceptives increased from 4,248 in 2003 to 4,566 in 2004, an increase of 7.5%.

Prenatal care is available to all prenatal clients. Most births were attended by trained health professionals at health institutions. All prenatal care clients also are offered HIV testing: between 2003 and 2005, there was a 20% increase of persons accepting testing.

The leading causes of death in this group include malignant neoplasms (22%), hypertensive disease (15.4%), and heart disease (12.7%), followed by diabetes mellitus and cerebrovascular disease. According to the 2003 Chief Medical Officer's report, there were 12 AIDS-related deaths (10 males and 2 females), representing 2.1% of all deaths.

During 2000–2003, there were 397 deaths in this age group, 250 males and 147 females.

Older Adults 60 Years Old and Older

At the end of 2003 there were 9,610 persons (4,183 males, 5,427 females) in this age group; 1.2% of the total population was over 85 years of age.

There were 1,574 deaths in this age group in 2000–2003, 746 males and 828 females. Research conducted in 2002 by the Dominica Council on Aging revealed that the main social problems facing older people are financial instability, lack of social support, loneliness among those who do not have extended families, and lack of community activities involving older persons. The main health problems experienced were hypertension, arthritis, eye problems, and diabetes. Women were more aware of their problems and seemed to have greater interaction with the health sector. Both males and females used prescription medications as well as home-prepared traditional medicines.

Family Health

Between 1991 and 2001 (the last two census years) the number of households increased by 10.9%. The Social Protection Review recorded that 34.0% of poor households were headed by single females; 45% of poor people lived in households headed by females.

According to the 2001 Population and Housing Census, female-headed households accounted for 36.9% of households. The average number of persons per household was 3.1, with 3.3% of households comprising more than eight persons. This includes 311, or 42.5%, households headed by women and 421 households headed by men. A higher number of women than men had lost spouses (3:1). This group of women continued to provide for themselves or depended on family, public support, or remittances, particularly those who had no pension earnings. More than three-quarters of heads of households only had primary-level education, although education levels in the country have improved for the population as a whole.

Teenage pregnancy levels were of great concern throughout the reporting period; rates were high despite the availability of free contraceptives at clinics. Drug use and alcohol consumption, especially among young males, also is a cause of concern.

The Disabled

Data for 2002–2005 show that a higher proportion of poor households had someone with a serious disability. Without social or family support, old age was clearly linked to ill health, disability, and poverty. The 2001 Population and Housing Census analyzed the percentage of the population with various disabilities: sight disabilities, 773 persons (1.1% of the total population); hearing disabilities, 320 persons (0.5%); speech disabilities, 475 persons (0.7%); mobility impairments, 1,131 persons (1.6%); mental retardation, 556 persons (0.8%); and all other disabilities, 1,046 persons (1.5%).

Indigenous Peoples

The Carib population is young, with 70% being under 30 years old and 40% being younger than 19 years old. Carib economic activity centers around mixed subsistence farming, craft production, and boat building. Caribs live in a demarcated area called the Carib Territory on the country's northeast. The prevalence of poverty among the Carib population was 70% in 2002 with almost half being indigent. The Caribs represent about 2,800 (4%) of the total population and 7% of the poor population (4).

In 2001, only 2.3% of the Carib population had water supplied by in-house connections, 4.6% had flushing toilets, 56.3% had electricity, and 63.0% used wood for cooking. These data reflect important disparities in living conditions between the Carib population and the rest of the population.

The Government is working to improve the efficiency, effectiveness, and quality of services delivered to the Carib popula-

tion. Plans include making an ambulance service available throughout the Carib Territory; improving the physical infrastructure of health facilities; implementing health promotion activities to foster healthy behaviors; and improving mental health through programs to prevent substance abuse including abuse of alcohol. The Carib Territory is served by two health districts, Castle Bruce and Marigot.

The 2002–2006 National Health Plan acknowledges the specific health needs of the Carib people. In 2001, specific initiatives were launched for the prevention of helminthiasis and tuberculosis in that community.

HEALTH CONDITIONS AND PROBLEMS

COMMUNICABLE DISEASES

Vector-borne Diseases

The vector-borne diseases of significance in the country are **dengue** and **leptospirosis**. The 2004 report of the Chief Medical Officer underscores vector control activities in light of troubling house indices[1] that ranged between 18% and 25%. There were five reported cases of dengue between 2001 and 2004. There have been no indigenous cases of **malaria** since the 1960s; the *Anopheles albimanus* mosquito, however, is endemic in three health districts. There was an increase in the number of persons who migrated to Dominica from countries where malaria is endemic.

Vaccine-preventable Diseases

In 2001–2005, the vaccination coverage of antigens included in Dominica's national immunization schedule (BCG, OPV, DPT, and MMR) varied between 95% and 100%. **Hepatitis B** vaccine is administered to health workers and others considered to be at high-risk for the disease. *Haemophilus influenzae* type b and hepatitis B vaccines are administered to infants only through the private sector. As part of the program to eliminate **rubella**, in 2000, 21,172 (94.1%) persons between 12 and 35 years old received the MMR vaccine, and 99.2% of children 1–5 years old received their second dose of MMR vaccine. Vaccination coverage of administered antigens in 2005 is as follows: BCG, 98%; MMR, 100%; third dose of OPV, 98%; and DPT, 98%.

The last case of **poliomyelitis** was in 1980 and the last case of measles in 1991. In 2000–2001, there were no reported cases of rubella, **congenital rubella syndrome, diphtheria, pertussis, tetanus,** or **neonatal tetanus**.

Dominica's immunization program was comprehensively evaluated and a five-year plan was developed in 2004.

---

[1]Percentage of houses infested with *Aedes aegypti* larvae or pupae.

Intestinal Infectious Diseases

Gastroenteritis was the leading intestinal infectious disease in the country in 2001–2005, with 740 reported cases in children under 5 years old and 712 cases among persons 5 years old and older. There were no deaths from gastroenteritis in the period. Five cases of **typhoid fever** were diagnosed in the period.

Chronic Communicable Diseases

The incidence of **tuberculosis** did not increase in the period, and protocols were developed to facilitate case finding, contact tracing, and treatment regimens.

The influenza incidence rate in 2003 was 605 per 100,000 population, an increase from 2002.

HIV/AIDS and Other Sexually Transmitted Infections

Between 1987 and 2005, there were 305 persons who tested positive for HIV infection. Eight persons tested positive for HIV in 2003, although this figure should be interpreted carefully because voluntary HIV testing was not widespread in the country. Men 25–44 years old were the most affected by HIV/AIDS. Since 1987, 120 persons have died from AIDS-related diseases. In 2005, 34 patients attended the infectious disease clinic: 23 males and 11 females. Among 37 patients who undertook CD4 tests, 24 started antiretroviral treatment. Men having sex with men were the leading mode of transmission of the disease.

The number and percentage of positive VDRL blood samples increased each year from 1998 to 2001.

Zoonoses

There was one confirmed case of **leptospirosis** in 2005.

NONCOMMUNICABLE DISEASES

Metabolic and Nutritional Diseases

Diabetes was a major public health problem, taking a heavy toll on morbidity and mortality. In 2002 diabetes accounted for 5,253 clinic visits at district health centers, 13.2% of total clinic visits. In 2004, there were 12,623 clinic visits for diabetes. In 2002–2003, anti-diabetic drugs accounted for 14.4% of the total drug budget. Among males, 50% of visits for diabetes were in the age group 65 years old and older; for females, 50% of visits occur in the age group 60 years old and older.

Cardiovascular Diseases

Cardiovascular diseases accounted for 474 deaths in 2000–2004. The male-female breakdown was 234 cases (49%) in males and 240 cases (51%) in females. Gender differences were greater in cerebrovascular diseases, where females accounted for 61% of total deaths. In 2004, 27,676 clinic visits were made for **hypertension**.

Malignant Neoplasms

Between 2000 and 2004, there were 583 deaths due to malignant neoplasms, for an annual average of 117 deaths. Males represented 60.9% of all deaths from malignant neoplasms. The sites most frequently reported were stomach, 75 (13%, 36 males and 39 females); prostate, 163 (28%); breast, 39 (7%); digestive system, 46 males and 45 females (16%); and cervix, 70 (12%). Persons 70 years old and older accounted for 46% of all deaths due to malignant neoplasms; 267 persons (172 males and 95 females) in that age group died from this cause. The number of deaths due to prostate cancer increased from 29 in 2000 to 41 in 2004.

OTHER HEALTH PROBLEMS OR ISSUES

Mental Health

The stigma and discrimination associated with mental illness remained a major concern. There were 318 admissions for mental illness in 2003. Inpatient psychiatric treatment is available in the capital, at the Princess Margaret Hospital.

Dominica's 2002 Action Plan for Health Care contemplates the establishment of a national health program designed to reduce the incidence of mental health disorders.

Oral Health

Oral health services are offered through a network of public and private health care facilities. The Government operates seven public health dental clinics that offer preventive, curative, and restorative dentistry.

RESPONSE OF THE HEALTH SECTOR

Health Policies and Plans

The Government's mission is to promote the well-being of all citizens of Dominica by providing preventive, curative, health promotion, and rehabilitation services that adhere to acceptable standards and that are affordable and sustainable.

The 2002 Strategic Plan continued to provide the framework for health. The Plan seeks to engage multisectoral collaboration and participation, strengthen partnerships between the public and private sector, and involve individuals and civil society. The Plan is flexible to accommodate adjustments in accordance with emerging challenges.

In 2002, the Hospital and Health Care Facility Act Number 21 was revised. A draft medical act was finalized and presented to the Minister of Health in 2003, but still awaited enactment by the end of 2005. A food safety act was drafted and national consultation held in 2005. Other draft regulations submitted for enactment covered construction; disposal of offensive matter; air, soil, and water pollution; and health standards for hairdressers.

In 2004, the Cabinet approved Dominica's participation in the WHO Framework Convention on Tobacco Control, and in June of that year, the country became a signatory and party to the Convention.

Health Strategies and Programs

The Government provides a social safety net through public assistance and social security programs, as well as through broader efforts to ensure that the poor have access to basic education and health care. The Government also is committed to introducing a national health insurance program.

The 2002 Action Plan for Health Care in Dominica targeted several objectives: for women's health, to reduce morbidity, disability, and mortality among women 25–59 years old; for reproductive health, to promote responsible sexual behavior and parenting skills among adults; for men, to reduce morbidity and mortality among young adult and elderly males; for the elderly, to implement programs enhancing their well-being; for persons with disabilities, to provide better access to health and public services; for marginalized persons, to harness resources for healthy living by fostering community involvement; for the Carib population, to improve efficiency and quality of services; and for oral health, to ensure improved oral health status in specific target groups. In terms of mental health, the objective is to establish a national health program to reduce the incidence of mental health disorders in relation to the demand and supply of drugs. In food and nutrition, the objective is to improve the nutritional status of pregnant and lactating mothers and infants. In the control of communicable diseases, the goal is to reduce morbidity and mortality.

Organization of the Health System

Health care delivery in Dominica is channeled into primary health care and social health care.

For delivering primary health care, Dominica is divided into seven districts, which, in turn, are grouped into two administrative regions, as follows: Region I includes Roseau, St. Joseph, and Grand Bay health districts, and Region II includes Portsmouth, Marigot, Castle Bruce, and La Plaine health districts. Each district has four to seven Type I health clinics and one Type III health center. Type I health clinics serve between 600 and 1,000 persons living within 5 mi of the clinic (there are 44 Type I clinics in the country as a whole). Type III health centers serve as the district's administrative headquarters. The clinics are the first point of contact with the health services and serve to minimize demand pressures on the health center and the secondary care hospital. Two district hospitals also are part of the primary health care system—Marigot and Portsmouth hospitals—which offer limited inpatient services. Primary care services are fully decentral-

ized and are provided free of charge. The direct managerial responsibility for the delivery of primary health care services lies with the Director of Primary Health Care and the Senior Community Health Nurses. The management of the district is supported by a multidisciplinary health team of professionals.

Secondary care services are provided at the 225-bed Princess Margaret Hospital. Secondary care is not decentralized; a payment schedule has been established for medical care at the hospital, indicating fees for specialist medical officers' visits, technical procedures, and hospitalization. There is a well-organized referral system in place: cases that cannot be managed at the primary level are referred to Princess Margaret Hospital.

Private health care services are limited to outpatient care provided by individual practitioners, who usually work on a part-time basis. The great majority of private practitioners work in the capital.

As of this writing, Dominica has no national health insurance scheme, although there are several procedures to assist patients who cannot afford medical care costs. The Social Welfare Division has a yearly budget of about EC$ 1 million to operate a program that provides a living allowance to those registered and to cover the cost of CT scans for those who qualify. A special allowance is given to severely handicapped children. Some mechanisms are in place at the Ministry of Health and Social Security and at Princess Margaret Hospital to, within some limits, assist financially or reduce/waive bills in order to facilitate access to medical services by the less fortunate. Dominica Social Security ensures short-term and long-term benefits for those who are employed in terms of pensions, sick leave benefits, and maternity grants.

Public Health Services

The Health Information Unit, led by the National Epidemiologist, is responsible for the surveillance of the country's health issues, especially communicable diseases. In 2001–2005 the Unit strengthened the surveillance of diseases of public health interest. Significant in this regard is the establishment of the National Public Health Surveillance and Response Team, which is a multisectoral, multidisciplinary committee that meets and reviews surveillance data on a weekly basis and initiates coordinated responses to perceived health threats. With technical assistance from the Caribbean Epidemiology Center (CAREC), the Canadian Society for International Health (CSIH), the United States Peace Corps, and the Japanese Overseas Cooperation Volunteers, the Unit upgraded surveillance systems for communicable diseases, including making improvements in computerized systems that have greatly improved analysis and reporting capability.

The Dominica Water and Sewerage Company, Ltd. (DOWASCO), is charged with controlling and managing the country's public water supply systems.

The Ministry of Health's Environmental Health Department ensures the delivery of safe, potable water. In 1990–2000, 924 water samples were submitted for analysis. On average, 85% of the samples analyzed were within standards established by WHO's Guidelines for Drinking Water. The Environmental Health Department also encourages the use of sanitary methods to slaughter animals sold for human consumption. In 2003–2004, 3,624 animal carcasses were inspected, 362 cattle, 554 pigs, 30 goats, and 2,696 poultry. The Department also held food hygiene education programs in all districts to inform registered food handlers on aspects of food sanitation, including personal hygiene, proper food handling techniques, methods of food storage, and the Hazard Analysis Critical Control Point Program (HACCP).

The Solid Waste Management Corporation, created and regulated by the 2000 Solid Waste Management Act, is responsible for storing, collecting, and disposing solid waste in the country. The Corporation's overall objective is to monitor and facilitate the effective implementation of a solid waste program by supervising and cocoordinating environmental health programs associated with solid waste management at the district and national levels.

In the second semester of 2003, the Solid Waste Management Corporation undertook joint educational activities with the Environmental Health Department and local village councils in Castle Bruce, LaPlaine, Tete Morne, Ma Bouche, Cochrane, Vieille Case, Wesley, and Woodfordhill. Residents were shown improved solid waste management practices and were informed on plans to serve these areas with curbside collection of solid waste. Several communities, especially along Dominica's northeast and east, remain without any established collection system. In areas where curbside collection had been implemented, residents complained of infrequent waste collection by the Solid Waste Management Corporation, which led to litter in the roadsides and, in some cases, the creation of indiscriminate dump sites.

Government laboratories performed both clinical and public health functions. They provided services in microbiology, serology, clinical chemistry, histopathology and cytology, hematology, and blood banking. Basic laboratory services are free of charge for residents who have been referred from the district clinics or from the accident and emergency department. HIV testing requested by a physician within the public sector is free of charge for pregnant women. In 2003, 32,581 persons were referred by both the public and private sector. There were 847 blood donors.

The Office of Disaster Preparedness coordinates disaster management.

Individual Care Services

Type I clinics are staffed by resident staff/midwives or primary health care nurses. Clinics offer a range of services, such as maternal and child health services, including deliveries and immunizations; medical care; cancer screening; diabetic and hypertensive clinics; health education; dental services; home visits; and environmental monitoring.

Type III health centers are staffed by a resident doctor, a family nurse practitioner, an environmental health officer, a pharmacist, community health nurses, registered nurse midwives, a dental therapist, and support staff. Type III health centers offer more complex and comprehensive services than Type I clinics; specialists in psychiatry and ophthalmology also provide services at the centers.

Princess Margaret Hospital, the only referral hospital providing secondary care in the country, provides inpatient, ambulatory, specialist, and diagnostic services, including internal medicine, dialysis, gastroenterology, surgery, ophthalmology, otolaryngology, obstetrics and gynecology, dermatology, psychiatry, pathology, oncology, radiology, anesthesiology, and pediatrics. Tertiary services are provided by visiting consultants or are acquired in neighboring islands; the cost is borne by the patient.

Health Promotion

The Government has adopted a health promotion strategy that is being carried out through various intervention programs.

The Healthy Community Initiative, for one, harnesses resources to foster healthy living by involving the community in a partnership with officers of governmental and nongovernmental departments and agencies, and with citizen volunteer groups. As part of this effort, the health promotion resource center provided training to district officers and community leaders; conducted community assessments and profiles for villages in all districts in preparation for healthy community initiatives; formulated terms of reference for the district coordinating committee to oversee the implementation and evaluation of the Healthy Community Initiative; established a partnership with the Ministry of Tourism to work on healthy tourism initiatives; and received a financial commitment from the Ministry of Tourism to grant Healthy Community Awards in 2005.

Human Resources

The Ministry of Health and Social Security undertook to substantially increase retaining health personnel by 2006. As part of this endeavor, the salary scales for specific occupations or professions, such as nurses, teachers, and computer technicians, were reviewed in 2004. Following the results of the salary survey, a decision was taken to increase by at least 15% the gross earnings of wage-earners and salaried employees that fell below US$ 110.00 per month. In 1999–2001, 20 mental health nurses were trained; they are the main channel for change within the health system.

Health Supplies

The Government strives to improve public- and private-sector pharmaceutical services. Dominica continued to participate in the Organization of Eastern Caribbean States Pharmaceuticals Procurement Service. Essential medicines are free of charge at district pharmacies but some medicines may not be available, depending on the current stock at the Central Medical Store.

Better Health Care Access for the Kalinago People

Dominica's 3,000 Kalinago (also known as Caribs) live in eight villages scattered in a 3,700-acre area along the country's east coast. The community's economic activity has centered on subsistence farming and boat building. Although Caribs represent only 4% of the total population, they account for 7% of the population living in poverty. Their access to health services has been less than that of the general population. The Government's 2002–2006 National Health Plan acknowledges the health needs of the Carib people, and the Government is working to improve the efficiency and quality of services for this population. In addition, nongovernmental agencies also provide health services to the Kalinago. One of these is The Salybia Mission Project, which is supported by the work of medical students from de School of Medicine of Ross University and is led by a physician who is himself a Carib.

Health Sector Expenditures and Financing

The Government of Dominica's total recurrent expenditure budget for 2005/2006 is EC$ 226.8 million. The Ministry of Health and Social Security's recurrent expenditure budget is EC$ 29.8 million, 14% of the total annual budget.

The lion's share of the budget for health goes to salaries and other benefits to nurses, doctors, and administrators. Personal emoluments and allowances accounted for 80% of the total health budget; the remaining 20% is for goods and services. Purchases of medical supplies represent the largest expenditure item under goods and services.

In terms of budgetary allocation by service, Princess Margaret Hospital accounted for more than half of the health recurrent budget (50.49%). Primary health care, which includes the Type I clinics and Type III health centers in the seven health districts, plus two hospitals in the northern part of the country, took up 26.21% of the total health budget.

Princess Margaret Hospital was broken down into seven programs, each with its own allocated budget. Administration accounted for 4%, general maintenance for 3%, medical services for 70%, support services for 8%, safety and security for 1%, the psychiatric unit for 8%, and laboratory services for 7%.

The Ministry's budget also consists of capital budget. The Government of Dominica's total capital expenditure budget for 2005/2006 was US$ 30 million. The Ministry of Health receives US$ 3.3 million, or 11% of the total capital budget. From the US $3.3 million allocated to health, US$ 2.3 million represents grant funds, US$ 0.8 million represents a loan, and US$ 0.1 million is government financing.

Technical Cooperation and External Financing

Technical and financial support came from the Global Fund to Fight AIDS, Tuberculosis, and Malaria (GFATM); the United Kingdom Department of International Development (DFID); the Clinton Foundation; Harvard Medical School; the Caribbean Epidemiological Center; the American Red Cross; the European Union; the Caribbean Development Bank; the Brenda Strafford Foundation, and the Pan American Health Organization. Cuba, Nigeria, the Republic of China, and Taiwan also provided assistance.

References

1. Caribbean Development Bank; Government of the Commonwealth of Dominica. Country Poverty Assessment. Final Report. Volume 1 of 2: Main Report. June 2003. Halcrow Group Limited; 2004.
2. Caribbean Community, Programme on Social Gender and Environment Statistics. Dominica Social Indicators and Millennium Development Goals (SIMDG) 2006.
3. Demographic Statistics, No. 4, 2004.
4. Government of the Commonwealth of Dominica. Medium Term Growth and Social Strategy (GSPS), April 2006.

DOMINICAN REPUBLIC

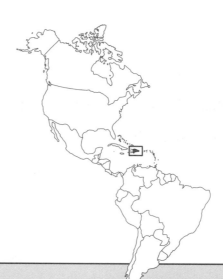

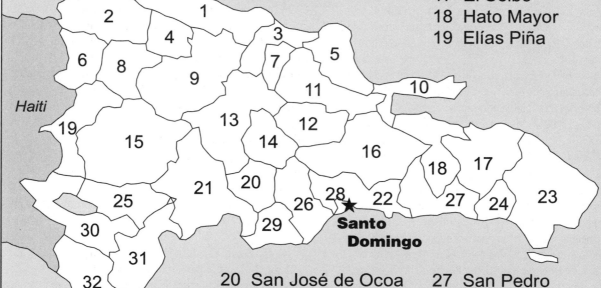

1 Puerto Plata
2 Monte Cristi
3 Espaillat
4 Valverde
5 María Trinidad Sánchez

6 Dajabón
7 Salcedo
8 Santiago Rodríguez
9 Santiago
10 Samaná

11 Duarte
12 Sánchez Ramírez
13 La Vega
14 Monseñor Nouel
15 San Juan
16 Monte Plata
17 El Seibo
18 Hato Mayor
19 Elías Piña

Haiti

Santo Domingo

20 San José de Ocoa
21 Azua
22 Santo Domingo
23 La Altagracia
24 La Romana
25 Bahoruco
26 San Cristóbal

27 San Pedro de Macorís
28 National District
29 Peravia
30 Independencia
31 Barahona
32 Pedernales

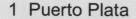

0   25   50 Miles

The Dominican Republic takes up two-thirds of the island of Hispaniola and lies between the Caribbean Sea and the Atlantic Ocean. The country has a land area of 48,442 km², an estimated population of 8.9 million (1), and a population density of 176.8 persons per km². It has 31 provinces and the National District.

GENERAL CONTEXT AND HEALTH DETERMINANTS

Social, Political, and Economic Determinants

Economic growth in the 1990s, fanned by the increase in free zones and tourism, had little impact in terms of social investment and human development (2), since urban poverty rose from 47.9% in 1992 to 66.5% in 1999 (3), and public investment in education, health, and social welfare remained unchanged at 5% of the gross domestic product (GDP) (2).

The country has high levels of inequity in income distribution. In 2002, the wealthiest 20% obtained 53% of gross income, while the poorest 40% obtained just 14% (4). The 2003 banking fraud caused losses of 20% of GDP, a fiscal deficit, and inflation of 42.7%. As a result, the country faced an economic and social crisis that affected the free zones, tourism, and construction, and the GDP was 0.4%. Between 2002 and 2005, GDP grew from US$ 21.7 billion to US$ 29.3 billion. In 2003, public social spending was 6.8% of GDP; public spending on health was 1.9% of GDP in 2002, 1.7% in 2003, and 1.2% in 2004. It has been estimated as 1.9% of GDP for 2006 (2, 5). In 2000, 54% of the population lived in poverty and 28% in extreme poverty. In 2003, these figures rose to 62% and 33%, respectively (6).

Presidential elections were held in May 2004. A new Standby Arrangement was signed with the International Monetary Fund in January 2005 which, coupled with other monetary policy measures, helped to overcome the economic crisis and contributed to GDP growth. The economy was affected by high costs, shortfalls in electric power supplies, and high oil prices.

The Dominican Republic is one of the seven pilot countries in the United Nations Millennium Project. The Presidential Commission on the Millennium Goals and Sustainable Development identified the interventions needed and the estimated cost of attaining the Millennium Development Goals (MDGs). That exercise became the foundation for the development of national and provincial plans, and for the mobilization, redirection, and rationalization of resources.

Between 2003 and 2004, unemployment rose from 17% of the economically active population to 18.4%, falling to 17.9% in 2005 (7). That year, women earned 30% less than men on average, and in some cases as much as 41% less, particularly in the free zones and in the tourism sector (7), even though women had higher levels of education (8). GDP grew by 9.3%, although the few jobs created were of poor quality, offered no social protection, and paid low wages (5).

Between 1996 and 2002, the percentage of people without elementary education fell from 20% to 10%, and the percentage of those with secondary and university education rose from 25% to 30%. Illiteracy among persons 10 years old and older declined from 15% to 13%, with women scoring better (12%) than men (13%), and rural areas scoring worse (19%) than urban areas (9.5%). Among children who enter first grade, 50% complete just four years of primary school, 22% complete eight years, and 10% complete secondary school (2). Teenage pregnancies are a contributing factor to school dropout rates; 19% of teenage girls have children and 23% have been pregnant at some point (8).

The percentage of the population with an average daily food intake of ≤ 1,900 kcal (undernourished) fell from 27% in 1990–1992 to 25% in 1999–2001. If this trend continues, the Millennium Development Goal of reducing the percentage of persons who suffer from hunger by half between 1990 and 2015 can be attained.

Between 2002 and 2005, the number of tourists rose from 2,308,869 to 3,088,247. In 2005, the National Health and Tourism Commission was established, which prepared a national plan to enable the country to continue being a healthy tourist destination.

Demographics, Mortality, and Morbidity

The country is in a stage of demographic transition. Between 1993 and 2002, the reduction in mortality, birth, and fertility rates led to changes in the population's age structure, with growth in the urban population (from 35% to 63.6%) also being a contributing factor (Figure 1).

The annual growth rate in 2005 was 1.8%. Between 2000 and 2005, the general fertility rate fell from 2.8 births per woman to 2.7; the gross birth rate declined from 24.5 per 1,000 population to 23.3 per 1,000; the gross mortality rate dropped from 5.9 per 1,000 population to 5.7; and life expectancy from birth rose from 68.6 years (70.8 for women and 66.5 for men) to 70 years (72.4 for women and 67.8 for men) (9).

FIGURE 1. Population structure, by age and sex, Dominican Republic, 1993 and 2002.

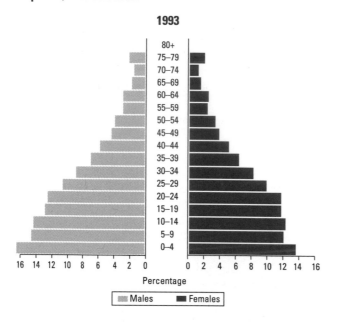

1993

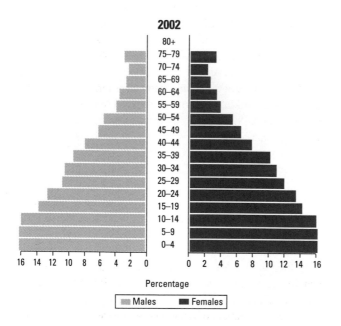

2002

The pace of emigration picked up between 1992 and 2002. Estimates place the number of Dominicans who live abroad at between 1 million and 1.5 million and the number of foreigners in the country at 1.2 million. There is a tendency toward the feminization of emigration; most emigrants come from urban areas (2).

Table 1 shows selected indicators of mortality. Underreporting was estimated at 52.5% in 2000 and at 50% in 2005 which,

TABLE 1. Estimated mortality rates, general, maternal, and for selected age groups, Dominican Republic, for years and periods between 1992 and 2005.

	Year or period	Rate
Maternal mortality (per 100,000 live births)	1992–2002	178[a,b]
	2005	120[c]
Infant mortality (per 1,000 live births)	2002	31[b]
	2005	32[c]
Neonatal mortality (per 1,000 live births)	1997–2002	22[a,b]
Postnatal mortality (per 1,000 live births)	1997–2002	10[a,b]
Mortality in children under 5 years old	1997–2002	38[a,b]
General mortality (per 1,000 population)	1995–2000	5.9[a,d]
	2000–2005	5.7[a,d]

[a]Average for the period.
[b]ENDESA, 2002.
[c]DIGEPI, 2005.
[d]ONAPLAN, 1999.

coupled with problems in filling out death certificates, affects the quality of the data.

Diseases of the circulatory system continue to be the leading cause of death in both sexes. External causes continue to rank second among men, with a proportional increase. Deaths from malignant neoplasms increased proportionally in both sexes. In 2002, external causes and communicable diseases had the largest impact on premature deaths (Table 2). The highest percentage of potential years of life lost in persons under 70 years old corresponded to external causes (24%).

HEALTH OF POPULATION GROUPS

Children under 5 Years Old

Infant mortality tended to decline, mainly driven by a drop in postneonatal deaths. The trend in neonatal mortality remained unchanged and is related to the poor quality of care during delivery and the perinatal period. The mortality rate among children under 5 years old tended to fall.

In 2002, reported infant mortality accounted for 9.9% of all deaths. Among children under 1 year old, the risk of dying fell from 45 per 1,000 live births in 1987–1992 to 38 per 1,000 in 1992–1997, and to 31 per 1,000 in 1997–2002. In 2002, the neonatal mortality rate was estimated at 22 deaths per 1,000 live births. In 2005, the leading causes of death in newborns were neonatal sepsis, respiratory distress syndrome, and prematurity, while the main causes of postneonatal death were septicemia, diarrhea and gastroenteritis, and pneumonia.

TABLE 2. Mortality by broad groups of causes and percentage of total deaths by cause, by sex, Dominican Republic, 1990 and 2002.

	Men		Women	
	1990	2002	1990	2002
1	Diseases of the circulatory system (27%)	Diseases of the circulatory system (29%)	Diseases of the circulatory system (33%)	Diseases of the circulatory system (35%)
2	External causes (17%)	External causes (21%)	Communicable diseases (17%)	Malignant neoplasms (16%)
3	Communicable diseases (16%)	Malignant neoplasms (14%)	Malignant neoplasms (11%)	Communicable diseases (12%)
4	Malignant neoplasms (9%)	Communicable diseases (11%)	External causes (6%)	Conditions originating in the perinatal period (8%)
5	Conditions originating in the perinatal period (5%)	Conditions originating in the perinatal period (7%)	Conditions originating in the perinatal period (5.5%)	External causes (7%)
6	Other diseases (25%)	Other diseases (18%)	Other diseases (28%)	Other diseases (23%)

Mortality in children 1–4 years old was 1.6% in 2002 and the risk of dying fell from 14 per 1,000 in 1987–1992 to 11 per 1,000 in 1992–1997, and to 7 per 1,000 in 1997–2002.

Breast-feeding is becoming increasingly less common. Only about 3.8% of children 4–5 months old are breast-fed exclusively (8) and 46% of newborns are given other food before being breast-fed.

Children 5–14 Years Old

In 1990–2002, mortality in children 5–14 years old declined; this age group represented 2.8% of deaths in 1986 and 1.6% in 2002.

Between 1993 and 2002, stunting among schoolchildren 6–9 years old dropped from 19% to 8%, with a larger decline in rural areas (11%) than in urban ones (8%). No up-to-date data are available on micronutrient deficiencies. The prevalence of goiter in schoolchildren was 5.3% and, based on urinary excretion of iodine, 74% of the school-age population (6–9 years old) was at risk. In 2002, urinary excretion of iodine fell to 34.3%. In its most recent assessment (1997), the Oral Health Program reported a decayed, missing, and filled (DMF) teeth index of 5.0 (10).

In 2002, 18% of children and adolescents 5–17 years old worked (27% of boys, 9% of girls), with the percentage being higher in rural areas (20%) than in urban ones (17%); 90% began working before age 15 and they mainly worked in service industries (11).

Adolescents 15–19 Years Old

In 2002, the percentage of teenage (15–19 years old) pregnancies was 23% (28% in rural areas and 21% in urban areas). Among pregnant teenagers, 64% had no education. One out of every five women who died from causes related to pregnancy or delivery was an adolescent, and the obstetrical risk among girls 15–19 years old was much higher than that for women 20–34 years old. In 2002, the fertility rate among urban adolescents was 104 per 1,000 girls; in rural areas, the rate was 145 per 1,000. Of adolescent pregnancies, 43% were unwanted (8).

According to a survey, some 25% of students 13–15 years old had used tobacco at some point (24.4%) in 2004. The prevalence of use (within 30 days prior to the survey) was 18%. Prevalence was higher among boys (21.5%) than among girls (14.2%). Fewer than 10% of youths use tobacco in the form of cigarettes; 12.3% use other forms, such as chewing tobacco, snuff, cigars, cigarillos, and pipes (12).

Adults

Absolute and proportional mortality in this group declined. In 2002, external causes were the leading cause of death in the group (44.2%), followed by communicable diseases (21.6%), mainly AIDS and tuberculosis.

Among women 15–49 years old, AIDS was the main cause diagnosed, accounting for 18.3% of deaths; traffic accidents ranked second; and undetermined events third. Among men 15–49 years old, the largest number of reported deaths were caused by traffic accidents and by undetermined events. AIDS ranked third.

In 2002, the general fertility rate was 3.0 births per woman (2.8 in urban areas and 3.3 in rural areas). Between 22% and 25% of women in the different age groups had their first child before they were 18 and between 40% and 45% did before they were 20; 75% had had at least one child by the time they were 25 (8). In 2002, 70% of married women used some form of contraception.

The maternal mortality rate did not decrease, which is related to the quality of medical care. The leading causes of maternal mortality are toxemia, hemorrhages, and abortion.

Older Adults (60 Years Old and Older)

The population older than 60 years old represents 6.1% of the country's total population and is increasing (*13*). Diseases of the circulatory system were the leading cause of death in this group, followed by malignant neoplasms, communicable diseases, and external causes. Between 70% and 80% of older adults live in urban areas; fewer than 10% live alone.

Workers

Occupational accidents climbed from 3,313 in 2004 to 3,717 in 2005 (54% in the National District, 23% in Santo Domingo West, and 3% in La Romana). Of all occupational accidents, 6.3% occurred in the services sector, 21.7% in manufacturing, 17.5% in industry, 13.1% in commerce, and 11.2% in construction; 79.4% of accidents occurred in the workplace, while 20.6% were traffic accidents that took place going to or from work.

Persons with Disabilities

In 2002, 4.2% of the population had some kind of disability; 51% were men and 60.5% lived in urban areas. The most frequent disabilities were motor limitations (24%), blindness (14%), and mental retardation (12%) (*14*).

HEALTH CONDITIONS AND PROBLEMS

COMMUNICABLE DISEASES

Vector-borne Diseases

Malaria mainly affects rural and suburban populations in provinces classified as having a high risk of transmission. The native parasite species is *Plasmodium falciparum*, which is sensitive to chloroquine. Outbreaks are associated with internal and external migration of temporary agricultural and construction workers; with the occurrence of natural phenomena that cause heavy rainfall, mainly hurricanes; and with limited response capacity at the local level. Between 2000 and 2004, the number of malaria cases averaged 1,490 a year, increasing to 2,354 in 2004 (incidence rate of 27.5 per 100,000 population). In 2005, there were 3,837 cases reported (64% in men); 10–49-year-olds were the most heavily affected (73.8% of cases); and 75% of cases were reported in rural areas.

Dengue fever is endemic, and all four serotypes circulated between 1997 and 2004. In 2003, 6,268 probable cases were reported (nearly double the 2002 figure), 2,478 in 2004, and 2,949 in 2005. This last figure represented an incidence of 29 per 100,000 population. Seropositivity to the dengue virus among probable cases was 45%. Of the dengue cases, 82% were reported as hemorrhagic dengue, causing 18 deaths, for a case fatality rate of 21.9%. The virus was not isolated in 2005.

Vaccine-preventable Diseases

In 1998–2001, there was an outbreak of **measles**, which required the activation of control activities; no cases have been reported since 2002.

In October 2000, there was an outbreak of **poliomyelitis** caused by virus 1 derived from the oral poliomyelitis vaccine (OPV) (14 cases), which mainly occurred in the country's central portion. The outbreak's possible cause was the circulation of the vaccine-derived virus in populations with low coverage or an immunodeficient patient. No cases of poliomyelitis have occurred since 2002. The pentavalent vaccine was introduced in 2001 and the triple viral vaccine (MMR) in 2004, which provides coverage for the 10 most importance vaccine-preventable diseases.

In 2005, vaccination campaigns were conducted against **tuberculosis**, **hepatitis B**, and poliomyelitis, with coverage of 100%, 92.5%, and 85.8%, respectively.

The incidence of invasive infections caused by *Haemophilus influenzae* type b (Hib) fell after the pentavalent vaccine was introduced. Cases of meningeal tuberculosis, **neonatal tetanus**, **whooping cough**, and **diphtheria** have been reported in the infant population, and **tetanus** cases have been reported in adults. During 2004–2005, there was a major outbreak of **diphtheria** in children under 15 years old. In 2004, seven cases of rubella were reported in the country.

Intestinal Infectious Diseases

Diarrheal diseases are a significant public health problem, mainly in children under 5 years old; between 2,000 and 5,000 cases a week are reported each year. In 2002, according to the National Demographic and Health Survey (ENDESA), 14% of children under 5 had suffered from diarrhea two weeks before the survey, with the hardest hit groups being children between 6 and 23 months old (24%) and infants under 6 months old (12.7%). In 1997–2002, mortality from this cause in children under 5 declined, dropping from 58 to 38 per 1,000 live births.

Chronic Communicable Diseases

Tuberculosis is a priority public health problem. The estimated incidence rate is among the highest in the Region, with close to 85 new cases per 100,000 population (7,000 new cases every year); 3,500 of those cases are pulmonary, confirmed by positive bacilloscopy (BK+) (*15*). Some cases were resistant to first-line antituberculotic drugs. The incidence rate varied from 57 per 100,000 population to 54 per 100,000 between 2003 and 2004 and climbed to 58.4 per 100,000 in 2005. The cure rate rose from 46% in 2000 to 85% in 2005, thanks to an increased reliance on the use of the Directly Observed Treatment, Short-course (DOTS) strategy. Tuberculosis is the leading opportunistic infection in people with HIV (close to 12.2%) and in 2005, 8.6% of TB cases were HIV positive.

Leprosy remains at under 1 case per 10,000 population. In 2002–2004, the annual incidence was 0.2 per 10,000 population and in 2005 it was 0.17, although there are still 13 municipalities whose rates remain higher than 1 per 10,000. Yuma, Bayaguana, Barahona, and Oviedo are among the municipalities with the highest rates. Between 2002 and 2004, 30 cases were reported in Santo Domingo, 13 in the National District, 15 in San Pedro de Macorís, 12 in Barahona, and 10 in Monte Plata (*13*).

Acute Respiratory Infections

In 2005, acute respiratory infections were the main cause of outpatient consultation by the general public; in 2001–2002, they were among the five leading causes of death. Every year, between 6,000 and 10,000 cases are reported each week. In 2002, acute respiratory infections accounted for 80% of morbidity among the population. In children 1–4 years old, acute respiratory infections were the leading cause of illness and reason for medical care in health establishments. According to the 2002 National Demographic and Health Survey, 19.6% of children under 5 years old had suffered from coughing accompanied by breathing difficulties in the two weeks prior to the survey. Of those children, 60% received medical care, with the figure declining with an increase in the child's age and the mother's level of education.

The probable cases of **meningococcal disease** reported in 1995–2002 averaged 132 a year and the incidence rate ranged from 0.5 to 2.9 per 100,000 people. During 2002–2004, there was a reduction in the number of cases reported (55% of the number expected). During 2005, 39 probable cases were reported.

HIV/AIDS and Other Sexually Transmitted Infections

HIV/AIDS is one of the leading causes of death in the population 15–49 years old. An estimated 88,000 people are infected with HIV, including adults and children. The disease's transmission is linked to tourism, the existence of free zones, the high migratory flow, port establishments, and poverty. The main form of transmission is heterosexual sex. Among 15–29-year-olds, seroprevalence is higher among women than men. According to the 2002 National Demographic and Health Survey, more than 50% of women do not think they are at risk of contracting the infection and 9% of sexually active women suffered from sexually transmitted infections in 2001. In 2002, HIV prevalence was 1% (1.1% for men and 0.9% for women) and in the substandard *bateyes* neighborhoods (the poorest areas in the country) it was 5% (4.7% for men and 5.2% for women). In 2003, an estimated 23,000 women 15–49 years old were HIV positive (*16*). The prevalence among pregnant women was 1.4% in 2004 and 2.3% in 2005.

In 2004, **hepatitis B** had a seroprevalence of 1.5% and **syphilis,** of 1%. The prevalence was higher in 15–29-year-olds, among the rural population, and among women with five-to-eight years of schooling.

Zoonoses

In 2005, there were 707 cases of **leptospirosis** reported; samples were taken in 588 cases and 50 were confirmed in the laboratory. The provinces that reported the largest number of probable cases were Santiago (42%), the National District (14%), Espaillat (13.3%), Puerto Plata (6.8%), and Santo Domingo (4.4%). The *L. pomona* serotype was most frequently found, affecting mainly men 20–39 years old who worked in agriculture. There were 21 deaths in the provinces of Puerto Plata and Santiago Rodríguez.

Between 2002 and 2004, there were four cases of human **rabies,** and it is believed that one of them was caused by an insectivorous bat (there are no hematophagus bats). The country has been free from human rabies since 2005; rabies in animals occurred in the Dajabón zone bordering Haiti and in the country's eastern part, mainly in San Pedro de Macorís, where there are large wild populations of mongooses, which are the second most important animal population after dogs implicated in rabies transmission. The country is free from **avian influenza, foot-and-mouth disease**, **bovine spongiform encephalopathy, anthrax**, and **African swine fever**.

In November 2002, 152 blood samples were taken from live migratory birds and resident birds in the Los Haitises (61) and Bahoruco (91) National Parks, which were studied at the United States Centers for Disease Control and Prevention (CDC) in Atlanta. Nine were positive for **flavivirus**, and **West Nile virus** antibodies were identified in two of the samples from Los Haitises. The virus was not isolated in the birds' tissue cultures, which indicates that the transmission occurred while they were alive.

NONCOMMUNICABLE DISEASES

Metabolic and Nutritional Diseases

Between 1996 and 2002, chronic malnutrition among children under 5 years old fell from 11% to 9%; the highest rate was among 12–23-month-olds, and was higher for boys (10%) than girls (8%) (*8*). The figure for acute malnutrition was 2% and for global malnutrition, 5%.

Among children with no schooling, 15% presented with chronic malnutrition, as did 13% of children whose mothers did not complete primary school. In urban areas, 8% of children presented with chronic malnutrition and 4% presented with global malnutrition. In rural areas, the figures were 11% and 7%, respectively. According to the 2002 national census, the height-for-age deficit, or chronic malnutrition, among schoolchildren 6–9 years old nationwide was 8%, which is lower than the level reported in 1993 (19%). The highest levels were reported in the provinces of Elías Piña (15.7%), La Vega (12.7%), and Bahoruco (11.2%). The provinces with the lowest levels of chronic malnutrition were La Altagracia (2.8%) and Santiago, La Romana, and San Pedro de Macorís (4%) (*17*). The prevalence of obesity among people over age 50 was 30%.

Cardiovascular Diseases

Diseases of the circulatory system accounted for more than 10% of medical consultations and more than 6% of emergency cases in the country's health establishments. Close to 80% of nonobstetric hospital admissions among adults are for cardiovascular problems (*18*). A study on cardiovascular risk factors conducted on 6,400 persons between 1996 and 1998 and adjusted to the 2004 classifications indicated a prevalence of obesity of 16.4%, and diastolic hypertension of 21.8% (33% in women, 36.7% in men, and 30% in people over 50). According to the study, 65% of people with hypertension were not receiving treatment, 55% had a family history of hypertension, 9.1% had hypercholesterolemia, and 24% had a cholesterol count higher than 200 mg/dl. The study also showed that 20% smoked at the time of the study and 22% had stopped smoking.

Malignant Neoplasms

Reported mortality from this cause increased in 2004 (*15*). **Breast cancer** ranked first in frequency (25.9%), followed by **cancer of the cervix** (21.2%) and prostate cancer (7%).

OTHER HEALTH PROBLEMS OR ISSUES

Disasters

The country's location exposes it to tropical storms and cyclones. Floods are the most frequent natural disaster, and they occur year round. The most vulnerable regions lie close to watersheds of the Yaque del Norte, Yaque del Sur, Yuna, and Soco rivers, and the riverbanks in the cities of Santo Domingo and Santiago. The country suffered from the effects of hurricanes David (1979), George (1998), and Jeanne (2004). Severe earthquakes have occurred in some parts of the country, as well as drought caused by poor watershed management, deforestation, and global climate change. Close to 70% of the population lives in high-risk areas vulnerable to emergencies and disasters.

Acute respiratory infections and acute diarrheic diseases are some of the illnesses associated with natural disasters. Injuries are also an important cause of morbidity during disasters, as are malaria and dengue fever.

Violence

According to the 2002 National Demographic and Health Survey, 9.5% of women 15–49 years old stated that they had suffered from physical violence. The figure was higher for women 20–29 years old (11.7%).

Environmental Pollution

Water pollution from untreated liquid waste, growing difficulties in the adequate management and treatment of the increasing quantity of solid waste, and the degradation of air quality due to particulate-matter pollution are the main environmental problems, and they are linked to urban and industrial growth. Agricultural-chemical contamination is a serious problem in areas where production is intensive. Between 1994 and 2005, carbon dioxide emissions increased from 15,000 tons to 16,649 tons.

RESPONSE OF THE HEALTH SECTOR

Health Policies and Plans

Two important laws were passed in 2001, mapping out a new direction for the national health system: the General Health Act (Law 42-01) and the Social Security Act (Law 87-01). The General Health Act separated the system's service delivery, leadership, and financing functions and created the National Health Council as the national body coordinating health matters. The act laid the groundwork for regulating public health and health-risk matters and charged the Secretariat of Public Health and Social Welfare with formulating the national 10-year health plans and performing essential public health functions. Law 87-01 created the Dominican Social Security System and established the sources and mechanisms for financing the national health system's assistance. The Dominican Social Security System is funded by prepaid, mandatory contributions, based on ability to pay and employment status; it guarantees public insurance for the poor and indigent population. Law 87-01 introduced family health insurance, which is mandatory and universal and entails a basic health plan for the three established regimes: contributive, subsidized contributive, and subsidized. In 2003, the Labor Risk Administration was created to prevent and cover occupational accidents and work-related diseases. By December 2005, the Labor Risk Administration had registered 30,531 companies and enrolled 1,218,737 workers (*19*).

Health Strategies and Programs

The national health system encompasses two subsystems: the individual care subsystem and the collective health subsystem, both operating under the direction of the Secretariat of Public Health and Social Welfare. The individual care subsystem is composed of public and private health service providers, with each sector organized into primary, secondary, and tertiary care levels. Public services are organized into Regional Health Services. These function as autonomous entities, have their own legal status, are duly accredited as health care providers with the Dominican Social Security System are financed by the National Health Insurance, and deliver health care under the basic health plan. The collective health subsystem includes a series of public health programs and programmatic networks aimed at health promotion and the prevention and control of priority health problems; their management is deconcentrated to provincial health directorates that are financed by the Government. The programs to prevent and control priority problems need to be reformed and financed: many operate with international donations and loans and receive Government funding in national emergencies, which limits their sustainability and effectiveness. Most programs of the Secretariat of Public Health and Social Welfare have had a vertical, centralized structure. Measures to decentralize and bolster the response capability of the provincial health directorates are being carried out, as a way to enable them to better manage programs in their geographic areas.

Organization of the Health System

In November 2002, family health insurance under the subsidized insurance regime was introduced in Region IV, in the country's southeastern portion, which entailed one of the largest transfers of funds and responsibilities to the local level. The subsidized regime has been extended to Regions III, IV, and V, with approximately 400,000 members in these four regions (4.3% of the total population). The introduction of family health insurance for the contributive regime (including public and private employees and their dependents) has been postponed nine times in the last five years by the National Social Security Council, preventing the estimated 30% of the population eligible for this regime from gaining access to the basic health plan. Implementation of family health insurance is being studied at the highest political level.

After the Secretariat of Public Health and Social Welfare was reorganized, that agency was charged with delivering collective health services through the general preventive programs established by the new legal framework. It will gradually shed the service delivery function, but not before organizing and empowering the regional health services so that they can link health care establishments and levels into a network and assure that persons can receive comprehensive and continuous care. The source of financing will be the per capita contributions paid by the Dominican Social Security System, through management contracts between public suppliers and the National Health Insurance.

The Secretariat of Public Health and Social Welfare chairs the National Health Council, the National Social Security Council, the National Health Insurance Council, the Presidential HIV/AIDS Commission, and the Executive Commission for Health Sector Reform, which are strategic venues for consolidating various leadership aspects (management and regulation, financial modeling, oversight of insurance, and harmonization of service delivery) and for directing efforts in accordance with national health priorities and objectives.

The National Health Council is chaired by the Secretariat of Public Health and Social Welfare (the highest national health authority) and encompasses the President's Technical Secretariat, the Secretariat of Labor, the Secretariat of Education, the Dominican Social Security Administration or the body in charge of social security (the National Social Security Council), the Military Medical and Health Corps of the Armed Forces and the National Police Force, the Dominican College of Physicians, the Association of Private Clinics and Hospitals, the Autonomous University of Santo Domingo, the Dominican Municipal League, the drinking water and sewerage sector, duly-accredited nongovernmental organizations working in the field of health, the Secretariat of the Environment and Natural Resources, the National Higher Education Council, and any other institution that the Secretariat of Public Health and Social Welfare or the National Health Council may invite temporarily.

The Dominican Social Security System is organized according to a separation of functions: the Government is responsible for direction, regulation, financing, and supervision, while the functions of insurance, risk management, and service delivery are the responsibility of duly-accredited public or private entities, or joint entities.

The National Social Security Council is composed of the Secretary of Labor, who chairs it, the Secretary of Public Health and Social Welfare, the Vice-President, the Director General of Social Security, the Director of the National Relief and Housing Administration, the Governor of the Central Bank, a representative of the Dominican College of Physicians, and representatives of other health professionals and technicians, employers, and employees.

The health sector is mixed in nature, with participation by public and private institutions and nongovernmental organizations. The Secretariat of Public Health and Social Welfare is still the main provider of public services and is organized along central, regional, and provincial levels. The central level encompasses the Secretary's Office, which is supported by five undersecretariats: Administration, Collective Health, Individual Care, Technical (in charge of institutional planning, health accounts, information systems, etc.), and Social Welfare. At the provincial level, the Secretariat has 30 provincial health directorates (one per province). The province of Santo Domingo and the National District are organized into eight health area directorates that have a decentralized leadership function.

Although provincial health directorates have mixed functions, they operate as central agencies responsible for providing leadership, participate in the administration of health services, and act as deconcentrated bodies in charge of local management of the health sector. Provincial health directorates are responsible for installing health facilities; evaluating quality, access, and performance of public and private service providers; and providing oversight of local insurance coverage and harmonization of delivery. They are required to ensure that these processes abide by the principles of equity, comprehensiveness of care, and universal access.

The organization of the local-level health service delivery network is the responsibility of each of the nine regional health directorates, which are responsible for the management and coordination of establishments providing different levels of care, that are formed into networks in each region, in the so-called regional health services. The Secretariat of Public Health has a network of 1,037 establishments that include 6 specialized hospitals, 8 regional hospitals, 107 municipal hospitals, 22 provincial hospitals, 615 rural clinics, 90 health posts, 30 health centers, and 159 physicians' offices (20). The Dominican Social Security Institute has a network of 210 establishments: 20 hospitals (3 national and specialized hospitals, 2 regional hospitals, and 15 general hospitals), 30 polyclinics, and 160 physicians' offices.

The Essential Medications Program and Logistics Support Center (PROMESE/CAL), which reports to the nation's President, also is one of the public health sector institutions.

Public Health Services

Programs for the prevention and control of communicable diseases that could feasibly be eradicated or controlled are the most highly structured. The programs for the eradication of diseases (immunizations and leprosy) are managed by the Secretariat of Public Health and Social Welfare and the Dr. Humberto Bogaert Díaz Dermatological and Skin Surgery Institute (a semiprivate institution). Disease control programs are administered by the Secretariat and include the programs to combat tuberculosis, HIV/AIDS, rabies, malaria, and dengue fever. All programs are being strengthened to boost their local level response capacity.

The programs for immunizations and for the prevention and control of tuberculosis, HIV, and dengue fever are progressing and being strengthened and are incorporating social communications and mobilization. Within the context of MDG objectives to strengthen health programs and improve the population's health indicators, in 2005 the Secretariat of Public Health and Social Welfare launched the Zero Tolerance Mobilization strategy intended to enlist civil society's participation in the Secretariat's efforts to reduce avoidable maternal mortality and mortality in children under 5, the number of cases of tuberculosis not being treated under the DOTS strategy, human rabies cases, deaths from malaria and malaria outbreaks in priority population groups and territories, deaths from dengue fever, and avoidable vertical transmission of HIV.

In 2005, the Government invested 2% of the national budget (7% of social spending) in seven food assistance programs. It has implemented programs for distributing vitamin A, folic acid, iron, and calcium supplements to pregnant women, women who have recently given birth, children under 2 years old, and school-aged children. It also has established programs for fortifying salt with iodine, sugar with vitamin A, and wheat flour with iron and folic acid.

The Directorate General of Epidemiology is responsible for epidemiological and health surveillance. It is supported by the Dr. Defilló National Laboratory in conducting serological diagnosis of dengue fever and HIV infection, tuberculosis cultures, and sensitivity tests; by the Central Veterinary Laboratory in the viral isolation and diagnosis of zoonoses; by the Robert Reid Hospital for conducting bacterial cultures and antibiotic sensitivity tests; and by the laboratory of the Center for the Control of Tropical Diseases for malaria.

In 2000, 48.3% of the population had water supply service. There are shortcomings in the treatment and disinfection of the water supply and in the operation and maintenance of the systems, particularly in rural areas—52% of liquid waste is not treated before being disposed of in bodies of water. This figure must be improved to attain target 10 of goal 7 of the MDGs (21).

In 2003–2005, the country played an increasingly active role in the creation and consolidation of the Central American and Dominican Republic Forum on Potable Water and Sanitation, which was developed under the framework of the Central American and Dominican Republic Meeting on Health (RESSCAD), a forum for coordinating member country primary care institutions. A reform project was presented to the Congressional Standing Committee on the Environment and Natural Resources to improve institutional organization in the water and sanitation sector.

Municipal solid waste management was deficient in 2002, since necessary technical and financial resources were unavailable. In 57% of municipalities, solid waste is disposed of in rivers and open-air dumps. Hazardous waste management, including biomedical waste (22), is not handled separately from municipal waste.

In 2003, an evaluation was performed in the country as part of the regional Latin American and Caribbean initiative for solid waste management. It generated policy and strategy proposals to strengthen the sector, some of which have been implemented in the cities of Santo Domingo and Santiago.

The Secretariat of Public Health, in coordination with the Directorate General of Quality Standards and Systems, prepared standards for food protection and control and established a Codex Alimentarius National Commission. There have been 37 technical committees established on food, pesticides, fertilizers, and veterinary waste, and 79 standards have been published related to food, which have been registered or adapted to Codex standards. In 2003, a national committee was established to apply the Agreement on Sanitary and Phytosanitary Measures and the Agreement on Technical Barriers to Trade of the World Trade Organization (WTO). Proposals to update agricultural health laws were prepared to facilitate compliance with those agreements.

The National Public Health Laboratory, the Central Veterinary Laboratory, and the Biotechnology and Industrial Innovation Institute Laboratory are the government laboratories responsible for supporting food surveillance and control. A national network of food laboratories and a quality assurance system are being established to obtain accreditation from a pertinent national or international organization.

The country is governed by national quarantine inspection rules and international rules of the World Organization for Animal Health (OIE), the International Plant Protection Convention, and the European Good Agricultural Practices (EUREGAP) standards in specific cases of exports of bananas and other products (23).

The National Emergency Commission and the Emergency Operations Center execute, with some limitations, the natural disaster prevention and mitigation plan; risk zones have been identified.

In cooperation with the Secretariat of Public Health's National Emergencies and Disasters Directorate, contingency plans for hospitals were developed in 11 municipalities in Cibao's central, north-central, and northeastern regions, which establish these hospitals' emergency plans. The Emergency Operations Center developed a training and education plan so that instructors in the supply system and hospital personnel can prepare hospital emergency plans. An interagency emergency and disaster plan was designed, coordinated by the Center and UNDP; the plan includes a health, water, and sanitation component. The country participated in the proposal for the strategic Central American disaster response and prevention plan for the drinking water and sanitation sector. This initiative led to the establishment of a water and sanitation sector group as a specialized unit within the Emergency Operations Center. A national plan was drawn up to reduce vulnerability to disasters.

Coordination of avian influenza surveillance and control has begun, particularly along the border. A National Avian Influenza Commission has been established and a national plan to combat the disease is being prepared.

Individual Care Services

In 2005, 86% of the Secretariat of Public Health and Social Welfare's 1,294 establishments and the Dominican Social Security Institute's 153 establishments provided primary level care. In emergency services in public hospitals, care is provided under different arrangements. The most common is the "doctor-on-call" service, with each doctor working a 24-hour shift; this arrangement does not involve additional payment for the medical professional. There is a public psychiatric hospital that has 62% of the 245 available psychiatric beds (28% in general hospitals and 10% in private health centers). The country has 117 psychiatrists (1.4 per 100,000 people) and 240 psychologists (2.9 per 100,000 people), mostly in the private sector.

The country's health care model leans more toward treating disease than promoting health, and is based on free demand. In 2005, public health establishments had 19,078 available beds (1 per 469 persons). The Secretariat of Public Health has 9,204 professional medical positions (20 per 100,000 population). Primary care units are responsible for providing primary care; the units' interdisciplinary teams consist of a general physician, a nursing assistant, a community health agent, and several health promoters, who are responsible for overseeing the health of approximately 500 families living in the catchment area. The primary care units rely on methods and tools that permit the identification and early capture of people at risk. The community, represented by neighborhood boards and health committees, coordinates activities and participates in local health management.

In 2002, 41.3% of the population visited a Secretariat of Public Health hospital for a first consultation, 11.5% visited an outpatient center (health post or rural clinic), 5.8% used Dominican Social Security Institute services, and 1.1% used a military hospital (8, 24). Among the poorest quintile, 68.3% used Secretariat of Public Health facilities for the first consultation, and 31.7%

used the services of other institutions; 53% used Secretariat establishments for hospitalization services. Use of Secretariat of Public Health services rose to 72% in the poorest quintile. Private clinics received 35% of the total population and 19% of the poorest-quintile population. Private sector health care service provision was concentrated in urban areas and was based on direct payment and prepaid medical plans known as the "igualas médicas," some of which combine medical care and insurance. In 2002, 21.1% of the population had insurance coverage (6.5% in the poorest quintile); insurance coverage in the wealthiest quintile was 44.1%.

Blood donation, processing, storage, and use are regulated by law. There is a national policy and a national commission drawn from the different sectors involved and users' representatives. A proposal has been made to centralize blood processing and donations. There are standards for the evaluation and selection of blood donors, rules for hygiene and security in blood banks and transfusion services, and a manual of procedures. According to the catalogue of establishments inventoried in 2005 in the geographic information system for the health sector, the organization of blood banks and storage centers, the dispensing of blood derivatives, and the quality of blood screening are flawed, and this issue must become a priority on the political agenda.

Of all schizophrenia patients, 50% remain in the community, with little opportunity to receive specialized care. Community mental health services are scarce and existing centers are located in urban areas. Standards for the national mental health program were updated and a mental health act has been enacted and is in the process of being regulated.

Health Promotion

In 2003–2005, the country progressed in developing health promotion policies legitimized by various laws, including policies on AIDS, on the control of drugs and controlled substances, on the environment and natural resources, and on banning smoking in enclosed spaces. Strategies for healthy municipalities and communities and health promoting schools have been implemented in five municipalities; the health promoting schools program promotes the prevention of pregnancies and HIV/AIDS among teenagers.

The Zero Tolerance Mobilization strategy is intended to mobilize public awareness to transform the population's health status. The strategy emphasizes health promotion, disease prevention, and control of priority health problems through social and intersectoral participation throughout all national health system levels. The new Dominican Social Security System allows users and society to participate in decision making. Users and different civil-society sectors are represented on the National Social Security Council and the National Health Council. The municipal selection and certification committees are required to validate information for enrolling in the subsidized family health insurance regime. While health committees and neighborhood boards continue to exist, their participation in local management remains limited. Intersectoral participation is promoted for disease prevention and control of priority health problems.

Health Supplies

In June 2005, the basic table of essential drugs for national use included 468 drugs and 871 pharmaceutical formulations. There are approximately 23,000 legally registered pharmaceutical specialties and 4,812 pharmaceutical establishments devoted to the manufacture or sale of drugs, 105 of which are production laboratories, 1,305 are distributors, 3,300 are private outpatient pharmacies, 51 are public hospital pharmacies, and 417 are low-cost drugstores (25). Exports of nationally produced pharmaceuticals grew by 50%. Approximately 99% of the raw material used to produce medications is imported.

There are four public warehouses for the deposit and distribution of drugs, including the Essential Drugs Program's warehouse (PROMESE/CAL). No inventory is available of private-sector or nongovernmental organization drug stocks. The public sector's drug purchasing system is centralized and is carried out through PROMESE/CAL. According to a cost analysis conducted in 2000 for the current purchasing and supply system, PROMESE/CAL supplied between 45% and 65% of the cost of medications and health materials used by hospitals and subcenters and procured them at prices that were, on average, 250% lower than the cost of purchasing the same products directly. At the end of 2000, a decree was promulgated transforming PROMESE/CAL into a center to provide logistical support for specific functions to procure medications for the health system, and it took over the low-cost drugstores. The Government signed an agreement to formalize its participation in PAHO's Regional Revolving Fund for Strategic Public Health Supplies, which will allow it to participate in joint procurements of essential drugs in the Region and will improve access to essential drugs and strategic inputs for health.

The Drug Regulatory Authority oversees the application of the country's 2005 pharmaceutical policy. The price of pharmaceuticals can be freely determined, with Government oversight. There are vast differences between the prices charged by private pharmacies and international reference prices (26).

Human Resources

In 2005, the country had 18,450 physicians (20 per 10,000 population), 3,603 professional nurses (3.9 per 10,000), 15,511 nursing assistants or nursing technicians (15.7 per 10,000), 2,946 bioanalysts (3.2 per 10,000), 8,320 dentists (9 per 10,000), and 3,940 pharmacists (4.3 per 10,000). Between 1994 and 2004, the number of Secretariat of Public Health physicians grew from 5,626 to 9,204, the number of nurses and nursing assistants from 8,600 to 11,333, dentists from 376 to 1,431, and pharmacists from 372 to

527. Only the public subsector produces information on the geographic distribution of human resources. In 2002, the numbers ranged from 5.6 physicians per 10,000 population in the province of Azua to 38.5 in the National District (27).

Requirements for the certification of universities, higher education institutions, schools, academic departments, and undergraduate and graduate programs are set by the Higher Education, Science, and Technology System. The Department of Higher Education, Science, and Technology oversees higher education, approving the establishment of schools and study programs and sanctioning their extension to other cities. There are 18 universities offering health-related degrees. There are 9 medical schools, 11 nursing schools, 6 bioanalysis programs, 11 dental schools, and 4 pharmacy schools. Enrollment in health programs rose from 30,360 in 2003 to 40,479 in 2005. In 2003, 78% of students were women; in 2005, 76% were women. Medicine had the largest number of students (24,186 in 2005) and has grown faster than other programs. There are more than 40 postgraduate programs for specialties and subspecialties. There are residency programs in 15 teaching hospitals, and programs that offer master's degrees in public health, bioethics, and health management, as well as specialized studies in health reform and social security, and in maternal and child health and adolescent health. There are active professional associations and organizations of health workers, consisting of professional colleges and associations, and unions.

Research and Technological Development in Health

The Department of Higher Education, Science, and Technology is in charge of health research and technology and has a program for competitively allocating nonreimbursable resources to finance science and technology research and innovation projects in universities and legally recognized, eligible research centers. By law, the Department's budget includes a National Science and Technology Innovation and Development Fund designed to promote scientific and technological research.

The main holdings of bibliographical information on human and environmental health are found in the universities, health sector NGOs, research institutes, official institutions, international agencies, and the network of hospital libraries. The network is composed of eight teaching hospitals and was developed under an agreement among the Secretariat of Public Health, the Autonomous University of Santo Domingo, the Santo Domingo Technology Institute, PAHO, and the European Union.

In 2002, an agreement was reached to develop the country's Virtual Health Library. Progress made in this initiative has led its consultative committee to consider that it now can safeguard the health sector's intellectual legacy and provide equitable access to that information, as well as publicizing and disseminating health information generated by the different member institutions. Fifteen institutions subscribe to the HINARI program (established by WHO and the main publishing houses from around the

Community Participation Assures Health

The "Zero Tolerance Mobilization strategy" is designed to harness citizen participation in improving the population's health. The strategy emphasizes health promotion, disease prevention, and the control of priority health problems. The new Dominican Social Security System also allows users and civil society to participate in decision making. Users and different civil-society sectors are represented on the National Social Security Council and the National Health Council. Intersectoral participation is actively sought in preventing disease and controlling priority health problems.

world), which offers free or virtually free electronic access to many journals in biomedicine and other topics in the field of social science to institutions in developing countries. New collective subscriptions are being arranged for public institutions that report to the Secretariat of Public Health and Social Welfare.

The Information and Knowledge Management Center at the PAHO/WHO Country Office constitutes the technical memory of the country's public health system and the reference center on this topic. There is a network composed of 12 PALTEX posts located in different regions that provide students and teachers with access to high-quality materials at low cost. The National Commission for the Information and Knowledge Society does important work in implementing the corresponding strategy. It recognized the Virtual Health Library as an example of a portal that includes content that achieves the proposed objectives.

Research conducted on human subjects must be reviewed and approved by a bioethics research committee that is nationally and internationally accredited. The National Bioethics Council created by the Secretariat of Public Health and Social Welfare acts as the regulatory agency for biomedical research in the country.

Health Sector Expenditures and Financing

In 2003, social spending accounted for 8.1% of GDP; per capita social spending was approximately US$ 213. In 2002, the public sector spent less than US$ 3.00 per capita on drugs (less than 9.4% of total spending on health reported that year). Estimates suggest that 21% of spending on health was financed by the public sector and 79% by the private sector, with 27% of this second figure coming directly from families' pockets (28).

In 2002, a report on national health accounts underlined the small percentage of funds that the public sector destined to health care, compared to the large percentage contributed by families. National per capita spending on health was US$ 191, with the Secretariat spending US$ 40 and households spending US$ 93. If the Dominican Social Security System is to fully develop as an alternative for extending social protection with equity, these proportions must be reversed.

Spending on medications is the largest item in health costs. They are financed under a mixed arrangement. The Government allocates a budget to SESPAS and PROMESE/CAL to subsidize the medications dispensed in the network of public establishments but there are no mechanisms to ensure that they reach the very poor. The Dominican Social Security System includes drug assistance as part of the pharmaceutical benefits for members under the different regimes. In the subsidized regime, patients receive medications free of charge; in the subsidized contribution regime they pay 30% of the cost and the government pays 70%; and in the contribution regime patients pay 30% of the cost and the supplier pays 70%.

Private suppliers, including pharmacies and providers of medical inputs, are the main beneficiaries in the market for goods and services, since they capture about 61% of national spending on health (29). In the public sector, the Secretariat is the main financial agent, administering 21% of total spending on health; followed by the Dominican Social Security Institute, with 6.4%; private insurance with 14%; and NGOs with 6.4%. Of Government spending, 5% goes towards public health programs; this figure is being increased to cover the Zero Tolerance Mobilization program. To finance the basic family health plan, public spending on health will have to be increased by 2% of GDP, which means that between 3.7% and 4% of GDP will be required to ensure that the plan has universal coverage and to finance the prevention and control activities (30).

Technical Cooperation and External Financing

International cooperation agencies working in the country include PAHO/WHO, the United Nations Food and Agriculture Organization, the World Food Program, the United Nations Development Program, the United Nations Population Fund, the United Nations Children's Fund, the Joint United Nations Program on HIV/AIDS, the United Nations International Research and Training Institute for the Advancement of Women, and the International Organization for Migration.

In 2005, the United Nations system prepared a joint analysis of the country (31), considering human rights, equity, gender, the life cycle, and the institutional framework as cross-cutting issues. This work was the result of a participative process of evaluation and analysis intended to define the situation, priorities, and strategies for technical cooperation with the country during 2007–2011. The budget was distributed along four thematic lines: democratic governance, growth and development with equity, quality social services, and sustainable environmental management; and managing risks in emergencies and disasters.

The World Bank will continue providing support until 2009 through programs to improve the living conditions of vulnerable groups; these programs focus on youths and women and are closely linked to the MDGs (*32*), which will help the country to develop and achieve social equity.

The Inter-American Development Bank provided US$ 75 million in financial support for a project to modernize and restructure the health sector, carried out in 1998–2006. The project is closely related to the Government's strategies for the health sector, including decentralization; reorganization of service delivery; the restructuring of the Secretariat of Public Health and Social Welfare and the Dominican Social Security Institute; reform of hospital administration; establishment of integrated information systems; and the design of policies, laws, and regulations to support institutional reform and modernization.

In June 2000, the Government signed the Cotonou Agreement with the European Union to reduce and eradicate poverty by promoting sustainable development. A National Office for European Development Funds was established, which is responsible for defining, administering, evaluating, and monitoring multilateral cooperation programs to execute the resources offered to the country through the agreement.

A Tripartite Committee on International Cooperation was established, composed of the Secretariat of Foreign Affairs, the President's Technical Secretariat, and the National Office for European Development Funds, to coordinate the various sources of cooperation. The European Union supported health sector reform through a program to strengthen the health system which began in 2000 and ended its first stage in 2005 with financial support amounting to a donation of €12 million, plus US$ 1.5 million arranged by the National Office for European Development Funds. The program to strengthen the health system had three components: institutional strengthening, human resource management, and drugs. The second stage is under way.

In 2002, USAID presented its five-year strategic development plan to advance priorities in the fields of economic growth, democracy and governance, and health. The Agency plans to invest US$ 100 million over that period. Its contribution to health will be targeted to the prevention and treatment of HIV/AIDS, infant survival, reproductive health/family planning, and health sector reform. The first phase of the project to reform and decentralize the health sector began in 2000 and concluded in 2005; it received a donation of US$ 13.3 million to support the management of local health services in the eastern region and at the Secretariat of Public Health's central level. A two-year extension of the project was approved in 2005 (*29*).

The Spanish Cooperation Agency has a master cooperation plan for 2005–2008, which is intended to support compliance with the MDGs (*33*). Scientific and technical cooperation agreements were signed in June 2005. The agency has supported reform initiatives since 1996 in the fields of justice and municipal development and strengthening.

In 2005, the German Cooperation Agency (GTZ) ended its support in the health area and turned to cooperation in local development, with a contribution of US$ 3 million until 2012 (*34*).

References

1. Centro Latinoamericano y Caribeño de Demografía; Comisión Económica para América Latina y el Caribe. Población total de la región por países y año calendario. Available at: http://www.eclac.cl/celade/proyecciones/basedatos_BD.htm.
2. Programa de las Naciones Unidas para el Desarrollo. Informe nacional de desarrollo humano 2005: hacia una inserción mundial incluyente y renovada. Santo Domingo: PNUD; 2005.
3. República Dominicana, Oficina Nacional de Planificación. Focalización de la pobreza en la República Dominicana 2005. Available at: http://www.onaplan.gov.do/publicaciones/Focalizacion%20de%20la%20Pobreza%20(Resumen%20Ejecutivo).pdf.
4. Fondo de las Naciones Unidas para la Infancia. Estado mundial de la infancia 2005: la infancia amenazada. New York: UNICEF; 2005.
5. República Dominicana, Banco Central. Estadísticas económicas, 1980 a 2005. Available at: http://www.bancentral.gov.do.
6. República Dominicana, Oficina Nacional de Planificación. Porcentaje de hogares pobres por provincias, 2002. Available at: http://www.onaplan.gov.do/publicaciones/Atlas%20De%20La%20Pobreza%20(Resumen%20Ejecutivo).pdf.
7. República Dominicana, Banco Central. Encuesta nacional de fuerza de trabajo. Available at: http://www.bancentral.gov.do/estadisticas_economicas/Mercado_de_Trabajo/tasa_desocupacion_anual.xls.
8. República Dominicana, Centro de Estudios Sociales y Demográficos. Encuesta de demografía y de salud: ENDESA 2002. Santo Domingo: CESDEM; 2003.
9. Organización Panamericana de la Salud; Fondo de las Naciones Unidas para la Infancia. Evaluación global de los servicios de agua potable y saneamiento 2000: informe analítico República Dominicana. Santo Domingo: OPS; 1999.
10. República Dominicana, Centro Nacional de Investigaciones en Salud Materno Infantil. Encuesta nacional de micronutrientes 1993: Excreción urinaria de yodo y consumo de sal yodada en escolares dominicanos, 2002.
11. Oficina Internacional del Trabajo. Encuesta nacional de trabajo infantil en República Dominicana. San José: OIT; 2004.

12. Organización Panamericana de la Salud. Informe sobre la encuesta mundial de tabaquismo en jóvenes: República Dominicana, 2004. Santo Domingo: OPS; 2005. [Unofficial report].

13. República Dominicana, Oficina Nacional de Estadística. Encuesta nacional de hogares de propósitos múltiples, ENHOGAR 2005: informe final. Santo Domingo: ONE; 2005.

14. República Dominicana, Oficina Nacional de Estadística. VIII Censo de población y vivienda 2002. Resultados definitivos. Santo Domingo: ONE; 2004. Available at: http://www.one.gov.do.

15. Organización Panamericana de la Salud. Situación de la tuberculosis en las Américas 2004. Washington, DC: OPS; 2005.

16. Programa Conjunto de las Naciones Unidas sobre el VIH/SIDA. Informe sobre la epidemia mundial de SIDA 2004: cuarto informe mundial. Geneva: ONUSIDA; 2004.

17. República Dominicana, Secretaría de Estado de Educación; Centro Nacional de Investigaciones en Salud Materno Infantil. Censo de talla y peso en escolares 2002. Santo Domingo: SEE; CENISMI; 2002.

18. República Dominicana, Secretaría de Estado de Salud Pública y Asistencia Social. Memorias 2004. Santo Domingo: SESPAS; 2005.

19. Instituto Dominicano de Seguros Sociales. ARL Salud Segura. Anuario 2005; marzo 2006.

20. República Dominicana, Secretaría de Estado de Salud Pública y Asistencia Social. Memorias 2002. Santo Domingo: SESPAS; 2003.

21. Organización Panamericana de la Salud. Evaluación regional de los servicios de manejo de residuos sólidos municipales: República Dominicana 2003. Santo Domingo: OPS; 2003.

22. República Dominicana, Oficina Nacional de Planificación. Las proyecciones de población en la República Dominicana, 1990–2025. Santo Domingo: ONAPLAN.

23. Análisis de situación del sistema nacional de inocuidad de los alimentos: informe de la República Dominicana. Presentado en: Conferencia Regional FAO/OMS sobre Inocuidad de los Alimentos para las Américas y el Caribe; 6–9 dic de 2005; San José, Costa Rica. Available at: ftp://ftp.fao.org/docrep/fao/meeting/010/af310s.pdf.

24. Rathe M. Salud y equidad: una mirada al financiamiento de la salud en la República Dominicana. Calverton: Macro International; 2000.

25. República Dominicana, Secretaría de Estado de Salud Pública y Asistencia Social; Universidad Autónoma de Santo Domingo; Organización Panamericana de la Salud. Perfil del sector farmacéutico de la República Dominicana 2005. Santo Domingo: SESPAS; 2005.

26. República Dominicana, Ministerio de Salud y Ambiente. Programa de Reforzamiento del Sistema de Salud (PROSISA). Estudio de precios de medicamentos esenciales: informe preliminar junio 2005. Santo Domingo: PROSISA; agosto 2005.

27. República Dominicana, Secretaría de Estado de Salud Pública y Asistencia Social; Organización Panamericana de la Salud. Indicadores básicos de salud, 2003. Santo Domingo: SESPAS; 2005.

28. República Dominicana, Secretaría de Estado de Salud Pública y Asistencia Social. Análisis de situación de salud de la República Dominicana 2003: documento preliminar. Santo Domingo: SESPAS; 2003.

29. Rathe M. Análisis de cuentas nacionales de salud en República Dominicana: informe final. Santo Domingo: Fundación Plenitud; 2005.

30. Lizardo J. Dime de cuánto dispones y te diré para cuánto te alcanza: la reforma de salud y seguridad social en la República Dominicana. En: Conferencia en el Instituto Dominicano para el Desarrollo Social; 2004.

31. Naciones Unidas. Análisis Común de País. Visión del Sistema de las Naciones Unidas sobre la Situación de República Dominicana, 2005. Santo Domingo: NNUU; 2005.

32. Banco Mundial. Asistencia del Banco Mundial a República Dominicana. Available at: http://web.worldbank.org/WBSITE/EXTERNAL/BANCOMUNDIAL/EXTSPPAISES/LACINSPANISHEXT/DOMINICAREPUBLICINSPANISHEXT/0,,menuPK:509093~pagePK:141159~piPK:51067387~theSitePK:500740,00.html.

33. Agencia Española de Cooperación Internacional. Documento de estrategia país 2005–2008 cooperación española: República Dominicana. Available at: http://www.aeci.es/03coop/2coop_paises/6coop_mex_acentral_caribe/ftp/DEP_rep_domin_2005_2008.pdf.

34. Castillo Levisón A. El rol de la cooperación en el proceso de reforma y modernización del Estado: caso dominicano. Presentado en: VIII Congreso Internacional del CLAD sobre la Reforma del Estado y de la Administración Pública; 28–31 oct de 2003; Panamá. Available at: http://www.clad.org.ve/fulltext/0047118.pdf.

ECUADOR

Galápagos

0   50   100 Miles

Colombia

Esmeraldas   Carchi

Imbabura

Pichincha   Sucumbíos

★ **Quito**

Manabí   Napo   Orellana

1

2   4

3   Pastaza

5

Guayas

Cañar   Morona-
Santiago

Azuay

El Oro   Peru

1 Cotopaxi
2 Los Ríos
3 Bolívar
4 Tungurahua
5 Chimborazo

Loja   Zamora-
Chinchipe

0   50   100 Miles

Ecuador is situated on the northwestern coast of South America and has a surface area of 256,370 km². The Andes mountain chain divides the country into geographic regions: coastal, mountain, Amazon, and island (the Galápagos Islands are located 1,000 km from the coast). The country is divided geopolitically into 22 provinces, which in are divided into 269 cantons; the latter are subdivided into parishes.

GENERAL CONTEXT AND HEALTH DETERMINANTS

Social, Political, and Economic Determinants

As a result of the economic crisis in 1999, Ecuador adopted the U.S. dollar as its official currency in 2000. Between 2001 and 2005, Ecuador's economy grew at an average rate of 4.9%. This performance resulted in a higher per capita gross domestic product (GDP), which expanded at an annual average rate of 3.5% during this period. The per capita GDP was US$ 2,743 by the end of 2005. In addition, inflation decreased significantly from an annual average of 37.7% in 2001 to 2.12% in 2005, making possible the recovery of real salaries (*1*). Unemployment also decreased: urban unemployment went from 10.9% in 2001 to 7.9% in 2005, and, according to the National Statistics and Census Institute (INEC), unemployment among the total population (246,085 women and 215,008 men) was 9.2% in November 2003 (*2*). In real terms, minimum salaries increased an average of 10% between 2001 and 2005. As a result of the 1999–2000 economic crisis, approximately one million people left Ecuador in 2001–2005 in search of better living conditions and economic opportunities. By 2005, more than US$ 1.7 billion per year entered the economy in the form of money sent from abroad.

These economic changes took place in the midst of domestic political instability, with three presidents between 2001 and 2005, even though the normal presidential term is four years. The health sector's fiscal budget—which includes the Ministry of Public Health (MSP), the Ecuadorian Social Security Institute (IESS), and other institutions—increased from 3.3% of the general budget in 2001 to 5.9% in 2005 (*3*). Other sources of funding included the Solidarity Fund for application of the Free Maternity and Child Health Care Law to strengthen the public network of the MSP.

In 2004, the Second Congress on Life and Health issued policies to promote interculturalism and recommendations for the structural reforms needed to implement a comprehensive (i.e., taking into account economic, psychological, social, cultural, and spiritual factors) and intercultural health care model with a gender and intergenerational approach (*4*). The 2005–2006 health agenda was proposed at the same Congress to complement these policies.

The INEC carried out a national survey to measure poverty in terms of consumption.[1] It found that 41.5% lived in poverty, and 8.5% lived in extreme poverty in 2003. The next year, the figures were 52% and 14%, respectively. During 2005–2006, the rate of poverty was 79% among the rural population and 39% among the urban population. That same year, the wealthiest 20% of the population represented 46.5% of total consumption, while the poorest 20% had access to 7.7%. The Government recognized, via Executive Decree 1619 of May 2004, that poverty is one of the most serious problems facing Ecuador, so it designed a national strategy to reduce poverty through sustained institutional reform processes that would make it possible to consolidate new management parameters in the production and delivery of public social services to the most vulnerable population.

In 2004, approximately 56% of women between 20 and 49 years of age did not engage in paid labor; this percentage was slightly lower in the mountain (51%) and island (54%) areas. Women have less voice than men in political and public spheres and hold, through popular election, 31% of executive posts and 25% of local posts.

According to the 2005 *Human Development Report* of the United Nations Development Program, Ecuador ranked 82 among the 159 countries included in the measurement of the Human Development Index (HDI).

A report published in 2005 set forth the national policy for meeting the Millennium Development Goals (MDGs) (*5*). The report examined social progress made during 1990–2003; detailed the major challenges, including a cost analysis of the first accounting period; and highlighted the primary issue of changing trends toward inertia in economic growth and social and public action. It was estimated that a real growth of 4.5% of the annual GDP would make it possible to achieve the levels of public invest-

---

[1] "Consumption poverty" is the number of poor people expressed as a percentage of the total population for a specific year. The "poor" are defined as those people from homes whose per capita consumption during a certain period is below the poverty line. The poverty line is the monetary equivalent of the cost of a basic basket of goods per person per time period (usually 2 weeks or a month).

ment needed to comply with the MDGs, provided that effective priorities were applied in social public spending for disadvantaged sectors.

The political instability from 2001 to 2005 caused problems in governance and social violence and increased corruption (*6*), administrative instability, and lack of continuity in public management (*7*). This situation affected the dynamics of the health sector and its potential reform. The repeated replacement of authorities (nine Ministers of Health between 2001 and 2005,) who inserted their own plans and programs in each administration—such as social protection in health, decentralization, extension of coverage, licensing of services, a comprehensive complementary and nutritional feeding program in the poorest parishes in Ecuador, and universal insurance, among others—weakened the national health authority, limiting the development and sustainability of more coherent reform processes. During the first phase of Universal Health Insurance (*8*), the goal was to achieve universal coverage by 2010 for the bottom two income quintiles (5,200,000 inhabitants). Also included were several initiatives for intersectoral educational and preventative actions to control epidemics (especially dengue and other communicable diseases) and comprehensive food and nutrition actions for the protection of the most vulnerable groups in the poorest urban and rural areas.

The general illiteracy rate for the population older than 15 years old was 9.0% in 2004: 9.3% in the mountains and east and 8.7% on the coast. In the provinces of Chimborazo, Cotopaxi, and Bolívar, where there is a high concentration of the indigenous population, these figures were 19%, 17.6%, and 17.5%, respectively. The rate was higher for women (10.3%) than for men (7.7%). This predominance of illiteracy among women was recorded in all provinces, except for Manabí (for example, the rate was 13.4% for men and 23.8% for women in Chimborazo). In 2005, 66.8% of the population had completed primary education (67.9% of men and 65.8% of women) (*9*). The proportion of women who did not enter the education system was 1% among 15- to 19-year-olds, compared with 10% among 45- to 49-year-olds. The rate of secondary and university education was 23% of women between 20 and 24 years of age, compared with 16% of those between 45 and 49 years old. Except for 15- to 19-year-olds, average schooling for women (national average = 8.7 years) decreased as age increased (*10*).

In its 2003 national water and sanitation policy, the Government identified the need for an investment of approximately US$ 150 million per year to eliminate the existing deficit in water and sanitation services for 2001–2010. It is estimated that US$ 42 million are required for this same period for the final disposal of solid wastes in 180 municipalities in the country.

In 2001–2005, two major border areas were identified for analysis and intervention by the Government as a whole and by the health sector and cooperation agencies in particular: the northern border with Colombia and the southern border with

Peru. The northern border comprises the provinces of Esmeraldas, Carchi, Imbabura, and Sucumbíos, all of which border Colombia, with the exception of Imbabura. They cover a surface area of 42,065 km^2 (16% of the national territory) and have 1,119,550 inhabitants (8.3% of Ecuador's population in 2005). In Esmeraldas, Imbabura, and Sucumbíos, there are 7 cantons (out of a total of 20) in which more than 90% of the population lives below the poverty line (measured by unmet basic needs), particularly in rural areas (*11*).

Conflict in Colombia led to the displacement of people from that country in search of refuge. The MSP and the United Nations High Commissioner for Refugees (UNHCR) registered an increase in refugee applications. There were 475 applicants in 2000, 11,515 in 2003, and 27,190 in the first half of 2004. As of the first quarter of 2006, 12,000 people had received refugee status, and they are primarily located in the provinces of Sucumbíos, Esmeraldas, Imbabura, Pichincha, Carchi, and Azuay.

Ecuador is at risk for natural disasters due to multiple threats (geographic faults, volcanoes, steep terrain, deforestation, floods, landslides, etc.), which interact with the vulnerabilities of a high percentage of the population. The Andes mountain range and highly volcanic islands have a group of 72 volcanoes with some risk factor; at least 13 of them represent a significant risk to the population. The most well known are Tungurahua, Guagua Pichincha, Reventador, Cotopaxi, Sangay, and Sierra Negra (in the Galápagos).

Demographics, Mortality, and Morbidity

In 2005, the total estimated population was 13,215,089, of which 6,586,721 (49.8%) were women (Figure 1). Population density is 49.3 inhabitants per km^2, and the majority of the population (63.4%) lives in urban areas. The population distribution is not homogenous and is concentrated in the most developed areas of the main provinces (Guayas 26% and Pichincha 15%), especially in the cities of Quito (12%) and Guayaquil (17%) (*12*). Ecuador is multicultural and multiethnic; according to the Sixth Population Census carried out by the INEC in 2001, 6.1% of the population over 15 years of age is considered to be indigenous, 5% Afro-Ecuadorian and mulatto, 77.7% mestizo, and 10.8% white. The indigenous population was concentrated in certain provinces; in 2005, it was as follows: Chimborazo 70%, Cotopaxi 60%, Imbabura 45%, Bolívar 40%, and Tungurahua 28% (*13*).

As per the 2001 population census, the annual population growth rate was 2.05% compared with 2.19% in 1990, with greater growth in the urban sector (3%) than in the rural sector (0.85%). According to various sources, the total fertility rate continued to decrease during 2001–2005. In 2001, it was 2.8 children per woman, and it was 2.7 in 2005 (*14, 15*). According to the INEC and the Latin American and Caribbean Demographic Center (INEC-CELADE), the total fertility rate was 2.8 children per woman during 2000–2005 and 3.1 during the previous period

FIGURE 1. Population structure, by age and sex, Ecuador, 2005.

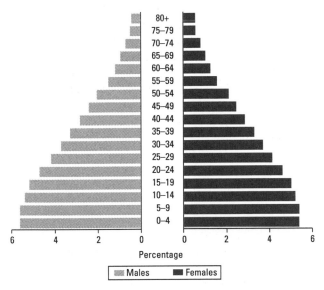

Source: Ecuador, Population Projections 1950–2025, INEC-CEPAL.

(1995–1999) (*16*), while the 2004 Demographic and Maternal and Child Health Survey showed that the total fertility rate was 3.3 for 1999–2004, with the highest rates in rural areas, 3.9 (urban 2.9); among the indigenous population, 4.9; and among mestizos, 3.1.

According to INEC-CELADE, the aging index for 2005 was 25% (adults over 60 years of age/0- to 14-year-old population). Life expectancy in the periods of 1995–1999 and 2000–2005 increased for both sexes from 72.3 to 74.2; for men the increase was from 69.6 to 71.3 and for women it was from 75.1 to 77.2 (*16*). There were 305,620 live births registered in 2004, of which 53.3% corresponded to births in that same year; the rest were late registrations (46.7%).

The estimated underreporting of mortality for 2000–2005 was 13.4%. The crude mortality rate (per 1,000 population) was estimated at 5.8 for 2001 (*14*) and at 5.0 for 2005 (*15*). The INEC reported in 2003 that death certificates were issued for 76.9% of deaths and that the causes for 12.6% of those deaths were ill-defined (*17*). Previously (in approximately 2000), the latter figure was 13.3% (*18*). In 2004, a total of 54,729 deaths were registered (31,292 men and 23,437 women); the main causes of death are detailed in Table 1.

In 2004, the causes of death were distributed differently among men and women. The rate for cirrhosis and other liver diseases was 8.0 per 100,000 population for women and 17.0 for men; for diabetes mellitus it was 23.0 for women and 18.0 for men; and for cardiac insufficiency, complications, and ill-defined diseases of the heart, the rate was the same for men and women, 31.0.

In 2004, the causes of violent death per 100,000 population were aggression (homicides), 18.0 (32.0 men, 3.0 women); traffic accidents, 14.0 (22.0 men, 7.0 women), and suicides, 6.0 (9.0 men, 4.0 women).

HEALTH OF POPULATION GROUPS

Children under 5 Years Old

In 2001, the estimated infant mortality rate per 1,000 live births was 24.9, and in 2004, it was 22.3 (*15*). In 2003, a total of 3,942 children died before their first birthday (2,241 boys and 1,701 girls), of which 3,121 were reported in urban areas, and 821 in rural areas. Most of the deaths occurred in the mountain region (2,100), and Pichincha was the province with the most deaths (1,061). The leading causes of infant mortality were complications related to the duration of gestation and fetal growth (14.8%, 340 boys and 244 girls), pneumonia and influenza (10.1%, 218 boys and 181 girls), bacterial sepsis in newborns (9.0%, 205 boys and 150 girls), other respiratory illnesses in newborns (6.1%, 143 boys and 99 girls), and respiratory difficulty in newborns (4.5%, 97 boys and 80 girls) (*19*). With regard to breast-feeding, 73% of women interviewed in 2004 breast-fed the first day after birth; at 3 months only 49% were breast-feeding exclusively. A total of 39.6% of infants under 6 months were breast-fed exclusively. The total average (not exclusive) was 16 months (*10*).

In 2003, there were 1,800 registered deaths of children between 1 and 4 years old (996 boys and 804 girls). The main causes of death were influenza and pneumonia (14.4%), followed by infectious intestinal diseases (11.2%), accidental drowning and submersion (5.4%), malnutrition and nutritional anemia (4.7%), and traffic accidents (3.4%) (*20*). In 2004, the MSP reported coverage of 20.6% in ambulatory care for this age group (*21*).

Children 5–9 Years Old

In 2005, this group constituted 21.1% of the population (with a similar proportion for males and females). In 2003, there were 1,364 registered deaths among those between 5 and 14 years old (787 boys and 577 girls). Traffic accidents were the leading cause of death (12.1%), followed by accidental drowning and submersion (6.0%); influenza and pneumonia (5.8%); malignant neoplasms in lymphatic, hematopoietic, and related tissues (4.8%); and urinary tract diseases (2.8%). Malnutrition and nutritional anemia were ranked tenth at 1.7% (*20*). A study carried out in 2001 found a 14% prevalence rate of overweight and obesity in 8-year-old schoolchildren (obesity 5% and overweight 9%) (*22*).

Adolescents 10–14 and 15–19 Years Old

According to INEC projections, in 2005 children and adolescents between 10 and 19 years old represented 20.7% of the total

TABLE 1. Mortality rate, by cause and sex, according to the condensed list of 103 groups of causes, ICD-10, Ecuador, 2004.

			Country total								
			Total			Males			Females		
		2004 estimated population	13,026,891			6,535,564			6,491,327		
		Total deaths	54,729			31,292			23,437		
		General mortality rate	420.1			478.8			361.1		
Code	ICD-10 codes	Causes of death	Number	Rate	%	Number	Rate	%	Number	Rate	%
068	I26–I51	Other heart diseases	4,014	30.8	7.3	2,010	30.8	6.4	2,004	30.7	8.6
074	J12–J18	Pneumonia	2,998	23.0	5.5	1,608	24.6	5.1	1,390	21.3	5.9
069	I60–I69	Cerebrovascular diseases	2,949	22.6	5.4	1,540	23.6	4.9	1,409	21.6	6.0
052	E10–E14	Diabetes mellitus	2,672	20.5	4.9	1,179	18.0	3.8	1,493	22.8	6.4
066	I10–I13	Hypertensive diseases	2,474	19.0	4.5	1,289	19.7	4.1	1,185	18.1	5.1
102	X85–Y09	Violence	2,315	17.8	4.2	2,104	32.2	6.7	211	3.2	0.9
067	I20–I25	Ischemic heart diseases	2,300	17.7	4.2	1,379	21.1	4.4	921	14.1	3.9
092	P00–P96	Certain conditions originating in the perinatal period	1,906	14.6	3.5	1,109	17.0	3.5	797	12.2	3.4
096	V01–V99	Transport accidents	1,873	14.4	3.4	1,451	22.2	4.6	422	6.5	1.8
080	K70–K76	Liver diseases	1,655	12.7	3.0	1,124	17.2	3.6	531	8.1	2.3
029	C16	Malignant neoplasm of stomach	1,484	11.4	2.7	822	12.6	2.6	662	10.1	2.8
076	J40–J47	Chronic diseases of the lower respiratory tract	909	7.0	1.7	529	8.1	1.7	380	5.8	1.6
101	X60–X84	Intentional self-inflicted harm	796	6.1	1.5	559	8.6	1.8	237	3.6	1.0
012	A40–A41	Septicemia	697	5.4	1.3	356	5.4	1.1	341	5.2	1.5
005	A15–A16	Respiratory tuberculosis	697	5.4	1.3	471	7.2	1.5	226	3.5	1.0
053	E40–E46	Malnutrition	646	5.0	1.2	315	4.8	1.0	331	5.1	1.4
040	C61	Malignant neoplasm of prostate	636	4.9	1.2	636	9.7	2.0	0	0.0	–
031	C22	Malignant neoplasm of liver and intrahepatic bile ducts	573	4.4	1.0	279	4.3	0.9	294	4.5	1.3
034	C33–C34	Malignant neoplasm of trachea, bronchi, and lungs	569	4.4	1.0	332	5.1	1.1	237	3.6	1.0
093	Q00–Q99	Congenital malformations, deformations, and chromosomal abnormalities	503	3.9	0.9	265	4.1	0.8	238	3.6	1.0
020	B20–B24	Human immunodeficiency virus (HIV)	495	3.8	0.8	404	6.2	1.1	91	1.4	0.3
098	W65–W74	Accidental drowning and submersion	467	3.6	0.9	391	6.0	1.2	76	1.2	0.3
045	C91–C95	Leukemia	458	3.5	0.7	237	3.6	0.7	221	3.4	0.8
049	D50–D64	Anemia	424	3.3	0.8	198	3.0	0.6	226	3.5	1.0
038	C54–C55	Malignant neoplasm of corpus uteri or uterus, part unspecified	409	3.1	0.7	0	0.0	–	409	6.3	1.7
030	C18–C21	Malignant neoplasm of colon, rectum, and anus	401	3.1	0.7	175	2.7	0.6	226	3.5	1.0
097	W00–W19	Falls	369	2.8	0.7	303	4.6	1.0	66	1.0	0.3
003	A09	Intestinal infectious diseases	334	2.6	0.6	178	2.7	0.6	156	2.4	0.7
036	C50	Malignant neoplasm of breast	312	2.4	0.6	8	0.1	0.0	304	4.7	1.3
032	C25	Malignant neoplasm of pancreas	256	2.0	0.5	122	1.9	0.4	134	2.1	0.6
056	F10–F19	Mental and behavioral disorders due to psychoactive substance use	251	1.9	0.5	228	3.5	0.7	23	0.4	0.1
079	K25–K27	Gastric and duodenal ulcers	247	1.9	0.5	156	2.4	0.5	91	1.4	0.4
043	C82–C85	Non-Hodgkin's lymphoma	239	1.8	0.4	136	2.1	0.4	103	1.6	0.4
037	C53	Malignant neoplasm of cervix uteri	235	1.8	0.4	0	0.0	–	235	3.6	1.0
042	C70–C72	Malignant neoplasm of meninges, brain, and other parts of the central nervous system	204	1.6	0.4	111	1.7	0.4	93	1.4	0.4
070	I70	Atherosclerosis	163	1.3	0.3	81	1.2	0.3	82	1.3	0.3
100	X40–X49	Accidental poisoning or exposure to harmful substances	156	1.2	0.3	125	1.9	0.4	31	0.5	0.1

(continued)

TABLE 1. Continued.

Code	CIE-10 codes	Causes of death	Number	Rate	%	Number	Rate	%	Number	Rate	%
083	M00–M99	Diseases of the musculoskeletal system and connective tissue	154	1.2	0.3	52	0.8	0.0	102	1.6	0.4
059	G00,G03	Meningitis	126	1.0	0.2	78	1.2	2.0	48	0.7	0.2
039	C56	Malignant neoplasm of ovary	111	0.9	0.2	0	0.0	–	111	1.7	0.5
089	010–092	Other obstetrical deaths	109	0.8	0.2	0	0.0	–	109	1.7	0.5
099	X00–X09	Exposure to smoke, fire, and flames	101	0.8	0.2	66	1.0	0.2	35	0.5	0.1
094	R00–R99	Symptoms, signs, and abnormal clinical and laboratory findings not classified elsewhere	6,363	48.8	11.6	3,338	51.1	10.7	3,025	46.3	12.9
		Other causes of death	9,679	74.3	17.7	5,548	84.9	17.7	4,131	63.2	17.6

Note: The information in the table includes the population in unmapped areas and includes 69 deaths of residents abroad; the rate is per 10,000 population.

population (more than 2.7 million), of which 46.9% were male, and 53.1% were female (*23*). In 2004, a study (*24*) found that 45% of adolescent deaths between 12 and 17 years of age were preventable, such as accidents or acts of violence. According to that same study, between 2000 and 2002 an average of 1,200 adolescents died per year from the same causes. It was also estimated that there were a total of 256 suicides (one every 4 days). In 2003, 32% of adolescents between 15 and 19 years old reported experiencing some form of violence (*25*).

In 2004, 27.0% of females between 15 and 19 years of age had had sexual relations, and 38.9% of those between 15 and 24 years of age had been pregnant—38.0% in urban areas and 40.3% in rural areas. Percentages by region were 43.0% on the coast, 42.9% in Amazonia, and 35% in the mountains. By province, Los Ríos had the highest percentage (50.8%) (*10*). The INEC reported in that same year that 78.6% of births were attended by a professional (*19*). In 2003, the INEC reported 30,489 abortions; this was the second leading cause for hospitalization of women at the national level (*16*). In 2004, the MSP reported 20,439 abortions and 21,358 dilation and curettage procedures (*21*).

Adults 20–59 Years Old

In 2005, the average age of the population was estimated at 24 years. The population between 15 and 29 years represented 27.7% of the total population, and adults between 30 and 59 years, 32%. In 2004, 13.5% of females between 15 and 24 years old who had had a sexual experience reported having used a contraceptive method in their first sexual relation. The national average of contraceptive use was 73%, and it was 47% among indigenous people. Condoms were the most frequently used method (6.7%). With regard to births, among females between 15 and 49 years old, 43.9% received care in MSP institutions, 20.1% in homes with or without midwives, 19.2% in semiautonomous institutions, and 16.8% in private institutions (*10*). That year, the MSP reported providing care in 130,524 births (estimated cover-

age of 36%). The provinces with the greatest number of attended births were Pichincha (31,091, 47.3% coverage), Guayas (19,666, 21.2% coverage), and Manabí (13,437, 34.3% coverage). Also in 2005, a total of 30,783 Cesarean sections were reported with the highest numbers by province in Pichincha (7,098), Guayas (4,484), and Manabí (3,918). The Ministry of Public Health registered 144,514 cervical-uterine cytologies in 2004 (estimated coverage of 8.3%) (*21*).

In 2001, the estimated maternal mortality ratio was 97 per 100,000 live births and in 2003, it was 77.8 (*15, 26*). In 2004, the INEC reported that the main causes of maternal death were: eclampsia and other hypertensive disorders (41.7%), complications during labor and birth (31.7%), pregnancy ending in abortion (6.5%), and complications primarily related to the puerperium (5.8%). In 2004, the national maternal mortality rate was 76.4 per 100,000 live births. In terms of rural and urban distribution, the Maternal Mortality Epidemiological Surveillance System stated there were more deaths among rural women living in high-poverty areas (65%), which coincides with the information provided by the Demographic and Maternal and Child Health Survey in 2004. In 2003, the INEC registered 12,089 deaths of people between 15 and 49 years of age (8,213 men and 3,876 women). The leading causes were homicides (12%, 1,346 men and 114 women), traffic accidents (9.7%, 988 men and 194 women), suicides (4.4%, 344 men and 186 women), accidental drowning and submersion (4.1%, 420 men and 78 women), and cerebrovascular diseases (3.4%, 247 men and 167 women). During that same year, 8,053 deaths were reported among people 50 to 59 years of age (4,821 men and 3,232 women). The leading causes of death were diabetes mellitus (8.3%, 345 men and 322 women), cerebrovascular diseases (6.0%, 277 men and 207 women), cirrhosis and other liver diseases (5.8%, 345 men and 121 women), ischemic heart diseases (5.4%, 296 men and 144 women), and hypertensive diseases (4.8%, 234 men and 155 women). In this age group, 193 deaths from malignant neoplasm of the uterus were reported (2.4% of the total) and 122 from female breast cancer (1.5% of the total). Traffic accidents (3.8%) fell to eighth place among this group, and malignant neoplasm of the stomach (3.6%) was ninth (27).

Older Adults 60 Years Old and Older

Based on the 2001 population census, the 2004 population projection for the 65-year-old and older age group was 724,658 (53.2% women), and for 2000–2005, it was estimated that there would be a 16.5% increase among this group (19). In 2003, 26,173 deaths were reported (13,317 men and 12,856 women). The leading causes of death were cardiac insufficiency, complications of heart disease, and ill-defined heart diseases (8.7%, 1,045 men and 1,220 women); cerebrovascular diseases (7.5%, 956 men and 1,011 women); hypertensive diseases (5.9%, 712 men and 823 women); ischemic heart diseases (5.8%, 859 men and 647 women); and diabetes mellitus (5.8%, 600 men and 905 women) (27). In 2005, the IESS reported 87,000 retired people who were members, of which 17,000 received social services to complement health services.

The Family

In terms of family composition, in 2003–2004, family groups had an average of 4.1 members in urban areas, with a difference between the poorest (5.4) and wealthiest quintiles (3.0). During the same period, per capita income per family group was US$ 177.70 per month—US$ 48.90 for the poorest quintile and US$ 555.60 for the wealthiest (28). Emigration had a significant impact on the structure of homes; in 2003, it was reported that an average of 15% of families in the main cities of Ecuador (Quito, Guayaquil, and Cuenca) had a family member who had emigrated. Emigrants were distributed equally by sex in the national total (50% for each), with the exception of Cuenca, where men predominated at 67%. The greatest concentration was among the 20- to 39-year-old age group (29).

Ethnic Groups

The average rate of chronic malnutrition in indigenous children from 0 to 59 months was 47%, while the national average for that age group was 23%. The global malnutrition rate among children under 5 was 9.4%; it was 15.3% among indigenous children, 11.6% among children of African descent, 8.7% among mestizos, and 6.3% among whites.

In 2004, the average percentage of women who are members of or who received benefits from public social security was 15.7%, and 13.7% of indigenous women. The percentage of indigenous women who reported being physically mistreated before their 15th birthday was 40.8% (national average 27.7%), and 34.7% reported being psychologically mistreated (national average, 24.9%) (30).

Displaced Persons

In 2004, a ministerial agreement ratified Ecuador's commitment to humanitarian assistance and care for the refugee population. Refugees were incorporated into the regular programs of the MSP, and it was established that they should receive health care under conditions equal to those of the local population. Care for pregnant refugee women was also integrated into the Free Maternity and Child Health Care Law. In that year, coverage for prenatal care for this group in provinces with refugees was 87.8% in Carchi, 79.2% in Imbabura, and 82.8% in Esmeraldas (national average of 80.6%). In terms of professional assistance at birth, Carchi reported 78.5%, Imbabura 60.4%, and Esmeraldas 51.8% (national average of 75.0%) (10). With regard to ambulatory care in MSP facilities in these provinces, the most common diseases were 15,058 cases of acute respiratory infections in Carchi (65.2%), 2,328 cases of acute diarrheal disease in Esmeraldas (65.9%), and 15,644 cases of acute respiratory infections in Sucumbíos (60.8%) (31).

HEALTH CONDITIONS AND PROBLEMS

COMMUNICABLE DISEASES

Vector-borne Diseases

With regard to **malaria**, in 2001, the annual parasite index (API) per 1,000 population was 22.5, and the provinces with the highest API, in order of frequency, were: Cotopaxi (54.7), Esmeraldas (54.7), Sucumbíos (53.5), and Pichincha (35.1). In 2005, the national API was 2.21, and the highest APIs were recorded in Esmeraldas (17.0), Pastaza (6.6), Pichincha (5.9), and Sucumbíos (5.0). That year, Esmeraldas was the province with the highest percentage of malaria cases with 29.0%. During 2001–2005, most malaria cases were transmitted by *Plasmodium vivax*, even though there were some cases transmitted by *P. falciparum*. In 2005, a total of 358,361 blood samples were examined from which 16,487 cases were diagnosed, of these 2,127 were positive for *P. falciparum*, and 14,360 were positive for *P. vivax*. The most affected age group was the economically active population (15 to 44 years), with 65% of the total cases. Therapeutic failure in 90% of patients after antimalarial treatment exceeded the recommended threshold of 25%. Incipient resistance to sulfadoxine with pyrimethamine was detected at levels of 8%. Susceptibility of *P. vivax* to the use of chloroquine remained at 100% (32).

With regard to the transmission of **dengue**, *Aedes aegypti* were found in tropical, Amazon, subtropical, and island areas of the country, and four serotypes of the dengue virus were identified. In 2003, there was a dengue outbreak with a total of 10,726 suspected cases of classic dengue and 206 confirmed cases of **hemorrhagic dengue**, of which 189 were in the province of Guayas, for a provincial rate of 5.44 per 100,000 population. The rate of incidence in the coastal region was 3.15 (33). In 2004, 6,057 cases were reported in Ecuador, of which only 1,111 were confirmed through examination. In 2005, there were 4,653 confirmed cases; the highest rates were seen in Napo, Zamora, and Manabí, with 268.0, 135.1, and 131.0 per 100,000 population, respectively. In 2004, there were 64 reported cases of hemorrhagic dengue in the entire country, primarily concentrated in the coastal provinces: 46 cases in Guayas, 10 in Manabí, 3 in Los Ríos, and 2 in El Oro (the rate for the coastal region was 0.9 per 100,000 population). In 2005, there was an outbreak of hemorrhagic dengue in the coastal region with 334 cases (rate of 4.9 per 100,000 population and a case fatality rate of 4.2%). The highest numbers of these cases were located in Guayas (225; 175 of them in Guayaquil), Manabí (75), and Los Ríos (14).

No cases of **yellow fever** were reported in 2001. Sentinel sites in place since 2003 made it possible to improve surveillance of the acute hemorrhagic febrile icteric syndrome related to yellow fever. Rapid monitoring was implemented for urban and rural coverage in Amazonia to improve coverage among the high-risk population (*34*).

During 2000–2004, there were 32 cases of **plague** and 3 deaths were reported. No cases were reported in 2005; however, risk factors continued to be observed (*35*).

Areas at risk for **Chagas' disease** included 183 cantons in 20 provinces. Of the approximately 8.4 million people living in these areas, 3 to 5 million were especially vulnerable because of their living conditions or poverty. The general prevalence of infection by *Trypanosoma cruzi* reached 1.3% of the general population (0.6% in the mountains; 1.9% on the coast, and 1.7% in Amazonia).

Ecuador was part of the regional initiative headed by the **Onchocerciasis** Elimination Program for the Americas. Within the framework of the regional strategy, effective, safe, and locally sustainable programs were also carried out to distribute ivermectin in endemic localities. In 2001, WHO distributed elimination criteria, and Ecuador initiated a certification process based on them. In 2002, two rounds of distribution and treatment were carried out, with a coverage rate of 94.8% in the eligible population. In 2005, the distribution of ivermectin as a strategy to eliminate the disease was carried out in 119 communities where **onchocerciasis** is endemic: 117 in the province of Esmeraldas and 2 in Pichincha (approximately 25,000 people at risk).

Vaccine-preventable Diseases

In 2006, the Expanded Program on Immunization (EPI) marked 16 years without **poliomyelitis**, 9 without **measles**, 4 without **yellow fever**, and 1 without **rubella** and managed to eliminate **neonatal tetanus** as a public health problem. The vaccine law, created in 1999 and amended in 2000, helped in obtaining these results and also made it possible to have budgetary allocations to finance the application of regular vaccines and to introduce new vaccines. Starting in 1999, a vaccine against yellow fever was introduced among the population under 1 year of age in the Amazon region. In 2000, a triple MMR (measles, **mumps**, and rubella) viral vaccine was introduced, and in 2003 a pentavalent vaccine was introduced (**diphtheria**, **tetanus**, **whooping cough**, **hepatitis B**, and *Haemophilus influenzae* **type b**) with three doses in children under 1 year. A monovalent vaccine against hepatitis B was also incorporated for school children in risk areas. Coverage levels remained above 90% in 2004–2005 (in that last year, for example, the three doses of the pentavalent reached 93.45%; the three doses of the poliomyelitis oral vaccine was 92.6%, and the MMR was 92.9%). The country increased its notification rate of flaccid paralysis from 0.5 per 100,000 children under 15 in 2004 to 1.0 in 2006 (as of epidemiological week 25).

Comprehensive surveillance of **measles** and **rubella** was strengthened, which increased notification of suspected cases. With regard to the elimination of rubella, Ecuador began applying vaccination strategies for MR (measles and rubella), suggested by PAHO since 2002, by vaccinating the population between 6 months and 14 years of age and increasing coverage. Between May and June 2004, a successful campaign was carried out to vaccinate adolescents and adults of both sexes against measles and rubella, covering 98% of the target population. Circulation of the rubella virus was interrupted in November 2004, when the last laboratory-confirmed case was reported.

Intestinal Infectious Diseases

A **cholera** outbreak of 25 cases was reported at the end of 2003 in the Zamora-Chinchipe province, which corresponded to a rate of 30.8 per 100,000 population in that province. No cases were reported during 2001, 2002, 2004, and 2005.

In 2003, 2004, and 2005 notification rates for **acute diarrheal diseases** were 2.0, 2.4, and 2.7 per 100,000 population, respectively. In 2005, the eastern region had the highest notification rate (5.9), which is twice the national rate. The highest rates in the country by province were: Pastaza, Morona, Napo, and Zamora (*36*).

Chronic Communicable Diseases

In 2004, **tuberculosis** was the 15th leading cause of death (5.0 per 100,000 population). It was more common among men (7.0 per 100,000 population) than women (3.0). The most affected group was those between 15 and 24 years of age with 1,254 cases, followed by the 25- to 34-year-old age group. Those least affected were in the 0- to 14-year-old age group and those 65 years and older (192 and 237 cases, respectively). That same year 5,557 cases of all forms of tuberculosis were reported (rate of 42.6 per 100,000 population); 4,340 cases had positive sputum smears, and 438 were extrapulmonary tuberculosis. In 2003 and 2004, there was an average of 226 annual cases of AIDS/tuberculosis coinfection (out of a total of 1,806 AIDS cases). Most coinfected people were from Guayas (76.5%), followed by Pichincha (8.0%); they were predominantly men (73.0%), and 60.6% were workers and laborers. In 2005, a study on antituberculosis drug resistance showed evidence of primary resistance (5%) and secondary resistance to multiple drugs (24.3%). Coverage for Directly Observed Treatment, Short-course (DOTS), in operating MSP facilities as of 2005 was 100% in Azuay, Pichincha, Guayas, Tungurahua, and El Oro, and 90% in Manabí (which in total represents 70% of the target population defined by the program).

There were 251 cases of **leprosy** reported in 2003, which translated into a rate of 2.0 per 100,000 population. During that year, 189 new cases were reported. In 2004, there were 144, and 116 in 2005 (rates of 14.0, 11.0, and 9.0 per 100,000 population, respectively). The group most affected was those over 15 years of age. Multibacillary cases predominated among men (78%) and paucibacillary cases were more frequent among women (58%).

Acute Respiratory Infections

In 2005, acute respiratory infections were the leading cause of outpatient visits to operating MSP facilities in all provinces, with the exception of Bolívar. The highest rates (26.6 and 18.7 per 100,000 population) were in Napo and Morona. That year acute respiratory infections were three times more frequent than acute diarrheal diseases during outpatient visits (36).

HIV/AIDS and other Sexually Transmitted Infections

As of 2006, Ecuador did not have a study on the prevalence of people infected with HIV. From 2001 to 2005, a total of 2,752 HIV-positive cases were reported (varying from 294 in 2001 to 1,027 in 2005); there were 1,902 cumulative cases of AIDS during that same period (varying from 318 in 2001 to 445 in 2005), and 884 people died. In 2005, 67.9% of people over 14 years old with AIDS were men, and the male-to-female ratio was 2:1, lower than the previous year (3:1). In 2005, the highest AIDS notification rates corresponded to the 30- to 34-year-old age group (8.9 per 100,000 population) followed by 35- to 39-year-olds and 25- to 29-year-olds (8.8 and 8.1, respectively). Among those under 15 years old, 1- to 4-year-olds had the highest rate (1.9 per 100,000 population), and in those over 60 years old it was 1.0 per 100,000.

In 2005, the highest percentage of HIV-positive women and women with AIDS corresponded to housewives (73.9%), followed by sex workers (5.5%). By province, the highest rate of AIDS notification in 2005 was in Guayas, with 6.6 per 100,000 population, followed by Manabí (5.2), Sucumbíos (3.9), Pichincha (3.87), and Cañar (3.17). As of March 2006, a total of 1,093 patients were receiving antiretroviral treatment (887 adults and 206 children). The INEC reported 399 and 422 deaths from AIDS in 2002 and 2003, respectively. In 2003, 82.4% of deaths corresponded to men, and 89.1% to the 15- to 49-year-old age group, followed by the 50- to 64-year-old age group with 9.3% (37).

The HIV/STI National Program began implementing syndrome management for sexually transmitted infections in 2005; as of 2006, there were no consolidated national data. In 2005, the

provinces that reported infections were Guayas, Pichincha, El Oro, Manabí, Loja, and Sucumbíos. The latter province reported a rate of 58 per 100,000 population for **gonorrhea**, 55 for primary and secondary **syphilis**, and 18 for **genital herpes**.

Zoonoses

In 2005, 23 herds (21 bovine and 2 porcine) were reported as being infected with type O virus **foot-and-mouth disease** (38, 39), with 4,089 animals endangered and 7 deaths; 78% of these incidences were reported in Manabí. As of 2006, Ecuador had no areas free of this disease. National vaccination was reported at 56.2% in 2005.

In 2001, 75 cases of canine **rabies** were reported; from 2002 to 2005, 6, 12, 11, and 2 annual cases were reported, respectively. From 2001 to 2003, the provinces with reported cases were Cañar, Azuay, Cotopaxi, and Tungurahua, and Guayas and Manabí in 2004. Vaccination coverage in 2004 was 82% of the estimated canine population for that year. In 2001, one case of human rabies was reported; no cases were reported during 2002–2004, and in 2005, there were two cases of human rabies caused by bat bites in the province of Pastaza (40).

NONCOMMUNICABLE DISEASES

Malignant Neoplasms

In 2004, the INEC death registry reported that the most frequent malignant neoplasms were stomach with 2.7% (1,484 total: 822 men and 662 women), followed by prostate, 1.2% (636); liver and intrahepatic bile ducts, 1.0% (total 573: 279 men and 294 women); trachea, bronchia, and lungs, 1.0% (569 total: 332 men and 237 women); uterus, 0.7% (409); colon, sigmoid colon, rectum, and anus, 0.7% (401 total: 175 men and 226 women); and female breast cancer, 0.6% (312) (16).

OTHER HEALTH PROBLEMS OR ISSUES

Disasters

Eruptions of the Tungurahua volcano in 1999 and their aftermath led to the evacuation of 25,000 people. Damages were estimated at US$ 17 million, and tourist industry losses at US$ 12 million. Various crisis periods between 1999 and 2006 followed that volcanic activity. The eruption of the Reventador volcano in November 2002 compromised close to 40,000 hectares of pastureland and damaged roads and services to access safe water. Lessons were learned about evacuating people in high-risk areas and the effects on the population's health as well as about intervention activities. In winter 2002, close to 28,000 people were affected: 25 died, 1,700 were left homeless, and 1,500 families were evacuated. There was also damage to 5,200 houses and 3,000 educational centers. The rainy season at the beginning of 2006 affected 29,818 families, 1,160 of them with injuries. There were 12 deaths, and five provinces in the coastal region were compromised by the increase in communicable disease morbidity. International support was mobilized to mitigate the impact on health.

Mental Health

In 2005, the main reasons for psychiatric consultations in the MSP per 100,000 population were violence and mistreatment (53.6), alcoholism (23.6), and suicide attempts (15.3) (36). The second national survey on drug consumption, carried out in 2005 by the National Council for the Control of Narcotics and Psychotropic Substances with the support from the Organization of American States (41) among students between 11 and 21 years old, reported that the lifetime prevalence was 61.6% for alcohol consumption, 54.5% for cigarettes, 7.0% for marijuana, and 6.1% for tranquilizers without a prescription. In addition, the age of first-time drug use was between 12.6 and 14.1 years.

Environmental Pollution

The production of flowers and nontraditional crops increased between 2001 and 2005, which caused an increase in the production, marketing, and use of pesticides. In 2004, an estimated US$ 115.8 million worth of pesticides were imported—2.6 times more than the figure reported for 1992 (42). This same study found in 2003 that the mortality rate of agricultural workers exposed to pesticides was 20.5 per 100,000 population. That year, the provinces of Carchi and Manabí listed acute pesticide poisoning as the ninth cause of morbidity. In 2004 and 2005, the notification rate in Carchi increased from 28.0 to 33.2 per 100,000 population, making it the 10th leading cause of morbidity. In 2005, the provinces of Tungurahua and Orellana reported 35.9 cases of acute poisoning per 100,000 population, making it the ninth leading cause of morbidity. In 2003, the INEC recorded 1,826 hospital visits due to pesticide poisoning; 49.2% of the cases were among the 20- to 44-year-old age group, followed by the 10- to 19-year-old age group with 26.1%. By sex, 48.4% of the cases were men, and 51.6% were women (43).

Oral Health

In 2004, the MSP recorded 1,850,010 dentist visits. In 1995–2003, estimates reported a DMFT (decayed/missing/filled teeth) index of 2.9 (15).

RESPONSE OF THE HEALTH SECTOR

Health Policies and Plans

Ecuador's Constitution, which has been in force since 1998, expresses the Government's decision to recognize health as a right that must be guaranteed, promoted, and protected, as well as permanent and uninterrupted access to health services by people who need them.

The National Health System Law (2002) structures the health system into national, provincial, and cantonal levels and provides for the operation of provincial and cantonal health councils. It also defines the scope of the health system in terms of its leadership, provision of services, and insurance and financing and establishes general rules concerning human resources in health, medications, inputs, and science and technology.

In May 2005, the MSP drafted and distributed its strategic plan for 2005–2006, which had the following objectives: to strengthen the leadership role of the MSP; to carry out the first phase of universal health insurance for the poorest population; to develop a national health system; to control diseases with high epidemiological, social, and economic impacts; to strengthen the services network, especially in the provinces and cantons that have the parishes where the poorest people live; and to carry out intersectoral actions to protect and promote health, primarily in areas related to the environment, schools, food, and nutrition.

The National Health System, through the National Health Council (CONASA), organized two national congresses in 2002 and 2004 on the subject of "for health, for life." These meetings had a great deal of social participation, and the Government's health policy was developed during them, as was the health agenda to implement it.

The Constitution establishes the State decentralization in Articles 225 and 226. The health decentralization process began in 2001 with issuance of Executive Decree 1616 and formulation of the National Decentralization Plan. The State Decentralization and Social Participation Act has been in force since 1997 and was amended in 2000 and 2003. The law reaffirms leadership strength at the central level and, in turn, promotes the operation of the health councils as coordination bodies to make decentralization a coherent and ordered process. Since March 2004, work has been under way on the draft version of the Health Act, which would substitute for the Health Code (1971).

Health Strategies and Programs

The national health policy is based on the principles of equity, universality, solidarity, quality, plurality, efficiency, ethics, and comprehensiveness. Its main objectives are to promote among citizens the guarantee, respect, promotion, protection, and demand of and for human rights in health for the exercise of a dignified and healthy life; to guarantee comprehensive health protection for the population, facilitating the means to promote both physical and mental health; and to prevent and to address diseases and their causes, mitigating their biological, economic, and social effects.

CONASA and provincial and cantonal governments promoted application of the law to develop the system through the formation of cantonal and provincial health councils and their respective health plans. As of 2006, the MSP was carrying out disease prevention and health protection activities along with providing care for prevalent morbidity; the Ecuadorian Social Security Institute and the Armed Forces and Police Health Services attended to their members, and the private sector focused on care for morbidity events. The legal framework to modernize the State and the National Health System Law expressly mentions social and community participation as a basic requirement for its implementation and development and recognizes all existing neighborhood and community organizations. Within this context, agreements have been made in the health arena since 2002 to empower the community in decision making in the health councils as well as in committees of users to ensure compliance with the maternal and child health care and family violence prevention laws.

In 2002, the National Health System Law was enacted, which established the general principles and rules for organization and operation of the National Health System. The Social Security Law, in force since November 2001, established the reference framework in this field. Along with approval of the new Constitution in 1998, amendments were made to the Free Maternity and Child Health Care Act in force since 1994. As per its provisions, it is a step toward universal health insurance by ensuring the right of all women to free and quality health care during pregnancy, during birth, and after birth; access to sexual and reproductive health care; and cost-free care for children from birth to 5 years. Ecuador has other specific laws, such as the Law on Patient Rights and Protection, the Law on HIV/AIDS Prevention and Comprehensive Care, the Law on the Provision and Use of Blood and its Derivatives, the Law on Organ and Tissue Transplants, and the Law on Food and Nutritional Safety, as well as amendments to the Health Code and official adoption by the National Commission of the *Codex Alimentarius*. In May 2006, the National Congress ratified the Framework Convention on Tobacco Control.

Organization of the Health System

The public health sector comprises the services of the MSP, which implements traditional health promotion and protection programs: the IESS, the Armed Forces and Police Health Services (divisions of the Ministries of Defense and of Government, respectively), health services for certain municipalities, the Guayaquil Welfare Board (JBG), the Guayaquil Child Protection Society, the Society to Combat Cancer (SOLCA), and the Ecuadorian Red Cross. The Ministry of Public Health is responsible for regulating, supervising, and controlling the sector and has a local office in every province, and, within each one, the Ministry of Public Health has specific sections that provide service in terms of geography and population and which largely coincide with the political and administrative divisions of the canton or municipality. The Ministry of Public Health also carries out a series of health promotion and protection programs and coordinates with the Ministry of Education in implementation of the healthy schools initiative.

The IESS has a personnel membership system, primarily geared toward protecting dependent workers in the public and private sectors. The social insurance system includes economic resources and medical care, which cover 10% of the population. The Farmers' Social Security system covers workers in rural areas and provides family coverage. It includes the provision of social services, such as death, disability, and pension benefits, as well as primary medical care, which are extended to the country's rural population (37% of the national population). It is estimated that 9.2% are covered. The Armed Forces and Police Health Services offer ambulatory care and hospitalization. The JBG is an autonomous social services agency financed primarily by the national lottery. It has four hospitals: two general and two specialized hospitals located in Guayaquil. SOLCA is a private social agency that covers part of the national demand for the diagnosis and treatment of cancer and is based in regional institutions in the country's main cities, where it operates with administrative and financial autonomy. It has five specialized hospitals. Municipal health services are responsible for health offices that address environmental health and sanitary control problems, with the exceptions of Quito and Guayaquil, which include certain private ambulatory and hospital services.

The private sector (which represents 15% of the country's health facilities) includes nonprofit entities (hospitals, clinics, dispensaries, medical offices, pharmacies, and health care insurance providers) as well as various NGOs, social service associations, and others. To operate, private bodies must be registered and authorized by the Ministry of Public Health. Prepaid medicine providers cover less than 3% of the middle- and upper-income population.

In compliance with the National Health System Law and the recommendations of the Second Congress on Life and Health, the National Office for the Health of Indigenous Peoples of the Ministry of Public Health, along with the Confederation of Indigenous Nationalities of Ecuador, and other private, public, and official agencies created traditional medicine commissions, as well as an intercultural commission to strengthen health care models (4). In 2006, there were activities focusing on interculturalism and development among health systems. Examples include the decentralized canton of Cotacachi in Imbabura; the quality assurance project in Tungurahua, applied in health areas and a provincial hospital (executed by an NGO); health promoters of the agriculture and livestock production cooperative in Napo and Orellana (supported by the Swiss Red Cross); the Borbón health post in the province of Esmeraldas; and the sustainable human development project located in the province of Morona in health areas three and five. In this context, there are also initiatives such as the Jambi Huasi comprehensive health center in Otavalo, Imbabura; the Alli Causai Hospital in Ambato, Tungurahua; and the Andean Alternative Hospital in Riobamba, Chimborazo. Likewise, indigenous health departments promoted works related to the use of ethnobotanic resources in Guayas, the intercultural health model in Azuay (Nabón), and vertical birth and birthing homes in Pastaza (Puyo). The Guamaní health area also provided traditional and alternative medicines and therapies in Quito.

Public Health Services

Various national forums brought together the ideas of the different actors in the sector, which focused on the need for more in-depth governmental reform based on strengthening the deconcentration and decentralization of the health structure, safeguarding the effectiveness of the national health system, strengthening the health authority, and broad and ongoing social participation in developing the family and community health model. In this context, the Ministry of Public Health defined and has been applying since June 2004 a new comprehensive care model based on primary health care.

Evaluation of the Ministry of Public Health epidemiological surveillance system in 2001 identified 47% underreporting of diseases of mandatory notification (44). In response to this underreporting, surveillance systems were developed by program (such as EPI, maternal death, food and nutrition, and vector-borne diseases), by disease (HIV/AIDS, tuberculosis, and leprosy), or by events (maternal deaths and family violence). However, the simultaneous and growing development of information systems (multiple and parallel) limited the comprehensiveness of information and surveillance systems. There were also difficulties and limitations in this area in the Ministry of Public Health's coordination with other institutions providing services, as well as in the systematization, analysis, and use of information for management.

In 2003, the Ministry of Public Health began implementing the comprehensive epidemiological surveillance system (SIVE), which, according to an end-of-year evaluation, covered 60% of the provinces. In 2004, SIVE-Alerta began to be implemented as a more developed system than the previous one. In 2005, the system covered 88% of Ministry of Public Health areas (150 of 169).

The Leopoldo Izquieta Pérez National Hygiene and Tropical Medicine Institute (INHMT), an agency assigned to the Ministry of Public Health, is headquartered in Guayaquil; it has 33 national laboratories and supervises 250 local laboratories. Its areas of action are: being the national center for reference laboratories; making definitive diagnoses in epidemiological surveillance; executing the health registry, which guarantees the quality of products used in Ecuador (medicines, natural products, cosmetics, hygienic products, processed foods, and pesticides); producing biologicals and vaccines; carrying out research in human and animal health; and ensuring the training and education of internal and external human resources. The Institute maintains a structured microbiology laboratory network for the diagnosis of tuberculosis, syphilis, HIV, dengue, plague, leishmaniasis, Chagas' disease, aspergillosis, chlamydiosis, meningococcemia, and others. The INHMT certified the processed food laboratory based on rule ISO 17025 and received certification from an external evaluation of the biochemical laboratory in human health during 2003–2005 (45).

Water, sanitation, and solid waste services are the responsibility of the Undersecretariat of Drinking Water and Basic Sanitation of the Ministry of Urban Development and Housing, which exercises the guiding role in this sector via the water and sanitation national policy. Within this framework and at the request of the Government, PAHO/WHO initiated an intersectoral discussion table on water and sanitation, whose objective was to manage the portfolio of projects to benefit the poorest populations. The Ministry of Public Health was responsible for coordination and the Ministry of Urban Development and Housing (MIDUVI) was in charge of the secretariat.

In 2006, MIDUVI, as the guiding agency in water and sanitation services, recorded national coverage levels of 67% in drinking water, 57% in sanitation, and 51% in solid waste (46). According to United Nations estimates, national coverage was 86% in 2002 (92% urban and 77% rural). The Government slated an investment of US$ 343 million during 2002–2006 to increase drinking water coverage by 6.5% and sewage services by 11.5% (47).

In 2005, the Hospital Waste Management Program was implemented in 891 public and private institutions. This program is subject to regulations covering management of infectious wastes in health institutions. In addition, the Ministry of Public Health trained and advised nearly 6,000 health workers and professionals on the management of hospital wastes. In 2001, the Stockholm Convention on Persistent Organic Pollutants (POPs) was signed, and, in 2004, it was ratified, carrying with it the responsibility to develop the National Implementation Plan for POP Management, whose goal is to protect the population and the environment from POPs. The plan proposes: monitoring the reduction of polychlorinated biphenyls (PCB), which in 2003 were calculated at 6,000 tons of contaminated oil; eliminating dioxins and furans, with an annual emissions rate of 97.57 g TEQ/y, and completing the elimination of POP pesticides, most of which have been eradicated in the country, although there are still 1,650.81 kg of residual DDT that need disposal.

In September 2005, the Government requested that the United Nations create a mission to examine the feasibility and types of study possible to evaluate the potential impact that spreading glyphosate by aircraft would have on health, the environment, and agriculture on the country's northern border. In response, the United Nations created an interinstitutional mission that began work at the beginning of 2006 and submitted its report during that year. It proposed five studies needed for scientific clarification of the scenario of eventualities that could harm health and the environment as a result of spreading glyphosate herbicides and its compounds by aircraft, as well as short-term projects geared toward improving the basic conditions for comprehensive socioeconomic development of the region.

The Ecuadorian Agricultural and Livestock Health Service (SESA), via the National Commission for the Elimination of Foot-and-Mouth Disease (CONEFA), is the body in charge of monitoring the health situation of Ecuadorian livestock. To this end, SESA has 51 national offices, with the support of 194 local CONEFA committees. The Ministry of Public Health and other sectoral institutions do not have a food safety surveillance system.

In 2003, to integrate programs and strategies on the subjects of food and nutrition, an executive decree was issued, via which the Comprehensive Food and Nutrition System (SIAN) was initiated. This system focused its actions on the poorest population and was formed by the National Food Program and Comprehensive Micronutrient Program of the Ministry of Public Health, the School Food Program of the Ministry of Education and Culture, and the Feed Yourself Ecuador Program of the Ministry of Social Welfare. In 2005, the Ministry of Public Health reformulated the system and designed a comprehensive complementary food and nutritional program to improve the nutritional state and food situation of the population in the 200 parishes in the country farthest behind in terms of unsatisfied basic needs (48). The strategy included integration and coordination with other programs and projects of the MSP, the Ministry of Education and Culture, and the Ministry of Social Welfare that had been created as social assistance strategies based on the delivery of food supplements. Evaluation of the national food program, in terms of the baby food product "Mi Papilla" geared toward children 6 to 24 months, showed that it improved nutritional status (improvement of weight-for-age) and provided micronutrients (iron, zinc, and vitamin A) (49).

The health sector provided timely responses and leadership in sectoral coordination in the floods in the coastal region (2002, 2005, and 2006) as well as during the eruptions of Reventador (2002) and Tungurahua (2006) and with regard to the continued flow of people over the northern border seeking refuge (2001–2005). The most complex hospitals in provinces at risk of flooding (Guayas and Manabí), volcanic eruptions (Chimborazo, Pichincha, Tungurahua, and Cotopaxi), and massive population flux (Sucumbíos, Imbabura, Carchi, and Esmeraldas) had disaster contingency plans, which helped them provide an appropriate response.

In 2001, the National Civil Defense System initiated, along with the appropriate rules and guidelines, the Emergency Operations Center, which encompasses the health sector. The response to emergencies included formation of situation rooms at the regional level and the creation of rapid-response multidisciplinary teams; the coordination of the teams is the responsibility of the disaster focal points in the provincial offices, which have been trained in methodologies to evaluate damages and analyze needs, which has facilitated timely care in emergency and disaster situations. In 2004, the Ministry of Public Health established a National Health Network for Addressing Emergencies and Disasters, led by the Office of Safety Planning for National Development, which is responsible for managing risks and planning the execution of mitigation, prevention, and health care actions in the event of emergencies and disasters.

From 2002 to 2006, PAHO/WHO executed five phases of the project for strengthening the health sector to provide care for the refugee population. A total of US$ 250,000 were mobilized from USAID, ECHO, and CIDA, in coordination with the Ministry of Public Health, local governments, NGOs, churches, and United Nations agencies (UNCHR and IOM). The project generated results in risk management for emergencies and disasters, hospital

planning, public health surveillance, information systems, comprehensive care for the refugee population, and improvement of the quality of drinking water in at-risk communities on the northern border. Working within the framework of the Bilateral Technical Health Committee, the governments of Ecuador and Colombia implemented the plan to develop the integrated border area in 2005. PAHO/WHO offered support to strengthen public health surveillance, with an emphasis on pesticides and water quality. Between 2004 and 2005, as part of the strengthening of the health sector response capacity and with financing from the Humanitarian Aid Office of the European Commission (US$ 400,000), PAHO/WHO developed a project on preparedness for volcanic eruptions for Ecuador and Colombia. The project's technical materials were later used by countries in Central and South America. During 2002–2006, United Nations bodies in Ecuador established an interinstitutional technical group to respond to emergencies caused by floods, volcanic eruptions, mass displacements, and related occurrences.

In 2005, a national contingency plan was developed to confront a possible influenza pandemic in Ecuador; the plan was interinstitutional in nature and included operating guides and strategies to address this threat during prepandemic and pandemic periods. The plan included specific coordination actions among ministries (Ministry of Public Health, Ministry of Agriculture, Ministry of the Environment, the Ecuadorian Agricultural and Livestock Health Service) and among sectors (Ministry of Governance, poultry businesses, and social communication media). It also received contributions from bodies of the United Nations system—particularly PAHO/WHO and FAO. The major components of the plan were: epidemiological surveillance, preparation of health services, and a strategic communication and social mobilization plan. In 2006, vaccination against seasonal flu was initiated (with resources allocated in the Ministry of Public Health budget) (50). National investment in this area began in 2006, and budgetary allocations were made for 2007. Before the entry in force of the International Health Regulations in 2007, health authorities assumed voluntary and immediate compliance with the provisions related to bird flu and a possible influenza pandemic.

Individual Care Services

The resolution capacity of the Ministry of Public Health's services is organized according to level of complexity. At level I (basic complexity), there are 434 posts, 1,122 subcenters (774 rural and 348 urban), and 153 health centers, which offer ambulatory care, health promotion, disease prevention, and health recovery; all promote basic environmental health and community participation actions, and the subcenters offer care during birth and emergencies as well as dental care. At level II (intermediate complexity), there are 90 basic hospitals and 23 general hospitals, which, in addition to level I care, provide short-term hospitalization. The basic hospitals provide ambulatory and hospital care in

Intersector Integration for Food Safety

The Comprehensive Food and Nutrition System (SIAN) was launched in 2003 to carry out integrated actions in the area of diet and nutrition to protect the most vulnerable groups in the neediest urban and rural areas. In 2005, the system was reformed and an integrated plan for food and nutrition supplements was designed, composed of the following programs:

- The Ministry of Public Health's Supplementary Food Program that assists pregnant and breastfeeding women and children under 3 years old with the food supplements "Mi Bebida" and "Mi Papilla."
- The Ministry of Public Health's Integrated Micronutrient Program, with subprograms for micronutrient supplements (iron, folic acid, vitamin A) and the subprogram to fortify wheat flour with micronutrients.
- The Ministry of Education and Culture's School Food Program which covers the school population from 6 to 15 years of age.
- The Ministry of Social Welfare's food program (Aliméntate Ecuador) that assists the child population between 4 and 5 years old, persons with disabilities, and older adults.

The evaluation of "Mi Papilla," (a precooked product that requires only the addition of clean drinking water to prepare, and provides 100% of the daily requirement of iron, folic acid, and zinc; 60% of the vitamin C, the vitamin B complex, and magnesium requirement; and 30% of the vitamin A, calcium, and phosphorus requirement) indicated that it has had a beneficial effect on nutritional and micronutrient status, principally iron, in the population under 2 years of age.

general medicine, gynecology and obstetrics, pediatrics, and emergency surgery; the general hospital also offers, in addition to those items mentioned, some specialization in keeping with the epidemiological profile of its area of influence and has auxiliary diagnostic and treatment services. At level III (high complexity), there are 14 specialty hospitals and 1 reference hospital for care of the local, regional, and national populations. They also provide educational training and carry out health research.

In terms of the functional organization of the Ministry of Public Health, there were three levels in 2005: health areas (169), the provincial level (22), and the national level (1). The health area comprises the management unit and operating units at the first and second levels, with the ability to resolve technical, administrative, and financial issues. The provincial level includes the provincial health office whose role to provide technical and administrative support to the area divisions and to the hospitals in its geographic jurisdiction. The guiding agency of the health sector is at the national level and incorporates the different processes responsible for creating and distributing technical, administrative, and financial rules applied at the national level. The IESS administers 5 level I hospitals, 10 level II hospitals, 3 level III hospitals, 25 ambulatory centers, 42 ambulatory units, and 348 rural social security dispensaries.

In 2003, there were 33 blood banks in Ecuador, and 79,204 units of blood were collected (29.9% were voluntary donations, and the rest were replacement donations), all of which were tested for *Trypanosoma cruzi*, syphilis, hepatitis C, hepatitis B surface antigen, and HIV. Prevalence of these markers was 0.36% for

T. cruzi, 3.90% for syphilis, 0.35% for the hepatitis C virus, 0.15% for the hepatitis B surface antigen, and 0.28% for HIV (*51*).

In 2006, the Ministry of Public Health requested that the country be incorporated into the CARMEN regional proposal for the control of noncommunicable diseases. That same year, there were no data on this group of diseases.

Health Promotion

In 2004, CONASA formed a health promotion commission to coordinate and guide intersectoral promotion actions. In 2006, discussion began on the national health promotion policy (*52*), with participation of the Ministry of Public Health, the Ministry of Education, the Ministry of Environment, the Association of Municipalities of Ecuador (AME), universities, certain local governments, NGOs, and other institutions. The Ecuadorian network of schools that promote health is coordinated by the Ministries of Education and Health and by PAHO; it is supported by other national and international organizations. In 2004, it registered more than 3,000 schools that promoted the development of ecoclubs. The network of ecoclubs promotes community participation and social communication in the control of dengue, malaria, and other diseases and risks (*53*).

The Loja project on healthy spaces ended in 2002. It generated local knowledge and experience in health promotion. In 2006, the network of healthy municipalities, coordinated by AME and the Ministry of Public Health and supported by PAHO, was made up of more than 20 municipalities. That same year, a ministerial agreement was approved to establish the promotion of physical activity and healthy eating, focused on regulating the places where food is provided in schools and on combating sedentary lifestyles.

Health Supplies

The basic lines of the medication national policy (1999) are geared toward guaranteeing availability, access, quality, rational use, and low prices of medicines. The Law on the Production, Importation, Marketing, and Sale of Drugs for Human Use of 2000 establishes rules geared toward expanding the use of generic medications, providing incentives for national production, and facilitating their registry through a uniform procedure for imported products. In 2004, the Ecuadorian pharmaceutical market (87% private and 13% public) had approximately 225 laboratories, 170 distributors, 5,000 pharmacies, and 6,439 products (1,539 of them generic) (54, 55). The private market grew 35.8% during 2001–2005 (from US$ 407,079 million to US$ 553,157 million) (56). The number of generic products increased from 16.2% in 2001 to 25.2% in 2005; sales volume in 2005 did not surpass 11.3% of the total, due, among other reasons, to a lack of trust among those issuing the prescriptions because there was no guarantee of the quality and safety of these products. In 2004, it was estimated that approximately 80% of medicines were obtained and consumed without a prescription. The National Commission on Medicines and Inputs of CONASA updates, publishes, and distributes the national list of basic drugs biannually. The fifth version was published in 2004, and, in 2006, the sixth was approved. The medicines included in that list are of mandatory use in all public health institutions and reference institutions for the private sector.

In 2006, the country produced vaccines against DPT (diphtheria, whooping cough, and tetanus), DT (diphtheria and tetanus), BCG (antituberculosis), rabies for human use and for veterinary use (modified suckling mouse brain vaccine), and antivenin serum (against poisoning by snakes of the genus *Bothrops*, and species *asper*, *atrox*, and *xantograma*). Good manufacturing processes were implemented that year.

In 2004, based on primary health care and the comprehensive health care model, the Ministry of Public Health coverage extension program developed and applied a licensing system for level I and level II health units in the 200 poorest parishes in the country (in terms of unmet basic needs), mobilizing financial resources (US$ 6,600,000) and updating and equipping the units (57). It also trained human resources at the technical and administrative support levels and identified the target population.

Human Resources

In 2001, the female-to-male ratio was 1.8:1 in schools of medicine, nursing, obstetrics, and medical technology. That year,

physicians and dentists tended to be concentrated in urban areas, while nurses and obstetricians were more often in rural areas. In 2003, for every 10,000 population, there were 15.6 physicians; 5.3 nurses; 1.7 dentists; 1.8 obstetricians; and 9.8 nursing assistants. That same year, the lowest rate of physicians was in Orellana (5.4) and the highest was in Azuay (26.6). In terms of nurses, the province of Orellana had the lowest rate (1.8) and Pichincha the highest (9.8). A 2004 study carried out in four universities in Quito and Cuenca concluded, at the time of the study, that of the total physicians and nurses trained in 2001, 9.8% had left the country, and 34.8% had plans to travel abroad (58). In 2005, there were 18 universities for training medical professionals, duly recognized and accredited by the National Higher Education Council. Between 2001 and 2005, 5 institutions for training dentists, 2 for nurses, and 1 for obstetricians were created. As of 2005, higher education centers that included intercultural subjects were Universidad Andina Simón Bolívar and the Universidad Intercultural de las Nacionalidades y Pueblos Indígenas Amawtay Wasi, both in Quito.

Since 2001, the National Health Human Resources Commission of CONASA has been responsible for the Human Resources Observatory in the country. In addition, this body created the draft law of the Health Career Law (2006), which was submitted to CONASA. As of 2006, the Ministry of Public Health was developing permanent health education projects and programs.

Given that, in 1992, the creation of posts in Ministry of Public Health services was halted, in 2003, the Ministry of Public Health employed 54.6% of physicians working in the sector; 59.6% of nurses, 68.8% of dentists, and 94.6% of obstetricians. In that same year, the distribution of health professionals working in the public sector corresponded to 49.95% of physicians, 81.86% of nurses, 91.82% of dentists, and 80.95% of obstetricians (59).

Research and Technological Development in Health

The MSP, through its scientific and technological processes, plays the guiding role in scientific and technological research and development in health. To this end, it has the support of the National Secretariat of Science and Technology, the National Science and Technology Commission of CONASA—which in 2006 formulated the health research policy considered by CONASA—the National Council of Universities and Polytechnic Schools, and other national and international organizations. The National Forum on Health Research brings together researchers and institutions related to health research and initiates research policies geared toward national priorities.

The investment in research and development in 2003 was 0.07% of the GDP. Because of its importance as an instrument for the country's social and economic development, the Government decided to invest in science and technology, which is why it appropriated 5% of existing funds in the Special Account for Productive and Social Reactivation—US$ 8 million in 2005 and US$ 26 million in

2006, in each case approximately 14% of the total for health—for activities related to science, technology, and innovation (*60*).

Since its inception in 1998 up to 2003, the Virtual Health Library (VHL) opened seven cooperating centers, which regularly receive and send information to expand the VHL database (*61*); in addition, an information network was organized with four centers located in different universities and a coordinating center for areas. In January 2006, the national policy on science, technology, and innovation was published (*60*).

Health Sector Expenditures and Financing

In 2004, 50.4% of total health spending came from the public sector (Ministry of Public Health, IESS, Armed Forces and Police Health Services, and sectional governments) and 49.2% from the private sector. Ninety percent of the total private health spending corresponded to direct household spending (61% for the purchase of medications and inputs; 24.3% for medical care; and 4.7% for laboratory exams, dental materials, and orthopedic devices); the remaining 10% is direct payment to medical providers. In terms of private expense, 74.7% was carried out in urban areas, and 25.3% in rural areas, where 37% of the population lives, more than 50% of which is poor. Public social spending in health as a percentage of the GDP went from 0.6% in 2000 to 0.8% in 2001, 1.2% in 2002, and 1.5% in 2004. In the public sector, health spending allocated 81.2% for curative care and 18.8% for preventative care. Moreover, spending on primary care was 34.1%, with 29.9% on secondary care, and 36% on tertiary care. Of this spending, 34.4% corresponded to the provision of hospital services, 29.3% to the supply of medicines, 23.6% to ambulatory services, 11.7% to public health, and 0.9% to research. Only 31.8% was geared toward the poor, and the rest received 68.2%. The MSP budget has been constantly increasing from 2001 (US$ 151.7 million) to 2006 (US$ 561 million), going from 2.8% of the general budget for the State in 2001 to 6.0% in 2006 (*3*). The proposed budget submitted for 2007 was US$ 845 million (8.3%) of the national budget.

Technical Cooperation and External Financing

In 2003, Ecuador received US$ 811 million in international cooperation, 79.6% in external loans and 20.4% in nonreimbursable funds. In 2004, this amount dropped to US$ 555 million, of which 67.3% corresponded to external loans, and 32.7% to nonreimbursable funds. The total amount of bilateral cooperation during 2003–2004 fluctuated between US$ 105 million in 2003 and US$ 102 million in 2004, while multilateral cooperation increased 40% from US$ 26 million in 2003 to US$ 36 million in 2004. Cooperation from nongovernmental organizations increased 23% from 34 million in 2003 to 42 million in 2004 (*62*). Multilateral cooperation primarily focused on the social welfare sector (nine cooperation partners); education, science, and technology (eight cooperation partners); and the environment, natural resources, health, and sanitation (seven cooperation partners). In terms of financing awarded for projects during 2003–2004, the European Commission was the main donor at 8.6% of the total amount (US$ 12.31 million).

During 2001–2005, PAHO/WHO cooperation focused politically and technically on strategic processes that contributed to health development. The most important achievements were approval of the National Health System Law and its later implementation. During implementation, the law supported the regulatory process, the development and strengthening of the CONASA board of directors and its technical commissions (intersectoral in nature), and cantonal and provincial health councils, as well as an increase in the public health budget.

In 2003, the pentavalent vaccine (diphtheria, whooping cough, tetanus, hepatitis B, and *Haemophilus influenzae* type b) was introduced. The vaccine against seasonal flu was incorporated for at-risk groups, and financing was approved for a vaccine against rotavirus for 2007. During this period, Ecuador remained free of poliomyelitis, and measles, diphtheria, rubella, congenital rubella syndrome, and neonatal tetanus stopped being a public health problem. PAHO supported the Ministry of Public Health in strengthening and decentralizing the National Malaria Program and in developing research on resistance to insecticides and antimalarials. There was intersectoral collaboration with regard to dengue, headed up by the Ministry of Public Health and involving the participation of the municipalities, the Ministries of Education, Governance, and Defense, and the organized community, which aided in the rapid control of outbreaks and a decrease in the number of deaths.

In addition, PAHO supported the response to emergencies and disasters caused by floods and volcanic risks. The Ministry of Public Health strengthened the decentralization of the National Disaster Preparedness, Response, and Mitigation Program. International resources were mobilized to mitigate disasters, primarily flooding on the coast, and interinstitutional work was encouraged for the coordinated response of the international community. Recognized leadership was developed by all the national and international actors, and intersectoral and interinstitutional work was promoted along the border with Colombia. Participants in the latter included the MSP, the Ministry of Housing and Urban Development, and the International Organization for Migration to ensure monitoring of water quality at treatment plants and in storage networks, and to guarantee drinking water for the population without access to it through the use of appropriate technology and community participation; this experience was also carried out among populations in the poorest parishes in the country. Ecuador was advised on the creation of national policies for compliance with the MDGs and implementation of universal health insurance, as well as the preparation of reports and practical plans related to the MDGs in general and to health in particular.

References

1. Banco Central del Ecuador. Boletín estadístico mensual. Available at: www.bce.fin.ec. Accessed May 15, 2006.

2. Ecuador, Instituto Nacional de Estadística y Censos. Encuesta Nacional de Empleo, Subempleo y Desempleo (ENEMDU). Serie histórica. INEC; diciembre 2006. Available at: www.inec.gov.ec. Accessed April 14 and May 15, 2006.

3. Ecuador, Ministerio de Economía y Finanzas. Estados financieros consolidados a diciembre 2005. Available at: www.minfinanzas.ec-gov.net. Accessed April 14 and May 15, 2006.

4. Ecuador, Consejo Nacional de Salud; Ministerio de Salud Pública; Organización Panamericana de la Salud/Organización Mundial de la Salud; Fondo de Población de las Naciones Unidas; Fondo de las Naciones Unidas para la Infancia. II Congreso Nacional por la Salud y la Vida, junio 2005.

5. Gobierno de Ecuador; Naciones Unidas, Secretaría Nacional de Objetivos de Desarrollo del Milenio. Informe ODM 2015: el futuro tiene fecha. 2005.

6. Transparencia Internacional. Barómetro Global de la Corrupción, 2004, Ecuador, septiembre 2005. Available at: www.transparencia.org.es. Accessed April 14 and May 15, 2006.

7. Sola J. Una desconcentración incompleta: la reforma de la salud en el Ecuador. Revista Ecuador Debate N° 61. Quito; 2004.

8. Presidencia de la República del Ecuador; Secretaría Nacional de los Objetivos de Desarrollo del Milenio. Sistema Nacional de Aseguramiento Universal en Salud; abril 2006. Available at: www.presidencia.gov.ec. Accessed April 14 and May 15, 2006.

9. Contrato Social por la Educación en el Ecuador. Indicadores de la situación educativa en Ecuador; 2005.

10. Ecuador, Centro de Estudios de Población y Desarrollo Social. Encuesta Demográfica y de Salud Materna e Infantil (ENDEMAIN) 2004. Informe final. Quito: CEPAR; octubre 2005.

11. Naciones Unidas. La frontera norte del Ecuador: evaluaciones y recomendaciones de la Misión Interagencial del Sistema de Naciones Unidas del Ecuador. Quito; junio 2004.

12. Ecuador, Instituto Nacional de Estadística y Censos. Proyecciones de población por provincias, cantones, áreas, sexo y grupos de edad, período 2001–2010.

13. Ecuador, Ministerio de Salud Pública. Informe de la Dirección Nacional de Salud de Pueblos Indígenas; 2005.

14. Organización Panamericana de la Salud. Situación de salud en las Américas. Indicadores básicos 2001. Washington, DC: OPS; 2001.

15. Organización Panamericana de la Salud. Situación de salud en las Américas. Indicadores básicos 2005. Washington, DC: OPS; 2005.

16. Ecuador, Ministerio de Salud Pública; Instituto Nacional de Estadística y Censos; Programa Anual de Inversiones (SEMPLADES); Secretaría Técnica de Frente Social. Indicadores básicos de salud del Ecuador, 2005. septiembre 2005.

17. Ecuador, Ministerio de Salud Pública; Instituto Nacional de Estadística y Censos; Secretaría Técnica de Frente Social; Organización Panamericana de la Salud/Organización Mundial de Salud; Fondo de las Naciones Unidas para la Infancia; Fondo de Población de las Naciones Unidas; Programa de las Naciones Unidas para el Desarrollo. Indicadores básicos de salud del Ecuador, 2004. agosto 2004.

18. Organización Panamericana de la Salud. Boletín Epidemiológico. 2003;24(4).

19. Ecuador, Instituto Nacional de Estadística y Censos. Anuario de estadísticas vitales, nacimientos y defunciones, 2004. Available at: www.inec.gov.ec. Accessed April 14 and May 15, 2006.

20. Ecuador, Ministerio de Salud Pública, Dirección de Mejoramiento y Control de la Salud Pública, Subproceso de Epidemiología-Vigilancia Epidemiológica. Situación de la salud del Ecuador. Quito; marzo 2006.

21. Ecuador, Ministerio de Salud Pública, Sistema Común de Información. Producción de establecimientos de salud, Ecuador 2004. Quito; mayo 2005.

22. Aguilar D, Alarcón E, Guerrón A, López P, Mejía S, Riofrío L. El sobrepeso y la obesidad en escolares de 8 años del área urbana. [Thesis.] Quito: Universidad Central del Ecuador; 2001.

23. Ecuador, Ministerio de Salud Pública; Organización Panamericana de la Salud/Organización Mundial de la Salud; Fondo de las Naciones Unidas para la Infancia; Fondo de Población de las Naciones Unidas. Proyecciones de la población por provincias, cantones y parroquias según grupos programáticos. Ecuador 2005. abril 2005.

24. Fondo de las Naciones Unidas para la Infancia, Observatorio de los Derechos de la Niñez y Adolescencia. Estado de los derechos de la niñez y adolescencia en el Ecuador, 2005. UNICEF; 2005.

25. Ecuador, Ministerio de Salud Pública, Proceso de Normatización del Sistema Nacional de Salud, Comisión de Salud y Derechos Sexuales y Reproductivos del CONASA. Quito; abril 2005.

26. Organización Panamericana de la Salud. Situación de salud en las Américas: Indicadores básicos 2003. Washington, DC: OPS; 2003.

27. Ecuador, Instituto Nacional de Estadística y Censos. Anuario de estadísticas vitales nacimientos y defunciones 2003. Available at: www.inec.gov.ec. Accessed April 14 and May 15, 2006.

28. Ecuador, Instituto Nacional de Estadística y Censos; Banco Interamericano de Desarrollo. Encuesta Nacional de Ingresos y Gastos de Hogares Urbanos 2003–2004. Resultados preliminares. Quito; abril 2004.

29. Facultad Latinoamericana de Ciencias Sociales, Sede Ecuador; Banco Central del Ecuador; Universidad de Guayaquil; Universidad de Cuenca. La emigración internacional en Quito, Guayaquil y Cuenca. Quito; enero 2004.

30. Ecuador, Centro de Estudio de Población y Desarrollo Social. Situación de salud de los pueblos indígenas en el Ecuador. In: ENDEMAIN 2004. 2006.

31. Gross M, Terán C, Terán J. Línea de base en temas del sector salud de provincias de la frontera norte del Ecuador. Quito; mayo 2006. Unedited document.

32. Ecuador, Ministerio de Salud Pública, Programa Nacional de Malaria; Instituto Nacional de Higiene. Estudio de drogo-resistencia a los anti-maláricos. Resultados preliminares. Ecuador 2004–2005.

33. Ecuador, Ministerio de Salud Pública. Informe anual Programa Nacional de Malaria, 2004.

34. Ecuador, Ministerio de Salud Pública. Informe Programa Ampliado de Inmunizaciones, 2005.

35. Ecuador, Ministerio de Salud Pública, Programa Nacional de Zoonosis, 2001–2005.

36. Ecuador, Ministerio de Salud Pública, Sistema Integrado de Vigilancia Epidemiológica, 2001–2005.

37. Ecuador, Ministerio de Salud Pública. Informe Programa Nacional de SIDA, 2005.

38. Ecuador, Ministerio de Salud Pública. Informe del Programa Nacional de Rabia, 2001–2006.

39. Terán G. Plaguicidas su impacto en salud. Ecuador 2005.

40. Ecuador, Instituto Nacional de Estadística y Censos. Egresos hospitalarios, 2003.

41. Consejo Nacional de Control de Sustancias Estupefacientes y Psicotrópicas; Organización de Estados Americanos, Comisión Interamericana para el Control del Abuso de Drogas; Naciones Unidas, Oficina contra la Droga y el Delito. II Encuesta Nacional sobre Consumo de Drogas en Estudiantes de Enseñanza Media. Ecuador, 2005.

42. Organización Panamericana de la Salud, Centro Panamericana de Fiebre Aftosa; Servicio Ecuatoriano de Sanidad Agropecuaria; Ministerio de Agricultura y Ganadería. XXXIII COSALFA: Informe anual de los países 2005. Working document. OPS; 2005.

43. Organización Panamericana de la Salud, Centro Panamericano de Fiebre Aftosa. Situación de los programas de erradicación de la fiebre aftosa: América del Sur. 2004.

44. Ecuador, Ministerio de Salud Pública, Dirección Nacional de Planificación y Financiamiento. Propuesta para la creación del sistema único de información con enfoque georeferencial para el Ministerio de Salud Pública y el sector salud. septiembre 2001.

45. Benites E. Instituto Nacional de Higiene y Medicina Tropical "Leopoldo Izquieta Pérez". Informe especial MT15-SSH.AC. junio 2005.

46. Ecuador, Ministerio de Vivienda y Desarrollo Urbano. Agenda de agua potable y saneamiento básico, 2006.

47. Ecuador, Ministerio de Vivienda y Desarrollo Urbano. Política nacional de agua y saneamiento, diciembre 2003.

48. Ecuador, Ministerio de Salud Pública; Organización Panamericana de la Salud/Organización Mundial de la Salud; Fondo de las Naciones Unidas para la Infancia; Programa Mundial de Alimentos de las Naciones Unidas. Plan integrado de alimentación complementaria y nutricional en las parroquias más pobres del Ecuador. Quito; 2005.

49. Lutter C, Sempértegui F, Rodríguez A, Fuenmayor G, Ávila L, Madero J, et al. Evaluación de impacto del Programa Nacional de Alimentación y Nutrición (PANN 2000). Washington, DC: OPS; mayo 2005.

50. Ecuador, Ministerio de Salud Pública; Ministerio de Agricultura y Ganadería; Servicio Ecuatoriano de Sanidad Agropecuaria; Ministerio del Ambiente. Plan nacional de contingencia para enfrentar posible pandemia de influenza en el Ecuador, diciembre 2005.

51. Organización Panamericana de la Salud. Medicina transfusional en los países del Caribe y Latinoamérica 2000–2003. Washington, DC: OPS; 2005. (Publicación técnica THS/EV-2005/005 E).

52. Ecuador, Consejo Nacional de Salud, Comisión de Promoción de la Salud. Política nacional de promoción de la salud. Versión preliminar; junio 2006.

53. Ecuador, Fundación Nacional de Ecoclubes. Ecoseñal: guía para la formación de ecoclubes. Guayaquil; noviembre 2004.

54. Paredes P, Romo H, Quevedo M. Estudio del mercado farmacéutico en el Ecuador. Quito; julio 2004.

55. Corporación de Estudios para el Desarrollo. Impacto económico sobre el sector farmacéutico ecuatoriano de la adopción de un capítulo sobre la protección de derechos de propiedad intelectual. Resumen ejecutivo. Quito; septiembre 2005.

56. Ecuador, Instituto Nacional de Salud. Auditoría mercado farmacéutico privado. Investigación de mercado en salud. Ecuador. 2001–2005.

57. Ecuador, Ministerio de Salud Pública; Organización Panamericana de la Salud, Proyecto Modernización y Desarrollo de Redes Integrales de Servicios de Salud (MODERSA). Programa de extensión de cobertura en salud en base a la estrategia de atención primaria y el licenciamiento de la red de servicios de salud. mayo 2004.

58. Ecuador, Consejo Nacional de Salud; Comisión Nacional de Recursos Humanos; Observatorio de Recursos Humanos de Salud en Ecuador; Ministerio de Salud. Migración de médicos y enfermeras recién graduados en Quito y Cuenca. Informe para el Proyecto Modersa. Elaborado por Merino C. Quito; 2004.

59. Merino C; Observatorio de Recursos Humanos en Salud en Ecuador; Comisión Nacional de Recursos Humanos. Empleo de los recursos humanos en salud en instituciones del sector público. Quito; 2006.

60. Ecuador, Secretaría Nacional de Ciencia y Tecnología, Fundación para la Ciencia y Tecnología. Memoria anual 2005. enero 2006.

61. Ecuador, Biblioteca Virtual en Salud. Available at: www.bvs.org.ec. Accessed May 15, 2006.

62. Ecuador, Instituto Ecuatoriano de Cooperación Internacional; Ministerio de Relaciones Exteriores. Cooperación para el desarrollo. Ecuador 2003–2004. Quito; 2005.

EL SALVADOR

Guatemala

Honduras

Santa
Ana

Chalatenango

Ahuachapán

1   2   Cabañas

Son-
sonate

San Salvador
★

Morazán

La
Libertad

San
Vicente

La Unión

La Paz

San
Miguel

Usulután

Nicaragua

1 San Salvador
2 Cuscatlán

0   25   50 Miles

El Salvador is in Central America. It has an area of 21,040.79 km² structured into 14 departments and 262 municipios for administrative purposes. It is a republic, with a decentralized, representative, democratically elected government composed of executive, legislative, and judicial branches.

GENERAL CONTEXT AND HEALTH DETERMINANTS

Social, Political, and Economic Determinants

Gross domestic product (GDP) at current prices grew from US$ 12.5 billion in 1999 to US$ 16.9 billion by 2005, at an average rate of 2.8% (1, 2). Total central government spending averaged 14.4% of GDP for 2000–2003 (2), peaking at 15% in 2003. Per capita GDP at current prices for 2005 was US$ 2,469, compared with US$ 1,220.50 at constant prices (real GDP). Real GDP grew at an average annual rate of 2.6% between 1996 and 2005 (from US$ 1.7 billion to US$ 2.3 billion). The Ministry of Economy put the annual inflation rate for 2005 at 4.7% (2).

According to the Human Development Index, the country ranks 104th out of 177 countries, with an index of 0.732 (3). Based on data from the 2002 Multipurpose Household Survey, the human development indexes for the departments of San Salvador (0.783) and La Libertad (0.752) were higher than the nationwide index. An estimated 183,874 persons were unemployed in 2004 (4).

As revealed in the 2004 Multipurpose Household Survey, the country's poverty rate is decreasing; the urban-rural divide has widened, however. According to survey data for 2002 and 2004, the percentage of households living in poverty dropped from 42.9% in 2002 to 34.6% in 2004. Of the latter group of households, 12.6% were living in extreme poverty or, in other words, were unable to cover the cost of the basic food basket. Survey data for 2004 put the share of rural households living in poverty at 43.7%, down 12.1 percentage points from 2002. The share of poor urban households went from 29.5% to 29.2% between 2002 and 2004. Of these 263,000 households living in poverty, 46% were concentrated in the San Salvador Metropolitan Area. Most of the population living in extreme and relative poverty without a health care safety net lived in the country's rural areas (19.3% and 24.4%, respectively) (4).

According to the 2004 Multipurpose Household Survey, anyone older than 10 years old in El Salvador is considered to be of working age. The working population accounted for 61.1% of the total population (60.4% were male and 39.6%, female). The nationwide unemployment rate was 6.8% (6.5% in urban areas and 7.2% in rural areas). The urban underemployment rate was 34.6%: 4.3% of workers were classified as openly underemployed (working fewer than the legal working hours) and 30.3% were hidden underemployed (working more than the legal working hours but earning less than the legal wage).

In 2005, El Salvador's Legislative Assembly approved the United States-Dominican Republic-Central America Free Trade Agreement (CAFTA), which was viewed as a tool for promoting development and the country's incorporation into the global market. This presented a major challenge, in that it required the country to undertake policy adjustments in such areas as competitiveness, copyright laws, and tax structure (5). Approving the Agreement also sought to expand employment, improve the country's trade balance with the United States, and strengthen the GDP by boosting domestic and foreign investment.

The number of Salvadorians living abroad jumped from 250,000 in 1970 to 2,778,286 in 2002. Of them, approximately 90% were living in the United States. El Salvador's Central Reserve Bank calculated that the income from remittances in 2004 amounted to US$ 2.5 billion, or 16% of GDP (US$ 15.8 billion) (1–3).

Total, urban, and rural illiteracy rates for 2004 for the population older than 10 years old were 15.5%, 9.6%, and 24.6%, respectively (4). The illiteracy rate for the San Salvador Metropolitan Area was 6.4%, one of the lowest in the country. A gender breakdown shows a higher female illiteracy rate (17.7%) compared with that of males (13.0%). The average number of years of schooling (the number of grades completed by persons older than 6 years old) was 5.6 (6.9 in urban areas and 3.7 in rural areas).

According to data from the 2004 Multipurpose Household Survey, 70.8% of dwellings were made of concrete, 37.9% had asbestos laminate roofs and 30% had metal laminate roofs, 58.1% had brick or cement floors, and 21.2% had dirt floors (4). Moreover, an estimated 96.5% of households had electricity and 65.5% had running water through individual house connections to a water supply system (80.9% in urban areas), while 109,129 households nationwide had no sanitary facilities, of which nearly 84% were in rural areas.

The growing number of natural disasters the country has experienced in the past several decades has left a rising death toll and increasing physical damage in disaster-prone areas. El Salvador is vulnerable to hydrometeorological events such as hurricanes that produce heavy flooding and landslides, severely damaging basic facilities and infrastructure, as well as loss of life, especially in low-lying river basins.

According to the Ministry of Public Health and Social Welfare's Disaster Unit, 5% of the nation's population lives in areas at a very high risk of yearly flooding, 80% lives in areas prone to seismic activity occurring at roughly 10-year intervals, and 1% lives in areas exposed to volcanic eruptions every 80 years (6).

Table 1 shows progress in the attainment of the Millennium Development Goals and remaining challenges.

Demographics, Mortality, and Morbidity

The Ministry of the Economy's Statistics and Census Bureau estimated the country's population in 2005 at 6,874,926 persons, 49.2% male and 50.8% female, with an estimated growth rate of 2.1% for 1991–2001 and a fertility rate of 3.0 children per woman. The population growth rate and the fertility rate have both come down, although they have yet to reach the replacement level (a fertility rate under 2.5 and/or a "zero" [1%] growth rate). At this rate of population growth, El Salvador's population will double in roughly 39 years (7).

Population density was 321 persons per km^2, with large disparities between different parts of the country. Thus, 46% of the country's population is concentrated in the Greater San Salvador Metropolitan Area—which includes San Salvador, El Paisnal, Aguilares, Guazapa, Tonacatepeque, Apopa, Ayutuxtepeque, Cuscatancingo, Ciudad Delgado, Ilopango, Mejicanos, Nejapa, San Marcos, San Martín, Soyapango, Santiago Texacuangos, Santo Tomás, Panchimalco, and Rosario de Mora—where the population density was 4,250 persons per km^2.

About 53% of the population was under 25 years old. Only 7.5% of the population was 60 years old and older (Figure 1), a

TABLE 1. El Salvador's progress toward the Millennium Development Goals, status in 1991, current status, and 2015 targets.

Indicator	1991[a]	Current[b]	2015 target
Population living on less than US$ 1			
Total	57.8	19.2 (2002)[c]	28.9
Urban	38.6	12.1 (2002)[c]	19.3
Rural	75.2	29.1 (2002)[c]	37.6
(Household) poverty gap			
Total	34	34.6 (2004)[d]	17
Urban	30	29.2 (2004)[d]	15
Rural	37	43.7 (2004)[d]	18
Population under the poverty line			
Total	10.3	49.2 (2002)	5.15
Urban	6.9	34.0 (2002)	3.45
Rural	13.2	55.8 (2002)	6.6
Malnutrition rate			
Total	11.2 (1993)	7.6[e]	7
Urban	9.1 (1993)		
Rural	13.2 (1993)		
Mortality rate for children under age 5	52 (1993)	24.6 (2004)	17
Infant mortality rate	41 (1993)	41.3 (2004)	14
Percentage of children vaccinated against measles	98 (1990)	99 (2005)	100
Maternal mortality rate	158 (1993)	172 (2002/03)[f]	118
		71.5 (MSPAS)	
Percentage of deliveries attended by health personnel	51	69.4 (2002/03)	100
Incidence of HIV/AIDS	2.46 (1991)	10.2 (2004)	1.43
Number of cases of HIV	96 (1990)	1,946	
Incidence of tuberculosis	1.9 (1990)	22.4 (2005)	
Number of cases of tuberculosis	2,367 (1990)	1,788 (2005)	

[a]www.digestyc.gob.sv.

[b]Estimates/Adaptation PAHO/El Salvador.

[c]United Nations Development Program, El Salvador. Human Development Report: El Salvador 2005. A Look at the New 'Us': The Impact of Migration. UNDP-El Salvador; 2005.

[d]El Salvador, Ministerio de Economía. Resultados económicos 2005 y Perspectivas 2006: Informe de gestión. Ministerio de Economía; December 2005.

[e]Ministerio de Salud Pública. Diagnóstico del estado nutricional (una vez al año) 2005. Only the population served by the Ministry of Public Health.

[f] El Salvador. Ministerio de Economía, Dirección General de Estadística y Censos. Encuesta de Hogares de Propósitos Múltiples, 2003. Ministerio de Economía; 2004.

figure that is expected to climb to 8.8% by 2015. The share of the total population aged 0–4 years old decreased from 14.2% in 1995 to 11.1% in 2005. The fastest growing age group was 25–29-year-olds, which jumped from 6.1% to 9.6%. Life expectancy at birth in 2004 was 69.5 years (66 years for males and 72.7 years for females).

There were 30,075 reported deaths nationwide in 2004 (for a mortality rate of 445 per 100,000 population) (7), of which 58% were males (Table 2). Of all reported deaths, 13.4% were classified as "ill-defined," up 2.7% from 2000, when this category accounted for 10.7% of deaths. The breakdown of mortality data was based on municipal death records which, in practice, are subject to underreporting that has not yet been measured. In any event, the crude general mortality rate has been declining for the past 10 years, falling 9%, or from 489.5 per 100,000 population to 445.1 between 1997 and 2004.

Of the leading causes of death, noncommunicable diseases accounted for 74.0% of deaths, and communicable diseases, for 25.8%. The five leading causes of death (Table 3) were cardiovascular diseases (81.61 per 100,000 population), whose most frequent complications were myocardial ischemia and heart failure; injuries from external causes (81.57 per 100,000), mainly homicides associated primarily with shootings, and pedestrian traffic accidents; malignant neoplasms (48.51 per 100,000), of which stomach cancer was the leading cause of death in both males and females; diseases of the respiratory tract (39.19 per 100,000), particularly pneumonia; and diseases of the genitourinary system (28.3 per 100,000) (7).

The leading causes of death from communicable diseases were pneumonia, septicemia, HIV infection, and acute respiratory infections. A gender breakdown of these deaths showed no major differences between the sexes. There were, however, higher numbers of male deaths from external causes, mental disorders and the use of psychoactive substances, diseases of the genitourinary system, and HIV infection.

The leading external cause of death was homicide, with 91% of homicides involving males and most involving adolescents and young adults, while most fatalities from traffic accidents involved older adults.

Males accounted for 74.2% of the 805,572 years of potential life lost (YPLL) to the 10 leading causes of death in 2004 (Table 4), with the remaining 25.8% involving females. The breakdown of YPLL by group of diseases, in descending order, was: external causes (33.0%), noncommunicable diseases (26.0%), infectious diseases (10.0%), mental diseases (3.0%), and other diseases (28.0%).

In contrast to data furnished by calculations of mortality rates for the leading causes of death, among which malignant neoplasms ranked fourth, computations of YPLL elevated malignant neoplasms to second place, due primarily to the fact that most deaths involved young and middle-aged adults. Females were hardest hit, accounting for 61.5% of all deaths.

FIGURE 1. Population structure, by age and sex, El Salvador, 1995 and 2005.

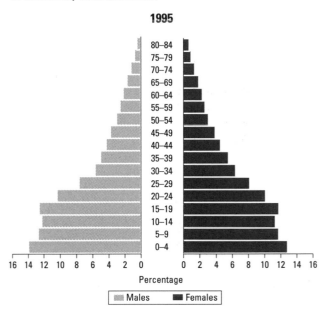

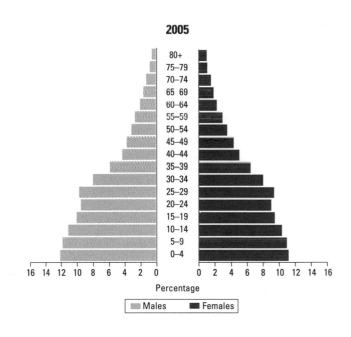

HEALTH OF POPULATION GROUPS

Children under 5 Years Old

According to the 2002–2003 National Family Health Survey, the infant mortality rate was 25 per 1,000 live births (Table 5) (8), down 10 deaths from the 1998 survey findings. This improvement was attributable to a decline in postneonatal mortality (from 18 per 1,000 to 12 per 1,000) and in neonatal mortality

TABLE 2. Number of deaths and mortality rates[a] for the 15 leading causes of death, by gender, El Salvador, 2004.

	Groups of causes	Males Deaths	Males Rate	Females Deaths	Females Rate	Total Deaths	Total Rate
1	Cardiovascular diseases	2,578	77.6	2,937	85.5	5,515	81.6
	Ischemic heart disease	917	27.6	939	27.3	1,856	27.5
	Congestive heart failure	434	13.1	591	17.2	1,025	15.2
	Cerebrovascular diseases	442	13.3	509	14.8	951	14.1
	Hypertensive diseases	157	4.7	222	6.5	379	5.6
2	Injuries from external causes	4,632	139.4	880	25.6	5,512	81.6
	Homicide	2,376	71.5	239	6.9	2,615	38.7
	Traffic accidents	1,406	42.3	354	10.3	1,760	26.0
	Suicide	349	10.5	117	3.4	466	6.9
3	Ill-defined symptoms	2,057	61.9	1,970	57.3	4,027	59.6
4	All malignant tumors	1,364	41.1	1,914	55.7	3,278	48.5
	Stomach	276	8.3	223	6,5	499	7.4
	Lungs	98	2.9	110	3.2	208	3.1
	Cervix	—	—	220	6.4	220	3.3
	Liver	81	2.4	114	3.3	195	2.9
	Prostate	175	5.3	—	—	175	2.6
	Breast	5	0.2	128	3.7	133	1.9
5	Diseases of the respiratory tract	1,388	41.8	1,260	36.7	2,648	39.2
	Influenza (flu) and pneumonia	798	24.0	687	20.0	1,485	21.9
	Chronic diseases of the lower respiratory tract	238	7.2	284	8.3	522	7.7
	Other acute infections of the lower respiratory tract	15	0.4	7	0.2	22	0.3
6	Diseases of the genitourinary system	1,340	40.3	575	16.7	1,915	28.3
	Chronic renal failure, unspecified	774	23.3	333	9.7	1,107	16.4
	Renal failure, unspecified	439	13.2	161	4.7	600	8.9
7	Diseases of the digestive system	890	26.8	584	17.0	1,474	21.8
8	Diabetes mellitus	402	12.1	572	16.6	974	14.4
9	Diseases of the liver	563	16.9	271	8.0	834	12.3
10	Mental disorders and use of psychoactive substances	802	24.1	28	0.8	830	12.3
11	Septicemia	397	11.9	325	9.5	722	10.7
12	Diseases of the nervous system	340	10.2	367	10.7	707	10.5
13	HIV	389	11.7	161	4.7	550	8.1
14	Disorders originating in the perinatal period	245	7.4	201	5.9	446	6.6
15	Congenital malformations/deformities/chromosomal abnormalities	187	5.6	157	4.6	344	5.1
	Total	17,594	529.7	12,481	363.3	30,075	445.1

Source: Dirección General de Estadística y Censos, mortality statistics, 2004.
[a]Rate per 100,000 population.

(from 17 per 1,000 to 13 per 1,000). Of all infant deaths, 56% occurred in the neonatal period (the first 28 days of life). The mortality rate in mothers getting five or more prenatal checkups was 19 per 1,000 live births, compared with 35 per 1,000 among mothers getting fewer than five checkups or no prenatal care at all. A breakdown by birthweight put infant mortality at 20 per 1,000 live births among infants weighing 2,500 g or more and at 40 per 1,000 for infants weighing under 2,500 g at birth. The neonatal mortality rate for full-term infants was 8 per 1,000 live births, compared with 72 per 1,000 for premature infants.

According to Statistics and Census Bureau data, the leading causes of perinatal mortality in 2004 were bacterial sepsis of the newborn (24.3%), respiratory distress syndrome (22.5%), and intrauterine hypoxia (11.0%) (7). There were 1,258 reported deaths among children under 1 year old in 2004, of which 35.4% were due to conditions originating in the perinatal period, 26.5% were due to noncommunicable diseases, and 25.0% to communicable diseases. The leading causes of death among noncommunicable diseases were unspecified congenital malformations (47.0%), congenital malformations of the heart (28.5%), and congenital hydrocephaly, unspecified (7.9%).

Ministry of Public Health data for 2005 established the five leading causes of morbidity in children under 1 year old as acute respiratory infections (67.8%), diarrhea (20.8%), pneumonia

TABLE 3. Ten leading causes of death, El Salvador, 1997 and 2004.

Groups of causes	1997	Ranking	2004	Ranking
Diseases of the circulatory system (I00–I99)	3,816	3	5,515	1
External causes of morbidity and mortality (V01–Y89)	4,932	2	5,513	2
Symptoms, signs, and abnormal clinical and laboratory findings not elsewhere classified (R00–R99)	5,478	1	4,027	3
Tumors (neoplasms) (C00–D48)	2,788	4	3,278	4
Diseases of the respiratory tract (J00–J98)	2,625	5	2,648	5
Diseases of the genitourinary system (N00–N98)	1,033	10	1,915	6
Certain infectious and parasitic diseases (A00–B99)	2,000	6	1,656	7
Diseases of the digestive system (K00–K92)	1,689	7	1,474	8
Endocrine, nutritional, and metabolic diseases (E00–E88)	1,126	8	1,343	9
Mental and behavioral disorders (F01–F99)	1,034	9	840	10
Other causes	2,401		1,867	
Total	28,922		30,076	

Source: Statistics and Census Bureau (DIGESTYC).

TABLE 4. Years of potential life lost (YPPL) for selected causes of death, El Salvador, 2004.

	Gender		
Cause of death	Males	Females	Total
All injuries from external causes	227,419	40,728	268,147
Assaults	127,810	12,622	140,432
Traffic accidents	60,612	15,439	76,051
Neoplasms	27,267	43,094	70,361
Pneumonia	34,195	25,668	59,863
Genitourinary diseases	31,395	13,376	44,771
Ischemic disease	14,520	26,237	40,757
Mental and psychoactive diseases	28,633	1,118	29,751
Liver disease	18,502	6,688	25,190
Septicemia	11,352	7,027	18,379
Diabetes	8,121	9,105	17,226
Cerebrovascular disease	7,528	7,116	14,644
Total YPPL	597,354	208,218	805,572

TABLE 5. Infant and maternal mortality, El Salvador, 1993 to 2002.

Survey and reference period	Maternal deaths per 100,000 live births	Infant mortality rate per 1,000 live births	Neonatal mortality rate	Postneonatal mortality rate
FESAL 2002/03 1993–2002	173	25	13	12
FESAL 98 1988–1998	120	35	17	18
FESAL 93 1983–1993	158	41	23	18

Source: FESAL 2002/03.

(5.7%), bacterial conjunctivitis (2.4), and mild malnutrition (1.0%). This age group accounted for 42,213 hospital discharges, and the main diagnoses at the time of discharge were pneumonia (18%), respiratory disorders specific to the perinatal period (12.6%), diarrhea of presumed infectious origin (11.0%), and fetuses and newborns affected by maternal factors and complications of pregnancy, labor, and delivery (9.2%). The most common causes of in-hospital mortality were certain conditions originating in the perinatal period (53.9%), congenital malformations, deformities and chromosomal abnormalities (20.0%), pneumonia (9.0%), and other intestinal infectious diseases (2.6%).

There were 405 reported deaths in 2004 among children 1–4 years old due to communicable diseases (31.0%), noncommunicable diseases (31%), external causes (18.5%), and ill-defined causes (16.3%) (7). Of deaths attributable to communicable diseases, 42.2% were due to pneumonia and bronchopneumonia, 35.5% to diarrhea and gastroenteritis of presumed infectious origin, 13.0% to unspecified septicemia, and 5.0% to bacterial meningitis, unspecified. Of deaths from external causes, 41.3% were due to traffic accidents, 29.3% to accidental drownings and submersions, 9.3% to accidents obstructing respiration, and 8.0% to assault and homicide.

According to Ministry of Public Health data, the leading causes of morbidity in this age group in 2005 were acute respiratory infections (71.7%), diarrhea (15.9%), pneumonia (2.8%), amebiasis or amebic dysentery (2.5%), and mild malnutrition (1.5%). There were 30,074 hospital discharges in 2005, with the most common diagnoses being pneumonia (21.8%), diarrhea (19.0%), asthma (4.8%), and other intestinal infectious diseases (4%). The leading causes of hospital deaths were pneumonia (19.8%), congenital malformations (10.8%), and malnutrition (5.1%).

Children 5–9 Years Old

There were 221 reported deaths among children in this age group in 2004: 45.7% were due to external causes, 9.5% were due to diseases of the respiratory system, 1.9% were due to diseases of the nervous system, 1.8% were due to malignant neoplasms, and 1.4% were due to congenital malformations. External causes of deaths included traffic accidents (63.4%), accidental drownings and submersions (22.8%), and assaults and homicides (5.0%).

According to Ministry of Public Health data, the leading causes of morbidity in 2005 were acute respiratory infections (79.2%), diarrhea (6.0%), amebiasis (4.5%), giardiasis (2.1%), and bacterial conjunctivitis (1.5%). There were 17,314 hospital discharges that year, in which the leading diagnoses were appendicitis (7.2%), fractures of the extremities (6.9%), pneumonia (5.6%), asthma (5.3%), and other traumas (5.3%). The leading causes of hospital deaths were head trauma (15.7%), pneumonia (10.1%), malignant meningiomas (6.7%), and other diseases of the blood and blood-forming organs (6.7%).

Adolescents 10–14 and 15–19 Years Old

Of the 1,069 reported deaths among adolescents in 2004, 68.0% were attributable to external causes, 5.6% to diseases of the respiratory tract, and 4.3% to malignant neoplasms. The leading external causes of mortality (at 51.4 per 100,000) were assaults, traffic accidents, and self-inflicted injuries.

The leading causes of morbidity in adolescents in 2005 were acute respiratory infections (74.3%), amebiasis (5.8%), diarrhea (5.6%), bites from rabid animals (2.2%), and giardiasis (1.8%). Adolescents accounted for 15.4% (52,527) of all hospital discharges reported by the Ministry of Public Health, with females making up 74.0% of this figure. Of hospital discharges involving adolescents 15–19 years old, 69.0% were associated with sexual and reproductive health problems. Adolescents accounted for 31.7% (28,943) of prenatal visits reported by the Ministry in 2005. Of the 72,293 deliveries attended by health professionals in 2005, 21,730, or 30.1%, involved adolescents.

Nearly 40% of females and 65% of males 15–24 years old had engaged in premarital sex. For females, the median age of their first pregnancy was 20 years, and their age at their first sexual experience was 18 years; on average, males had their first sexual experience at 16 years old.

Adults 20–59 Years Old

In 2004, the 10,490 reported deaths in this age group were due to external causes (36.2%, or a rate of 116.4 per 100,000), malignant neoplasms (10.1%, or a rate of 32.6 per 100,000), diseases of the circulatory system (8.6%, or a rate of 27.8 per 100,000), and communicable diseases (7.5%, or a rate of 24.1 per 100,000). Males accounted for 88.5% of deaths from external causes (3,802 cases). The leading external causes of death were assaults and homicides (54.0%), traffic accidents (29.2%), and self-inflicted injuries (9.2%). The most frequently reported sites for malignant neoplasms (1,065 total cases of malignant neoplasms) were the stomach (12.2%), the cervix (11.6%), and the breast (6.5%). Diseases of the circulatory system (907 cases) included ischemic heart disease (36.2%), cerebrovascular disease (19.7%), and hypertensive disease (8.4%). The most common communicable diseases were HIV infection (63.0%); septicemia, unspecified (26.0%); and diarrhea and tuberculosis (both with a 4.0% share). Males accounted for 70.1% of these deaths. The most common causes of morbidity in this age group in 2005 were acute respiratory infections (65.1%), diarrhea (9.4%), amebiasis (5.0%), anxiety disorders (3.6%), and vulvovaginal candidiasis (2.5%). The leading diagnoses associated with hospital discharges of adults 20–24 years old were sexual and reproductive health problems (71.0%), other traumas to specified areas (3.3%), and appendicitis (2.2%). The leading diagnoses associated with the 112,733 reported discharges of adults 25–59 years old were sexual and reproductive health problems (30.6%), colelithiasis and colecystitis (3.4%), diabetes mellitus (3.3%), other and unspecified traumas (3.3%), and other genitourinary disorders (3.0%). The three leading causes of hospital deaths were AIDS (9.8%), intracranial trauma (9.2%), and liver disease (7.9%).

According to findings from the 2002–2003 National Family Health Survey, the maternal mortality rate in 1993–2002 ranged between 106 and 239 deaths per 100,000 live births, with a median value of 173. The Ministry of Public Health is working to develop a nationwide baseline for measuring maternal mortality.

According to an assessment of the availability and use of emergency obstetric care in El Salvador dating back to the year 2003 (9), the leading causes of maternal morbidity and mortality were hypertension, pre- and postpartum hemorrhaging, sepsis, and complications of abortion. The leading causes of death in 54% of reported deaths were misdiagnoses, mismanagement, procedures performed by unqualified personnel (anesthesia and surgery-related), shortages of supplies and equipment, and belated and improper patient referrals. Another 33% of maternal deaths were caused by the failure of the woman in question and her family to recognize complications, which delayed seeking medical care or the services of a midwife. An examination of the number of deaths reported by the Statistics and Census Bureau between 1997 and 2004 revealed a 43% underreporting in the Bureau's maternal mortality statistics, compared with the statistical data reported by health facilities, which jumped to more than 90% between 2003 and 2004 (9).

Older Adults 60 Years Old and Older

There were 16,449 reported deaths in this age group in 2005, accounting for 54.7% of all deaths nationwide, of which 27.4% were caused by diseases of the circulatory system, 12.8% by malignant neoplasms, 10.8% by diseases of the respiratory tract, and 5.1% by genitourinary disorders. The leading causes of death among diseases of the circulatory system were ischemic diseases (33.4%), heart failure (24.4%), pulmonary circulatory disorders (17.7%), cerebrovascular disease (16.8%), and hypertensive disease (6.5%). The most common sites for malignant neoplasms were the stomach (17.4%); the prostate (7.9%); the trachea, bronchial tubes, and lungs (6.9%); the liver and intrahepatic bile ducts (6.8%); and the cervix (4.5%).

Acording to the Ministry of Public Health's epidemiological report for 2005, the five leading causes of mortality were acute respiratory infections (60.1%), arterial hypertension (9.3%), diarrhea (8.9%), amebiasis (4.2%), and diabetes mellitus (3.6%). There were 47,770 hospital discharges reported that year, and the leading diagnoses were diabetes (8.1%); bronchitis, emphysema, and other chronic obstructive pulmonary diseases (5.0%); pneumonia (4.7%); heart failure (3.9%); and renal failure (3.8%).

The Family

An estimated 62.7% of households were headed by men and 37.3% by women (8). Female-headed households made up a larger share of urban households (43.2%) than of rural households (30.7%). The Ministry of the Economy's Statistics and Census Bureau found women caught in a vicious circle of poverty and lack of education. In fact, the most common reason given by women for dropping out of school was "economic problems" (cited by 31.3% of women), which, added to the statement that "they had to work" (10%), indicates that at least one of every 10 women had left school as the result of a low income. Other reasons cited for dropping out of school were pregnancy, a first marriage (12.9%), and other unspecified family problems (11.3%).

Workers

To date, there has been no comprehensive assessment of the state of workers' health. It is a well-known fact that the level of coverage by the Salvadorian Social Security Institute is quite low (roughly 13% to 15% of the workforce). Moreover, there are reports of complaints of poor working conditions by workers in the country's more than 85,000 "maquilas," although many of these complaints are not well documented.

Persons with Disabilities

According to the 1992 Population Census, there were 81,721 persons with disabilities (1.6% of the total population), of which 53.3% were male and 46.7% were female. The 2000–2001 nationwide sample survey of persons with disabilities conducted as part of a joint WHO/German Technical Cooperation Agency (GTZ)/Universidad Don Bosco (UDB) project put the general prevalence of different types of disabilities at 6.6%. As of January 2005, the National Registration Office for Individuals, which is charged with keeping records on all persons older than 18 years old, showed 153,583 registered persons with disabilities (4.1%). According to the WHO/GTZ/UDB survey, the five most common types of disabilities among respondents were impaired vision (41.9%), impaired mobility, including difficulty walking, climbing, jumping, or standing (31.2%), difficulty grasping, lifting, and carrying objects (15.5%), hearing loss (15.2%), and speech problems (11.9%) (10). The age group 21–50 years old accounted for the largest share of persons with disabilities (35%), followed by the age group under 20 years old (30%), the age group 51–70 years old (22%), and the age group 71 years old and older (13%). A gender breakdown put the share of disabled females at 49.9% and the share of males with disabilities at 50.1%, while a breakdown by geographic area showed 61% of persons with disabilities living in rural areas and 39%, in urban areas. According to the same survey, disease was the leading cause of disabilities, with a 48.4% share (with no breakdown by type of disease).

The second most common cause was congenital abnormalities (27.1%), with common accidents in third place (9.8%), and "other" causes ranking fourth, including but not limited to chronic degenerative diseases like arthritis, diabetes, hemophilia, and senile dementia of unknown origin.

Ethnic Groups

The indigenous population is estimated to be 687,492 persons (10% of the total population). The largest ethnic group is the Nahuat, which accounts for 94.4% of the country's indigenous population, followed by the Lenca (4.1%) and the Cacaopera (1.5%). These ethnicities are found in seven of the country's 14 departments, namely in Ahuachapán (in 4 municipios), Sonsonate (14), La Libertad (5), San Salvador (4), La Paz (8), Morazán (3), and Santa Ana (1). Their main language is Nahuatl (11). They live from subsistence farming, growing corn, beans, and other crops on small, mostly leased, parcels of land. The working life of members of the indigenous population begins at age 8 and goes to age 59; 38.3% of indigenous households are living in abject poverty, and 61.1% are living below the poverty line (11). There is no current disaggregated data on the health of members of ethnic groups, the most recent data being from 1999. According to a 2003 World Bank report, entitled "El perfil de los pueblos indígenas en El Salvador" [Profile of Indigenous Peoples in El Salvador], only 3.2% of indigenous peoples had health insurance coverage by the Salvadorian Social Security Institute. Only 2% of female heads of household used any form of contraception, and the fertility rate was 3.5 children per woman. Indigenous women of childbearing age accounted for 20.8% of the total population, and only 0.5% of all indigenous women of childbearing age used birth control. The infant mortality rate was 42.5 per 1,000 live births, 73% of children had been vaccinated, and 27% had full vaccination coverage. In indigenous communities, 91.6% of the population drew water from rivers, springs, or wells; 30% of households dumped their garbage near their homes, 20.9% dumped their garbage far away from their homes, and 40.8% either buried or burned their garbage; 37.2% of households defecated outdoors, 59.7% had latrines, and 3.1% had sanitary facilities with running water.

HEALTH CONDITIONS AND PROBLEMS

COMMUNICABLE DISEASES

Vector-borne Diseases

Malaria has been on the decline. The number of reported cases of malaria in each year from 2000 to 2005 was 753, 362, 117, 85, 112, and 67, respectively; 2 were from imported *Plasmodium falciparum* and the rest from *P. vivax*, with an annual parasite index of 0.011. There have been no reported indigenous cases of *P. falciparum* malaria for more than 10 years. In the past few years, there have been small outbreaks associated with imported cases from neighboring countries, such as Guatemala and Honduras, where the incidence of malaria has been on the rise.

There were 70,945 suspected cases of **dengue** between 2000 and 2005, with an average 20% of the cases reported each year involving hospitalization. There were more than 28,352 laboratory-confirmed cases, of which 95% were classified as classic dengue and 5% as hemorrhagic dengue. The number of deaths dropped from 26 in 2000 to a single death in 2004. The laboratory tested more than 72,000 samples of IgM for dengue, confirming the circulation of all four serotypes during the reference period.

Dengue is endemic in the country, with epidemic outbreaks in the last six years and with the number of cases of hemorrhagic dengue on the rise. There were two epidemics in the last six years. The first was in 2000, caused by serotype 2, producing 16,963 suspected cases of classic dengue, including 491 suspected cases of hemorrhagic dengue and 26 deaths; 2,824 cases of classic dengue and 409 cases of hemorrhagic dengue were laboratory-confirmed. The second epidemic broke out in 2002, with 18,267 suspected cases of dengue and 5,076 laboratory-confirmed cases, of which 4,671 (92%) were classic dengue and 405 (8%) hemorrhagic dengue, causing 11 deaths. There was an average of over 7,000 reported cases of dengue in both 2004 and 2005. There is ongoing active dengue transmission in 46% of the country's municipios, with only 8% of municipios reporting no cases of dengue during the reporting period. The risk of contracting the disease was 6 to 8 times greater during the rainy season.

There are an undetermined number of cases of **Chagas' disease** every year. The epidemiological surveillance system for Chagas' disease has a serious underreporting problem, making it impossible to establish the real incidence of the disease and, thus, to take timely, effective prevention and control measures. The Ministry of Public Health recorded 101 suspected cases of acute Chagas' disease in 2005, of which 75 (74.2%) were laboratory-confirmed; 87% of the cases were treated through outpatient visits. Half the cases involved children under 10 years old, and the disease affected both sexes equally. A geographic breakdown put 58% of the cases in rural areas and 42% in urban areas. The departments of Sonsonate, Santa Ana, and Ahuachapán (in the western reaches of the country, close to the Guatemalan border) reported the largest number of cases (46.5% of the country's total) and the highest infestation indexes. Sonsonate Department, for example, which has had a Japanese International Cooperation Agency (JICA) assistance program in place since 2003, had an infestation index of 33.3%. Serologic studies confirmed 1,311 and 1,292 cases in 2000 and 2005, respectively. Of 76,096 blood specimens in blood banks subject to screening (a 100% screening rate), 1,826 tested positive, for a seropositivity rate of 2.40%. The number of blood donors went down to 38,725 in 2005, with an equal number of blood specimens screened for Chagas' disease, of which only 956 tested positive, with a seropositivity rate of 2.46%.

Vaccine-preventable Diseases

El Salvador has made great strides with respect to the eradication, elimination, and control of vaccine-preventable diseases. It has been free of **poliomyelitis** since 1987; the last confirmed indigenous case of **measles** was in 1996; and **diphtheria** (for more than 20 years) and **neonatal tetanus** (at less than 1 case per 1,000 live births) have been virtually eliminated. The endemic chain of **rubella** virus transmission was broken in 2004, thanks to a mass vaccination campaign targeting 2,694,763 individuals 15–39 years old (97.5% of the goal for this age group); only four isolated cases were reported in 2006, which may have been imported from other countries where the disease is still endemic. There have been no reported cases of congenital rubella syndrome since 2004, but active case-finding needs improvement.

According to the 2005 epidemiological report, incidence rates for chickenpox were 278 per 100,000 population, 28 for hepatitis A, 8 for mumps, 3.4 for acute flaccid paralysis in children under 15 years of age, 3.4 for hepatitis B, 0.4 for rubella, and 0.1 for tetanus. There were no confirmed cases of diphtheria, poliomyelitis, or measles, suggesting that the at-risk population is adequately protected. There were two confirmed imported cases of measles in 2001; they were not included in the national case load because their incubation period occurred in Europe, meaning that these persons were infected on that continent. Active case-finding for flaccid paralysis was up in 2005, with 130 reported cases compared with 105 the previous year. Laboratory testing isolated other enteroviruses in 27.0% of the specimens studied.

There was a **whooping cough** outbreak in 2004. The reference pediatric hospital reported 52 cases and 5 deaths, with a 9.6% case-fatality rate. Females accounted for 31 of the cases. The mean age was 5.2 months for females and 3.6 months for males. *Bordetella pertussis* was isolated in one of the specimens tested, which led to the strengthening of epidemiological and laboratory surveillance activities, the updating of treatment protocols, the training of health personnel, and an assessment of the vaccination program.

Intestinal Infectious Diseases

Gastrointestinal diseases are one of the three leading causes of morbidity reported in El Salvador. There are two seasonal surges, one each in the dry and in the rainy seasons: the first is associated primarily with viral infections and the second with bacterial infections. A study conducted at Benjamín Bloom Children's Hospital between May 2001 and April 2002 found **rotavirus gastroenteritis** to be seasonal, with most cases occurring in the dry season, and associated with vomiting and dehydration. Children suffering from rotavirus gastroenteritis were younger (with median age of 9 months) than children infected by other agents (the median age was 13 months for bacteria and 16 months for parasites). The Ministry of Public Health began to conduct viral surveillance for rotavirus at various sentinel sites in the country in 2003, sampling children under 5 years old.

The last reported case of **cholera** dates back to October of 2000. *Vibrio cholerae* has not been detected anywhere in the country in the reporting period, despite the fact that there is ongoing surveillance in humans and in sources of drinking water for humans.

The mean annual number of recorded cases of **intestinal parasitic diseases** between 2000 and 2005 was 193,000. The incidence rate in 2005 was 2,670 per 100,000 population, down 15% from the 2000 figure. The highest incidence rates were associated with children under 10 years old. Protozoan infections (amebiasis and giardiasis) accounted for 93% of reported cases of intestinal parasitic diseases, with 7% attributable to helminthic infections (uncinariasis or ancyclostomiasis and cestode infections).

Chronic Communicable Diseases

Between 1997 and 2005 there were 63 diagnosed cases of **leprosy** nationwide. The disease's prevalence has been declining, from 0.03 per 10,000 population (20 cases) in 1997 to 0.001 per 10,000 in 2005 (1 case). As of this writing, there are 14 cases under treatment, 71% of which are in the northern and central parts of the country (Santa Ana, Chalatenango, San Salvador, and La Libertad).

The incidence of **tuberculosis** has been declining for the past several years, going from 70.0 per 100,000 population in 1994 to 25.6 per 100,000 in 2005. In fact, a comparison of data for 1990 and 2005 shows a reduction in the number of reported cases from 2,367 to 1,758. The mortality rate for tuberculosis dropped by 49%, from 2.35 per 100,000 population in 1997 down to 1.20 per 100,000 in 2004. According to the latest estimates (2005), the annual risk of tuberculosis infection was 0.6%, which is equivalent to a smear-positive case rate of 32 per 100,000 population.

The success rate in treating tuberculosis is high, nearly 88%, which exceeds the PAHO/WHO target rate of 85% for 2005. There was sizeable improvement in the dropout rate for patients undergoing treatment for tuberculosis between 1997 and 2004, which went from 11.3% down to 4.1%. These patients are believed to be facing problems such as alcoholism or poverty that make it difficult to administer and oversee their treatment. Coverage for the Directly Observed Treatment, Short-course (DOTS) strategy first introduced in 1997 in Ministry of Public Health facilities, the social security system, and correctional facilities is currently 100%. The average share of patients diagnosed as co-infected with HIV and tuberculosis rose from 3.6% to 8.5% between 2002 and 2005, with a 167% jump in the number of cases.

Acute Respiratory Infections

Acute respiratory infections are one of the leading causes of illness and death in El Salvador. There were 1,895,819 reported cases in 2004 in all age groups, for an incidence of 34,509 per 100,000 population. Females accounted for 58.7% of all cases. A breakdown by age group showed 184,151 cases in children under 1 year old (139,544 per 100,000), 515,101 cases in children

1–4 years old (763,313 per 100,000), 404,739 cases in children 5–9 years old (63,499 per 100,000), and 92,303 cases in adults 60 years old and older (22,710 per 100.000). Children under 5 years of age accounted for 36.9% of all treated cases. The morbidity rate for this type of disease in adults over 60 years of age has been quite low, although the mortality rate in this age group was 200.6 per 100,000 population, compared with a rate of 116 per 100,000 live births for children under 1 year old.

A **pneumonia** epidemic in 2003 was responsible for the more than 50% jump in the number of cases of this disease as compared with previous years; the incidence was 130 per 10,000 population. Children under 5 years old accounted for 77% of outpatient visits. This age group had the highest incidence (832 per 10,000 population), followed by adults over 60 years of age (103 per 10,000) (*12*). The mortality rate for pneumonia and bronchopneumonia was 22.0 per 100,000 population in 2004, which marked the beginning of sentinel surveillance programs at two sites for identification of the respiratory virus associated with these diseases.

HIV/AIDS and Other Sexually Transmitted Infections

Since the occurrence of the first AIDS case in 1984, 16,343 cases of HIV infection had been reported as of December 2005. Of these, 7,339 were AIDS cases, for an annual incidence of 2.5 per 100,000 population in 1991 to 10.2 in 2004, then dropping again to 6.2 in 2005. Most cases have occurred in urban areas (73% of cases were urban, 24% rural, and 3% unspecified); the epidemic is spreading into the center of the country. The annual incidence jumped from 2.5 per 100,000 population in 1991 to 20.0 in 2004, falling back to 17.3 in 2005. It should be noted that the Joint United Nations Program on HIV/AIDS (UNAIDS) annual report released in May 2006 estimated underregistration between 40% and 50%, which could put the number of people infected with HIV as high as 30,000 nationwide. According to the epidemiological classification scheme proposed by UNAIDS, El Salvador is a country with a low-prevalence epidemic concentrated in high-risk population groups such as homosexual males and sex workers (*13*). An estimated six people a day were infected with HIV in 2004, versus 4.4 in 2005 (*14*).

In 2004, HIV infection/AIDS ranked thirteenth among the causes of general mortality in El Salvador, and was the second leading cause of death in adults 20–30 years old and the fifth leading cause of death in adults 20–59 years old. HIV/AIDS mortality is on the rise. From 258 reported deaths in 1997 (a rate of 4.32 per 100,000 population), the number of deaths jumped to 549 by 2004 (8.14 per 100,000). There were 1,611 recorded hospital deaths from AIDS between 1998 and 2004, representing the leading cause of death in adults 20–59 years old. The highest concentration of cases was found among adults 20–34 years old, at 36% of the total figure for that age range. Males accounted for 63% of all cases. There were 1.3 infected males for each infected female in 2005. The main transmission mechanism was through sexual contact, which accounted for 85% of all cases, compared with 7.0% for mother-to-child transmission. A breakdown by the reported sexual orientation of the carrier/patient put the share of HIV/AIDS cases associated with homosexual and bisexual relations at 5.0% and 3.0%, respectively. The latest available data (*15*) shows 21.6% of street children infected with the HIV virus in 1997. San Salvador had the largest share of cases, with 56%, compared with 8% for Sonsonate, 6% for La Libertad, and 6% for Santa Ana.

Other sexually transmitted infections (STIs) have one of the highest contagion indexes nationwide. There were more than 313,000 reported STI cases between 2000 and 2005, with an average of 52,000 cases a year. The incidence of certain STIs went up over this same period. Diseases such as trichomoniasis and genital candidiasis have higher prevalence rates than the five classic venereal diseases (syphilis, gonorrhea, chancroid [soft chancre], venereal lymphogranuloma, and inguinal granuloma), which appear to be on the decline. According to Ministry of Public Health data for 2005, the incidence of sexually transmitted infections, in descending order, was 909 per 100,000 population for vulvovaginal candidiasis, 126 for urogenital trichomoniasis, 22 for gonorrhea, 17 for genital herpes, and 16 for condyloma acuminatum (genital warts). There was a 55.0% decline in the nationwide incidence of acquired syphilis between 2000 and 2005, from 18.0 per 100,000 population to 8.1. The Minstry of Public Health reported a total of 433 cases of congenital syphilis between 2000 and 2005, or an average of 72 cases a year. The number of reported cases of syphilis dropped slightly beginning in 2002, with 45 reported cases, for an incidence of 0.38 per 1,000 live births in 2005.

Zoonoses

El Salvador has been successful in controlling rabies. There were many cases of human rabies in the early 1990s—19 cases in 1992, for example. That year marked the beginning of a gradual decline in the disease, which bottomed out in 1999, a year in which there were no reported cases, followed by a single case in the year 2000. There were four reported cases of human rabies in 2001, increasing to six the following year, for a mortality rate of 0.10 per 100,000, 10 times greater than the rate for Latin America and the Caribbean. The numbers held in 2003. The incidence of human rabies began to come back down in 2004, with three cases reported that year and a single case reported in 2005. There were 39,329 reports of people attacked by animals between January 2005 and June 2006, 57.8% of which came out of the departments of San Salvador, La Libertad, and Santa Ana. Of these attacks, 16,506 victims were treated for rabies, 67.3% of whom were from the departments of San Salvador, La Unión, San Miguel, and Usulután.

There were 1,314 reported cases of animal rabies between 1999 and 2005, nearly 90% of which involved urban pet dogs and cats. There was a 3.7-fold spike in animal rabies cases between

Coordination for Disaster Prevention and Mitigation

The natural disasters that have buffeted the country in the past several decades have left a rising toll in human life and material losses in El Salvador's disaster-prone areas. The country is vulnerable to hydrometeorological events, such as hurricanes, which produced heavy flooding and landslides, severely damaged basic services and infrastructure, and left behind many dead, particularly in low-lying river basins. In 2005, the Santa Ana Volcano, also known as Ilamatepec, erupted without warning. That same year, tropical storm Stan pounded the country for six straight days—the storm's rainfall led to flooding that claimed 69 lives and caused heavy physical damage. The Economic Commission for Latin America and the Caribbean (ECLAC) put the cost of these two 2005 events at US$ 355.7 million. The National Civil Defense System, established under the 2005 Civil Defense and Disaster Prevention and Mitigation Act, is charged with ensuring the safety of at-risk communities and with coordinating disaster prevention or response efforts with other agencies and organizations (government agencies, NGOs, private enterprises, relief agencies, among others).

1999 (68 cases) and 2004 (253), dropping to 175 cases in 2005. During this same period, 52% (136) of the country's municipios had at least one confirmed case of animal rabies. A nationwide survey of the dog and cat population conducted in 2002 put the number of animals at roughly 1,176,000. Vaccination coverage rates for 2005 against canine and feline rabies were 60.4% and 47%, respectively.

NONCOMMUNICABLE DISEASES

According to Ministry of Public Health records for 2005, the incidence of noncommunicable diseases, in descending order, was 639 per 100,000 population for arterial hypertension, 36 for chronic renal failure, 33 for cervical cancer, and 9 for breast cancer. Chronic diseases are the second leading cause of years of potential life lost (YPLL) nationwide.

Metabolic and Nutritional Diseases

Diabetes ranked eighth among the leading causes of general mortality. However, according to the Ministry's Morbidity and Mortality System, it was the second leading cause of hospital deaths and the eighth most common diagnosis in hospital discharges.

The 2002–2003 National Family Health Survey (8) showed that the rate of **stunting** (as measured by the height-for-age indicator) in children 3–59 months old was 18.9% (down 4.4 percentage points from the 1998 figure), affecting males and females almost equally (18.3% and 19.7%, respectively). The rural rate (25.6%), however, was 2.3 times higher than the urban rate. There is a direct correlation between childhood stunting and the mother's level of education. In El Salvador, this indicator was 31.7% for boys and girls whose mothers had no formal schooling, five times higher than that for children whose mothers had 10 or more years of schooling.

A look at trends in wasting among children under 5 years old (low weight-for-height [≤2.00 SD]) shows that El Salvador has had a low prevalence of wasting (2.1%) since 1988 and up to the last reported figure for 2002–2003, which compares favorably with the 2.3% figure expected in industrialized countries. Low weight-for-age in children under 5 years old is still a major problem, with a prevalence rate of 10.3% in 2002–2003, down 1.5% from 1998 (8).

The 2002–2003 National Family Health Survey found that 19.8% of children 12–59 months old suffered from **anemia**, compared with a figure of 18.9% in 1998, indicating that the problem had worsened slightly. The prevalence of anemia in rural areas (23.1%) was greater than in urban areas (15.8%). The same survey found that, nationwide, 8.8% of mothers of children under 5 years old also suffered from anemia, with no major differences between urban (8.5%) and rural (9.1%) rates. Of the 195,013 children under 5 years old treated by the Ministry of Public Health in 2005, only 7.6% suffered from some degree of **malnutrition**. Nonetheless, the mortality due to malnutrition jumped from 3.07 per 100,000 population (200 deaths) in 2002 to 3.30 per 100,000 (223 deaths) in 2004 (8); of all such deaths, 92 involved children under 5 years old (59 males and 33 females).

In urban areas, 5.1% of children under 5 years old were **overweight**, a figure that is 2.2 times the norm (2.3%) and that points to the fact that this condition is beginning to pose a problem. The national prevalence rate in the same age group was 3.6%. This marks the beginning of what could become an overweight epidemic in the country's future generations. The prevalence of overweight in urban areas (5.1%) was 2.1 times greater than in urban areas (2.4%). Overweight does not appear to have any correlation with the mother's level of education; the highest prevalence rates of overweight were seen in households in the top socioeconomic brackets (40%) and households in which the mother had no fixed income and did not work outside the home (37.2%). The age group 15–19 years old had the lowest prevalence of overweight and **obesity** (27.2% and 9.1%, respectively). Adults 30–34 years old had the highest prevalence of overweight

333

(43.3%) and adults 40–44 years old had the highest prevalence of obesity (25.0%). Among women 15–49 years old, 35.8% were overweight and 18.4% were obese. The 2002–2003 National Family Health Survey found overweight or obesity in over 60% of persons older than 18 years old. This is not a public nutrition problem but, rather, could be the result of changes in eating habits related to the environment, access to foods high in calories, and insufficient physical exercise (8) in the absence of safe, convenient facilities for engaging in physical activity.

Cardiovascular Diseases

According to 2004 data from the Statistics and Census Bureau, there were 5,515 recorded deaths associated with diseases of the circulatory system, for a mortality rate of 81.6 per 100,000 population; 53% were among women. The largest share of deaths were attributable to ischemic heart disease (33.6%), cardiovascular diseases (17.2%), and hypertensive diseases (6.9%). Adults 60 years old and older accounted for 82% of all such deaths, with a mortality rate of 903 per 100,000 population.

Malignant Neoplasms

There were 3,278 recorded deaths from malignant neoplasms in 2004, for a mortality rate of 48.5 per 100,000 population (41.1 per 100,000 for males and 55.7 per 100,000 for females), 58% of which involved women. Malignant neoplasms were responsible for 12.5% of all deaths nationwide. Adults 60 years old and older were hardest hit, with a mortality rate of 118.83 per 100,000 population. There was a large gender gap in mortality from this cause in persons 80 years old and older, among whom the cancer mortality rate for men was 1.4 times greater than for women (284.07 per 100,000 for females and 403.52 per 100,000 for males). The main sites of malignant neoplasms were the stomach (15.2%); the digestive organs and peritoneum (14.3%); the cervix (6.7%); and the trachea, bronchial tubes, and lungs (6.3%).

OTHER HEALTH PROBLEMS OR ISSUES

Disasters

There were two devastating earthquakes in El Salvador in 2001. The death toll was 1,259, with another 8,864 persons injured and 1,616,782 left homeless, with injury and death rates of 140 and 20 per 100,000 population, respectively; the first earthquake was responsible for 75% of the fatalities, 63% of the injuries, and 84% of the property damage. The first earthquake affected 71% of the country, and the second, 28%. In both cases, men and women older than 70 years old were hit hardest. After the first earthquake, 33% of victims were hospitalized, compared with 38% following the second quake; in both cases, traumas were the main cause of hospitalization (accounting for 47% and 52% of hospital admittances, respectively) (6).

The Santa Ana Volcano, also known as Ilamatepec, erupted in 2005, causing two fatalities; more than 5,014 residents evacuated to shelters in the face of the imminent risk of a second eruption (6). Table 6 shows the country's number of fatalities and extent of damage and economic losses caused by natural disasters between 1998 and 2005.

Also in 2005, Tropical Storm Stan pounded the country for six straight days. The storm's intermittent rainfall caused serious flooding, claiming 69 lives and causing severe material losses. The departments of La Libertad, Sonsonate, San Salvador, La Paz, San Vicente, and Santa Ana were the hardest hit, accounting for 81.5% of the injured and 87% of the fatalities. More than 1,500 multidisciplinary health workers were assigned to the shelters. The Health Assistance Fund (FOSALUD) provided financial support to the Ministry of Public Health to help hire 200 health professionals to address the needs of residents of disaster areas. The Ministry of Education suspended classes, as some 269 school buildings were used as shelters and another 86 schools were damaged by the rains. According to the Ministry of Public Health, 80 health facilities were damaged (64 health units, three hospitals, six "casas de salud" or home-based microclinics, and seven administration buildings). Total damage was assessed at US$ 15.6 million, including US$ 9.7 million in damages to health units.

The Economic Commission for Latin America and the Caribbean (ECLAC) put the economic impact of the Santa Ana Volcano eruption and tropical storm Stan at US$ 355.7 million, including US$ 196.2 million in direct damages (capital losses) and US$ 159.5 million in indirect damages (losses in flows).

Violence and Other External Causes

According to 2004 general mortality statistics furnished by the Statistics and Census Bureau, all types of injuries from external causes were the second leading cause of general mortality nationwide, with a rate of 81.6 per 100,000 population (5,512 deaths), up from 71.9 per 100,000 (4,687 deaths) in 2002. Homicide was the leading external cause of death (at 38.7 per 100,000 population), followed by traffic accidents (26.0 per 100,000) and suicide (6.9 per 100,000). Males accounted for 90.8% of all homicides, 79.1% of traffic accidents, and 74.9% of suicides in 2004. In terms of years of potential life lost (YPLL), homicides ranked first, accounting for a total of 140,432 YPLL, or 52.4% of the total number of years of potential life lost to all deaths from external causes (see Table 4).

According to Ministry of Public Health data for 2005, the incidence of injuries from external causes was, in descending order, 331 per 100,000 population for workplace accidents, 74 for traffic accidents involving motor vehicles, 68 for injuries from cutting and thrusting weapons, 49 for injuries from firearms, 19 for physical abuse, and 2 for sexual assault.

The Statistics and Census Bureau reported a rise in the total number of fatalities caused by traffic accidents, from 1,415 in

TABLE 6. Fatalities, damages to homes, and economic losses from natural disasters, El Salvador, 1998–2005.

Event	Fatalities	Families left homeless	Economic losses (US$)
Hurricane Mitch	240	10,000	398 million
2001 earthquakes	1,159	316,500	1.660 billion
Eruption of the Santa Ana Volcano and tropical storm Stan	69	14,525	355.7 million

1997 to 1,760 in 2004. Moreover, the Ministry of Public Health's hospital network reported these types of traumas as the third leading cause of hospitalization, accounting for 5,327 reasons for hospital discharges, with a fatality rate of 8.6%.

Ministry physicians reported 438 cases of domestic violence, of which 103 (23.5%) involved children 0–9 years old and 151 (34.5%) involved women 20–59 years old.

There were more than 15,000 reported cases of acute pesticide poisoning between 1996 and 2004, with an average of 1,700 incidents per year (and an incidence of 28 per 100,000 population), 67% of which involved males and 98% of which were treated in hospitals. The main symptoms were digestive (49%) and systemic (37%), and the case-fatality rate was 12%. The leading cause of poisoning was attempted suicide (46%), and the main pesticide used was phosphine. There were also cases of accidental (28%) and occupational (26%) poisoning.

Mental Health

The Ministry of Public Health's National Mental Health Program data for 2005 shows incidence rates for mental health problems at 715.1 per 100,000 population for anxiety disorders, 132.6 for depression, 34.1 for alcoholism, 7.7 for attempted suicide, and 1.7 for drug addiction. The first two disorders affect mostly women. Alcohol-related mental and behavioral disorders were the reasons for 2,912 hospital discharges; 209 involved the use of psychoactive substances, and mood disorders accounted for another 406. There were 840 recorded deaths from mental and behavioral disorders in 2004, for a rate of 12.4 per 100,000 population. The leading cause of death was the use of psychoactive substances (mainly alcohol consumption). The departments of Cuscatlán (22.3), San Vicente (14.8), and La Paz (11.1) had the highest mortality rates.

Addictions

The 2002–2003 National Family Health Survey found that 70% of males 15–59 years old had smoked, 85% had consumed alcoholic beverages, and 33% had had 1–4 drinks a week. According to the 2006 Preliminary Report on the First National Study of Drug Use in the General Population of El Salvador (16), of 4,819 subjects surveyed, 61.6% of males and 20.7% of females reported having used tobacco at some time. The survey also found that 66.5% of male respondents and 31.0% of female respondents had consumed alcohol, 5.0% of all respondents had taken tranquilizers, and 3.1% of male respondents and 0.1% of female respondents (virtually none) had used inhalants. The survey revealed that nearly 150,000 Salvadorians had used some type of illegal drug and that illegal drug use was more prevalent among males (15.2%) than among females (0.5%). The main drug used (by 14.3% of males and 0.2% of females) was marihuana, followed by cocaine (4.0% of males and 0.2% of females), and hallucinogenic drugs (used by 1.3% of males and 0.007% of females). There was very little usage of any other types of drugs. The survey found that most respondents reporting having used these drugs were in the 12–29-year-old age group. According to respondents (71% of males and 65% of females), it was relatively easy or very easy to get hold of any type of drug, and their main source of information on drugs was the television.

Environmental Pollution

The Ministry of Public Health's hospital network reported 310 cases of pesticide poisoning, 71.6% of which involved males, with females accounting for the remaining 28.4%. It is noteworthy that 123 (39.7%) of these cases were classified as pesticide poisoning inside the home. There were 20 fatalities among poisoning victims admitted to hospitals, 13 of which involved males. Age groups 15–19 and 20–24 years old had the highest rates of pesticide poisoning (6.8 and 7.8 per 100,000 hospital admittances, respectively). Moreover, the fatality rate rises with the victim's age. A geographic breakdown of cases of pesticide poisoning showed different patterns depending on the type of substance involved. For example, organophosphate poisoning was more prevalent in the departments of Usulután, Ahuachapán, and Santa Ana, while poisoning with herbicides and fumigants was more common in the departments of La Unión, Usulután, La Libertad, and Morazán.

RESPONSE OF THE HEALTH SECTOR

Health Policies and Plans

El Salvador is stepping up implementation of a health reform program geared to the rights and obligations of the general public and the Government's role to provide free health care for the poor. Within this reform framework, the concept of health is viewed from a comprehensive, intersectoral perspective, and is grounded in the need to promote the general welfare from the bottom up, ensuring quality of life, a social safety net, and good family health within the framework of a sustainable environment (17). Thus, it is important to bolster health sector integration and establish integrated health service networks that make the best possible use of ever-scarce resources, ensuring equitable and timely access to health care for the Salvadorian people and implementing strategies for expanding the health care safety net (17). Numerous efforts have been made to modernize health sector institutions by promoting decentralization in search of efficiency and better coverage.

Health system reforms aim to redefine the roles of different institutions, separating oversight, regulatory, financial, and health delivery functions as a way to optimize the health sector's efficiency (17). The National Comprehensive Health Care Reform Monitoring Council, consisting of the Minister of Health, the director of the Salvadorian Institute of Social Security, and representatives of NGOs, health trade associations, health professionals, consumers, and health manpower training institutions, seeks to build consensus and establish lines of action within the health sector to serve as national health policy guidelines. It has issued a health care reform proposal that the Executive Branch has submitted to the Legislative Assembly for deliberation and approval. The national policy envisions an integrated health care system with effective intrasectoral coordination; a health care model that minimizes overlap and that coordinates and synchronizes the three levels of care; and a management model based on decentralization and social participation and that optimizes the use of available resources, and that amends the legal framework according to national realities (17). The Monitoring Council has four subcommittees: Human Resources, Financing, Reform Modeling, and Social Participation.

The comprehensive health care reform proposal establishes nine guidelines (17): (1) strengthen the national health care system; (2) bolster a health care model based on health promotion, disease prevention, and primary health care; (3) consolidate a mixed health delivery model; (4) develop a management model based on the Ministry of Public Health's steering role; (5) institutionalize social participation as a cornerstone of the health care system; (6) promote decentralization as a cornerstone of the health care system; (7) invest in human resources for health as the pivotal force for change in the health system and for its management; (8) strengthen cross-sector coordination as a synchronized social response to health challenges; and (9) assure universal basic health services.

Health Strategies and Programs

The Health Assistance Fund (FOSALUD) was created as one of the central government's main strategies for the country's health sector; it is a building block of the Presidential Plan known as *Plan Oportunidades*. FOSALUD is helping to expand basic health service coverage in rural and urban areas, as well as emergency care and emergency medical services, by mounting special programs to strengthen public health care. FOSALUD services, which have been operational since August 2005, are free, and they benefit 3.8 million persons nationwide. To date, the Fund operates 66 health units that provide round-the-clock service, including weekends and holidays. FOSALUD uses Ministry of Public Health facilities to maximize its resources. A gradual, phased reform of the national health care system designed to reduce disparities in access to health care by expanding comprehensive health care coverage, reducing inequities in health care for different social groups, and modifying health delivery and health management models based on new approaches with the emphasis on comprehensive, decentralized, managed health care implies many, multifaceted changes. These include changes in the organization and operation of health institutions; in the roles of health officials and workers; in goal-setting, targeting, and planning processes and in corresponding management procedures; in conflict resolution procedures; in decision-making procedures based on relevant information; in moral, professional, and financial incentive systems; and in procedures for monitoring, evaluating, and expanding the reform process.

The Ministry of Public Health conducted two exercises to measure the performance of essential public health functions to help steer needed health sector reforms in El Salvador; both were based on national and local experiences. The first evaluation (May 2001) was conducted with multisectoral, multidisciplinary participation, and it provided an overview of the current situation in terms of optimal standards to be attained. The second evaluation workshop (April 2005) was the product of an inter-organization effort by the Ministry of Public Health and PAHO/WHO, and it raised the need for framing a national plan for improving performance. The Ministry of Public Health carries the greatest weight nationwide for the performance of essential public health functions. It cannot fully function as a National Health Authority, however, because it depends on the functions and attributes of other institutions within and outside the health sector.

Functions more strictly related to "health intelligence" or, at any rate, to institutional capacity-building designed to improve efficiency and effectiveness scored better. The best scores went to health monitoring and analysis functions; public health surveillance, research, and risk and damage control functions; policy-making and planning functions in support of public health programs and national health authority oversight functions; institutional capacity-building functions for health regulation and control; and functions dealing with disaster and emergency mitigation, all of which scored in the above-average and best performance quartiles.

The functions of health promotion; social participation and citizen empowerment in health; evaluation and promotion of equitable access to health services; human resource development and training in public health; quality assurance in public health services and services targeted to individuals; and innovative problem-solving scored in the lowest performance quartile (0.0%–0.25%).

There have been major improvements in some indicators of essential public health functions, while progress in others has been piecemeal due to the fragmentation of the health care system. Overall, improving essential public health functions depends on budget appropriations, inter-agency and intersectoral efforts, and the attitudes and practices of civil society.

The Ministry of Public Health plans to mount programs within the framework of the Solidarity Alliance (*Alianza Solidaria*) and Alliance for Security (*Alianza por la Seguridad*) to help raise the standard of living and the level of health of Salvadorians. To this end it promotes efficiency, effectiveness, equity, quality, and compassion in the delivery of health care services, pursues a comprehensive approach to health care, and bolsters the active involvement of all social stakeholders. Another strategy is the establishment of integrated basic health systems (SIBASIs), whereby health facilities are organized into mutually supporting networks to improve their ability to meet the public's needs (*18*). Each SIBASI serves a clearly delineated geographic area and population, which ensures the equitable allocation and efficient use of available resources to effectively meet, on an ongoing basis, the health needs of its target population (*18*). The country is divided into 28 SIBASIs, whose operations are coordinated by five technical area teams.

Together, SIBASIs constitute the basic structure for the local-level organization and operation of national health system facilities, subject to the Ministry of Public Health's oversight. This structure provides an integrated health care model that operates through a well-organized network of complementary health care providers, which prevents overlapping and duplication of efforts by efficiently and effectively using available resources and by facilitating the monitoring and evaluation of all corresponding activities in terms of their impact on the health of the population served by the SIBASI (*18*). According to the Integrated Basic Health Systems Act enacted in late 2005 that entered into effect in April 2006, the responsibility for the technical/administrative management of all resources allocated to the SIBASIs is vested in regional headquarters, with the SIBASI, in turn, charged with providing full primary health care coverage, particularly to the poor. The SIBASI system coordinates the services of different health care providers to solve problems identified at the local level. To this end, it relies on an integrated health care model and the delivery of individual, family, community, and environmentally based health promotion, disease prevention, and treatment and rehabilitation services to attain a standard of health that fosters social development. To serve its target population, the SIBASI system synchronizes its primary health care services with those of secondary and tertiary health facilities. A referral and counter-referral system ensures that the health care that is delivered is comprehensive and ongoing. In order for the SIBASIs to operate optimally will require that the coordination and sharing of responsibility by all social and economic stakeholders be ongoing. This, in turn, requires social participation and intersectorality, or a cross-sector approach, to help solve problems and ensure transparent management (*18*).

Organization of the Health System

The health sector is made up of four subsectors: the public subsector, the social security system, independently operated health care services, and the private subsector. The main players in the public health care system are the Ministry of Public Health and Social Welfare, the High-Level Public Health Council, the Salvadorian Social Security Institute, the Military Health System, the Teachers' Health and Welfare System, and the Salvadorian Rehabilitation Institute for the Disabled.

The 1987 Health Code, whose revision is to be submitted to Congress, gives the Ministry of Public Health policy-making, regulatory, program management, financial, technical/administrative assistance, and direct health service delivery functions (theoretically, serving 80% to 85% of the population).

The High-Level Public Health Council has numerous functions, particularly in the policy-making, regulatory, and operational arenas.

The Salvadorian Social Security Institute, an independent agency within the Executive Branch attached to the Ministry of Labor and Social Insurance, has policy-making, health program management, financial, technical/administrative assistance, and service delivery functions, serving insured workers and retirees and their dependents (16% of the population).

The Military Health System provides preventive health services and treatment care to members of the Armed Forces, retired military personnel, and their families. For the past few years it has been providing health care services to the general public on a fee-for-service basis to optimize infrastructure use (serving 3% of the population).

The Salvadorian Rehabilitation Institute for the Disabled is an independent agency that provides rehabilitation services at various facilities specialized in caring for the disabled and the elderly.

The Teachers' Health and Welfare System provides health care to teachers and their families by contracting out services that are funded by member contributions and a government subsidy.

Although for many years it has claimed that it covers 80% of the population, the Ministry of Public Health actually provides health care coverage for about 50% of the population (*4*). The last Health Service Demand Survey (dating back to 1988) found that the Ministry met roughly 40%–45% of demand for outpatient care and as much as 75% of nationwide demand for in-hospital care. According to Ministry data for 2004, it treated 527,902 children under 1 year of age; performed 709,923 check-ups of children 1–4 years old; performed 341,974 prenatal examinations; attended 73,447 deliveries; provided family planning services to 222,142 clients, including sterilization procedures, with an estimated 206,310 active acceptors between 15 and 49 years old; processed 331,825 hospital discharges; and performed 93,099 major surgeries, with an 85.2% hospital occupancy rate (*12*). As stipulated in El Salvador's Constitution, the Ministry of Public Health's target population is the poor, and the general public in the event of disasters or epidemics. In practice, however, the Ministry provides health care to anyone in need, regardless of their socio-economic status or insurance coverage (*19*), which prevents it from concentrating its resources and efforts on the poor, who have the greatest need for its services.

The Salvadorian Social Security Institute serves roughly 1,099,988 insured workers and retirees and their dependents, or 16% of the country's total population. However, only 11% of the sick or injured were treated at the Institute's facilities (*4*). In general, workers with social security coverage are employed in the economy's formal sector.

The Military Health System serves members of the Armed Forces and their families; there are no reliable figures on its coverage. The Teachers' Health and Welfare System provides services exclusively to members of the teachers' union and their families. Existing data puts its coverage rate at somewhere around 1.6% of the total population. El Salvador does not have a well-established private insurance system. In fact, at most, only 1% of the population has group insurance coverage. The private not-for-profit subsector serves 0.1% of the population and the private for-profit subsector serves just over 1% of the population. A sizeable percentage of the population (18%) turns to traditional healers, pharmacists, and other practitioners to solve their health problems (*4*). Roughly 12% of the population has no public or private health insurance coverage.

Public Health Services

Other important milestones include the introduction of new vaccines such as the triple diphtheria/whooping cough/tetanus vaccine introduced in 1997; the hepatitis B vaccine introduced in 1999; the yellow fever vaccine for travelers introduced in 2000; the pentavalent vaccine against diphtheria, pertussis, tetanus, hepatitis B, and *Haemophilus influenzae* type b introduced in 2002; the flu vaccine for children aged 6–23 months old and adults older than 60 first introduced in 2004, followed up by three nationwide vaccination campaigns to date; and the measles/rubella vaccine for adults 15–39 years old. The country laid the groundwork for introducing a vaccine against rotavirus in October of 2006 through a fiscal strategy that established a new sales tax on alcohol and tobacco and set up the Health Assistance Fund, known as FOSALUD, to hold the corresponding revenues.

Surveillance indicators for acute flaccid paralysis have consistently exceeded international minimum standards, with rates higher than 1 case per 100,000 in persons older than 15 years old. Measles/rubella surveillance indicators have all exceeded 80%, except for the adequate case-finding indicator, which has been consistently below this figure for the last six years. As far as rotavirus surveillance is concerned, the country has seven sentinel hospitals detecting circulating serotypes of rotavirus since 2003 (G1P8), 2004 (G1P8 and G9P8), 2005 (G9P4), and 2006 (G2P4 and G9P8), which should help assess the impact of the introduction of the rotavirus vaccine.

On average, 41% of the country's municipios have vaccination coverage rates of 95% or better, while 59% of municipios (156 of 262) are still trying to reach coverage of 95% or above by using all available biologicals, which means scaling up inoculation programs and epidemiological surveillance activities. The immunization program information system is scheduled to be modified shortly so it can supply coverage data broken down by gender and by rural/urban area; this will help correct inequities between municipios by targeting stepped up vaccination efforts.

According to Ministry of Public Health data, antiretroviral therapy was first administered to HIV/AIDS patients in 2001 (73 cases). By December of 2005, 2,235 patients were receiving this therapy, with an impressive jump in the number of patients with free access to these drugs. Antiretroviral therapy was also administered to 94 pregnant women in 2006 (between January and June) as a prophylactic measure against mother-to-child transmission, and to 104 newborns as a post-perinatal exposure prophylaxis. Ministry statistics show that the use of antiretroviral therapy has been stepped up every year since it was first administered back in 2001 (to 73 patients), particularly in 2004 and 2005 (with 731 new courses of therapy started in 2004 and another 980 in 2005). According to data from the National Strategic Plan for the Prevention, Treatment and Control of HIV/AIDS and Sexually Transmitted Infections, 44% of patients are receiving antiretroviral therapy, a far better rate than WHO's recommended 25% and a reflection of the country's progress in this area.

Of all HIV tests administered in 2005, 48.5% were given to pregnant women, 0.14% of whom tested positive for HIV. That same year, antiretroviral drugs were reportedly administered to 242 women as post-exposure prophylaxis and to 242 newborns as post-perinatal exposure prophylaxis. According to the statistics, there was a sizeable drop in the number of cases of HIV infection/AIDS in children under 1 year old between 2001 (with 142 reported cases) and 2004 and 2005 (with 20 cases each year), which is another major achievement for the country. This improvement was attributable to the stepping up of nationwide efforts to prevent mother-to-child HIV/AIDS transmission in 2003 by offering free testing in laboratory-equipped health units around the country, providing training to Ministry line personnel, and conducting an intensive educational media campaign. The number of screening tests went from 98,393 in 2001 to 217,748 in 2005 (a jump of over 100%) with the decentralization of diagnostic services and the use of rapid testing methods. Only 20.3% of males and 5.6% of females reported having used a condom in their last sexual contact (*8*).

The water supply and sanitation sector consists of the National Water Supply and Sewerage Authority, which serves 151 municipios; another 110 municipios are served by city governments and other service operators. Cuisnahuat, in the Department of Sonsonate, is the only urban area without a water supply system. Rural communities operate their own water services. The country has no national water resources policy, and there is no clear or logical separation of regulatory, policy-making, and service delivery functions.

According to existing data on water service coverage, 65.5% of Salvadorian households have individual house connections to a water supply system, 11.2% draw water from wells, and 10.4% get their water from public standpipes or fountains. In urban areas, 80.9% of households have individual house connections and 10.1% get their water from public standpipes or fountains. In contrast, only 39.5% of rural households have piped water anywhere on their property, 24.9% draw water from wells, and 19.7% get their water from a spring. Most households in the San Salvador Metropolitan Area have individual house connections (80.2%). Public standpipes or fountains are the second leading source of supply (7.6%), including shared taps (7).

Reforms to the water supply sector are still ongoing. Existing proposals include new water legislation that focuses on watershed management and the sustainable development of the water supply and sanitation subsector, a national rural water supply and sanitation policy, and a proposed policy package promoting land use planning and the establishment of a national water resources council. The Ministry of Public Health is still conducting its disinfection program for drinking water, to which end it produces and promotes the use of a 0.5% sodium hypochlorite solution known as PURIAGUA. It also undertakes to keep its 250 generators in running order, fosters community participation, develops educational strategies to promote the use of PURIAGUA, and endeavors to strengthen health stakeholder commitment.

In October 2004, the Ministry of Public Health issued official technical sanitary standards for the installation, use, and upkeep of no-flush pit latrines, regulating the different types of latrines used for sanitary excreta disposal in the country's periurban and rural areas.

Ministry of Environment data for 2005 put daily refuse production at 2,715.3 tons (2,258.4 tons in urban areas and 456.9 tons in rural areas), for an annual production figure of 991,084.5 tons, half of which was produced in the San Salvador Metropolitan Area, which has a proper refuse collection and disposal system and a sanitary landfill that meets minimum sanitary engineering requirements for handling 1,500 tons of refuse per day. Waste disposal has improved nationwide, as reflected by the addition of 10 new manual and mechanized sanitary landfills. Regular municipal solid waste collection service coverage went from 73.7% in 2003 to 81.0% in 2005, with 211 municipios nationwide operating some type of trash collection service. In addition, 88% of municipios subsidize trash collection with locally generated revenues, which means either that user charges are extremely low or that, nationwide, people are paying nothing towards the cost of average per capita daily refuse production (0.62 kg), and this has implications for the sustainability of municipal trash collection services. Moreover, as of yet there is no national integrated waste management program, although some progress has been made in establishing a regulatory framework for integrated solid waste

management that sets waste collection and transportation standards and environmental standards for waste transfer, treatment, and final disposal sites.

According to the Salvadorian Foundation for Economic and Social Development, there were 1.25 million tons of pollutant emissions released nationwide in 2003, consisting mostly of carbon monoxide (CO), 36%, and volatile organic compounds (VOCs), 28%. San Salvador (with 300,000 tons) is the department with most air pollution emissions, followed by La Libertad (152,000 tons) and Sonsonate (140,000 tons). The main sources of pollutant emissions are motor vehicles and the burning of firewood for cooking. Motor vehicles account for 51% of pollutant emissions in the Department of San Salvador. The most polluted areas are San Salvador (the downtown area), Soyapango, Apopa, and Santa Tecla. The main source of pollution in the departments of Santa Ana and Sonsonate is burning of firewood for cooking, which accounts for 49% and 47% of total emissions in these departments, respectively. One of the contributing factors in air pollution is the age of the vehicle fleet. Data for 2003 showed 35% of motor vehicles were already more than 20 years old and responsible for 50% of all pollutant emissions. Vehicles manufactured between 1998 and 2003, which made up 20.6% of the vehicle fleet, were responsible for only 5.25% of total pollutant emissions.

The share of air pollutant emissions released by solid waste disposal sites using open burning and composting methods is 13.4%, compared with 81% for sanitary landfills.

To improve hospital solid waste management, all 30 national hospitals adhere to the separation of regular and hazardous wastes at the source point, which has lowered the risk of workplace and environmental contamination. With assistance from the German Cooperation Agency (GTZ), two national hospitals (Nueva Guadalupe in San Miguel and Santiago de Maria in Usulután) and 21 health units in the Cojutepeque, La Paz, and Santiago de María SIBASIs have been equipped with devices for crushing and destroying sharp objects (needles contaminated with body fluids) as a source reduction and waste disposal control measure. A total of 196 Ministry of Public Health employees have benefited from technical training and capacity-building activities, including the members of hospital infection control committees in all 30 national hospitals and environmental engineers, epidemiologists, and nursing personnel attached to the 28 SIBASIs. The Ministry's efforts to regulate the management of infectious biological waste have been noteworthy: it has issued a mandatory standard (NSO: 13.25.01:05, published in Volume 370 of the Official Gazette, on February 2, 2006) and also has developed a management model for the sanitary handling of infectious biological waste. Of the 7.58 tons of waste generated daily, 3.85 meet the sanitary requirements set by this standard.

El Salvador does not manufacture pesticides, but it does have maquilas that process pesticides formulation for marketing firms; these formulations account for 5% of the pesticides sold in the country. The rest are imported, generally in 200 l containers or 25 kg packages.

According to Ministry of Agriculture data on pesticide use, vegetable crops account for the highest pesticide spending (anywhere from 13.9% to 30.8 %). The share of spending on pesticides for different agroindustrial crops is similar, 3.6% for coffee, 4.7% for sugar cane, and 8.6% for staple grain crops. The most popular pesticides for vector control are deltamethrin, permethrin, bendiocarb, kaothrin, and temephos. There is legislation banning the use of products from the so-called "dirty dozen" list (which includes DDT; aldrin; dieldrin; chlordane; heptachlor; 2,4-D; and parathion).

The Ministry of Public Health is committed to keeping the surveillance system in place and to crafting a plan to strengthen the Central Laboratory so it can begin monitoring pesticide levels in water. It also will provide ongoing training at all Ministry levels and in local communities on how to care for poisoning patients so as to reduce the morbidity and mortality from pesticide poisoning.

The Ministry of Public Health is bolstering several food security and nutritional initiatives. For example, the Comprehensive Health and Nutrition program is a community-based effort to promote good health and nutrition by monitoring weight gain in pregnant women and in children under 2 years old, using volunteers (parents) and local health workers, mainly health promoters. Other initiatives include the Feeding with Love program, which, in conjuction with the National Secretariat for Family Affairs, local governments, NGOs, and local community members, has provided nutritional counseling, food, and protein supplements to children under 5 years old, pregnant women, and nursing mothers since 2000. Finally, the Nutritional Assistance Plan targets mothers and children in municipios hardest hit by the crisis in the coffee industry.

The nationwide Processed Food Fortification Program directed at all segments of the population is designed to ensure that the public gets an adequate supply of vitamins and minerals. The program provides four fortified foods, namely iodized salt; sugar fortified with vitamin A; wheat flour fortified with iron, folic acid, and B-complex vitamins; and cornmeal enriched with iron, folic acid, and B-complex vitamins.

El Salvador has a National Civil Defense System (established under the Civil Defense and Disaster Prevention and Mitigation Act of August 30, 2005) charged with protecting at-risk communities and coordinating with other agencies and organizations (government agencies, NGOs, private enterprise, relief organizations, etc.) in preventing or responding to disasters.

Individual Care Services

There is a network of 623 public health facilities (30 hospitals, 367 health units, 170 small clinics (*casas de salud*), 51 rural nutrition centers, 3 clinics, and 2 emergency care centers). There are four tertiary referral hospitals (maternity, pediatric, pulmonary, and specialty hospitals) (*12*). The Salvadorian Institute of Social Security has 273 health care facilities nationwide—11 hospitals, 65 health units (33 community clinics and 32 medical units), and 197 clinics in private companies (*12*).

As part of efforts to modernize the health care system, the National Blood Program and the Council for El Salvador's National Blood Bank Network (including the Ministry of Public Health, the Social Security Institute, the Military Health System, the Red Cross, and private hospitals) are involved in various activities designed to ensure the efficient and timely supply of safe blood and blood products.

Overall, the National Blood Program follows PAHO/WHO resolutions and strategic guidelines regarding blood safety, and has advanced in the training of personnel involved in all phases of this process. Pertinent legislation has been amended, and new regulations governing transfusion medicine and blood banks await the President's signature. New policy manuals for donor selection and transfusion medicine also have been issued. The Ministry of Public Health's Max Bloch Central Laboratory and other such facilities are still taking part in outside performance evaluation programs sponsored by PAHO/WHO. Implementation of a strategic zoning plan as part of the continuous quality improvement program for the health sector is being expedited, in line with a proposal for the regionalization of blood banks.

According to a report by the Max Bloch Central Laboratory covering January through December of 2005 (*20*), 32 blood collection centers collected 80,142 units of blood, of which only 9.5% was donated by volunteers, with the remaining 90.49% provided by patients' friends and relatives. Of the total units of blood, 0.09% tested positive for HIV, 0.28% for hepatitis B, 0.019% for hepatitis C, 1.02% for syphilis, and 2.4% for Chagas' disease; 95.3% of the units of blood were separated into blood components.

As part of reform and modernization efforts in mental health, mental health units were put in place at San Juan de Dios Hospital in Santa Ana; at Dr. José Antonio Zaldaña Pulmonary and Family Medicine Hospital and San Juan de Dios Hospital in San Miguel; and San Rafael Hospital in La Libertad. By systematically bringing mental health services to these hospitals, the overload at the National Psychiatric Hospital has been alleviated and a specialized care area has been created in these facilities. Guidelines have been issued for establishing mental health units in general hospitals, as a way to harmonize standards for the operation of mental health services. Regulatory instruments establishing mental health care guidelines also have been disseminated, including: (1) standards for comprehensive mental health care; (2) clinical guides for the treatment of common mental health problems; (3) clinical guides for the treatment of individuals whose behavior is consistent with addiction to psychoactive substances; and (4) a crisis intervention model for disasters and emergencies that encompasses all necessary elements for the delivery of timely psychological assistance and the referral of cases requiring specialized care in the event of a disaster or emergency.

There is a proposal for decentralizing health care services for epileptics that is scheduled to go into effect in 2007; it will lead to an official comprehensive health care guide for epileptics.

Health Promotion

Government agencies and nongovernmental organizations are following guidelines established under the Government's 2004–2009 "Safe Country" Program, whose lines of action pertaining to health (quality and universal coverage), strengthening of society and the family (social cohesion), and public security (better quality of life) are designed to improve living conditions for the population (18). To this end, the strengthening of institutional modernization and decentralization processes, health promotion, disease and environmental threat and damage prevention, and rehabilitation are all part of the Health Ministry's institutional policy for improving the standard of human and environmental health through a primary care approach (18). There are ongoing efforts to develop an integrated health care model designed to serve as a package of health promotion policies, standards, interventions, and instruments through the operation of various programs, including "Feeding with Love," safe motherhood, health promoting schools, rural nutrition centers, mental health, the Integrated Management of Childhood Illnesses (IMCI) strategy, STIs/HIV/AIDS, and the National Tuberculosis Prevention and Control Program.

The Salvadorian Social Security Institute is a link between promotion and prevention, implementing these strategies through community-based clinics that bolster the health care delivery model defined as "networking alternatives for public and private health care providers, ensuring access to health system benefits with quality, equity and continuity of care" (17).

A National Declaration on Health Promotion, signed in 2001, puts forward a plan to implement public policies that foster social participation, investment in health, mutual responsibility, research in health, and strengthening of municipal governments. So far, there is a proposal for a national health promotion policy formulated with the active involvement of representatives of agencies and organizations conducting health promotion activities (18). Focus areas under health communication and/or education strategies include healthy lifestyles, environmental health, and vaccination-related issues.

There are ongoing efforts to promote participation and partnerships between civil society and various sectors, primarily as a basis for the development, implementation, and evaluation of health promotion policies or programs. Examples include the formation of community-based social consultation committees; the implementation of projects in conjunction with local governments, universities, intersectoral committees, mayors' offices, the National Civil Police, the Ministry of Public Health, and nongovernmental organizations, among others; and the development of consensus- and consultation-based policy-making, rule-making, and planning, which served as a basis for the designing of a health promotion policy.

The main problems hampering implementation of the health promotion policy are a lack of a specific budget, a lack of standard procedures for the replication of successful experiences, a lack of sharing of information about each sector's promotional activities, lax enforcement of existing legislation and regulations, and a shortage of trained professionals. According to the Ministry of Public Health, the main challenges in expanding and strengthening health promotion over the next five years are to monitor implementation of the provisions of the National Declaration on Health Promotion; to approve and institutionalize the health promotion policy framed in December of 2005; to craft health promotion programs, plans, and projects; to improve health communication, information, and education strategies; to provide proper financial management ensuring human resource development and sustainability; to devise health-promoting public policies and refine current legislation; to systematize and share successful experiences in health promotion; to lay the groundwork for community participation in health promotion activities; to steer international cooperation toward health promotion projects; to establish a National Council for Health Promotion and strengthen health promotion networks; and to promote public and private intersectoral participation.

Human Resources

As of 2005, El Salvador had 10,694 registered physicians. The physician-patient ratio went from 14.1 to 15.5 per 10,000 population between 2002 and 2005. There has been a similar pattern of growth in other health professions, though the numbers are somewhat smaller. The ratio of registered nurses to physicians went from 0.5 to 4.9 between 1999 and 2003, only to slightly slip down to 4.7 in 2005. The largest increase in specialists was in the field of public health, with the three specialized programs of study offered in this area for the past several years turning out about 100 public health experts in each graduating class (19). The largest increase in manpower has been in nursing personnel of all types, whose numbers went from 13,784 in 2003 to 15,191 in 2005.

Health Sector Expenditures and Financing

According to El Salvador's National Health Accounts, the share of current GDP spent on health between 1999 and 2004 was 7.8%, with a low of 7.7% of GDP in 2003; per capita health expenditures rose from US$ 161 in 1999 to US$ 184 in 2004. By these figures, the country has an average-to-low level of health care spending in the context of Latin America (1).

Moreover, a look at the composition of health care expenditures (which is as important if not more important than total spending) shows three main drivers: households, employers, and the Government. According to national health account data, a large share (over 50%) of national expenditures for health care is in the form of direct out-of-pocket household spending, although the Government's share of total health spending has gradually increased over the past few years. The large share of direct household spending on health care is an important indicator of the skewed composition of national health expenditures, dictating a need for the development of health financing schemes in which the priority is on providing financial protection for Salvadorian families.

As the collection agency and administrator of national Government revenues, the Ministry of Finance performs a financial macrofunction (the mobilization, allocation, and administration of public or private funding for the delivery of health services). The Ministry of Public Health's budget went from US$ 231.99 million in 2002 to US$ 313.07 million in 2006, which, in relative terms, is a 35% increase (US$ 81 million) from the budget appropriation for 2002. Despite the growth in the absolute and current value of the Ministry's budget over the past few years, it has never once topped 1.8% of GDP.

Likewise, the Teachers' Health and Welfare System finances procurements of health services for members of the teachers' union and their families; the Military Health System provides health care services for members of the Armed Forces.

Technical Cooperation and External Financing

International cooperation has been instrumental in assisting the Ministry of Public Health, bolstering the implementation of high-priority national plans, programs, and projects, and helping the institution deal with emergencies created by epidemics, earthquakes, and floods between 1999 and 2004. In 2005, international cooperation funding helped provide comprehensive health care coverage in at-risk areas. Strategic interventions included the promotion of programs to strengthen quality; efforts to decrease in maternal and child mortality rates; the delivery of comprehensive health care under programs for the prevention, treatment, and control of HIV/AIDS and STIs; health care programs for adolescents and older adults; nutrition programs; and disaster management and basic sanitation programs. External financing also has supported the design of renovation and equipment projects for the country's network of health facilities to improve their operating capacity, and has furnished technical assistance and training services for health personnel. Data supplied by the External Cooperation Office (attached to the Ministry of Public Health's Planning Department) put the value of external funding for 2005 at US$ 15.4 million. The World Bank provided a US$ 142.6 million loan for the rebuilding of physical hospital infrastructure in the wake of the 2001 earthquake. Direct donor assistance in 2003–

2004 totaled US$ 16,672,114. Projects undertaken with this type of funding included the National Epidemiological Information and Surveillance System (with US$ 1,325,766 in USAID funding); the rebuilding of health infrastructure (with US$ 2,343,541 in USAID funding and US$ 271,285 in Government funding); the strengthening of primary health care, water quality, and environmental sanitation (with US$ 3,255,590 in European Union funding); the HIV/AIDS and tuberculosis program (with US$ 6,593,932 from the Global Fund); and a health program in the eastern portion of the country (with US$ 2,882,000 in funding from the Grand Duchy of Luxembourg). PAHO/WHO technical cooperation for 2004–2005 amounted to US$ 4,644,003, allocated to epidemiology, environmental health, human security, and quality of service.

References

1. Meerhoff R. Análisis del financiamiento del sector salud de la República de El Salvador y de la producción de servicios del MSPAS y del ISSS. OPS; 2005.
2. El Salvador, Ministerio de Economía. Resultados económicos 2005 y Perspectivas 2006: Informe de gestión. MINEC; 2005.
3. Programa de las Naciones Unidas para el Desarrollo, El Salvador. Informe sobre el desarrollo humano: El Salvador 2005. Una mirada al nuevo nosotros. El impacto de las migraciones. PNUD; 2005.
4. El Salvador, Ministerio de Economía, Dirección General de Estadística y Censos. Encuesta de Hogares de Propósitos Múltiples 2003. MINEC; 2004.
5. El Salvador, Ministerio de Economía. Available at: www. minec.gob.sv.
6. Organización Panamericana de la Salud. Informe final. Flash Appeal: Atención a emergencias. OPS; 2005.
7. El Salvador, Dirección General de Estadística y Censos. Available at: www.digestyc.gob.sv.
8. Asociación Demográfica Salvadoreña. Encuesta Nacional de Salud Familiar. FESAL 2002–2003. El Salvador; 2004.
9. Organización de las Naciones Unidas para la Educación, la Ciencia y la Cultura. Evaluación de disponibilidad y uso de cuidados obstétricos de emergencia en El Salvador, 2003.
10. Organización Mundial de la Salud; Cooperación Técnica Alemana; Universidad Don Bosco. Encuesta para Personas con Discapacidad; 2000–2001.
11. Banco Mundial. Perfil de los pueblos indígenas de El Salvador; 2003.
12. El Salvador, Ministerio de Salud Pública y Asistencia Social. Boletín sobre indicadores de salud. MSPAS; 2004.
13. Programa Conjunto de las Naciones Unidas sobre el VIH/SIDA. 2006 Informe sobre la epidemia mundial de SIDA. Geneva: ONUSIDA; 2006.

14. El Salvador, Ministerio de Salud Pública y Asistencia Social. Boletín informativo sobre la situación del VIH/SIDA en El Salvador; junio 2006.
15. Pan American Health Organization. Health in the Americas 2002. Washington, DC: PAHO; 2002.
16. Sistema Interamericano de Datos Uniformes sobre Consumo de Drogas. Primer estudio nacional sobre consumo de drogas en población general de El Salvador: Informe preliminar. SIDUC; 2006.
17. El Salvador, Ministerio de Salud Pública y Asistencia Social. Informe de El Salvador sobre los logros en promoción de la salud con respecto a los compromisos en la declaración de México. MSPAS; 2002.
18. El Salvador, Ministerio de Salud Pública y Asistencia Social. Memoria de labores 2005–2006.
19. El Salvador, Ministerio de Salud Pública y Asistencia Social. Memoria de labores 2003–2004.
20. El Salvador, Ministerio de Salud y Asistencia Social; Organización Panamericana de la Salud. Marco conceptual y operativo para el desarrollo del Sistema Básico de Salud Integral (SIBASI).

FRENCH GUIANA, GUADELOUPE, AND MARTINIQUE

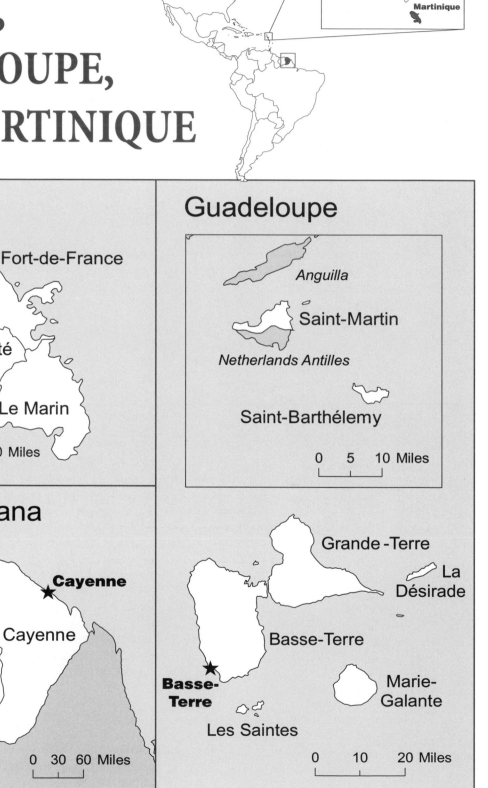

Guadeloupe
Antigua and Barbuda
St. Kitts and Nevis
Montserrat
Guadeloupe
Dominica
Martinique

Martinique

Fort-de-France

Saint-Pierre

La Trinité

Fort-de-France

Le Marin

0 10 20 Miles

Guadeloupe

Anguilla

Saint-Martin

Netherlands Antilles

Saint-Barthélemy

0 5 10 Miles

French Guiana

Suriname

Cayenne

Saint Laurent du Maroni

Cayenne

Brazil

0 30 60 Miles

Grande-Terre

La Désirade

Basse-Terre

Basse-Terre

Marie-Galante

Les Saintes

0 10 20 Miles

The islands of Guadeloupe and Martinique in the Lesser Antilles, and French Guiana, located on the northern coast of South America between Suriname and Brazil, are the three French overseas *départements* in the Region of the Americas that have been an integral part of France since 1946. Despite their geographical distance from France, their political and administrative organization into departments and regions coincides with that of the rest of France.

GENERAL CONTEXT AND HEALTH DETERMINANTS

The archipelago of Guadeloupe, covering an area of 1,703 km², is the largest of the two islands. It comprises, in addition to Guadeloupe proper—which is actually two separate landmasses, Basse-Terre and Grande-Terre, bisected by a seawater channel—the islands of Marie-Galante, Les Saintes, La Désirade, Saint-Barthélemy, and the French section of Saint-Martin. Martinique occupies an area of 1,128 km², and French Guiana, 83,534 km². Guadeloupe and Martinique enjoy a tropical climate tempered by trade winds, but are often buffeted by tropical storms between July and October, whereas the climate in French Guiana is equatorial. Even though French Guiana is the largest of the three French Overseas Departments in the Americas, 94% of its land is dense Amazonian forest crisscrossed by rivers of all sizes.

Social, Political, and Economic Determinants

As part of France, French Guiana, Guadeloupe, and Martinique belong to the European Union (EU), and the euro is the official currency. The economy of the French Overseas Departments shares a number of problems common to small island entities: insufficiently competitive exports, a tendency to specialize in services, a strong reliance on tourism and natural resources, environmental fragility, and vulnerability to natural disasters. Additionally, the Departments' economic and political stability is accompanied by heavy financial dependence on metropolitan France and limited economic exchanges with the rest of the world. Only 9% of imports from the three Departments come from the Caribbean, and barely 3% of exports go to markets in that subregion.

The economy of French Guiana includes two peculiarities. The first is a space center built by the French Government in the mid-1960s as a base from which to launch its satellites. Located in the small coastal town of Kourou, once known only as the headquarters for the infamous Devil's Island penal colony, the center's impact on GDP varies from year to year. The second is gold panning, the leading export activity (along with space-related activities),

but also a source of illegal employment and widespread trafficking. In Guadeloupe and Martinique, the banana production and exportation sector is hampered by constant fluctuations in market conditions.

In terms of per capita GDP, despite a marked improvement over the past few years, the French Overseas Departments rank lower than all regions in metropolitan France. In 2002, GDP per capita was 15,622 euros in Martinique, 14,108 euros in Guadeloupe, and 12,858 euros in French Guiana. Compared to most of their geographical neighbors, the French Overseas Departments have a relatively high standard of living, due to susidies and imports from the French Government, but their performance in employment and foreign trade places them at or near the bottom of the Caribbean group, and their GDP is less a reflection of wealth and internal productive activities than it is of their unique departmental status.

The unemployment rate in 2005 was very high throughout the French Overseas Departments: in French Guiana, 26.5% of the working-age population was without a job; in Guadeloupe, this figure was 26%; and in Martinique, it was 21.8%. Although these rates have remained constant over the past several years, the situation has improved somewhat compared to that of 1998, when unemployment peaked at 30% in the Antilles (Guadeloupe and Martinique). Those hardest hit by unemployment are the young, especially the least skilled in this group, and women. Unemployment on this scale is largely the product of a sharp increase in the size of the economically active population since the 1980s and the shift from farming to tertiary services. In French Guiana, the unemployment issue is even more acute, since the marked increase in workforce size has not been offset by the generation of sufficient job opportunities; the level of training available is lower, and employers are unable to find qualified staff. The unemployment situation is further compromised by the presence of illegal workers willing to work for low wages.

The available indicators show that the socioeconomic environment in the French Overseas Departments is less favorable than that found in other French regions, even though the overall standard of living is higher than in most neighboring countries. In France, a mechanism was devised in 1988 called the *Revenu Min-*

imum d'Insertion (RMI), or Minimum Integration Income, which provides persons aged 25 or over with a minimum amount of resources, access to certain social benefits, and assistance with social and/or professional integration. The percentage of RMI beneficiaries is much higher in the French Overseas Departments than in the regions of metropolitan France. On 31 December 2005, there were 80,000 RMI beneficiaries in the French Overseas Departments, representing 13% of the population between the ages of 20 and 59 in French Guiana, 14% in Guadeloupe, and 15% in Martinique.

A 2001 French National Institute of Statistics and Economic Studies (INSEE) survey found a larger percentage of poor households in the French Overseas Departments than in metropolitan France. It also showed that of the three departments, French Guiana fared the worst, with 20.7% of all households living below the poverty line,[1] compared to 12.5% in Guadeloupe and 12% in Martinique. The differences are even more marked when child poverty is measured: 32% of children in French Guiana live below the poverty line, compared to 16% in Guadeloupe and 13% in Martinique, as opposed to 8% in metropolitan France.

To ensure access by the entire population to health care, the French Government has implemented a measure called universal basic health coverage, which provides access to health insurance for anyone who has lived in France for at least three months and who does not otherwise already have health insurance coverage. The plan also includes supplementary health insurance coverage, which, unlike basic universal health insurance, provides additional health care free of charge—that is, with no deductible and without having to pay an out-of-pocket reimbursement. Supplementary health insurance coverage is targeted towards the neediest populations. A high percentage of the population in the French Overseas Departments is covered by these basic and supplementary universal health insurance arrangements. In 2005, one-quarter of the population in the Antilles and one-third of the population in French Guiana had supplementary universal health insurance coverage.

The availability of housing is growing, due in part to tax measures that encourage new housing construction as well as a greater supply of low-cost rental accommodations. Despite the progress made, there is still a heavy demand for housing due to growth in the population and the total number of households and a decreasing tendency for extended families to live under one roof. Housing conditions are improving, along with the trend toward a reduction in substandard dwellings.

The impact of urban policy on the most precarious and poorest districts of French Guiana, Guadeloupe, and Martinique was somewhat mixed in the 1990s. On the one hand, the government's efforts to improve housing and living conditions are evident. On the other, the residents of those districts were the first to be hit by the rise in unemployment, despite the incentives designed to generate jobs.

School attendance is obligatory for children ages 6 to 16. Thus nearly all children ages 3 to 6 attend school. At the start of the 2005–2006 school year, the school population in the French Overseas Departments totaled almost 275,000. Over half of the pupils were in nursery and elementary (primary) schools, one-quarter attended junior high school, and one-fifth (aged 15 to 18) were enrolled in schools preparing them for the baccalaureate (*lycée*).[2]

Baccalaureate pass rates are improving; in 2004, 72% of students in French Guiana, 75% in Guadeloupe, and 79% in Martinique passed the general baccalaureate. These rates still lag behind those of metropolitan France, and the percentage of nongraduates is relatively high, particularly in French Guiana, with the rate increasing with the age bracket.

The French Overseas Departments had 19,050 university students during the 2004–2005 school year, 60% of whom were enrolled at the University of the Antilles French Guiana. After marked growth in the 1990s, the number of students has stabilized in recent years. Not all courses of study are available locally, forcing some young people to continue their studies in metropolitan France or other countries.

Various characteristics of the environment may affect the health of the inhabitants of the French Overseas Territories. In the Antilles, natural hazards, such as earthquakes, tropical storms, and volcanic eruptions, are taken into account in the development of major risk prevention plans. Moreover, the use of organochlorine pesticides over a number of years in Guadeloupe and Martinique has negatively affected the natural environment (water bodies, river sediment, and soils). Several studies have been conducted or are currently under way to gauge the health risks for the inhabitants of these regions.

In French Guiana, the principal environmental health issues are water supply and gold panning. The pillaging of gold deposits takes place both on the fringes of authorized mining sites and in the jungle interior. The environmental impact has manifested itself dramatically through deforestation, the decimation of wildlife, mercury pollution of rivers, and malaria transmission. Due to its geographical features, French Guiana is unable to supply all of its inhabitants with safe water. This is particularly the case for inland populations and for certain segments living along riverbanks or in marginal urban and periurban districts without the availability of running water.

---

[1] A person is considered "poor" if he or she lives in a household whose standard of living is below the poverty line, with the latter being defined as half the median standard of living. The median standard of living divides the totality of households in a given geographical area into two equal halves. This definition is both monetary and relative, since the poverty line is a function of its position on the income ladder of a set of households. This explains why the poverty line differs from one territory to another and why these lines are calculated separately for the French Overseas Territories and metropolitan France.

---

[2] Secondary school education (or *deuxième degré*) follows pre-elementary and elementary school (*premier degré*) and is provided in junior high schools and *lycées*.

Demographics, Mortality, and Morbidity

From the 1960s to the 1980s, the population of the French Overseas Departments held stable, despite a high birth rate, due to emigration to metropolitan France where there was a shortage of labor. In the mid-1980s, emigration flows began to slow down, spurring population growth in the French Overseas Departments. Furthermore, the populations of Guadeloupe and, to an even greater extent, French Guiana were boosted by an influx of immigrants. Thus, the population of Guadeloupe doubled in 50 years (it had 229,000 inhabitants in 1954) while that of French Guiana multiplied seven-fold in the same period (from 28,000 in 1954).

From the time of the 1999 census to the end of 2004, the population grew by 4.5% in Martinique and 7.5% in Guadeloupe, whereas in French Guiana it grew by 22.5%. On 1 January 2005, Guadeloupe had the largest population (453,029 inhabitants), followed by Martinique (397,820 inhabitants) and French Guiana (190,842 inhabitants). Given its small land area, Martinique is the most densely populated territory, with 353 inhabitants/km² in 2005. That same year, there were 266 inhabitants/km² in Guadeloupe, while in French Guiana, despite the relative vastness of its territory, the population density was only 2 inhabitants/km².

The population distribution differs from one Department to another. In the Antilles, the population is still young, but aging. With 17% of its population being age 60 or older in 2005, Martinique has the highest share of older adults. In contrast, French Guiana has the youngest population, with 44% being under the age of 20. The population distribution in 1990 and 2005, by age and sex, for French Guiana, Guadeloupe, and Martinique is presented in Figures 1, 2, and 3, respectively.

The population of the French West Indies is mainly the product of intermarriage among the Amerindian, Black, White, and Indian populations that have inhabited them for centuries. Unlike some other Caribbean islands, there are no survivors of an ethnically pure indigenous (Amerindian) population. French Guiana's population is a mosaic of influences. Amerindians were joined by Europeans and the descendants of Black African slaves beginning in the 17th century. In the 19th century, penal colonies and the first gold rush led to an increase in the population. Finally, in the 20th century, there were inflows of Chinese and Lebanese traders, as well as settlement by a community of Hmong farmers from Upper Laos.

In Martinique, the minority population of external origin remains stable at 1% of the total population. It consists mainly of nationals of Haiti and Saint Lucia. In Guadeloupe, immigrants accounted for 5% of the population in the 1999 census, and almost half of them were from Haiti. The Saint-Martin municipality accounts for half of all foreign nationals in Guadeloupe. In French Guiana the largest immigrant contingents are from Suriname (39%), Haiti (30%), and Brazil (15%). Officially, the population of external origin accounts for 33% of the population, but

FIGURE 1. Population structure, by age and sex, French Guiana, 1990 and 2005.

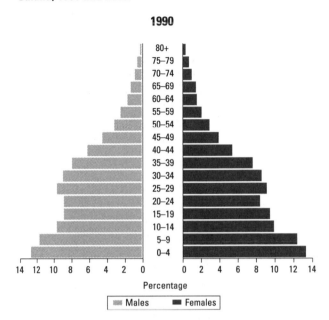

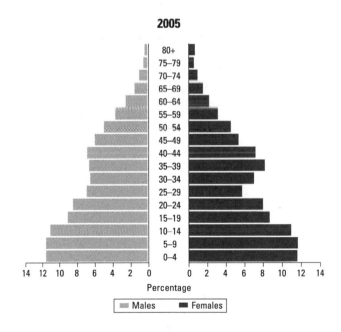

the sheer length of the territorial borders, the ease with which borders defined by the Maroni and Oyapock Rivers may be crossed, and activities such as gold panning all promote clandestine immigration. The number of foreign nationals is underestimated, thus indicating that official figures for the total population are lower than they would be if accurate numbers on this group were available.

FIGURE 2. Population structure, by age and sex, Guadeloupe, 1990 and 2005.

1990

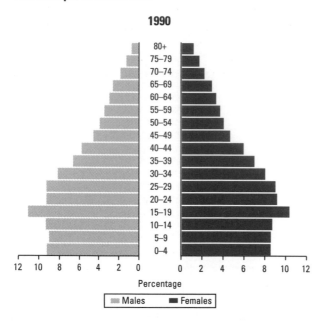

2005

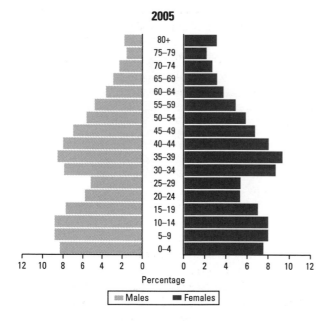

FIGURE 3. Population structure, by age and sex, Martinique, 1990 and 2005.

1990

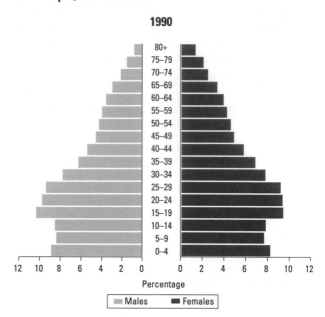

2005

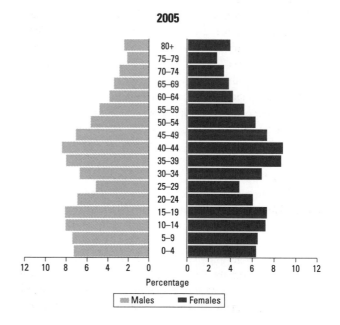

There are 34 municipalities in Guadeloupe and Martinique and 22 in French Guiana. In Guadeloupe, over 40% of the population lives in Pointe-à-Pitre, the economic capital located on Grande-Terre, while only 10% live in the administrative center of Basse-Terre on the island of the same name. In Martinique, more than one-third of the population lives in the administrative center, Fort-de-France. In French Guiana, most of the population

lives along the coast; the dense rainforest cover renders inland municipalities more difficult to reach.

In Guadeloupe and Martinique, health conditions generally reflect those of developed countries. The situation in French Guiana is more mixed, however, with some indicators resembling those of developed countries, such as chronic disease incidence and relative wealth, while at the same time exhibiting other characteristics typical of developing countries, such as a young population, high perinatal mortality, and a high incidence of infectious and parasitic diseases. Obstacles in French Guiana include its geography (sizeable remote areas and the challenges these pose for timely communication and accessibility), its sociodemographic indicators (a rapidly growing population, fragile economy, and migration flows), and its lack of human resources and infrastructure (too few health professionals and a chronic shortage of medical equipment). Despite these challenges, the health status of the population has improved over the past 30 years. In Guadeloupe, the principal indicators show an improvement over the past 15 years, with a decline in infant mortality, an overall improvement in the standard of living, and progress in medical care and the development of health services delivery. Despite progress in these areas, certain health problems have proven to be especially intractable in Guadeloupe and the other two French Overseas Departments, including high blood pressure, stroke, diabetes, mental health problems (including alcohol and crack addiction), prostate cancer, and HIV infection. At the same time, all three regions continue to record troubling perinatal indicators, and Martinique and Guadeloupe, with older populations than that of French Guiana, are increasingly facing public health issues related to aging.

Life expectancy at birth is highest in Martinique. In 2003, it was 81.7 years for women and 75.9 years for men. Guadeloupe follows closely behind, with 81.6 years for women and 75.3 years for men. Life expectancy was lowest in French Guiana, with 79.7 years for women and 71.3 years for men.

The above figures indicate progress being made since 1990, when life expectancy at birth was 79.6 years for women and 73.3 years for men in Martinique; 78.5 years for women and 70.8 years for men in Guadeloupe; and 76.1 years for women and 67.2 years for men in French Guiana.

In 2004, the overall birth rate was 13.3 births per 1,000 inhabitants in Martinique, 16.2 in Guadeloupe, and 28.8 in French Guiana. Women of childbearing age (15–49 years old) accounted for 50% of the female population in the Antilles and 52% of the female population in French Guiana. The fertility rate was 53 births per 1,000 women of childbearing age in Martinique and 62 in Guadeloupe, but it was twice as high in French Guiana, with 113 in 2004. The estimated fertility rate was approximately 2 children per woman in the Antilles, and nearly 4 children per woman in French Guiana.

The aging of the population and a decline in the birth rate explain why the actual number of births is declining in the Antilles, whereas in French Guiana there has been a sharp increase. In 2004, there were 7,273 births reported in Guadeloupe, 5,255 in Martinique, and 5,312 in French Guiana.

As expected, because of the aging of the population, both the number of deaths and the total morality rate are increasing in the Antilles. For instance, in Martinique, deaths averaged 2,200 to 2,300 per year during the 1990s, whereas the number is now 2,700.

Nearly 6,000 deaths are registered each year, with 52% of these occurring among males and 48% among females. The principal mortality cause in all three Departments is cardiovascular diseases, followed by neoplasms and external causes of trauma. In French Guiana, infectious and parasitic diseases rank fourth, while in the Antilles, endocrine, nutritional, and metabolic disorders—primarily diabetes mellitus—are the next leading cause of death.

HEALTH OF POPULATION GROUPS

Children under 1 Year Old

Although there have been health improvements achieved among this age group (for instance, with respect to infant mortality), perinatal indicators in the French Overseas Departments are still a cause for concern and remain inferior to those recorded for metropolitan France. While slight improvements have been recorded in the Antilles, progress in French Guiana has been both slow and intermittent.

In 2003, the infant mortality rate was 6.1 deaths per 1,000 live births in Martinique, 7.9 per 1,000 in Guadeloupe, and 10.4 per 1,000 in French Guiana. In 1990, the rates had been 7.2, 10.2, and 18.1, respectively. The steady decline witnessed in the infant mortality rate over the past several decades is a consequence of an improved standard of living, medical advances, better access to health care, and the organization of prevention campaigns.

The pattern for perinatal mortality for the Antilles and French Guiana is similar to that for infant mortality. In Martinique, perinatal mortality increased from 14.6 per 1,000 total births in 2000 to 19 in 2002. In 2002, more than 16 children per 1,000 total births were stillborn. Early neonatal deaths have declined: 3 out of every 1,000 babies born alive died during their first week of life in 2002, compared to 4.6 in 2000. The persistence of a high stillbirth rate is probably due to poor monitoring of pregnancy, while the death rate for newborn babies has decreased due to better sanitation and medical advances. In Guadeloupe, perinatal mortality declined up to 1992, then rose again because of the increase in stillbirths. The trend has fluctuated from year to year, reaching 19.2 deaths per 1,000 total births in 2002. Even though the overall trend with this indicator over the past 20 years has been satisfactory, it is worth emphasizing that the downward trend still needs to be consolidated. According to health professionals, the two leading causes of perinatal mortality have been maternal-fetal infections and maternal high blood pressure.

In French Guiana, the perinatal mortality rate declined throughout the 1990s from 25.8 per 1,000 total births in 1990 to 16.1 in 2000, after which it held steady between 17 and 18 in the early 2000s. This decline is explained mainly by the drop in the stillbirth rate, from 20 per 1,000 total births in 1990 to just over 13 per 1,000 in 2002. The early neonatal mortality rate, on the other hand, has hardly declined at all. In 2002, it stood at the same level as in 1990 (approximately 6 deaths per 1,000 live births) and had even increased in the mid-1990s, peaking at 10.8 in 1995. In French Guiana, the distance from health centers for some women about to give birth hampers their ability to seek adequate and regular prenatal care. Table 1 presents period-specific mortality rates for the under-1 age group for the 2001–2003 period.

In the French Overseas Departments, 10% to 12% of all births are premature. The two leading causes of maternal death are hemorrhage in childbirth and maternal high blood pressure.

Age Group 1–14 Years Old

This age group averaged 78 deaths a year during the 2000–2002 period, or approximately 1% of all deaths. These deaths were mainly the result of trauma or poisoning in all three regions, representing 40% of all deaths in this age group. In French Guiana, a third of all deaths were due to trauma or poisoning, followed by 17% due to infectious and parasitic diseases. In Guadeloupe and Martinique, 40% of all deaths were due to trauma or poisoning, followed by 10% which were due to diseases of the respiratory system.

Age Group 15–34 Years Old

In 2000–2002, an average of 320 deaths per year occurred in this age group, or 5% of all deaths. Traffic accidents and other forms of violence were the leading causes in all three French Overseas Departments. In Guadeloupe and Martinique, these were followed by neoplasms and diseases of the circulatory system, while in French Guiana a considerable number of deaths were caused by infectious and parasitic diseases. The leading chronic conditions among both sexes in this age group are mental disorders, diabetes mellitus, and cardiovascular diseases (Table 2).

TABLE 1. Mean annual period-specific mortality rates[a] for the population under age 1, French Overseas Departments, 2001–2003.

Rates	Guadeloupe	French Guiana	Martinique
Stillbirth	15.6	12.0	15.5
Perinatal mortality	18.4	17.3	18.8
Early neonatal mortality	2.9	5.3	3.3
Late neonatal mortality	1.8	2.2	1.1
Post-neonatal mortality	2.4	4.2	2.2

[a]For stillbirth and perinatal mortality rates, per 1,000 total births; for all other rates, per 1,000 live births.

Source: French National Institute of Statistics and Economic Studies (INSEE).

TABLE 2. Leading causes of admission to long-term care for the population aged 15–34 years, by sex, French Overseas Departments, 2003.

MEN	Number	%
Mental disorders	252	44
Diabetes mellitus, types 1 and 2	49	8
Cardiovascular diseases	46	8
Other	229	40
Total	**576**	**100**

WOMEN	Number	%
Mental disorders	119	20
Diabetes mellitus, types 1 and 2	78	13
Cardiovascular diseases	58	10
Other	342	57
Total	**597**	**100**

Source: CNAMTS and CANAM study, World Health Organization.

While the average age of mothers at first birth is increasing in Martinique and Guadeloupe, the number of teenage pregnancies is very high in French Guiana; in 2002, one birth in every six was by an adolescent mother. At 52 births per 1,000 women, the fertility rate in French Guiana is higher than that for 19-year-olds in Guadeloupe and Martinique. Fertility for women in French Guiana increases with every year of age thereafter, until peaking at 151 births per 1,000 women at age 19.

Nearly 9,000 elective abortions were performed in 2004 in the three French Overseas Departments: 40 per 100 conceptions in Guadeloupe, 32 in Martinique, and 24 in French Guiana.

Adults 35–64 Years Old

During the 2000–2002 period, an average of 1,450 deaths per year occurred within this age group, or 25% of all deaths. Neoplasms and cardiovascular diseases were the leading causes of mortality for the three French Overseas Departments, followed by traffic accidents and other forms of violence in both Guadeloupe and Martinique. Among both women and men in the 35–64-year-old age group, the leading chronic conditions are cardiovascular diseases, diabetes mellitus, and neoplasms (Table 3).

Older Adults 65 Years Old and Older

Long considered islands with young populations, Guadeloupe, and to an even greater extent Martinique, are now increasingly facing issues associated with an aging population. The population size of those aged 65 years old and older in Martinique almost tripled between the 1967 and 1999 censuses, increasing from 16,000 to 47,000. In 2005, this population was estimated at 52,645, or 13% of the total population. In Guadeloupe, this age group consisted of 50,500 persons, or 11% of the total population in 2005. At the other extreme, for French Guiana the proportion

TABLE 3. Leading causes of admission to long-term care for the population aged 35–64 years, by sex, French Overseas Departments, 2003.

MEN	Number	%
Diabetes mellitus, types 1 and 2	1,292	36
Cardiovascular diseases	973	27
Neoplasms	504	14
Other	805	23
Total	**3,574**	**100**

WOMEN	Number	%
Cardiovascular diseases	1,646	38
Diabetes mellitus, types 1 and 2	1,246	28
Neoplasms	536	12
Other	976	22
Total	**4,404**	**100**

Source: CNAMTS and CANAM study, World Health Organization.

TABLE 4. Leading causes of admission to long-term care for the population aged 65 years and older, by sex, French Overseas Departments, 2003.

MEN	Number	%
Cardiovascular diseases	1,411	41
Neoplasms	916	27
Diabetes mellitus, types 1 and 2	536	16
Other	560	16
Total	**3,423**	**100**

WOMEN	Number	%
Cardiovascular diseases	2,080	52
Diabetes mellitus, types 1 and 2	872	22
Mental disorders	395	10
Other	648	16
Total	**3,995**	**100**

Source: CNAMTS and CANAM study, World Health Organization.

of those aged 65 and older represents only 4% of the population, or 7,500 people.

The incidence of major health problems is highest after age 65 and leads to more frequent care-seeking for health issues. The frequency of comorbidities increases, such as high blood pressure with diabetes, significantly impacting on the quality of life. For the group 85 years of age and older, the prevalence of physical and/or psychological dependence rapidly increases.

After age 65, the first two leading causes of death are diseases of the circulatory system and neoplasms, respectively. In Guadeloupe and French Guiana, endocrine, nutritional, and metabolic disorders—primarily diabetes mellitus—are the third leading cause of death. In Martinique, the third leading cause of death is respiratory diseases. For males in this age group, the three leading chronic conditions requiring long-term care are cardiovascular diseases, neoplasms, and diabetes mellitus, respectively. In women, the three leading chronic diseases requiring long-term care are cardiovascular diseases, diabetes mellitus, and mental disorders, including dementia and Alzheimer's disease, respectively (Table 4).

The Family

Household size has continued to decline during the review period; while the decline is less marked in French Guiana, household size in the case of Guadeloupe and Martinique currently stands at fewer than three persons per household. Family structure in the French Overseas Departments also shows a pronounced shift toward single-parent households, with approximately 40% of families in Guadeloupe and Martinique and one-third in French Guiana being headed by a single parent. In nine out of ten cases, these households are headed by a woman, reflecting both tradition (matriarchal societies) and more recent social trends (less permanent unions).

Persons with Disabilities

In each of the three French Overseas Departments, the Departmental Commission on Special Education is responsible for reviewing all requests for placement of children under the age of 20 with disabilities, as well as requests for financial assistance by their families. As of 31 December 2005, there were 2,673 children benefiting from the special education allowance, which means that there were eight beneficiaries for every 1,000 young persons under the age of 20.

For adults over the age of 20 with disabilities, the Technical Commission for the Guidance and Professional Reclassification of Disabled Persons is the body responsible for assigning individual disabled status, providing employment guidance, reviewing the allocation of financial assistance, and directing candidates to specialized institutions. In the French Overseas Departments, as of 31 December 2005, there were 16,031 adult beneficiaries of the disabilities allowance, or 29 beneficiaries for every 1,000 individuals between the ages of 20 and 59 years.

For the most part, adults with disabilities live with their families or in their own homes. Very few are cared for in specialized institutions because of limited space. There is more specialized institutional care available for children.

HEALTH CONDITIONS AND PROBLEMS

COMMUNICABLE DISEASES

Vector-borne Diseases

Martinique and Guadeloupe report an annual average of 10 imported cases of **malaria**, while in French Guiana the disease is much more widespread. The annual number of cases in the

French Guiana provinces with endemic malaria held stable at approximately 4,000–5,000 reported cases until 1999. That number declined to approximately 3,000 cases each in 2002 and 2003, but then increased again in 2005, with 4,414 reported cases.

Since the end of 2001, along the coastal areas of French Guiana there have been troubling increases in the number of malaria cases in the Régina and Cacao municipalities and the more interior Camopi municipality. The uncontrolled development of gold mining activities and constant migration and mobility among the population over vast remote areas make malaria control a particularly daunting task in French Guiana.

There were no reported cases of yellow fever in French Guiana, Guadeloupe, and Martinique during the 2001–2005 period. All travelers to French Guiana are required to provide proof of yellow fever vaccination.

In French Guiana, there were three **dengue** epidemics (in 2001, 2002, and 2004–2005), all of them associated with serotype 3. A new dengue serotype 2 epidemic that began at the end of 2005 affected more than 15,000 people and was responsible for four registered deaths between December 2005 and July 2006. Two dengue epidemics broke out in Guadeloupe and Martinique in 2001 and 2005. The first was due to serotype 3 and the second mainly to serotype 4. In Martinique, serotype 2, which is frequently associated with severe forms of dengue, was also isolated in the course of this epidemic. In Martinique, the 2001 epidemic is estimated to have affected approximately 25,000 people, leading to 400 hospitalizations and four deaths. Some 14,500 people were affected in 2005 (4% of the island's population), with 200 hospitalizations and four deaths. In Guadeloupe, nearly 9,000 people are estimated to have consulted a town doctor due to suspected dengue during the 2005 epidemic.

Réunion, the French Overseas Department located in the Indian Ocean, was stricken by a widespread **Chikungunya fever** epidemic in late 2005 and early 2006. Three confirmed cases of Chikungunya fever imported from Réunion were detected in Martinique in the first quarter of 2006, as well as three cases in French Guiana and one in Guadeloupe. To prevent the disease's establishment in the French Overseas Departments, health authorities activated surveillance and early warning and response systems for all travelers returning from Réunion and other Indian Ocean islands and employed mosquito eradication programs.

Vaccine-preventable Diseases

Many years have passed since the last cases of **acute flaccid paralysis**, **poliomyelitis**, and **diphtheria** were reported in the French Overseas Departments. In contrast, epidemics or isolated cases of **whooping cough** are regularly reported. There have been no cases of neonatal **tetanus** since the late 1970s. A few cases are found in older adults whose immunity through vaccination has weakened and who were never revaccinated. Very few cases were reported between 1993 and 2003: nine in Guadeloupe, five in Martinique, and none in French Guiana. However, in 2005,

French Guiana reported two cases. During the 2001–2005 period, only one suspected case of **measles** was reported by the sentinel network in Martinique, and none were reported in Guadeloupe. In French Guiana, measles surveillance has been coupled with dengue surveillance since 2001. All suspected cases of dengue with a rash are tested for measles and German measles immunoglobulin M (IgM). No case has tested positive to date. France has embarked on a policy of eliminating measles and congenital rubella syndrome by 2010.

While vaccination coverage levels among the young in the Antilles are generally satisfactory, the situation is less positive in French Guiana, with lower levels in the isolated interior and higher levels in the developed coastal areas. In 2000, MMR vaccine coverage along the coast at 24 months of age was 69%, compared to coverage levels ranging from 43% to 61% in the country's interior. DPT 3 vaccine coverage at one year of age was 68% on the coast, compared to a range of 9%–60% for the interior.

Intestinal Infectious Diseases

There is a year-round high incidence of viral **gastroenteritis** epidemics, and these represent the leading cause of **diarrhea** in the Antilles. In French Guiana, the distribution of gastroenteritis is uneven due to water supply contamination for certain population segments. The incidence of enteric diseases exceeds 10% in some inland municipalities.

Every year an average of 10 outbreaks of food poisoning are recorded in each of the three French Overseas Departments. A few cases of ciguatera poisoning are regularly reported in the Antilles, and in June 2006, two ciguatera outbreaks were reported; one occurred in Guadeloupe and the other in Martinique.

Due to improved hygiene and prevention and detection activities led by local health authorities, there has been a sharp decline in the number of cases of **ancylostomiasis** and **strongyloidiasis** in the Antilles over the past 20 years.

Chronic Communicable Diseases

In 2004, 30 cases of **tuberculosis** were reported in Guadeloupe, 17 in Martinique, and 51 in French Guiana.

Hansen's disease remains endemic in the French Overseas Departments but the incidence is declining. There are fewer than 10 cases reported annually in each of the three regions. In Guadeloupe, the number of cases detected fell from 14 in 1997 to 9 in 2004. In French Guiana, the incidence rate of 3.29 cases per 10,000 inhabitants in 1984 declined to 0.57 case per 10,000 inhabitants in 2001, representing approximately 10 new cases per year. Each of the French Overseas Departments has a referral center for Hansen's disease that screens patients, offers consultations with a physician and social worker, and conducts home visits.

Sickle cell disease is the leading genetic disease in the French Antilles. Newborns are routinely screened, and on average, one newborn in 300 is born each year with one sickle cell trait lead-

Changes in French Public Health Policy Extend To The Overseas Departments

In 2004, France's legislature enacted three laws—one on local freedoms and responsibilities, one on public health policy, and one on health insurance—that radically changed the country's health governance. Subsequently, French Guiana, Guadeloupe, and Martinique, which as overseas departments of France have the same political and administrative structure as the rest of the country, each drew up a regional public health plan for 2006–2010. The plans share the overall objectives of preventing avoidable deaths, lowering the incidence of diseases and disabilities, reducing inequities by addressing the social determinants of health—education, nutrition, access to health services, and environmental health—and enlisting the public's engagement in public health. At the heart of each plan is a commitment to achieve health for all the French citizens living in the departments in the Americas.

ing to a major sickle cell syndrome (SS, SC, or S/b thal). Guadeloupe and Martinique have specialized facilities that provide medical care and offer preventive activities. As a result of improved management, sickle cell disease now poses problems similar to those of other chronic diseases, with increased numbers of active patients, longer life expectancy, and complications that accompany aging.

Acute Respiratory Infections

During the winter season, the French Overseas Departments regularly experience outbreaks of **bronchiolitis**. Based on a survey conducted in Martinique from November 2005 to February 2006, it was estimated that between 115 and 230 newborns or infants were affected by bronchiolitis each week.

From 1998 to 2003, three cases of **Legionnaires' disease** were reported in Guadeloupe, and one each in Martinique and French Guiana.

HIV/AIDS and Other Sexually Transmitted Infections

HIV/AIDS is more prevalent in French Guiana and Saint-Martin than on the islands of Guadeloupe and Martinique. During the 2001–2005 review period, the stigmatization of those with HIV-positive status, as well as discrimination and other forms of exclusion, remained major obstacles for early screening and detection, access to treatment and care, and thus control of the infection. The situation is more precarious for vulnerable groups such as injection drug users, commercial sex workers, and illegal immigrants.

From the start of the epidemic through 30 September 2005, 2,885 cases of HIV/AIDS had been reported in the French Overseas Departments, with 1,074 being from French Guiana, 1,175 from Guadeloupe, and 636 from Martinique. Women accounted for 35% of the cases, and the population aged 50 and older accounted for 20% of all cases. In 71% of the cases, the infection was contracted through heterosexual contact. Since the start of the epidemic, 1,492 people have died, representing a case fatality rate of 52%. Due to the availability of antiretroviral drugs, the

AIDS death rate remained relatively stable during the 2001–2005 period.

Following the introduction of the triple drug regimen in 1996, the prevalence of people living with HIV has increased and the progression to full-blown AIDS is primarily among HIV seroconverters not receiving treatment. In March 2003, the reporting of HIV diagnoses became mandatory. This notification affords better insight into the HIV-positive population and facilitates the tracking of HIV infections. Between March 2003 and September 2005, 735 newly detected cases of HIV seropositivity were reported (343 in French Guiana, 239 in Guadeloupe, and 153 in Martinique). Challenges for health care personnel in the provision of effective HIV/AIDS care in the French Overseas Departments include overcoming language barriers and social, cultural, and religious restraints among those seeking treatment, as well as dealing with discrimination and stigmatization issues. Monitoring and evaluation were implemented in 2002 to find and apply solutions to these problems.

Treatment for persons living with HIV is handled by HIV information and care centers (*Centres d'informations et de soins de l'immunodéficience humaine*). There are seven patient centers: one in Fort-de-France for Martinique, three in Guadeloupe (Pointe-à-Pitre, Basse-Terre, and Marigot on Saint-Martin), and three in French Guiana (Cayenne, Kourou, and Saint-Laurent-du-Maroni). Between January and December 2004, the centers monitored and provided services to 2,862 individuals with HIV infection in the French Overseas Departments. Female patients are proportionately overrepresented in the Saint-Martin and French Guiana centers, with a male-to-female ratio of 0.7 and 0.8, respectively, while in Guadeloupe and Martinique, the male-to-female ratio is 1.2 and 1.6, respectively. In more than 90% of cases, transmission is via sexual contact, primarily heterosexual. In Martinique, sexual relations between men account for 22% of all transmissions. There is little or no transmission via injecting drug use. Patients who are non-French nationals are especially numerous in Saint-Martin and French Guiana; French patients account for just 24% and 20% of active cases visiting these clinics, respectively, while in Guadeloupe and Martinique the proportion is 69% and 89%, respectively. Seventy-five percent of the patients monitored received antiretroviral drugs in 2004.

HIV screening is carried out at medical laboratories and screening centers; this service is anonymous and free of charge. There have been renewed outbreaks of syphilis, first in Guadeloupe in 2001 and then in Martinique in 2004. In Guadeloupe, a cluster of 13 cases of primary and secondary syphilis was reported at the University Hospital Center in Pointe-à-Pitre in early 2001. Among a higher-risk, mostly unemployed population, a survey identified 38 cases of syphilis in 2001. Coinfection with HIV was found in approximately a quarter of the cases. The 2004 epidemic in Martinique largely affected persons living with HIV. Eight out of 14 patients were men who have sex with men. These 14 cases of recent syphilis were diagnosed at the University Hospital Center in Fort-de-France between January 2004 and September 2005, and 11 of them were diagnosed between April and September 2005.

Zoonoses

Leptospirosis is a commonly reported disease in Guadeloupe and Martinique. The incidence of confirmed leptospirosis cases is much higher in Guadeloupe than Martinique. In Guadeloupe, the incidence was 16.5 confirmed cases per 100,000 inhabitants in 2003, with the incidence of confirmed cases peaking in January and December. In 2004, the incidence rate was 21 cases per 100,000 inhabitants in Guadeloupe. In Martinique, leptospirosis incidence peaked in July and October–December in both 2003 and 2004. For those two years, the annual incidence rate was 7.3 and 6.9 per 100,000 inhabitants, respectively. In French Guiana, leptospirosis cases have been reported regularly over the past 30 years. The main serogroups found in both animals and humans in the Antilles are *icterohaemorrhagiae* and *ballum* (or *castellonis*). However, some 10 other serogroups are also found, including *australis, cynopteri, canicola, panama, sejroë,* and *grippotyphosa*.

There were no suspected cases of **avian influenza** in the French Overseas Departments during the 2001–2005 period.

Chagas' disease is not found in Guadeloupe or Martinique. Between 1939 and 1989, only nine cases of Chagas' disease were reported in French Guiana. Between 1990 and 2004, 15 clinical cases of Chagas' disease, including six acute and eight chronic cases, were diagnosed in French Guiana, with two deaths attributed to the disease. Infection in the areas around the Maroni and Oyapock Rivers was the source of nine indigenous cases, while some imported cases have been detected in the coastal region. In late 2005, a cluster of eight confirmed cases, one probable case, and one suspected case of acute Chagas' disease occurred in the Iracoubo municipality in French Guiana.

Deforestation, uncontrolled migration, and importation of the Chagas vector have increased the risk of disease in French Guiana.

The distribution of **schistomiasis** in the French Overseas Departments is uneven. Surveys conducted between 2001 and 2005

in Martinique's watercress fields and aquatic environments confirmed the successful eradication of the *B. glabrata* snail, the principal intermediate host for schistosomiasis. In the past few years, rare residual cases of schistomiasis have been detected. The absence of active transmission of the parasite for more than 20 years and the elimination of the principal intermediate snail host, which was confirmed in 2001, suggest that as of 2005 schistosomiasis was eradicated in Martinique.

In Guadeloupe, the swamps are home to large populations of black rats heavily infested with schistosomiasis, supporting an endemic of the parasite. Although these areas constitute a danger for cattle breeders and farmers who frequent them, the current extent of transmission in humans remains unknown.

In French Guiana, only imported cases of schistosomosis have been detected. Active transmission of the parasite has never been confirmed. The acidic waters of French Guiana are highly unfavorable habitats for the intermediate snail hosts of schistosomiasis.

NONCOMMUNICABLE DISEASES

Metabolic and Nutritional Diseases

Social and economic improvements, changes in lifestyle, and the growing availability of fast foods have altered dietary habits in the French Overseas Territories, and in recent years diseases linked with poor dietary habits and overeating, such as obesity, diabetes, and hypercholesterolemia, have garnered increasing importance as public health concerns.

Approximately 260 deaths due to **diabetes** are registered in the French Overseas Departments each year, representing some 4%– 5% of all deaths. The majority of diabetic deaths occur among older women.

According to a survey conducted in Martinique in late 2003 and early 2004 among those aged 16 or older, the prevalence of reported diabetes was 6.5% (8.1% for women and 4.7% for men). This prevalence increased with age, being 1.7% in the 16–44-year-old age group, 10% in the group aged 45–64, and 18% in those aged 65 or older.

In Guadeloupe and Martinique, there is a high number of chronic renal insufficiency cases, with an estimated incidence of 200 cases per one million inhabitants in Guadeloupe. Diabetes is the primary cause for dialysis (one-third of all those on dialysis are diabetics), the second leading cause of blindness, and the third leading cause for amputation. Since late 2004, kidney transplants on patients with renal insufficiency in the three French Overseas Departments have been offered in Guadeloupe. Approximately 50 transplants were performed in the first 18 months following the availability of this new service.

The proportion of the population that is **overweight** or **obese** is growing in Guadeloupe and Martinique. A 2003–2004 survey revealed that almost one child in every four (24%) in Martinique is affected by either overweight (16%) or obesity (8%). In the case of adults, these conditions are 33% and 20%, respectively. Obesity is more common among women (26%) than men (14%). Findings from surveys in Guadeloupe have yielded similar results. Studies in schools conducted in all three of the French Overseas Departments indicate that far fewer children in French Guiana suffer from overweight than in Guadeloupe and Martinique.

Cardiovascular Diseases

Cardiovascular diseases are the leading cause of death in the French Overseas Departments, accounting for 1,800 deaths per year, or 30% of all deaths. The figures are higher for women than men. The share of cardiovascular diseases in overall mortality increases with age, becoming particularly high after age 65.

Compared to regions in metropolitan France, the French Overseas Departments are characterized by a higher incidence of **cerebrovascular diseases**, while **ischemic heart diseases** are less common. Among diseases covered for long-term care, cardiovascular diseases account for 38% of annual admissions. Most cases involve hypertensive and cerebrovascular diseases.

Hypertension is common among the population of the French Overseas Departments. According to a 2003–2004 survey, the incidence of high blood pressure in the population aged 16 or older is 22% (20% among men and 25% among women). The incidence increases with age, from 5% in the 25–34-year-old age group to 65% among persons aged 65 or older. Of those diagnosed with high blood pressure, 73% were receiving treatment at the time of the survey. The percentage of those receiving treatment is lower for men (55%) than it is for women (84%).

Patients with cardiovascular diseases are likely to suffer from such comorbidities as high blood pressure, diabetes, and high cholesterol, leading to serious complications that include stroke, amputation, renal insufficiency, and blindness.

Malignant Neoplasms

On average, slightly more than 1,300 deaths from malignant neoplasms are registered annually in the French Overseas Departments. This cause accounts for one death in every four among men and one in every five among women. After age 65, neoplasms account for almost one death in every four.

In men, the most common forms of cancer are prostate cancer, followed by stomach cancer and cancer of the lips, mouth, and pharynx. Among women, the most common cancers are breast cancer, followed by colon or rectal cancer and cervical cancer.

Systematic screening for breast cancer has been in place in all three French Overseas Departments since 2005. Martinique provides cervical cancer screening as well. However, the fact that Guadeloupe is an archipelago whose population is scattered across several islands and that many of French Guiana's inland municipalities are isolated presents formidable obstacles to providing universal cancer screening and health care.

OTHER HEALTH PROBLEMS OR ISSUES

Violence and Other External Causes

There were 954 road traffic accidents in Guadeloupe in 2003; 1,383 persons suffered injuries, and 83 in this group died. In Martinique every year there are approximately 700 traffic accidents, leaving some 800 injured and 50 dead. In French Guiana, there are nearly 800 accidents a year, with about 1,000 persons injuried. The annual number of deaths ranges between 30 and 40.

Mental Health

A survey conducted among the general population of Guadeloupe and Martinique in the late 1990s found that the most frequent pathologies were depression, suicidal tendencies, and general anxiety. The leading causes of hospitalization were schizophrenia, psychoses with delirium, and addiction-related disorders.

Suicide and suicidal behavior are addressed in a national plan covering each region in France. In the French Overseas Departments, the average annual number of deaths from suicide is 85, and the majority of these occur among men and the population over age 35. While the annual number of deaths from suicide is under surveillance, there is no periodic collection of data on attempted suicides. However, in a 2000 mental health survey conducted in Martinique, 4.1% of adults reported that they had attempted suicide at least once in their lives. In a school survey carried out in Martinique in 2003–2004, 13% of young people aged 14–19 reported thinking fairly often or very often about killing themselves over the previous 12 months, and 11% reported having attempted suicide once or more than once during their lifetime. More girls (15%) than boys (6%) had attempted suicide one or more times. Of those who had attempted suicide one or more times, only 15% had been hospitalized for that reason.

Addictions

Guadeloupe and Martinique are traditional producers of rum, and while consumption of this product may be declining, consumption of other alcoholic beverages such as wine, champagne, whisky, and beer is on the rise.

A survey of the patients of general practitioners conducted in late 2000 and early 2001 found that out of the 26 French regions, Martinique ranked third, French Guiana fourth, and Guadeloupe fifth in prevalence of alcoholism among men. Surveys conducted periodically in Martinique and French Guiana also point to a growing prevalence of alcohol consumption by the school-age population.

By contrast, tobacco use in the French Overseas Departments is relatively low; this translates into reduced morbidity and mortality from respiratory illnesses and cardiovascular diseases related to this risk factor. According to a 2003–2004 survey, 87% of those aged 16 or older in Martinique do not smoke; of this group, 77% are nonsmokers and 10% are former smokers. Ten percent of those surveyed said they were habitual smokers, and 3% reported being occasional smokers. More men than women were smokers, and the largest proportion of current smokers were between the ages of 25 and 34 years.

Illegal substances abuse in the French Overseas Departments is characterized by predominantly high rates of cannabis consumption and, since the mid-1980s, an increasing prevalence of crack cocaine usage. The surge in crack use has had a significant impact on society in the French Overseas Departments, in terms of increasing criminal activity and the likelihood that persons using crack will become homeless.

Among schoolchildren, cannabis is the most frequently used substance; in fact, there is very little use of other illegal substances. There are, however, age and sex-related differences, such as increased experimentation and/or more regular use as children grow older and greater use by boys. According to the findings of a survey regularly conducted among 18-year-olds, as of 2003 regular use of cannabis appeared to be slightly more frequent among young people in Guadeloupe and French Guiana (7% and 6%, respectively) than in Martinique (3%). To address the rising use of cannabis and identify interventions better tailored to youth, cannabis consultations were organized in each of the French Overseas Departments in 2005.

The majority of those with an addiction to illicit substances are users of crack cocaine, male, and between the ages of 25 and 39 years. Addictions are among the priority health concerns in each of the French Overseas Departments.

Environmental Pollution

Two leading agencies are responsible for environmental health concerns in the French Overseas Departments, the *Cellule Interrégionale d'Epidémiologie d'Intervention Antilles-Guyane* (Antilles-French Guiana Interregional Epidemiology Unit), known as CIRE and which primarily directs interventions and responses to address environmental threats to health, and the French National Health and Medical Research Institute, which focuses on conducting research addressing these issues.

Protecting the population's health from contamination of foodstuffs is a priority. In 2002–2003, the French Agency for Food Safety (*Agence Française de Sécurité Sanitaire des Aliments*, or AFSSA) was directed by the ministries responsible for agriculture and fisheries, regulations related to consumption, and health to assess the harmful effects to health of exposure to the organochlorine pesticide chlordecone in Martinique. The foods found likely to contribute to chronic chlordecone exposure were commonly consumed and included taro, sweet potatoes, yams, cucumbers, carrots, tomatoes, melons, and chicken skin.

Based on AFSSA survey data and studies, 3% of Martinique's population, or some 12,700 individuals, showed exposure levels to this pesticide in excess of the established safety benchmark value for repeat exposure. Given these results, a pesticide exposure prevention program is currently being developed.

Other studies have been conducted or are under way in Guadeloupe and Martinique to examine the health risks posed by the presence of organochlorine pollutants in the environment and associated occupational risks. These studies are examining the association of pesticide exposure with male fertility, prenatal and postnatal development, and prostate cancer.

One of the studies examining chlordecone exposure among pregnant women in Guadeloupe detected chlordecone in 90% of blood samples taken from the mother and the umbilical cord, in 100% of abdominal fat samples taken from the mother, and in 40% of breast milk samples taken within 72 hours of delivery.

Studies from the 1990s established that mercury used in gold panning in the interior of French Guiana was contaminating river fish which in turn were being consumed by the population. Some interior Amerindian populations, among whom consumption of river fish is high, showed high levels of mercury exposure. Further studies of mercury exposure by the Antilles-French Guiana Interregional Epidemiology Unit (CIRE) in 2001, 2002, and 2004 confirmed that the most exposed population groups were those living along the upper reaches of the Maroni and Oyapock Rivers whose diet was largely based on the consumption of fish. A 1997 survey revealed that 57% of women of childbearing age from the interior area of Haut Maroni exceeded established safety limits of mercury, while a 2004 survey found 8%–21% of women living in villages along the Oyapack River to similarly have reached unsafe levels.

RESPONSE OF THE HEALTH SECTOR

Health Policies and Plans

Metropolitan France has 22 regions and 96 departments (*départements*), all of which have the same status. Overseas France, which was restructured in 2003, is legislatively split into two distinct entities: (1) the four overseas departments (*Départements d'Outre-Mer*) created in 1946 (Martinique, French Guiana, Guadeloupe, and Réunion), which are subject to the same legislature as the *départements métropolitains*, and (2) the other partially autonomous overseas *collectivités territoriales* (e.g., New Caledonia, French Polynesia), which are subject to special legislative regimes.

Each French Overseas Department is an administrative region that has two authorities, each with its own assembly elected by popular vote: the General Council (*Conseil Général*) for the Department and the Regional Council for the Region.

The French Overseas Departments are considered "ultraperipheral regions" of the EU, and as such they benefit from special protective measures and structural funding from this entity.

The constitutional reform of 2003 proposed amendments that replace departmental authority with individual partially autonomous authority. After consultation with and agreement from their electorates, Guadeloupe, French Guiana, and Martinique maintained their department status, but the islands of Saint-Martin and Saint-Barthélemy elected to separate from Guadeloupe and with passage by the French Parliament will form partially autonomous *collectivités territoriales*.

In a *Département*, the *Préfet*, who is appointed by the President of France, is the government representative who exercises sole authority of the State. State administration is centralized, but at the French Overseas Departments level it includes several layers of delegated authority known as decentralized government departments (*services déconcentrés de l'état*).

Public health is the responsibility of the French Government. Three laws passed in August 2004 radically altered health policy in France. Law 809, on local freedoms and responsibilities, recentralized numerous prerogatives of the *Conseil Général*. Health responsibilities of the *Conseil Général* are now limited to social action policy and health protection for families and children (maternal and child health and family planning). Law 810 on health insurance aims to achieve better control over health sector expenditure. A regional health mission, composed of the regional agency for hospitalization and regional association of health insurance funds, determines guidelines for changes in the territorial distribution of private health professionals, the organization of mechanisms for continuing care, and the annual program of action to improve coordination among the various regional components of the health care system for delivering the preventive, diagnostic, and curative services covered by health insurance.

Finally, law 806, focusing on public health policy, places prevention at the forefront of collaborative efforts and seeks to strengthen the role of the State in coordinating the activities of the various players in the health sector, the actions undertaken, and their funding. The way the health sector is now organized validates both the regional input in health policy and a volunteerism approach to prevention and health promotion through the linking of preventive strategies and health care. Regional organization of the health sector is based on utilization of the Regional Public Health Plan (PRSP) as the framework for public health planning, the Regional Public Health Group as the policy implementation body, and the Regional Health Conference as a consultative body. During 2005–2006, each of the three French Overseas Departments established priorities within the corresponding PRSP.

In Guadeloupe, 11 public health priorities were identified: (1) to ensure that everyone has access to information promoting good health; (2) to promote the health of schoolchildren; (3) to combat social inequalities in health care; (4) to promote behaviors favoring a balanced diet and adequate physical activity; (5) to prevent, screen, and monitor chronic diseases and their complications; (6) to combat the HIV/AIDS epidemic; (7) to promote the population's sexual and reproductive health and improve maternal and perinatal health care; (8) to prevent and screen for sickle cell disease; (9) to prevent and control cancer; (10) to combat addictions; and (11) to develop and implement an environmental health plan.

In French Guiana, the PRSP identified core strategies to focus on the following nine priority areas: (1) HIV/AIDS, (2) cancer, (3) health education, (4) vaccine-preventable diseases, (5) addictive behaviors, (6) infectious diseases, (7) the Upper Maroni-Upper Oyapock Health Program, (8) environmental health, and (9) access to health promotion strategies and care for the disadvantaged.

In Martinique, seven public health areas for action were selected: (1) nutrition, (2) risk behaviors, (3) vulnerable social groups, (4) preventive health care, (5) rare diseases, (6) environmental health, and (7) health alerts and emergency management.

The overarching challenges that the PRSPs of the three French Overseas Department share are overcoming social and territorial inequalities in health care, preventing avoidable diseases and reducing associated mortality, promoting a healthy environment, increasing public health knowledge and rendering it multidisciplinary, and fostering community participation in public health issues.

Complementing the PRSP, the Regional Hospital Agencies in each of the French Overseas Departments published the third edition of the Regional Health Care Organization Plans (*Schémas régionaux d'organisation sanitaire*) in March 2006.

Public Health Services

Epidemiological surveillance is performed by the Health and Social Development Directorates in partnership with the Antilles-French Guiana Interregional Epidemiology Unit (CIRE), established in 1997. It acts in tandem with the National Health Watch Institute to strengthen the work of the decentralized departments of the Ministry of Health in two major areas: infectious diseases and health risks linked with the environment.

As in all regions of France, 27 communicable diseases have been identified for mandatory reporting to public health authorities. This reporting is supported by a network of physicians participating in a sentinel surveillance system, who on a weekly basis report suspected cases of dengue, influenza-like conditions, gastroenteritis, measles, chicken pox, gonorrhea, and other STIs, among others. The sentinel surveillance network has existed for several years in Guadeloupe and Martinique, but was not created in French Guiana until 2006. This system is reinforced by reports from public and private laboratories, including the Pasteur Institute in Pointe-à-Pitre, Guadeloupe, which specializes in mycobacteria, and another in Cayenne, French Guiana, which is a referral center for arbovirus and influenza viruses.

Given new potential threats to public health and heightened security concerns in response to the current global environment, strengthening early warning and response systems is a priority for the French Ministry of Health. The Plan for Alarm Systems and Health Emergency Management strengthens local and regional health watch and warning facilities in the French Overseas Departments.

The Antilles-French Guiana Interregional Epidemiology Unit (CIRE) and the Health Watch Units of the Health and Social Development Directorates maintain the regional health watch and warning systems. CIRE brings its scientific expertise to bear on public actions undertaken by the *Préfets* of the three French Overseas Departments by coordinating with the Health Watch Unit, the operational level of the early warning and response system. Through this structure, with recently updated procedures and new human and technological resources, the French Overseas Departments are not only strengthening their capacity to respond rapidly and effectively to local public health threats, but are also contributing to the forging of a Caribbean and international health surveillance system that is essential in today's globalized world.

In collaboration with the Health Watch Units and numerous other players, the Antilles-French Guiana CIRE began work on the development of its Dengue Epidemic Surveillance, Early Warning, and Management Program in 2005. This initiative establishes dengue surveillance and control strategies for different epidemic risks. The Program's four principal areas of activity are: (1) epidemiological and entomological surveillance and research; (2) mosquito eradication through insecticide use and social mobilization strategies; (3) information-sharing with health professionals, political and administrative leaders (Health and Social Development Directorates, hospitals, *Préfets*, *Conseil Général*, and mayors' offices), and the public at large; and (4) development and dissemination of patient care and treatment protocols. These actions require the well-coordinated participation of numerous additional players in the areas of epidemiology, entomology, mosquito eradication, clinical medicine, biology, and mass media. Program development was finalized in 2006.

A National Environmental Health Plan was adopted in June 2004 to reduce the incidence of diseases linked with the environment and improve natural habitats. The Plan includes 45 objectives to be pursued at the national and/or regional level. Utilizing the Plan as its framework, each of the French Overseas Departments has drawn up its own regional environmental health plan. Certain goals are shared by the three, such as protecting the health and well-being of populations living in unhealthy habitats, preserving water catchment areas, eradicating disease vectors, combating Legionnaires' disease, and reducing the harmful effects of pesticides on the environment and human health.

Drinking water in Guadeloupe and in Martinique is bacteriologically safe, except during periods of special weather conditions. In French Guiana, universal access to safe water remains a challenge. Solid waste disposal is also a problem; numerous untreated dump sites exist, incinerators handle only a portion of the refuse, and recycling is still in its early stages. Efforts are under way to bring current dump sites up to standards before resorting to closure and major rehabilitation. The dumping of various kinds of waste materials in the natural environment also has a negative impact on the development of tourism and urban improvement projects.

Establishment of a ceiling of 0.1 g/L of chlordecone in drinking water has led to the closure of certain catchment areas in Guadeloupe and Martinique. Prefectorial decrees issued in 2003 have been directed primarily toward preventing vegetables grown in contaminated soils from reaching public markets. Based on scientific study and review, in October 2005 provisional contamination ceilings for chlordecone concentrations in various foodstuffs were set to protect consumers.

Individual Care Services

Health care is provided by hospital complexes and private clinics. Unlike the other two French Overseas Departments, French Guiana has health centers. These facilities are designed to respond to the needs of geographically isolated residents and represent the only access to health care for the scattered and isolated communities that make up 20% of French Guiana's population.

Previously under the management of the *Conseil Général*, since 2000 these health centers have been separated into two groups, based on whether the provision of care is curative or preventive in nature. Curative care is undertaken by 10 health centers and 11 health posts under the supervision of the hospital complex in Cayenne and includes medical consultations, routine care, nursing services, and dispensing of medications. Disease prevention activities are the focus of some 20 vaccine and maternal and child health centers that remain under the general management of the *Conseil Général*.

Facilities in the short-term care sector are generally satisfactory, but inadequate in the area of follow-up care and psychiatry. The lack of facilities for older adults with special needs is evident, especially in Guadeloupe and Martinique. Currently, there are insufficient alternatives to hospitalization, even though home hospitalization initiatives are beginning to emerge and health care networks have begun to participate in this alternative strategy. Health care networks have been or are in the process of being established for such conditions as hypertension, gerontology, perinatal care, oncology, addictions, diabetes, and asthma. The availability of beds for various types of care at short-term facilities is shown in Table 5.

Health Promotion

The PRSP in each of the three French Overseas Departments underscores the importance of health education for the public and the need to strengthen efforts in this area. In 2004, Guadeloupe and Martinique drew up their Regional Education for Health Plan, although it has not yet been completely implemented in Martinique. French Guiana has yet to draw up a plan. Guadeloupe and Martinique each have a committee working in

TABLE 5. Beds per 1,000 population at short-term health care facilities, French Overseas Departments, 2005.

Type	Guadeloupe	French Guiana	Martinique
Medicine	2.09	1.50	2.32
Surgery	1.08	0.96	1.39
Obstetrics and gynecology	0.48	0.69	0.53

tandem with the National Institute for Prevention and Health Education. They are the Guadeloupian Committee for Health Education and the Martinican Committee for Prevention and Health Education. In addition, numerous associations, including entities at the national, district, and municipality levels and patients' groups, play an essential role as partners in prevention of disease, bringing their expertise to bear in such areas as HIV/AIDS, substance abuse, sickle cell disease, and cancer.

Human Resources

The shortage and equitable distribution of health professionals are a challenge in all three Departments, but particularly in French Guiana. With respect to physicians, the lack of specialists is even more pronounced than the lack of generalists (Table 6). This applies to all types of medical specializations. At the Cayenne hospital complex, numerous positions remain vacant or are filled by physicians who do not possess adequate qualifications for hospital practice.

In Guadeloupe and Martinique, there are sufficient midwives and nurses to meet current needs (Table 7), but for all other career categories the density rates are far below those found in metropolitan France. This shortage is expected to worsen in the years to come, given the increase in demand for health services due to the population's aging in Guadeloupe and Martinique and the demographic growth occurring in French Guiana. Medical and paramedical schools have substantially increased the number of training programs available and of students being trained, but the output of new professionals has remained insufficient to meet the demand.

TABLE 6. Number and density of physicians per 100,000 population, French Overseas Departments, 1 January 2005.

Type	Guadeloupe	French Guiana	Martinique
General physicians			
Number	542	195	536
Density	121	106	136
Specialists			
Number	434	147	450
Density	97	80	114
Total number of doctors	**976**	**342**	**986**

TABLE 7. Number and density of health professionals other than physicians per 100,000 population, by type, French Overseas Departments, 1 January 2005.

Type	Guadeloupe	French Guiana	Martinique
Dentists			
Number	162	43	155
Density	36	23	39
Midwives			
Number	160	51	167
Density	36	28	42
Nurses			
Number	2,159	573	2,365
Density	482	311	599
Physical therapists			
Number	257	58	260
Density	57	31	66

The third year of medical studies and the first year of medicine are taught in the French Overseas Departments (in the case of Guadeloupe and Martinique, only the first year). Training for various other medical and paramedical professions is also available in the French Overseas Departments, including one school for midwives, one school for massage and physical therapists, three schools for nurses (one in each of the French Overseas Departments), one school for pediatric nurses, one school for surgical nurses, one school for nurse-anesthetists, one school for biomedical technicians, three schools for child care auxiliaries, and three schools for nursing auxiliaries. Training for the other health professions is available in metropolitan France. Certificates were awarded in 2004 to 14 midwives, 116 nurses, 9 surgical nurses, 19 pediatric nurses, 64 child care auxiliaries, and 81 nursing auxiliaries who completed their training in the French Overseas Departments.

Health Supplies

There are a total of 340 pharmacies in the French Overseas Departments, excluding medical dispensaries in health centers. Of these, 153 are found in Guadeloupe (one for every 2,960 inhabitants), 150 are in Martinique (one per 2,650 inhabitants), and 37 are located in French Guiana (one for every 5,150 inhabitants). All pharmaceuticals are imported from France, with delivery from the manufacturer to the pharmacist taking place through the wholesale distributor or dealer. A "third-party payer" system is widely used in the French Overseas Departments, especially by public hospitals and pharmacies, in which the health care provider receives reimbursement directly from the universal health insurance plan, after the payment of any deductibles. Prices are fixed by the French public health authorities for reimbursable medications. In the French Overseas Departments, drug prices are subject to a markup to cover shipment costs from France. There is no local production of vaccines in the French Overseas Departments; all vaccines are likewise imported from France.

Health Sector Expenditures and Financing

Expenditure on health care and medical products continued to increase during the period under review. In 2004, health expenditures totaled nearly 1,879 million euros for all three French Overseas Departments (Table 8). Annual expenditure is approximately 2,000 euros per inhabitant in Martinique, 1,800 euros per inhabitant in Guadeloupe, and 1,400 euros per inhabitant in French Guiana. These variations are due in part to the different age structures of the respective populations. Hospitals, especially public hospitals, account for the bulk of the expenditure. In addition to these outlays, major sums are disbursed each year by the State or the *Conseil Général* in the social sector for special groups, including the elderly and persons with disabilities.

TABLE 8. Total health insurance expenditure and distribution by category, French Overseas Departments, 2004.

Category	Guadeloupe	French Guiana	Martinique
Total health insurance expenditure (in millions of euros)	805.3	268.4	804.8
Hospitalization	50%	68%	57%
Ambulatory care	18%	11%	17%
Drugs	16%	10%	15%

Technical Cooperation and External Financing

Apart from partnerships, programs, and financing mechanisms that have been developed with other EU members, the French Oversees Departments do not receive cooperation funds from abroad from international institutions such as the World Bank and United Nations entities.

On the other hand, between 2001 and 2005 the three regions developed a number of activities with neighboring countries and provided technical expertise as needed. For example, the staff at the University Hospital Center in Fort-de-France, Martinique, provided training in pathology to Caribbean physicians and technicians for cervical cancer screening and in the maintenance of biomedical equipment. There was also bilateral cooperation between the hospital complex in Lamentin, Martinique, and a hospital in Cuba. The Pasteur Institute's mycobacteria reference laboratory in Guadeloupe provided technical expertise on laboratory development and infrastructure to Haiti and other Caribbean countries. Professionals from Martinique and Guadeloupe helped train those responsible for treating HIV/AIDS patients in Haiti and other countries. In French Guiana, the Pasteur Institute conducted regional cooperation activities in connection with its role as the national referral center for arbovirus and influenza viruses.

Exchanges in expertise, medical equipment, and patients took place between French Overseas Departments' facilities in heart surgery, kidney transplants, oncology, and other areas. The university hospitals are also attracting patients from neighboring countries. The University Hospital Center at Fort-de-France handles an annual average of 400 to 500 hospitalization cases involving patients who reside outside the French Overseas Departments. In 2004–2005, one-third of the hospitalizations were cancer-related, followed by cardiovascular and osteoarthritic conditions.

GRENADA

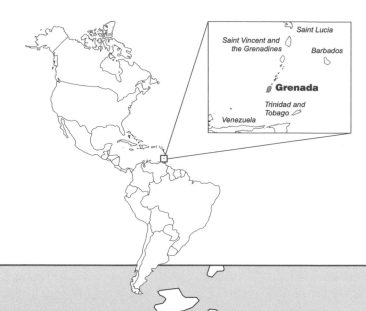

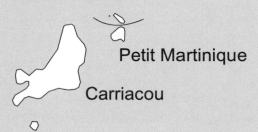

Saint Vincent and the Grenadines

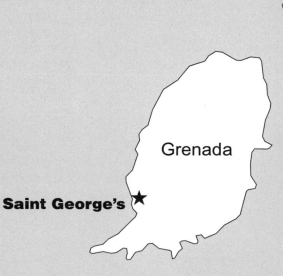

Petit Martinique

Carriacou

Ronde Island

Grenada

Saint George's ★

| 0 | 5 | 10 Miles |

The State of Grenada includes the islands of Grenada, Carriacou, and Petit Martinique and covers a land area of 344 km². Grenada lies at the southern end of the Windward Islands, about 100 miles north of Venezuela and 90 miles southwest of Barbados.

GENERAL CONTEXT AND HEALTH DETERMINANTS

Social, Political, and Economic Determinants

Grenada is governed as a parliamentary democracy. The legislative branch is made up of a bicameral legislature composed of a 15-member elected House of Representatives and a 13-member appointed Senate. Executive powers are vested in the Prime Minister, as head of government, and in the Cabinet. The chief of state is the Governor General, who represents the British Crown. The country has several active political parties, and general elections are held every five years.

Since 1983, Grenada has enjoyed a stable political climate, which has paved the way for sustained economic growth and development, despite the country's small and open economy being vulnerable to the effects of global economic recession and natural disasters. According to data from the Ministry of Economic Affairs, after Grenada's decline in economic growth following the events of September 11, 2001, in the United States, the country began to experience economic recovery. In 2002 and 2003, the economy showed positive growth of 0.8% and 5.8%, respectively.

The results of the 2005 Core Welfare Indicators Survey show an adult literacy rate of 96%. Less than half of households with primary school-age children have easy access to primary schools and 24% have access to secondary schools. Access to schooling is defined in terms of time taken to reach a primary or secondary school; households within 15 minutes of a facility are defined as having easy access. According to the survey, urban households have easy access, while less than 30% of poor students from the rural areas have access. However, despite limited access enrollment figures exceed 90%.

Grenada's economy was dealt serious blows by hurricanes Ivan in 2004 and Emily in 2005. Hurricane Ivan, in particular, caused significant damage, especially to the housing sector where damages were estimated at US$ 5.2 billion, or 58% of all damages sustained by the country. About 90% of the buildings were damaged and many persons lost their homes. There were 37 confirmed deaths and more than 300 injuries reported. Ivan's damage had important implications for Grenada's economy; as a result the agriculture and tourism sectors sustained negative growth of 6.9%. The health sector, as were most other sectors, was severely affected by hurricanes Ivan in 2004 and Emily in 2005. The over-

all estimated cost of damages to the health sector was US$ 4 million, and many health facilities were damaged. Despite these setbacks, the Government continued to provide affordable, quality health care services to the population. By 2005, most of the damaged facilities had been repaired, refurbished, and recommissioned, with financial assistance from donor agencies, organizations and institutions, other governments, civic organizations, and individuals.

In 2005, the economy experienced a significant growth of 12.9%, and it was projected to grow by 7.4% in 2006. This robust performance was due to increased activities in construction, mining and quarrying, and tourism industries, which registered growth rates of 7.6%, 10.2%, and 54.5% respectively.

The average inflation rate for 2005 was 3.5%, driven mainly by recent increases in fuel prices. Fiscal performance in 2005 improved compared to that in 2004. Recurrent expenditures, on the other hand, fell by 10.6%, to US$ 109 million, mainly due to lower interest payments. Savings on interest accounted for US$ 18.4 million in 2005.

The active labor force represents two-thirds of the population. Unemployment is highest among the poor and the 15–29-year age group.

Prior to Hurricane Ivan the unemployment rate was 13%. With many persons losing their jobs as a result of the hurricane, the unemployed rate increased sharply thereafter. According to the 2005 Core Welfare Indicators Survey, the unemployment rate was 18.8% that year, and it was higher among women. In urban areas, female unemployment more than doubles the male rate. Nearly one-third of youths are unemployed, again with higher rates among females.

A waste inventory conducted in 2003 indicated that there were an estimated 30,000 tons of waste generated in Grenada. A breakdown by sector showed that organic waste accounted for 46.4% and 43.7% of waste generated by rural and urban residents, respectively; waste paper accounted for 17.9% and 19.5%, respectively. Rural areas generate more organic waste that is less damaging to the environment. Some urban waste may generate environmental hazards, but this impact has yet to be fully investigated. Based on the current per capita waste generation rate of 2.2 kg per person per day, it is projected that waste generation would be approximately 38,000 tons per annum by the year 2016. The projected level of waste generation poses a challenge to the government in finding new/alternative disposal sites. Grenada has a very small land mass, and its hilly topography makes it extremely difficult to find alternative waste disposal sites.

A UNDP-sponsored Core Welfare Indicator Survey conducted in 2005 revealed that 87% of households have access to safe drinking water; 70% have access through publicly supplied water piped into the dwelling; 8.4% through publicly supplied water piped into the yard; and 8.5% through public standpipes.

In rural areas, 60.3% of the population has access to safe excreta and sewage disposal and sanitation services; 88.3% of urban households do. Septic tanks are used in 54.4% of households; 36.3% rely on pit latrines; 5.4% flushing toilets; and 0.7% have no access at all.

Of total households, 97% have access to a waste collection system. The Government's collection service offered by the Grenada Solid Waste Management Authority serves 87% of households; 1.1% of households rely on burning and crude dumping.

Demographics, Mortality, and Morbidity

In 2001, Grenada's population was estimated at 103,137. In 2005, the estimated population was 105,892, with an estimated growth rate of 2.6%. The population group under age 15 years represented 32% of the population and the group older than 64 represented 9%, for a dependency ratio of 71.5. (See Figure 1 for the country's population structure.)

In 2002, life expectancy was estimated at 71 years. Preliminary data show that between 2003 and 2005 the estimated average life expectancy increased to 73 years. An expected 10% increase in the group 65 years and older in the next decade will place added demand on health services, which may require large expenditures from the national budget. Consequently, the health systems will be required to develop supportive environments and appropriate services for this age group. In addition, the public health delivery system overall faces many development challenges, in part due to an increased demand for new technology with its escalating costs; additional challenges include health sector reform, health financing, and health information.

The number of recorded deaths in 2001–2005 was 3,230, for an average of 807 annual deaths. In 2002, the leading causes of death were diseases of the circulatory system (including diseases of pulmonary circulation and other forms of heart and cerebrovascular diseases), malignant neoplasms, diseases of the respiratory system, and parasitic diseases. Preliminary data from the General Hospital indicated that between 2003 and 2005 the leading causes of death were similar to those of the previous years. The number of deaths due to malignant neoplasms was 151 (24% of total deaths) in 2003, 45 (24%) in 2004, and 47 (21%) in 2005. Other leading causes of death in the period were due to endocrine and metabolic diseases, ischemic heart disease, diseases of the genitourinary system, and accidents and injuries.

FIGURE 1. Population structure, by age and sex, Grenada, 1990 and 2005.

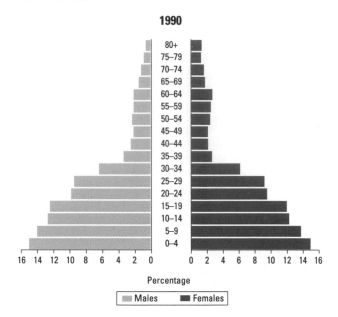

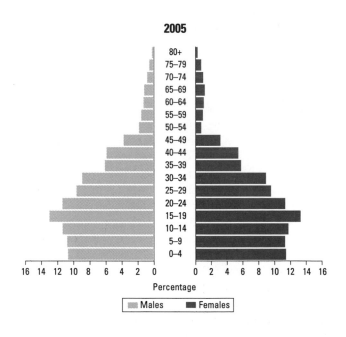

HEALTH OF POPULATION GROUPS

Children under 5 Years Old

During 2002–2005, there were 107 infant deaths recorded, representing 27 annual deaths or 15 deaths per 1,000 live births. In the same period there were 50 neonatal deaths, averaging 12 annual deaths, or 7 deaths per 1,000 live births. Between 2003 and 2005, 3,683 (49%) of all acute respiratory infection cases occurred in the age group 0–4 years old. Cases of gastroenteritis recorded for the same period (488) represented 45% of total cases. There were 18 infant deaths recorded in hospital records between 2004 and 2005. The leading causes of death among them were hypoxia, birth asphyxia, and respiratory conditions (8), acute respiratory infections (5), congenital heart disease (2), septicemia (1), broncho-aspiration (1), and diseases of the genitourinary system (1).

Community health reports indicate that between 2003 and 2005, 1,224 infants under 1 year old were seen at the country's clinics. Of that number, 450 (37%) were breast-fed exclusively for at least three months. In the same period, an average of 3% of these infants were found to be underweight or overweight. Among children aged 1–4 years, only 0.3% of 18,444 visiting clinics were underweight or overweight.

Children 5–9 Years Old

Two deaths were reported in this age group in 2004. One death was due to cerebrovascular disease; the other was due to disease of pulmonary circulation. No deaths were reported in 2005.

Adolescents 10–14 and 15–19 Years Old

The estimated population of 10–14-year-olds and 15–19-year-olds was 23,504 in 2005. Most attended school and appear to be in good health. Hospital data show that in 2004 there were no recorded deaths in these age groups. In 2005 one death was reported in the 15–19 age group, due to a malignant neoplasm. Between 2003 and 2005, the number of teenage mothers was 444, or 23% of total live births in 2003, 28% in 2004, and 32% in 2005.

Adults 20–59 and 60–64 Years Old

Grenada's labor force falls entirely in this age group, making it the most productive segment of the population. Hospital records indicate that between 2004 and 2005, there were 100 deaths in this age group, 61% males and 39% females. The three main causes of death were malignant neoplasms (27%), followed by diseases of the respiratory system (15%) and cerebrovascular diseases (13%).

Older Adults 65 Years Old and Older

The Ministry of Social Development is charged with providing services for Grenadians 65 years old and older. There are 11 homes for older adults in the country. The four homes owned and operated by the Government are Richmond Home, Grand Anse Home for the Aged, and Cadrona Home on mainland Grenada, and Top Hill on Carriacou. The Ministry of Social Development gives a monthly subsidy to the remaining privately owned and operated homes. Older adults are primarily affected by chronic diseases such as diabetes, hypertension, and coronary or cardiovascular diseases and their complications.

In 2005, it was estimated that 9% of the population was older than 65 years, and this group is expected to increase by more than 10% in the next decade. As this population group increases in the coming years, the management of chronic diseases will pose a major challenge, as the demand grows for hospital services and services in the community. Grenada observed an International Day against the Abuse of the Elderly in 2006. A national policy on caring for the elderly has been drafted. This policy will protect the rights of older persons, ensuring that they can live with dignity and respect. It will also guarantee their involvement in national and community development and other social issues affecting their lives.

The Family

In 2003, 5,057 women received contraceptive injections and 1,557 received oral contraception at public health clinics. In 2004, 1,300 received injections and only 421 received oral contraceptives, representing a 74% and 73% decrease, respectively. This sharp drop is likely attributed to the disruption in services following Hurricane Ivan. The Grenada Planned Parenthood Association also provides reproductive health services. In 2004, 6,570 visits were recorded for services other than receiving contraceptives. Of these, 505 were for Pap smears, of which 12 were treated for minor infections and 45 were referred to a physician for follow-up care. That same year, 906 pregnancy tests were conducted; 283 were positive. In terms of contraceptive use, 241 new acceptors were recorded in 2004, compared to 216 in 2003; 149 of these were oral contraceptives and 77, injectable contraceptives. The intrauterine device (IUD) and other barrier methods are not widely used. There were 9,596 condoms distributed.

Workers

Data from the national insurance scheme indicates that between 2001 and 2005 a total of 16,323 new persons registered, at an average of 3,265 persons per annum. During 2002–2005 there were a total of 1,518 reported injuries. Of these, 478 (32%) occurred in construction, 333 (22%) in social and related services, 160 (11%) in the wholesale/retail sector, and 153 (10%) in restaurant and hotel services. In the same period, there were 403 trauma injuries, 226 lacerations, and 218 fractures reported. Of all injuries reported, 59% occurred between 2004 and 2005. This may be attributed to the increased activities in the construction industry to repair damage from Hurricane Ivan.

Persons with Disabilities

It is estimated that 10% of Grenada's population has some form of disability. In 1985, the Grenada National Council for the

Disabled was established to provide a forum where persons with disabilities could voice concerns and seek ways to address them, to sensitize the public about the plight of disabled persons, and to advocate for persons with disabilities. The Council is funded by the Government of Grenada and receives a subsidy through the Ministry of Social Development, which is charged with looking after the needs of and providing services to persons with disabilities. The Dorothy Hopkins Home and Bel Air Home, both in Saint George's, cater to children with disabilities.

Through its "Spice Project," the National Children's Home Action for Children provides day care and school services for children with disabilities in St. Mark's parish. There are also two special education schools, one in St. George's and one in St. Andrews. There is a school for the deaf in the St. George parish.

HEALTH CONDITIONS AND PROBLEMS

COMMUNICABLE DISEASES

Vector-borne Diseases

The Ministry of Health's Environmental Health Department aims to reduce the incidence of **malaria** and **dengue** through the control of their vectors, *Anopheles* and *Aedes aegypti* mosquitoes, respectively. One imported case of malaria was reported in 2005. Before that, the last two imported cases were confirmed in 1998. There is no active surveillance for the *Anopheles* mosquito, although some surveillance is conducted at sentinel sites, such as the General Hospital. In 2004, the house index[1] for the *Aedes aegypti* mosquito was 13.9%. By October 2005, the house index had dropped slightly, to 11.5%. In 2002, there were 310 confirmed positive dengue cases, for a rate of 3 per 100,000 inhabitants. This upsurge was due primarily to the introduction of Serotype 3 into the island and the commensurate increase in surveillance activities. In 2003, there were only four confirmed cases; in 2005, there were two.

Vaccine-preventable Diseases

The Ministry of Health continues to give priority to the country's immunization program. In 2001 *Haemophilus influenzae* **type b** and **hepatitis B** vaccines were introduced into the national immunization schedule through use of the pentavalent vaccine (DPT/HepB/Hib). During 2001–2005 there were no cases of **diphtheria**, **rubella**, **tetanus**, **neonatal tetanus**, or *Haemophilus influenzae* type b.

The vaccination coverage in 2001 to 2005 held above 90%, with the exception of 2004, when all programs were disrupted by Hurricane Ivan. In 2004, the coverage for the third dose of DPT, hepatitis B, and *Haemophilus influenzae* type b; OPV3; and MMR

vaccines was 84%, 84%, and 75%, respectively. In 2005, vaccination coverage was 100% for all three vaccines.

Intestinal Infectious Diseases

Throughout 2001–2005 the reported incidence of **gastroenteritis** continuously decreased. There were 1,566 cases of gastroenteritis reported in 2003, 1,376 in 2004, and 1,065 in 2005; 24% of cases occurred among the 5–14 age group.

Chronic Communicable Diseases

The incidence of bacilloscopy-positive **tuberculosis** cases in 2001–2005 was 12 per 100,000, compared to 4 per 100,000 in 2000. There were 7 cases of tuberculosis recorded in 2005; 2 each in 2002, 2003, and 2004; and 1 in 2001. There were three reported deaths due to the disease, one each in 2002, 2003, and 2004. The rise in the incidence of tuberculosis in 2005 may have been due to deteriorating living conditions after Hurricane Ivan. The majority of cases (8) fell within the age group 25–64 years old.

There were two confirmed cases of **leprosy** in 2001–2005, one male and one female in the same family. Both completed a regimen of Rifampicin, Clofloxamine, and Dapsone over 18 months, and are under surveillance to observe any resurgence of the infection.

Acute Respiratory Infections

Acute respiratory infections are one of the main causes of morbidity in Grenada. Hospital sources indicate that there were 9,170 reported cases in 2003, 8,605 in 2004, and 7,852 in 2005.

HIV/AIDS and Other Sexually Transmitted Infections

There were 75 persons who tested positive for **HIV infection** for the first time (49 males, 26 females) and 59 newly confirmed cases of **AIDS** (39 males, 20 females) between 2001 and 2005. The cumulative total up to 2005, since the first case was confirmed in 1984, stood at 277. Of these, 179 were males and 98 were females. The male to female ratio is 1.6:1. The most affected population group is persons between the ages of 15 and 45, the most productive population group. There were 158 AIDS-related deaths. Between 2000 and 2005, 12 infants were born to 10 HIV-infected mothers. Since then, three mothers have died and two of the children have tested HIV-positive. There are nine children living with AIDS.

According to hospital data, 319 cases of **gonorrhea** were reported between 2003 and 2005, 133 in 2003, 119 in 2004, and 67 in 2005. In 2005, persons aged 15–44 were the most affected by the disease, 31 cases in the 15–24 group and 25 in the 25–44 group. The numbers of cases in these groups were similar in 2003 and 2004.

There were 150 cases of **syphilis** reported in 2004 and 35 in 2005. Those most affected by this disease in 2005 were persons 65 years old and older (15) followed by the age group 25–44 (8).

---

[1]The ratio of the number of positive houses to total number of houses inspected.

Zoonoses

There were two cases of **leptosperosis** confirmed in 2004 and seven in 2005; the disease is of public health importance in the country. **Animal rabies** remains endemic in the mongoose population throughout Grenada. No human rabies cases have been reported since 1970.

NONCOMMUNICABLE DISEASES

Metabolic and Nutritional Diseases

According to results from the 2005 Grenada Food and Nutrition Council nutritional assessment of government-run and government-assisted day care centers, **underweight infants** ranged from a high of 6.6% in 2002 to a low of 1.8% in 2005; **overweight infants** ranged from 5.3% in 2002 to 9.0% in 2005.

There is a high prevalence of **iron deficiency** among children in Grenada. Iron deficiency tests conducted among one-year-olds showed that of those screened in 2003, 2004, and 2005, 65%, 62%, and 56%, respectively, were anemic, with hemoglobin levels under 11 g; more than 60% of these required iron supplementation. The prevalence of anemia among pregnant women screened at prenatal clinics during the same period showed that 14.3% had iron levels under 10 g in 2003, 9.6% did in 2004, and 15.1% did in 2005. Women whose iron levels ranged between 8 g and 10 g were 12.5% in 2003, 9.6% in 2004, and 13.5% in 2005; those whose iron levels were under 8 g were 2%, 6%, and 1.6% for those same years. During the same period, postnatal women with hemoglobin levels under 10 g were 3.2%, 5.2%, and 6.4%. The highest prevalence of anemia among pregnant women and one-year-old children was recorded in the parish of St. Andrews.

In 2004 and 2005 there were 35 deaths due to endocrine and metabolic diseases.

There were 1,726 cases of **diabetes** in 2003–2005.

Cardiovascular Diseases

According to hospital statistics, of the 8,061 cases of noncommunicable diseases recorded between 2003 and 2005, 1,407 were due to **hypertensive disease**. In 2004 and 2005, the leading causes of death were **cerebrovascular disease** (82 deaths), followed by **diseases of the pulmonary circulatory system and other forms of heart disease** (52), and **ischemic heart disease** (36). Cerebrovascular diseases represent 20% of all deaths recorded at the hospital. The age group 65 years old and older is the most affected.

Malignant Neoplasms

Between 2003 and 2005, there were 634 reported cases of malignant neoplasms, for an average of 211 cases per year. Most cases fell among persons aged 45 years old and older. In 2003, there were 41 cases of malignant neoplasm of the digestive system (24 males and 17 females); in 2004 there were 37 (32 males and 5 females) and in 2005, 28 (19 males and 9 females). In 2005,

there were 36 cases of malignant neoplasm of the hematopoietic and lymphatic system (19 males and 17 females); 29 cases were reported in 2004 (13 males and 16 females) and 28 in 2003 (19 males and 9 females).

In males 45 years old and older there is an increased prevalence of prostate cancer; 45 cases were reported in 2003 and 44 in 2004.

In females 45 years and older, there were 26 cases of malignant neoplasm of the uterus and 21 cases of malignant neoplasm of the breast reported for 2003; the numbers of malignant neoplasms of the uterus and of the breast were 21 and 19, respectively, in 2004, and 27 and 17, respectively, in 2005.

Violence and Other External Causes

Hospital discharges due to accidents and violence include accidental poisonings, falls, firearm accidents, road traffic accidents, homicides, and self-inflicted injuries. Data suggest that males are more frequently admitted to hospitals for accidents and violence.

Among total hospital discharges for males for 2001–2004, accidents and injuries increased from 9,695 (2.1% of the total) in 2001 to 10,928 (6.3%) in 2004. In 2003, there were 348 reported cases of accidents and injuries; the numbers for 2004 and 2005 were 336 and 512, respectively. The number of road traffic accidents was 1,321 in 2001, 1,484 in 2002, and 1,506 in 2003. The number of injuries in those same years was 236, 269, and 239, with 10, 6, and 8 fatalities. In 2003, there were 88 accidents due to motor vehicle and other transport; in 2004 there were 91. In 2005, the number rose to 129, an increase of 30%. This rise is due mainly to an increase in motor vehicles and other transport, as well as to improvements in road conditions. Reported accidents due to falls were 183 in 2003, 138 in 2004, and 223 in 2005. The spike in 2005 may be due to an increase in construction and home and building repairs after hurricanes Ivan and Emily. In 2005, accidental poisoning and punctures caused by machinery accounted for 25 and 22 cases, respectively. In 2003, 15 cases of suicide and self-inflicted injury were recorded; there were 10 in 2004 and 9 in 2005. In 2003–2005, the most cases were seen among young women 15–24 and 25–44 years old.

Oral Health

Dental services at the centers are provided mainly to persons 65 years old and older and to children. In 2003, 2,238 children and youth (5–19 years old) were examined for the first time: 99% of them were identified as having problems, 95% (2,023) of which received treatment. In 2003 and 2004, visits to dental services by persons 65 years old and older and younger adults were 6,318 and 5,015, respectively. Extractions and some restorative work are offered, but these services are constrained by a lack of regular equipment maintenance and supply shortages. Apart from the salt fluoridation program launched in the 1990s, the country has no caries prevention or dental health promotion programs.

RESPONSE OF THE HEALTH SECTOR

Health Policies and Plans

The Ministry of Finance, Planning, and Development coordinates Grenada's national development, guided by a three-year Medium Term Economic Strategic Plan that responds to economic considerations, including social development issues such as health care and gender equity. The Plan is prepared by the Ministry of Finance in collaboration with various ministries, including the Ministry of Health. The Ministry currently is guided by the 2006–2008 Medium Term Economic Strategic Plan.

Open discussions are being held with a wide range of stakeholders to establish a management information system that will more effectively monitor the country's social development and progress. The system's indicators focus on human resource development, quality health care, poverty reduction and elimination, rural development, sustainable use of the physical environment, and gender equity.

Although the Ministry of Health is responsible for providing health services to the population, the Ministry of Finance has final authority over all expenditures. The Department of Human Resources, under the Prime Minister's office, approves all public service staffing. The Public Services Commission selects, appoints, and determines terms and conditions of employment for all staff.

The Agency for Reconstruction and Development was established to foster cooperation among ministries, statutory bodies, the private sector, civil society, and international organizations in several activities aimed at restoring the population's livelihood after Hurricane Ivan. Various sectors of the economy participated in this effort, dubbed "Building Back Better."

The Ministry continues to update the regulatory framework for the control and improvement of the public health system. The most recent legislation enacted is the 2001 Waste Management Act, which provides for waste management in conformity with the best environmental practices. The law also provides for the development of a national waste management strategy.

The Road Traffic Act was amended in 2001, regulating the use of seatbelts in all public and private vehicles; the Act requires all persons sitting on the front seats of any vehicle to wear seatbelts. The Act also requires persons riding or driving a motorcycle to wear a protective helmet.

The 2002 Dog Registration and Control Act regulates the keeping of dogs and controls the importation and keeping of dangerous dogs or dogs kept for dangerous purposes.

The 2005 Noise Control Act regulates and controls excessive and unreasonable noise.

Health Strategies and Programs

Since 1998 the Government has embarked on a health sector reform program which continues today; it aims at improving ef-

ficiency and effectiveness of the health services provided to the population. The reforms were mainly intended to deal with structural and institutional problems in the health care delivery system.

To cope with the escalating costs of providing acute care services, the Government will give greater emphasis to primary prevention by carrying out health promotion and educational activities. This effort is designed to encourage healthy lifestyles in the population, which will ultimately reduce the burden of disease and the demand for acute and rehabilitation services.

A new mental health policy and plan are also being developed to improve these services. Priority will be given to integrating the community mental health services into the primary care services. Emphasis will also be given to training personnel to staff mental services.

In 2002, the Government of Grenada received a grant from the Caribbean Development Bank for strengthening the hospital management system, including the review and development of policies and procedures manuals. An executive-agency model proposed for managing hospital services is now being gradually implemented. An executive management account was created for procuring goods and services. There is a Director of Hospital Services who manages all hospitals. The first phase of the hospital development project was completed and commissioned in January 2003. Work on the second phase of the project will begin soon.

In 2005 the Government began the process of developing a five-year national strategic plan for health under the theme "Health for Economic Growth and Development." This plan is expected to chart the way forward in health for the period 2006–2010. A health situational analysis has already been completed and priority areas identified that will serve as a baseline in the planning process.

An Environmental Affairs Department was established within the Ministry of Health in 2001, and an Environmental Protection Officer was appointed. The department is charged with facilitating the coordination, collaboration, and cooperation among stakeholders in the management of activities pertaining to Grenada's natural resources. The department is responsible for enforcing the institutional framework for environmental management and sustainable development to minimize indiscriminate potential adverse effects on human health and national development. It will also increase the level of public awareness on environmental issues in Grenada and facilitate the development of attitudes and skills necessary for community-based activities of environmental management.

The 2005 National Environmental Policy and Management Strategy complements and builds upon existing environmental policies and instruments to address environmental quality and sustainability issues. A draft environmental management bill is designed to enhance the efforts and scope of the 2001 Solid Waste Management Act. The legislation mainly relates to abating solid waste pollution. Part of the bill addresses environmental man-

"Building Back Better" after Hurricane Ivan

Grenada is especially vulnerable to hurricanes. Hurricane Ivan in 2004 proved to be one of the worst, leaving a toll of 37 deaths and more than 300 injured. Almost every structure sustained some damage, much of it severe. Damages to housing exceeded US$ 5 billion. Countless Grenadians lost their homes. The agriculture and tourism sectors sustained damages, which seriously dampened the economy. Many health facilities also were struck, with damages to the health sector estimated at US$ 4 million. In response to Hurricane Ivan's devastation, the Government established the Agency for Reconstruction and Development in September 2004. Working under the motto "Building Back Better," the agency served as an umbrella, coordinating the reconstruction work of ministries, statutory bodies, and elements of the private sector, civil society, and international organizations.

agement activities pertaining to marine issues, the movement of hazardous wastes, climate change, and marine-related conventions to which Grenada is a signatory (the Basel Convention on the Trans-boundary Movement of Hazardous Wastes and the Montreal Protocol, among others).

Organization of the Health System

The Ministry of Health, Social Security, the Environment, and Ecclesiastic Relations is responsible for the overall management of the health sector; it discharges its responsibilities through a centralized management. Within this structure, the Minister functions as the political head, the Permanent Secretary is the administrative head, and the Chief Medical Officer is the principal technical advisor on medical services. The Ministry is divided into three functional areas—Administration, Hospital Services, and Community Health Services. The Ministry's administrative role is to formulate policies; enforce regulations; provide direction to programs; and oversee health and vital statistics, expenditures, inventory control, and personnel. The hospital services area comprises four acute care hospitals: General Hospital, Princess Alice Hospital, Princess Royal Hospital in Carriacou, and Mount Gay Psychiatric Hospital. Community Health Services, referred to as the primary/preventive care services, are provided at the district level. It is the first point of contact for anyone requiring health care services.

Grenada is divided into seven health districts—St. Andrews, St. George's, St Johns, St. Mark's, St. Patrick's, St. David's, and Carriacou—six of which have a health center as their main primary care facility. There also are 30 medical stations distributed throughout the country, which are usually the first point of contact with the public health system. Every person has access to a health facility within a three-mile radius of his or her residence.

Each health district is managed by a District Medical Officer, various categories of nurses, dentists and dental auxiliaries, pharmacists, environmental health officers, and community mental health workers. Some facilities provide specialty services, such as pediatrics, psychiatry, and chronic disease management. Grenada's public sector hospitals include General Hospital in St. Georges; Princess Alice in St. Andrews; Princess Royal in Carriacou; and Mount Gay Psychiatric Hospital in St. George's.

The Ministry of Health is responsible for the social security and national insurance scheme. Some persons have private individual or group health insurance, where contributions are made by both employer and employee. The Government is considering introducing a national health insurance scheme, offering a basic package of services as an alternative financing option.

Public Health Services

In 2002, the National AIDS Program was extended to include other sexually transmitted infections, and a national HIV/AIDS Prevention and Control project was launched under a National AIDS Directorate. A National Infectious Disease Control Unit also was established that year. In 2003, the Unit launched a counseling and testing program to prevent mother-to-child transmission, and a clinic was opened to conduct the testing. Antiretroviral drugs also were made available at no cost that year.

Grenada continues to implement strategies to control the spread of HIV/AIDS. As part of that effort, a volunteer counseling and testing program was established in 2005 to encourage persons infected with HIV to have checkups and tests to determine their health status. Since the program began, 34 persons have been trained to help carry out this activity.

In terms of controlling vector-borne diseases, chemical control of mosquitoes, focusing on high-risk areas, and health education programs are the two main thrusts of the effort. The widespread use of insecticides such as Malathion and Temephos over the last five decades or so continues to play an integral role in the control of *Aedes aegypti* mosquitoes.

The Environmental Health Department continues to work to reduce the incidence of animal rabies by conducting annual country-wide vaccination campaigns of domestic animals. In 2005 approximately 7,000 animals were vaccinated, representing a success rate of just over 87% of the 8,000 animals targeted in the rabies vaccination program.

In addition, mongooses are trapped and laboratory-tested to estimate the incidence of rabies in animal communities, thereby maintaining the established barrier of rabies transmission from mongoose to man.

In 2005, the Department continued to ensure the availability of safe water through the water quality monitoring program that was instituted in 1998. In addition, reports of weekly bacteriological sampling conducted by the National Water and Sewerage Authority are reviewed and analyzed. Reviews of these bacteriological results show a general adherence to the water quality according to established standards.

The Environmental Health Department also continues to be responsible for overall sanitation; however, efforts are being made to relieve the Ministry of Health of these traditional roles and to function more in a monitoring and regulatory capacity.

One of the main functions of the Grenada Solid Waste Authority is to control all aspects of solid waste management in the country, with emphasis on efficiency and due regard to ecological and environmental factors.

The Government is revising the imposition of an environmental levy on imported filled and empty containers as a way to reduce the level of importation into the country. Consideration is also being given to the practice of reusing and recycling as a means of waste management.

The Environmental Health Department is responsible for controlling water pollution; improving wastewater treatment, ensuring that safe drinking water is delivered to the population; and identifying risks to health and safety within water catchment areas. The Department also is responsible for improving systems for the disposal of excreta and other harmful substances to humans, animals, and plants, as well as food hygiene.

Food safety activities continue to concentrate on the inspection of food service facilities, meats, and other foods, as well as providing ongoing education of food handlers. Plans are under way to strengthen the epidemiological surveillance of food-borne illnesses through improvements in the collection, collation, analysis, and interpretation of data. It should be noted that street food vending and the proliferation of itinerant food vendors in urban centers pose new challenges to Grenada's traditional method of inspecting food establishments. In 2004, there were approximately 600 itinerant food vendors registered with the Environmental Health Department. This sector of activity remains largely unregulated and new food safety practices, such as the application of Hazard Analysis Critical Control Principles (HACCP), are yet to be understood and adopted by the street vendors. Moreover, outbreaks of food-borne diseases are generally underreported. In the third quarter of 2002, for example, 56 cases were reported; only 10 were reported during the same period in 2003. No substantial changes occurred for the first quarter of 2004 (16 cases) and 2005 (15 cases).

The Grenada Food and Nutrition Council works closely with the ministries of Health and of Agriculture to implement joint programs to foster healthier eating habits and other lifestyle practices; it also monitors iron deficiency in pregnant women and children.

The events of September 11, 2001, underscored the vulnerability of Grenada's fragile economy to external influences. In response, the Government of Grenada put in place a food security program through the Ministry of Agriculture that was implemented in 2002. The program aims at ensuring some measure of self-sufficiency by increasing food production and the consumption of locally produced food—it is estimated that 90% of the food consumed in Grenada is imported. Farmers were provided with planting materials and livestock. Technical assistance and training were provided, including instruction on land preparation, use of fertilizers, types of animal feed, and other issues important to increased food and livestock production. Although most farmers were involved in the production of traditional crops, many new persons became involved and food production appears to be on the increase.

Individual Health Care Services

Individual health care services are provided mainly through public facilities, which offer outpatient, emergency, and inpatient services. The 198-bed General Hospital is the main referral hospital; it offers 24-hour accident and emergency and specialist services, including pediatric, surgical, internal medicine, obstetrics/gynecology, ophthalmic, oncology, psychiatric, orthopedic, and neurology services. Support services include laboratory, imaging, physiotherapy, rehabilitation, and social services. A 20-bed acute psychiatric unit that is part of General Hospital is the main admission unit for all patients requiring psychiatric services. The hospital also offers dietary and nutrition and ambulance services. The services are managed by an executive management team comprising a Director of Hospital Services, a Director of Medical Services, a Director of Nursing Services, and health services administrators from the Princess Alice Hospital, Princess Royal Hospital, and Richmond Hill Hospital.

In 2003–2005, 76,133 persons were seen at the General Hospital's accident and emergency department; 20,977 were admitted to the hospital, with an average length of stay of six days and an occupancy rate of 95%. Admissions and discharges are categorized by services. Of the total number of admissions in 2005, 2,107 (1,137 males, 970 females) were admitted to the medical wards, 1,785 (1,185 males, 600 females) to the surgical wards, 750 to gynecology, 1,653 to obstetrics, 1,364 (841 males, 523 females) to the pediatric ward, and 208 (123 males, 85 females) to ophthalmology; 1,183 were newborns.

The 60-bed Princess Alice Hospital is located in the rural parish of St. Andrews. It was seriously damaged by Hurricane Ivan and now has a reduced capacity of 20 beds. It provides secondary health care services with an emphasis on low-risk obstetrical, general medical, and minor surgical services, as well as stabilization of emergencies. The total number of persons seen at the accident and emergency department in 2004 and 2005 was 21,919; there were 2,820 admissions.

Princess Royal Hospital, a 40-bed secondary-care facility located on the island of Carriacou, also serves residents of Petit Martinique. It provides services similar to those provided by Princess Alice Hospital, as well as limited diagnostic services. Between 2003 and 2004, 5,892 persons were seen at the accident and emergency department, resulting in 1,002 hospital admissions.

The 80-bed Mt. Gay Hospital is the only long-stay mental health facility in Grenada. It provides psychiatric, psychotherapy, occupational and recreational therapy, and individual and family counseling services. Community mental health services are offered at various health centers throughout the country and provide follow-up and reevaluation of patients. Community mental health workers are assigned to each health district to provide follow-up care and treatment and ensure patient compliance and stability. There were 1,011 admissions to Mt. Gay Hospital between 2002 and 2005. Diagnostic categories are not available.

Carlton House is a 16-bed facility and the only substance-abuse treatment and rehabilitation center. This facility was severely damaged by Hurricane Ivan in 2004 and services have been suspended as a result. Between 2000 and 2004, 242 persons were admitted to Carlton House, 235 (96%) males and 7 (4%) females. Alcohol abuse was the reason for 43% of all admissions, while 31% were for multiple drug use, 16% for crack cocaine use, and 9% for marijuana abuse.

Specialty clinics in psychiatry, gynecology, chronic diseases, and sexually transmitted diseases are conducted at the hospitals and at the district level. In 2005, 9,475 patients were seen at General Hospital's specialty clinics. There were 3,184 patients admitted for obstetric/gynecological services, 2,303 for surgical-urological services, 1,860 for orthopedic services, 1,587 for medical services, 399 for maxillofacial services, and 142 for neurosurgery services. A range of services, mainly targeted to children, are provided by a visiting medical team from a United States organization, Children's Health Organization Relief and Educational Services (CHORES). The team comes to Grenada twice yearly to see new patients and provide follow-up care. In 2005, 163 patients were seen, 53.4% females and 46.6% males.

An oncology clinic staffed by a visiting oncologist was started in May 2005; between May and December 2005, 255 patients were seen at the clinic; 70% were females and 30% were males.

District Medical Officers refer persons seeking care in other specialties to the general hospital but there are long waiting times for such services. Referrals from other hospitals and health care facilities for admission are usually made via General Hospital's accident and emergency department. There is no formal system for follow-up and referral for patients discharged from General Hospital.

Mental health services provide treatment and rehabilitation for persons admitted to the Mental Hospital.

Health Promotion

The Ministry of Health's Health Promotion Department is responsible for coordinating the development, implementation, and evaluation of health promotion activities at the national, community, and organizational levels by strengthening health education efforts in the health sector and other sectors. The Department also provides leadership, technical expertise, and resources to strengthen community activities. The Department works closely with the Royal Grenada Police Force's Traffic Department to increase awareness of road safety. A workshop introducing the concepts of health education and health promotion was held for representatives from non-governmental organizations to encourage social participation which is critical to the advancement of health initiatives. A directory is now being developed to foster networking among community groups, non-governmental organizations, and related agencies. A teaching guide was produced to help teachers deliver information on sensitive issues and make them aware of innovative teaching methods.

Interventions have been applied to reach the various target populations through consultations on health issues, questionnaires, and various forms of mass communication activities. Healthy lifestyles were promoted through health screening programs, health walks, and school-based competitions. In addition, a study was conducted on the attitudes and the level of satisfaction of workers throughout the health system. The results of the study will help to plan appropriate programs to address problem areas.

Human Resources

In 2002, Grenada had 8.1 physicians per 10,000 population, the same ratio it had in 1997. The ratios of nurses (19.5 per 10,000) and dentists (1.1 per 10,000) also have remained at 1997 levels. In 1998, there were 6.9 pharmacists per 10,000 and 0.75 nutritionists per 10,000 population. Graduates of the schools of pharmacy and of nursing continue to come into the health system. In 2001, the Government implemented a policy of zero growth in the public service as part of a cost containment strategy. Special provisions are made for the employment of medical and nursing personnel on a contractual basis as needed.

Health Supplies

The Procurement Unit is responsible for obtaining, storing, and distributing pharmaceutical, medical and surgical, dental, x-ray, laboratory, domestic, and other health supplies needed for administrative functions. The Unit has developed a systematic and coordinated procurement process to ensure the cost-effectiveness of obtaining supplies, given that health supplies account for between 20% and 25% of total expenditures for hospitals and community services. The purchase of drugs is centralized through the Regional Organization of Eastern Caribbean States Pharmaceutical Procurement Services (OECS/PPS), based in Saint Lucia, which allows for drugs to be purchased at competitive prices. About 85% of the drugs used in the public health sector are obtained through this service, based on a regional formulary which Grenada adapts as its national formulary. The formulary is updated every 18 months with agreement from national formulary committees of all member states. Procedures also are in place for requesting non-formulary drugs. All drugs and other supplies are stored at the Central Medical Supplies Department and are distributed through requisitions from the various departments. A donations policy is also in place to provide guidance for better collaboration and coordination with donors, to ensure that Grenada derives the greatest benefit possible from donations, and to maintain standards for the supply, delivery, and receipt of donated goods and for professional and technical services.

All high technology equipment is located at General Hospital, the main acute care hospital. The biomedical and the main maintenance unit also are located at General Hospital; the other hospitals have smaller maintenance units. These units are responsible for conducting preventive maintenance of all the country's health facilities. The second phase of construction of General Hospital is about to begin; the new facilities will be outfitted with modern equipment.

The public health laboratory is fully equipped; it and the imaging department are to be housed in a new facility.

The private sector provides some laboratory services; it is the sole provider of CT scans. Both the public and private sectors offer ultrasonograms, electrocardiograms, and mammograms.

Most public sector facilities are in reasonable condition. About 20% still need repairs, which will be completed over the next three years.

Health Sector Expenditures and Financing

The Ministry of Health receives its funding from general taxation through the Ministry of Finance's consolidated fund. International donor agencies, governments, charitable organizations, and individuals also help fund projects and programs. The management of public financing for health is the joint responsibility of the ministries of Health and of Finance, under the direction of Parliament and the Cabinet; it is part of the annual budgetary process.

Total public sector expenditure in 2003, 2004, and 2005 was US$ 105 million, US$ 121.3 million, and US$ 108.5 million, respectively. Health expenditures for the same period were US$ 14.5 million in 2003, US$ 14.6 million in 2004, and US$ 16.1 million in 2005. Data on expenditures show that health and education continue to consume, on average, 11.6% and 16.7%, respectively,

of the total recurrent budget. The estimated recurrent expenditure for 2006 is US$ 120.8 million, with expenditures on health estimated at 12.09%. That same year, the per capita expenditure on health was US$ 1,033. Hospital services receive a subsidy grant of approximately EC$ 8 million annually for the provision of goods and services. Services provided at the hospitals are generally free, with nominal user fees for the use of private wards, operating theatres, diagnostic services, and prescription drugs for private bed patients; all fees collected are deposited into the consolidated fund.

External Technical Cooperation and Financing

The Ministry of Health continues to receive significant technical and financial assistance from PAHO/WHO, the Caribbean Development Bank through the Basic Need Trust Fund, USAID, Project Hope, the World Bank, and countries such as Cuba, New Zealand, Qatar, and Venezuela.

PAHO provides most of the technical and financial support towards health reform, environmental health, health promotion, and disease prevention. The Organization also provides short- and long-term fellowships. During hurricanes Ivan and Emily, PAHO mobilized funds to reconstruct the country's only public facility for the elderly, which had been severely damaged. Emergency funding also was provided for procuring supplies for the clinical laboratory and the vector control unit.

Project Hope made available US$ 80,000 for a continuing education program for nurses and for acquiring computers, textbooks, and other supplies for the Grenada School of Nursing.

The Government of Cuba provides ongoing support for the General Hospital's biomedical department through trained biomedical engineers and technicians. However, because the Ministry has limited funds for preventive maintenance, the service provided by this department is curtailed by a lack of equipment and inadequate funding. Various funding agencies have provided financial assistance to refurbish both primary health and hospital facilities, especially in the aftermath of hurricanes Ivan and Emily.

USAID provided US$ 340,000 to repair 11 community health facilities. The Government of New Zealand also provided funds to complete the construction of the Grenada School of Nursing, and the Caribbean Development Bank financed the refurbishment and reconstruction of six community health facilities. The Government of Venezuela has committed US$ 13.5 million towards completing the construction of General Hospital's second phase.

Through the World Bank, funds were reallocated from HIV/AIDS to replace much needed equipment for the laboratory and for Woburn and Crochu Medical Stations and nurses' quarters at St. David's Health Center.

St. George's University has signed a memorandum of understanding with the Ministry of Health whereby the University awards five scholarships to Grenadians each year—two in medicine and three in the masters in public health program. The University also provides US$ 150,000 annually to hospital services for purchasing medical equipment. The University also cooperates with General Hospital in research and in providing medical assistance in specialist areas.

In 2005, Dalhousie University consultants undertook a review of the country's mental health services, with a view toward developing a national mental health policy and plan that will be part of the Five Year National Strategic Plan for Health.

GUATEMALA

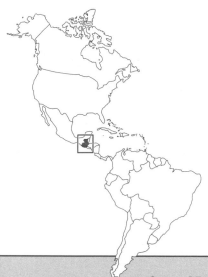

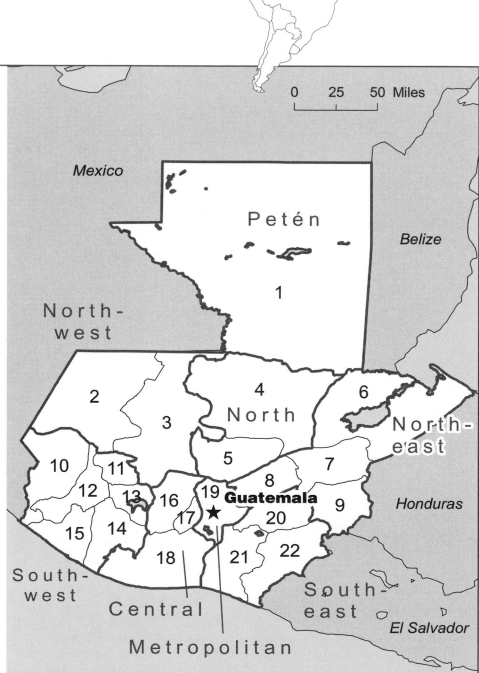

1. Petén
2. Huehuetenango
3. Quiché
4. Alta Verapaz
5. Baja Verapaz
6. Izabal
7. Zacapa
8. El Progreso
9. Chiquimula
10. San Marcos
11. Totonicapán
12. Quezaltenango
13. Sololá
14. Suchitepéquez
15. Retalhuleu
16. Chimaltenango
17. Sacatepéquez
18. Escuintla
19. Guatemala
20. Jalapa
21. Santa Rosa
22. Jutiapa

0 25 50 Miles

Mexico

Belize

Petén

1

North-
west

2

3

North

4

6

North-
east

5

7

10

11

8

Guatemala

12

13

16

19

9

Honduras

17

14

20

15

18

21

22

South-
west

South-
east

Central

El Salvador

Metropolitan

The Republic of Guatemala is bordered on the north and northwest by Mexico; on the east by Honduras, El Salvador, and Belize; and on the southwest by the Pacific Ocean. It covers an area of 108,889 square kilometers, divided into 22 departments and 331 municipios with 20,485 towns and villages for administrative purposes (*1*).

GENERAL CONTEXT AND HEALTH DETERMINANTS

Of the total population, 56.2% (6,397,903 persons) lives in poverty (with a daily income of less than US$ 1.60), and 15.7% (1,786,682 persons) lives under conditions of extreme poverty (with a daily income of less than US$ 0.70) (*2*). The incidence of poverty is much higher in rural areas (74.5% of the population) than in urban areas (27.1%). Poverty rates among indigenous peoples (77.3% of the population) are higher than for the non-indigenous population (41.0%). The human development index (HDI) was 0.663 in 2005, up from 0.640 in 2002 (*3*). The HDI in the nation's capital (0.795) is quite a bit higher than in the interior (0.457 in Sololá department, where 96.4% of the country's indigenous population lives) (*3*). The poorest regions also have the highest rates of malnutrition; 80% of children suffering from chronic malnutrition live below the poverty line (*2*). Poor women have a higher total fertility rate, or an average of two more children than non-poor women (with an average of four children) (*2*). The incidence of chronic malnutrition among indigenous peoples (69.5%) is nearly double the figure for the nonindigenous population (35.7%) (*4*). The allocation of arable land continues to be a major problem in all parts of the country, hitting indigenous groups particularly hard. In fact, half of all farmers nationwide are members of indigenous groups, who control a mere 24% of the land they farm (including both leased and personally owned land) (*3*).

Social, Political, and Economic Determinants

To achieve the first Millennium Development Goal (MDG 1), to eradicate extreme poverty and hunger by the year 2015, the country will need to turn around recent setbacks, with the share of national income going to the poorest fifth of the population slipping from 2.7% in 1989 down to 1.8% in 2004 (*3*). This is reflected, in part, in the share of the population living on less than a dollar a day, which went from 20.0% in 1989 to 21.5% in 2004.

There are 4,791,512 workforce members, of whom 20.8% are between 10 and 18 years of age, 31.2% are between the ages of 19 and 30, 33.9% are between 31 and 50, and 14.0% are over 50 years of age. The labor force participation rate for the nonindigenous population is 55.2%. Moreover, 71.3% of the working population is employed in the informal sector (*5*), 86.8% of them have no employment contract, and 59.6% work more than 40 hours a week. Only 18% of the working population is registered with the Guatemalan Social Security Institute (*5*). The agricultural sector generates the most employment (40.1%), followed by commerce (21.8%) and the manufacturing industry (15.5%). There are 108,050 unemployed, of whom 60.3% are male and 47.0% are between 19 and 30 years of age.

The country's economic reforms and macroeconomic stabilization policies are responsible for its poor economic performance, giving rise to short periods of economic growth followed by a slowdown in growth rates and a stagnating gross domestic product (GDP) per capita, which steadily declined between 1999 and 2003, rallying slightly in 2004 and 2005, with a moderate expansion in economic activity. GDP grew by 2.7% in 2004 and by even more (3.2%) in 2005, outstripping the rate of population growth in both years, at 2.5% (*6*). GDP per capita went from US$ 1,823.40 to US$ 2,204.70 between 2001 and 2004 (*3*).

Since 2002, family remittances have outstripped income from exports of traditional products (green coffee, bananas, sugar, and cardamom). The value of remittances was estimated at US$ 2.998 billion in 2005 (*3*). Family remittances help 3.4 million individuals, or 774,000 recipient households (31.2% of all households nationwide) (*3*). The fiscal deficit went from –1.9 in 2001 to –1.0 in 2004 (*7*). Guatemala has low taxes, which represented roughly 10.1% of GDP in 2005. A 1.5% tax increase has been proposed to help meet commitments under the Peace Accords and MDGs. A breakdown of spending shows 2.4% of GDP going to education, science, and culture and 1.2% going to health (*7*). The government has established monitoring and auditing mechanisms for government agencies such as the Integrated Financial Administration and Auditing System, the Information System on Government Procurements and Contracts (Guatecompras), the National Public Investment System, the Government Targets System, the Integrated Accounting System, and the Integrated Municipal Financial Administration System as part of its battle against corruption. In 2005, against a backdrop of social and labor discord and unrest, the Guatemalan Congress ratified the Central America–Dominican Republic–United States Free Trade Agreement, looking to strengthen the small and medium enterprise sector. Physical infrastructure development, institutional infrastructure building through small farmer organizations, and the sharing of technology by small farmers should all be considered as strategies geared to preventing growth from benefiting a mere handful of large-scale exporters rather than promoting local market development as a whole (3).

The small share of income going to the poorest 20% of the population is a reflection of the vulnerability of the poorest segments of society. The ratio of the income of the top quintile of the population to that of the bottom quintile rose steadily between 1984 and 2004, from 19.3 to 34.2. The extreme inequity in income distribution is reflected in a Gini coefficient of 0.57 for the country as a whole. Guatemala has one of the world's highest inequality indexes. It is ranked 13th out of 111 countries evaluated by the United Nations Development Program (UNDP), with indexes ranging from 0.20 to 0.61 (3). The Peace Accords signed by the government of Guatemala and the Guatemalan National Revolutionary Unity movement call for an integrated approach to health care, in line with the MDGs. The country's health priorities are to control malnutrition as a way of combating extreme poverty and expand environmental sanitation services to ensure environmental sustainability. Another priority is to reduce maternal and child mortality by expanding and strengthening primary health care services targeted at these high-risk groups. These are all examples of common ground between the peace agreement and the MDGs. Other elements of the peace accords such as agreements on drugs, supplies, and equipment and on preventive health issues should also help further MDG 5 (combat HIV/AIDS, malaria, and other diseases).

The budding activism following the signature of the Peace Accords in 1996 was marked by: (1) a wavering but growing effort to organize and empower indigenous groups, strengthening the participation of the indigenous population; (2) the emergence of agencies and organizations (not necessarily indigenous) furnishing assistance, training, and information to disadvantaged groups and filing complaints and taking action on their behalf; and (3) an ignorance on the part of government and other social stakeholders of how to formulate a comprehensive plan and build a pluralistic State in a multiethnic nation (3).

According to projections based on the 2002 Population Census, the adult literacy rate is 69.1%, with the 15- to 24-year age group showing the most improvement in this area (1); their literacy rate jumped from 76% in 1994 to 82.2% in 2002. The rise in the literacy rate for rural women by nearly 9 percentage points between 1994 and 2002, or from 59.8% to 68.2%, and the even sharper rise in the literacy rate for the young indigenous population during the same period, by 11 percentage points, or from 60.4% to 71.5%, are especially noteworthy. Of the illiterate popu-

lation, 60% entered first grade but dropped out of school before learning to read and write (3); the remaining 40% never entered first grade. Two-thirds of all illiterates are female. As of 2002, there was still no change in traditional patterns of school enrollment, with males completing more years of school than females across all age groups and the nonindigenous population completing more grades than the indigenous population (8). Urban dwellers also had more years of schooling than residents of rural areas. Figure 1 compares adult (15 years and older) literacy rates for 1994 and 2002, broken down by gender and ethnic origin.

The average truancy rate among the population between 7 and 14 years of age was 28.9%, and 26% of the secondary-school-age population was enrolled in school. The average number of years of schooling completed by youths between the ages of 15 and 24 went from 4.5 in 1994 to 5.4 in 2002 (8). There were large disparities in figures for the indigenous population (2.7 years in 1994 versus 3.8 years in 2002) and the rest of the population (5.8 and 6.5 years, respectively). A breakdown by gender and ethnic origin shows nonindigenous males with the most education in 2002 (an average of 8.2 years) and indigenous females with the least education (an average of 4.4 years) (8).

The country has made progress in furtherance of the second MDG (achieve universal primary education), as reflected in the rise in the net primary school enrollment rate from 71.7% in 1989 to 92.3% in 2004. The share of pupils entering first grade who go on to complete sixth grade went from 43.7% in 1989 to 65.1% in 2004.

According to data on nutritional status, 23% of the population (the equivalent of 2.8 million people) is undernourished (consuming less than the minimum dietary energy requirement) (4). The monthly incomes of over 60% of Guatemalan households are too low to cover the cost of the basic food basket. The fortification of

FIGURE 1. Comparative adult (age 15 and older) literacy rates, by sex and ethnic origin, Guatemala, 1994 and 2002.

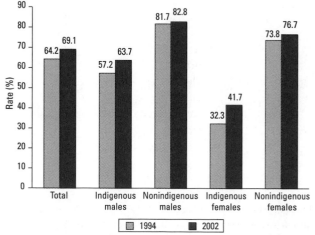

Source: Guatemala, Ministerio de Educación.

food products is the main strategy for reducing and controlling micronutrient deficiencies. Wheat is fortified with iron and folic acid to prevent anemia, salt is fortified with iodine to prevent hypothyroidism, and sugar is fortified with vitamin A to prevent blindness. Some progress has been made with respect to MDG 1 aimed at reducing the number of people suffering from hunger, as reflected in the drop in the percentage of underweight children less than 5 years of age from 34% to 23% between 1987 and 2002 (3).

Studies of air pollution and its health effects found several locations in Guatemala City with annual levels of total suspended particulates as high as 681 $\mu g/m^3$ (compared with the WHO guideline of 80 $\mu g/m^3$). Levels of particulates with diameters of less than 10 μm (PM_{10}) (breathable particulates) were as high as 192 $\mu g/m^3$ (versus the WHO guideline calling for an average annual level of 50 $\mu g/m^3$). Nitrogen dioxide levels reached 80 $\mu g/m^3$, with an average annual level of 57.43 $\mu g/m^3$ for the year 2000 (compared with the WHO guideline of 40 $\mu g/m^3$). The average annual ozone level in the year 2000 was 30.17 $\mu g/m^3$ (versus the WHO guideline calling for an average annual level of 60 $\mu g/m^3$). The average annual concentration of carbon monoxide in the city center was 2.83 ppm (versus the WHO guideline of 9 ppm over 8 hours).

The use of fuelwood has been cut back over the last 15 years as an environmental and air pollution prevention and control measure. However, measurements of carbon dioxide emissions per capita show a rise in emission levels (from 0.47 metric tons in 1990 to 0.73 metric tons in 2005). Approximately 75% of the rural population is exposed to indoor air pollution from smoke produced by biomass combustion (the burning of wood, straw, dung, coal, etc.) (3).

The country is struck by an average of 200 natural disasters per year. The most common phenomena with the largest impact are earthquakes, floods, and landslides. Other events include volcanic eruptions, severe cold spells accompanied by snow and hail, explosions, and forest fires. There are 1,733 high-risk human settlements with a total of 219,821 residents. The departments with the largest number of endangered villages and residents are Escuintla, Zacapa, Santa Rosa, and Petén.

Approximately 30% of the population lives in an earthquake zone. There are 641 villages with 84,000 residents located close to major faults. There were 37,698 reported earthquakes in Guatemala over the period between 1977 and 2003. Its 38 volcanoes and four tectonic faults have turned the country into a seismic zone with a high likelihood of multiple eruptions. An area of approximately 5,500 km^2 (representing 5.1% of the country's land area) is considered to have a high or very high risk of drought.

Demographics, Mortality, and Morbidity

In 1980, the country had a population of 7,013,435 inhabitants, of which 50.5% was male, 45.3% was under the age of 15, 40.1% was between 15 and 44, 10.8% was between 45 and 65, and 2.9% was 65 and older (Figure 2). By 2002, Guatemala's popula-

FIGURE 2. Population structure, by age and sex, Guatemala, 1980 and 2005.

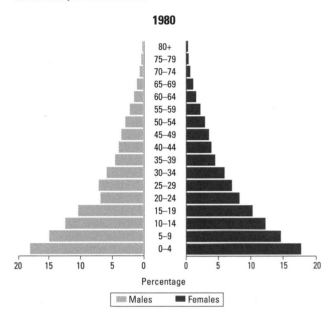

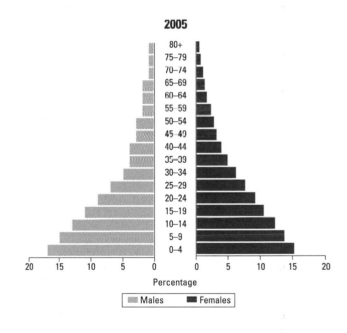

tion had grown to 11,237,196 inhabitants, of which 2,541,581 (22.6%) lived in the capital (9). By 2005, it had 12,700,611 inhabitants (9) and an average population density of 103 inhabitants per km^2, ranging from a high of 1,196 inhabitants per km^2 in the capital to a low of 10 inhabitants per km^2 in Petén department, with males making up 51.1% of the population (9).

A look at the population pyramid shows a high proportion (43%) of young people under the age of 15, with 15-to-44-year-olds representing 42% of the population, 45-to-65-year-olds representing 10% of the population, and adults over 65 years of age accounting for only 4% of the population (*1*). Population growth rates in Guatemala are among the highest in the region, with intracountry disparities and different total fertility rates (average number of children per woman) for each region and ethnic group. The sharpest declines in fertility rates are associated with nonindigenous women with a secondary education who live in rural areas, as illustrated in Figure 3 (*4*).

Life expectancy at birth for the total population was 68.9 years (65.5 years for males and 72.5 years for females) for the 5-year period 2000–2005. The crude birth rate in 2004 was 30.97 per 1,000 population (32.16 for males and 29.82 for females) (*1*). The share of the total population living in urban areas went from 35% to 46% between 1994 and 2002.

In 2002, 11% of the population was living in a department other than that of their birth as a result of internal migration. The departments of Guatemala, Sacatepéquez, Escuintla, Petén, and Izabal all had positive net migration rates. Six percent of the households surveyed had at least one family member permanently residing in another country in the 10-year period prior to the 2002 census. In 2002, 46% of the total population was living in an urban area (*1*).

Guatemala has a rich cultural, ethnic, and linguistic heritage. Indigenous Mayan, Xinka, and Garifuna peoples make up 41% of its total population. The three largest of the 21 Mayan groups are the K'iche' (28.8%), Q'eqchi' (19.3%), and Kaqchikel (18.9%); 68.3% of the Mayan population and 44.3% of the nonindigenous population live in rural areas. According to the 2005 National Human Development Report, 43.4% of the Mayan population is monolingual, able to speak only one of 21 Mayan languages (rather than Spanish) (*3*).

Table 1 lists the 10 leading causes of death by broad groups of causes in 1990 and 2001–2003. The general mortality rate for the period 2001–2003 was 5.71 per 1,000 population (*10*). The leading causes of general mortality for both sexes were influenza and pneumonia (14.7% of the total) and diarrhea (6.6%) (*10*). The male mortality rate was 6.74 per 100,000. The top cause of death was pneumonia, with a rate of 105 per 100,000, followed by events of undetermined intent (50.2 per 100,000), homicide (44.8 per 100,000), conditions originating in the perinatal period (48.4 per 100,000), and intestinal infectious diseases (47.8 per 100,000). The next highest ranked causes of death were cirrhosis, malnutrition and nutritional anemias, mental and behavioral disorders due to psychoactive substance use, ischemic heart diseases, and cerebrovascular diseases. The female mortality rate was 4.73 per 1,000 (*10*). The five leading causes of death among females were influenza and pneumonia (with a rate of 86.1 per 100,000), intestinal infectious diseases (38.2 per 100,000), conditions originating in the perinatal period (34.9 per 100,000), malnutrition and nutritional anemias (25.9 per 100,000), and diabetes (22 per 100,000). These were followed by cerebrovascular diseases, complications of heart failure, ischemic heart diseases, events of undetermined intent, and cirrhosis. According to the epidemiological surveillance system attached to the Ministry of Public Health and Social Welfare (MSPAS), 64.4% of deaths were certified by physicians, 8.9% by traditional birth attendants or midwives, and the remainder (26.7%) by other officials (*11*).

HEALTH OF POPULATION GROUPS

Children under 5 Years Old

The infant mortality rate for 2002 was 39 per 1,000 live births. The neonatal mortality rate was 22 per 1,000 live births and the

FIGURE 3. Total fertility rate, by educational level, ethnic origin, and region, Guatemala, 1987, 1995, 1998–1999, and 2002.

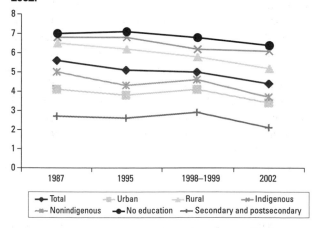

Source: Guatemala, Ministerio de Salud y Asistencia Social e Instituto Nacional de Estadística. Encuesta Nacional de Salud Materno Infantil (ENSMI), 1987–2002.

TABLE 1. Leading causes of death, by broad groups of causes, Guatemala (1990 and 2001–2003).

	Leading causes of death	
	1990	2001–2003
1	Acute diarrheal syndrome	Influenza and pneumonia
2	Bronchopneumonia	Intestinal infectious diseases
3	Measles	Conditions originating in the perinatal period
4	Malnutrition	Events of undetermined intent
5	Fevers	Assaults (homicides)
6	Unknown	Malnutrition and nutritional anemias
7	Senility	Cirrhosis and other liver diseases
8	Fluid and electrolyte disorders	Cerebrovascular diseases
9	Injuries from other unspecified causes	Diabetes
10	Low birthweight	Ischemic heart disease

postneonatal rate was 17 per 1,000 (*4*). The infant mortality rate came down from 48 per 1,000 in 1997 to its more recent levels, with the sharpest rates of decline in postneonatal mortality and very little improvement in neonatal mortality rates. Infant mortality rates are higher in rural areas (48 per 1,000 live births) than in urban areas (35 per 1,000) and higher for the indigenous population (49 per 1,000) than for the rest of the population (40 per 1,000). The highest infant mortality rates are associated with the southeastern (66 per 1,000), central (55 per 1,000), northeastern (53 per 1,000), and northern (51 per 1,000) regions of the country (*4*) and are closely correlated with rural living, poverty, and the share of indigenous peoples. Children under 1 year of age accounted for 18% of all deaths over the period 2001–2003 (*10*). The leading causes of death in this age group were conditions originating in the perinatal period (38.9%), pneumonia (26.9%), and diarrhea (11.8%). The infant mortality rate was 32 per 1,000 live births for both sexes, 35.3 per 1,000 for males, and 28.5 per 1,000 for females (*10*). According to data for 2002, 50% of live-born children accounted for 60% of all infant deaths, reflecting a 1.5-fold jump in inequality from the period prior to the survey.

Live-born children in Region V (Chimaltenango, Sacatepéquez, and Escuintla) face a 1.7 times greater risk of death in the first year of life than children born in Region I (the Metropolitan region). Thus, the risk of live-born children dying before reaching their first birthday in Region V is 24.54 per 1,000 live births more than the risk faced by children born in Region I. If all regions had the same infant mortality rate as the region with the lowest total rate (Region I, with a rate of 36.54 per 1,000 live births), the total infant mortality rate for all eight regions would have been lowered by close to 30%, preventing some 18,000 deaths among children under 1 year of age out of the approximately 61,000 deaths reported by the three surveys. The risk of children born in Region V (with the highest infant mortality rate) dying before reaching their first birthday is nearly twice that of children born in Region I (with the lowest infant mortality rate). Thus, there are 24.54 more deaths per 1,000 live births in Region V than in Region I (*12*).

Deaths of children between 1 and 4 years of age accounted for 7.4% of all deaths over the period 2001–2003 (*10*). The mortality rate for this age group was 59 per 1,000 live births (*4*). The leading causes of death in this age group were pneumonia, diarrhea, and malnutrition (*10*), and the main causes of morbidity were respiratory infections and diarrhea (*11*).

The net preprimary school enrollment rate for males and females in this age group is 45.2% (*8*). Significant progress has been made in furtherance of MDG 4 (reduce child mortality), as reflected in the decline in the child mortality rate from 121 per 1,000 live births in 1989 to 59 per 1,000 in 2004.

Children 5–9 Years Old

This age group made up 14.4% of the nationwide population in 2004. The leading causes of death were pneumonia, diarrhea, and accidents (unspecified polytraumas) in the case of males, and pneumonia, diarrhea, and malnutrition in the case of females (*10*). The net school enrollment rate in 2004 was 94.7% for males and 90.1% for females (*8*). The estimated dropout rate for this age group was 7%.

Adolescents 10–14 and 15–19 Years Old

This age group made up 24% of the population in 2005. Of this figure, 31.3% had access to a secondary education and 17.5% had access to a comprehensive secondary education. The gender breakdown was 32.6% and 17% for males and 30% and 18.1% for females (*8*). Seven percent of the population was enrolled in a university (7.0% of males and 4.8% of females), compared with rates of only 1.6% for indigenous males and 0.8% for indigenous females (*3*).

The leading causes of morbidity were injuries and accidents, which accounted for 91.3% of total morbidity (66.3% of which involved males) (*13*). The number of deaths among 15- to 19-year-olds (797) was three times the figure for the 10- to 14-year age group (273) (*10*). The leading causes of death among 10- to 14-year-old and 15- to 19-year-old males were infections and gunshot wounds, respectively.

This age group accounted for 5,868 reports of abuse and assaults in 2002 and 2003, of which 40% involved physical abuse; 27% involved rape; 11% involved abandonment; 9% involved sexual abuse and indecent acts; 8% involved assaults, injuries, and threats; 3% involved neglect; 3% involved attempted rapes; and 0.2% involved incest.

In 2002, the median age of adolescent females and males in urban areas at the time of their first sexual experience was 18.8 and 16.4 years, respectively (*4*), compared with figures of 17.7 and 16.9, respectively, for rural areas and 17.3 and 17.9, respectively, for the indigenous population. Moreover, 1.8% of youths of both sexes reported being raped in their first sexual encounter. This figure jumps to 18% among youths who had their first sexual experience before the age of 13 (*4*). Fifteen percent of 15- to 19-year-old girls were already mothers, and only 7.2% had used any form of birth control. Among women under 29 years of age, 28.2% had inter-pregnancy intervals of less than 24 months (*4*). As of June of 2004, there were 270 reported cases of AIDS among youths between 10 and 19 years of age (representing 3.8% of all AIDS cases).

Approximately 4,000 youths between the ages of 13 and 15 were living on the street (*14*). The main reasons these youths gave for living on the street were abuse, abandonment, and poverty; 20% of street kids reported having frequent suicidal thoughts. Sexual exploitation is a common phenomenon among street kids.

Adults 20–59 Years Old

According to the findings of the 2002 National Maternal and Child Health Survey (ENSMI), 84% of pregnant women reported having some type of prenatal checkup (*4*). The actual share of women receiving prenatal care varied according to their level of education (from 76% of women with no formal education, to 87% of women with a primary education, and 97% of women with a secondary or higher education). The percentage of pregnant women receiving at least one dose of tetanus toxoid in the course of their pregnancy was 64% nationwide (60% of indigenous women and 68% of nonindigenous women) (*4*).

Trained personnel attended 41.4% of all deliveries (with 37% of deliveries attended by physicians and 4.4% by nurses), and 47.5% of deliveries were attended by midwives. A breakdown by ethnic origin shows 16.4% of deliveries by indigenous women attended by trained personnel, compared with 52.0% of deliveries by nonindigenous women. On average, 11.4% of all deliveries nationwide, 18.8% of deliveries in urban areas, and 7.7% of deliveries in rural areas were by cesarean section (*4*). Among nonindigenous women, 15.8% of deliveries were by cesarean section, compared with 5.2% of deliveries by indigenous women. During the postpartum period, 20% of women nationwide, 12% of rural women, and 26% of urban women got postpartum care and 43% of newborns received follow-up care (*4*).

Of women living in free unions, 43.3% (23.8% of indigenous women and 52.8% of nonindigenous women) used some type of birth control method (34.4% used modern birth control methods and 8.8% used traditional methods). The most popular modern methods of birth control were female sterilization, hormone injections, the pill, condoms, IUDs, and male sterilization (*4*).

The year 2000 maternal mortality baseline put the maternal mortality rate at 153 per 100,000 live births, with an underregistration rate for maternal deaths of 44% nationwide (*15*). Maternal mortality rates came down by 30% over an 11-year period, from 219 (in 1989) to 153 per 100,000 live births (in 2000) (*15*). The highest maternal mortality rates were associated with the departments of Alta Verapaz (266.15 per 100,000 live births), Sololá (264.53), and Huehuetenango (245.83), all of which have a large rural, poor, indigenous population with limited access to health care. A breakdown by cause of death shows 53% of maternal mortality attributable to hemorrhaging during labor, 14% to septicemia, 12% to pregnancy-induced hypertension, 9.5% to abortions, and 11.5% to other causes. Of all maternal deaths, 66.5% involved women with no formal education. The risk of death for indigenous women was three times greater than for nonindigenous women and 1.38 times the national average. According to the findings of the same 2000 survey, the inequality in the regional distribution of maternal mortality is 2.3 times that of the pattern of infant mortality according to the at-risk population. As in the case of the dissimilarity index with respect to the distribution of infant mortality, 466 maternal deaths (or 23.6% of all deaths) would have to be redistributed among the different regions of the country in order to get the same maternal mortality rate (463.25 per 100,000 live births) in each region (*12*). Bearing in mind the reported maternal mortality rates in

each region, if all regions had the same maternal mortality rate as the region with the lowest rate (Region I, the Metropolitan region), the maternal mortality rate could have been lowered by 73.6%, preventing approximately 1,500 of the 2,000 reported maternal deaths, or roughly eight of every 10 maternal deaths. The largest number of preventable maternal deaths is associated with Region VI, the southwest, both in percentage terms and in absolute figures.

The risk of maternal death in Region VI (the southwest) was nearly seven times greater, or 722.76 per 100,000 live births more than in Region I (the Metropolitan region) (*12*). The progress made toward the attainment of MDG 5 ("improve maternal health") is reflected in the reduction in the maternal mortality rate from 248 per 100,000 live births in 1989 to 153 per 100,000 live births in the year 2000.

Cervical cancer is the leading cause of death among women of reproductive age (*16*). In 2003, 67.6% of women reported having taken a Pap test at some point in their life (77.0% of urban women versus 58.1% of rural women, and 42.3% of indigenous women compared with 73.7% of nonindigenous women).

The general mortality rate for males between 25 and 44 years of age was 5.94 per 1,000. The leading causes of death were homicide, with a rate of 95 per 100,000; events of undetermined intent (93 per 100,000); mental and behavioral disorders due to psychoactive substance use (56.4 per 100,000); cirrhosis (55.2 per 100,000); influenza and pneumonia (41.3 per 100,000); and HIV/AIDS (23.1 per 100,000) (*10*).

Older Adults 60 Years Old and Older

The size of the population aged 60 and above has been steadily growing for the past several decades. In 2002, this age group made up 6.3% of the total population (*1*), 5% of the rural population, and 4% of the urban population. An estimated 6% of older adults live alone and have no family support network. They have limited access to health care and very little social security coverage, with only 12.2% receiving any pension or retirement benefits. The leading causes of death for males over the age of 65 were influenza and pneumonia, cerebrovascular diseases, malnutrition, nutritional anemias, ischemic heart diseases, and complications of heart failure. The five leading causes of death for women aged 65 and above were influenza and pneumonia, cerebrovascular diseases, malnutrition and chronic anemias, diabetes, and complications of heart failure.

The Family

There are 2,200,608 households in Guatemala, of which 23% are headed by women. Of all heads of household, 45% reported having successfully completed at least one year of primary school (*4*). A breakdown of the population by marital status shows 35% married, 19% living in free unions, 40% single, and 3.7% divorced, separated, or widowed (4). Records for 2004 show 53,860 marriages and 1,888 divorces (17, 18).

Workers

There are an estimated 4,791,512 workforce members (10 years of age and older), of whom 63.7% are male. An estimated 69.1% of males and 75.3% of females are employed in the informal sector of the economy. The findings of the 2002 National Employment and Income Survey (ENEI) show 68.2% of male and 44.8% of female respondents in jobs with a work week of more than 40 hours (5). Only 19.2% of working males and 15.9% of working females were registered with the Guatemalan Social Security Institute (5). An estimated 34.1% of children between 7 and 14 years of age were working (53.9% as laborers, 38.2% as unpaid family workers, and 7.7% as self-employed workers).

The share of children between 7 and 9 years of age in the workforce is 2.7%. Child labor is a complex phenomenon in Guatemala, with numerous causes such as poverty, adult unemployment and underemployment, the lack of universal basic social services, and cultural acceptance of the concept of child labor (19). Examples of the types of jobs performed by children in this age group include firework-making and stone cutting.

Persons with Disabilities

There were an estimated 401,971 persons with some type of disability in 2005, for a rate of 37.4 per 1,000 population for both sexes, a male rate of 39.2 per 1,000 and a female rate of 35.6 per 1,000 (20). An estimated 65.9% of persons with disabilities are members of the nonindigenous population, and 52.8% of disabled males and 34.6% of disabled females are married. Moreover, 56.5% of disabled males reported knowing how to read, compared with only 42.6% of females. The most common types of disabilities are visual (27%), musculoskeletal (22.8%), auditory (18.1%), and mental (12.6%); 42.6% of disabled persons reported having never gotten any medical treatment for their disability, with most respondents giving a lack of money as the reason for not having been treated.

Ethnic Groups

Indigenous peoples make up 41.2% of the nationwide population, and the Maya account for 95.7% of the indigenous population. The departments with the largest proportions of indigenous peoples are Totonicapán (98%), Sololá (96%), Alta Verapaz (93%), and Quiche (89%) (1, 3).

There are discernible differences in the health status of the indigenous and nonindigenous populations. Infant mortality is higher among indigenous groups (49 per 1,000) than in the nonindigenous population (40 per 1,000), as is child mortality, with rates of 69 per 1,000 for the indigenous population compared

with 52 per 1,000 for the nonindigenous population (with virtually no change in this gap since 1995).

Most maternal deaths involve indigenous women as a result of their strained economic circumstances, higher fertility rates (with two to three more children than nonindigenous mothers), and poorer health care. The maternal mortality rate for indigenous women was three times that of nonindigenous women (211 per 100,000 live births versus 70 per 100,000 live births). Fewer indigenous women use contraceptives than nonindigenous women (23.8% versus 52.9%).

The share of the indigenous population with water service coverage varies according to the ethnic group in question (ranging from 62.0% to 77.8%). Likewise, the level of sanitation service coverage ranges from 64.9% to 79.2% (3).

Migrant Population

Every year, there is a significant volume of seasonal migration by farm workers, primarily from the northwest and parts of the east to farming areas for export crops (sugar cane and coffee). Of the 881,324 members of the country's migrant population in 2004, 18,894 received health care (21). The leading health problems affecting this population group are pesticide poisoning, vector-borne diseases, insect and snake bites, gastrointestinal diseases caused by the lack of a safe water supply and basic sanitation services, and poor food access.

HEALTH CONDITIONS AND PROBLEMS

COMMUNICABLE DISEASES

Vector-borne Diseases

Malaria is present mostly in the northern part of Guatemala. There were a total of 39,571 laboratory-diagnosed malaria cases in 2005, with an annual parasite index (API) of 4.94 per 1,000 population. A breakdown of these cases puts 53.3% in Alta Verapaz department, 25.85% in Petén department, and 5% in Ixcán (22, 23). Moreover, 17.1% of malaria cases involved children under 5 years of age, 32% involved children between 5 and 14 years of age, and 40% involved the population aged 15–49. There is a higher incidence of malaria among males, who accounted for 54% of all cases. The main causative agent was *Plasmodium vivax*, which accounted for 96% of all cases. The vectors present in malaria transmission areas were *Anopheles albimanus*, *A. pseudopuntipennis*, and *A. darlingi*. Case finding and treatment are community based. There were seven deaths from malaria in 2003 and a single death in 2004 (11, 21). The API for the country as a whole was 7.37 per 1,000 in 2002 and as high as 44.66 per 1,000 in high-risk areas. Of a total of 197,113 blood slides examined in 2002, 35,540 tested positive (18.03%) (23). The malaria morbidity and mortality index went from 0.4 in 1990 up to 3.1

per 1,000 in 2002 (nearly an eightfold jump). Given the relevance of this indicator in evaluating progress in furtherance of MDG 6 (combat HIV/AIDS, malaria, and other diseases), the country will need to redouble its efforts to attain this goal.

Dengue is present in 80% of the country, although 57% of all cases are concentrated in the Guatemala, Alta Verapaz, Escuintla, Zacapa, and Petén North health areas. There were a total of 828 laboratory-diagnosed cases of dengue in 2003, compared with 688 cases in 2005 (*24*). Most cases involved the population aged 15–30. There were four cases of hemorrhagic dengue and a single reported fatality in 2003. Males accounted for 52% of all cases. All four serotypes are in circulation in Guatemala. There are centralized serological diagnostic testing services based at the National Health Laboratory.

There are seven high-risk areas for infection with **Chagas' disease** in Guatemala (Huehuetenango, South Guatemala City, Santa Rosa, Escuintla, Sololá, Chimaltenango, and Suchitepéquez). The prevalence rate in children under 14 years of age is 5%. All blood used in transfusions is screened for Chagas' disease. In 2001, *Rhodnius prolixus* was found in 241 communities nationwide. By 2005, two rounds of spraying in 1,996 or 100% of all infested communities had effectively eliminated this vector. The house infestation index for *Triatoma dimidiata* was brought down to 2.7% in 2005. The seroprevalence rate for *Trypanosoma cruzi* among blood donors was 1.4% in 2004 and 0.011% in 2006 (*25*).

Onchocerciasis is present in nine of the country's health areas (Chiquimula, Zacapa, Jalapa, Jutiapa, El Progreso, Huehuetenango, Santa Rosa, Baja Verapaz, and Quiché). The main intervention strategy is treatment with Mectizan. There were 160,418 eligible recipients in 2003, or 320,836 treatments administered in 518 endemic communities (*26*). Guatemala had exceeded its 85% coverage target by 2002, reaching 91% of patients with the first round of treatment and 95% in round two. By 2003, the coverage rate for both rounds of treatment was as high as 96%.

Vaccine-preventable Diseases

The country's high and constantly improving vaccination coverage rates have helped lower the incidence of vaccine-preventable diseases. In fact, the last reported case of paralytic **poliomyelitis** was in 1990, and the last laboratory-confirmed case of **measles** was reported in 1997. **Diphtheria** has disappeared, and neonatal **tetanus** has not been a public health problem since the 1990s. The number of cases of **tuberculous meningitis** is also way down, and the number of cases of **pertussis** or whooping cough and related fatalities is lower than ever, with all outbreaks concentrated in a handful of municipios. These achievements have all helped further MDG 4, which is to reduce child mortality. Country-wide vaccination coverage rates for children under 1 year of age in 2005 were 2% for the DTPw-HB/Hib pentavalent combination vaccine (against diphtheria, pertussis, tetanus, hepatitis B, and *Haemophilus influenzae* type

b), 92% for the OPV (Sabin oral polio vaccine), 96% for the BCG (bacillus Calmette-Guérin) vaccine, and 93% for the MMR (triple viral vaccine against measles, rubella, and mumps) for children between 12 and 23 months of age. The country is compliant with most acute flaccid paralysis surveillance indicators and integrated measles and rubella surveillance indicators.

A retrospective study conducted in 2005 identified 45 cases of defects consistent with congenital **rubella** syndrome and five confirmed cases, projecting a total of 2,225 cases over the next 15 years. A vaccination drive aimed at administering the MR vaccine (the double viral vaccine against measles and rubella) to 7.4 million recipients was scheduled for early in 2007.

The pentavalent combination vaccine was introduced in 2005 during Vaccination Week in the Americas, increasing the number of antigens in the basic vaccination scheme from eight in 2001 to 10 in 2005. Introduction of the flu vaccine in 2007 and the rotavirus vaccine is also being considered. The 2003, 2004, and 2006 immunization drives conducted as part of Vaccination Week in the Americas focused on reaching inaccessible rural, indigenous, and poor urban communities and improving coverage in problem municipios. The challenges facing this program include raising fiscal revenues to ensure its sustainability, attracting funding to strengthen the cold chain, introducing new vaccines, and achieving and sustaining high coverage levels in most municipios.

Intestinal Infectious Diseases

Intestinal diseases, defined as "intestinal parasitosis" and "acute diarrheal disease," were the second and third leading causes of general morbidity (accounting for 17.2% of all illness) and of morbidity within the 1- to 4-year age group in 2003 (accounting for 22.8% of the total) (*11*). Acute diarrheal syndrome was ranked second, and intestinal parasitosis was ranked sixth among causes of morbidity in children under 1 year of age. A total of 408,973 cases were reported in 2003. The general morbidity rate from this cause was 3,383 per 100,000 population. There were 3,636 reported deaths from acute diarrheal disease in 2004, of which 51% involved males and 24% involved children under 1 year of age. The general mortality rate from diarrhea was 42.9 per 100,000 population.

Chronic Communicable Diseases

There were 3,727 new cases of all forms of **tuberculosis** diagnosed in 2005 (for a rate of 27.23 per 100,000 population), which is equivalent to only 23.7% of the expected number of cases based on World Health Organization (WHO) estimates, suggesting the need to improve case finding and detection (*27*). There were 2,420 laboratory-diagnosed cases of tuberculosis based on positive sputum smears, for a rate of 17.75 per 100,000 population, or 48% of the expected number of cases based on WHO estimates. The number of new cases of all forms of tuberculosis (pulmonary tuberculosis with acid-fast bacilli or AFB-positive sputum smears, extrapulmonary tuberculosis, and pediatric tuberculosis) has leveled off in the last 14 years, at rates of from 19.80 (2001) to 27.33 (2005) per 100,000 population for all forms of tuberculosis and from 14.30 (2001) to 17.75 (2005) for AFB-positive tuberculosis (27). Case detection rates in health facilities are low (48%), cure rates are fair (75%), and suggested global and national targets are still unattainable (a 75% case detection rate and 85% cure rate). Laboratory networks are poorly organized. The increase in the number of cases of tuberculosis is partially attributable to tuberculosis-HIV/AIDS coinfection present in 25% to 30% of HIV-positive patients. The rate of primary multidrug resistance is 3% (27). There has been visible progress with respect to MDG 6 (combat HIV/AIDS, malaria, and other diseases), measured by the morbidity rate associated with tuberculosis, which came down from 32 to 24 per 100,000 population between 1990 and 2001.

Leprosy diagnoses are made in response to spontaneous demand in facilities not run by the Ministry of Health. There has been only one diagnosed case a year for the last four years.

Acute Respiratory Infections

Acute respiratory infections are the leading cause of morbidity and mortality in Guatemala. There were 1,306,255 cases of acute respiratory infection in 2003, for a rate of 1,059 per 10,000 population (107), of which 60% involved children under the age of 5. The general mortality rate for pneumonia was 9.19 per 10,000 population, with higher rates in rural areas and among children whose mothers have less education. The general mortality rate for acute respiratory infections was 95.4 per 100,000 population (10). Acute respiratory infections were the third leading cause of death in the adult population aged 15–44 and the top cause of death among adults aged 45 and above.

There was an outbreak of influenza in 2002 among schoolchildren in the capital, in which the influenza A H1N1 New Caledonia virus as well as influenza B/Brisbane/32/2002-like viruses were detected.

HIV/AIDS and Other Sexually Transmitted Infections

There were 8,685 reported cases of AIDS between January of 1984 and August of 2005 (for a rate of 79.4 per 100,000 population based on reported cases of the disease) (28), with 77% of all cases concentrated in the departments of Suchitepéquez (with a rate of 150.1 per 100,000 population), Guatemala (149.5), Izabal (136.8), Escuintla (128.2), Retalhuleu (127.1), and Quetzaltenango (109.7). The male-female ratio went from 8:1 in 1988 to 2:4 in 2005, dropping sharply beginning in the year 1997. The AIDS epidemic is spreading in the general population. The population aged 15–49 accounts for 83.2% of all cases, and 52.1% of all AIDS cases involve members of the 20- to 34-year age group. The most common route of transmission is through sexual intercourse, which accounts for 94.4% of AIDS cases, with 5% of AIDS cases involv-

ing mother-to-child transmission (28). There are no reports of any cases of AIDS transmission attributable to intravenous drug use. The main transmission route is through sexual intercourse and, according to studies, the highest prevalence rates for AIDS are associated with men who have sex with other men (MSM) and female sex workers (FSW), who have become bridge populations for its transmission to heterosexuals and women not employed in the sex industry, which has also boosted the number of cases of vertical transmission. The coverage rate for antiretroviral treatment was 68% among the adult population. There has been visible progress in furtherance of MDG 6 in terms of the indicator measuring the rate of contraceptive use, which jumped from 4.5% in 1987 to 57% in 2002.

Other sexually transmitted infections are treated in health facilities in response to spontaneous demand. According to one-off studies, the prevalence of syphilis is 13% among MSM and 10% among FSW. The prevalence rate for all other sexually transmitted infections among female sex workers is 21.9%. Efforts to expand the coverage of sexually transmitted infection syndrome management approaches at the local level have been unsuccessful.

Zoonoses

There were 20 cases of seropositive animals exhibiting no clinical symptoms of **West Nile virus** in 2004, in which it was impossible to isolate the virus. There is active and passive surveillance of all symptomatic cases through the epidemiological surveillance system for animal diseases attached to the Policy and Regulations Unit of the Ministry of Food, Agriculture and Livestock (MAGA) (29).

The incidence of **brucellosis** jumped from 10 to 49 cases between 2002 and 2005. The MAGA is working with animal health brigades and veterinary epidemiologists in all parts of the country. Milk monitoring activities in processing plants for dairy products based on the milk ring test yielded a 9% positivity rate for 808 sampled farms (29).

Sampling for **bovine tuberculosis** started in 2005 led to the detection of 12 cases of the disease, resulting in the restriction of 171 herds, with no herds declared free of the disease. The MAGA has its own monitoring and control program (29). There is ongoing surveillance for **leptospirosis**, including searches for cases with related symptomatology. There were no reported cases of the disease in Guatemala during the period between 2001 and 2005, although a number of seropositive animals were found, prompting the recommendation of preventive vaccinations for the equine population (29).

Though there have been no reported cases of **foot-and-mouth disease**, there is ongoing surveillance of all cases with similar symptomatology, since foot and mouth disease can be confused with vesicular stomatitis, which is present in Guatemala (29). With reports of low-pathogenicity H5N2 avian influenza present in Guatemala, all suspected cases are monitored under the Poultry Health Program (29).

Addressing Health Care Gaps among the Indigenous People

Indigenous peoples make up 41% of the population of Guatemala, and there are evident differences in the health status of the indigenous and nonindigenous population. Infant mortality is higher among indigenous people (49 per 1,000 live births) than in the nonindigenous population (40 per 1,000), as is child mortality, 69 per 1,000 among indigenous people and 52 per 1,000 in the nonindigenous population, with virtually no change in this gap since 1995. Most maternal deaths involve indigenous women as a result of their more precarious economic circumstances, higher fertility rates—two or three children more than nonindigenous mothers—, and more limited access to health care.

The Mayan population, the country's largest indigenous population, has access to community-based traditional and alternative health care services offered by a number of nongovernmental organizations. There is a popular, traditional and alternative medicine program within the Health Ministry with treatment regimens based on the use of medicinal plants. The Ministry's Coverage Extension Program designed to provide health care coverage for people without access to other health care services is targeted specifically at the 12 departments with the largest indigenous populations.

Although there are no records of any cases of **bovine spongiform encephalitis** in Guatemala, there is ongoing active surveillance for this disease. There have been reports of seropositive animals for Venezuelan equine encephalitis, with one reported case of the disease in 2004 and another in 2005. There is ongoing active surveillance for this disease, and preventive vaccinations for the equine population are recommended (29).

There were no reported cases of human **rabies** over the period between 2002 and 2004. There was one reported case in 2005 in a child from a periurban area of Guatemala City, caused by a dog bite. Most cases of animal rabies involve dogs and cattle. The number of cases leveled off between 2002 and 2004, with approximately 93 dogs and 6 head of cattle testing positive in laboratory tests. Canine vaccination coverage levels were consistently in the 62% to 70% range over the period between 2002 and 2005.

NONCOMMUNICABLE DISEASES

Metabolic and Nutritional Diseases

The percentage of children between 3 and 59 months of age with chronic **malnutrition** in 2002 was 49.3%, compared with rates of 46.4% and 57.9% in 1998 and 1987, respectively, with 21.2% of this age group suffering from severe chronic malnutrition. Chronic malnutrition is a more serious problem in indigenous (69.5%) than nonindigenous (35.7%) children (4) and up to three times more prevalent in children with uneducated mothers (64.8% of mothers of malnourished children had no formal education, and only 18.4% of mothers with a secondary or postsecondary education had children suffering from malnutrition) (4). Children from families with less than 14,000 square meters of land (1.4 hectares) were found to have a 3.2 times greater risk of malnutrition than children from families with more than 35,000 square meters (3.5 hectares) of land.

Moreover, 22.1% of pregnant women with children under 59 months of age were anemic. A geographic breakdown put the share of anemic mothers in urban areas at 18%, compared with 24.1% in rural areas. Only 14.4% of mothers with a secondary or postsecondary education were affected by anemia, compared with 21.8% of uneducated mothers.

The share of schoolchildren suffering from chronic malnutrition was as high as 48.8%. Studies of the diets of school-age children found only 16% of this group eating enough calories, 35% eating enough protein, and barely 2% getting enough iron. Among children under 3 years of age, 38% had blood levels of iron below 11 g/dl. The incidence of **anemia** is significantly higher in younger children. The share of children under 5 years of age with a vitamin A deficiency (blood-serum retinol concentrations of less than 20 µg/dl) was 15.8% (30). Moreover, 49% of first-grade pupils showed signs of **stunting** (31).

The body mass index (BMI) of 1.9% of the female population between 15 and 49 years of age is below 18.5. The Petén (4.1%), southeastern (3.8%), and central (3.1%) regions have the highest percentages of underweight women (4). As of 2002, the average height of Guatemalan women was 149.2 centimeters, and 25.4% of women fell short of the critical threshold value of 145 centimeters. Moreover, 47.5% of indigenous women measured less than 145 cm, compared with 15.2% of nonindigenous women. On average, women with a secondary and postsecondary education were 7 centimeters taller than women with no education. Iron deficiency anemia was present in 22.1% of pregnant women and 20.2% of nonpregnant women.

The rate of breast-feeding is inversely correlated with the age of the child. Only children up to five months of age are exclusively breast-fed. Breast-feeding is more widespread in rural areas (58.5%) and among indigenous peoples (63.3%), compared with urban dwellers (34.7%) and the nonindigenous population (40.4%). It is also more widespread in the northwestern and southwestern regions (70.8% and 62.9%, respectively) and less common in the Metropolitan (36.2%) and northeastern regions (36.4%) (*4*).

Diabetes was the eighth leading cause of general mortality over the period from 2001 to 2003, with a rate of 19.9 per 100,000 population. It was the fifth leading cause of death in the female population, with a rate of 22 per 100,000. A 2002 study in a peri-urban area of Guatemala City (Villa Nueva) put the prevalence rate of diabetes at 8.4% for both sexes among the population over 40 years of age. Of the study population, 80% was **overweight**, 44% suffered from obesity, and 54% did not get enough physical exercise.

Cardiovascular Diseases

Cerebrovascular diseases and **ischemic heart diseases** were ranked seventh and ninth among the leading causes of general mortality for the period 2001 to 2003, with rates of 20.7, 19.9, and 18.8 per 100,000 population, respectively. Male mortality rates for ischemic heart disease and cerebrovascular diseases were 21.4 per 100,000 and 20.9 per 100,000, respectively. Cerebrovascular diseases were the sixth leading cause of death among the female population, with a rate of 20.6 per 100,000, and the female mortality rate for ischemic heart diseases was 16.4 per 100,000 (*10*). A breakdown by region shows large disparities in the geographic pattern of chronic diseases, which are more common in Regions I and III (the Metropolitan and the northeast) and less common in Regions VI and VII (the southwest and the northwest).

A 2002 study in a periurban area of Guatemala City (Villa Nueva) put the prevalence of arterial **hypertension** at 13%, with very little difference between the sexes or between different over-40 age groups.

Malignant Neoplasms

The National Cancer Registry (a non-population-based registry), which keeps records of all cancer cases treated by the National Cancer Institute, reported a total of 2,303 cases of cancer in 2003 (1,444 involving women and 559 involving men) (*32*). The most common cancer sites were the cervix (47.5%), breast (14.7%), and skin (7.3%) in women, and the prostate (13.1%), skin (12.3%), and stomach (10.0%) in men (*32*).

OTHER HEALTH PROBLEMS OR ISSUES

Disasters

There were 564 floods between 1996 and the year 2000, mostly on the Pacific slope. In October of 2005, tropical storm Stan claimed 1,514 lives, left another 2,723,000 homeless (*33*), and caused approximately US$ 988.03 million in economic losses, of which 42.6% involved capital losses, with the remainder in the form of post-disaster losses in economic flows. The infrastructure (45%), productive (27%), and social (15%) sectors absorbed

most of the impact. The hardest hit departments were San Marcos and Retalhuleu (*13*).

Violence and Other External Causes

The Guatemalan people put a premium on public safety. There were 29,436 crimes reported in 2003 nationwide (including physical assaults and violations of laws), of which 85.9% involved males and 14.4% (4,237) were homicides (*34*), with 43.3% of all homicides committed in Guatemala City (*34*). There were also reports of assaults, crimes against property, sex crimes, and unlawful restraint. There has been a wave of murders of young women since 2001, which has prompted an investigation into gender-based homicides (Figure 4). There was a 56.8% jump in female homicides between 2002 and 2004.

According to the report on crimes against women in Guatemala (*35*), of female crime victims, 17.5% were under the age of 13, 11.9% were between the ages of 14 and 17, 25.5% were between 18 and 25 years of age, 44.5% were from 26 to 59 years of age, and 5.8% were 60 and above.

Road safety statistics put the number of traffic accidents at 4,680 in 2004 and 5,127 in 2005. Traffic accidents claimed 692 lives and left 4,336 people injured in 2002, with 581 dead and 2,586 injured in 2004. There are approximately a million motor vehicles on the nation's roads, and this figure is growing at an annual rate of 30%.

Addictions

Fifty-two percent of youths between 12 and 19 years of age consumed alcohol, 42% smoked cigarettes, 18% took tranquilizers, 8% used stimulants, 4% smoked marihuana, 2% used inhalants, 2% used cocaine, 1% smoked crack, and 1% took ecstasy (*36*). Among youths consuming alcohol, 44% had at least one alcohol-related problem and 18% had gotten intoxicated. Fifteen

FIGURE 4. Number of complaints filed and homicide prosecutions by the Special Prosecutor's Office for Crimes Against Women, Guatemala, 2001–2004.

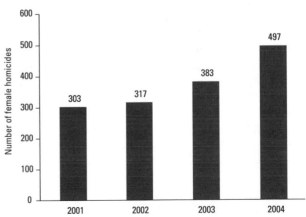

Source: Guatemala Instituto Nacional de Estadística. Crime statistics for 2003.

percent of all youths had problems involving the use of other types of drugs (*36*). The average age at the time of their first experience with alcohol, cigarettes, and inhalants was 12.5 to 13.5 and one or two years older at the time of their first experience with other types of drugs. There is a high correlation between alcohol consumption and the use of illicit drugs, with drinkers eight times more likely to use illegal drugs.

Environmental Pollution

The country visibly stepped up its imports of pesticides between the year 2000 and 2002, from 10,429.22 to 11,277.57 tons. There were 1,116 reported cases of pesticide poisoning in 2002, for a poisoning rate of 9.3 per 100,000 population, and 238 deaths, for a mortality rate of 1.98 per 100,000. The fatality rate from pesticide poisoning was 21.3% (*37*). Of the 1,043 reported cases of pesticide poisoning in 2004, the most common types of poisoning were from organophosphates and herbicides. Males accounted for 71% of all poisonings, with 2% involving children under the age of 5. Occupational poisonings accounted for 43.4% of all cases (*21*).

Oral Health

The decayed, missing, and filled teeth (DMFT) index for 12-year-olds was 4.9% for males and 5.5% for females in 2002. According to Dean's index, 2.7% of males exhibited mild dental fluorosis, 2.5% had moderate fluorosis, and 0.3% had severe fluorosis. The figures for females were 3.8%, 2.0%, and 0.4%, respectively.

RESPONSE OF THE HEALTH SECTOR

Health Policies and Plans

The Government Plan for 2004–2008 sets out basic lines of action and health policies. Current health policies are aimed at strengthening the oversight role of the Ministry of Public Health and Social Welfare, meeting public health needs, stepping up the deconcentration and decentralization process, ensuring timely procurements and stores of health supplies, streamlining the Ministry of Public Health and Social Welfare's administrative-financial management and planning system, strengthening human resource management and development for health, promoting environmental sanitation measures improving the quality of life of the Guatemalan people, and protecting the public from hazards associated with the consumption of and exposure to foods, drugs, and substances with adverse health effects (*38*).

The Guatemalan Social Security Institute's (IGSS) strategic plan for 2004–2008 is designed to make basic reforms in the IGSS geared to improving its competitiveness, efficiency, and institutional work quality while promoting ethics, stability, and growth. Its strategic objectives are to oversee the delivery of timely, efficient, high-quality services to meet the needs of corresponding beneficiaries, strengthen its human resources, ensure transparent financial management, trim spending, and make timely pension and benefit payments. There is also a sixth internal objective aimed at improving its institutional image (*39*).

The third health policy alluded to above involves stepping up the deconcentration and decentralization of authority, responsibility, resources, and decision-making power to health areas and hospitals as established in the Basic Internal Regulations. These regulations are implemented by the Ministry of Health based on a new administrative-financial management and planning model defining the management authority of Health Area Offices. The Integrated Health Care System (SIAS) extended coverage by a basic health service package to 3.2 million rural residents who previously had no access to these health care services (*40*).

The findings of the evaluation of essential public health functions (EPHF) in 2002 and 2003 showed improvements in EPHF 1 (monitoring, evaluation, and analysis of the health situation), EPHF 2 (public health surveillance, research, and control of risks and threats to public health), and EPHF 11 (reducing the impact of emergencies and disasters on health).

The Health Code, Decree 90-97 organizing and regulating health-related activities, is the legal framework governing all operations in the health sector. There are also other legislative texts governing the health industry. Table 2 outlines the main pieces of legislation governing activities in the health sector (*41*).

Health Strategies and Programs

The major health strategies for the period 2004–2008 include strengthening the oversight role of the Ministry of Health and streamlining its management, improving the quality control system for spending, optimizing existing financial and human resources, human resource development, decentralization and deconcentration, public participation, implementing the current legal framework, intra- and extrasectoral coordination, extending service coverage to at-risk groups, technical and financial cooperation, and providing adequate supplies of drugs (*38*).

The country's 17 health priorities were set based on its vulnerability and risk profile and include maternal and neonatal mortality; malnutrition; communicable diseases, including respiratory infections, water-, food-, and vector-borne diseases, vaccine-preventable diseases, zoonoses, tuberculosis and sexually transmitted infections (HIV/AIDS); noncommunicable diseases (accidents and violence, chronic and degenerative diseases, addictions, pesticide poisoning, oral-dental health problems, and mental health problems); disasters; and demand response, all of which focus on the most vulnerable and highest risk population groups.

Organization of the Health System

The Ministry of Public Health and Social Welfare is the oversight agency for the health sector and one of its main service

TABLE 2. Major health legislation and provisions, Guatemala.

Type of legislation	Date passed	Objective
Social Development Act	October 2001	Establish a legal framework for the institution of legal proceedings and public policies for the promotion, planning, coordination, implementation, monitoring, and evaluation of State and government social, family, human, and environmental development programs, with the emphasis on special needs groups.
General Decentralization Act	April 2002	Fulfill the State's constitutional duty to systematically promote economic and political decentralization for effective national development.
Urban and Rural Development Councils Act	March 2002	Strengthen the development councils system as the main participation mechanism. Views the development councils system as the main mechanism for engaging the Mayan, Xinka, and Garifuna peoples and the nonindigenous population in public policy making as the basis for a democratic development planning process guided by principles of national, multiethnic, pluricultural, and multilingual unity geared to the country's diverse population.
Food and Nutritional Security Act	2005	Implement policy measures reducing abject poverty and strengthening food and nutritional security at the country level.
Signature of the Framework Agreement on Tobacco Control	November 2003, ratified in November of 2005	Protect present and future generations from the harmful effects of tobacco. First international public health treaty with the unanimous backing of 192 countries.
Patent and Trademark Act	2000, as subsequently amended	Protect intellectual creativity with business and industrial applications. Addresses the definition of a "new product" and upholds the five-year protection period for clinical trial data.
Implementing Regulations for the Transfusion Medicine Services and Blood Banks Act	2003	Facilitate the establishment of a Blood Bank Program, which later became the Transfusion Medicine and Blood Bank Program under Ministerial Order AM955-2006.
Ministerial Order Renewing the Primary Health Care Commitment	2004	Renew the commitment to achieve health for all by strengthening primary health care services under the Peace Accords.
Law for the Prevention, Punishment, and Eradication of Domestic Violence and Violence against Women	1996	Govern the implementation of necessary measures to protect the life, physical safety, security, and dignity of victims of domestic violence. Afford special protections for women, children, youths, the elderly, and the disabled, in keeping with their specific circumstances. The implementation of these protective measures is independent of specific penalties established under the Penal Code and Code of Criminal Procedure for felonies or misdemeanors.
HIV/AIDS Act	December 2000	Establish a legal framework for the implementation of necessary mechanisms for HIV/AIDS education, prevention, epidemiological surveillance, research, treatment, and follow-up and guarantee, promote, protect, and defend the human rights of persons with HIV and AIDS.

providers. Other stakeholders in the public health sector include the municipalities, the universities, the Ministries of Government and Defense, social funds, and the National Fund for Peace. The Guatemalan Social Security Institute (IGSS) serves members of the working population and their beneficiaries, retirees, and pension holders under Accident, Disability, Retirement, and Survivorship programs in 22 departments around the country and Maternity and Common Disease programs in 19 departments (39). The private health sector consists of private diagnostic facilities, hospitals, and physicians' practices and clinics.

The Ministry of Public Health and Social Welfare serves approximately 70% of the population. The IGSS covers 18.4%, and the private sector serves a small segment of the population (approximately 12%).

The Ministry of Public Health and Social Welfare is broken down into 29 Health Area Offices. Health Area Offices and hospitals are in charge of budget implementation. Health care services are delivered through health provider networks with varying levels of sophistication and resolution capacity. The IGSS has a deconcentrated service network geared to its health programs.

There are private for-profit and nonprofit health care services. For-profit services are delivered through a hospital services network, 50% of which is concentrated in the department of Guatemala. The nonprofit sector consists of nongovernmental organizations.

According to estimates for 2004, women accounted for 18.3% of the IGSS insured population. There is very little private insurance coverage. Only comprehensive insurance providers offer health care services backed by a provider network. Certain physicians' groups and hospital centers have set up prepayment schemes (42).

As far as health care for the indigenous population is concerned, a number of nongovernmental organizations are providing community-based traditional and alternative health care services to the Mayan population. There is a popular, traditional, and alternative medicine program within the Health Ministry with treatment regimens based on the use of medicinal plants (43). The Ministry of Public Health and Social Welfare's Coverage Extension Program designed to provide health care coverage for people without access to other health care services is targeted at the 12 departments with the largest indigenous populations (4).

Public Health Services

Health service coverage has been expanded to deliver free health care to the country's most underprivileged population groups in the form of a package of 26 basic health services. The health care model is geared to the country's demographic features: multilingual, multiethnic, and pluricultural. In 2005, these services were offered in 184 municipios with 394 jurisdictions, each with approximately 10,000 residents, with indigenous peoples accounting for 60% of the population served. The basic geographic unit is a jurisdiction serviced by a basic health team consisting of physicians, a nurse, and community workers. Social Security offices in two departments (Escuintla and Suchitepéquez) have also implemented the coverage extension strategy expanding service coverage to the general population through health promotion, development, and preventive health programs.

The Ministry of Public Health and Social Welfare has programs for maternal and child health, communicable diseases, noncommunicable diseases, social problems (violence and addiction), and food security and nutrition in all health care facilities, according to their level of sophistication. Social security programs include disease-prevention activities relating to reproductive health, accidents, and common diseases, as well as counseling and educational activities for different groups of patients.

The Epidemiology Department attached to the Ministry of Public Health and Social Welfare has a nationwide network of epidemiologists based in hospitals and health areas (44). It also has laboratories at the secondary health care level in charge of performing basic clinical laboratory procedures. Tertiary level care is bolstered by chemical, hematological, and bacteriological technology. Epidemiological surveillance activities are backed by the National Reference Laboratory, whose duties include performing specialized diagnostic tests, setting standards, monitoring, and supervision.

According to information on access to a clean water supply and sanitation services, Guatemalan households have water service only 16.7 hours a day (only 13.1 hours a day in the Metropolitan region). As of 2002, 92.4% of Guatemalan households had a drinking water supply less than 15 minutes from their home (on foot), compared with 91.9% in 1995 (4). National Census data from 2002 (45) showed 75% of the population with access to an improved water supply (60% of the rural population and 90% of the urban population) and 47% with access to improved sanitation services (77% in urban areas and 47% in rural areas). Levels of bacteriological and physical/chemical pollution affecting raw water quality in most surface water sources are unacceptable. Groundwater resources and headwaters protected by local communities are of better quality. There is no oversight or regulatory agency for water supply and sanitation services. Each municipality is responsible for regulating and setting rates for these services under the provisions of the Municipal Code. Water supply and sanitation services are operated by both public and private service providers.

Solid waste management services are decentralized, with each municipality responsible for providing refuse collection service. Municipal or private solid waste collection services are used by 58.3% of urban households and 4.5% of rural households (1). The Ministry of Public Health and Social Welfare approved and issued Hospital Solid Waste Management Regulations in 2003.

Central America agreed to restrictions and bans on a list of 12 pesticides headed by Paraquat in the year 2000.

Food safety and control measures include regulations and standards compliance monitoring through a company registration system and national staff of technicians conducting inspections of major food manufacturers.

The National Food and Nutritional Security Council (CONASAN) headed up by the Vice President of Guatemala includes representatives of government agencies, the business sector, civil society, and the Food and Nutritional Security Program (PROSAN). It is a technical regulatory body responsible for implementing health measures designed to strengthen food and nutritional security in the public interest. The government has been pushing forward with a National Program for Combating Chronic Malnutrition targeted at pregnant and breast-feeding women and children under 3 years of age since 2005.

The National Disaster Relief Coordination Center (CONRED) is the agency in charge of coordinating, planning, setting up, and mounting all activities designed to mitigate the effects of natural, socionatural, or anthropogenic disasters and avoid new threats through disaster prevention, mitigation, and response efforts.

Individual Care Services

The Ministry of Public Health and Social Welfare delivers health care through a service network. The IGSS and the Ministries of Defense and of Governance also provide health care services. The Health Ministry has 1,301 health facilities around the country, and the IGSS has another 97 facilities (*39, 46*). The Ministry of Health also operates 1,244 hubs, 926 health posts, and 300 core units at the primary health care level. There are three integrated maternal and child health care centers (CAIMI), 32 type A health centers, 249 type B centers, 16 canton-level maternity centers, 3 satellite clinics, and 32 comprehensive care centers at the secondary level. The tertiary level consists of 43 hospitals, including 2 national referral hospitals and 7 specialty, 8 regional, 16 departmental, 5 district, and 5 contingency hospitals. In sum, there are 6,030 hospital beds in Health Ministry hospitals.

The IGSS has 145 health facilities, including 23 hospitals, 30 outpatient clinics, 59 comprehensive health care units, and another 33 health posts, polyclinics, satellite clinics, and comprehensive health care centers, with 50% of its services concentrated in 6 departments (*39*).

The country has clinical, reference, anatomical pathology, and imaging laboratories and blood banks based mainly in secondary and tertiary level facilities run by the Ministry of Public Health and Social Welfare, IGSS hospitals, and a private health care providers network duly accredited by the Health Ministry. The National Health Laboratory consists of the Unified Food and Drug Control Laboratories and Central Reference Laboratory. The National Transfusion Medicine and Blood Banks Program has legal backing for the framing of national policies aimed at ensuring a safe national blood supply.

The Mental Health Program has stepped up the deconcentration of services previously based at the National Mental Health Hospital and has been working to incorporate a mental health component as part of the integrated health care system (SIAS), with the emphasis on an integrated approach to the treatment of victims of the armed conflict and on services aimed at reducing levels of public psychosocial vulnerability during natural disasters.

Health Promotion

Health promotion strategies have been implemented at the municipal level since the year 2000 as part of so-called "municipios for development" initiatives, in keeping with ongoing social reforms. A total of 41 municipal health commissions have been formed and charged with implementing healthy schools and adolescent-friendly health services strategies. The Health and Education Ministries crafted a joint healthy schools plan in 2004, establishing guidelines for the integration of multisectoral projects and programs (*47*). Four universities in Guatemala City are implementing the tobacco smoke-free environments strategy.

Health Supplies

There are 77 private, domestically funded laboratories and three multinational enterprises in Guatemala, 15 of which are the source for 60% of all government procurements, with all remaining supplies purchased from importers of generic and brand name products, mainly from the United States, Mexico, the European Union, Colombia, and Argentina (*48*). The Ministry of Health is in charge of drug monitoring and quality control activities, issuing marketing permits, licensing pharmaceutical firms, monitoring good manufacturing practices, and performing physical/chemical and/or microbiological analyses at the National Health Laboratory. According to the 2005 inspection report, 81% of laboratories meet established standards for good manufacturing practices.

All immunobiologicals are imported from drug companies licensed to supply drugs to the private market.

Clinical diagnostic reagents are procured in accordance with the provisions of the Government Contracting Act, which are marketed by duly licensed firms.

Most equipment is imported, and health equipment is subject to registration with the Registration and Inspection Department for Drugs and Related Products.

Human Resources

As of the end of 2005, the country had a total of 12,273 licensed physicians (*49*), of whom 71% were male and 29% female. There has been a gradual increase in the share of female physicians over the last 10 years. Of the country's 2,346 dentists, 60.5% were male and 39.5% female (*50*). There are no data for nursing personnel but, according to estimates based on information from the country's main national service delivery agencies (the Ministry of Public Health and Social Welfare and the IGSS), there are four physicians and six nursing aides for each professional nurse. The population-to-physician ratio was 9.7 per 10,000 in 2005, ranging from a high of 30.8 per 10,000 in urban areas to less than 2 per 100,000 in rural areas. Figures for dentists are similar, with a ratio of 1.9 per 10,000 population, ranging from a high of 6.6 per 10,000 in the department of Guatemala to less than 1 in 18 of the other 21 departments.

Training programs for health professionals are university based. Five of the country's 11 universities train physicians and surgeons in four programs offered in the capital and two in the interior. The health sector added 188 Cuban-trained Guatemalan physicians to its ranks in 2006. The only training programs in dentistry are at the national university and two private universities in the capital. There are training programs for nursing personnel at three different academic levels turning out degreed nurses (with a *"licenciatura"* or bachelor's degree), university technicians, or professional nurses and nursing aides. There are six national schools for nursing aides as well as private schools accredited by the Ministry of Health, including the IGSS. Two universities offer master's degree programs in different public health specialties. There are technician training programs in different areas offered by schools operating under the aegis of the Ministry of Health and by private establishments. A total of 44 radiology technicians, 23 clinical laboratory technicians, 13 respiratory therapy technicians, 6 cytology technicians, and 49 rural health technicians were licensed in 2005. There are four university training programs for nutritionists, as well as a MANA (Master's in Diet and Nutrition) program.

There are Continuing Education Committees in each health area with decentralized functions at different stages of development. In 2006, the IGSS mounted an effort to strengthen and solidify continuing education approaches for its own manpower training activities.

The two agencies with the most personnel are the Ministry of Public Health and Social Welfare and the IGSS. The Health Ministry has 21,592 employees in all categories, of which 85% are budgeted personnel. There are a total of 38,801 individuals involved in the delivery of community-based health care services, including 367 traveling physicians, 37 nursing aides, 461 institutional facilitators, 3,920 community facilitators, 24,248 volunteers, 261 educators, and 9,874 traditional birth attendants. The Social Security Institute has 12,333 employees, of which 88% are full-time budgeted personnel. The other 12% are short-term, temporary staff.

Research and Technological Development in Health

The Technical Secretariat (SENACYT) of the National Science and Technology Council (CONCYT) is the agency in charge of research in Guatemala and the umbrella organization for all agencies and organizations performing research.

There is no national information system on scientific output in Guatemala. According to the CONCYT, since 1996, health project funding has lagged behind other areas (agriculture and technology).

In 2005, the government kicked off its 10-year National Science and Technology Plan for 2005–2014 designed to improve scientific research conditions, refurbish laboratories around the country, and improve competitiveness, to be implemented through the National Science and Technology Council.

There is limited access to scientific literature in Guatemala. Professionals, scientists, and students use technical library resources. Though many users read and understand English, scientific publications in that language are not readily available. There

are very few specialized scientific publications in university libraries due to budget problems. In the last five years, PAHO/WHO has been working with various public and private agencies and organizations to expand the Virtual Health Library.

Health Sector Expenditures and Financing

Public health spending for 1999–2003 came to US$ 2.2 million, accounting for 40% of total spending on health. A breakdown of total public expenditures shows 46.4% made by the government and 53.6% by the Social Security Institute. Total health care spending as a percentage of GDP for the period 1999–2003 (Figure 5) ranged from 4.7% to 5.5%, trending downwards (*51*). The pattern of Health Ministry funding for different levels of care has changed. The new trend is to bring spending for primary and secondary level health care in line with expenditures at the tertiary level (Figure 6).

Aggregate spending on drugs for the period 2000–2004 came to approximately US$ 1.464 billion, with 38% of this figure coming from the public health sector and 62% from the private sector (*39*). There has been no change in the pattern of health spending in the last five years, with most outlays in the Metropolitan region, where there is significantly less poverty and a larger percentage of the population is covered by social security.

Private financing agents include households with out-of-pocket costs, private insurers, and nonprofit organizations serving households (nongovernmental organizations). Spending channeled through these agents for the period 1999–2003 came to US$ 3.413 billion, with households accounting for 90% of all

FIGURE 5. Total health spending as a share of GDP, Guatemala, 1990–2004.

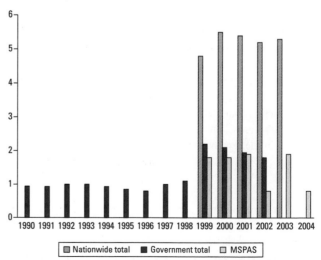

Source: Guatemala, Cuentas Nacionales de Salud, 1990–1995. Programa de las Naciones Unidas para el Desarrollo. Informe nacional de desarrollo humano, Guatemala, 1999–2003.

FIGURE 6. Allocation of Ministry of Public Health and Social Welfare resources by level of health care, Guatemala, 1999–2003.

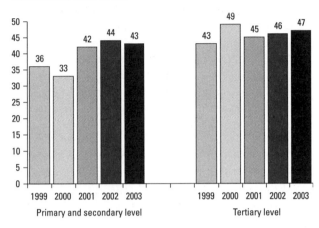

Source: Guatemala, Ministerio de Salud y Asistencia Social.

such spending, followed by nongovernmental organizations, with a 5.7% share, and private insurers, with a 4.3% share. The largest expenditures are in the form of out-of-pocket spending, most of which (72.7%) goes for drugs, tests, and doctors' visits, according to the national living standards survey (ENCOVI).

There are four sources of health financing: households (contributing 65.2%), government (19%), business (10.5%), and international cooperation (2.9%). According to different sources, health financing grew by an average of 10.7% a year between 1999 and 2003. Funds flow in 2003 was 65% greater than in 1999 (*51*).

Public health financing grew by 4.7% a year in absolute terms. The share of private financing went from 70.5% to 76.7% between 1999 and 2003, with household or out-of-pocket spending accounting for 86% of this figure. External financing brought in US$ 1.2 million over the period 1999–2003, of which 37% was allocated to the social sector and 17.4% to the health sector (US$ 446.1 million and US$ 209.8 million, respectively), according to the Planning and Programming Department attached to the Office of the President (SEGEPLAN).

Technical Cooperation and External Financing

Technical and financial cooperation resources for health came to US$ 2.3 million for the last five-year period, of which 37% was in the form of nonreimbursable cooperation resources. Bilateral as well as multilateral cooperation in the health sector has been trending downward, with multilateral bank lending on the rise. Together, various countries and humanitarian organizations furnished a total of US$ 34 million in direct technical and financial assistance in 2005 in response to the emergency created by Hurricane Stan, affecting 45% of the country, of which US$ 12.550

million was contributed by Japan, the Republic of China (Taiwan), the Central American Bank for Economic Integration (CABEI), and the Organization of American States (OAS), to be administered directly by the government, and US$ 21.074 million was contributed by various cooperation agencies, to be administered by different U.N. agencies, funds, and programs.

References

1. Guatemala, Universidad de San Carlos, Centro de Estudios Urbanos y Rurales. Mapa de división político-administrativa. Available at: http://www.usac.edu.gt/~usacceur/mapas.htm. Accessed July 2006.
2. Guatemala, Instituto Nacional de Estadística, Programa de Mejoramiento de las Encuestas de Condiciones de Vida. Encuesta Nacional de Condiciones de Vida 2000. Perfil de la Pobreza en Guatemala. Ciudad de Guatemala; 2002.
3. Programa de las Naciones Unidas para el Desarrollo. Diversidad étnico-cultural y desarrollo humano: la ciudadanía en un Estado plural. Informe Nacional de Desarrollo Humano: Guatemala 2005. Ciudad de Guatemala; 2005. (Documento oficial P964).
4. Guatemala, Ministerio de Salud y Asistencia Social; Instituto Nacional de Estadística. Encuesta Nacional de Salud Materno Infantil 2002: Mujeres. Ciudad de Guatemala; 2003.
5. Guatemala, Instituto Nacional de Estadística, Programa de Mejoramiento de las Encuestas de Condiciones de Vida. Encuesta Nacional de Empleo e Ingresos 2002. Ciudad de Guatemala; 2002.
6. Banco de Guatemala. Algunas variables macroeconómicas años 1950–2004. Available at: http://www.banguat.gob.gt/inc/ver.asp?id=/indicadores/hist03&e=13980. Accessed July 2006.
7. Guatemala, Ministerio de Finanzas Públicas. Estructura: análisis y estudios económicos y fiscales, 1997–2004. Available at: http://www.minfin.gob.gt/. Accessed July 2006.
8. Guatemala, Ministerio de Educación. La educación en Guatemala 2004: el desarrollo de educación en el siglo XXI. Informe nacional. Ciudad de Guatemala; 2004. Available at: http://www.ibe.unesco.org/international/ICE47/English/Natreps/reports/guatemala.pdf. Accessed July 2006.
9. Guatemala, Instituto Nacional de Estadística. Proyecciones de Población. Censo 2002. Ciudad de Guatemala; 2004.
10. Guatemala, Instituto Nacional de Estadística. Defunciones de porcentajes por causas definidas y tasas estimadas por 100.000 habitantes para las diez principales causas de defunción por país, por grandes grupos de edades y sexo: Período 2001–2003. Ciudad de Guatemala; 2004.
11. Guatemala, Ministerio de Salud Pública y Asistencia Social, Departamento de Epidemiología, Vigilancia y Control Epidemiológico. Memoria Anual de Vigilancia Epidemiológica.

Indicadores Básicos de Análisis de Situación de Salud. Ciudad de Guatemala; 2003.

12. Organización Panamericana de Salud. Análisis de la mortalidad infantil de la mortalidad materna por regiones de Guatemala según resultados de las encuestas de mortalidad infantil y materna. Ciudad de Guatemala; 2006.

13. Guatemala, Secretaría de Planificación y Programación de la Presidencia; Naciones Unidas. Efectos en Guatemala de las lluvias torrenciales y la tormenta tropical Stan 2005. Ciudad de Guatemala; 2006.

14. González Izas M. La explotación sexual comercial de niñas, niños y adolescentes en Guatemala: ¿Un problema nuestro? Guatemala: UNICEF; 2006.

15. Guatemala, Ministerio de Salud Pública y Asistencia Social. Informe final: línea basal de mortalidad materna para el año 2000. Ciudad de Guatemala; 2003.

16. Guatemala, Ministerio de Salud Pública y Asistencia Social. Lineamientos Nacionales para la Prevención y Control del Cáncer del Cuello Uterino. Ciudad de Guatemala; 2003.

17. Guatemala, Instituto Nacional de Estadística. Estadísticas vitales: divorcios por año de ocurrencia, según departamento de ocurrencia del divorcio. Período 1995–2004. Ciudad de Guatemala; 2005.

18. Guatemala, Instituto Nacional de Estadística. Estadísticas vitales: matrimonios por año de ocurrencia según departamento donde se efectuó el matrimonio. Período 1995–2004. Ciudad de Guatemala; 2005.

19. Organización Panamericana de la Salud. Perfil de la situación ambiental de las niños de Guatemala, 2003. Available at: http://www.ops.org.gt/ADS/PERFIL%20DE%20SITUACION%20AMBIENTAL%20NI%C3%91EZ-GUATEMALA%20Versi%C3%B3n%203%20ab%20 2003.pdf. Accessed July 2006.

20. Guatemala, Instituto Nacional de Estadística. Encuesta Nacional de Discapacidad 2005. Versión Interactiva. Ciudad de Guatemala; 2005.

21. Guatemala, Ministerio de Salud Pública y Asistencia Social, Departamento de Epidemiología, Vigilancia y Control Epidemiológico. Memoria Anual de Vigilancia Epidemiológica. Indicadores Básicos de Análisis de Situación de Salud. Ciudad de Guatemala; 2004.

22. Guatemala, Ministerio de Salud Pública y Asistencia Social, Programas de Enfermedades Trasmitidas por Vectores. Informe de la situación de malaria 2002. Ciudad de Guatemala; 2003.

23. Organización Panamericana de la Salud. Situación de malaria: datos generales de área y población 2005. Ciudad de Guatemala; 2006.

24. Guatemala, Ministerio de Salud Pública y Asistencia Social, Departamento de Epidemiología, Vigilancia y Control Epidemiológico. Memoria Anual de Vigilancia Epidemiológica.

Indicadores Básicos de Análisis de Situación de Salud. Ciudad de Guatemala; 2005.

25. JICA/PAHO. (Japan International Cooperation Agency). Basic entomological and epidemiological information on Chagas disease control in Central America. 2006.

26. Programa para la Eliminación de la Oncocercosis en las Américas. XIII Conferencia Interamericana sobre Oncocercosis 2003. Sesión 1: Cómo van nuestras coberturas de tratamiento. Guatemala; Ciudad de Guatemala; 2004.

27. Organización Panamericana de la Salud. Análisis Situacional de la Tuberculosis en Guatemala, 2000–2005. Ciudad de Guatemala; 2006.

28. Guatemala, Ministerio de Salud Pública y Asistencia Social, Programa Nacional Prevención y Control del VIH/SIDA. Análisis situacional del VIH/SIDA 2005. Ciudad de Guatemala; 2006.

29. Guatemala, Ministerio de Agricultura, Ganadería y Alimentación, Departamento de Vigilancia Epidemiológica Zoosanitaria. Informe sobre programas, acciones, observaciones, y número de casos de enfermedades de 2005. Ciudad de Guatemala; 2006.

30. Guatemala, Ministerio de Salud Pública y Asistencia Social. Encuesta Nacional de Micronutrientes. Informe Ejecutivo, 1995. Ciudad de Guatemala, 1996.

31. Guatemala, Ministerio de Educación. Censo Nacional de Talla en Escolares de Primer Grado, 2002. Ciudad de Guatemala; 2003.

32. Guatemala, Instituto de Cancerología; Liga Nacional Contra el Cáncer. Informe de los casos de cáncer registrados en el Instituto de Cancerología durante el año 2003, por el registro de cáncer de Guatemala. Ciudad de Guatemala; 2005.

33. Guatemala, Coordinadora Nacional para la Reducción de Desastres. Boletines informativos de inundaciones en Guatemala. Available at: http://www.conred.org/boletines/boletines_antiguos.php. Accessed July 2006.

34. Guatemala, Instituto Nacional de Estadística. Hechos Delictivos, 2003. Cuadro 3: Total de homicidios cometidos, por tipo de arma utilizada o causa de muerte según departamento. Ciudad de Guatemala; 2005.

35. Chile, Amnistía Internacional. Informe de crímenes contra mujeres en Guatemala. Santiago de Chile; 2005. Available at: http://web.amnesty.org/report2006/. Accessed July 2006.

36. Guatemala, Secretaría Ejecutiva Comisión contra las Adicciones y Tráfico Ilícito de Drogas; Embajada de los Estados Unidos de América en Guatemala, Sección de Asuntos Narcóticos. Estudio nacional sobre la desregulación psicológica y su relación con el consumo de drogas en jóvenes adolescentes guatemaltecos: principales hallazgos. Ciudad de Guatemala; 2003.

37. Guatemala, Plaguicidas en el Istmo Centroamericano. Vigilancia sanitaria de plaguicidas: experiencia de plaguicida en Centroamérica. 2003. Ciudad de Guatemala; 2004.

38. Guatemala, Ministerio de Salud Pública y Asistencia Social. Lineamentos estratégicos de la Agenda Nacional de Salud. Documento preliminar. Ciudad de Guatemala; 2006.

39. Guatemala, Instituto Guatemalteco de Seguro Social. Informe Anual de Labores 2004. Available at: http://www.igssgt.org/downloads/Informe%20de%20Labores%202004%20-%20IMPROBADO.pdf. Accessed July 2006.

40. Guatemala, Ministerio de Salud Pública y Asistencia Social, Unidad de Provisión de Servicios de Salud. Aplicación Censo Neto 2005.

41. Guatemala, Congreso de la República de Guatemala. [Various laws]. Available at: http://www.congreso.gob.gt/. Accessed July 2006.

42. Guatemala, Ministerio de Salud Pública y Asistencia Social, Dirección General del Sistema Integral de Atención en Salud. Protección Social en Salud: Guatemala. Informe Final 2002. Available at: http://www.lachealthsys.org/documents/extension/ infoguatemala.pdf. Accessed July 2006.

43. Guatemala, Ministerio de Salud Pública y Asistencia Social, Programa de Medicina Popular Tradicional y Alternativa.

44. Guatemala, Congreso de la República; Ministerio de Salud Pública y Asistencia Social. Acuerdo Ministerial SP-M-946-2006. Available at: http://www.congreso. gob.gt/gt/mostrar_acuerdo.asp?id=16419. Accessed July 2006.

45. Guatemala, Instituto Nacional de Estadísticas. XI Censo Nacional de Población; VI Censo Nacional de Habitación. Ciudad de Guatemala; 2002.

46. Organización Panamericana de la Salud, División de Desarrollo de Sistemas de Servicios de Salud. Perfil del Sistema de Servicios de Salud en Guatemala. Available at: http://www.lachsr.org/documents/perfildelsistemadesaludde guatemala-ES.pdf. Accessed July 2006.

47. Guatemala, Ministerio de Salud Pública y Asistencia Social; Ministerio de Educación. Plan Nacional de Escuelas Saludables de Guatemala, 2004. Ciudad de Guatemala; 2005.

48. Guatemala, Ministerio de Salud Pública y Asistencia Social, Departamento de Regulación y Control de Productos Farmacéuticos y Afines. Informe Anual de 2006. Ciudad de Guatemala; 2006.

49. Guatemala, Registro de Colegio de Médicos y Cirujanos de Guatemala 2006. Available at: www.colmedguatemala.org/noticias/item?item_id=18752. Accessed July 2006.

50. Guatemala, Registro de Colegio Estomatológico de Guatemala 2006. Available at: http://www.cio.com.gt/colestgua. htm. Accessed July 2006.

51. Guatemala, Ministerio de Salud Pública y Asistencia Social. Situación de la salud y sufrimiento. Tercer informe. Período 1999–2003. Ciudad de Guatemala; 2004.

GUYANA

1 Pomeroon-Supenaam
2 Essequibo Islands-
  West Demerara
3 Demerara-Mahaica
4 Mahaica-Berbice

Venezuela

Barima-Waini

1

Georgetown

2

3

4

Cuyuni-Mazaruni

Upper
Demerara-
Berbice

Potaro-
Siparuni

Suriname

Brazil

Upper Takutu-
Upper Essequibo

East Berbice-
Corentyne

0   50   100 Miles

uyana is located on the northeastern coast of South America, where it is bordered by Venezuela to the west, Brazil to the south, and Suriname to the east. It is the only English-speaking country in South America. The country covers an area of approximately 215,000 km^2 and has an estimated population (mid-year 2006) of 767,000, the majority of whom live along the coastline.

GENERAL CONTEXT AND HEALTH DETERMINANTS

Social, Political, and Economic Determinants

A former British territory, Guyana gained independence in 1966 and became a republic in 1970. The country is a democratic republic functioning under a Westminster system of government. The legislative branch is represented by a unicameral National Assembly comprised of 12 nonelected members and 53 members elected under a system of proportional representation. An Executive President is both the Head of State and Government. The country is divided into 10 administrative regions. The local government structure consists of 10 Regional Democratic Councils (RDC), 65 Neighborhood Democratic Councils (NDC), 6 municipalities, and 76 Amerindian Village Councils. Both regional and local governments play an important role in the provision of public services in Guyana. The RDCs are administratively responsible for the delivery of services such as health and education to their respective populations. Because of its historical and cultural development, Guyana is linked to the English-speaking Caribbean and is a Caribbean Community and Common Market (CARICOM) member, as well as part of the British Commonwealth of Nations.

The economy is based on natural resources. Agriculture, forestry, and fishing accounted for 30.3% of gross domestic product in 2005, with sugar being the main contributor; mining and quarrying accounted for 10.5%, followed by manufacturing (8.0%) and engineering and construction (6.2%). The remaining 45% of the GDP was accounted for by services. During the last five years, Guyana has experienced a number of external and internal shocks that significantly weakened the economy. These setbacks included a continuing decline in export prices for bauxite, gold, timber, and rice, as well as a depreciation in the euro that resulted in reduced values of preferential sugar exports, a public services strike, and rising oil prices. Agricultural production was severely impacted by heavy rains and flooding during the first quarter of 2005. The economy has potential for diversification, and the country depends on the production and export of raw materials, which have very little added value.

The Government seeks to restore confidence in the domestic economy by generating sustained growth, creating new employment opportunities, and protecting the environment. It currently is pursuing a privatization program aimed at improving the efficiency of enterprises, reducing public sector financial and administrative burden, redeploying scarce public resources, and increasing modernization through better management, technology, and new investments.

The country has a high debt burden. In 2001, debt stood at G$ 32 billion, or 23.4% of GDP. Having qualified for debt relief under the Highly Indebted Poor Countries (HIPC) Initiative, G$ 3.3 billion was erased by the International Monetary Fund in December 2005 and has been reallocated to health, education, and poverty alleviation programs. Political priorities on the health agenda include providing adequate funding for primary health care programs and basic drugs, low income housing, and water and sanitation infrastructure.

The 10 administrative regions have varying topographical features, population distributions, and levels of development, which in turn influence health status. According to the Economic Commission for Latin America and the Caribbean, almost 90% of Guyana's population lives along a narrow strip of the coastline, which is the administrative, agricultural, commercial, and industrial hub of the country.

The capital city of Georgetown, with 156,000 people, comprises 20.7% of the total population. The interior is sparsely populated with limited health infrastructure. Regions 7 (Cuyuni-Mazaruni) and 8 (Potaro-Siparuni), where much of the mining and quarry sector is located, share the same population density but have populations of 14,682 and 6,000, respectively. Household size declined from 4.7 persons per household in 1991 to 4.1 persons in 2002, indicating a large increase in standing houses. Also, while the household population has grown only 3.3%, the number of households has grown by 20.5%. The largest increase in housing has been in the coastal region that includes Georgetown.

The risk groups most affected by poverty are Amerindians, who are mostly located in the country's undeveloped interior; those of mixed race (a combination of Amerindian, African, Indian, and/or

European ancestry); and women. Amerindians recorded the highest level of poverty among ethnic groups, while the prevalence of poverty is higher among women than men. In particular, women are paid lower wages and salaries, face major difficulties in accessing credit, experience more serious health problems than do men, and have higher rates of illiteracy.

Poverty reduction is a government priority. The 2002 Poverty Reduction Strategy Paper (PRSP) examined how determinants of health outcomes affect the poor and proposed policies to address them. It also evaluated investments and policies for improving the health of the poor. Health and nutrition are key components within the PRSP. The role of health in development is emphasized in both the PRSP and the National Development Strategy.

The size of the working-age population has continued to grow steadily and accounted for two-thirds of the population in 2002. Almost one-third of this population is involved in duties in and around the home, while 7% attend school. Although males comprise a little more than one-half of the total population, they account for 49.7% of the working-age population. Of working-age males, approximately 7% are attending school, 5% perform home duties, and 2% form part of the institutional population. By contrast, for females of working age, a little over one-half perform home duties, and 7% attend school. The female institutional population is also very small (0.6%) compared to males. Twenty-two percent of the male working-age population is not engaged in any type of activity to earn formal income, compared with 66% of females.

Education is a legal requirement for children from 5 years and 9 months of age to age 14. Approximately 60% of the school-age population (i.e., up to age 18) currently attends school, up from 55% at the previous (1991) census. The highest percentages of school-age children who actually attend school are in the 5–9- and 10–14-year-old age groups. Just over 90% of children in these age groups attend school, which indicates that the Millennium Development Goal (MDG) target for primary school enrollment has been surpassed.

Housing has become increasingly modernized. According to the 2002 census, the percentage of households without toilet facilities stood at 2%, compared to the 3.1% recorded in the 1991 census. Despite the increased use of toilet facilities, these are usually linked to cesspits or septic tanks, given the higher costs associated with the installation and maintenance of sewer systems. Two-thirds of all households, however, continue to use pit latrines, considered by MDG indicators to be an improved sanitation facility. Nearly 80% of all households have access to a source of improved drinking water as defined by the MDG target (i.e., household connection, public standpipe, borehole, protected dug well, protected spring, or rainwater collection). These improvements corroborate estimates by the World Health Organization/United Nations Children's Fund (WHO/UNICEF) Joint Monitoring Program, which estimated that by 2002, 83% of the Guyanese population would have access to improved drinking

water and 70% to improved sanitation. Significant inequities exist, however, as regards urban versus rural access to adequate water and sanitation facilities. For every urban dweller without water coverage, there are 1.7 rural dwellers. In the case of sanitation, for every one urban dweller without sanitation means, there are 4.9 rural dwellers. The quality of water supply and sanitation in Guyana is poor. Major problems with services safety, continuity, and reliability persist both along the coastal area and in the severely underserviced hinterland regions. In many distribution systems, water disinfection procedures do not achieve the minimum amount of free chlorine at point of use as recommended by WHO guidelines, resulting in the risk of microbiological contamination. In 2004, water service availability averaged only about 4.3 hours per day. Additionally, the lack of periodic inspection of household connections has allowed inadequate pipe systems to cross-trench with polluted water.

The Government's strategy for the water and sanitation sector is to improve the services level, increase efficiency, and achieve financial sustainability. In 2002, the Guyana Water Authority and the Georgetown Sewerage and Water Commissioners were merged into Guyana Water Incorporated (GWI). In January 2003, a five-year performance-based management contract for GWI was initiated. Since then, GWI's performance has been below target level, although some progress has been achieved in the performance targets for non-revenue water and collection efficiency, customer relations, and commercial services. Numerous challenges to meeting the proposed standards remain due to inherent difficulties in the present system. These include inadequate maintenance procedures and stresses on the system due to overconsumption and wasting. Additionally, the presence of large amounts of iron in the water hampers the chlorination process, clogs pipes, increases the potential for contamination, and raises the pressure needed for water delivery.

Guyana has experienced a prolonged period of violence in which political conflict, race and ethnic tensions, and the narcotics industry all interact. Civilian violence has included that of civilian against civilian, civilian groups against the country's security forces, and security force violence against civilians. The number of murders up to the end of March 2003 (58) was more than triple the figure for the same period in 2002 (17). This upsurge in violence has had economic, political, and social effects that are national in scope.

Guyana's worst natural disaster occurred in January 2005, marked by torrential rains that led to extensive flooding in the capital city and surrounding areas. Fifty-two inches fell—more than seven times the average coastal rainfall (7.3 inches) for January over the past 100 years—affecting almost 85% of the population, and 37% severely. From one to seven weeks, residents along the coast lived in three to five feet of water, in deteriorating environmental conditions that included the accumulation of solid waste and sewage from pit latrines and septic tanks, carcasses of livestock and household pets, and a contaminated drinking water distribution system, all factors which heightened the risk of transmission of water- and vector-borne diseases. The disruption to human life and social development resulted in a GDP loss of 59.5%.

In recent years, the number of safety and quality inspections of fish, poultry, and red meat products for human consumption has increased. In 2005, 582 fishing vessels and large poultry processing establishments were audited and inspected for sanitary conditions and certified. Sixteen fishery establishments were audited, inspected, and monitored, along with a number of small dry shrimp and fish processing facilities and small and medium poultry plants. The Ministry of Health's Food and Drug Department Laboratory conducted microbiological testing on 195 fish and water samples. Daily inspections of poultry meats took place during slaughter days at two large poultry processing plants. Fish and meat products exported and imported through the national airport and other port facilities were monitored and inspected, and foods served to airline passengers were subject to safety inspections.

Demographics, Mortality, and Morbidity

The 2002 census recorded a population of 751,223, compared to the 1991 census of 723,673. There has been a consistently slow growth rate over the last 15 years. Four of the 10 administrative regions have urban centers; the combined population of these towns and the capital city of Georgetown totaled 213,705 (28.4%) of the population in 2002. The remaining 71.6% of the population is clustered in villages, mostly along the coastal belt, as well as a few other settlements scattered deep in the country's hinterland. The non-Guyanese-born population increased from 0.5% in 1991 to 1.3% in 2002. The majority are from Suriname (27%), Brazil (13%), Venezuela (12%), three countries of the eastern Caribbean—Barbados, Saint Lucia, and Trinidad and Tobago (10.7%)—the United States (7.4%), China (6.8%), the United Kingdom (3.4%), and Canada (2.4%).

Comparisons of 1980 age distribution data with that of the latest census show that the population is beginning to age. Fertility rates based on available data substantiate this, showing total fertility rates approaching the replacement level. The overall male-female ratio is nearly 1:1. The population distribution of Guyana in 1991 and 2002, by age and sex, is presented in Figure 1.

Guyana has a multiracial population. The 2002 census indicated that Indo-Guyanese represent 43% of the population, Afro-Guyanese account for 30%, and Amerindians account for 9%. There has been a growth in the population of persons of "mixed" heritage (a combination of Indian, African, Amerindian, European, and/or Chinese ancestry), comprising 17% of the population. The remaining population, less than 1%, include those of European and Chinese descent.

The population composition by religious affiliation is led by Hindus (28.4%); others are Pentecostals (16.9%) and other

FIGURE 1. Population structure, by age and sex, Guyana, 1991 and 2002.

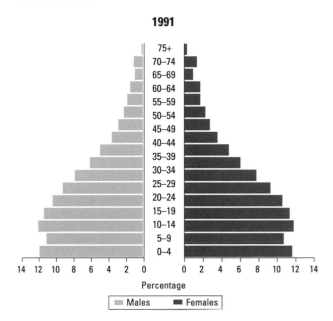

1991

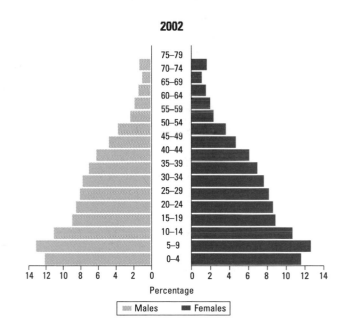

2002

Christians (17.9%), Roman Catholics (8.1%), Muslims (7.2%), Anglicans (6.9%), Seventh-Day Adventists (5.0%), Methodists (1.7%), Jehovah's Witnesses (1.1%), Rastafarians (0.5%), Bahai (0.1%), no religious affiliation (4.3%), and other (1.3%).

The 2005 total fertility rate stood at 2.5, down from 3.1 in 1999. In 2004, approximately 20% of all births were to women under 20 years of age, with 3% to girls under 16. The Multiple Indicator Cluster Survey (MICS), conducted in 2000 by the

Guyanese Bureau of Statistics with funding from UNICEF, showed that birth registration of the under-5 population stood at 96.5%. The proportions of children registered show some variation by age of children and mother's education. Children in the country's interior had lower proportions of registration (86%) compared with the urban coast (99%) and rural coast (98%).

The lack of a sustained growth rate in the Guyanese population reflects the continuing impact of external migration to other CARICOM member countries, the United States, Canada, and the United Kingdom. Data on emigration is difficult to accurately measure, due to violations of visa conditions and undocumented travel across Guyana's overland borders. Thus, actual emigration rates are believed to be higher than those officially reported. There also has been an increase in internal migration from urban to hinterland areas, due primarily to an increase in job-generating activity in the mining and quarrying sector.

Over the 2001–2003 period, there was a total of 14,687 registered deaths (57% of them male and 43% female). Among those with defined causes (98.9%), cerebrovascular diseases ranked first (10.9%), followed by ischemic heart diseases (10.3%), HIV/AIDS (8.8%), diabetes (7.5%), hypertensive diseases (4.2%), suicide (4.0%), conditions originating in the perinatal period (3.8%), heart failure and complications (3.8%), and cirrhosis or other disorders of the liver (2.9%).

The leading causes of death among children under age 5 were conditions originating in the perinatal period (47.3%), intestinal infectious diseases (11.6%), congenital malformations (10.0%), influenza and pneumonia (6.3%), HIV/AIDS (4.6%), malnutrition and nutritional anemias (3.2%), septicemia (2.1%), events of undetermined intent (1.4%), fluid/electrolyte disorders (1.0%), and land transport accidents (1.0%).

Among children 5–9 years old, land transport accidents accounted for 18.9% of deaths, followed by HIV/AIDS (17.0%), congenital malformations (8.5%), events of undetermined intent (7.5%), and accidental drowning (4.7%).

Suicide was the leading cause of death in the 10–19-year-old age group (17.8%). This was followed by land transport accidents (14.0%), assault (homicide) (7.8%), HIV/AIDS (6.2%), events of undetermined intent (6.2%), congenital malformations (5.0%), vector-borne diseases and rabies (3.7%), influenza and pneumonia (2.8%), accidental drowning (2.5%), malignant neoplasms of lymphoid tissue (2.2%), and status epilepsy seizure (2.2%).

HIV/AIDS (17.7%) was the leading cause of death among adults aged 20–59 years, followed by ischemic heart diseases (7.5%), suicide (7.4%), cerebrovascular diseases (6.6%), diabetes (6.5%), assault (homicide) (5.5%), cirrhosis or other disorders of the liver (4.8%), land transport accidents (4.0%), influenza and pneumonia (2.5%), and events of undetermined intent (2.5%).

Adults 60 years old and older carry the greatest burden of chronic diseases. The leading causes of death in this age group

were cerebrovascular diseases (17.8%), ischemic heart diseases (15.5%), diabetes (10.3%), hypertensive diseases (7.1%), heart failure and complications (6.4%), influenza and pneumonia (5.2%), malignant neoplasms of the prostate (2.6%), cirrhosis or other disorders of the liver (1.8%), chronic lower respiratory disorder (1.7%), and fluid/electrolyte disorders (1.5%).

Overall, these causes accounted for 339,480 years of life lost. HIV/AIDS accounted for the most (14.5%), followed by conditions originating in the perinatal period (12.1%), suicide (6.4%), homicide (4.6%), ischemic heart diseases (4.6%), cerebrovascular diseases (4.3%), land transport accidents (4.2%), diabetes (3.9%), influenza and pneumonia (3.6%), and intestinal infectious diseases (3.4%).

HEALTH OF POPULATION GROUPS

Children under 5 Years Old

This age group accounted for 12% (87,907) of the population in the 2002 census. There has been a decline in the number of live births over the past five-year period, with an estimated 18,537 live births in 2001 and 16,391 in 2004. Trained health personnel attended over 95% of these births, and approximately 90% took place in government hospitals and health centers. The crude birth rate in 2003 was 23.1 per 1,000 population. The most prevalent diseases reported were respiratory tract infections (39.2%), acute diarrheal diseases (18.8%), skin diseases (11.0%), worm infestations (8.9%), accidents and injuries (2.6%), eye infections (2.0%), asthma (1.3%), other oral problems (0.5%), and abscess (0.5%).

The infant mortality rate was 24.7 per 1,000 live births in 2004, with 340 registered deaths among children under age 1. In 2001–2003, an average of 203 infant deaths was registered per year. The infant mortality rate was listed at 17.5 per 1,000 live births in 2003. For the 2001–2004 period, hypoxia (22%), intestinal infections (18%), other perinatal conditions (13%), acute respiratory infections (11%), and congenital anomalies (9.8%) were the leading causes of mortality. The main causes of infant deaths are conditions originating in the perinatal period and respiratory problems of the newborn.

For the 2003–2004 period, the leading causes of infant deaths were respiratory disorders in the perinatal period (33%), bacterial sepsis of the newborn (11%), congenital malformations (11%), hemorrhagic and hematological disorders of fetus or newborn (6.5%), acute respiratory infections (5%), slow fetal growth (4.1%), intestinal infectious diseases (5.6%), newborns affected by obstetric complications (4.3%), nutritional deficiencies and nutritional anemia (2.8%), HIV-related conditions (2.9%), and all other causes (13.6%).

The neonatal mortality rate was 15 per 1,000 live births in 2004, with 72.3% of babies who died in the first year of life dying within 28 days of birth. Low birthweight is the greatest risk factor for neonatal mortality. In Guyana's primary referral hospital, the Georgetown Public Hospital Corporation, 12.7% of all newborns were of low birthweight (< 2,500 g), 1.5% of the newborns were of very low birthweight (< 1,500 g), and 0.6% had extremely low birthweight (< 1,000 g). The percentage of low-birthweight newborns declined from 18% in 2001 to 15% in 2004. The most recent five-year analysis of neonatal mortality at this hospital showed a 10% decline.

Premature babies made up 4% of all births, and neonatal sepsis occurrence in hospitals was low (0.7%). In 2004, the main reasons for infant visits to outpatient clinics at hospitals and health centers were acute respiratory infections (53.1%), skin disorders (8.1%), and scabies (7.0%).

The mortality rate for children under age 5 was 72 per 1,000 live births. The number of children in this age group who died during the 2001–2004 period was 414. The leading causes of death among 1–4-year-olds during the 2003–2004 period were intestinal infectious diseases (13%), acute respiratory infections (10.2%), undetermined injury (6.1%), congenital malformations (10.7%), HIV/AIDS (10.8%), and land traffic accidents (6.3%). Among 1–4-year-olds, acute respiratory infections (42%), helminthiasis (13%), skin conditions (8.0%), and accidents (5.5%) were the main reasons for visits to outpatient clinics.

The prevalence of moderate malnutrition from 2000 to 2004 was slightly lower in the age group of 0–11 months (12%) than in the age group of 12–23 months (15%). Only 0.8% in the first age group and 0.4% in the second age group were severely malnourished.

Children 5–14 Years Old and Adolescents 15–19 Years Old

There were 95,723 children (12.9%) in the 5–9-year-old age group in the 2002 census; adolescents aged 10–14 years accounted for 10.8% (80,140), while 15–19-year-olds accounted for 8.9% (66,042). The 2004 Global School-based Student Health Survey focused on students in both primary and secondary schools. Fifty-one percent of those surveyed were females, and 49.0% were males. Results showed that 8.9% were overweight, with no difference between female and male students. The majority of those affected by this problem were in the 13–15 years age category. As many females as males (11.4% of all students surveyed) were at risk of becoming overweight. Three in four students practiced good dietary behavior. Hunger, though a small problem among these students (7.8%), was higher among male students (8.0%) than females (7.4%), but more pronounced among younger students (ages 13–15).

On an average, one in four students reported finding themselves in situations involving violent behavior (bullying, threats, use of weapons, physical fights). Many more males (1 in 3) than females (1 in 5) reported they had directly experienced a confrontation. One in two students was severely injured as a result of accidents.

The incidence of cigarette smoking and the use of other tobacco products were relatively low, being 7.0% and 8.0%, respectively; the male-to-female ratio was 3:1. One in two students attempted to quit smoking. Nearly one in three students consumed alcohol, while one in nine used drugs. One in two males and one in four females consumed alcohol, while one in six males and one in 17 females used drugs.

Only 69% of students (with more females (73%) than males (65%)) were taught about the benefits of a healthy diet, and only 47% of students were taught the importance of washing their hands.

Twenty-five percent of students had had sexual intercourse; 23% had had their first sexual experience between the ages of 13 and 15, and 39% had done so by age 16 or older. In addition, 16% of students had had sexual intercourse with multiple partners, with almost half of the females and three-quarters of the males surveyed having more than one partner. While the condom was the most common form of contraception (74%), overall contraceptive use was 76% among adolescents under age 15 and 71% among those 16 or older. Other methods of birth control were used, but the rate was relatively low (5.4%) and they were more frequently used by younger students than by older ones. In spite of the overall high rate of use of condoms and other methods of birth control, one in 26 female students became pregnant, while one in 10 male students claimed that they had made their partner pregnant.

Adults 20–59 Years Old

The leading causes of death among males ages 20–59 for the 2001–2003 period were HIV/AIDS, with 653 deaths, or 16.4% of the total deaths defined by cause among males in this age group; followed by suicide, with 382 deaths (9.6%); ischemic heart diseases, with 324 deaths (8.1%); diabetes, with 168 deaths (4.2%); events or injuries of undetermined intent, 128 deaths (3.2%); and tuberculosis, 122 deaths (3.1%). The leading causes of death among females ages 20–59 years of age for the same period were HIV/AIDS, with 456 deaths, or 20.1% of the total deaths defined by cause among females in this age group; diabetes, with 237 deaths (10.4%); cerebrovascular diseases, with 181 deaths (8.0%); ischemic heart diseases, with 146 deaths (6.4%); malignant neoplasms of the uterus, with 91 deaths (4.0%); suicide, with 83 deaths (3.7%); heart failure, with 68 deaths (3.0%); malignant neoplasms of the breast, with 65 deaths (2.9%); hypertensive diseases, with 61 deaths (2.7%); and cirrhosis of the liver, with 58 deaths (2.6%).

Older Adults 60 Years Old and Older

This age group increased from 3.9% in 1980 to 5.4% in 2002, another indication that the population is aging. The leading causes of death defined by cause among males 60 years old and older for the 2001–2003 period were cerebrovascular diseases, with 595 deaths, or 17.7% of the total deaths among males in this age group; ischemic heart diseases, with 539 deaths (16.0%); diabetes, with 254 deaths (7.6%); hypertensive diseases, with 194 deaths (5.8%); heart failure, with 188 deaths (5.6%); influenza and pneumonia, with 182 deaths (5.4%); malignant neoplasms of the prostate, with 170 deaths (5.1%); cirrhosis and other diseases of the liver, with 91 deaths (2.7%); chronic lower respiratory diseases, with 71 deaths (2.1%); and tuberculosis, with 54 deaths (1.6%). The leading causes of death defined by cause among females 60 years of age and older for the same period were cerebrovascular diseases, with 562 deaths, or 17.9% of the total deaths among females in this age group; ischemic heart diseases, with 471 deaths (15.0%); diabetes, with 419 deaths (13.3%); hypertensive diseases, with 268 deaths (8.5%); heart failure, with 226 deaths (7.2%); influenza and pneumonia, with 154 deaths (4.9%); disorders of fluids and electrolytes, with 56 deaths (1.8%); malignant neoplasms of the uterus, with 50 deaths (1.6%); malignant neoplasms of the breast, with 46 deaths (1.5%); and diseases of the urinary system, with 41 deaths (1.3%).

The Family

Nearly three-quarters of all households are headed by males. Family planning services are offered at health facilities, and contraceptives are available at all maternal and child health clinics. However, prevalence of contraceptive use among women aged 15–49 who are married or in long-term, single-partner relationships remains low at 37.5%. The Guyana Responsible Parenthood Association Report for 2004 indicated that oral contraceptives are the most frequently dispensed contraceptive in the country's maternal and child health clinics (58%), followed by condoms (23%), injections (17%), intrauterine devices (1.3%), and spermicides (0.6%).

According to the MICS, overall 81% of pregnant women received antenatal care from skilled personnel, with 90% of women from the coast—particularly the urban coast—receiving this care and only 49% of women in the hinterland areas. Approximately 95% of all deliveries were conducted or attended by trained personnel. Again, there was significant regional disparity, with only 43% of all births in the interior being attended by a trained professional.

Of the 46 deliveries by HIV-positive pregnant women, 61% (28) of the women and 78% (36) of the babies received nevirapine. Of the 46 babies born with HIV/AIDS during the reporting period, 29 (63%) received breast milk substitutes, 2 were breast-fed, 2 received mixed feeding (breast milk and formula), and the feeding choice for 9 babies is unknown. There was one stillbirth and 3 deaths from other causes.

There was a decline in the maternal mortality ratio over the 2000–2004 period from 133.3 per 100,000 live births (25) to 115.9 per 100,000 live births (19). For the 2000–2005 period, approximately 119 deaths of women due to obstetric complications were reported. The leading causes of maternal death in the two largest maternity wards in Guyana, which represent the majority of the maternal deaths recorded in this country, were: hemorrhages (32%), hypertensive diseases of pregnancy (21%), puerperal sepsis (13%), ectopic pregnancy (2%), and malaria (2%). There were 19 registered deaths reported by hospitals, attributed to hemorrhage during pregnancy and/or childbirth, hypertensive disorders during pregnancy, complications of labor and the puerperium, and existing medical conditions prior to pregnancy, including cardiac and respiratory problems.

While abortions are legal in Guyana, no services are available in public hospitals for elective abortion. The hospitals will provide care to patients with incomplete abortion in progress, proceeding with evacuation. There is also a relatively high number of women who seek health services with complaints of vaginal bleeding due to self-medication with prostaglandins (Cytotec). Maternal death rates due to abortion are low due to the ability of hospital maternity ward staff to effectively manage abortion situations. Between January and April 2005, a situational analysis was carried out at each of the country's two largest maternity wards. Findings revealed hospital deficiencies in the follow-up and complete utilization of protocols and in the standards and procedures for the management of pregnancy, childbirth, puerperium, and newborn care.

Breast-feeding is a traditional practice. For more than 90% of deliveries attended in the maternity wards, mothers begin breast-feeding within the first hour after giving birth. Seventy percent of newborns are exclusively breast-fed during the first month of life, while only 47% are exclusively breast-fed at four months. Ensuring skin-to-skin contact immediately following delivery is another traditional practice that occurs in nearly all births in both maternity wards.

Workers

A 2004 survey of 133 working children in eight commercial communities found that most were involved in marketplace vending, agricultural, or fishing activities. While most appeared to be in reasonable health, a variety of the tasks they were required to perform raised safety and health issues. For example, the regular lifting of heavy objects increased their risk of back disorders and other injuries. They additionally reported being subjected at times to physical and sexual abuse, in the latter case thereby increasing their exposure to HIV/AIDS and other sexually transmitted infections. The children generally only sought medical care when their health problem had become a serious concern, indicating that many less pressing health issues went undetected and thus untreated.

In 2004, the total number of accidents reported to the Ministry of Labor's Occupational Safety and Health Division was 2,202, including 2,198 nonfatal accidents. The fatal accidents ranged from

14 in 2000 to 4 in 2004. Ninety-five percent of the nonfatal accidents in 2004 occurred in the agricultural sector, and about 2% occurred in the manufacturing sector. Despite the lack of data regarding work-related exposure to toxic pesticides, the extensive use of chemicals in agricultural enterprises indicates that this poses a significant threat to workers' health. Inadequate procedures for waste disposal, including chemicals, represent another risk factor to the health of Guyanese workers. Informal recycling takes place at the main landfill in Georgetown, which employs 121 persons who are exposed to a variety of safety risks and unhealthy conditions.

Persons with Disabilities

The 2002 census identified 10,876 persons living with a disability (2.2% of the total population). A survey conducted in four of the country's administrative regions and based on a sample of 1,500 persons with disabilities found that 14% were totally socially excluded. Access to health services differed by type of impairment; those with physical and hearing impairments had better access to services (72% and 55%, respectively) than those with a hearing/speech impairment (44%) or learning impairment (27%). The survey also showed barriers in accessing health services in the hinterland (only 20–40% of the respondents in these regions had access to any type of rehabilitation services).

Ethnic Groups

Amerindians, the predominant population group throughout most of the country's interior, are also the poorest social sector and exhibit some of the lowest health indicators in Guyana. Malaria is a serious health concern; 60% of all reported cases occur among the Amerindian population. Other health problems disproportionately affecting this group include dental caries, snake bites, scabies, worm infestation, substance abuse, and HIV/AIDS. At the same time, Amerindian women are at a higher risk of poor maternal health since fewer births in the interior are attended by trained health care workers. Community health workers are often the only type of providers serving the interior's population, and their work is hampered by transportation difficulties, lack of refrigeration, and staff shortages.

Other Groups

Gold mining communities, located in Guyana's remote interior, are characterized by rapid population growth due to the influx of miners and those who provide services to them, as well as the lack of basic sanitary and waste disposal facilities. These conditions create the ideal setting for the emergence of vector-borne and other diseases.

Mining impacts on the physical and social environments of all surrounding areas and adversely affects population health. Some of these factors are directly related to mining activities, such as chemical runoff into the water supply and the presence of unfilled pits of water that encourage mosquito breeding, while others are related to the social circumstances surrounding mining, such as temporary living accommodations without adequate sanitary facilities and transient relationships involving risky sexual behaviors. The social impact of mining is further seen in the imbalance of males to females in all mining communities, in the weakness of the family structure manifested by the high levels of unattached adults, and in the relative poverty that persists in the face of wealth generated in mining activities.

More than 50% of miners are affected by malaria. Campsites and housing for mining operations are usually situated in remote, forested areas, often otherwise uninhabited and with very difficult and often dangerous access. Despite these circumstances, antimalarial drugs are easily available through mining concessions.

HEALTH CONDITIONS AND PROBLEMS

COMMUNICABLE DISEASES

Vector-borne Diseases

Malaria is a major public health problem and remains endemic in the interior regions, particularly affecting the Amerindian population. For 2005, a total of 38,984 new cases were reported, of which *Plasmodium falciparum* represented 39% and *P. vivax* 54%. The average annual parasite index in 2005 was 173.95, while the percentage of malaria risk areas stood at 21.5%.

Since 2003, *P. malariae* strains have been diagnosed, corresponding to approximately 3% of all new cases. The majority of these cases (73%) occur in male adults. Malaria often goes untreated, especially in children, and many people have multiple episodes per year. Bed nets are used by 61% of children under age 5, but only 11% of the nets are treated with insecticide. Malaria is also thought to be a major contributory factor to anemia in women and children.

Since 2000, surveillance of **dengue fever** has improved, although weaknesses remain in overall case reporting and in reporting of circulating serotypes. In 2002, the largest number of cases (202) was recorded, and serotype 3 was identified. Information on the circulating serotypes for 2003 is not available. There have been only 2 reported cases of **dengue hemorrhagic fever** (DHF), both occurring in 2002. For the 2001–2005 period, there were no registered deaths due to DHF.

There were no reported cases of **leishmaniasis, schistosomiasis**, or **Chagas' disease** during the 2001–2005 review period. Clinical observations in some patients with cardiomegaly suggest the possible existence of cases of Chagas' disease; however the vector's presence has not been demonstrated, especially in the coastal areas where the greatest percentage of the population is concentrated.

Surveys in 2001 demonstrated that more than 90% of Guyana's population is at risk of infection with **lymphatic filariasis**. In 2003, sentinel sites were established to monitor the effectiveness of salt fortified with diethylcarbamazine (DEC) in reducing transmission and prevalence of lymphatic filariasis. Evaluation of the two sentinel sites with the highest prevalence of lymphatic filariasis, using a baseline circulating filarial antigen card, showed 35% for Georgetown and 18% for New Amsterdam, while microfilaremia prevalence for these two areas was 11.4% and 2.6%, respectively.

Vaccine-preventable Diseases

The immunization program in Guyana—which includes BCG, DPT, OPV, and MMR—has been very successful, with more than 80% of children receiving all the recommended vaccinations (excluding MMR) during the first 12 months of life. MMR vaccine is administered between 12 and 23 months of age, and an average of 91% of all children received it before age 23 months during the 2001–2005 period. DPT3 average coverage was 90% for the same period. Among children under age 1, BCG and OPV3 coverage averaged 94% and 92%, respectively, between 2001 and 2005. The pentavalent vaccine of DPT, hepatitis B, and *Haemophilus influenzae* type b (Hib) was introduced in 2001, and average coverage over the same five-year period was 90%.

There have been no confirmed cases of **measles**. The vaccination coverage for MMR and yellow fever was over 88%. Yellow fever vaccine continues to be part of the routine immunization schedule for children aged 12–23 months. The Expanded Program on Immunization national coverage from January 2004 to December 2005 revealed that coverage of children under age 1 for all antigens was more than 90%. **Poliomyelitis** has been eliminated, and there have been no confirmed cases of **neonatal tetanus**.

Intestinal Infectious Diseases

Statistical data from the Ministry of Health indicate that sections of the population in all 10 of Guyana's administrative regions are infected with **intestinal worms**. There have been no reported cases of **cholera** since the 1992–1993 outbreaks.

Chronic Communicable Diseases

The incidence of **tuberculosis** (TB) has continued to increase, particularly since 2000. Coverage with the Directly Observed Treatment, Short Course (DOTS) strategy increased from 6.0% in 2000 to 42% in 2004; however, decentralization of the TB control program to the primary care level has not been achieved.

Mortality rates have also increased, from 3.6 in 2001 to 5.3 in 2004, as seen in Figure 2; this situation has been associated with TB/HIV coinfection. The TB notification rates and HIV prevalence rates in adults for the 1984–2004 period are presented in Figure 3.

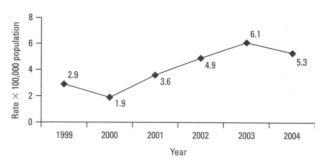

FIGURE 2. Tuberculosis mortality rates, Guyana, 1999–2004.

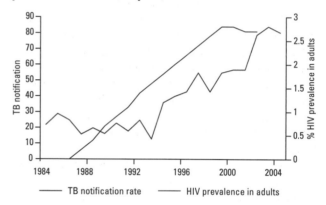

FIGURE 3. Tuberculosis notification rate and HIV prevalence in adults, Guyana, 1984–2004.

The incidence rate is significantly greater in males, and the most affected age group is the 25–44-year-old population, with men contributing 57.7% of the cases and women 48.3% in 2004.

The TB new cases detection rate with ss + is still low, only reaching 27% in 2004. The cure rate of the case cohort under DOTS coverage in 2003 reached only 57%, diminishing in comparison with the rates for the two previous years, which had been 90% and 85%. In the areas not covered with the DOTS strategy the cure rate in 2003 was 50.9%, higher than that reached in the two previous years.

The prevalence of **Hansen's disease (leprosy)** increased from 0.9 in 2000 to 1.2 in 2004; the incidence rate also increased from 0.4 in 2000 to 0.5 in 2004, both increases in the indicators due to multibacillary forms. An average of 12% of the new cases presented with degree II disabilities at the time of diagnosis, indicating a late diagnosis. Self-referred cases accounted for 44.7% of the cases diagnosed; 21% were diagnosed through examined contacts; and 14.7% were patients referred by other health services for leprosy consultation.

Acute Respiratory Infections

Acute respiratory infections (ARI) continue to play an important role in Guyana's morbidity and mortality patterns, occupying first place in terms of the demand for health care services. Around 50,000 ARI cases are recorded annually; of these, more than 2,000 require hospitalization, and an average of 200 people die annually from ARIs. In 2003, 48,629 first visits to care were recorded, representing a rate of 6,553 per 100,000 population. In 2004, the number of visits increased to 53,262, with a rate that increased to 7,111 per 100,000 population. ARI mortality rates were 23.8 per 100,000 population in both 2003 and 2004. ARIs were the seventh leading cause of mortality in the under-1-year-old age group in 2003 and the fifth leading cause for this age group in 2004. They were the third leading cause in children ages 1–4 in 2003–2004.

HIV/AIDS and Other Sexually Transmitted Infections

By the end of 2004, there were 7,512 officially recorded cases of persons testing positive for HIV, and the Joint United Nations Program on HIV/AIDS estimated that there was an adult prevalence of HIV infection of about 2.5% (range: 0.8%–7%) at that time. The findings of surveillance studies conducted among vulnerable populations suggest a stabilization of the epidemic. This is supported by reported cases and incidence data for the period between 1987 and 2004. With greater accessibility to health care centers offering voluntary counseling and treatment, more testing for HIV is being carried out by both the public and private sectors and nongovernmental organizations. Underreporting was a serious problem in the early years of the epidemic, and while significant underreporting remains a problem, this issue is gradually being addressed. In spite of increased testing, the number of new recorded cases remained relatively stable between 2001 and 2005. Data demonstrate that while men were more affected than women in the epidemic's early years, there is an increasing feminization of the epidemic, and today more women are recorded as being HIV positive than men, especially in the 15-to-24-year old age group, which is the only one that recorded more female than male HIV infections during 2001–2004. More than 90% of the recorded cases occur among those between the ages of 15 and 49.

A government-sponsored program to prevent mother-to-child transmission of HIV (PMTCT) began in 2001 at 11 pilot sites and has grown to 56 sites in 8 of the country's 10 administrative regions. Since November 2001, more than 21,000 women have been offered testing and more than 18,000 have accepted. Uptake increased from 67% in 2002 to 94.6% in 2005. Almost 50% of pregnant women have access to PMTCT.

In 2005, the number of persons accessing the antiretroviral treatment program accelerated, rising from 13 per month at the beginning of the year to 23 per month by the end of the year, with a total of 986 persons on treatment in the national program. Laboratory services have expanded to include CD4 and viral load testing. These improved testing services have contributed to more informed decision-making and have resulted in significant clinical and immunological improvement for HIV-positive patients and those diagnosed with AIDS.

The number of annual AIDS-related deaths has slowed down and appears to have stabilized. Following a sharp upturn in the number of deaths between 1999 and 2000 (302 to 483), the crude death rate decreased to 49.8 in 2003, with the number of deaths remaining stable at 314.

Zoonoses

A suspected human case of **rabies** was reported in 2001. In 2003 and 2004, 22 clinical diagnoses of rabies in cattle were reported. No cases in dogs were reported for those years. In May–June 2004, an outbreak of equine encephalitis was detected. Approximately 25 animal deaths were reported, and 3 human cases with symptoms were confirmed by the Caribbean Epidemiology Center laboratory. A vaccination campaign was implemented as a control measure. Guyana was certified free of foot-and-mouth disease in 2002.

NONCOMMUNICABLE DISEASES

Metabolic and Nutritional Diseases

The following risk groups have been identified in terms of food security: low income families, the indigent and homeless population, children 0–5 years of age, adults over age 65, and those infected with communicable diseases or affected by one or more noncommunicable chronic diseases. A 2003 nutrition and anthropometric survey conducted in nursery schools showed that 9.7% of children ages 3–4 were **underweight** for their age and 6.5% had **growth retardation (stunting)**. These indicators were 11% and 8.5%, respectively, in children ages 4–5. For the 5–6-year-old age group, 14% were underweight, 9.8% showed stunting, and 27% presented **anemia**, which was a marked improvement from previous study results. In 2002, a community consultation concluded that there was a generally high intake of macronutrients (energy, protein, and fats); it also noted differences by sex, geographic region, ethnicity, and age group; a high prevalence of **overweight**; and high intake levels of sugar and sodium. In a 2002 survey on physical activity, 69% of the participants were sedentary, with the index being greater among women and urban dwellers; only 20% said they exercised, with this practice being more frequent among men, as well as young professionals. A 2002 nutrition survey found that 6.4% of the respondents were underweight, 31% were overweight, and 19% were obese. **Obesity** was more frequent among women and people living in urban areas.

For the 2001–2004 period, an annual average of 8,433 new **diabetes** cases were reported. There were 6,832 persons, or 74% of the total population with diabetes, aged under 65 years, and some 2,400 (26%) were older than age 65. Available statistics indicate that twice as many females as males are affected; this may be due to the more sedentary lifestyles observed among females and more health-promoting behaviors seen among males. Unless effective prevention strategies are implemented, the incidence of diabetes in Guyana will continue to rise, increasing the already high socioeconomic burden on families and the health system.

Cardiovascular Diseases

In Guyana ischemic heart diseases were the second leading cause of death among both sexes. The number of deaths due to this cause was 1,491, comprising 10.3% of all deaths defined by cause for the 2001–2003 period. During the same time, the number of deaths among males from ischemic heart diseases was 866, or 10.4% of all deaths among males defined by cause; for females there were 625 deaths, or 10.1% of all deaths among females defined by cause.

Malignant Neoplasms

The incidence rate of recorded cases of cancer (2,236) for the 2001–2005 period was 301.3 per 100,000 population. The annual incidence rate tended to increase over the period, which can be attributed to improvements in the case registry system. Breast cancer contributed 15.4% of the total incidence, prostate cancer 14.6%, and cervical cancer 12.9%. Other most-frequent cancer types were of the colon, stomach, lung, uterus, and liver, varying from 5.6% to 3.1%. These locations contributed 64% of the total number of recorded cases between 2001 and 2005. Of all the recorded cases, 1,295 (57.9%) were females, reflecting a high number of patients with breast and cervical cancer. The cumulative incidence rates for females were 352.8 per 100,000 population and for men, 251.1 per 100,000 population. Prostate, colon, and lung cancer were most common among males, while breast, cervix, and colon cancer were most common among females.

The cumulative cancer incidence rate in the infant population was very low—20.3 per 100,000 population, with 53 cases—for the 2000–2004 period. The main sites were the bone marrow, kidneys, blood, long bones of the lower limbs, and lymph nodes of the head, face, and neck.

Incidence rates are much higher in some areas than in others; this is particularly true along the coastline. This phenomenon might be attributable to the fact that in some regions health services are of higher quality and the levels of case investigation, diagnosis, and registration are higher in comparison with other lesser-served areas.

OTHER HEALTH PROBLEMS OR ISSUES

Disasters

A major widespread outbreak of leptospirosis occurred during the extensive flooding in 2005. Based on daily field surveillance by some 40 Ministry of Health mobile medical teams and hospital surveillance, 87 leptospirosis cases were reported. To prevent the disease's further spread, the Ministry provided weekly doxycycline prophylaxis for three weeks to the entire age-appropriate population. There were 23 confirmed leptospirosis deaths registered during the flood disaster. There were 12 other deaths due to the flooding.

Environmental Pollution

Due to the agricultural sector's high economic importance and its continued growth, the use of pesticides predominates and is consistently increasing as synthetic chemical pest control is promoted to enhance productivity. There is growing concern in the Ministries of Health, Agriculture, and Labor regarding the magnitude of acute pesticide poisonings. A 2005 workshop highlighted several occupation-related problems, such as the lack of safety education and use of protective equipment, the persistent use of various highly toxic pesticides, and the scarce resources available with which to implement regulation. A 2000 survey found that 66.9% of suicides are committed via ingestion of liquid poison, which is the predominant method chosen in heavy agriculture areas. Little is known about domestic poisonings and environmental exposure to pesticides.

Gold mining also impacts negatively on the physical and human environment due to traditional mining practices. Empirical surveys conducted during the mid-1990s confirm mercury contamination of soils, river sediments, rivers, fish, and residents of hinterland communities in both mining and adjacent nonmining areas. A major obstacle is that mining is a hinterland activity, thereby complicating environmental monitoring efforts for the Environmental Protection Agency (EPA) and the Guyana Geology and Mines Commission (GGMC), the agencies charged with the regulation of mining activities. The principal factors associated with elevated mercury levels include the lack of use by miners of specialized equipment designed to trap mercury vapor in the mines; amalgam burning and improper mercury storage in the home, which affects the health of miners' families; diet (consumption of fish three or four times weekly); and length of residence in a mining or adjacent non-mining community (residents of more than five years were seven times more likely to have mercury levels above 10 ppm). Goldsmiths also exhibit symptoms of mercury contamination due to inadequate use of safety gear, insufficient knowledge about chemicals and materials used in the workshops, and lack of adequate ventilation systems. Mercury exposure is significantly associated with hearing loss and paresthesia. There is no association between mercury concentration and sex or age.

Oral Health

In 2005, 73,309 patients were seen nationwide in the public health system by a total workforce of 110 comprised of 22 dentists, 1 maxillo-facial specialist, 24 dental aides, 32 dentexes, 15 administrative and support staff, and 16 community dental therapists providing primary oral health services to schoolchildren and communities. Clinical preventive procedures, such as tooth cleaning, polishing, and topical fluoridation, have continued to increase. Of importance was the introduction of pit and fissure sealants in Georgetown to prevent dental caries. The delivery of restorative care (tooth fillings) continued to grow, nationwide, with a total of 13,013 teeth filled in 2005, compared with 10,500 in 2004 and 6,774 in 2003. Health promotion continued to be a major focus; over 40,000 pupils nationwide were exposed in the classroom to relevant oral health messages; and mass promotion during Oral Health Month was sustained and consolidated in the administrative regions.

Schools and community outreach clinics have remained two key strategies to reach persons in need of dental care. The Rotary Club of Georgetown Central's School Program Mobile Unit allowed over 6,000 children of Regions 3 (Essequibo Islands-West Demarara) and 4 (Demarara-Mahaica), the latter of which includes Georgetown, to receive free dental care, including tooth extraction, prophylaxis, and fillings.

Efforts continued on the consolidation of the public oral health workforce with the recruitment of more dentists and the training of 27 dental auxiliary personnel. In May 2005, consolidation of cross-infection control in government clinics was achieved with the delivery and distribution to various clinics, including regional/district clinics, of 15 autoclaves.

The shortage of preventive/restorative materials and supplies has persisted, with no procurement made in 2005. At the same time, the absence of electricity in some isolated locations and the scarcity of portable generators have impeded the delivery of preventive and restorative care during outreach visits to rural and hinterland areas.

There are no available data on oral health in the private health sector.

RESPONSE OF THE HEALTH SECTOR

Health Policies and Plans

The overall objectives of the National Health Plan 2003–2007 are to improve the nation's health; to support the Poverty Reduction Strategy, the goals of the National Development Strategy, and the MDGs; and to achieve good value for money in the health sector. The National Health Plan focuses on the modernization and rationalization of health services, the decentralization of public health programs to Health Management Committees as semiautonomous providers, the establishment of workforce development and human resources management systems, and the implementation of a national quality framework.

The Plan identifies the following national priority programs: family health, communicable diseases, STI/HIV/AIDS, chronic noncommunicable diseases, oral health, and environmental health. Between 2003 and 2005, the Ministry of Health drafted a number of specific national policies, plans, and strategies to address priority health areas. They include the National Strategic Plan for the Reduction of Maternal and Neonatal Mortality in Guyana, the National Mental Health Policy and Plan, the National Framework for Quality Care, the National Nursing Strategy, the National Blood Transfusion Policy, the National Strategy for Blood Safety, the National Plan for HIV/AIDS, and the Patient Charter of Rights and Obligations.

The Regional Health Authorities Act for the decentralization of services management, the Ministry of Health Act, and the Pharmacy Practitioners Act were passed during the 2003–2005 period. In addition, the Health Facility Act, indicating minimum standards for public and private health care facilities, was prepared by the Ministry of Health; the Water and Sewerage Act was passed in 2002; and the draft of the Health Protection and Promotion Act was submitted to Parliament by the Ministry of Health in 2005.

Organization of the Health System

The main public institutions in the health sector are the Ministry of Health and the Ministry of Local Government and Regional Development. The overall responsibility for the population's health rests with the Minister of Health as the Ministry of Health's political head. The Permanent Secretary is the accounting officer and administrative head of the Ministry. The Chief Medical Officer oversees all technical and professional aspects. The Ministry of Health's sectoral responsibilities include policy formulation, standard setting, monitoring, evaluation, and the implementation of vertical programs. The Ministry of Local Government and Regional Development is responsible for financing and providing services at the regional level through the Regional Democratic Councils. The Ministry of Health provides technical support and some of the human resources to this effort. The private sector functions independently, but there is legislation through the Private Hospitals Act that provides for the licensing of private hospitals. Nongovernmental organizations are actively involved in services delivery, especially in the area of HIV/AIDS.

The Ministry of Health includes several entities with regulatory responsibilities. The Pharmacy and Poisons Board regulates pharmacies and pharmaceuticals, while the Government Analyst/ Food and Drug Department is the regulatory authority for various aspects of food and drugs. Laboratory capacity for drug quality monitoring and potable water analysis was recently strengthened. The EPA has overall responsibility for the protection of the environment. The Directorate of Standards and Technical Services is responsible for the development of standards and quality control in clinical, pharmacy, radiography, laboratory, and blood transfusion services. The Guyana National Bureau of Standards regulates laboratories and blood banks, and preparations for accreditation of laboratories are in place. The professional councils (medical, dental, nursing, and pharmacy) regulate professional health practice, and continuing medical education is required for the annual registration of doctors. The Ministry of Health has a drug formulary and an Essential Drugs List, which is regularly updated.

The structure of Guyana's public health care system is highly decentralized. Administrative control over health resources in the regions rests with the Regional Executive Officers of the 10 Regional Democratic Councils (RDC). Each RDC has a Regional Health Officer who reports administratively to the Regional Executive Officers, but receives technical and professional guidance from the Ministry of Health. Experiences over the past decade have shown that the necessary health management skills available at the regional level are limited. The national referral hospital in Georgetown functions under the Public Corporation Act as a semiautonomous body with its own board.

The St. Joseph Mercy Hospital is a private facility that also offers treatment and care under the Ministry of Health's program. Care and treatment are offered free of charge to persons living with HIV/AIDS.

Guyana does not have a national health insurance system. The National Insurance Scheme operates a social insurance program for employees. Participation in the Scheme is mandatory for employed persons between the ages of 16 and 60, including the self-employed. The Scheme provides illness, maternity, medical care, and job-related injury benefits. Medical coverage is provided, on a reimbursable basis, for such selected services as hospitalization, eyeglasses, dental care, surgery, and the purchase of drugs, with limits on the reimbursement amount. Some employers provide additional contributory or non-contributory insurance for their employees. In other cases, individuals purchase health insurance from private insurance companies.

Public Health Services

Guyana's health care system is based on the primary health care principles of equitable distribution of health services, intersectoral collaboration, and community participation. A major challenge is to ensure equitable access to health care for populations residing in small remote riverside and hinterlands settlements and to provide culturally appropriate intervention approaches for a wide range of ethnic groups. In collaboration with the Ministries of Amerindian Affairs and of Local Government and Regional Development, the Ministry of Health introduced the concept of community health workers (CHWs) in the late 1980s to strengthen the link between isolated villages and the formal health care system. Operating from small health posts, CHWs are often the only locally available health worker, forming a bridge with other levels of care. They are trained and supported by the Ministry of Health to provide community health promotion education and simple treatment and medications for common illnesses, in addition to child vaccinations.

The Ministry of Health is collaborating with donor agencies and the Pan American Health Organization (PAHO) to implement a lymphatic filariasis national elimination plan. The main strategies are public education, collaboration with salt manufacturers in the distribution of DEC-fortified salt, community-mapping, and use of a more rapid diagnostic procedure for surveillance. After two years of preparation, DEC salt was launched in July 2003 with financial support from the Bill and Melinda Gates Foundation.

The Partners for Parasites Control was formed in 2001. Its participants include the PAHO/WHO Member Governments of countries in which helminthic infections are endemic, the United Nations Children's Fund, WHO, World Food Program, World Bank, universities, philanthropic foundations, and pharmaceutical companies. In May 2001, WHO World Health Assembly Resolution WHA 54.19 endorsed a strategy for the control of schistosomiasis and soil-transmitted helminths in high transmission areas. One of WHO's targets is the "regular treatment of at least 75% of all school-age children at risk of morbidity for schistosomiasis and soil-transmitted helminth infections by 2010." A draft proposal for the National Deworming Program for school-aged children was written in 2005 for implementation during 2006–2007.

As regards the country's HIV/AIDS program, treatment with antiretroviral medications (ARVs) commenced in April 2002 at one treatment center (the GUM Clinic). At the end of 2005, there were eight public health centers offering treatment and care, including the provision of ARVs and CD4 testing. Private physicians and hospitals also provide treatment, but these private arrangements have not yet become part of the national surveillance system.

A National Diabetes Strategic Plan has been developed with the aim of diabetes prevention, improving diabetes care, and decreasing the disease's burden in Guyana. The Plan describes priority areas for action in the current health care system; proposes goals, rationales, objectives, and evaluation measures for each of the areas; and provides an overall framework to guide diabetes prevention and control efforts for the 2007–2015 period.

The Government's water and sanitation sectoral strategy seeks to improve service level, increase efficiency, and achieve financial sustainability. Following initiation of GWI's five-year performance-based management contract in January 2003, considerable progress has been made towards implementing key institutional and regulatory water and sanitation reforms. The Public Utilities Commission, established as an independent regulatory body for the sector, requires capacity-strengthening to perform its functions. The National Water Council is not yet operational. The Ministry of Health and EPA have signed a Memorandum of Understanding to jointly develop water quality standards. At the same time, GWI, under license from the government, is required to supply safe drinking water in accordance with WHO standards. With PAHO support, the Ministry of Health plans to implement a region-by-region Water Safety Plan in Guyana.

Regarding the institutional framework of the solid waste management sector, the main stakeholders are the Georgetown Mayor and City Council, the other five existing municipalities (New Am-

Prioritizing Equitable Environmental Services for All Guyanese

The Government of Guyana is giving priority to improving water and sanitation. The challenge is formidable, in large measure because of the population's geographic distribution and the state of the infrastructure. Nine in 10 Guyanese live in a narrow strip along the coast and one in five resides in the coastal capital of Georgetown; the remainder lives in the mostly remote underserved rural hinterland. Urban dwellers have significantly greater access to both water and sanitation services, although water quality throughout the country falls short of the minimum quality levels recommended by WHO. To redress these deficiencies, the Government passed a Water and Sewerage Act in 2002 and subsequently launched a National Health Plan for 2003–2007 that identifies environmental health as a key target to address.

sterdam, Corriverton, Anna Regina, Rose Hall, and Linden), and the NDCs. At the national level, entities involved in solid waste management are the Ministries of Health, Local Government and Regional Development, and Finance, along with the EPA. Nongovernmental organizations and private contractors also play important roles in this sector.

Policy-making is a shared responsibility between the Ministry of Health and the Ministry of Local Government and Regional Development. The Ministry of Health and EPA share responsibility for the public health and environmental aspects of solid waste management. Through its Environmental Health Unit, the Ministry of Health is responsible for approving sanitary facilities and providing guidance to households, municipalities, industries, and other groups regarding adequate solid waste collection and disposal. The Ministry of Local Government and Regional Development is responsible for formulating national policy on solid waste management and providing financial support to municipalities and NDCs. At the current time, however, this institutional framework is not adequately coordinated and needs further strengthening. The Ministry has released a draft national solid waste policy, but institutional weakness has impeded the implementation of a technically sound and publicly supported policy.

The 2004 Sectoral Analysis of Solid Waste showed that many municipalities have deficient solid waste collection systems. Although coverage varies from 62% to 100%, the frequencies of collection rarely exceed the once-a-week minimum standard, and treatment/sanitary disposal is only performed on special restricted wastes.

It is estimated that 102,900 metric tons/year of solid waste will require adequate solid waste disposal if collection is to cover the entire population. However, only 63,700 metric tons of waste are deposited at the main landfill annually. The waste not delivered to the landfill is burned, buried, or disposed of in empty lots, canals, and approximately seven community dumpsites. There is no information on solid waste management in areas outside the capital city.

While the municipality of Georgetown possesses a Solid Waste Management Program, the other five municipalities have weak technical, administrative, and financial capabilities that are reflected in their inadequate waste collection and disposal. There are no recycling and composting activities in the country.

Special wastes, such as those from hospitals and slaughterhouses, are treated by burning, either in the open air in most municipalities or in a highly inadequate incinerator located in Georgetown. Since none of the methods are acceptable, there is an urgent need to implement technically sound and sustainable methodologies for hazardous wastes disposal.

There are several national initiatives under way to address the issue of mercury contamination and the destructive nature of mining activities. One notable example is the Guyana Environmental Capacity Development Mining Project aimed at strengthening the environmental management capacities of key stakeholders in the mining sector.

Air pollution has not been a priority issue in Guyana, though pollution from bauxite mining leads to chronic obstructive lung diseases among residents of mining and nearby communities.

The Veterinary Public Health (VPH) Unit of the Ministry of Health is responsible for setting standards and for monitoring, inspecting, and certifying the quality and safety of the production, processing, and distribution of all meat, seafood, milk, and related products, whether these are destined for local consumption, imported, or prepared for exportation. The Ministry of Health's Environmental Health Unit is responsible for ensuring that proper standards are maintained by regional-level food protection and control services. Food service inspections are carried out by Environmental Health Officers attached to municipalities and regional health departments.

The VPH Unit works in collaboration with the Ministry of Agriculture to establish and maintain epidemiological surveillance of zoonoses and minimize risks through appropriate disease control and eradication measures. The Unit also collaborates with the Environmental Health Unit; EPA; Georgetown's Mayor and City Council; other Town Councils; Government Analyst/ Food and Drug Department; Institute of Applied Science and Technology; Ministry of Fisheries, Crops, and Livestock; and the Guyana National Bureau of Standards. Collaborative efforts include providing prophylactic treatment to susceptible animals, raising public awareness, environmental monitoring, and inspection of supermarkets and marketplaces. There is also sharing of technical information, regulations, and laboratory facilities among these agencies. The VPH Unit establishes and maintains surveillance management over animal-derived foods and the detection of waterborne diseases; it also educates food handlers and processors about their important role in food protection and safety during all activities leading up to the consumer. Sanitary inspections and monitoring of fishing vessels are conducted twice annually. Implementation of the quality and safety assurances action plan for small- and medium-sized fish plants continues, and there is daily monitoring and evaluation of landing dock sanitary conditions and of raw fish products at the four major seafood establishments by VPH Unit inspectors.

Personnel assigned to landing dock sites and other fishing personnel received training on proper fish handling, and improvement of health facilities at these locations was carried out jointly with the European Union and the Caribbean Program for Economic Competitiveness. The VPH Unit provided training to seafood processors, landing site personnel, and fish handlers on Good Manufacturing Practices, Sanitation Standard Operating Procedures, and Hazard Analysis Critical Control Point systems, as well as orientation on new fishery regulations.

The VPH Unit and Guyana National Bureau of Standards held a joint meeting with poultry producers on the implementation of two poultry standards: Specifications for Poultry Meats and Poultry Products and Grading and Quality Requirements for Table Eggs.

The VPH coordinated a Food and Agriculture Organization project on the strengthening of the food control system in Guyana in which the Ministry of Agriculture serves as the implementing agency and the Ministry of Health as project coordinator. Technical work continued with the Guyana National Bureau of Standards to develop food standards.

A Healthy Market Project was initiated in 2005 with the Mayor and City Council of Georgetown for a small public market located on the capital's outskirts serving a diverse community of primarily medium to low income earners. A task force was established among stakeholders, including government and nongovernmental organizations, vendors, and private sector representatives, to address food safety, water, and sanitation issues.

Since its creation in October 2005, the National Committee on Influenza Preparedness has monitored the global spread of avian influenza. Led by the Ministry of Health, the Committee's other members include the Ministries of Agriculture, Home Affairs, and Education; University of Guyana; and Guyana Poultry Association, among others. The National Influenza Preparedness Plan focuses on minimizing and/or eliminating unwanted and unfore-

seen social disruption and economic consequences resulting from any possible pandemic influenza outbreak and on maximizing the effectiveness of the national response. As part of this effort, the national communication plan targets the general public, mass media, health workers, schools, workplaces, ports of entry, and communities. The Committee networks with other countries in the Region of the Americas to share information, identify funding sources, and establish a working group within the Global Framework for the Progressive Control of Transboundary Animal Diseases, a joint initiative of the Food and Agriculture Organization and the World Organization for Animal Health.

In response to the heavy flooding of early 2005, a Health Task Force was formed by the Ministry of Health in an effort to prevent the outbreak of diseases. The health response was guided by a syndromic surveillance system specially implemented during the flood. In February 2005, the Ministry introduced a mass chemoprophylaxis campaign, delivering some 450,000 courses of doxycycline (200 mg/day for 5 days) to residents of flood-affected areas. The local media reinforced this effort with comprehensive disease prevention messages targeted to vulnerable communities. Syndromic surveillance case report forms were revised to identify possible cases, and persons hospitalized with suspected leptospirosis were interviewed to assess clinical presentation and possible risk factors associated with the disease.

More than 5,000 persons were housed in 45 shelters run by the Guyana Defense Force (GDF), the Guyana Relief Council, and private organizations, with support from the World Food Program, Red Cross, and civil society and religious organizations such as Rotary Clubs. The Joint Services (JS) command center provided more than 146,000 hot meals, and more than 78,000 food hampers were distributed by government workers; 6,000 hampers were delivered to 22 mosques by the Central Islamic Organization. The Ministry of Health, JS, private contractors, Oxfam International, and international agencies supplied potable water to the affected communities through a network of water tanks, bottled water supplies, and community standpipes. The Ministry of Health and EPA organized an emergency water monitoring exercise to ensure safe water distribution. The GDF and Red Cross distributed 32,613 cleaning kits, which included soap powder, a scrub brush, washing soap, and bleach. Solid waste and sanitation responses were coordinated by a task force including the Ministry of Health, Ministry of Local Government and Regional Development, and the Georgetown Mayor and City Council. The relief assistance response from the international community was swift and amounted to greater than US$ 3.7 million.

Individual Care Services

Health services in the public sector are provided through a five-tiered, upward-moving referral system. Level I includes 188 health posts; level II, 136 health centers; level III, 20 district hospitals; level IV, 4 regional hospitals; and level V, the Georgetown

Public Hospital Corporation, which serves as the general hospital for the capital and surrounding areas and as the tertiary referral hospital for the country as a whole. Other level V care facilities include the national psychiatric hospital, the leprosarium, and the geriatric hospital. In the private sector, five hospitals and a variety of health and diagnostic centers and pharmacies exist. The vast majority of private facilities are located in Georgetown and other urban centers. There are 4.23 hospital beds per 1,000 population (3.77 in the public sector and 0.46 in the private sector). There is no organized ambulance service for the general population. The Georgetown Public Hospital Corporation, all of the regional hospitals, and some of the private hospitals provide ambulances for patient transport. Some private security firms also provide hospital ambulance services to their clients.

Public sector laboratories are located at the Georgetown Public Hospital Corporation, the four regional hospitals, and most of the 20 district hospitals. There are a limited number of private independent laboratories, some of which are combined with diagnostic imaging services. The National Blood Transfusion Service (NBTS) is governed by a semiautonomous board. In 2005, about 5,526 units of blood were collected countrywide; this filled approximately 64% of physicians' requests. In 2005, the NBTS, with support from the Red Cross, collected 82% of the blood supply, while the regional hospitals collected 13% and the private hospitals 5%. The NBTS tests all the units issued for transfusion for HIV, HBV, HCV, syphilis, and malaria. There is no screening for Chagas' disease.

Pursuant to the 2003–2007 National Health Plan, in 2004 the Ministry of Health's Division of Disability and Rehabilitation Services created a strategic plan to develop strategies for the provision of preventative, therapeutic, and rehabilitative services to the population. The Rehabilitation Services Program is comprised of the following components or sub-programs: Administration, Regional Physiotherapy, Occupational Therapy, Speech Therapy, Audiology, a home for the blind, and the National Vocational Training Center. Staffing in the rehabilitation services has been hampered by a high attrition rate of physiotherapists and assistants. The current profile indicates that services are mainly centrally based; the greatest proportion of the staff are mid-level workers known as Rehabilitation Assistants and Audiology Practitioners. There are a limited number of professional staff, mainly physiotherapists, the majority of whom are non-nationals. In 2004, there were 41 vacant positions, of which 52% were for technical personnel.

Health Promotion

Guyana's health promotion framework is based on the Caribbean Charter for Health Promotion. At the same time, the new directions called for in the Bangkok Charter for Health Promotion (2005)—including greater policy coherence and the creation of partnerships across government sectors, the private sector, and civil society—continue to be progressively integrated into national development programs at the ministerial level. A diversity of multisectoral alliances have been established among public and private agencies and faith- and community-based organizations.

Within the Ministry of Health, health promotion strategies have been mainstreamed into the program areas of communicable and noncommunicable diseases, immunizations, maternal and child health, integrated management of childhood illness, adolescent health, and STI/HIV/AIDS. In addition, policies have been developed and implemented in these areas. In a new initiative, community health advocates were introduced to the health system following training in the early detection of diseases and in health promotion and prevention techniques that will allow them to address community health concerns such as diabetes and hypertensive diseases.

The Healthy Municipalities and Communities Program continues to expand with the inclusion of new communities in the hinterland and the establishment of health promotion committees tasked with developing, coordinating, and supporting various healthy setting initiatives in remote areas populated primarily by Amerindian groups. The health concerns of hinterland and suburban communities alike are increasingly being addressed through new intersectoral collaborations that enable the Program's strengthening.

The Ministry of Health established a Health Promotion Unit within the Adolescent and Young Adult Health and Wellness Unit to coordinate health promotion and healthy setting programs within the Ministry, and to support the Health Sciences and Education Division, focusing on addressing the determinants of adolescent health, particularly tobacco control and accidents and injury prevention. Health promotion in school curricula has been adapted by the Ministry of Education as a complementary framework for its Education for All by 2015 mandate. This has facilitated rapid assessments of schools conducted by teachers, students, parents, and other school community partners, as well as the development of action plans and the mobilization of resources to address the issues identified.

The Adolescent and Young Adult Health and Wellness Unit holds direct responsibility for the Ministry of Health's School Health Program, which is divided into two sub-programs; the first targets nursery and primary schools for children ages 3–12, and the second targets secondary and tertiary institutions with students ages 12 and over. In the latter case, a nationwide network of Health Clubs has been formed comprised of teachers and students who jointly address health issues within their individual schools, including tobacco control and reproductive health.

The School Health Program was initiated in 2001 as part of the Caribbean Network for Health-promoting Schools and has been adapted by the Ministry of Health as a strategy to improve the nation's health. Its participants include teachers, students, parents, and other school community partners who have fostered recognition of the need for healthy public policies in schools. Among the group's achievements are formulation of a smoke-free schools policy and improvements in facilities in 35 schools located in areas affected by the 2005 floods.

A school-based Vision Screening Program was developed with the goal of reducing childhood blindness due to uncorrected refractive errors. Teachers, health care workers, and parents were trained to conduct screening activities at their respective schools. Referrals and assessments were made primarily at the Georgetown Public Hospital Corporation. Of 2,428 students screened during the 2005–2006 school year, 262 were referred for further assessment, and 36 of the 191 seen were prescribed eyeglasses and corrective lenses. This experience has provided valuable input for the implementation of other basic screening programs in auditory and oral health.

As a result of advocacy surrounding the observance of World Health Day 2004 and its slogan "Road Safety Is No Accident," the Ministry of Home Affairs spearheaded the resuscitation of the National Road Safety Council, which developed a national road safety program based on alliances among governmental ministries, nongovernmental organizations, and the private sector.

Human Resources

External migration of health professionals—in all categories, including managers and health teachers/tutors—has created a serious workforce shortage in the health care field and placed constraints on health services provision to the population. In the public health sector, vacancy rates range between 25% and 50% in most professional categories. A geographical imbalance of professional staff also exists; 70% of the country's physicians are located in Georgetown, where only 25% of the population resides. For the medical specialties, Guyana relies largely on non-nationals, who fill more than 90% of the medical speciality positions in the public sector.

Another challenge is the low ratio of professionals to non-professionals. For nurses, this ratio was 0.60 in 2003 due to a high attrition rate of professional nurses. The professional nursing attrition rate in the public sector in the country's two most populous regions was 13% of the staffing level, while it was only 3%–4% for non-professional nursing. In some instances retired nurses are being rehired. The Ministry of Health has introduced various low- and mid-level cadres as a response to these challenges and as a way to ensure equitable access to care despite limited human resources.

The University of Guyana has a Faculty of Health Sciences with a School of Medicine and other departments which offer Bachelor of Science degrees in medical technology and nursing, and associate degrees in pharmacy, environmental health, and radiography. The University also plans to open a School of Dentistry. There are three public nursing schools—one in Georgetown and one each in the country's two other largest towns (Lin-

den and New Amsterdam)—as well as one private school at the St. Joseph Mercy Hospital in Georgetown.

The Ministry of Health Department of Health Sciences Education trains the lower- and mid-level cadres who serve primarily in rural areas. Training lasts 12–18 months and is provided for rural midwives, x-ray technicians, multipurpose technicians, community dental therapists, laboratory assistants, rehabilitation assistants, environmental health assistants, and for the medex (mid-level physician assistants).

Health Sector Expenditures and Financing

In 2005, total government expenditure in health was approximately US$ 34.2 million, or US$ 45 per capita. This represents 7.9% of the total government expenditures (all sectors) and 4.4% of the GDP. Recurrent expenditure of the total government health expenditure was approximately US$ 29.7 million, or 86.7%, in 2005, and capital expenditure was around 13.3%. Employment costs are about 38% of total government expenditure in health, and drugs and medical supplies are about 20.2%. No recent estimates of the total private expenditure in health are available.

From the recurrent government health expenditure, about 36.7% was allocated to the Georgetown Public Hospital Corporation and about 40% to the Regional Health Services. Most of the Regional Health Services are related to primary health care. However, the expenditure on these services includes an unspecified percentage of spending on secondary health care services that is provided through regional hospitals in some regions. Under the assumption that the expenditure on primary health care is at least one-third of the total expenditure in the regions (both through regional budgets and Regional Health Services), then primary health care expenditure represented at least 17% of total recurrent expenditure (public) in health in 2005, and 8% of the total capital expenditure (public) in health.

Health care is provided free of charge to the public. There are no data or information on financing in the private health sector.

Technical Cooperation and External Financing

The municipality of Georgetown's Solid Waste Management Program has been financed by the Inter-American Development Bank since 2000. In 2005, PAHO provided technical support to the Ministry of Local Government and Regional Development in the development of final disposal/transfer sites of solid waste in the flood-affected areas along the east and west coasts of the Demerara River.

PAHO is also supporting the Ministry of Health in the development of an action plan to enhance the Environmental Health Unit's capacity and to review functions among other agencies in Guyana involved in environmental health issues. The Government Analyst/Food and Drug Department has also received support to perform water quality analysis in the majority of parameters included in the WHO Guidelines for Drinking-water Quality.

Since 1999, the Rotary Club of Georgetown Central has been providing free dental services to schools and surrounding communities, utilizing one dentist, two dentexes, and a community dental therapist provided by the Ministry of Health. Intersectoral cooperation for health was strengthened during 2005. Colgate Palmolive and the Rotary Club of Georgetown Central have remained key partners, along with PAHO, which supported the participation of Ministry of Health dental personnel in two international conferences and in various activities related to Oral Health Month in 2005. Various overseas and local nongovernmental organizations continue to provide valuable support to the country's dental care delivery system through periodic outpatient clinic visits and financial contributions.

Bibliography

Beckles F. Incidence of suicide in Guyana. 2000.

Economic Commission for Latin America and the Caribbean.

Guyana, Bureau of Statistics; International Labor Organization. Child Labour Survey. 2004.

Guyana, Bureau of Statistics. Multiple Indicator Cluster Survey (MICS), 2000.

Guyana. Global School-based Student Health Survey. 2004.

Guyana, Ministry of Education. Strategic Plan 2003–2007.

Guyana, Ministry of Foreign Affairs; United Nations Children's Fund. Mid-term review (MTR) report. 2003.

Guyana, Ministry of Health. Human resources recording and reporting system.

Guyana, Ministry of Health, Mecanismo de Coordinación de País (MCP).

Guyana, Ministry of Health, Regional Health Services Unit. 2004.

Guyana, Ministry of Health, Veterinary Public Health Unit.

Guyana, National Blood Transfusion Service. 2005.

Guyana Responsible Parenthood Association. Report 2004.

Joint United Nations Programme on HIV/AIDS. 2004.

Pan American Health Organization. Basic Indicators. Washington, DC: PAHO; 2005.

Situation analysis of hospital maternity wards. January–April 2005.

World Health Organization; United Nations Children's Fund, Joint Monitoring Program. Country, Regional and Global Estimates on Water and Sanitation.

HAITI

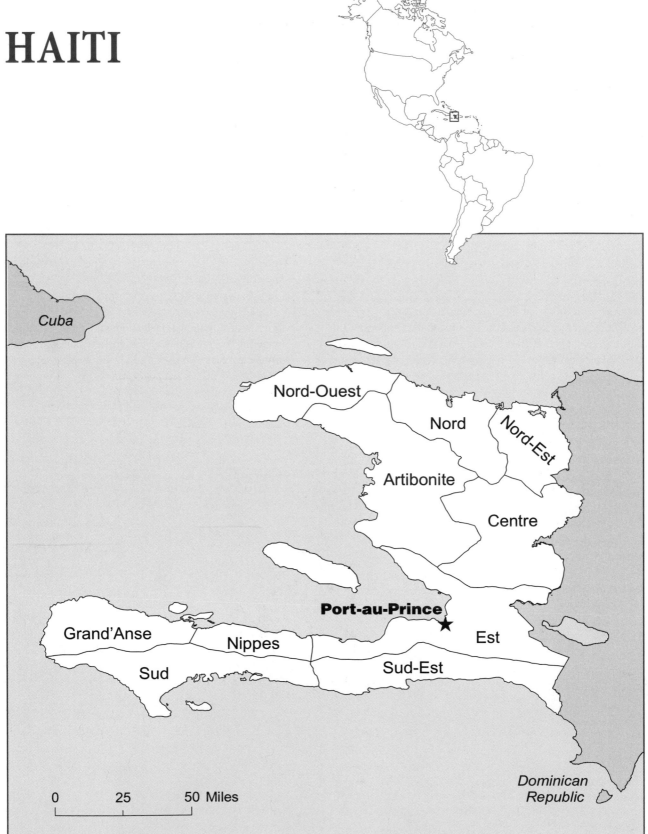

Cuba

Nord-Ouest

Nord

Nord-Est

Artibonite

Centre

Grand'Anse

Nippes

Port-au-Prince

Est

Sud

Sud-Est

Dominican
Republic

0   25   50 Miles

aiti's 27,700 km² take up the western half of the island of Hispaniola, which it shares with the Dominican Republic. Haiti is divided into 10 departments (Nippes became the 10th in 2004), 41 *arrondissements* (similar to districts), 135 *communes* (similar to parishes), and 565 communal sections.

GENERAL CONTEXT AND HEALTH DETERMINANTS

Social, Political, and Economic Determinants

In 2004, Haiti—the first black nation and the first country to gain independence in Latin America—celebrated its independence bicentennial. After nearly two centuries of dictatorship and intermittent attempts at democracy beginning in the late 1980s, the country has suffered recurrent periods of political instability. To summarize political events in the period under review, Jean Bertrand Aristide returned to Haiti in 2001. He again left the country in February 2004, and in March 2004 a transitional government was installed with the support of the United Nations Stabilization Mission, paving the way to normalization and efforts to strengthen the country's institutions and to presidential and parliamentary elections in February 2006.

The vast majority of Haitians continue to live under precarious conditions, in poverty and marginalization. Haiti is considered to be the poorest country in the Americas. The country's unequal income distribution (4% of the population has 66% of the nation's wealth, while 10% has practically nothing) forces the poor to turn to nature for survival. Deficient farming practices on steep terrain have accelerated soil erosion, as the run-off from tropical rains flushes arable land toward the sea, obstructing urban drainage systems in its wake. Surface water is polluted by ineffective excreta and household waste management.

According to the 2001 Haiti Living Conditions Survey, 55% of the population lives in households that are below the extreme poverty line of US$ 1 per person per day, and 71%—more than six million people—live below the poverty line of US$ 2 per person per day. That same survey shows that poverty is far worse in the country's rural areas and involves 82% of the country's population.

According to the 2003 General Population and Housing Census, more than 61% of the population aged 10 and older is literate (53.8% of females and 63.8% of males), a figure that is much higher in urban areas (80.5%) than in rural ones (47.1%). According to the 2001 Haiti Living Conditions Survey, the gross primary-school enrollment ratio is 120%, a figure that indicates that many overaged students are still enrolled in primary school. The net enrollment rate in primary school for children 6–11 years old is 60% nationwide. Slightly more than one of every two children in this age group attends primary school in rural areas, compared with upwards of 7 of every 10 in urban areas. There is no important difference in net primary enrollment rates for girls and boys.

This is not the case with secondary-school enrollment, where the gross enrollment ratio for girls is 37%, while that for boys is 45%. There is a wide gap in the gross secondary-school enrollment ratios of children from more affluent households (71%) compared with those from households in the lowest income quintile (23%). The country's official languages are Creole and French, but only 10% of the population speaks French, mainly those who have completed secondary schooling.

Access to basic health care is inadequate. According to the 2005–2010 National Strategic Plan for Health Sector Reform published in November 2005, less than 40% of the population has access to basic health services in certain departments (among them, Ouest, Nord, and Nord-Est); 80% seeks care from traditional healers. For many Haitians, the need to pay before receiving treatment precludes their getting any health care. Some organizations are promoting the idea of offering free services to increase access to treatment. Health costs (consultations, hospitalization, medical care, and drug purchases), too, have risen precipitously and can no longer be borne by people of limited means.

Forty-seven percent of the population lacks access to basic health care; 50% lacks access to basic drugs. A medical consultation that cost 25 Haitian Gourdes (HTG) in the late 1980s now costs 1,200 HTG—48 times more.

For the past two decades, the country's social and political crisis has had serious socioeconomic consequences. Haiti's GDP has generally decreased, translating into an average annual growth rate of –0.3% in 1986–2004.

From 2000 to 2004, the country experienced negative growth, along the order of –1.1% per year. Per capita GDP has been falling even more precipitously, at around 2.8% annually, mainly due to the rapid population growth (2.5% per year) between 1982 and 2003.

In August of 2000, the exchange rate of the HTG was 22 to 1 US$; it depreciated to HTG 42 per US$ 1 in 2005.

The qualitative and quantitative increase in food production in Haiti since the late 1950s has not been able to keep up with the population's needs, although food availability varies widely from

413

department to department. The population's nutritional status is eroded by inaccessibility to highly nutritional food and a lack of access to enough food.

Unsanitary preparation of food sold on the street is undoubtedly linked to high morbidity.

According to the Food and Agriculture Organization (FAO), 3.8 million people in Haiti, most of them living in rural areas, experience hunger; 23% of children under 5 years old suffer from chronic malnutrition. More than 40% of households experience food insecurity, and a high proportion of women (12%) are below the critical threshold for chronic energy deficiency.

The nutritional manifestations of food insecurity are numerous in Haiti. Worth citing among them are low birthweight; protein-energy malnutrition; micronutrient deficiencies, such as iron and folic acid deficiency, that lead to anemia in women and children; and vitamin A and iodine deficiency.

The decline in agricultural production has likewise intensified in recent years, at an annual rate of –1.2% between 2000 and 2004. The impact has been twofold. First, the nutritional status of children has deteriorated; recent surveys indicate an alarming increase in malnutrition in urban areas. Second, the widening of the trade deficit due to a rise in imports, notably food products, has been largely responsible for the devaluation of the country's currency and an increase in the cost of living.

The climate of insecurity has recently reached critical, even explosive, levels. It poses real challenges to private investment and has led to chronic unemployment and underemployment. The 2003 census indicates that 33%, or one-third of the economically active population, reported that it was out of work. This is but a baseline, of course, and real unemployment and underemployment most likely are far higher.

These circumstances easily explain the high incidence of extreme poverty in the country. Moreover, with structural adjustment programs calling for cutbacks in public expenditure, the supply of basic social services, notably in health and education, cannot meet demand. And, as the private sector takes over health and education services, prices tend to rise further.

Government workers account for 46% of the economically active population (50.4% of men; 42.2% of women). Workers in agriculture, forestry, animal husbandry, hunting, and fishing comprise 49.6% of the economically active workforce, which is dominated by men (93.3% in rural areas). "Wholesale and retail trade" ranks second, at 25.3%, and is dominated by women.

The country's political instability and insecurity slowed investment and economic growth after 2000. Real GDP fell in 2000–2003, plummeting from HTG 23.9 billion in 1987 to HTG 12.9 billion in 2003—a 48% drop. The average inflation rate was 17% (including a rise in the cost of basic goods), and the budget deficit (not including donations) represented 3.1% of GDP, on average.

The United Nations has referred to these dire circumstances as "the silent emergency."

The economic impact of events such as the 2004 floods, coupled with insecurity, material losses, and economic disruption

caused by political unrest early that year, contributed greatly to the estimated 5.5% drop in GDP.

In 2005, the economy stabilized, private sector activity rebounded, and foreign trade returned to pre-crisis levels. Inflation, too, shows signs of abating, and the Gourde has held stable, at around HTG 37/US$ 1.

In 2003, only 53.3% of the population—some 1,709,081 people—had access to safe drinking water. Drinking water coverage rates in 2000–2004 showed a modest 2.7% increase.

Drinking water supply coverage in urban areas in 2003 reveals that only 52% of the rural population, or around 2.4 million persons, had access to safe drinking water. This represents a 4.8% reduction in the population served since 2001.

In urban areas, 1.8 million people, or 58% of the population, have no access to excreta disposal services, and in rural areas, the figure is 3.6 million, or more than three-quarters of the rural population. In sum, roughly 5.5 million people, or 69% of Haiti's total population, do not have access to excreta disposal services.

Haiti is often buffeted by hurricanes, and the damage can be severe because of the country's degraded environment and precarious housing, often poorly constructed and built on unstable soil on very steep terrain, in marshlands, and along riverbeds. Given Haiti's pervasive deforestation, even normal rains can precipitate floods in Port-au-Prince and other urban areas.

Haiti is also extremely vulnerable to earthquakes. The country has eight fault lines, two of the most important located as follows: one in the far north and the other crossing east to west. Seismic activity in Haiti in 2003–2005 has revived the specter of a possibly major earthquake (7–8 on the Richter Scale), which experts have been forecasting for several years. The extremely high rate of urbanization that has left the metropolitan region of Port-au-Prince *commune* with slightly more than two million inhabitants (10,000–18,000 persons per km^2) will worsen the damage.

Demographics, Mortality, and Morbidity

According to the 2003 General Population and Housing Census, Haiti's annual population growth rate was 2.5%. According to that same census, the country has a population of 8,373,750 persons and a population density of 302 inhabitants per km^2. Three departments account for almost two-thirds of the population: Ouest, for 37%; Artibonite, for 16%; and Nord, for 10%. About 40% of the population is urban.

Haiti's population is young—60% was under 24 years old in 2003 and 36.5% was under the age of 15. Analysis of death certificates from 2003 shows that 4% of deaths in the country were in the age group 0–24 years old.

The birth rate remains relatively high, at 25 per 1,000 in urban areas; 30 per 1,000 in rural areas; and 28 per 1,000 for the country as a whole. The average number of children per woman has declined from 4.7 to 4.0, averaging 5 in rural areas, 3 in urban areas, and 2.4 in the capital. Life expectancy at birth is 52.7 years for males and 56.8 years for females. Around half of the population is single. Women represent 51.8% of the population (86 men per 100 women in urban areas and 98 men per 100 women in rural areas), a situation explained by factors related to population shifts—overwhelmingly, women migrate from rural areas to the cities, while the reverse is true for men. (See Figure 1 for the country's population structure.)

Out-migration is significant in Haiti, be it temporary or permanent, legal or illegal, or what is termed "brain drain." The Ministry for Haitians Living Abroad estimates that the total number of émigrés is 1.5 million: 700,000 are in the United States of America, 550,000 in the Dominican Republic, 100,000 in Canada, 70,000 in neighboring French overseas departments and territories, and 40,000 in the Bahamas. Many Haitian professionals and skilled technicians who live outside Haiti provide an important source of revenue for the country.

The first published analysis of death certificates in Haiti dealt with deaths in 1997. At that time, death certificates were filled out for only 6.3% of deaths. Coverage increased to 10% in 2003. However, a precipitous drop in death certificate coverage occurred in 2004 and 2005. At the same time, the way in which death certificates are completed improved (the percentage of death certificates with an ill-defined cause of death fell from 48% in 1999 to 26% in 2002). Immediate and effective feedback was put in place at the central and departmental levels. Given this poor coverage, mortality data should be interpreted with caution. Table 1 shows the 10 leading causes of death in 2003. The data come from an analysis of death certificates from the country's 10 departments.

Diabetes mellitus ranks as the 11th cause of death, and is implicated in 2.8% of deaths. Maternal mortality ranks 12th (the 7th leading cause of death in women).

According to the 2000–2001 Mortality, Morbidity, and Service Utilization Survey (EMMUS III), maternal mortality was 523 per 100,000 live births, representing a 15% increase over the figure from the 1991 national survey, which reported a rate of 457 per 100,000 live births. An analysis of the causes of maternal mortality in 2003 shows that complications in childbirth, such as hemorrhage, are the leading causes of death (29%), followed by problems linked with hypertension and eclampsia (26%). Abortion was implicated in 13% of cases. According to 2000–2001 Mortality, Morbidity, and Service Utilization Survey (EMMUS III), 54.4% of all women and 63.2% of pregnant women are anemic.

HEALTH OF POPULATION GROUPS

Children under 5 Years Old

Infant mortality estimates in Haiti are based on data from the Morbidity, Mortality, and Service Utilization surveys (EMMUS). Table 2 shows the infant mortality indicators from four surveys.

According to the preliminary report of the 2005–2006 Mortality, Morbidity, and Service Utilization Survey (EMMUS IV), 1 in 12

FIGURE 1. Population structure, by age and sex, Haiti, 1990 and 2005.

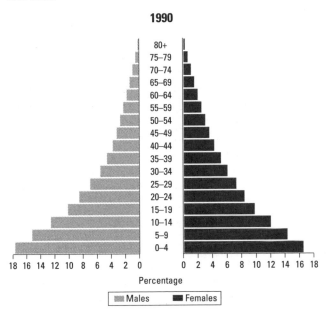

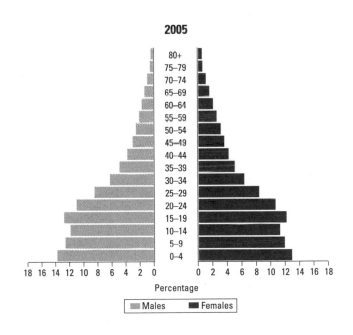

Haitian children die before their fifth birthday. The survey also found that acute respiratory infections and acute diarrheal diseases continue to be the most common health problems in children—40% of children under 5 years old had acute respiratory infection symptoms or fever in the two weeks preceding the survey. However, only 20% of children had been taken for a consultation or to get help (20% in urban areas versus 18% in rural areas; and 28% among children whose mother had a secondary education

TABLE 1. Ten leading causes of death in rank order, by sex, total deaths from leading causes, and percentage of total deaths by cause, Haiti, 2003.

Rank	Cause of death	Female deaths	Male deaths	Total deaths	% by cause
1	Diseases of the circulatory system	829	561	1,390	24.4
2	AIDS	219	271	490	8.6
3	Infectious intestinal diseases	219	268	487	8.6
4	Pneumonia and influenza	160	169	329	5.8
5	Malignant neoplasms	157	135	292	5.1
6	Tuberculosis	118	148	266	4.7
7	Malnutrition	117	132	249	4.4
8	Infections specific to the perinatal period	128	117	245	4.3
9	Accidents	77	142	219	3.8
10	Assault	28	145	173	3.0
	Total deaths with other defined causes	781	775	1,556	27.3
	Total deaths from defined causes	2,833	2,863	5,696	100
	Ill-defined causes	1,043	1,272	2,315	

Source: Haiti, Ministry of Public Health and Population. Analysis of causes of deaths, 2003.

TABLE 2. Infant mortality rate, by age group, as estimated by the first four Mortality, Morbidity, and Service Utilization surveys (EMMUS I–IV), Haiti, 1987–2006.

	EMMUS I 1987	EMMUS II 1994–1995	EMMUS III 2000–2001	EMMUS IV 2005–2006[a]
Infant mortality (0–1 years old)	99	74	80	57
Neonatal mortality (0–28 days old)	40	31	32	25
Postnatal mortality (1–11 months old)	59	43	48	32
Young child mortality (1–4 years old)	66	61	42	31
Infant and young child mortality (0–4 years old)	158	131	119	86

Source: Institut Haïtien de l'Enfance.
[a]These are preliminary results.

versus 15% among those whose mother had no schooling). Moreover, 24% of children under 5 years old had had one or more episodes of diarrhea in the two weeks preceding the survey, and 57% had been treated with oral rehydration therapy—an important increase in the use of this treatment as compared with the previous survey period (2000–2001), in which the figure was 41%.

The 2000–2001 survey (EMMUS III) found that 65.3% of preschoolers were anemic in 2000.

Children 5–9 Years Old

According to data from the 2003 census, the estimated population 5–9 years old accounts for 13% of the total. With the country's level of poverty and the fact that 89% of the schools are private, 17% of school-aged children do not attend school and 12.5% have never even been enrolled. In this latter group, 42% were younger than 10 years old and 54% were girls.

Infectious and parasitic diseases were responsible for 27% of recorded deaths in this age group. Tuberculosis, diarrheal diseases, malnutrition, HIV/AIDS, and malaria are the five leading causes of death, with no differences between the sexes. Also noteworthy is the importance of external causes in the mortality of children in this age group (8%). A more detailed study of the causes of death, based on data from 2000, reveals that boys are more likely to be the victims of traffic accidents and girls are more often victims of accidents in the home.

A national survey conducted in 2002–2003 on the prevalence of helminth infections in children 6–12 years of age (complemented with surveys on the prevalence and intensity of intestinal geohelminth infections in the departments of Sud and Grand' Anse) reveals that one-third of the children had parasites, with substantial variation from department to department. The department of Grand'Anse had the highest rate (74%), followed by Nord (46%). A deparasitization campaign was launched there by the Ministry of Public Health and Population and the Ministry of National Education, Youth, and Sports as part of a PAHO/WHO regional program and the Communicable Disease Prevention and School Health project. A single 400 mg dose of albendazole was administered every six months. The campaign was expanded to the departments of Nord and Nord-Est and to Artibonite.

Adolescents 10–14 and 15–19 Years Old

The 10 leading causes of death in these groups include AIDS, physical assaults, accidents, tuberculosis, typhoid, and maternal causes; services for adolescents are mainly provided by nonprofit organizations. According to the 2005–2006 Mortality, Morbidity, and Service Utilization Service Survey (EMMUS IV), the fertility rate among 15–19-year-old women is 69 per 1,000, with wide disparities between the metropolitan region (46 per 1,000) and rural areas (86 per 1,000). One of every five women aged 15–19 years old has access to modern contraceptives. Condom use was low in this group (7%) in 2005–2006.

In 2005, there were 1,002 deliveries among girls 10–14 years old, and 6,090 among women 15–19 years old. Violence and sexual abuse are more common among 10–19-year-olds than in any other age groups.

Adults 20–59 Years Old

This age group—which includes women of childbearing age and most persons in the workforce—represents 40% of the total population. According to the 2005–2006 survey (EMMUS IV), the fertility rate among women of childbearing age has declined from 4.7 children per woman in 2000 to 4.1 in 2003, with variations depending on area of residence (five children in rural areas, and three in the metropolitan area). Information on at least one modern family-planning method has been given to 99% of women. The modern methods most commonly used by women who are in a relationship are injections (11%), condoms (5%), and the pill (3%). Only 2% opt for sterilization in both urban and rural areas, and 2%, for IUDs.

Analysis of the causes of death in 2003 reveals that AIDS is the leading cause among 20–49-year-olds, resulting in 14.5% of deaths with a specific diagnosis. Cardiovascular disease ranks second (10%), followed by assaults (5%), maternal causes (4.4%), accidents (3.9%), and tuberculosis (3.7%).

Older Adults 65 Years Old and Older

According to the 2003 Population and Housing Census, the population older than 65 years old represents 5.1% of the total population. Some 72% of this group lives in rural areas, and 7.7% indicated that they had at least one disability. Women account for 53% of the age group. Approximately 78% of the elderly do not know how to read or write.

The analysis of the causes of death in 2003 for that age group reveals a predominance of noncommunicable diseases (in descending order, cardiovascular disease, stroke, neoplasms, lung disease, diarrheal disease, and diabetes mellitus).

There is no health care program for the elderly. According to Haitian tradition and culture, the elderly live at home and are cared for by their families. However, this situation is changing, and private nursing homes for elder care are beginning to appear, although their high cost (on the order of US$ 600 per month) makes them inaccessible to all but a minority of the population. Certain *communes* have nursing homes for the poorest among the elderly (communal nursing homes of Cap Haïtien, Port-au-Prince); other facilities are run by religious groups (the Catholic Church has a facility in Cayes); certain associations also operate homes for the elderly.

The Family

Constant relocation and emigration has contributed to a breakdown in the family structure in urban and rural areas. In major cities, a single home may house several families, either because members have emigrated or because children have lost their parents. In urban areas, 48% of single parent households are headed by women, compared to 33.3% in rural areas. Only 45% of children under 18 live with both parents. It should be noted that the Ministry of Public Health and Population has a Bureau of Family Health, which works with UNFPA to ensure, among other things, that family planning supplies reach outlying warehouses.

Prenatal check-ups with a health professional (doctor, nurse, or nursing auxiliary) are steadily increasing, with 85% coverage of pregnant women, in contrast to 67.7% coverage in 1995. Again according to the 2005–2006 survey (EMMUS IV), 60% of deliveries nationwide are attended by a professional or a skilled midwife (74% in urban areas and 53% in rural areas), in contrast to 46% in 1994. The fact that there are still so many women who die in childbirth should be cause for reflection, including concerns about the skills of the personnel involved. The fact that only 24.7% of deliveries take place in health facilities (2000–2001 survey [EMMUS III]) is probably more indicative of the real situation than the figure of deliveries attended by skilled personnel.

The Institute for Social Welfare and Research of the Ministry of Social Affairs and Labor provides some services to disadvantaged and handicapped children.

Workers

The employment rate is very low (46%). The informal sector, comprised mainly of women workers, and the agricultural sector together employ 96% of the workforce. A national vocational assistance program to promote productive employment and fight social exclusion, under the aegis of the Ministry of Planning and External Cooperation and with support from UNDP and ILO, has financed an inventory of organized groups from Haiti's informal sector that extend some form of social protection to their members or adherents. The program, offered by microfinancing institutions or health NGOs, reaches only around 2% of Haiti's population and generally covers illness and death. The social assistance systems that have been set up are similar to insurance or mutual insurance. They cover groups of 400 to 115,000 individuals and are managed by their members or by health care providers. Access to health services is linked to a low premium paid periodically by subscribers. These initiatives respond to the desire of groups in the informal sector to have insurance mechanisms to cover their basic needs. In addition, the Ministry of Social Affair and Labor's Institute for Social Welfare and Research provides some services to female sex workers.

Another study shows that state-sponsored social protection covers 1%–3% of the formal sector. The law grants three months' maternity leave for working pregnant women. Government employees and their families (about 215,000 people) are covered by a specific insurance system but services are considered unsatisfactory, particularly outside the capital.

Coverage for private-sector employees is provided by the Office of Labor, Illness, and Maternity Insurance, a decentralized autonomous agency that runs a hospital offering basic services and some specialized services, such as trauma and obstetrics and gynecology. In addition to medical care, beneficiaries are paid an indemnity for temporary or permanent disability. Some 43,000 people regularly receive benefits from this system. Certain companies offer protection to their day workers or regular staff.

Persons with Disabilities

According to the 2003 census, 1.5% of the population, or 125,600 people, had a handicap; 11% were under 15 years old, 57% were 15–64 years old, and 32% were 65 years old and older. More than 65% lived in rural areas and around 70% had no schooling. The most commonly reported disability was blindness; an estimated 1% of the population was blind and between 75,000 and 200,000 people were visually impaired as a result of trauma, glaucoma, cataracts, corneal infections, and diabetic retinopathy.

The disabled are often the poorest of the poor in Haiti. Deprived of financial resources, they have little access to curative care (three permanent and two temporary facilities provide prosthetics in Haiti, but only one-quarter of amputees have been able to obtain a prosthetic, whose cost is prohibitive for most disabled persons). In 2005, 28 national institutions or associations and 10 international institutions or associations were working in this area in Haiti.

Highly Vulnerable Children

Orphans, street children, and children working as domestic servants are particularly vulnerable. The 2005–2006 Mortality, Morbidity, and Service Utilization Survey (EMMUS IV) estimates that 11% of children under 18 have lost their father and/or mother. The most recent study on children living on the street (those who sever ties with the family home) and children who work on the street (those who maintain ties and stay in more or less regular contact with their families or return home to sleep or bring the fruits of their labors) dates to 1999 and was conducted by Quisqueya University's Unit for Research on Children in Difficult Situations. According to the study, there are between 6,226 and 7,833 children 5–17 years old living in such precarious situations in Port-au-Prince, 163 in Cap-Haïtien, and 41 in Jacmel. Often abused by the police, who regard them as delinquents, they are prone to diseases and stomach problems. According to these sources, as many as 300,000 children and adolescents live with so-called "foster families," in a situation known as restavèk ("stay with"); 81% live in rural areas, 75% are girls, and the majority are between the ages of 7 and 14. Only 55% attend school.

Prisoners

An analysis of medical statistics on the care of inmates in three metropolitan prisons in 2005 shows that, out of a total of 10,969 visits, the leading reasons for consultation were headaches, gastric problems, urogenital infections, hypertension, fever, scabies, arthritis, acute respiratory infections, and diarrhea. There were 75 cases of beri-beri reported during this period and 65 pregnancies. The Ministry of Public Health and Population provides tuberculosis treatment in 17 prisons, which covers more than 4,000 prisoners.

HEALTH CONDITIONS AND PROBLEMS

COMMUNICABLE DISEASES

Vector-borne Diseases

Malaria (*Plasmodium falciparum*) is endemic in Haiti, with higher transmission rates in certain communal sections after the rainy seasons from March to May and October to November. In 2003, 109 deaths were attributed to malaria (63 females and 46 males), 12% of whom were children under 5 years old. There were 86,768 cases of malaria reported in 2004, of which 24,205 were laboratory-confirmed. The figures for 2005 are 106,152 and 26,021, respectively. (There are 50 operational sentinel surveillance sites in the country.)

A five-year project (2004–2009) financed by the Global Fund to Fight AIDS, Tuberculosis, and Malaria (US$ 14.8 million) is under way, aimed at reducing morbidity to less than 10% and eliminating mortality from malaria by 2010.

Dengue hemorrhagic fever has not yet been documented in Haiti. All four serotypes (I–IV) circulate in the country, but no structured treatment program is in place. Suspected cases of dengue hemorrhagic fever are regularly reported by the routine surveillance system. *Aedes aegypti* is found throughout the country, especially in urban areas, where the presence of larval breeding sites facilitates its propagation, especially during the rainy seasons.

Lymphatic filariasis is found in both urban and rural areas, especially in the Nord department, on the Gulf of Gonâve, where it is a major public health problem. The entire country is at risk of the transmission of this disease by the *Culex quinquefasciatus* vector, which tends to multiply in urban areas and leeward coastal regions. In cities such as Léogâne, Arcahaie, Plaine du Nord, and Limbé, more than 20% of the population is infected with microfilaria. Certain *communes* in the Nord and Centre departments have positivity rates of over 30%.

A national prevalence study of 22,058 students aged 6–10 years old in 10 departments was conducted in three phases (November/December 1999, May/June 2000, and January/May 2001). The 898 children with a positive immunochromatographic card test (ICT) were treated with Diethylcarbamazine (DEC) at a dosage of 6 mg/kg. A 2003 project financed by the Bill and Melinda Gates Foundation, with assistance from PAHO/WHO, aims at the elimination of this disease by 2010 and has begun to bear fruit.

Following Hurricane Jeanne in September 2004, surveillance for mosquito-borne diseases in Gonaïves identified three patients with malaria, two with acute dengue infections, and two with acute **West Nile virus** infections among 116 acutely febrile patients.

Vaccine-preventable Diseases

Haiti's immunization program covers the following diseases: tuberculosis, poliomyelitis, diphtheria, tetanus, whooping cough, and measles (see Table 3). Vaccination coverage for infants 12–23 months is 41.3% (EMMUS IV). **Measles** is on the way to elimination. A total of 990 measles cases were confirmed in 2000, and the last epidemic was in 2001, with 158 confirmed cases, and no case of measles has been confirmed since.

In Haiti, a single laboratory-confirmed case of a non-wild poliovirus type 1 originating from a laboratory was reported in an inadequately vaccinated 2-year-old child; paralysis onset was August 30, 2000. Despite intensive case-finding activities, no additional cases have been identified.

There also was a **diphtheria** epidemic in 2004, with 801 suspected cases, 101 of which were investigated; 27 of them were confirmed by laboratory and 10 by epidemiologic contact. In 2005, data available to the Ministry of Public Health and Population indicated that there were 495 cases that year. Among the 17 reported cases that were investigated, 9 were confirmed, with 8 deaths. **Neonatal tetanus** remains a major public health problem. Despite concerted efforts to control the disease, 119 cases of tetanus were reported in 2005, 71 of which were neonatal; of these, 46 were investigated. Certain *communes* currently have neonatal tetanus rates in excess of 1 case per 1,000 live births. According to the 2005–2006 Mortality, Morbidity, and Service Utilization Survey (EMMUS IV), in almost three-quarters of births in the last five years (74%), the mother had received one dose of

TABLE 3. Expanded Program on Immunization coverage rate (%), by antigen, Haiti, 2001–2005.

Antigens	Year				
	2001	2002	2003	2004	2005[a]
BCG	49	45	54	43	62
Polio1					55
Polio2					45
Polio3	53	41	48	61	65
DPT1					57
DPT2					47
DPT3	52	39	50	62	68
Chickenpox	53	34	52	57	59
TT2+	ND	ND	ND	ND	19

[a]The percentages provided for polio 1–3 and DPT 1–3 in 2005 are based on data for multiple years, rather than for a single calendar year.
Source: Ministry of Public Health and Population, Expanded Program on Immunization, PAHO/WHO, administrative data.

tetanus vaccine during pregnancy. With regard to **whooping cough**, all cases are not reported or investigated. Available data show 4 cases in 2004 and 21 cases investigated out of the 697 reported by the Ministry of Public Health and Population in 2005.

Intestinal Infectious Diseases

Intestinal infectious diseases continue to rank high as a cause of infant morbidity and mortality. According to the 2005–2006 Mortality, Morbidity, and Service Utilization Survey (EMMUS IV), 24% of children under 5 years old had had one or more episodes of diarrheal disease in the two weeks preceding the survey. Of these children, 40% had been treated with a packet of oral rehydration therapy (ORT) and 7% had been treated at home with a solution prepared by the mother. At the national level, 57% also received fluids during a diarrhea episode, a net increase over the rate estimated for 2000 (41%). It should be pointed out, however, that ORT use is more prevalent in the cities (72% in the metropolitan area) than in the countryside (52%).

In terms of prevalence, children aged 6–11 are the most affected (41%), followed by infants 12–23 months old (38%). All the other age groups also are affected.

These pathologies ranked third, behind AIDS, on the list of leading causes of death in 2003, for all age groups and sexes combined (or 8.6% of deaths with a defined cause). Typhoid fever is responsible for 2.8% of deaths in children aged 5–9, 8.9% in the 10–14 age group, 3.2% in the 15–19 age group, and 1.5% in the 20–49 age group.

Chronic Communicable Diseases

Tuberculosis, which is endemic in Haiti, is the seventh leading cause of death according to the analysis of death certificates from 2003. Tuberculosis tends to strike persons in their productive years, between the ages of 15 and 44 years old.

The estimated incidence of tuberculosis was 12,632 (all forms) in 2005 and from 6,828 to 7,340 for sputum-smear positive cases. The objectives of the national tuberculosis program (70% detection and 85% cure) have not yet been met. The detection rate was estimated at 49% in 2006 and the cure rate, in the neighborhood of 70% in 2004.

In 1997, the cornerstone of a structured national tuberculosis program was laid with the application of the Directly Observed Treatment, Short Course (DOTS) strategy. An 8-month regimen was introduced, along with a National Tuberculosis Plan for 2001–2006. Between 2001 and 2005, the percentage of tuberculosis-infected individuals who were defined as "cured" ranged from 62% in 2001 to 70% in 2005. In 2005, 198 facilities participated in the program, four of them sanatoriums. Patients receive drugs free of charge. Haiti's HIV epidemic has greatly exacerbated the country's tuberculosis situation, making tuberculosis the leading opportunistic infection in people living with HIV. Available epidemiologic information indicates a TB/HIV co-infection rate of 29%.

Efforts to combat **leprosy** have been under way in Haiti for more than a century; the Ministry of Public Health and Population has declared leprosy elimination a priority.

Between 1998 and 2002, 1,718 cases of leprosy were detected and 75% of them were treated. Furthermore, more than 1,000 health professionals received training. The closing of the Gonaïves center[1] in the wake of tropical storm Jeanne in September 2004 led to a drastic reduction in the number of new cases detected, which fell from 56 in 2000, to 26 in 2004, and 24 in 2005. After 2004, the Ministry of Public Health and Population created a program office for leprosy and drew up a new strategic plan for 2006–2008. The Ministry signed a cooperation agreement with the Fame Pereo Institute and entered into an understanding with Fontilles, a Spanish NGO devoted to caring for leprosy patients.

In 2005, the Falciform Anemia League (LAAF), created in 1989 in Port-au-Prince, identified 706 individuals with **sickle-cell disease** in 679 families, 27 of which had two or three children with the malady. Among them, 540 (or 76% of those detected) were of the SS genotype. The distribution by age was 16% in the age group 0–10, 41% in the age group 11–20, 26% in the age group 21–30, and 16% in the age group older than 30. The highest morbidity was observed in subjects aged 0–24 (sequelae of stroke/ seizures, deafness, mutism, or priapism in 5% of young men over the age of 15; open leg ulcers in 4% of SS sickle cell patients older than age 12 years, with no clear preponderance in either sex). In May 2005, in the *commune* of Mirebalais (Central Plateau), a preliminary study provided a series of tests for 412 of the 900 people who had sought medical care (pa-

tients aged 22–45). Cellulose acetate electrophoresis of hemoglobin, followed by the falciformation test, identified 115 people with abnormal hemoglobin S and C (13.3% heterozygotic for hemoglobin S and 3.6% for hemoglobin C), percentages close to those observed in the capital. A high percentage (9%) of S, + thalassemia was observed in this region, calling for more systematic investigation (family study, neonatal detection, quantitative electrophoresis of hemoglobin).

Acute Respiratory Infections

According to the mortality, morbidity, and service utilization surveys, in 2005–2006, no less than 40% of children under 5 years old had had fever or symptoms compatible with ARIs in the two weeks preceding the survey. Only 20% of them had been formally examined to obtain treatment (26% in the cities, 18% in the countryside). The mother's schooling level also is associated with whether or not treatment is sought (28% with a secondary education versus 15% when the mother has had no schooling).

Analysis of the death certificates from 2003 reveals that mortality attributable to acute respiratory infections in children ranks just behind the number of deaths from malnutrition or diarrhea.

HIV/AIDS and Other Sexually Transmitted Infections

HIV/AIDS and sexually transmitted infections (STIs) are common in Haiti. Estimates put HIV prevalence at 2.2%, or 2.3% among women aged 15–49 and 2% among men aged 15–59 (EMMUS IV)—Haiti is in the throes of a generalized HIV epidemic. The virus strikes men and women of reproductive age, leads to death at a very young age, and leaves vulnerable orphans in its wake.

An estimated 40,000 HIV-positive persons needed antiretroviral therapy in 2005. Starting in 2003, antiretroviral therapy has been available in Haiti, chiefly through centers run by two organizations: the Haitian Group for the Study of Kaposi's Sarcoma and Opportunistic Infections (GHESKIO), and Zanmi Lasanté, a nongovernmental organization.

The number of treatment sites has substantially increased and the number of people receiving antiretroviral therapy rose from 5,500 in January 2006 to 9,412 in September 2006 (43% men and 57% women, for a male-to-female ratio of 1:1.3).

The vast majority of patients receive antiretroviral therapy at GHESKIO centers and the Zanmi Lasané network. Other patients are treated at 24 other treatment sites throughout the country, but coverage is still highly inequitable.

The number of treatment sites designed to prevent mother-to-child transmission has substantially increased, from 40 in 2003 to 74 in September 2006; effective care for pregnant women and their babies has yet to be achieved, however. Between October 2004 and September 2005, around 53,000 pregnant women were screened for HIV, and between October 2005 and September 2006, over 70,000 or just over 80% of pregnant women were seen in these centers. The HIV prevalence rate in this selected group

---

[1]On 26 September 2004, tropical storm Jeanne left 3,000 people dead, among them Father Olivier, who had devoted his life to leprosy patients in Artibonite. He was swept away while trying to bring help to patients in the flooded Hôpital de la Providence in the city of Gonaïves.

was 3.3%, and 91% of the women tested returned for their results and received post-testing counseling on site. But only 10% of these seropositive women and their babies received antiretroviral therapy to prevent mother-to-child transmission.

In 2005–2006, approximately 180,000 persons were tested for HIV (M:F ratio of 1:1.9) in 98 voluntary screening centers, with a positivity rate of 9.3% (10.7% for men and 8.6% for women).

In the 2005–2006 Mortality, Morbidity, and Service Utilization Survey (EMMUS IV), virtually all respondents had heard of HIV/AIDS, and 75% of the women and 85% of the men said that there was a way of preventing it; responses varied widely from department to department. Irrespective of these responses, condom use is very limited (11% of women and 23% of men who had had sexual relations in the 12 months prior to the survey had used them in their last sexual encounter). Singles stated more often that they used condoms (38% of women and 42% of men), and condom use was more common among young people (26% of girls and 33% of boys aged 15–19 years, versus only 6% or less among women over 30 and men over 40). Educational level also influences condom use (24% of women and 40% of men with a secondary education used them, versus 2% of women and 3% of men who had not attended school). People with HIV/AIDS continue to be stigmatized and discriminated against, and may even be rejected by their own families.

Noncommunicable Diseases

Metabolic and Nutritional Diseases

The 2000–2001 Mortality, Morbidity, and Service Utilization Survey (EMMUS III) revealed high levels of **anemia** in children (65%), women in general (54%), and pregnant women (63%).

Moreover, in 2005, the Haitian Children's Institute (l'Institut Haïtien de l'Enfance [IHE]) conducted a study on the prevalence of **vitamin A and iodine deficiencies**. One-third of children 6–59 months old had plasma retinol levels of ≤ 0.70 μm/L and suffered from vitamin A deficiency (essentially of nutritional origin) and 1.47%, from severe deficiency (≤ 0.35); there was no difference between the sexes. Children 24–35 months old were the most affected. Haiti can be considered a country with mild iodine deficiency (median 84 μg/l): 24% of the population suffers from moderate deficiency, and a very small fraction from severe deficiency. Rural areas are the ones with most of the severe iodine deficiency, but even the metropolitan area has pockets of severe deficiency. This deficiency has had an adverse effect on the health of pregnant women and children.

From September 2002 to May 2003, the Haitian Foundation for Diabetes and Cardiovascular Disease conducted a cross-sectional study of 1,620 adults older than 20 years old in metropolitan Port-au-Prince. The age-adjusted prevalence of **diabetes** was 4.8% in men and 8.9% in women, with 70.6% of cases already known. **Hypertension** was found in 48.7% of men and 46.5% of women. The rate in the group older than 40 was 69.1% in men and 67.2% in women.

Cardiovascular Diseases

Based on a review of a sample of death certificates for the years 2000 to 2003, cerebrovascular disease accounted for one-third of all deaths. Heart disease, diabetes, and hypertensive diseases were also important causes of death.

Malignant Neoplasms

In 2003, malignant neoplasms ranked fifth as the specific cause of death in Haiti, accounting for 5.1% of all recorded deaths with a certified diagnosis. A total of 292 cases of malignant neoplasms, 157 in women and 135 in men, were reported at that time. In women, the areas most affected were: the reproductive system (28% of malignant tumors), the digestive system (26%), the breast (18%), the respiratory system (9%), the blood and lymphatic system (7%), and the aerodigestive tract (5%). There is no systematic screening for cervical, breast, or prostate cancer.

Zoonoses

There were 21 cases of **human rabies** confirmed between 2001 and 2005, nine in 2001, four in 2002, four in 2003, three in 2004, and one in 2005. Most cases were in the metropolitan area. Currently, many foci that are reported are not investigated, due to the inadequacy of the epidemiological surveillance system.

Anthrax is endemic in the Nord, Sud-Est, Nippes, and Artibonite departments. These four departments are active foci.

Other Health Problems or Issues

Natural Disasters

Torrential rains flooded the cities of Cayes in 2002 and Saint-Marc in 2003. In 2004, the rural areas of Mapou and Fonds Verrettes also were hard hit by floods. In the latter, 1,800 deaths were reported and two villages were completely destroyed by mudslides. In September 2004, tropical storm Jeanne flooded the cities of Gonaïves and Port-de-Paix, resulting in 2,000 deaths and leaving 100,000 families homeless; eight hospitals and several clinics were destroyed.

The 2005 hurricane season was especially intense. Storm activity was more than twice as great as the average, with 26 storms and 14 hurricanes. Heavy rains and violent winds from these storms swelled most of the rivers and flooded several regions. Tidal waves were reported in some coastal areas in the departments of Sud and Grand'Anse.

Violence and Other External Causes

Accidents and violence contribute significantly to morbidity and mortality in Haiti, especially among the economically active population and adolescents and young adults. In 2003, 6% of deaths in the group aged 15–19 and 5% in the 20–49 age group were connected with assaults. In 2006, data were gathered by different agencies, such as the Police, the United Nations Stabilization Mission in Haiti, the Ministry on the Status of Women and Women's Rights, the National Network for the Defense of Human Rights, and Doctors without Borders. A review of these data showed that almost 90% of emergency care was treatment for assault with a deadly weapon and 10% for sexual assault or domestic violence.

Since opening its doors, the center operated by Doctors without Borders, France (MSF/F), has treated an average of 700 emergency cases each month, 200 of them the result of violence. MSF/F statistics show that there were an average of 232 victims of traffic accidents each month (70% among 19–49-year-olds, with an M:F ratio of 1.8:1, and 20% under the age of 18) and 414 monthly patient consultations due to accidents in the home. Kidnappings for ransom are another form of violence: in December 2005 alone, there were 237 cases of kidnapping for ransom.

Addictions

A Government study commissioned in 2000 that interviewed 778 children living in difficult situations and 4,317 students in secondary schools in metropolitan Port-au-Prince showed that there is easy access to psychoactive substances in Port-au-Prince. The number of individuals who consider access to be easy, however, varies with the substance in question: cigarettes (98%); alcohol (97%); analgesics (72%); tranquilizers (39%); and inhalants (paint thinner) (31%). Alcohol is the most common drug used (55% of the sample), with use beginning at the age of 14; it is followed by amphetamines (29%), sleeping pills (15%), and tranquilizers (11%). Boys who were questioned in the survey said that they had started using marijuana at around age 17, girls reporting starting around age 11.

The Association for the Prevention of Alcoholism and other Chemical Addictions offers rehabilitation services that follow the 12-step approach of Alcoholics Anonymous during 12 months. Between 2001 and 2006, the Association treated 143 persons, 88% of them men and 61% who had been addicted for more than five years. The breakdown of addictions by type of substance is as follows: alcohol (27%); marijuana (19%); crack cocaine (30%); Juicy Lucy (marijuana plus crack cocaine) (6%); and tobacco, prescription drugs, and heroin (8%).

RESPONSE OF THE HEALTH SECTOR

Health Policies and Plans

In 2005, the Ministry of Public Health and Population published a national strategic plan for health sector reforms to be carried out in 2005–2010. The plan identifies health as a basic human right of all Haitians, without discrimination, and underscores the direct link between health and human development and the necessary respect for the principles of solidarity, equity, and social justice.

Haiti's health policy's main mandate calls for strengthening the Ministry's steering role in planning, executing, and evaluation of health programs. Community Health Units are decentralized administrative entities responsible for carrying out health activities of guaranteed quality, in partnership with public and private health organizations and with the community's participation, in each Unit's assigned geographical area.

Traditional medicine, which is widely accepted regardless of social class or religious affiliation, is practiced by various healers ("doktè-fèy," midwives, voodoo priests, masseurs, bonesetters, herbalists, spiritualists).

In 2006, a decree created a Pharmacy, Drug, and Traditional Medicine Bureau within the Ministry of Public Health and Population. It is responsible for ensuring that a national policy on traditional medicine and drugs is developed and that research in this area is promoted.

The development of strategies and the execution of activities to guarantee basic services are hampered by a deficient, outdated legal framework and inadequate institutions. The absence of basic laws and a lack of consistency in the existing services have led to a state of anarchy in which the Government has been unable to regulate, direct, or monitor the quality of services and supplies offered.

As of the end of 2005, Haiti had no national drug policy.

In 2002, the Ministry of Public Health and Population launched a program to restructure and rationalize the national health system, including functionally decentralizing the Ministry based on the concept of Community Health Units. Decentralization is still in the early stages—11 Community Health Units in 5 departments were up and running by 2006. The development of an effective financing system, the strengthening of community participation, inter- and intrasectoral coordination, the development of a human resources policy compatible with Ministry needs, and the amendment of health legislation to safeguard the interests of the greatest number of people are other important strategies.

Organization of the Health System

Haiti's health system is made up of the public sector, the private for-profit sector, the mixed nonprofit sector, and the traditional sector. The public sector consists of the Ministry of Public Health and Population and the Ministry of Social Affairs. The private for-profit sector includes all health professionals in private practice, working on their own or in clinics. The mixed nonprofit sector consists of Ministry of Public Health and Population staff who work in facilities run by the private sector, by nongovernmental organizations, or by religious organizations.

The Ministry of Public Health and Population is headed by the Minister and the Director-General; it encompasses ten national bureaus and four coordinating units, each one dealing with infectious and communicable diseases, the Expanded Program on Immunization (EPI), nutrition, and hospital safety. There are also 10 departmental health bureaus, one for each of the country's 10 departments, which are headed by a Departmental Health Director, assisted by the professionals who oversee the national programs. The Community Health Units report to the departmental health bureaus. The number and location are dictated by the size of the population under their jurisdiction and their geographical location. The most recent organic law is from 2005–2006, but new structures have been created since its enactment, pursuant to the resolutions adopted by the country following international health and development conferences. Pending matters include the passage of the health and drug laws by the New Parliament and the creation of a Health Commission to support these processes.

All health system facilities are overseen and coordinated by the Ministry of Public Health and Population as part of the Ministry's regulatory role. The Ministry has not been able to fully assume this role, however. International cooperation resources have been directed more to the nonprofit private sector and, therefore, some private facilities have acquired greater capacity than the public sector. The Ministry of Social Affairs is theoretically responsible for workers' health in the formal private sector. To that end, several decentralized agencies fall under its responsibility, the most important of which are the National Old-age Insurance Office; the Insurance Office for Workplace Accidents, Illness, and Maternity; and the Social Welfare and Research Institute.

The private, for-profit sector is concentrated in the metropolitan area, where most professionals work. Private facilities, including clinics, laboratories, and pharmacies, operate without restriction but do not participate in the national health programs and epidemiological surveillance of diseases subject to mandatory notification.

The health services are distributed into first-level health services, communal referral hospitals, and departmental referral hospitals. The public sector encompasses about 35.7% of the health infrastructure; the mixed private sector, 31.8%; and the private sector, 32.5%. Under the old nomenclature, there were 402 dispensaries, 198 health centers with no beds, 54 centers with beds, and 63 hospitals, found primarily in the main locations of the departments. Some of the hospitals are specialized—in particular, the Hospital of the State University of Haiti, which is the national referral hospital, although its operations are often affected by budget constraints and repeated strikes. Certain *communes* have health centers, but they cannot meet the needs of their populations. An estimated 40% of the population lacks access to health services. Around 80% of the general population has

access to traditional medicine; most live in rural areas, where 13% of the population lives more than 15 km from the nearest health center.

Concerted efforts to set up a social security system are still incipient, despite the Government's efforts to provide a pension to employees over age 55 years with 25 years of service through the Ministry of Finance. The National Office for Old-age Insurance, created in 1965, covers employees in the private sector, but a very small percentage of the population is covered and the sums provided are often paltry.

Public Health Services

The Ministry of Public Health and Population relies on the primary health care strategy to attend to the health needs of the population. Care is delivered through a basic package of services, including child, adolescent, and women's health; emergency medical and surgical care; communicable disease control; health education; environmental health; and provision of drinking water and essential drugs. The provision of this basic package is still experimental, and limitations in national health programs prevent them from providing maximum coverage.

Priority is given to programs to combat HIV/AIDS and tuberculosis; these programs receive support from financial institutions working in the health sector. In addition, networks of NGOs and public and private health services have been developed to ensure better compliance with the strategies and activities in effect. These networks are too incipient to guarantee an effective national coverage, however. With regard to AIDS prevention, public-private cooperation with NGOs is under way in aspects that range from the implementation of five-year plans to serological sentinel surveillance and the prevention of perinatal transmission. As a result of a lack of organization and the absence of a performance evaluation system, the Expanded Program on Immunization was unable to prevent the accumulation of a large number of susceptibles, which was associated with a 2001 measles epidemic.

Since 1991, the Ministry of Public Health and Population has conducted epidemiological surveillance of HIV. Four sentinel studies of pregnant women yielded prevalence rates of 6.2% in 1993, 5.9% in 1996, 4.5% in 2000, and 3.1% in 2004. The decline in the prevalence rates over the last decade does not necessarily mean that the risk itself has decreased. It is also noted that the percentage of women under 20 years of age infected with the virus rose between 1996 and 2004.

A lymphatic filariasis program has demonstrated that it is possible to meet the regional objective of eliminating lymphatic filariasis by the year 2010.

In 2004 and 2005, two joint vaccination campaigns to combat canine rabies were carried out by the Ministry of Health and the Ministry of Agriculture. Some 100,000 dogs and cats were vaccinated in the capital, the Ouest department, and part of the Central

Plateau, where the alert had been sounded. (Brazil offered 5,000 doses of the vaccine and PAHO/WHO furnished the logistics.)

The Ministry of Agriculture has sponsored vaccination efforts against anthrax, although activities have been sporadic and have had little community participation. In 2004–2005, nearly one million animals were vaccinated against anthrax (FAO financing, implementation by VETERIMED).

In 2005, a national public health laboratory was built. It began functioning in 2006, albeit with insufficient physical resources or skilled human resources.

Two pilot initiatives for sustainable development were launched in Port Salut and Aquin; public sanitation and solid waste disposal systems were developed in the two *communes*, benefiting some 250,000 people. In the Lison neighborhood in north Port-au-Prince, a public sanitation and storm drainage system was constructed. The Ministry of Public Health and Population now has a Bureau for Health Promotion and Environmental Protection.

To improve sewage disposal, a project was initiated in 2005–2006, which provides technical and financial assistance to the community for building latrines.

Individual Care Services

In 1986, the Ministry of Public Health and Population decreed that the Haitian Red Cross would be in charge of blood transfusion services. In 2004, with support from the United States President's Emergency Plan for AIDS Relief project, the Ministry launched a national blood transfusion safety program and prepared a draft decree aimed at reorganizing the national blood safety system. The program involves the creation of blood transfusion posts and blood banks in every department in the country. Substantial improvements have been made in the collection of blood and the appropriate use of whole blood and blood products; this improvement is due primarily to the shift from a system based on replacement blood donors to one based on regular, volunteer, altruistic blood donation (volunteer blood donations increased from 5% in 2004 to 27% in 2006). Nevertheless, coverage is generally inadequate; the blood transfusion center in Port-au-Prince was able to meet only 47% of the demand in 2004 and 60% in 2005; the only blood bank set up outside the capital in 2006 is located in Miragoâne. In 2005, the screening of about 11,000 units of blood found 1.6% positive for HIV, 4% for hepatitis B, 0.7% for hepatitis C, 1% for HTLV-1, and 3% for syphilis.

The mental health sector is the responsibility of the Bureau of Health Promotion and Environmental Protection. The Centre de Psychiatrie Mars et Kline and the Hôpital Psychiatrique Défilé de Beudet are the government-run facilities in metropolitan Port-au-Prince. No public institution offers mental health services outside the capital, but several small, private centers have emerged. Available mental health care cannot keep up with demand, which has been exacerbated by the country's persistent stress and violence.

Health Promotion

In 2005, a new health promotion strategy was instituted in the country: ecoclubs were created to foster youth leadership and improve environmental conditions by promoting clean and green spaces, safe drinking water, sanitation, and vector control. In 2006, more than 500 young people were trained to work in a national network. Other initiatives, such as the promotion of healthy cities, also have emerged.

Human Resources

There are not enough human resources to meet demand and they are distributed unequally throughout the country.

In the past, only the public sector provided training for health personnel through its institutions—a medical school, a pharmacy school, a dental school, a medical technology school, and four national nursing schools in Port-au-Prince, Cap-Haïtien, Cayes, and Jérémie. In the past 10 years, private schools have proliferated, creating accreditation problems. Only two of the four private medical schools are officially recognized by the Government. Several schools for nurses and nursing auxiliaries operate without authorization, and others have not even been registered. In 1998, nine nursing schools were officially recognized and nine others were being evaluated.

In 2000, a school for nurse-midwives opened; it is currently training its sixth class of 30 students. In 2000–2005, the University of Haiti's Medical School graduated 463 doctors; the University's Pharmacy School graduated 153 pharmacists and 38 lab technicians. For these graduates to obtain a license to practice in Haiti, the government requires that they perform one year of social service in a rural public health facility. The lack of a national exam or any other official certification is a major obstacle to the regulation and standardization of competencies in the various medical professions in the country. The Ministry of Public Health and Population has developed and implemented a nursing school curriculum. Since 1998, with aid from France, the Public Health Administration Information and Training Center (CIFAS) has trained hospital administrators and directors for the public sector every year. The State University of Haiti trained 100 managers between 2001 and 2005. During that same period, the Haitian Foundation for Diabetes and Cardiovascular Disease offered basic training for health personnel in early diagnosis and treatment of diabetes and hypertension.

Health Supplies

There are four private-sector pharmaceutical laboratories that are officially authorized to manufacture drugs for national use. Their combined production covers some 30%–40% of the Haitian market. Since Haiti has no national drug quality control laboratory, it must resort to quality monitoring carried out through PAHO/WHO. There is no medical materials manufacturer, and

Hope in Haiti

Haiti is in the thick of a generalized HIV epidemic. Fanned by rampant poverty, illiteracy, and years of political and social turmoil, the country's HIV prevalence rates are the highest in the Region. Against this dismal background rises a story of success and inspiration—a story of preventing and fighting disease, treating the sick, and bringing hope to those who have lost hope. Zanmi Lasanté (meaning Partners in Health in Haitian Kreyol) is bringing first-rate comprehensive health care to the country's Central Plateau; it is the only provider of comprehensive primary care to the impoverished populations in the Plateau. The nongovernmental health care provider has come a very long way since it established the Clinique Bon Sauveur, a two-room clinic in the village of Cange, in 1985. In 1998, Zamni Lasanté pioneered a program providing antiretroviral therapy to 50 patients suffering from advanced AIDS. Among other ventures, today Zanmi Lasanté operates a 104-bed full-service hospital that encompasses two operating rooms, adult and pediatric inpatient wards, an infectious disease center, an outpatient clinic, a women's health clinic, clinics for ophthalmology and general medicine, a laboratory, a pharmaceutical warehouse, a blood bank, radiographic services, and a cluster of schools. In partnership with Haiti's Ministry of Health, Zanmi Lasanté has expanded to other sites besides Cange, where it trains and pays community health workers and complements Ministry of Health personnel. Its hallmark approach, however, is the training of *accompagnateurs*, health foot soldiers who march into the community to prevent illness, monitor medical and socioeconomic conditions, and deliver quality care to people with chronic diseases. Zanmi Lasanté currently provides health care to half a million persons in the Central Plateau. It has become a model for how to provide effective health care to the poorest of the poor.

one agency produces laboratory reagents locally. In August 2004, a census found 42 agencies that import pharmaceuticals and 6 offices authorized to handle their distribution. Added to these are some NGOs and institutional partners that import drugs and distribute them directly. In 2004, Haiti had 215 official pharmacies; the country also has an informal distribution system in which drugs are freely sold on the street, in the markets, and in malls.

The public sector has an essential drugs program, as well as a decentralized logistical system that operates nationwide, guaranteeing the availability of drugs and their distribution in public, private, and mixed nonprofit establishments.

In 2005, the total value of drugs and health supplies distributed to the country's health institutions through PAHO's Essential Drug Program (PROMESS) was US$ 4,315,326, broken down as follows: US$ 1,328,043 for drugs sold under the cost-recovery policy; and US$ 2,987,283 for drugs subsidized by the priority programs of the Ministry of Public Health and Population, including vaccines, contraceptives, and drugs for treating tuberculosis, malaria, and AIDS. This figure has fallen dramatically since 2001, when the value of drugs was US$ 7,748,907 for drugs and supplies distributed to health institutions by PROMESS; US$ 1,861,123 for drugs sold under the cost-recovery policy; and US$ 5,887,784 for drugs subsidized by the priority programs of the Ministry of Public Health and Population. Government outlays for drug procurement are extremely low, even when it is not expressed as a percentage of the total budget of the Ministry of Public Health.

Although the national list of essential drugs was drawn up by the public sector in 2003, it has numerous inadequacies and should be revised. To a certain extent, the basic markets for health technology, drugs, and other supplies are under the control of the Ministry of Public Health and Population.

Research and Technological Development in Health

The Bureau of Epidemiology, Laboratories, and Research, created in 2006 under the responsibility of the Ministry of Public Health and Population, is charged with planning and conducting research that contributes to the development of policies and programs on disease prevention and control. Financial constraints, along with a shortage of trained personnel, have prevented the Bureau from exercising this mandate. Several private and public facilities conduct research, but their studies are not always authorized or overseen by the Ministry's Committee on Bioethics and Protection of Human Subjects. The 11-member Committee has issued rulings on 23 research projects since it was created in 1999; most research projects reviewed were related to HIV/AIDS and vaccine trials.

Health Sector Expenditures and Financing

Public health expenditure represents only 0.8% to 1% of GDP. While the government regularly increases the health budget (HTG 661,121,148 per year in 2003–2004; HTG 871,239,000 in 2004–2005, or 3.5% of the national budget), it is not enough to cover the population's health needs. Since the national budget is very small, the funds currently disbursed are lower in real terms than in the 1980s, taking inflation and the depreciation of the Gourde against the US$ into account. Most of the funds go to salaries; priority programs and investment costs must be funded by multilateral and bilateral international cooperation. Decentralized resource management is beginning to emerge with the creation of the Community Health Units: the sluggishness observed in the disbursement of funds, rendering outlying facilities inoperable, is beginning to ease, making way for more rational execution of departmental operating plans.

Clearly, the issue of health financing is at the heart of the problem of access to care. Some studies argue for a policy of free care. Other initiatives, such as the debt forgiveness one with the International Monetary Fund and the World Bank, envisage using earmarked funds to offer a basic package of free services to the poorest population and, in the medium term (10–15 years down the road), putting a social protection system in place. Health financing in Haiti should be viewed from a macroeconomic perspective; to address it, various initiatives have been implemented in the formal and informal sectors, using microfinancing and microinsurance mechanisms to improve financial access to quality services at an acceptable price for users.

Technical Cooperation and External Financing

External aid to the health sector dropped from US$ 48 million in 1998–1999 (when it reached its highest level between 1997 and 2005) to US$ 28 million in 2001–2002 (the lowest level between those same years). The main providers of multilateral funds are the Global Fund to Fight Aids, Tuberculosis, and Malaria (with US$ 66.9 million over five years, beginning January 2003) and the IDB (with US$ 22.5 million in four years, beginning in late 2003). After providing critical support for the establishment of the Community Health Units, the European Union virtually suspended aid after the political crisis of 2000. Nine specialized United Nations agencies have representative offices in Haiti, and six of them work in the health sector (PAHO/WHO, UNICEF, FAO, WFP, UNAIDS, and UNFPA). A representative of the United Nations Secretary-General deals chiefly with political matters, in close collaboration with the Coordinator of the International Civilian Support Mission in Haiti. The health sector has been designated as a priority by bilateral cooperation agencies from countries including Canada, France, Japan, Spain, and the United States.

PAHO's Essential Drug Program (PROMESS) plays a key role in procuring drugs, essential supplies, laboratory products, and medical consumables in the international market and overseeing their distribution to Haiti's public health facilities, 12 outlying warehouses, and 2 drug banks, which together constitute the national drug distribution network.

The Minister of Public Health and Population and the Ministry of Planning and External Cooperation coordinate health activities with bilateral, multilateral, and private cooperation agencies. The United Nations agencies have been specifically involved in health sector reform, reproductive health, child health, family planning, immunization, nutrition, drinking water and sanitation, health services development, AIDS and sexually transmitted infections, gender issues in health, and essential drugs. The 2000–2005 period has been extremely difficult in Haiti. International aid has not always responded to the country's specific needs, and the Government's lack of liquidity has not allowed it to coordinate aid needs. Regional integration has been strengthened since Haiti joined CARICOM.

Several cooperation agreements have been signed with the Dominican Republic. Among them is the 2005 binational tuberculosis control project supported by PAHO/WHO; results have been meager, however. Another effort, a 2005 technical cooperation project for preventing and controlling rabies transmitted by dogs, has seen good results in both countries.

Several intercountry projects have been carried out. Highlights include a 2003–2005 project with support from Cuba (US$ 144,247) and a 2004–2005 project with Paraguay in environmental health that involved solid waste management and training in Haitian institutions in engaging the community's participation for installing drinking water and sanitation systems.

Bibliography

Bureau international du Travail, Programme STEP; Financial Services Network for Entrepreneurial Empowerment (DAI/FINNET). Louis dit Guerin O, Viau J. Mise en place d'un système d'assurance santé à l'hôpital Albert Schweitzer. Etude de faisabilité. Draft. October 2001.

Coalition Nationale Pour les Droits des Haïtiens. Non Au Système Restavek. Vers l'élimination de l'esclavage de l'enfant en Haïti. April 2002.

de Rochars MB, Kanjilal S, Direny AN, Radday J, Lafontant JG, Mathieu E, et al. The Leogane Haiti demonstration project: decreased microfilaremia and program cost after 3 years of mass drug administration. Am J Trop Med Hyg. 2005; 73(5): 888–94.

Facultad Latinoamericana de Ciencias Sociales; Organización Internacional para las Migraciones. Encuesta sobre Inmigrantes Haitianos en República Dominicana. Santo Domingo, March 2004.

Facultad Latinoamericana de Ciencias Sociales; Organización Internacional para las Migraciones. Las migraciones: la incapacidad de ofrecer una vida digna. In: Informe nacional de desarrollo humano 2005. Chapter V. p. 119–44.

Fleurival J. L'anémie falciforme à l'usage des généralistes et des étudiants en sciences de la santé en Haïti. Port-au-Prince, Imp. Collection Procédure. March 2006.

Fonds des Nations Unies pour la population; Unissons-nous pour les enfants. Evaluation des dépôts périphériques. Rapport consolidé. November 2005.

Gaillard EM, Boulos L-M, Cayemittes MPA, Eustache L, Van Onacker JD, Duval N, et al. Understanding the reasons for decline of HIV prevalence in Haiti. Sex Transm Infect. 2006 Apr;82 Suppl 1:i14–20.

Haïti, Association pour la prévention de l'alcoolisme et autres accoutumances chimiques; Institut Haïtien de l'Enfance; Programme des Nations Unies pour le controle international des drogues. Etude Connaissances, Attitudes et Comportements des élèves et des enfants des rues de la région métropolitaine de Port-au-Prince. November 2000.

Haïti, Conseil National pour la Réhabilitation des Handicapés; Ministère des Affaires sociales et du Travail; Programme des Nations Unies pour le développement. Vers l'élaboration d'une stratégie nationale d'intégration des personnes à besoins spéciaux. Port-au-Prince: Ed. des Antilles S.A.; May 2005.

Haïti, Groupe d'Appui aux Réfugiés et Rapatriés. Available from: www.garr-haiti.org.

Haïti, Groupe d'Appui aux Rapatriés et Réfugiés; Mouvement des Femmes Dominicano-Haïtiennes. En quête de la vie. Une étude sur les femmes haïtiennes impliquées dans la migration en République Dominicaine. February 2005.

Haïti, Groupe d'Appui aux Réfugiés et Rapatriés. Rapport migration haïtienne et les droits humains à la frontière haïtiano-dominicaine en 2004. April 2005.

Haïti, Institut Haïtien de l'Enfance; Macro International Inc. Enquête Morbidité, Mortalité et Utilisation des Services (EMMUS-III), Haïti 2000/2001. Calverton (Maryland), 2001.

Haïti, Institut Haïtien de l'Enfance; Macro International Inc. Enquête Morbidité, Mortalité et Utilisation des Services (EMMUS-IV), Haïti 2005/2006. Résultats préliminaires. Pétion-Ville, 2006.

Haïti, Institut Haïtien de Statistique et d'Informatique; Bureau du Recensement Général de la Population et de l'Habitat; Fonds des Nations Unies pour la population; Union Européenne; Coopération japonaise; Banque Interaméricaine de Développement; Région Wallonne. 4ème Recensement Général de la Population et de l'Habitat 2003 (RGPH-2003). Résultats définitifs. March 2005.

Haïti, Ministère de la Planification et de la Coopération Externe; Banque Interaméricaine de Développement. Carte de pauvreté d'Haïti. Version 2004.

Haïti, Ministère de la Planification et de la Coopération Externe; Programme des Nations Unies pour le développement; Bureau international du Travail. HAI.01.001. Expérience de promotion de micro-assurance santé: Le cas ASPAKO. Appui au développement d'un partenariat pour l'intégration économique et sociale et l'implantation d'un programme national de promotion d'emplois productifs et de lutte contre l'exclusion sociale. Port-au-Prince.

Haïti, Ministère de la Planification et de la Coopération Externe; Programme des Nations Unies pour le développement; Bureau international du Travail. HAI/99/001. Mathieu S. Etat des lieux en matière de protection sociale gouvernementale en Haïti. Etude de référence 4 dans le cadre du Projet d'Assistance préparatoire pour la promotion d'emplois productifs et la lutte contre l'exclusion sociale. January 2000.

Haïti, Ministère de la Planification et de la Coopération Externe; Programme des Nations Unies pour le développement; Bureau international du Travail. HAI/99/001. Ponticq F. Etat des lieux en matière d'extension de la protection sociale en milieu communautaire en Haïti. Etude de référence 5 dans le cadre du Projet d'Assistance préparatoire pour la promotion d'emplois productifs et la lutte contre l'exclusion sociale. April 2000.

Haïti, Ministère de la Santé Publique et de la Population, Consultance en Santé Publique, VIIIème FED. Programme d'appui au développement des ressources humaines dans le secteur de la santé. Rapport final. Port-au-Prince, October 1999.

Haïti, Ministère de la Santé Publique et de la Population, Direction Centrale de Pharmacie et de Contrôle des Substances chimiques, Direction de la Santé de la Famille; Haïti, Ministère de la Santé Publique et de la Population. Analyse du Secteur de la Santé pour la Réforme.

Haïti, Ministère de la Santé Publique et de la Population; John Snow Inc. Données sanitaires de routine 2004, 2005. Port-au-Prince.

Haïti, Ministère de la Santé Publique et de la Population; Les Centres pour le Développement et la Santé; Fonds des Nations Unies pour la population. Projet bi-national Haïti-Dominicanie. Etude sur les besoins en services de santé reproductive et sexuelle. Port-au-Prince, May 2006.

Haïti, Ministère de la Santé Publique et de la Population. Liste des institutions sanitaires. Port-au-Prince, September 2005.

Haïti, Ministère de la Santé Publique et de la Population; Ministère de l'Education Nationale de la Jeunesse et des Sports; Organisation panaméricaine de la Santé/Organisation mondiale de la Santé. Rapport de l'enquête sur la prévalence et l'intensité parasitaire dans le Département du Sud. March 2005.

Haïti, Ministère de la Santé Publique et de la Population; Nations Unies; Commission Européenne; Banque Mondiale; Banque Interaméricaine de Développement. Cadre de Coopération Intérimaire (CCI) 2004–2006. Rapport de synthèse, July 2004. Port-au-Prince, 2004.

Haïti, Ministère de la Santé Publique et de la Population; Organisation panaméricaine de la Santé/Organisation mondiale de la Santé. Analyse des causes de décès Haïti 1999. Port-au-Prince, March 2002.

Haïti, Ministère de la Santé Publique et de la Population; Organisation panaméricaine de la Santé/Organisation mondiale de la Santé. Analyse des certificats de décès. République d'Haïti 2001, 2002 et 2003.

Haïti, Ministère de la Santé Publique et de la Population; Organisation panaméricaine de la Santé/Organisation mondiale de la Santé. Etude sur la situation de la Médecine Traditionnelle en Haïti. Port-au-Prince, April 2003.

Haïti, Ministère de la Santé Publique et de la Population; Organisation panaméricaine de la Santé/Organisation mondiale de la Santé. Haïti 2004. Situation de Santé, Indicateurs de Base. Port-au-Prince.

Haïti, Ministère de la Santé Publique et de la Population; Organisation panaméricaine de la Santé/Organisation mondiale de la Santé. Plan stratégique pour le développement de l'épidémiologie en Haïti. 2001–2004. Port-au-Prince, March 2002.

Haïti, Ministère de la Santé Publique et de la Population; Organisation panaméricaine de la Santé/Organisation mondiale de la Santé. Saint Preux A. Rapport d'expertise. Répertoire des textes législatifs régissant la santé publique en Haïti, 2002.

Haïti, Ministère de la Santé Publique et de la Population; Organisation panaméricaine de la Santé/Organisation mondiale de la Santé. Tétanos maternel et néonatal en Haïti. Situation et dilemmes stratégiques de l'élimination. February 2006.

Haïti, Ministère de la Santé Publique et de la Population. Plan stratégique de lutte contre la tuberculose en Haïti 2001–2006.

Haïti, Ministère de la Santé Publique et de la Population. Plan Stratégique National pour la Réforme du Secteur de la Santé 2005–2010. Port-au-Prince, August 2005.

Haïti, Ministère de la Santé Publique et de la Population, Programme National d'Elimination de la Filariose Lymphatique. Nicolas MCE, St Jean Y, Milord MD, Beaude-Rochars M, et al. Résultats de l'enquête nationale de prévalence sur la filariose lymphatique. Port-au-Prince, undated.

Haïti, Ministère de la Santé Publique et de la Population, Programme National d'Elimination de la Filariose Lymphatique: Plan d'action pour l'élimination de la Filariose Lymphatique en Haïti (2003–2008). Port-au-Prince, 2004.

Haïti, Ministère de la Santé Publique et de la Population; Programme National de Lutte contre la Tuberculose; Secrétariat d'Etat à la Santé Publique et à l'Assistance Sociale; National Tuberculosis Control Program, Organisation panaméricaine de la Santé/Organisation mondiale de la Santé. Plan binational Haïti–République Dominicaine de lutte contre la tuberculose 2005–2006, final version. June 2005.

Haïti, Ministère de la Santé Publique et de la Population, Unissons-nous pour les enfants; Institut Haïtien de l'Enfance. Enquête sur la prévalence de la carence en Vitamine A et de la déficience en iode en Haïti. July 2005.

Haïti, Ministère de la Santé Publique et de la Population. Voltaire HC. Les Unités Communales de Santé. Principes et Orientations Stratégiques. Port-au-Prince, June 1999.

Haïti, Ministère de l'Economie et des Finances; Institut Haïtien de Statistique et d'Informatique; Programme des Nations Unies pour le développement. Enquête sur les conditions de vie en Haïti (ECVH-2001). Port-au-Prince, January 2004.

Haïti, Ministère des Affaires sociales et du Travail. Les fondements de la pratique de la domesticité des enfants en Haïti. Programme des Nations Unies pour le développement; Unissons-nous pour les enfants; Organisation internationale du Travail/Programme de lutte pour l'éradication du travail des enfants; Save the Children. July 2002.

Haïti, Ministère des Affaires sociales et du Travail; Programme des Nations Unies pour le développement; Unissons-nous pour les enfants; Organisation internationale du Travail/Programme de lutte pour l'éradication du travail des enfants; Save the Children. Domesticité des enfants en Haïti. December 2002.

Hallett TB, Aberle-Grasse J, Bello G, Boulos L-M, Cayemittes MPA, Cheluget B, et al. Declines in HIV prevalence can be associated with changing sexual behaviour in Uganda, urban Kenya, Zimbabwe, and urban Haiti. Imperial College.

Initiative Développement; Alter Santé Internationale et Développement. Vinard P, Boecker C, Malherbe P. Analyse de l'impact des paiements et de la gratuité sur l'accès aux soins: L'expérience d'Ennery en Haïti. Poitiers, October 2005.

Jean-Baptiste ED, Larco P, Charles-Larco N, Vilgrain C, Simon D, Charles R. Glucose intolerance and other cardiovascular risk factors in Haiti. Prevalence of diabetes and hypertension in Haiti (PREDIAH). Diabetes Metab. 2006 Nov;32(5 Pt 1): 443–51.

Joint United Nations Program on HIV/AIDS, UN Theme Groups Haiti and Dominican Republic. Interagency and bilateral project. Haiti–Dominican Republic. Prevention of HIV/AIDS on the northern border of Haiti. October 2004.

Junot F. Ministère de la Santé Publique et de la Population. Planification stratégique du système d'information sanitaire pour l'intégration des données du VIH/SIDA. Projet Measure Evaluation. Second draft. Port-au-Prince, July 2006, p.16.

Médecins Sans Frontières. Accès aux soins dans l'Unité communale de santé de Petite rivière, Verrettes, La Chapelle, Haïti. Résultats de deux enquêtes épidémiologiques concernant la mortalité et l'accès aux soins. September 2005.

Milord MD. Lymphatic filariasis elimination in the third America [Presentation]. Regional Program Manager's Meeting. Port-au-Prince, 4–6 September 2002.

Organisation panaméricaine de la Santé/Organisation mondiale de la Santé. Lacapère F. Mortalité des enfants d'âge scolaire en Haïti. Analyse des certificats de décès (2000). [PowerPoint presentation].

Pan American Health Organization. Press release. Outbreak of poliomyelitis in Dominican Republic and Haiti: low vaccination coverage with oral polio vaccine allows Sabin-derived vaccine to circulate. December 2000.

Programa de las Naciones Unidas para el Desarrollo. Proyecto interagencial y binacional. Haití–República Dominicana. Prevención del VIH/SIDA en la frontera norte de Haití. Informe de un taller de planificación operativa. Dajabon (República Dominicana), 31 May–1 June 2005.

Programme des Nations Unies pour le développement. Plan d'urgence, 2005.

Programme des Nations Unies pour le développement. Rapport sur le Développement humain, 2005.

Proposition de loi modifiant certaines dispositions du Code Pénal relatives aux agressions sexuelles (attentat à la pudeur, viol, harcèlement sexuel, inceste). Port-au-Prince, December 2005.

Rapport de l'étude sur la prévalence et l'intensité des géo-helminthiases intestinales chez les écoliers du Département de la Grand'Anse.

République d'Haïti. (2006). Décret portant sur l'organisation et le fonctionnement du MSPP, signé le 17 novembre 2005 paru au Moniteur, 5 January 2006.

République d'Haïti. Proposition de Décret sollicitant la création d'un système national de sécurité sanguine sous tutelle du MSPP, avec un Programme national de sécurité transfusionnelle, une Commission nationale de sécurité transfusionnelle et un réseau des services de médecine transfusionnelle.

Réseau Associatif National pour l'Intégration des Personnes Handicapées; Mission spéciale de l'OEA en Haïti. Convention interaméricaine pour l'élimination de toutes les formes de discrimination contre les personnes handicapées. (French/Creole bilingual version). Port-au-Prince: Le Natal; January 2002.

Système des Nations Unies, République d'Haïti. Programme Intégré de Réponse aux Besoins Urgents des Communautés et des Populations Vulnérables (PIR). March 2003.

United States Agency for International Development, Policy Project. Smucker GR. Les orphelins et les autres enfants vulnérables en Haïti: un rapport de terrain. April 2005.

Université Quisqueya; Unité de Recherche sur les Enfants en Situation Difficile. Bernier M, Ponticq F. Planification d'interventions. 1999.

Vorbe C. Les droits fondamentaux et le VIH/SIDA en Haïti. January 2006.

HONDURAS

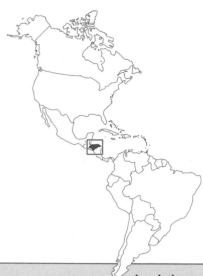

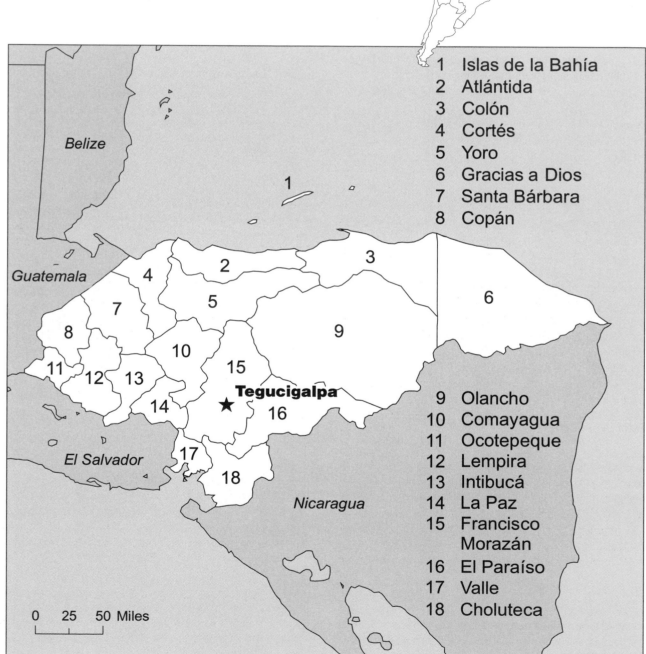

1 Islas de la Bahía
2 Atlántida
3 Colón
4 Cortés
5 Yoro
6 Gracias a Dios
7 Santa Bárbara
8 Copán

Belize

Guatemala

Tegucigalpa

El Salvador

Nicaragua

9   Olancho
10 Comayagua
11 Ocotepeque
12 Lempira
13 Intibucá
14 La Paz
15 Francisco
    Morazán
16 El Paraíso
17 Valle
18 Choluteca

0   25   50 Miles

H onduras has an area of 112,492 km^2 consisting mostly of mountainous terrain, with 19 river basins. The country lies in the heart of Central America. It is bounded on the north by the Caribbean Sea, on the south by the Gulf of Fonseca (the Pacific Ocean) and El Salvador, on the east by Nicaragua, and on the west by El Salvador and Guatemala. Administratively, it is divided into 18 departments, 298 municipalities, more than 3,000 villages, and more than 30,000 *caseríos* (hamlets, or settlements with fewer than 1,000 residents each).

GENERAL CONTEXT AND HEALTH DETERMINANTS

Social, Political, and Economic Determinants

Honduras is an independent, democratic republic with three branches of government: the executive, the legislative, and the judicial. The President of Honduras is also the Head of State. Each department is headed by a governor appointed by the President. The municipalities are governed by a municipal corporation headed up by the mayor, whose members are elected by popular vote.

The country has a centralized government, but is currently in the process of gradually transferring power to municipal governments under the Municipalities Act. Each cabinet ministry, or *Secretaría de Estado*, is in charge of a different sector of activity, and some are decentralized along geographic lines into a network of regional offices. The Ministry of Finance administers government revenues, overseeing tax collection activities through its regional offices. The Minister in charge of the Office of the President coordinates development planning and management efforts on the advice of an economic cabinet and a social cabinet consisting of the Ministers of Health, Education, and Labor. The social cabinet is in charge of making proposals to the President for social policy measures. As a local government authority, each municipality is free to formulate and manage its own development programs. Health policy is incorporated in national programs through strategic plans and programs. In general, the needs of the Honduran population are met by central or municipal government services, autonomous government enterprises, private for-profit enterprises, and nonprofit organizations.

With an external debt burden of more than US$ 4 billion up until 2005, Honduras was included in the Heavily Indebted Poor Countries (HIPC) initiative. That year, several governments forgave close to 15% of Honduras' debt, with the possibility of another 45% being waivered, on the condition that these funds be reallocated to projects within the country's Poverty Reduction Strategy (PRS) framework (*1*).

The Government, elected in November 2005 placed high priority on implementing the PRS established in August 2001, with the objective of ending the country's long historic cycle of poverty and inequality. Implementation of the PRS has presented a number of challenges, the most important of which involve securing sufficient support from national stakeholders and the uncertainty over the progress of program implementation. On the other hand, the PRS has engendered major improvements in budget management, thereby increasing the feasibility of the poverty reduction goal (*2*). The program area for increased and better access to health care services accounted for 22% of anti-poverty spending under the PRS in the first quarter of 2005, or the equivalent of 1.8% of GDP (*3*).

With a per capita gross national income of US$ 1,030 in 2004 (*4*), slightly more than two-thirds of the country's population was living in poverty and half of the population was living in conditions of extreme poverty. The situation was even worse in rural areas, where 75% of the population was living in extreme poverty (*5*). The ratio between the incomes of the richest and poorest quintiles in 1999 was 59:3 (*6*).

The limited access of rural farmers to productive resources and basic services fuels poverty, food insecurity, and internal and international migration. Open unemployment, which went from 3% to 6% between 1999 and 2004, and high levels of "invisible" underemployment (full-time workers earning less than the minimum wage), peaking at 29.6% in 2004, also help perpetuate poverty (*7*). The maquiladora assembly industry; the sector of micro-, small-, and medium-sized enterprises; and remittances from family members in the United States are three important sources of income and food security. Maquiladoras employed close to 130,000 workers in 2004, 80% of whom were women (*8*). Likewise, annual remittances from the United States jumped from US$ 883 million in 2003 to nearly US$ 1.82 billion in 2005 (*9*).

According to an unmet basic needs assessment conducted in 2001, 10.7% of all households surveyed had children not attending primary school, 18.0% had no household connection to a water supply system, 31.7% lacked proper sanitation facilities, 16.8% were living in overcrowded conditions, and 21.2% had no livelihood (*10*). These averages for national indicators mask the even lower values associated with municipalities in western Honduras and the La Mosquitia area (department of Gracias a Dios).

Despite an improvement in many social indicators over the past 10 years, it is uncertain whether the country can achieve the Millennium Development Goals (MDGs) and its PRS objectives. One stumbling block is the pervasive corruption at all levels of the public and private sectors, which the public perceives as an obstacle to good governance and socioeconomic development (*11*).

While the adult literacy rate is 80% nationwide and 72% in rural areas, there are no figures available regarding functional literacy. The average number of years of primary school attendance is 6.2 at the national level and 4.5 in rural areas. However, there are significant disparities in these indicators from one department to another, with the lowest values once again being associated with western Honduras (*10*). The school attendance rate at the primary level was 65.9% in 2003.

The main sources of insecurity are drug traffickers and criminal gangs engaged in kidnapping, stealing vehicles, and "settling scores." There are no anti-gang policies in place, only reactive measures such as the Anti-Gang Act of 2003 which, while initially effective in lowering the number of homicides, includes no strategies to ensure long-term sustainability.

Demographics, Mortality, and Morbidity

The country's population grew by more than 600,000 inhabitants between 2001 and 2005, by which time it had topped the 7 million mark. Despite the steady decline in the annual rate of population growth, Honduras expects to add nearly 1 million inhabitants by the year 2010 and projects life expectancy to steadily increase while the share of its rural population continues to de-

cline (Table 1). The structure of the population in 1988 and 2005, by age and sex, is presented in Figure 1; it depicts a high proportion of young people and growing numbers of older adults (even though the dependency ratio remains high).

According to the 2001 census, the total fertility rate ranged from 3.2 children per woman in Francisco Morazán Department, which includes Tegucigalpa, the nation's capital, to 6.3 in Lempira, one of the country's poorest departments. The declining birth and general mortality rates rank the country's demographic transition as moderate (*10*).

The crude mortality rate for 2005 put the number of annual deaths at approximately 35,000. According to data developed by the National Statistics Institute based on information from the National Registry of Individuals (Vital Statistics for 2003–2005, internal documentation), the non-reporting rate for mortality data, which hovered around 50% for decades, dropped to 42% in 2004 and to 37% in 2005, with departmental margins of difference of anywhere from 15% in Choluteca to 85% in Gracias a Dios for the last year of the reference period (personal communication, 25 July 2006). However, the coverage and quality of the medical registry for causes of death are still poor, making it difficult to establish national and by age and by sex mortality profiles. The only available profiles are based on mortality registries from the Ministry of Health and Honduran Social Security Institute (IHSS) hospitals, representing only 20% of the estimated annual number of deaths nationwide (Table 2).

The country has a long history of natural disasters such as hurricanes, droughts, seismic events, floods, and landslides that have resulted in thousands of deaths, heavy infrastructure damage, and obstacles to development. Approximately 20% of the population lives in disaster-prone areas. The areas most vulnerable to hurricanes and flooding are the Atlantic islands and northern coastal lowlands, where there has been a heavy concentration of new settlements over the past few years. The eastern and west-

TABLE 1. Selected demographic information, Honduras, 2001, 2005, and projections for 2010.

	2001	2005	2010
Total population (number of persons)	6,530,331	7,197,303	8,045,990
Under 15 years of age	2,722,205	2,911,873	3,087,979
Over 64 years of age	239,994	278,762	332,554
Rural population (%)	53.7	51.3	48.7
Annual growth rate (%)	2.5	2.4	2.1
Total fertility rate	4.1	3.79	3.4
Crude mortality rate	5.2	4.9	4.6
Crude birth rate	32.8	30.8	27.8
Life expectancy at birth (years)	70.8	72.1	73.6
Men	67.5	68.7	70.1
Women	74.3	75.7	77.2
International migration rate	−2.5	−2.2	−2.2

Source: Instituto Nacional de Estadísticas (INE). Proyecciones de Población 2001–2015. Tegucigalpa: INE; 2004.

FIGURE 1. Population structure, by age and sex, Honduras, 1988 and 2005.

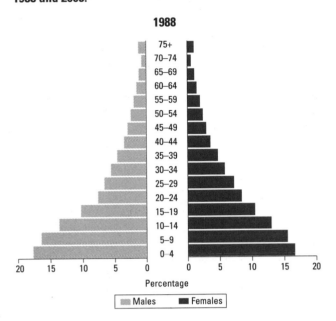

1988

Percentage

Males Females

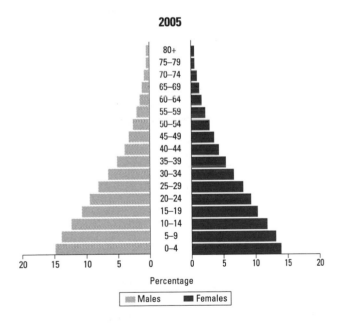

2005

Percentage

Males Females

TABLE 2. Leading causes of mortality[a], Honduras, 2004.

Causes	% total deaths[a,b]
Certain conditions originating in the perinatal period	18.8
Congenital malformations, deformations, and chromosomal abnormalities	6.3
Diabetes mellitus	5.6
Cerebrovascular diseases	5.0
Events of undetermined intent	4.6
HIV disease	4.4
Influenza and pneumonia	4.3
Chronic lower respiratory diseases	4.0
Cirrhosis and other diseases of the liver	3.6
Ischemic heart diseases	3.1

[a]Based on Ministry of Health and IHSS hospital data only.
[b]Represents only 20% of estimated annual number of deaths nationwide.
Source: Pan American Health Organization/World Health Organization-Honduras.

groundwater resources and the imposition of harsh rationing measures. The risk of drought may be heightened by unregulated human activity, which speeds up soil erosion and watershed degradation. More than 80,000 hectares of forest lands are lost every year, mainly in the southern and western parts of the country but also, to a lesser extent, in the central and eastern regions.

HEALTH OF POPULATION GROUPS

Children under 5 Years Old

Population projections based on the 2001 census put the infant mortality rate at 34 per 1,000 live births in 2001 and 30 per 1,000 live births in 2005 (*12*). Figure 2 illustrates the steady trend in infant mortality for both sexes that took place between 1990 and 2005. There are large variances between municipalities, with figures ranging from 17 per 1,000 live births in José Santos Guardiola (Islas de la Bahía) to 82 per 1,000 in Dolores Merendón (Ocotepeque) (Figure 3). The last census and recent family health surveys all show a high correlation between infant mortality levels and the mother's level of poverty and education. Thus, according to the findings of the 2001 National Epidemiological and Family Health Survey, the reduction in infant mortality rates during the final 15 years of the 20th century was achieved at the cost of a decline in so-called "high" socioeconomic status (with household socioeconomic status measured by a goods and services index consisting of nine household features or possessions: piped water, a toilet, electricity, a radio, television, refrigerator, telephone, personal vehicle, and an electric or gas stove. Household status was classified as "low" in the case of households possessing zero to two of these items, "medium" in the case of households with three to six items, and "high" in the case of households

ern parts of the country have also sustained earthquake damage. Tegucigalpa, and, to a lesser extent, the northern and western reaches of the country, are at the highest risk of landslides caused by heavy rains and by severe environmental degradation.

Droughts have had a severe negative impact on the Honduran household economy, particularly in the southern part of the country. Their impact on water supply is felt nationwide, with the drawdown and, in some cases, total depletion of surface and

433

FIGURE 2. Infant mortality trends, Honduras, 1990–2005.

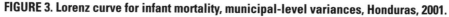

FIGURE 3. Lorenz curve for infant mortality, municipal-level variances, Honduras, 2001.

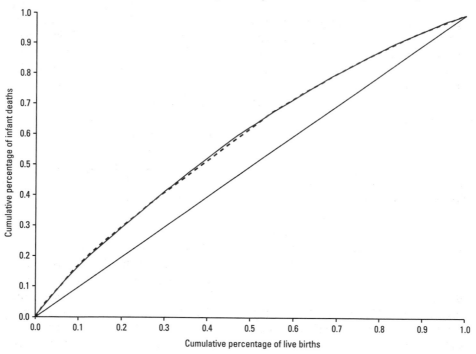

with seven to nine items) (*13*). The survey also found that the decline in infant mortality rates came at the cost of the post-neonatal mortality component, with no change in the level of the neonatal component.

According to 2001 census data, mortality rates for children under age 5 were higher in municipalities in the western part of the country. An extrapolation of the pattern of mortality for children in this age group since 1988 shows that, more than likely, at the current rate of decline, Honduras should meet the infant mortality target established by MDG 4 (reduce by two-thirds the mortality rate for children under age 5) by the year 2015. In the absence of vital statistics data, population surveys identify the leading causes of death as trauma/asphyxiation and low birthweight during the neonatal period, acute respiratory infections and acute diarrheal diseases during the postneonatal period, and acute diarrheal diseases and acute respiratory infections among children ages 1–4 (*13*). This mortality profile is consistent with health services statistics, which identify acute respiratory infections and diarrheal diseases as being the leading causes for seeking health care for the under-5 age group (*14*). The 2001 National Epidemiological and Family Health Survey found nearly one in five children under the age of 5 suffering from diarrhea that year, with an upward trend in prevalence rates over the previous 10-year period. The highest prevalence rates were associated with children aged 12–23 months and children of mothers without formal schooling or of mothers with only a primary-level education (*13*). Exclusive breast-feeding rates during the first five months of life were as high as 35%, even though 10% of infants in this age group were never breast-fed. A third of all children under age 5 suffered from iron deficiency and chronic malnutrition (*13*).

Children 5–9 Years Old

Stunting (low height for age) was present in slightly more than a third of schoolchildren ages 6–9 in 2001, affecting more males than females, and disproportionately affecting 9-year-olds and children living in rural areas. The rate of severe stunting in schoolchildren was 11.8%, ranging from a low of 0% in the municipality of Guanaja (Islas de la Bahía) to a high of 59.4% in San Francisco de Opalaca (Intibucá) (*15*).

Adolescents 10–14 and 15–19 Years Old

The median age of adolescents at the time of their first sexual experience was 18 for females and 17 for males. Nearly one-third of teenage girls were pregnant in 2001. The fertility rate for 15–19-year-old girls was 137 births a year per 1,000 population up to the year 1999 and had remained unchanged since 1986 (*13*).

Adults 20–59 Years Old

In 2001, women in the 20–24- and 25–29-year-old age groups had the highest fertility rates, at 229 and 202 children per 1,000 women, respectively (*13*). The use of contraceptive methods has been on the rise over the past several decades, particularly by women, with a sizeable percentage of males aged 15–44 adhering to their traditional gender-influenced role in matters of sexual and reproductive health and in household decision-making (*16*).

Data for 2001 showed 85% of pregnant women were receiving prenatal care; half of these services were being performed in Ministry of Health facilities, and 56% of intakes of pregnant women for prenatal care took place during the first trimester of pregnancy. Anemia was present in 15% of nonpregnant women and a third of pregnant women, but only 41% of this latter group took iron supplements and 32% took folic acid (*13*). The share of women with access to Pap test screenings increased from 50% to 61% between 1996 and 2001; the largest increase was recorded among women in rural areas. However, challenges remain regarding the timely availability of test results, particularly in rural areas (*13*).

The most recent data available put maternal mortality rates for 1990 and 1997 at 182 and 108 per 100,000 live births, respectively (*17*). According to maternal mortality surveillance system data, most deaths in 2004 and 2005 involved young women between 19 and 35 years of age without formal schooling or with only a primary-level education and occurred during labor or the immediate puerperium (*18*). The leading causes of maternal mortality were hemorrhaging and hypertensive disorders, and a study of the proximate causes of death showed serious limitations as regards access to quality health care. These factors indicate that Honduras will need to overcome significant obstacles if it is to achieve MDG 5 (improving maternal health) by the year 2015.

Persons with Disabilities

There were 177,516 individuals (25.5 per 1,000 population) affected by some type of disability in 2002. The most common disabilities were related to mobility, dexterity, and vision (*19*). There were large differences in the numbers of men and women with upper-limb amputations, dementia, and chronic depression, with more males affected than females. The leading causes of disabilities were common diseases, congenital disorders, accidents, and violence. The age group most affected by disabilities was the population aged 18–64, including both males and females, with the western departments of Ocotepeque, Santa Bárbara, Lempira, and Copán reporting the largest number of persons with disabilities.

Ethnic Groups

Over half a million Hondurans are of indigenous or African descent. There are nine culturally differentiated ethnic groups: the Lenca, Chortí, Tolupán, Tawahka, Garífuna, English-speaking Black, Pech, Náhuatl, and Miskito. The health status of these groups reflects their impoverishment, lack of access to basic services, and limited social participation. Of special concern are the high prevalence of Chagas' disease among the Tolupán in central Honduras, the Lenca in the southwest, and the Chortí in the northwest; the surge in the incidence of HIV/AIDS among the Garífuna on the country's northern coast; and the high prevalence of accidents due to unprotected immersion among the Miskito people of Gracias a Dios.

HEALTH CONDITIONS AND PROBLEMS

COMMUNICABLE DISEASES

Vector-borne Diseases

After a surge in 2002 to nearly 32,000 cases, mostly in large cities, the number of cases of **dengue** fell and stabilized at approximately 19,000 per year in 2004 and 2005; 10% of the cases were identified as **hemorrhagic dengue fever**.

Malaria, largely that spread by the *Plasmodium vivax* vector, is endemic in Honduras, primarily affecting the northern and eastern parts of the country. There are 25 municipalities with a combined population of close to 350,000 showing rates of more than 1,000 cases per 100,000 population.

Of the nearly 1,000 cases of **leishmaniasis** reported in 2004, 96% involved cutaneous leishmaniasis; the remainder was associated with the mucocutaneous and visceral forms of the disease. The departments of Olancho, Choluteca, and Colón accounted for 66% of all cases (*20*).

There has been a significant improvement in the differentiation of *Rhodnius prolixus*- and *Triatoma dimidiata*-transmitted **Chagas' disease**. According to National Chagas' and Leishmaniasis Program data for 2004, a serologic survey of blood samples from schoolchildren under 15 years of age yielded a seroprevalence rate of 29% in La Paz and figures of from 3% to 7% in Copán, Lempira, Intibucá, Yoro, and Santa Bárbara (personal communication, 2 July 2005). Data produced by the Central Reference Laboratory for Chagas' Disease and Leishmaniasis, the Laboratory and Blood Bank Network, and the Honduran Red Cross put the seroprevalence rate in blood donors at just over 1% (personal communication, 2 July 2005).

Vaccine-preventable Diseases

The decline in the number of cases of vaccine-preventable diseases in the last two decades of the 20th century was impressive, particularly as regards diseases prevalent among children under the age of 5. This decline is directly related to the gradual introduction of new vaccines as part of the national immunization program and the high vaccination coverage rates for children, women, and other at-risk groups. Table 3 presents a breakdown of vaccines introduced over the 1977–2003 period, along with the corresponding target population. Despite this progress, areas remain with a high prevalence of **rubella, mumps**, and **hepatitis A**. There has been an impressive decline in the incidence of **neonatal tetanus** in recent years. No cases of **diphtheria** have been reported since 1981, no cases of **polio** since 1989, and no cases of **measles** since 1996.

Intestinal Infectious Diseases

Of all reported cases of **acute diarrhea** each year, 77.0% involve children under the age of 5, with a prevalence rate of 22.5% in this age group and even higher rates in urban areas excluding Tegucigalpa and San Pedro Sula and rural areas, particularly La Mosquitia (Gracias a Dios). The most affected age group is that of children ages 6–23 months. Most children under age 5 suffering from diarrhea are treated with drugs (41.5% with pills, 37.1% with antidiarrheal medications, and 19.6% with antibiotics). During the last outbreak of diarrhea in 2001, 29.6% of children were given oral rehydration salts (Litrosol). That year, just over half the children suffering from diarrhea were fed less or prevented from eating certain solid foods during the diarrheal episode (*13*).

Chronic Communicable Diseases

Tuberculosis-associated morbidity slowly declined from 72 per 100,000 population in 1993 to 50 per 100,000 population in 2004; 54% of all cases occurred among males. However, the frequency of respiratory symptoms detection doubled over this same period. The incidence of **tuberculous meningitis** has remained under 1% since 1992. According to National Tuberculosis Control Program data from a 2004 assessment, the incidence of **HIV/tuberculosis coinfection** has been on the rise since 1986.

TABLE 3. Vaccines included in national vaccination program, by year of introduction, Honduras, 1977–2003.

Year	Vaccine	Target population
1977	BCG, OPV, DPT, measles	Children under age 1
1977	Tetanus toxoid (TT)	Pregnant women
1990	TT	Females ages 12–49
1994	Hepatitis B	At-risk groups
1995	Yellow fever	International travelers
1997	Measles, mumps, rubella (MMR)	Population aged 12–23 months
1998	Td (in lieu of TT vaccine), measles and rubella (MR)	Females ages 12–49
1999	*Haemophilus influenzae* type b (Hib)	Children under age 1
2000	DPT/HepB/Hib	Children under age 1
2001	IPV and DT, pediatric	At-risk groups
2003	Influenza	At-risk groups

FIGURE 4. New AIDS cases, by year and sex, Honduras, 1985–2005.

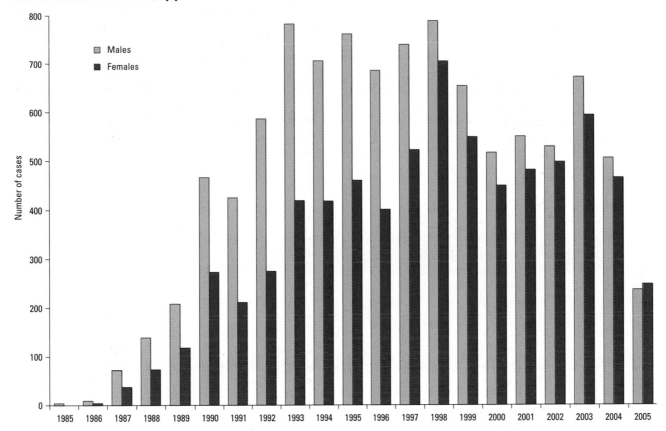

After a two-year hiatus, the National Leprosy Program reinitiated its activities in 1998 and, by late that year, had followed up on 78 patients, 13% of whom were still receiving multidrug therapy. The number of cases dropped to 72 the following year and stood at 35 by 2003.

Acute Respiratory Infections

Acute respiratory infections, including **pneumonia**, are still a leading cause of morbidity in children under age 5, particularly in the poorest municipalities in the country's western region. According to the findings of a 2001 survey of mothers who had lost children under 5 years of age, acute respiratory infections accounted for one out of every three deaths of children between the ages of 1 and 11 months and one out of every five deaths of children between 1 and 4 years of age (*13*).

HIV/AIDS and Other Sexually Transmitted Infections

AIDS has been present in Honduras since 1985. As of the end of 2005, there were just over 17,000 cumulative AIDS cases, with 970 new cases diagnosed in the year 2004 (for an incidence rate of 138 per 1 million population). San Pedro Sula and Tegucigalpa accounted for 40% of the new AIDS cases reported in 2005. The male-female ratio went from 2:1 to 0.95 at the beginning of the

last decade. Figure 4 shows the number of new AIDS cases, by year and sex, for the 1985–2005 period. The most affected age group was the population 25–34 years old, and the principal mode of transmission was heterosexual relations (88%). Nine percent of all new cases were due to perinatal exposure.

Zoonoses

The importance of **rabies** as a public health issue has steadily declined over the past decade due to high canine vaccination coverage. There have been no reported cases of canine rabies since 2003 and no cases of human rabies since the year 2000. There have been reports of isolated cases of rabies in cattle (one case in 2004 and another in 2005) (*21*).

NONCOMMUNICABLE DISEASES

Metabolic and Nutritional Diseases

A third of all Honduran children under age 5 are suffering from **iron deficiency** and from **chronic malnutrition** (*13*). The country was certified as virtually free of iodine deficiency disorders in 2002.

Various studies conducted between 2001 and 2004 found 2%–4% of children under age 5 suffering from **obesity**. Another survey of schoolchildren in Tegucigalpa found 20% affected by overweight and obesity problems. Meanwhile, a study of risk factors associated with **diabetes mellitus** and arterial hypertension in the adult population of Tegucigalpa in 2003 and 2004 found 36% of the subjects suffering from overweight and another 23% suffering from obesity (22). The study put the prevalence rate for diabetes mellitus at 7.8%, meaning that there were nearly 39,000 residents with diabetes in the nation's capital, 42% of whom were not even aware of their condition. The Ministry of Health put the incidence of diabetes in 2004 at 593 per 100,000 population.

Cardiovascular Diseases

The same study of risk factors associated with diabetes and hypertension found 19% of Tegucigalpa's adult population suffering from arterial hypertension, 53% with elevated total cholesterol levels, 37% with high LDL cholesterol levels, 34% with low HDL cholesterol levels, and 29% with elevated triglyceride levels. According to Ministry of Health data records, the incidence of hypertension in 2004 was 1,681 per 100,000 population.

Malignant Neoplasms

The National Cancer Program identified the leading cancer types in 1998 as being uterine, breast, skin, stomach, and ovarian. Data for 1998–2003 from the Emma Romero de Callejas Cancer Center, half of whose cases come from the department of Francisco Morazán, identified the most frequently occurring malignant cancers as being cervical (24.4%), breast (13.9%), brain (5.2%), and lymphoid leukemia (3.5%). Most cases of cervical cancer involved women between the ages of 35 and 54 who were in stages II or III, while 60% of breast cancer cases involved women between the ages of 40 and 59 in stages II or III. A population-based cancer registry was recently established by the Cancer Center with the goal of improving the capacity to monitor trends and patterns over time and thus better understand and address the national cancer burden.

OTHER HEALTH PROBLEMS OR ISSUES

Disasters

Since Hurricane Mitch in 1998, which affected countless lives and household economies, Honduras has not experienced another natural disaster of similar magnitude. However, numerous smaller hurricanes and storms cause fatalities and leave thousands of residents homeless every year. The most notable of these events were hurricanes Adrian and Beta, which struck in May and October of 2005, respectively, destroying homes and crops in Gracias a Dios, Atlántida, and Colón.

Violence and Other External Causes

Social insecurity, including homicides, suicides, traffic accidents, and gender-based violence, continued to rise during the 2001–2005 review period. According to the Criminal Investigations Bureau (DGIC), the largest numbers of complaints filed in 2003, in descending order, involved crimes against women, crimes against minors, and attempted homicides. Reports by the DGIC and the Department of Forensic Medicine attached to the Attorney General's Office show most violent deaths occurring in large cities, with 43% caused by gunshot wounds and involving mostly males and young adults aged 20–35 (23).

According to the DGIC, 8,877 complaints of domestic violence were filed between January and November of 2004. In 95% of the complaints, women were the victims; and in 94% of the complaints, the aggressors were male. Violence between intimate partners was responsible for 49% of the reported incidents, and in 74% of the cases, the violence occurred in the home. Many cases of domestic violence are believed to go unreported, although the establishment over the last few years of specialized prosecutors' offices for dealing with domestic violence cases has boosted the number of reported cases. During January and November of 2004, 394 women died as a result of instances of domestic violence.

The availability of data on accidents and other injuries is extremely limited and the data itself fragmented in nature. A recently established violence observatory bases its information on injuries from external causes on data from the Teaching Hospital in Tegucigalpa, where 3,704 injuries of this type were recorded during the first quarter of 2006; 51.3% of the injuries were accidental, 12.2% were caused by traffic accidents, 8.2% were intentional or caused by violence, 0.6% were self-inflicted, and 27.6% were of unspecified origin. A breakdown by gender revealed that 67.5% of all such injuries involved males and 32.5% involved females. The 5–14-year-old and 15–24-year-old age groups were the two groups most affected by injuries. Most intentional injuries were caused by a sharp object (34.4%), firearms discharge (24.9%), or a blunt object (23.3%), with most assaults being associated with attempted robberies (36.1%) or fights (24.9%) (24).

RESPONSE OF THE HEALTH SECTOR

Health Policies and Plans

Article 145 of the Honduran Constitution recognizes the public's right to health protection and establishes the State's responsibilities in this area. Other relevant national legislation includes the Civil Service Act, the Health Code and its accompanying regulations, the Environment Act and its implementing regulations, the Children's and Adolescents' Code, the Domestic Violence Act, the Equal Opportunities Act for Women, and the Special HIV/AIDS Act.

The Health Code stipulates that the health sector consists of public and private and national and international institutions and organizations providing health-related services. The Ministry of Health governs and regulates the sector, coordinates all health-related activities, sets health priorities, and charts the course of development efforts in the public and private subsectors. It formulates national plans and programs, establishes essential public health functions, issues regulations, and oversees and evaluates compliance with these, particularly as regards foodstuffs, beverages, drugs, cosmetics, hazardous substances, and medical facilities.

The current regulatory framework accords the Ministry of Health rather broad, detailed legal authority to effectively exercise its oversight functions. However, existing regulatory instruments are extremely fragmented, and the scope of the current Health Code is somewhat limited in light of the challenges presented by health sector reform and its implementation process. Clearly, there is a need for updated legislation and a more comprehensive legal framework better aligned to health sector reform priorities and goals.

Since 2005, the main functions of the Health Regulation Department have been the monitoring and regulation of health-related products, services, and facilities. To this end, it serves as the focal point for standard-setting, overseeing health system facilities, and enforcing applicable sanctions under existing regulations. The evaluation of essential public health functions underscored the existence of sound basic and subsidiary standards while, at the same time, highlighting the extent of noncompliance with these standards due, in part, to a lack of trained human resources. Areas considered especially weak were professional cer-

tification and facilities accreditation procedures, performance monitoring procedures for contracts with private services providers, and air and water quality control procedures.

Health Strategies and Programs

A number of policies and strategies formulated over the past few years have sought to improve health services coverage and otherwise extend the social safety net through health protection strategies. However, a large percentage of the population is still excluded from health services coverage, due to barriers to services access, inadequacies in continuity and the provision of viable and financially sustainable services, and/or the lack of culturally appropriate services which recognize and respect traditional ethnic values. Excluded population groups include the poor, rural residents, the indigenous population, and the unemployed, the underemployed, and workers in the informal sector. Table 4 presents the leading indicators of exclusion in health.

The Poverty Reduction Strategy has been unsuccessful in addressing the contributing factors to social exclusion. The most recent PRS progress reports show extremely slow progress in addressing poverty, health, water supply, and sanitation issues, indicating the need to revamp existing programs in these areas.

Likewise, policies designed to expand the social safety net have yet to make significant progress toward ensuring this type of protection for targeted population groups. While the IHSS has seen a sizeable expansion in its contributing base, the size of its beneficiary population increased by only around 3% between 2002 and 2004. Moreover, underemployment and informal

TABLE 4. Leading indicators of exclusion in health, by type, Honduras, 2004.

	Percentage
Coverage	
Population without health care	30.1
Population without health insurance	83.1
Financial and work-related accessibility	
Households living under poverty line	64.5
Population with per capita income under US$ 1/day	41.1
Workers employed in the informal sector	55.9
Cultural accessibility	
Illiteracy among ethnic population	38.1
Average number of years of formal schooling among ethnic population	2.2
Structure	
Number of physicians per 1,000 population	0.8
Number of beds per 1,000 population	0.6
Processes	
Home deliveries	45.6
Pregnant women without health care during first trimester of pregnancy	43.6
Households without indoor plumbing	26.0

Source: Pan American Health Organization. *Exclusion in Health in Latin America and the Caribbean.* Washington, D.C.: PAHO, 2004.

employment levels continue to rise to the detriment of the formal employment sector.

The Ministry of Health conducted a second national evaluation of essential public health functions in March 2003. The functions in which performance was judged to be best were EPHF11 (reducing the impact of emergencies and disasters on health), EPHF2 (public health surveillance), and EPHF10 (public health research). The functions in which performance was deemed to be poorest were human resources development and training in public health (EPHF8), ensuring quality in personal and population-based health services (EPHF9), development of policy, planning, and managerial capacity to support public health efforts (EPHF5), capacity-building for public health regulation and enforcement (EPHF6), and evaluation and promotion of equitable access to basic health services (EPHF7). Performance was determined to be intermediate as regards EPHF4 (social participation and empowerment of citizens in health-related issues), EPHF1 (health situation monitoring and analysis), and EPHF3 (health promotion).

The Ministry of Health is responsible for the framing and implementation of major health strategies at the national and local levels. To this end, its central headquarters regularly carries out health programs, oversees regulatory issues, and provides technical support to its own regional offices, the IHSS, and the private subsector.

Strategies geared to preventing and controlling major health problems include reduction of infant and maternal mortality and malnutrition rates, measles eradication, rubella elimination, ensuring the continued eradication of polio, control of transfusional transmission of diseases, increased emphasis on comprehensive child health care and expansion of the Integrated Management of Childhood Illness (IMCI) component within child health services, participation in the Roll Back Malaria and Stop TB initiatives spearheaded by the Pan American Health Organization/World Health Organization (PAHO/WHO), and control of sexually transmitted infections and Chagas' disease. The synchronization and coordination of efforts by different international cooperation agencies and the Ministry of Health in controlling Chagas' disease, with the PAHO/WHO-Honduras country office serving as the technical secretariat of this effort, has been particularly noteworthy and led to significant achievements.

Despite the successes recorded to date, a persistent obstacle is the country's medicalized health care model with an emphasis on recuperative care and only a very limited preventive health component; this is, in turn, a byproduct of the educational and training models that continue to be used for incoming health professionals and those updating their skills.

Organization of the Health System

The health sector consists of the Ministry of Health, the Honduran Social Security Institute, and the private subsector, with weak functional links between these entities. Until 2004, for administrative purposes, the Ministry of Health had been organized into eight health regions which, in turn, were subdivided into health districts, with the latter holding jurisdiction over outpatient facilities such as physician- and dentist-manned health centers, and rural health centers, and hospitals (with the exception of the six national hospitals attached directly to the Ministry's central headquarters). In May 2004, the Ministry was reorganized along functional lines and 18 Departmental Health Regions were created to coincide with the country's political-administrative subdivisions. In addition, two Metropolitan Health Regions were created: one in the municipality of the Distrito Central, of which Tegucigalpa forms a part, as the departmental capital of Francisco Morazán, and one in the municipality of San Pedro Sula, capital of the department of Cortés.

The IHSS is a decentralized government agency governed by a board of directors consisting of government representatives, employers, workers, and one member from the Honduran Medical Association and managed by an executive director. Its central level is divided into three national management offices, corresponding to the types of benefits administered: maternity health; disability, retirement, and death; and workers' compensation. IHSS coverage is in the process of being expanded through a network of public and private service providers and a national procurement office for outsourced services.

The IHSS central headquarters in Tegucigalpa has operational jurisdiction over the Central-Southern-Eastern Region including Danlí, Juticalpa, Choluteca, San Lorenzo, Tegucigalpa, Comayagua, Siguatepeque, and La Paz. The service area of its Northwest Regional Office based in San Pedro Sula includes San Pedro Sula, Puerto Cortés, Copán, Choloma, Villanueva, La Ceiba, Tela, Tocoa, Roatán, and Trujillo.

The IHSS delivers health care through in-house and outsourced services on three different levels: the primary level, providing family and community health services to enrolled social security beneficiaries; the secondary level providing outpatient and hospital care by referral; and the tertiary level consisting of the Tegucigalpa and San Pedro Sula specialty hospitals, treating patients referred by lower levels.

While only limited data are available, it is widely recognized that the health sector is highly segmented. According to a recent survey, 47% of the population visited a health facility when feeling ill; of this group, 58% sought care at a Ministry of Health facility, 7% went to an IHSS facility, 30% went to a private health facility, and the remainder consulted community health workers and pharmacies (25).

As stipulated in Resolution No. 895, the purpose of the 2004 Ministry of Health restructuring program was "to strengthen the administrative capacity of the . . . locally based health services system." Initially, the changes made in its administrative system were designed to decentralize or, more specifically, to "deconcentrate" management. The Ministry of Health is mounting programs geared to preparing local authorities to eventually take over decentralized powers and functions. Deconcentration based on a regionalization model transfers power mainly from the central to the subnational level, with very limited transfers of power to the local level. The public hospital network and operational levels have financial management authority over a specified share of financing to meet selected needs and are in charge of managing supplies and equipment. Some cooperation and investment projects have delegated responsibilities to health units at the local level, assigning them the necessary funding for such purposes. As the core policy for health sector reform, decentralization is possible only as part of a democratic process building solidarity and, more importantly, strengthening social participation and community empowerment. To this end, an effort is being made to strengthen channels of communication between the central, subnational, and local levels. The municipalities are beginning to undertake local health situation assessments with the involvement of all segments of the local community and to formulate integrated development plans.

Approximately 11% of the Honduran population and 37.1% of the working population is covered by the IHSS public health insurance subsystem. The IHSS provides health benefits to contributing wage earners covering all health risks, and maternity care and health care for children up to the age of 5 to indirect or noncontributing social security beneficiaries. There is no private social security coverage. There are 10 private insurance companies selling insurance plans covering medical care and hospitalization which are financed out-of-pocket by plan members; no data is available regarding the percentage of the population currently covered under such plans. There are no public funding mechanisms for private health insurance.

Public Health Services

Even though at one time Honduras was considered a model for the implementation of the primary health care strategy, currently major inequities in health care exist, community health workers and promoters are being called upon to complement or substitute for the limited availability of health services in some areas, and with few exceptions, there is no inter-agency or cross-sector coordination at any level. Moreover, large segments of the population are excluded from reaping the benefits of appropriate health technologies at an affordable cost.

Major ongoing health programs by the Ministry of Health include the HIV/AIDS Prevention Program, whose primary focus is on prevention and education, and, more recently, on the provision of antiretroviral drug therapy; the Sexually Transmitted Infections Control Program, which also includes a major educational component and administers standardized treatment protocols; the Tuberculosis Control Program, whose chief components are early detection based on screening tests and standardized treatment protocols and case follow-up; the Cervical Cancer Control Program, which similarly emphasizes the importance of early detection through screening interventions; the National Oral Health Program, whose primary focus is community education and awareness-raising through nationwide campaigns promoting the use of fluoride and sealers and the provision of dental checkups to schoolchildren and pregnant women; and the Expanded Program on Immunization, which has achieved and sustained national vaccination coverage rates above 95% over the past several years. The Ministry of Health's Comprehensive Family Health Care Department administers women's health programs (prenatal care, deliveries, postpartum care, and family planning services), as well as those for children under the age of 5 and adolescents.

The weakness of the health information system in capturing epidemiological surveillance, health services, and vital statistics data is a serious problem in Honduras. The only available data for measuring morbidity comes from Ministry of Health reports and population surveys, while mortality weights are established based on special studies. Major improvements in the National Registry of Individuals helped reduce the underreporting of births from 32% in 2002 to 8% in 2005. However, the problem of underregistration of deaths persists, with a rate that stood at 37% in 2005.

Most health information comes from routine data reporting systems within the health services network, which includes outpatient as well as hospital services. The result is fragmentary data originating from a variety of intra- or interinstitutional sources. The Ministry of Health has various subsystems for the recording and transmission of data whose processing places additional pressures on health services, with the same item of data sometimes taking different routes up to the central level. Most data are compiled and transmitted in printed form, which hinders their interpretation at higher levels. The variety of different data formats and sources hampers data disaggregation, comparison, and other statistical processes. Health surveillance is based solely on data reported by Ministry of Health services, on the so-called epidemiological warning or "telegram" system, and on monthly transmissions of data regarding the status of 46 diseases or events requiring obligatory reporting.

The second highest rated essential public health function in 2003 was that of public health surveillance (EPHF2), due largely to the development of guides, the level of professional expertise, and the support and assistance available at the subnational level. However, health situation monitoring and analysis (EPHF1), and in particular, the development of technology, experience, and methodologies for the management, interpretation, and communication of information to those responsible for public health decision-making, health care providers, and the population at large, were shown to be areas where improvements needed to be made.

The Health Surveillance Office is establishing epidemiological analysis units at the national, subnational, and local levels to serve as data processing, data analysis, and decision-making entities. As part of this effort, the teams who will staff these units are receiving capacity-building training and being provided with the necessary geo-referenced data analysis tools. Mapping of communicable disease risks is being undertaken, as well as the development of a municipal health needs index for assessment of six dimensions: access to water and sanitation services, urban development (overcrowding), human capital (primary education), access to health services (vaccination coverage), the supply of health services (physician-patient ratio), and health status (stunting in schoolchildren).

As regards the current status of water supply and sanitation services, most of the general population has access to a safe water supply, but less than half consumes properly disinfected water and more than 90% of all water supply systems provide only intermittent service. The coverage and quality of services delivery to the country's scattered rural and poor urban population are lacking. There are very limited wastewater treatment facilities despite the efforts made in several mid-size cities to build waste stabilization ponds. Two-thirds of the nationwide population has some type of excreta disposal facility, primarily latrines (35%), which are oftentimes the only solution available in rural areas (26).

The Ministry of Natural Resources and the Environment and the Pollutant Research and Control Center have an appropriate legal framework in place and have been endeavoring to strengthen environmental management by streamlining their procedures and promoting decentralization. However, capacity-building efforts for the monitoring and surveillance of health-related environmental factors need to be stepped up to bolster decentralization, intersectoral coordination, and institutional capacity. Until now, the coordination of these two entities with the Ministry of Health has been more the result of special circumstances than the product of a collective policy framed in conjunction with top decision-making authorities and implemented by intermediate- and local-level officials.

In order to ensure sustainability, there is a real need for an integrated surface and groundwater resources protection and management plan. This requires institutional restructuring in keeping with the provisions of the recently enacted Sector Framework Law, along with a financing policy and a financially sustainable services structure. Until the enactment of the Framework Law, there was no oversight or regulatory agency in this sector. There was, however, a wide variety of service providers, including the National Autonomous Water Supply and Sewerage Service, municipal government agencies and enterprises, semipublic enterprises, and a single private enterprise (in San Pedro Sula). Service providers in rural areas include municipalities and the Ministry of Health.

With municipal governments scheduled to take over responsibility for services delivery beginning in 2008, local water and sanitation authorities will need to build the necessary capacity, particularly in the case of the smallest municipalities. Utility companies will need to rectify their current lack of preventive maintenance procedures to reduce the vulnerability of water supply and sanitation infrastructure.

In the wake of the devastation caused by Hurricane Mitch in 1998, an effort was made to better organize sector mechanisms for the prevention and mitigation of emergencies and disasters. The health sector has established good inter-agency coordination for alliance-building and adequate advisory assistance to the subnational levels of government, and has developed a disaster mitigation plan with appropriate policies and procedures. The Ministries of Health and Agriculture are heading up efforts to frame a National Influenza Pandemic Preparedness Plan.

The growth in international trade and travel has heightened the risk of disease importation, particularly from neighboring countries with which there is heavy freight, animal, and passenger traffic. Over the past few years, Honduras has been on alert against the possible introduction of SARS (severe acute respiratory syndrome), West Nile fever, and Venezuelan equine encephalitis into the country. The global avian influenza threat could have a serious impact on food safety and the national economy and, in the event of an influenza pandemic, human morbidity and mortality would likely far exceed the national response capacity.

Individual Care Services

According to data from a 2002 survey of health facilities, the Ministry of Health has the country's largest health facilities network, with 28 hospitals and 1,241 outpatient or maternal and child health care facilities. In addition to the two specialty hospitals located in Tegucigalpa and San Pedro Sula, the INSS has 10 outpatient facilities, with plans for further expansion. In the private subsector, nongovernmental organizations (NGOs) and other agencies and organizations operate 108 hospitals and 820 outpatient facilities. As of 2002, the country had 6,659 beds (0.97 beds per 1,000 population); of these, 4,656 beds were located in Ministry of Health facilities; 250 in IHSS facilities; 1,652 in the private for-profit subsector; and 101 in facilities run by NGOs and other agencies and organizations.

A National Blood Council was established in 1997 and charged with setting up a national blood system to ensure the population's access to an adequate supply of blood and blood products of acceptable quality. The regulations issued under the National Blood Policy, enacted in 1998, contain general policies and guidance for the utilization of blood and guidelines for the organization of a national blood system, with the National Blood Council, the National Blood Program, the Blood Bank Department within the Ministry of Health, and the public and private hospital transfusion services network serving as its implementing agencies. The network includes 22 blood banks (16 public, 2 run by the Honduran Red Cross, and 4 private) and 45 public and private transfusion services. That same year, the Ministry of Health designated the Honduran Red Cross as the agency in charge of the establishment, operation, and expansion of the National Blood

Improving Health through Cooperation and the Sectoral Approach

More than half of the population of Honduras lives in poverty. The two most vulnerable population groups are the indigenous and those of African descent, among whom obvious inequalities and disadvantages exist as regards economic condition, level of education, and access to services. The situation is even worse in rural areas, where 75% of the population is living in conditions of extreme poverty. The formation of sectoral committees as a tripartite discussion forum for government, civil society, and cooperation agencies was designed as a tool to improve the efficiency and effectiveness of efforts to monitor progress in the national reconstruction and reform process and implementation of the Poverty Reduction Strategy. The goal is to harmonize and improve planning, implementation, and management mechanisms and strengthen and ensure the rational financial management of resources in the education, health, water supply and sanitation, and agricultural sectors. The Ministry of Health and other interested stakeholders feel that the transition to a sector-wide approach (SWAp) is the best strategy for efficient budget management of health sector funding. Moreover, the Ministry of Health has framed the National Health Plan 2021 and National Health Policy 2006–2010 to serve as the blueprint for SWAp implementation.

Program (i.e., in charge of donor recruitment and selection, the preparation of blood components, the performance of immuno-hematological tests, the detection of infectious agents, and the storage and shipment of blood and blood products). Technical standards for the proper handling of blood and blood products were approved in 1999.

The screening of 100% of blood donations nationwide in 2002 and 2003 revealed the continued prevalence of HIV (0.3% for both years), hepatitis B (0.5% and 0.34%), hepatitis C (0.7% and 0.95%), and syphilis (1.2% and 1.31%). Screening tests for *Trypanosoma cruzi* yielded a seroprevalence rate of 1.4% among blood donors in 2003.

The country has high-tech laboratory and imaging diagnostic services located mainly in private facilities in large cities. The only specialized public facilities are the Thorax Hospital and the Santa Rosita Psychiatric Hospital.

Health Promotion

In the 2003 essential public health functions evaluation, health promotion (EPHF3) was considered to be an area in which national performance needed to be improved. While efforts continue to promote healthy behaviors and lifestyles, many challenges have resulted due to limited technical support at the subnational and local levels, insufficient alliances-building capacity, and weaknesses in planning and coordination of information and education strategies.

The formation of sectoral committees as a tripartite discussion forum for government, civil society, and cooperation agencies, designed as a tool to improve the efficiency and effectiveness of efforts to monitor the national reconstruction and reform process and implementation of the Poverty Reduction Strategy, has proven its efficacy over time. The goal is to harmonize and

improve planning, implementation, and management mechanisms and strengthen and ensure the rational financial management of resources in the education, health, water supply and sanitation, and agricultural sectors. The Government has decided to chart national policy at the sector level, based on long-term country programs rather than individual projects as it had been doing in the past, in line with its series of Health Sector Policies for 2002–2006, the Government Plan for 2002–2006, the Poverty Reduction Strategy, the MDGs, and the National Health Plan 2021 and has set for itself the challenge of structuring all future planning on the so-called "sector-wide approach" (SWAp).

The Ministry of Health and other interested stakeholders feel that the move to this approach is the best strategy for efficient budget management of health sector funding. In their view, other essential steps will include the designing of management tools to facilitate efforts to monitor and evaluate progress, the implementation of sectoral strategies, the establishment of procedures to ensure accountability, compliance with established standards for each strategy, budget performance monitoring for national and international cooperation funding, and an impact assessment of this new work modality.

The Ministry of Health has framed the National Health Plan 2021 and National Health Policy 2006–2010 to guide Ministry of Health and IHSS operations. These two tools are designed to serve as the blueprint for implementation of the SWAp approach, whose adoption is intended to ensure the most efficient use possible of available health sector funding and achievement of the MDGs through the Poverty Reduction Strategy.

Human Resources

One of the country's lowest-scoring essential public health functions was that of human resources development and training in public health (EPHF8). The most critical issues were the lack of a workforce classification system and, more specifically, of a staffing needs assessment, as well as a dialogue among academic training facilities, other national government authorities, and civil society for the framing of a national policy in this area. Other shortcomings included the absence of a performance evaluation system for public health personnel and the lack of job stability, incentives, and continuing education opportunities.

The ratios of physicians, professional nurses, and dentists per 10,000 population are estimated at 8.7, 3.2, and 2.2, respectively, taking into account the sum of human resources in public and private health facilities. As the institution overseeing the country's largest health facilities network, the Ministry of Health would be expected to possess the largest share of human resources. However, its ratios of physicians, professional nurses, and dentists per 10,000 population are a mere 2.4, 1.2, and 0.2, respectively. There are also large geographical disparities in health personnel deployment by department, with physician-patient ratios varying from 5.6 per 10,000 population in Francisco Morazán to as low as 0.9 in Santa Bárbara.

Health Supplies

There are 16,000 drugs currently available, most of which are imported brand-name drugs. There has been some improvement in the regulation of drugs, with all regulatory functions currently being exercised solely by the Ministry of Health. Health surveillance has been stepped up, particularly with respect to supervision of pharmaceutical establishments and the enforcement of penalties, including the shutdown of pharmacies without adequate management. Very few of the 67 existing pharmaceutical firms are in compliance with Good Manufacturing Practices requirements. To address drug supply problems, the Ministry of Health plans to restructure the entire system, focusing particularly on storage and inventory control issues.

Research and Technological Development in Health

As measured by the publication of scientific and technical health information and data, there is very little output from scientific activity. Contributing factors include limited funding for scientific activity and inadequately trained health researchers. The efforts mounted by various institutions forming part of the National Virtual Health Library Committee and headed up by the National Autonomous University of Honduras Medical Library to improve scientific and technical health information management and make such information available to students, health professionals, and researchers are commendable.

While there is a special agency in charge of developing a public health research agenda, the lack of political, technical, and financial support has hindered progress. The main source of funding is external cooperation. Similar challenges are faced by the other agencies created by the Government to help promote health research, resulting in this function being left to individual professionals and academic institutions, whose research does not necessarily help build health knowledge or uphold the ethical principles governing such research.

Technical Cooperation and External Financing

International technical and financial cooperation plays a pivotal role in the Honduran economy and in the success of efforts to promote economic and social development within the framework of the Poverty Reduction Strategy and the MDGs. The Technical and International Cooperation Secretariat (SETCO) is a specialized agency in charge of setting government investment and spending program priorities and targets and monitoring progress toward the achievement of these. It is also responsible for the framing, negotiation, and monitoring of international cooperation policies and strategies. Sector projects and programs are identified, appraised, and selected by SETCO based on the Government Plan for 2002–2006 and the priorities established under the Poverty Reduction Strategy (27).

The flow of international technical and financial aid in the area of health increased significantly in the wake of Hurricane Mitch. However, the adequate channeling of funds to the population groups most in need and the capacity to maximize impact for recipient groups are still somewhat elusive goals.

External financing, including external grants and loans, accounts for close to 30% of the total budget. Figure 5 breaks down

FIGURE 5. Health budget, by financing source, Honduras, 2004.

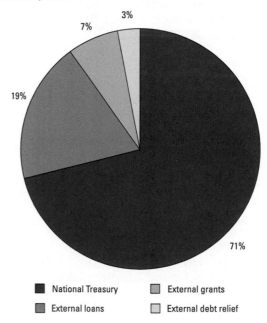

- National Treasury
- External loans
- External grants
- External debt relief

TABLE 5. Health projects, by funding type, Honduras, 1998–2003.

Country/agency/organization	Type of financing	Commitment (in US$)
Total nonreimbursable funding		**198,460,641**
United States	Bilateral	47,760,000
Japan	Bilateral	23,272,425
Sweden	Bilateral	9,000,000
Canada	Bilateral	4,730,525
Germany	Bilateral	1,182,000
United Kingdom	Bilateral	849,000
Spain	Bilateral	11,716
	Total bilateral	86,805,666
WFP	Multilateral	55,891,452
European Union	Multilateral	30,381,454
UNDP (Global Fund)	Multilateral	20,842,930
UNESCO	Multilateral	4,177,811
Catholic Relief Services	Multilateral	200,000
	Total multilateral	111,493,647
World Vision	NGO	161,328
	Total NGO	161,328
Total reimbursable funding		**92,400,000**
IDB	Multilateral	36,000,000
Spain (AEIC)	Bilateral	29,300,000
World Bank	Multilateral	27,100,000

Source: Honduras. Secretaría del Despacho de la Presidencia. *Hacia un Programa Sectorial Ampliado.* Tegucigalpa, June 2004.

the health budget for 2004 by source of funding. The pattern of financing has not changed over the last several years and, according to data supplied by various international agencies, the volume of aid is expected to remain more or less the same over the next five years.

Between 1998 and 2003, Honduras signed 54 health agreements for a total of nearly US$ 300 million (Table 5). Of the more than US$ 198 million in nonreimbursable health project funding, the largest share comes from multilateral organizations such as the World Food Program (WFP), European Union, and the United Nations Development Program (UNDP), and U.S., Japanese, and Swedish cooperation agencies. Reimbursable project funding from sources such as the Inter-American Development Bank (IDB), Spanish International Cooperation Agency (AECI), and World Bank amounts to more than US$ 92 million. It is difficult to find current, detailed, official data on cooperation in Honduras, and there are serious underreporting problems with respect to the amounts involved and numbers of participating organizations.

There are a number of international cooperation discussion forums, including various United Nations inter-agency coordination committees, bringing together stakeholders on a regular basis. In addition, the health sector has several discussion and study groups, including the Health Sector Committee and the CESAR (Rural Health Care Centers) Committee, addressing nationwide health issues on an ongoing basis.

References

1. Honduras, Secretaría de Finanzas. Informe de la deuda pública, período enero–diciembre 2005. Available at: http://www.sefin.gob.hn. Accessed on 24 July 2006.

2. Cabezas M. La manera hondureña de presupuestar la ERP. La Haya: Institute of Social Studies; 2005.

3. Honduras, Secretaría del Despacho Presidencial, Unidad de Apoyo Técnico. Informe de avance de la ERP, primer trimestre 2005. Vol. 2, N° 1. Tegucigalpa: Secretaría del Despacho Presidencial; 2005.

4. World Bank. World Development Indicators 2005. Available at: http://devdata.worldbank.org/data-query. Accessed on 3 March 2006.

5. Honduras, Instituto Nacional de Estadística. Encuesta de Hogares de Propósitos Múltiples. Tegucigalpa: INE; 2004.

6. World Bank. World Development Indicators 2005. Available at: http://devdata.worldbank.org/wdi2005/Section2.htm. Accessed on 8 July 2005.

7. Honduras, Instituto Nacional de Estadística. Mercado laboral. Encuesta de Hogares de Hogares de Propósitos Múltiples. Available at: http://www.ine-hn.org. Accessed on 6 October 2004.

8. Pratt L. El sector maquila de Honduras y riesgos ambientales y sociales. Available at: http://www.ecobanking.com. Accessed on 20 July 2006.

9. Honduras, Banco Central de Honduras. Honduras en cifras 2003–2005. Available at: http://www.bch.hn. Accessed on 27 July 2006.

10. Honduras, Instituto Nacional de Estadística. Censo de Población y Vivienda 2001. Tegucigalpa: INE; 2003.

11. Mercaplan Centroamérica. Encuesta Nacional sobre Percepción de Corrupción en Honduras 2001. Available at: http://www.worldbank.org/wbi/governance/honduras/results.html. Accessed on 20 July 2006.

12. Honduras, Instituto Nacional de Estadística. Proyecciones de población 2001–2015. Tegucigalpa: INE; 2003.

13. Asociación Hondureña de Planificación de Familia. Encuesta Nacional de Epidemiología y Salud Familiar 2001. Tegucigalpa: ASHONPLAFA; 2003.

14. Honduras, Secretaría de Salud, Departamento de Estadística, Unidad de Planeamiento y Evaluación de la Gestión. Boletín de Estadísticas Ambulatorias, año 2004. Tegucigalpa: SS; 2005.

15. Honduras, Programa de Asignación Familiar. Octavo Censo de Talla en Niños de Primer Grado, 2001. Tegucigalpa: PRAF; 2001.

16. Pantelides E. La salud sexual y reproductiva: también un asunto de hombres. Buenos Aires: Organización Panamericana de la Salud; 2005.

17. Meléndez JH, Ochoa JC, Villanueva Y. Investigación sobre mortalidad materna y de mujeres en edad reproductiva en Honduras. Informe final 1997. Tegucigalpa; 1999.

18. Quiroz C. Mortalidad materna en Honduras 2004–2005. Trabajo presentado en el Taller sobre Vigilancia de Mortalidad Materna, Centro Latinoamericano de Perinatología y Desarrollo Humano/Organización Panamericana de la Salud, 29 de marzo de 2006.

19. Honduras, Instituto Nacional de Estadística. La discapacidad en Honduras: análisis de los resultados de la XXVI Encuesta de Hogares de Propósitos Múltiples, 2002. Tegucigalpa: INE; 2003.

20. Honduras, Secretaría de Salud, Departamento de Estadística. Informe de enfermedades transmisibles (TRANS) 2004. Tegucigalpa: SS; 2005.

21. Organización Panamericana de la Salud, Centro Panamericano de Fiebre Aftosa. Sistema de Información Epidemiológica. Available at: http://siepi.panaftosa.org.br/Painel.aspx. Accessed on 20 September 2006.

22. Palma R, Pineda E, Fernández E, Amándola L. Prevalencia de diabetes mellitus e hipertensión arterial y factores asociados en Tegucigalpa 2003–2004. Preliminary data. In press.

23. United Nations, Joint Programme for the Support of Human Security in Honduras 2005–2006. Concept paper; 2004.

24. Universidad Autónoma de Honduras, Observatorio de la Violencia. Lesiones. Boletín trimestral enero–marzo 2006. Edición N° 2, mayo 2006.

25. Honduras, Instituto Nacional de Estadística. Encuesta de Condiciones de Vida 2004. Tegucigalpa: INE; 2006.

26. Honduras. Análisis del Sector de Agua Potable y Saneamiento. Tegucigalpa; 2003.

27. Honduras, Secretaría de Finanzas. Nuevo Financiamiento Cooperación Internacional en el Marco del Grupo Consultivo Período 2004–2006. Tegucigalpa: Secretaría de Finanzas; 2005.

JAMAICA

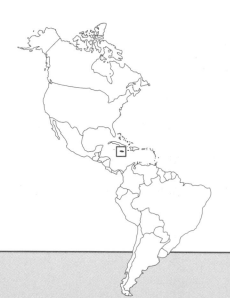

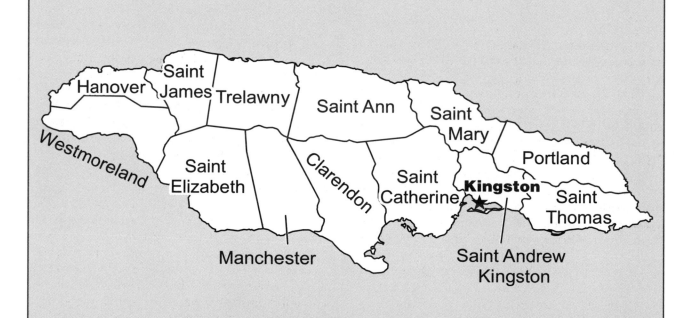

Hanover

Saint James

Trelawny

Saint Ann

Saint Mary

Portland

Westmoreland

Saint Elizabeth

Clarendon

Saint Catherine

Kingston

Saint Thomas

Manchester

Saint Andrew
Kingston

0   25   50 Miles

With a land area of 11,424 km², Jamaica is the largest English-speaking island in the Caribbean Sea. It is located 150 km south of Cuba and 160 km west of Haiti. The country is divided into 14 parishes. Its largest city is Kingston, the country's capital on the southeast coast. Other major population centers are Spanish Town, Portmore, and Montego Bay. Its estimated population in 2005 was 2,651,000.

GENERAL CONTEXT AND HEALTH DETERMINANTS

Social, Political, and Economic Determinants

Jamaica has been a stable constitutional democracy in the Commonwealth of Nations since its independence from Great Britain in 1962. Political governance is by a parliamentary system based on the Westminster/Whitehall model and a bicameral legislature. The Cabinet of Ministers forms the executive arm of the government and is headed by the Prime Minister.

The Jamaican economy reported its seventh consecutive year of real GDP growth (1.4%) during 2005 (1). The economy is heavily dependent upon services (71% of GDP) and continues to derive most of its foreign exchange from tourism, remittances, and bauxite-alumina. A study by the United Nations Environment Program (2), nonetheless, shows tourism "leakage" to be at 40% in Jamaica (i.e., the amount of tourism expenditure that remained in the country after taxes, profits, and wages paid outside the region are taken into account and imports are purchased). The economy faces serious long-term problems of high interest rates, increased foreign competition, a pressured exchange rate, a sizable merchandise trade deficit, large-scale unemployment, and a growing internal debt. Between June 2001 and September 2005, the exchange rate increased from J$ 45.7 = US$ 1 to J$ 62.5 = US$ 1. The government faced the difficult challenge of seeking to achieve fiscal discipline in order to maintain debt payments while simultaneously attacking a serious and growing crime problem that is hampering economic growth. Attempts by the government to control the budget deficit were derailed by Hurricane Ivan in September 2004, which resulted in damages costing an estimated US$ 599 million (3), while in 2005, a real GDP growth of 1.4% was achieved despite hurricanes Dennis and Emily, which caused damage to infrastructure and productive assets amounting to approximately US$ 96.9 million (1). Tropical storm Wilma in 2005 caused additional damages to agriculture, forestry, and fishing amounting to US$ 7.3 million.

According to the Jamaica Survey of Living Conditions conducted in 2003 by the Planning Institute of Jamaica (4), the poverty rate stood at 19.1%. The survey determined the poverty line to be J$ 63,717.17 per year for an individual and J$ 240,816.57 per year for a family of five. Incidence by region revealed higher levels of poverty in rural areas (24.2%), while other towns had the second-highest level at 15.8%, followed by the Kingston metropolitan area at 9.5%. According to a 2004 Millennium Development Goals (MDG) report prepared by the Planning Institute of Jamaica (5), half of the country's poor were children under age 18 and 10% were elderly. Two-thirds of all female-headed households were living at or below the poverty line. Despite lower poverty rates among the urban population, poverty was extreme in some inner-city areas.

The employment rate in 2005 was 63.9%, with a male participation rate of 72.9% and a female participation rate of 55.4%. The average unemployment rate for that year was 11.3%, down from 15.5% in 2000. Disaggregation by gender showed that the female unemployment rate (15.8%) continued to be more than twice that of males (7.6%) (1, 6).

Literacy rates for the population 15 years and older in 2005 stood at 88.7% (85% for males and 92.3% for females). Jamaica achieved universal access to primary education (MDG 2) before the start of the last decade. The gross enrollment rate for 2004–2005 in public primary schools was 96% with an estimated 75.8% full attendance rate (1). Student enrollment in public secondary education for the same school year was 86.2%. Males have shown significantly lower levels of educational achievement than females, and this gap widens at the tertiary level (7). The higher educational achievements of females have led to increasingly higher numbers of women who are qualified and well placed to take advantage of economic opportunities (8). Despite higher unemployment rates among females in the general population, the number of women in Parliament increased by 50% between 1990 and 2004. Out of 14 Cabinet Ministers, in 2006 three were females, including the Prime Minister.

Jamaica's geographical proximity to both North and South America places the island in a strategic position as regards international drug markets and underground economic activity based on the trade of criminalized commodities (9). In 2004,

45.4% of the 4,240 deportations to the island (primarily from the United States, United Kingdom, and Canada) were due to drug-related offenses. Half of those deported were between 16 and 25 years of age (6). The number of deportees steadily increased from 2,529 in 2001 to 4,240 in 2004. Women are disproportionately used as drug couriers, and many end up incarcerated either in Jamaica or abroad.

Violence has reached epidemic proportions, with a homicide rate of 63 per 100,000 population in 2005, compared to 39.8 in 2002. The increase has affected all age groups. The homicide rate for males was approximately eight times that recorded for females, and in 2002 homicide was the leading cause of death for males. According to the Green Paper of the Ministry of Labour and Social Security (revised in 2006) (10), the high incidence of homicide and violence is attributable primarily to domestic violence, drug- and/or gang-related conflicts, reprisals and mob killing, political tribalism, and a breakdown in the social order.

In 2004, 68.2% of the population had access to safe piped water on the premises, and 9.5% to safe water collected from standpipes (with 29.6% of this latter group having to walk a distance of more than 460 meters). The remaining 22.3% of the population received water from wells, rivers, or water distribution trucks (with 36.1% walking a distance of greater than 460 meters). With regards to sanitation, 21.9% of Jamaican households had toilet facilities connected to a sewer, 41.9% had a toilet not linked to a sewer, and 36.1% used pit latrines (11).

Demographics, Mortality, and Morbidity

Males comprise 49.3% and females 50.7% of the 2,651,000 total estimated 2005 population. The country's most recent census (2001) found that 52.0% of the population was urban, an increase of 2% over the previous census (1991) (12). The island is in an advanced stage of demographic transition, as reflected in a declining 0–14-year-old age group, and an increasing working age population (15–64 years old) and dependent elderly age group (65 years old and older). The country's population distribution by age and sex for 1990 and 2005 is presented in Figure 1.

High levels of emigration (17,900 in 2004) continue to impact on family life, as is evidenced by the phenomenon of the "barrel" children (i.e., those left to be raised on their own or by relatives); on the labor market (through the so-called "brain-drain," or emigration of well-educated, high-income, and qualified adults); on remittances (a major contributor to foreign exchange earnings); and on population structure (through low net rates of population growth). The age dependency ratio declined from 82.8% in 1982 to 73.9% in 1991, then to 73.1% in 2001 and 61.5% in 2004 (13); it is projected to continue declining over the coming years (6). The aging of the Jamaican population has implications for chronic disease prevalence and management, and utilization of health care services.

FIGURE 1. Population structure, by age and sex, Jamaica, 1990 and 2005.

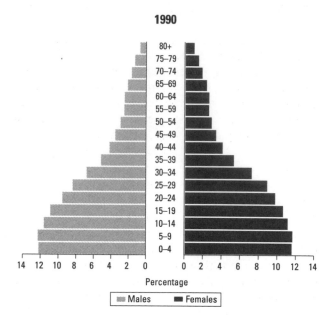

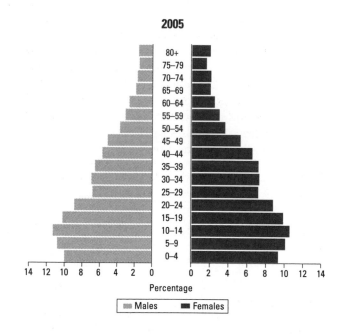

According to the 2005 Economic and Social Survey (1), life expectancy at birth was 73.3 years with the gap between males and females widening to 4.1 years (70.9 for males and 75.0 for females). Total fertility rates decreased from 2.8 in 1997 to 2.5 in 2002, and crude birth rates declined from 20.6 per 1,000 population in 2001 to 17.6 in 2004. Crude death rates showed a mild fluctuation from 6.2 per 1,000 population in 2001 to 6.0 in 2004, and registered net out-migration remained high at 17,900 in 2004. The annual rate of population growth was 0.6% in 2001 and 0.5% in 2005.

Mortality rates, which are calculated from Vital Statistics Reports from the Registrar General's Department (RGD), are limited in their utility and interpretation due to difficulties associated with the registration process. A study by McCaw-Binns and colleagues (14) found that 89% of deaths registered in 1998 occurred in that year, 4% occurred in the previous year, and 6% occurred two or more years prior to being registered. Only 49% of fetal deaths and 64% of infant deaths were registered, compared to 96% of deaths in adults 60 years and over in 1998. In addition, 38% of deaths from external causes were not registered. Data from the Jamaica Constabulary Force for assaults and transport accidents and from the National Surveillance Unit of the Ministry of Health for HIV disease were substituted for registrations from the RGD in order to establish the leading causes of death (Table 1).

A number of distinctions appear when data are analyzed by gender. Malignant neoplasms, when aggregated, are the leading cause of death for both males and females, with the rate for males being 1.4 times higher than for females. When disaggregated by type of cancer, ranking for the 10 leading causes of death changes quite significantly, introducing prostate cancer for males with an increase from 29.3 per 100,000 population in 1999 to 40.5 in 2002, and cancer of the breast and cancer of the cervix uteri for females, with the latter pointing to insufficient efforts in screening. Cerebrovascular diseases rank first as a cause of death among females and second among males. The death rate for diabetes mellitus is 1.6 times higher for females than for males. Males are at a significantly greater risk of dying as a result of homicides and transport

accidents than females. The homicide rate for males was approximately eight times the rate for females and homicide is the leading cause of death for males. Three-and-a-half times as many males as females die as a result of transport accidents.

Chronic noncommunicable diseases accounted for half of the total reported annual deaths. The main risk factors as captured in the Jamaican Healthy Lifestyle Survey Report 2000 (15), based on a sample of 2,013 persons ages 15–74 years, were sedentarism in 42% of the population aged 40 and older, hypertension in 20%, overweight and obesity in 30% of men and 60% of women, and diabetes in 8% of the population 15–74 years of age.

The HIV/AIDS epidemic in Jamaica is classified as a generalized epidemic with an adult prevalence rate of 1.5% and a male-to-female ratio of 1.3:1. HIV death rates doubled for females between 1999 and 2002—15.8 per 100,000 population to 30.7—and increased from 26.9 per 100,000 population to 44.9 in males. The principal risk factors fueling the epidemic are unprotected sex, multiple sex partners, history of sexually transmitted infections (STIs), sex with sex workers, men having sex with men, and crack/cocaine use (16).

The epidemic poses a serious threat to the productive sector, since the majority of HIV/AIDS cases occur among the working and reproductive age group.

HEALTH OF POPULATION GROUPS

Children under 5 Years Old

In 2002, the infant mortality rate was estimated at 19.9 per 1,000 live births; this rate was maintained through 2004 and was approximately 4 deaths per 1,000 live births less than in 2000 (17).

Research by McCaw-Binns and colleagues (17) determined the neonatal mortality rate to be 15.3 per 1,000 live births and the post-neonatal death rate to be 4.6 per 1,000 live births. Perinatal death rates did not show any significant change and stood at 31.2 per 1,000 total births (live births + stillbirths) in 2005. The early neonatal death rate was 10.9 per 1,000 live births in 2004 and fetal deaths were 16.8 per 1,000 births in 2004. Both figures have shown little fluctuation during the period under review (Table 2).

Causes of infant mortality are presented in Table 3, where certain conditions originating in the perinatal period are shown to be the leading cause by a significant margin. The rate of low birthweight (< 2,500 g) stood at 10% in 2004, and this figure has remained stable during the period under review (18). Of the total number of births in 2004, 98.2% were hospital births. The number of mothers exclusively breast-feeding their children at 6 weeks of age declined from more than 60% in 2001 to 45% in 2004.

HIV disease was the leading cause of death in the 1–4-year old age group in 2002 (Table 4). However, there have been fewer pediatric deaths from this cause since 2000, declining from 81 cases that year to 61 in 2004. This is attributable to improvements

TABLE 1. Ten leading causes of death, by rank, Jamaica, 2002.

Disease category	Total number	Rate per 100,000 population
Malignant neoplasms	2,686	102.3
Cerebrovascular diseases	1,905	72.6
Heart disease	1,774	67.6
Diabetes mellitus	1,477	56.3
Assault (homicide)[a]	1,045	39.8
HIV disease[b]	989	37.7
Hypertension	784	29.9
Acute respiratory infections	479	18.2
Chronic lower respiratory diseases	437	16.6
Transport accidents[a]	408	15.5

[a]Data from the Jamaica Constabulary Force substituted for registrations.
[b]Data from the Ministry of Health National Surveillance Unit substituted for registrations.
Source: Ministry of Health epidemiological profiles of selected diseases and conditions 2003 and 2005. Vital Statistics Report 2002, Registrar General's Department.

TABLE 2. Perinatal, early neonatal, and fetal mortality rates, Jamaica, 2000–2004.

Year	Perinatal mortality rate[a]	Early neonatal mortality rate[b] per 1,000 live births	Fetal mortality rate[b] per 1,000 live births
2000	29.7	11.5	18.4
2001	31.0	12.4	18.8
2002	31.1	12.5	18.9
2003	29.5	11.7	18.0
2004	27.4	10.9	16.8

[a]Per 1,000 deliveries.
[b]Per 1,000 live births.
Source: Ministry of Health.

TABLE 3. Five leading causes of infant death, Jamaica, 2002.

Disease group	Total number	Rate per 100,000 population
Certain conditions originating in the perinatal period	335	73.8
Congenital malformations, deformations, and chromosomal abnormalities	51	11.2
HIV disease[a]	20	4.4
Acute respiratory infections	4	0.9
Malignant neoplasms	3	0.7

[a]Data from the Ministry of Health National Surveillance Unit substituted for registrations.
Source: Ministry of Health epidemiological profiles 2003 and 2005. Vital Statistics Report, Registrar General's Department.

in the care and treatment of HIV-infected children and a decrease in mother-to-child transmission.

The gastroenteritis case fatality rate in the under-5 age group remains low (< 1%) but continues to be an important cause of morbidity. Respiratory diseases are the leading cause given in hospital discharge diagnoses for this age group, followed by injuries and infectious/parasitic diseases. Accidents and emergency (A&E) outpatient visits for asthma in this age group represent about 60% of all A&E asthma visits. Children under age 5 accounted for the majority of the burns and poisoning cases presenting to hospital A&E departments. The rate of undernutrition in children under age 3 has not changed and remains at approximately 3.4%, with severe malnutrition below 1%. According to Ministry of Health reports, the rate of obesity among children in this same age group is 6.7% (*19*).

Children 5–9 Years Old

Injuries and respiratory tract diseases, including asthma, were the main conditions affecting this age group in 2004. New cases of rheumatic fever continue to be reported every year: 112 cases

TABLE 4. Five leading causes of death in children aged 1–4 years, Jamaica, 2002.

Disease group	Total number	Rate per 100,000 population
HIV disease	47	22.0
Congenital malformations, deformations, and chromosomal abnormalities	35	16.4
Land transport accidents	12	5.6
Malignant neoplasms	12	5.6
Acute respiratory infections	10	4.7

Source: Ministry of Health epidemiological profiles 2003 and 2005 from Registrar General's Department, National Surveillance Unit, and Jamaica Constabulary Force.

were reported in 2005; of these, 4 were confirmed cases. The activities register for this disease counted 822 persons in 2004 (*18*). Completed reports are not available, but the coverage for secondary rheumatic fever prophylaxis stands at approximately 57%. This is of concern as the number of patients developing rheumatic heart disease is not declining. An estimated 120 or more children under the age of 18 years were orphaned by the loss of one or both parents to AIDS in 2003. The number of child abuse cases among the population ages 0–18 reported to the police increased from 346 in 2001 to 459 in 2004. The majority (90%) was due to carnal abuse (sexual assault) and affected principally females.

Adolescents 10–14 and 15–19 Years Old

One in every five Jamaicans is an adolescent. In general, this age group enjoys good health, accounting for only 2% of the deaths in 2003. Poor health, disability, and death among adolescents are usually related to high-risk behaviors. Intentional and unintentional injuries and reproductive health conditions (including HIV disease) are common among adolescents and are among the leading causes of death in this age group (Table 5).

The total fertility rate has been falling over the past decades, reaching 2.5 children per woman in 2002 (*20*). While birth rates have been falling and adolescent fertility rates reached 79 live births per 1,000 women aged 15–19 in 2002, the percentage of teenage pregnancies remains at 20%. One in every four girls aged 15–19 years is sexually active, and 12% of the female population aged 15–19 has had two or three pregnancies. Twelve percent of girls ages 15–19 who are sexually active report having been pregnant. Of those pregnancies, 30% did not end in a live birth (*21*). A 2002 study funded by the United Nations Population Fund (UNFPA) and the United Nations Children's Fund (UNICEF) indicated that abortion, despite its illegal status, was accessible to Jamaican adolescents (*22*). A 2005 study by UNFPA and the European Union on demand for emergency contraception among female adolescents between the ages of 15 and 30 ($n = 1,524$)

TABLE 5. Five leading causes of death in adolescents aged 10–19 years, Jamaica, 1999–2002.

Disease group	Total number	Rate per 100,000 population
Assault (homicide)	108	20.4
Unintentional injuries (transport accidents)	55	10.4
HIV disease	18	3.4
Malignant neoplasms	29	5.5
Heart disease	13	2.5

Source: Ministry of Health epidemiological profiles 2005 from Registrar General's Department, National Surveillance Unit, and Jamaica Constabulary Force.

showed that the 15–19-year-old age group is the one most frequently accessing abortions and the abortion incidence ratio in this age group was 21 per 100 pregnancies. Only 40% of the respondents indicated that they knew about the Emergency Oral Contraceptive (EOC), which was introduced as an over-the-counter drug in 2003. Access to the EOC was mainly through local pharmacies. The 2002–2003 Jamaica Reproductive Health Survey (20) indicated that condoms are the contraceptive method most widely used by adolescents aged 15–19 years. Contraceptive use at first intercourse in this age group was 76% for females and 44.9% for males. These contraceptives were obtained most frequently at shops or supermarkets, followed by pharmacies, according to respondents. Of the total postnatal clinic attendees accepting a family planning method in 2004, 20% were adolescents. The average age of sexual initiation was 15.8 for females and 13.5 for males. In the same survey, in 2002, 20% of the women between 15 and 19 years of age reported having been forced into sexual intercourse, compared to 25.9% in 1997. Females in the 10–19-year-old age group had a two-and-a-half times higher risk of HIV infection than males of the same age group in 2004. This difference may be related to social factors involving girls having sexual relations with HIV-infected older men. According to the Jamaican Healthy Lifestyle Survey Report 2000 (15), 11.6% of adolescents reported physical abuse, and 2.7% reported engaging in a fight with a weapon. Adolescents accounted for 26% of all persons with injuries from violent acts who were treated at the A&E departments of all hospitals.

Adults 20–59 Years Old

Visits to curative, family planning, STI, dental, casualty (emergency), and outpatient services, with a male-to-female ratio of approximately 1:2.3 for these visits, have allowed closer monitoring and earlier diagnosis of health conditions in women. In 2004, men accounted for 32.9% of visits made to primary care curative services and for 7.7% of visits made to family planning services. Reproductive health conditions are the main reason for women's contact with all levels of the health system. Other important

health problems include STIs, diabetes, hypertension, and cancer. Women's reproductive health is monitored through a network of prenatal and postnatal clinics. According to Ministry of Health reports, in 2004, 58.9% of pregnant women made an average of 4.4 visits per pregnancy to prenatal clinics in government health centers (compared to 67% of women averaging 4.3 visits per pregnancy in 2000). Pregnant women are routinely screened for anemia, sickle cell, syphilis, and HIV. In 2005, testing of antenatal clients stood at 80.2% for syphilis and approximately 90% for HIV. The seropositive rate for syphilis was 1.3%, and for HIV it was 1.5%. However, the timeliness of screening and of the results' availability continues to be a problem, and thus treatment of positive cases was low (46.8% for syphilis and approximately 57% for HIV). There were 12 cases of congenital syphilis reported through the active hospital surveillance system in 2004. Testing of 80.9% of pregnant women revealed an anemia level (Hb < 10 g/dL) of 15.8%, similar to the 2001 level. Postnatal visits by mothers to clinics represented a coverage of 69.7% of the estimated births in 2005, a slight decrease compared to 2000 (73%). Of postnatal clinic attendees, 71.1% were recruited as family planning acceptors. Fifty-three percent of women aged 15–44 years interviewed in the Jamaica Reproductive Health Survey 2002–2003 (20) were current users of a contraceptive method. Condoms and the contraceptive pill have maintained their position as the two most frequently used methods, at 33.6% and 24.5%, respectively. Although 98.2% of babies are born in hospitals, the acute shortage of trained nurse midwives affected the quality of care given to women. Cesarean section rates remained fairly constant at approximately 14%. The maternal mortality ratio has remained unchanged over the past decade and stood at 94.8 per 100,000 live births for the 2001–2003 period (17). Direct obstetric deaths, although still responsible for most of the deaths, are declining, and indirect causes are increasing. Gestational hypertension remained the leading direct obstetric cause of maternal death, while HIV/AIDS was the leading cause of death of indirect obstetric mortality. The growing contribution of indirect causes, such as HIV/AIDS, cardiac disease, sickle cell disease, diabetes mellitus, and asthma, suggests the need for clinical guidelines and improved collaboration with medical teams to provide targeted care to women with chronic disease conditions who become pregnant (17).

Violence has been responsible in the last few years for a number of coincidental maternal deaths.

Maternal mortality surveillance has improved since the development in 2002 of regional committees, and as a result, 47 maternal deaths were investigated in 2005. This measure was undertaken as a way to improve preventive interventions and treatment and evaluate their results; at the same time, it provides input for future policy and program development.

Partographs were introduced in 2005 in all hospitals that perform deliveries. The Jamaica Reproductive Health Survey 2002–2003 (20) showed that 59% of women had had at least one Pap smear in their lifetime, compared to only 50% in 1997. The survey (20) also found that 20% of women in the sample had at some point in their life been sexually assaulted by being forced into sexual intercourse. No difference was found between age groups or geographical location, and in most cases, the perpetrator was someone they knew.

HIV/AIDS and STIs are the second leading cause of death for both men and women in the 30–34-year-old age group in Jamaica. The rate of HIV infection is increasing more steadily among women than among men. One in four men and one in 10 women reported having had a sexually transmitted infection, and one in two men and two in 10 women reported having had more than one sexual partner in 2003. In addition, one in two persons reported not using a condom in their last sexual act (15).

Older Adults 60 Years Old and Older

Malignant neoplasms were the leading cause of death in this age group in 2002, followed by diseases of the circulatory system, heart diseases, diabetes mellitus, and hypertension. Communicable diseases, including HIV/AIDS, ranked sixth in the leading causes of death, indicating the growing importance of HIV/AIDS among the older population as a public health issue. The main causes of disability remain arthritis and visual impairment. The mental health issues of loneliness and social isolation have been identified as requiring special attention in the development of social policy approaches to healthy aging. As reported by the World Health Organization (WHO) Collaborating Center for the Aged (23), in 2003–2004 there were 263,000 persons (10%) over 60 years of age in Jamaica, and this figure is projected to double over the next two decades.

There is a feminization of aging, with more frail older females than males. Most of the population 60 years old and older is supported by families (65%) and the remainder by self-generated wages and other financial means. Pension coverage levels are low, as are levels of insurance coverage, while costs are high.

The Family

Of the 744,700 households identified by the 2001 census (12), 59% were headed by males and 41% by females. While 62% of male-headed households involved common law or married unions, only 27% of female-headed households fell into this category. Women also accounted for the greater proportion of large-sized households.

Persons with Disabilities

In the 2001 census (12), 6.2% of persons reported having a disability. Restricted activities were reported by 44.4% of this group. The five main disabilities reported were: visual impairment only (31%), physical disability (20%), hearing impairment

only (9.8%), mental illness (9%), and multiple disabilities (6.3%). Of the 444,400 persons (17%) reporting a chronic illness, 15% indicated that they additionally had a disability which limited their activities.

Displaced Populations

In 2004, following political turmoil in Haiti, Haitians arrived by boat in successive waves, totaling 881 by 2005.

HEALTH CONDITIONS AND PROBLEMS

COMMUNICABLE DISEASES

Vector-borne Diseases

Monitoring of mosquitoes continues as an important initiative to control the *Culex, Aedes aegypti,* and *Anopheles* species. All **malaria** cases in the period under review were imported. In 2004, 141 cases were confirmed, and in 2005 there were 79 such cases. The majority of these were linked to the displaced Haitian population that began arriving in 2004. Special vector control interventions were devised to interrupt possible transmission of malaria and **filariasis**. There were 27 cases of **dengue fever**. The last dengue outbreak occurred in 2002, with 102 confirmed cases. The national *Aedes* Household Index remains well over 5% (range: 6.0%–45%). The 2004 indices for the country's two international airports, Montego Bay Sangsters and Kingston Norman Manley, were 4% and 0.75%, respectively (24).

Vaccine-preventable Diseases

In 2001 to 2005, no cases of **measles, polio, diphtheria, rubella, congenital rubella,** or **neonatal tetanus** were reported. There were 8 cases of suspected **pertussis** and 13 **non-neonatal tetanus** cases reported in 2005.

Preliminary results of a 2005 vaccination coverage survey revealed that 95% of the 12–23-month-old age group were adequately immunized, while by age 1, 89–90% were vaccinated. The immunization coverage at age 1 for 2005 by antigen using corrected target populations is: 94.5% for **tuberculosis** (TB); 83.6% for polio; 87.5% for diphtheria, pertussis, and tetanus; 88.6% for *Haemophilus influenzae* **type b** (Hib); and 87.2% for **hepatitis B**. Coverage for measles, mumps, and rubella for the 12–23-month-old age group is 84%. Hepatitis B and Hib vaccines were introduced as a combination pentavalent (DPT/HepB/Hib) vaccine in June 2003 (25). A comprehensive evaluation of the immunization program, together with the development of a five-year plan, took place in October 2003.

There were 307 laboratory-confirmed cases of hepatitis B in 2004. The number has increased over the last few years due to improved data collection.

Intestinal Infectious Diseases

No **cholera** cases have been reported in Jamaica for many decades. **Typhoid** is endemic, and three cases of typhoid fever were confirmed in 2005 and eight in 2004. There were outbreaks of **gastroenteritis** in 2003 and 2004; the case fatality rate remained at less than 1%.

Chronic Communicable Diseases

The national **tuberculosis** (TB) incidence rate in 2004 was 4.4 per 100,000 population, similar to the rate of 4.5 in 2000, but with an increase of case numbers in urban areas. Four pediatric cases were reported in 2004, compared to 17 in 2001; three of the four cases were HIV-coinfected. TB/HIV comorbidity increased from 14.2% in 2000 to 40% in 2003, but decreased to 27% in 2004. Coinfection rates were higher in urban areas compared to rural ones. Sixty-six percent of the 117 pulmonary-positive cases converted to sputum-negative in three months. Only 44% of the cohort of 117 successfully completed the course of treatment. The case fatality remains high at 22 per 100 sputum smear-positive cases. Drug compliance stood at 85% in 2000, but declined to 55% in 2004. A national assessment of the TB program carried out by the Pan American Health Organization (PAHO) in May 2005 concluded that despite the low incidence rate, TB is not under control, as evidenced by the high incidence in children, the high TB/HIV coinfection rate, and the high proportion of sputum smear-positive cases. The absence of sustained Directly Observed Therapy, Short Course (DOTS) was also deemed a constraining factor (26).

Ten new cases of **Hansen's disease** (leprosy) were confirmed in 2005, compared to eight in 2004. The prevalence rate was 0.05 per 10,000 population. Leprosy control is fully integrated in the primary health care services. Currently, 14 active cases are registered for chemotherapy; 13 of these cases are multibacillary, which highlights the infectious reservoir in the local population. At the end of 2004, 54 cases were registered for surveillance (27).

In 2005, 15,917 newborns, or approximately 30% of all live births, were screened for **sickle cell**. Of these, 118, or 0.8%, had an electrophoretic pattern suggestive of hemoglobin SS, SC, or CC disease. The Sickle Cell Unit at the University of the West Indies (UWI) offers counseling, education, and health maintenance checks. It also operates an ambulatory clinic and a day care ward where complications such as acute painful crises, acute febrile illness, and acute anemia are managed. Over 90% of patients with acute painful crises are managed as outpatients, and this model of aggressive acute day care has served as a model for sickle cell disease treatment centers elsewhere. Outreach clinics for health maintenance checks are also conducted in two other regions of the country. At last estimates, the median survival for sickle cell patients in Jamaica was 53 years for men and 58.5 years for women (28).

Pulmonary Infections

Respiratory tract diseases (RTDs), including **asthma**, accounted for 17% of total curative visits in 2002, highlighting the importance of this health condition. The number of visits for RTDs increased from 79,000 in 1990 to 108,000 in 2002. Asthma accounted for half of the visits to A&E departments in 2002. A weekly pulmonary clinic began operating at the national pediatric hospital (Bustamante Children's Hospital) in 2000 and drastically reduced RTD morbidity and hospitalizations in 85% of the children who attended the clinic for at least one year (0–1 outpatient visits, compared to 5–22 visits prior to 2000). Asthma protocols have been developed and training organized in all parishes. **Bronchitis**, **emphysema**, and other obstructive pulmonary diseases accounted for 11% of RTD discharge diagnoses in males and 6% in females.

HIV/AIDS and Other Sexually Transmitted Infections

According to Ministry of Health reports, an estimated 22,000 adults in Jamaica were living with HIV in 2004. The AIDS incidence rate in 2005 was 505.13 per 1 million population. Of the estimated 8,000 children and adults in need of antiretroviral treatment, only some 1,500, or 19%, were receiving it at the end of 2005 (29). Despite the initiation of a plateau in the annual number of mortality cases, the introduction of antiretroviral therapy, and other advances in care and treatment strategies, HIV/AIDS remains a growing public health concern in Jamaica.

Knowledge regarding HIV/AIDS and its routes of transmission is high in Jamaica (30). Despite this fact, 24% of men and 34% of women having sex with a non-regular partner do not use a condom (31). The Ministry of Health estimates that 65% of those infected with HIV in Jamaica are unaware of their status. In 2003, the Ministry of Health established voluntary counseling and testing (VCT) sites at all major health centers and antenatal clinics. Approximately 90% of antenatal clinic attendees and over 50% of STI clinic attendees were receiving VCT services in 2006 (32).

A Jamaican Ministry of Health estimate in 2002 indicated that 19.4% of all HIV/AIDS cases were linked to sex work. A 2005 behavioral surveillance survey on HIV and female sex workers found stark differences between HIV-positive and -negative female sex workers. Those who were HIV-positive generally were found to be older, have fewer years of education, earn significantly less money per client, and be more likely to be street-based than those who tested negative for HIV. Additionally, the HIV-positive female sex workers reported having taken in significantly more regular paying partners in the seven days prior to the survey interview and reported significantly less condom use at last sex, particularly with local (Jamaican) clients. This group was also twice as likely to report no condom use at last sex with a non-paying partner (33).

The prevalence of STIs varies significantly by age and sex. A 2004 study on knowledge, attitudes, practices, and beliefs found that 34.3% of males ages 25–49 reported having an STI compared to 15.0% of females in the same age group. In the 15–24 age group, the figure was 9.8% for males and 8.2% for females (*34*).

Zoonoses

There was a sharp increase in the number of reported **leptospirosis** cases in 2005 following heavy rains during the hurricane season. Of the 921 suspected cases, 328 were confirmed. Zoonoses surveillance continued for the following diseases: leptospirosis, **bovine brucellosis**, **bovine tuberculosis**, **West Nile virus**, **bovine spongiform encephalopathy**, and *Salmonella enteritidis* contamination.

NONCOMMUNICABLE DISEASES

Metabolic and Nutritional Diseases

Diabetes mellitus is an important cause of morbidity and mortality in Jamaica and represents a significant burden on health services. The average length of stay was 8.3 days for diabetes in 2002, compared to 6.3 days for all conditions. In the Jamaican Healthy Lifestyle Survey Report 2000 (*15*), diabetes was found in 6.3% of males and 8.2% of females. There was a sharp increase with age. Awareness of diabetes among those classified as diabetic by the survey was 76.3%. Almost one-third of those classified as diabetic were not being treated, and 60% of those who reported being on medication did not have their condition controlled.

Cardiovascular Diseases

Hypertension and other diseases of the circulatory system remain an important cause of morbidity and mortality and create a major burden on health care services. Primary health care curative visits for diabetes and hypertension in 2002 represented 25.9% of all curative visits to government health centers, with a male-to-female ratio of 1:4.

In 2002, diseases of the circulatory system accounted for 7.7% of all government hospital discharge diagnoses, compared to 5.9% in the previous decade. This was the third leading cause of morbidity among hospital discharge diagnoses in 2002. The male-to-female ratio was 1:1.2 among these patients. The average length of stay for treatment of cardiovascular diseases was 8.7 days, compared to the 2002 average for all diseases of 6.9 days. Circulatory system diseases accounted for the third leading proportion of hospital care costs in all four of the country's health regions in 2002 (*35*). The Jamaican Healthy Lifestyle Survey Report 2000 (*15*) noted a prevalence of hypertension of 19.9% among males and 21.7% among females; prevalence increased with age in both rural and urban populations and in both sexes. Among persons known to be hypertensive, 42% were on treatment, and of this group, 37.7% had been able to lower and maintain their blood pressure at 140/90 or less.

Malignant Neoplasms

In 2002 there were 3,769 public hospital discharge diagnoses (4% of total discharge diagnoses) for malignant neoplasms with an equal gender distribution. The types of neoplasms involved for males, in order of decreasing frequency, were: trachea, bronchus, and lungs; prostate; leukemia; and non-Hodgkin's lymphoma, representing 56% of all cancers. For females, the order was as follows: breast; cervix uteri; other malignant neoplasms of female genital organs; trachea, bronchus, and lungs; leukemia; and non-Hodgkin's lymphoma, together representing 56% of all cancers. The Cancer Registry operates out of UWI and collects data mainly from the Kingston-Saint Andrew region. A 2003 study (*36*) found that gynecological cancers in this region represented 26.8% of all types of cancers found among females there. Cervical cancer accounted for 62% of these gynecological cancers, with an incidence of 27.9 per 100,000 women and a mortality rate of 15.8%.

OTHER HEALTH PROBLEMS OR ISSUES

Natural Disasters

Jamaica is vulnerable to a variety of natural hazards (hurricanes, floods, draughts, landslides, and earthquakes), and current efforts are concentrated on vulnerability reduction. This paradigm shift from preparedness to risk reduction is being achieved through staff training in new risk reduction concepts and the use of technology available to minimize such risks. Vulnerabilities were exposed during the recent experiences with hurricanes Charlie (2004), Ivan (2004), Dennis (2005), and Emily (2005), with economic losses reaching millions of US dollars.

Violence and Other External Causes

Jamaica has experienced an alarming upward spiralling of its crime rate, with homicides moving from a low of less than 200 per annum in the early 1970s to 1,674 in 2005, or 63 per 100,000 population. The increase has affected both sexes and all age groups, but particularly children, the elderly, and women. The Economic and Social Survey of 2005 (*1*) reported 1,292 major crimes committed against children between ages 0 and 19 years; of these, 573 were committed against children 14 years of age and under. Major crimes, including homicide shootings, rape, sexual offenses, and robbery, were committed by 53 children ages 12–14 years in 2005 (compared to 25 in 2003). In 2005, 188 women lost their lives in crime-related events, compared to 109 in 2001. Homicides against children (ages 0–20) increased from 145 cases in 2001 to 172 (ages 0–19) in 2005.

When obstetrics are excluded, injuries remained the leading hospital discharge diagnosis for the 1999–2002 period, representing 11% of all discharge diagnoses. When disaggregated by age group, injuries were in the top three leading causes given in discharge diagnoses in the 1–4-, 5–14-, 15–25-, and 26–44-year-old age groups, highlighting the impact of this condition on hospital services. Data from the Jamaican Injury Surveillance System, which is based in hospital A&E units, revealed that males accounted for 59% of outpatient visits in 2005. Fights/arguments were responsible for 76.4% of the cases. The major weapons used to inflict injury included blunt objects (40%), sharp objects (35%), and firearms (7%); injuries involving the last category increased 3.1% over the previous year.

The cost burden due to intentional and unintentional injuries has continued to grow, resulting in expenditures of US$ 11.3 million in 1996, US$ 21.3 million in 1999, and US$ 22.6 million in 2002. Nearly half of this last figure was concentrated in the South East Region (including Kingston). It is estimated that up to half of the total injury costs resulted from intentional injuries. In order to attend to those requiring immediate care for their injuries, health personnel had to curtail other types of non-emergency services previously scheduled; delays were also caused for emergency patients whose injuries were less serious.

A total of 1,846 persons were killed in motor vehicle accidents during the 2001–2005 period. The largest group of fatalities was among pedestrians, followed by private automobile passengers, private automobile drivers, and bicyclists and motorcyclists. In 2004, 14,046 persons utilized the A&E departments for injuries resulting from road traffic collisions, representing a 20% increase over 2000 figures.

The health care cost for road traffic accidents in 2005 was estimated to be US$ 8.8 million. That year, 10,339 road collisions resulted in 326 fatalities, with male drivers accounting for 81% of these collisions. An island-wide study on knowledge, attitudes, practices, and beliefs was conducted among 500 male drivers in 2005. Preliminary results indicated that 12% of the respondents bypassed the official driving test. One-third of the respondents reported having had at least one road traffic collision since receiving their driver's license. Among those who were involved in a major collision, 16.7% of the 18–29 age group admitted to having had two or more major collisions; this number rose to 36.9% for the group 60 years of age or older, suggesting a pattern of repeat collisions. Half of the interviewees admitted to disobeying speed limits, 42% said that they did not always wear their seat belts, and 28% admitted to drinking and driving.

Morbidity data revealed that in 2004 the major diagnoses in clients seen in public community mental health clinics were schizophrenia/psychotic disorder (59.1%), mood disorders (26.7%), substance abuse (6.1%), disorders of childhood and adolescence (4.3%), and anxiety disorders (3.8%). With respect to mental health clinics, gender analysis showed that 60% of the clients diagnosed with schizophrenia and 95% of those diagnosed with substance abuse were males, while 71% of those suffering from mood disorders were females. A year-long study was carried out during 2005 at two major hospitals on 147 cases of attempted suicide. Two-thirds of the cases were females with a mean age of 28 years, even though a significant number of the

cases were from the 15–19 age group. Drug overdose was the method of choice.

According to the Jamaican Healthy Lifestyle Survey Report 2000 (15), current cigarette smoking was reported by 29% of men and 8% of women, while 25% of the men and 4% of the women said they smoked marijuana.

Environmental Problems

In 2003, there were 1,127 clients seeking care for poisoning at the A&E outpatient departments of public hospitals. The under-5 age group remained the largest group affected, representing 54.3% of the cases. This trend has remained unchanged over the years. The most common poisons are bleach, kerosene, and pesticides. Eleven cases of lead poisoning in children were reported during the review period; seven of the cases were possibly linked to soil contamination through improper disposal of battery components.

Diseases Transmitted through Blood

All collected blood units are tested for the following infection markers: HIV, human T-cell lymphotropic virus type 1 (HTLV), hepatitis C surface antigen (HBsAg), hepatitis C virus (HCV), and syphilis. The positivity rate (%) in 2005 was 2.3 for syphilis, 1.59 for HTLV, 0.6 for HBsAg, 0.47 for HIV, and 0.43 for HCV. All markers showed a declining trend, with the exception of HCV (+0.13) and syphilis (+0.4).

RESPONSE OF THE HEALTH SECTOR

Health Policies and Plans

Jamaica is party to all of the international human rights conventions that recognize health as a human right. During 2004, the Ministry of Health focused on the three Millennium Development Goals whose scope of activity calls for a direct role by the health sector: MDG 4 (reduce child mortality), MDG 5 (improve maternal health), and MDG 6 (combat HIV/AIDS, malaria, and tuberculosis). A national report prepared by the Planning Institute of Jamaica noted that according to U.N. targets, Jamaica is "far behind" in achieving the child mortality reduction and maternal health goals and is "lagging" in relation to the target for HIV/AIDS, indicating that overall, insufficient progress was made during the 1990s to be able to attain the target values by 2015 (5). The government's commitment to achievement of the MDGs is to be bolstered by specific policy measures adopted during the period of the Medium-Term Social and Economic Policy Framework (MTSEPF). The MTSEPF 2004–2007 is buttressed on the two pillars of poverty reduction and economic growth, and its section on health issues focuses on strategies to achieve MDGs 4, 5, and 6.

The Ministry of Health's National Health Policy (2006–2015) and accompanying strategic plan for the 2006–2010 period take into consideration the gaps and strengths identified in the previous plan's evaluation. The indicators are outcome-oriented, and the 2006–2015 priorities are selected based on national needs and the island's disease burden and take into account MDG 8, which focuses on the creation of global partnerships for development. Through these health inputs and the forging of strong partnerships, the National Health Policy seeks to maintain the gains of previous years, regain lost ground for some indicators, move ahead in decreasing the major threats to population health—such as HIV/AIDS and other lifestyle diseases—and improve some of the development indicators.

The HIV/AIDS National Strategic Plan 2002–2006 outlined the policy framework for Jamaica's response to the global pandemic. In May 2005, the National HIV/AIDS Policy was officially launched; it incorporates a human rights approach in the multisectoral response to HIV. In 2003, the Cabinet mandated five key public sector ministries to prepare and implement HIV/AIDS work programs within their respective sectors and to report regularly to the Cabinet on progress. In 2005, the number of ministries involved expanded to 11, thereby involving all government ministries in integrating HIV/AIDS issues into their operations at the appropriate levels (1).

During the 2001–2005 period, legislation was introduced and/or amended to promote and protect the rights of children (The Child Care and Protection Act), to provide enhanced protection for victims of domestic violence and abuse (The Domestic Violence Amendment Act), and to safeguard the property rights of women and men in the event of a breakdown in a marriage or union lasting longer than five years (The Property Rights of Spouse Act). Other achievements of note taking place during the study period include the National Framework of Action for Children (2004), a national policy on children, a national youth policy, and the Early Childhood Act.

Progress also was made in phasing in implementation of the National Policy for Senior Citizens, the drafting of the National Assistance Bill to replace the Poor Relief Act, and regarding the Disability Bill to strengthen implementation of the National Policy for Persons with Disabilities. The following environmental legislation was also introduced: the Water Policy and Implementation Plan; Regulations for the Management of Septage and Sludge; Hazardous Waste Regulations; promulgation of regulations regarding hygiene standards in barber shops, hair salons, and related public establishments; and amended public health regulations regarding tourist attractions and swimming pools. The WHO Framework Convention on Tobacco Control was ratified by Jamaica in July 2005.

Health Strategies and Programs

Protection of vulnerable population groups from the risks associated with limited access to public services and of those possessing insufficient means to fulfill basic human needs remained a high government priority. The Social Safety Net Reform Program, which began in 2000, continued to streamline the delivery of welfare and social security benefits to needy families and individuals in a more structured, targeted, and efficient manner. Since 2002, the Poverty Alleviation through Health and Education (PATH) program has provided cash benefits to poor families with children, individuals living in extreme poverty, pregnant and lactating women, the elderly, and persons with disabilities, and links these benefits to preventive health care (primary care clinic attendance) and education. The National Health Fund (NHF), established in 2002 as a statutory body and whose budget is funded from government taxes, provides two categories of benefits. NHF Individual Benefits provide assistance for the purchase of specific prescription drugs used in the treatment and management of designated chronic illnesses. NHF Institutional Benefits provide assistance to private and public sector organizations for health-related projects. Within this category, the Health Promotion and Protection Fund provides financial assistance for initiatives supporting primary health care, with special emphasis on health promotion and disease prevention.

The older population suffering from chronic diseases benefits from the Jamaican Drugs for the Elderly Program and NHF assistance. Additionally, the National Council for Senior Citizens acts in an advisory capacity to the Ministry of Labour and Social Security and provides input on all matters relating to the socioeconomic welfare of the population 60 years of age and older.

Organization of the Health System

Health services delivery in the public sector is provided through a network of primary, secondary, and tertiary care facilities consisting of 24 hospitals, including the University Hospital of the West Indies. Hospitals are classed as "A," "B," "C," or "Specialist," depending on the level of complexity of the services offered. There are three type A hospitals, all located in large urban areas and providing the most specialized services; of the three, one offers specialized obstetrics services and another specialized children's services. The four type B hospitals, as the type A hospitals, are mostly situated in urban areas. They provide inpatient and outpatient services in general surgery, internal medicine, obstetrics and gynecology, and pediatrics, and support referrals from type C facilities, of which there are currently 11 in the country. These hospitals are usually found in rural population centers, provide general outpatient and inpatient services, and refer complex cases to type B and A facilities. There are currently four specialist hospitals, with one providing psychiatric services, another cancer care, a third rehabilitation services, and the fourth specialist pulmonary services. In 2005, the bed complement was 4,736, and there were 1.8 hospital beds per 1,000 population.

A major strategy of the health sector reform process was the decentralization of government health services. The passage of the National Health Services Act in 1997 led to the formation of four Regional Health Authorities (South East, North East, Western, and Southern). Each region has direct managerial responsibility for the delivery of public health services within a geographically defined area. A 2003 evaluation (37) of the impact of decentralization found minimal levels of improvement in health planning, services delivery, accountability and transparency, and community involvement. While moderate success was shown in the area of cost containment, negative effects were shown in the areas of personnel capacity, financial management, and organizational capacity. An evaluation of essential public health functions carried out in December 2001 identified the following as the weakest functions: quality assurance, health promotion, research, and human resources development and planning. Special emphasis was given to strengthening these four areas in the drafting of the new national strategic health plan.

Public Health Services

Jamaica has pursued the primary health care approach since the 1970s, and its achievements utilizing this strategy include a reduction of undernutrition, infant mortality, and fertility rates; an increase in immunization coverage; the elimination of polio and measles; improved sanitation status; the creation of a strong health centers network and of a new cadre of health workers (examples include the community health aide and the nurse practitioner); and strong local government engagement in health services.

Primary care facilities comprise 316 health centers, ranging from type 1 to type 5 and offering progressively more complex services, from maternal and child health services only in type 1 clinics, to curative, dental, STI, and mental health services in the others. Public sector hospitals provide more than 95% of hospital-based care on the island. The private sector dominates pharmaceutical and diagnostic services and provides about half of the ambulatory care through an extensive network of professionals offering specialist and general practice services. Nongovernmental organizations and other groups provide health services at a nominal fee.

Eleven hospitals (representing 70% of the public patient population) have a computerized Patient Administration System (PAS) in place. The basic information system for secondary care is supported by the PAS. The primary care system is not computerized. There is a multiplicity of databases for various programs resulting in fragmentation of the health information system. A vital statistics commission appointed by the Cabinet in 2004 has received the mandate to ensure the production of timely and accurate vital statistics. To that end, an audit was facilitated by PAHO in 2005, and recommendations currently are being implemented.

Disease surveillance is conducted using both active and passive systems, and includes public and private sentinel primary care facilities, hospitals, laboratories, and selected hotels. There is syndromic sentinel surveillance for fever, fever and rash, gastroenteritis, and accidents and violence. Data obtained from the various surveillance systems are disseminated nationally via weekly bulletins and internationally via weekly reports to the Caribbean Epidemiology Center (CAREC). In 2004, on-time reporting was over 95%. The class I surveillance system geared at reporting communicable diseases also includes events such as maternal deaths, rheumatic fever, accidents, and poisoning. The Jamaica Injury Surveillance System continues to operate from the major public hospitals. Surveillance for HIV/AIDS cases is carried out by case-finding and active and passive surveillance. Active surveillance is carried out by contacting laboratories, hospitals, hospices, and public and private physicians. Collaboration continued with the National Public Health Laboratory, the University Hospital of the West Indies, and CAREC for confirmation of cases of diseases.

Drinking water in Jamaica is provided mainly through such public agencies as the National Water Commission (71%) and the parish councils (rural water supplies) and by various private companies. Monitoring of water quality is the joint responsibility of the Ministry of Health, the National Water Commission, and the Office of Utilities Regulation. A water surveillance program was established jointly between the Ministry of Health and the National Water Commission. The Ministry determines residual chlorine levels, and, to a lesser degree, conducts bacteriological analysis, while monitoring by the National Water Commission is of a more frequent and complex nature.

A 2004 PAHO report (38) raised concerns regarding how water quality monitoring is carried out at the parish level, in terms of ratio of quantity of sampling versus population served, the frequency of sampling, and the disparity of standards used between parishes.

The 2001 national census (12) indicated that approximately 20,000 households (2.6%) were not provided with excreta disposal facilities, while approximately 119,000 households (15.9%) did not have a hygiene facility (shower, sink) in their home.

While there was a 50% increase in the number of cases of diarrheal diseases in the under-5 age group for the year 2003 compared with 2002, national efforts to deal with these diseases are focusing on the curative aspects and health education, and not on water quality and sanitation. Solid waste management in Jamaica is legislated under the 2001 National Solid Waste Management Act with its corresponding regulations for licensing, rates, recycling, and management of hazardous waste. The National Solid Waste Management Authority is the governmental regulatory agency overseeing this sector and four wastesheds in a shared solid waste disposal system. The collection of solid waste is subcontracted to private enterprises through a public-private sector arrangement. While there are four landfills island-wide, none satisfy the minimum requirements necessary to qualify as sanitary landfills. The 2002 PAHO Regional Evaluation of Solid Waste Management in Latin America and the Caribbean (39) reported that Jamaicans produce 2,670 tons of domestic waste daily (56% organic in composition). Coverage for municipal solid waste collection was reported at 63%.

According to a 2001 State of the Environment Report prepared by the Statistical Institute of Jamaica (40), mining and quarrying activities are responsible for more than 50% of air emissions in Jamaica. The 2001 census (12) indicates that 43% of all households burn their solid waste. The four landfills for solid waste disposal on the island are frequently on fire, thereby contributing to air pollution and producing other environmental effects detrimental to the health of nearby residents.

With more than 150 licensed hotels and 13,500 rooms, Jamaica is heavily dependent upon tourism. Mass tourism in particular has been promoted and developed. In 2004, the island's visitors, including cruise ship passengers, totaled 2.5 million, nearly equaling the total national population. The tourism and economic sectors are in turn highly dependent upon the country's natural resources and thus vulnerable to any degradation of coastal resources. During recent decades, negative impacts from improperly planned urban and tourism developments, including the introduction of inadequate sanitation and solid waste disposal practices, have affected water quality and near-shore ecosystems, especially in the important northern and northwestern tourism destinations (41). According to a 2000 study on the negative effects of tourism on Jamaica's ecology, tourists consume 10 times as much water and produce three times as much solid waste as the average resident (42), and ship-generated waste (cruise and commercial) is usually discharged at sea.

Some positive initiatives have been taken by the government with support from international agencies and local nongovernmental organizations. Among these is the introduction of Green Globe Certification in 2005, with the first five hotels in the world to receive Green Globe 21 Certification being located in Jamaica. (Green Globe 21 is a global affiliation, benchmarking, and certification system aimed at stimulating sustainable, ecologically responsible tourism and is based on the Agenda 21 principles for sustainable development endorsed by 182 Heads of State at the U.N. Rio de Janeiro Earth Summit in 1992.) The results have been significant in reducing water, chemical, and energy consumption, as well as solid waste output (41). Blue Flag certification, an international voluntary certification program, was introduced in Jamaica in 2005 as an environmental tool to stimulate proper planning and management of coastal recreation. Under the award system, beaches that fulfill a number of exacting criteria regarding such factors as bathing water quality, cleanliness, and safety are given the right to fly the Blue Flag; five beaches achieved this distinction in 2005 (1).

Nearly a decade ago, travelers' diarrhea (TD) was recognized as a major health problem affecting tourists visiting Jamaica. A survey carried out between March 1996 and May 1997 (43) indicated that one in every four tourists to Jamaica experienced TD during their stay. Interventions to reduce TD in hotels in Negril

and Montego Bay have been implemented by the Ministry of Health in collaboration with the Ministry of Tourism and hotel associations and have been progressively extended to all parishes offering tourism attractions. These included Hazard Analysis Critical Control Points (HACCP) training for hotel managers and supervisors, hotel food handlers' certification, and hotel certification. A surveillance system reporting on diarrhea, acute respiratory infections, and accidents among guests and staff was established in 34 hotels in seven parishes. Currently, all four major tourist regions report to local public health departments and the Ministry of Health and the national TD incidence rate stands below 5%. Accident rates have also declined for both staff and guests in recent years; where rates remain proportionately high, local public health departments work with individual hotels to identify and resolve safety issues.

HACCP training is seen as a priority to reduce the risks of foodborne diseases in the hospitality industry. Investigations carried out in collaboration with CAREC and the U.S. Centers for Disease Control and Prevention following an increase in reports of hotel-based foodborne disease outbreaks following Hurricane Ivan in 2004 resulted in interventions to monitor the quality of eggs. A new policy and procedures manual for the training of food handlers was used to operate 65 food handler training sites island-wide in 2004. This resulted in a 38% increase in the number of food handlers trained between 2003 (25,281) and 2004 (34,808).

In 2005, 116 occupationally related accidents were reported to the Ministry of Labour and Social Security, an increase of 16% over the previous year. Of these cases, 66% qualified for investigation. There were six deaths related to on-the-job incidents. There is, however, severe underreporting in this area.

Subsequent to the 2004 hurricane season, the Jamaican government commissioned the upgrading of the national building code. The 2005 hurricane season further highlighted Jamaica's vulnerability to flood and landslides. Risk-reduction measures are being promoted to help ensure the operation of essential services during hurricane and tropical storm events.

In 2003, a national program for the surveillance of West Nile virus was launched. Jamaica is also on high alert with regard to a potential introduction of avian influenza in the local wild bird and commercial poultry populations. Avian influenza surveillance was introduced in 2005 in collaboration with the Ministry of Agriculture and the Poultry Association. To date, there has been no appearance of highly pathogenic avian influenza (HPAIV) in the commercial poultry population. The introduction of HPAIV would have serious consequences for the national economy and directly impact on food security, since 86% of the population's protein consumption comes from poultry.

All pharmaceutical products containing ingredients of animal origin are screened for bovine extracts. A ban was placed on imported beef and beef products from several countries in 2003 and continues in some cases.

Promoting Healthy Lifestyles among Jamaican Youth

Three of the leading causes of mortality among adults in Jamaica are chronic noncommunicable diseases, which account for half of all deaths each year; HIV/AIDS, with a 1.5% prevalence rate among adults and ranking as the second leading cause of death among both men and women 30–34 years old; and homicides, which reached epidemic proportions in 2005, with a rate of 63 deaths per 100,000 population. To help combat the burden from these causes, the government has formulated a National Policy for the Promotion of Healthy Lifestyles that brings together public, private, and nongovernmental sectors to encourage young children, adolescents, and young adults to adopt good habits such as physical exercise, good nutrition, and responsible sexual behavior and acquire skills such as self-esteem and resilience.

Individual Care Services

During the period 2001–2005, attention was focused on the restructuring of mental health services. At the current time, emphasis is placed on deinstitutionalization, integration of the mental health component into general health care, and the training and retraining of mental health workers and their reassignment in the community. Mental health care is delivered through secondary and outpatient services. There is one psychiatric hospital (Bellevue) and two psychiatric units. Eleven of the general hospitals also offer psychiatric services. There are presently 111 mental health clinics operating island-wide, either through primary health care centers and/or the outpatient clinics of general hospitals. In addition, several churches provide community mental health services. In 2005, Bellevue Hospital saw its acute inpatient days decrease to 14 days for females and 28 days for males, compared to more than 60 days prior to 1998. This achievement has been part of an ongoing effort to reintegrate patients as quickly as feasible into their families and communities.

Mental health services targeted to children and adolescents have expanded from three locations in the South East Region to a decentralized network of clinics in all four Regional Health Authorities. In addition to clinical services, technical guidance and support, including training in the management of children and adolescents with mental health problems, are provided by the central level to the regions. Guidelines for the management of child abuse were developed in 2005, and 100 health workers received training in this area.

The mandate of the National Council on Drug Abuse is the alleviation of drug abuse through the development and implementation of effective drug prevention programs. Target populations include youth with both high and low literacy levels, parents, the community at large, the workplace, and service clubs. Activities include the generation of evidence-based information on substance abuse, training and health promotion, social mobilization, and advocacy. In 2005, a Caribbean database information network on poisons and poisonous substances was launched and will operate out of the University of Technology.

Rehabilitation services offered in the public sector include physiotherapy, social work, speech therapy, and occupational therapy. Private therapists provide a variety of services, although these are usually available only in the larger urban centers. The 71-bed Sir John Golding Rehabilitation Center located in Kingston offers short- and long-term rehabilitative services. Nongovernmental organizations at the Center provide support for those with disabilities by making prostheses, shoes, and wheelchairs; operating a crafts workshop; and assisting with the provision of schooling, skills training, and housing.

Dental services are essentially provided through primary care. Dentists principally perform extractions while the work of dental nurses is focused mainly on the 0–18-year-old population segment and includes restorative and preventive procedures.

Oncology treatment, intensive care, and renal dialysis are offered in the three type A hospitals. Intensive care additionally is offered at the specialist Bustamante Children's Hospital in Kingston. Two private and one nongovernmental facility offer dialysis services.

Public health laboratories provide testing services in the major public hospitals. The Kingston-based National Public Health Laboratory is a referral facility offering services in microbiology, cytology, hematology, chemistry, histology, immunology, and environmental testing.

The National Blood Transfusion Service serves both public and private clients and receives blood from 10 collection centers. Collection in 2005 reached an all-time low of approximately 22,000 units, insufficient to meet national demand, and representing a decline of 6% over 2004's collection levels. The majority (90%) of the units are collected from family and replacement donors. Only 10% of the donors are considered to be voluntary. In response to the national blood shortage, successful new partnerships have been forged with the private sector, the media, and academic institutions at the secondary and tertiary level to encourage voluntary blood donation.

A broad intersectoral approach has been adopted by many other programs within the Ministry of Health, as well, including

HIV/AIDS, mental health, health promotion and healthy lifestyles, environmental health, nutrition, and violence prevention. Partners include governmental and nongovernmental organizations, academic institutions, and community groups, among others.

Health Promotion

The 2004 National Policy for the Promotion of Healthy Lifestyles in Jamaica incorporates the public and private sectors, government and nongovernmental organizations, and communities in an intersectoral approach to address national health priorities. The policy's goal is to decrease the incidence of chronic diseases (heart disease, diabetes, hypertension, obesity, and cervical cancer), as well as discourage the practice of high-risk sexual behaviors and those leading to violence and injuries through the adoption of health-promoting behaviors by the general population and, particularly, young children, adolescents, and young adults. Other key behavioral elements promoted through the policy's strategic plan include physical activity, healthy nutritional habits, smoking prevention and/or cessation, and the building of self-esteem, resiliency, and life skills.

During the 2001–2005 review period, the Ministry of Health oversaw and/or facilitated various programs and interventions to address violence-related issues. These included the community-based Healthy Lifestyle Initiative in the violence-prone Mountain View area of the South East Region, and CAMP Bustamante (Child Abuse Mitigation Project), a UNICEF-supported initiative operating out of Bustamante Children's Hospital that identifies children in the community who have been victims of physical and sexual abuse and/or neglect and carries out interventions targeting these children and their parents or caregivers.) Progress also continued during the review period as regards the Change From Within program, which is funded by UWI and promotes a child-centered approach to teaching in which schools address children's emotional needs and social development and support synergistic positive change at four levels: individual, parents and home, the school environment, and the community as a whole. In November 2004, the Jamaican chapter of the Violence Prevention Alliance (VPA) was launched. International in scope, the VPA is an intersectoral nongovernmental initiative that promotes violence prevention through information-sharing and the strengthening of policies related to this issue.

Encouraging male participation in both preventive and curative health care services remains a challenge in Jamaica. Family planning materials specifically targeting males were developed and disseminated in 2005. An integrated approach to family health following a life cycle approach has been initiated by the Ministry of Health and is reflected in the new draft family health manual. During the 2001–2005 period, efforts were geared at integrating adolescent health and care for the elderly within the primary health care level of services.

Human Resources

The health sector continues to be faced with a severe shortage of health personnel in many key categories, with the exception of medical doctors. The total vacancy for registered nurses increased from 17% in 2003 to 26% in 2004. Vacancy rates for enrolled assistant nurses and public health nurses increased by 12% and 13%, respectively. Shortages also exist among registered pharmacists, radiographers, community mental health workers, health educators, and public health inspectors. The chief reasons cited for the chronic shortage of public health services professionals are emigration to Canada, the United States, and Great Britain and to the local private sector, in addition to a general dissatisfaction with working conditions. There are also salary and emolument disincentives to staff working in primary versus secondary health care, which ultimately skews the available services away from the more preventive aspects of health care. Inequalities in staff distribution also exist between rural and urban areas, with the majority of health personnel opting to work in the country's larger cities. Even though the government has embarked on a program of recruitment of health professionals from other countries, such as Cuba and Nigeria, this is considered to be only a short-term solution. Training programs are offered for all categories of health personnel at the basic and post-basic levels, with the availability of several nursing schools and universities. However, due to ongoing reductions in the availability of training funds, many students are unable to begin and/or continue their intended course of studies. In addition, there are more applicants than available places. This results in insufficient numbers of graduates each year in several disciplines. In 2003, the Ministry of Health reported 8.5 public sector physicians and 16.5 public sector nurses per 10,000 population.

Health Supplies

There is limited drug production in Jamaica from imported raw materials. The Ministry of Health's Standards and Regulations Unit provides information regarding the quantities of drugs imported and by whom to the International Narcotics Control Board as part of the Unit's reporting relationship for precursor chemicals and controlled substances. The importation of raw materials, drugs, vaccines, and laboratory reagents is regulated, monitored, and controlled through drug registration and import permit approval by the Ministry of Health. Jamaica has a thriving private drug distribution (retail trade). Local distributors register drugs and obtain import permits on behalf of the manufacturers. The procurement and distribution of pharmaceuticals and medical supplies for the public health sector is carried out through Health Corporation Limited, an agency of the Ministry of Health with statutory status. There is a system of pharmacovigilance in place to ensure quality maintenance. Quality assurance support is also provided by the Government Chemist and the Caribbean Drug Testing Laboratory. Over 90% of the vaccine supplies for the national immunization program are procured through the PAHO Revolving Fund for Vaccine Procurement. The Vital, Essential, and Necessary (VEN) list was updated in 2005 and guides public sector prescribing, while the National Drug Formulary, also designed by the Ministry of Health, is for wider use in the private sector.

Research and Technological Development in Health

Numerous linkages with UWI, the Caribbean Health Research Council, and other regional and international organizations have guided research initiatives and training within the Jamaican health services. The first-ever Caribbean Research Ethics Conference, organized by UWI, the University of Miami, and PAHO, was held in 2005 at UWI. The use of laparoscopic techniques for diagnosis and treatment has increased service delivery options and contributed to decreased morbidity and length of stay for many surgical conditions. Computerized axial tomography (CAT) scanning is now available in the public sector. Additionally, other machines such as magnetic resonance imaging (MRI) and top-of-the-line radiotherapy facilities are available in the private sector. CD4 count and polymerase chain reaction (PCR) testing were introduced in the public sector in 2005.

Health Sector Expenditures and Financing

Financing of the health sector comes primarily from governmental budgetary allocations that are supplemented by user fees and inputs from nongovernmental organizations and international development partners. During fiscal year 2004–2005, there was a 13.7% increase in the total governmental budgetary expenditure over 2003–2004, with the Ministry of Health receiving US$ 245 million, representing 4.5% of the government overall budget. Approximately 83.0% of the increase in the health allocation went toward paying accumulated outstanding statutory deductions. User fees, which are collected from clients at health centers, hospitals, and various other government facilities, represented 14% of the government's budgetary allocation and are therefore an important source of income for the Regional Health Authorities. US$ 215 million, or 90.4% of the Ministry of Health's recurrent budget, was supplied to the four Regional Health Authorities and the University Hospital of the West Indies to provide health services to the population (25). Pharmaceutical expenses accounted for 20% of total health expenditure. The public health sector's budget represented 2.7% and 2.6% of GDP at current prices in 1999 and 2002, respectively (44). Government expenditure on health (i.e., the sum of outlays for health maintenance, restoration, or enhancement paid for by government entities as a percentage of total health expenditure) was 56.7%, while private expenditures accounted for 43.3%. Net out-of-pocket household expenses for health care were 63.6% of private health expenditures. Expenditure data from fiscal year 2004–2005 revealed that human resources cost was 82.6% of the total recurrent expenditure for the Regional Health Authorities, compared to 79.3% in 2003–2004, which is indicative of a clear risk that non-wage health expenditures are being squeezed, affecting service delivery. In addition, the total government expenditure on health remained virtually the same between 1998 and 2004, during which time the expenditure percentage ranged from 45.7% to 58.6%, with a mean of 52.2%. During this period, there has also been a steady devaluation of the Jamaican dollar from J$ 37.2 = US$ 1 to J$ 61.4 = US$ 1, a devaluation of 63%. This has further impacted on the government's ability to provide adequate health services to the population.

Technical Cooperation and External Financing

During the 2001–2005 review period, Jamaica received assistance from the U.S. Agency for International Development, Inter-American Development Bank, United Kingdom Department for International Development, World Bank, and European Union, among others. Up to the end of 2005, new Official Development Assistance totaled US$ 19.8 million.

In 2002 the World Bank granted the Jamaican government a loan of US$ 15 million for its HIV/AIDS control program. This support was followed in 2003 by a US$ 23 million grant from the Global Fund to Fight AIDS, Tuberculosis, and Malaria.

References

1. Jamaica, Planning Institute of Jamaica. Economic and Social Survey 2005.
2. United Nations Environment Program. Economic impacts of tourism Web site.
3. Planning Institute of Jamaica; Economic Commission for Latin America and the Caribbean; Caribbean and United Nations Development Program. Macro-socio-economic and environmental assessment of damage done by Hurricane Ivan, 10–12 September 2004. Kingston; 2004. [Unpublished report].
4. Jamaica, Planning Institute of Jamaica. Survey of Living Conditions. 2003.
5. Jamaica, Planning Institute of Jamaica. Millennium Development Goals, Jamaica. April 2004.
6. Jamaica, Planning Institute of Jamaica. Economic and Social Survey Jamaica 2004.
7. World Bank. Millennium Development Goals: Jamaica Country Profile.
8. Planning Institute of Jamaica. Jamaica Draft Medium Term Socio-economic Policy Framework 2004–2007. February 2005. Page 32.
9. United Nations Development Program. Chapter 6: Crime and Globalization in Jamaica. In: Human Development Report: Jamaica 2005.

10. Jamaica, Ministry of Labour and Social Security. Green Paper. Revised in 2006.
11. Jamaica, Planning Institute of Jamaica. 2004 data.
12. Jamaica, Statistical Institute of Jamaica. Population Census 2001.
13. Jamaica, Planning Institute of Jamaica. Survey of Living Conditions. 2001; 2004.
14. McCaw-Binns A, Holder H, Spence K, Gordon-Strachan G, Nam V, Ashley D. Multi-source method for determining mortality in Jamaica: 1996 and 1998. Consultant report to the Pan American Health Organization. August 2002.
15. Figueroa JP, Ward E, Walters C, Ashley DE, Wilks RJ. Jamaica Healthy Lifestyle Survey Report 2000. [Unpublished survey].
16. Jamaica, Ministry of Health, National HIV/STI Control Programme. Jamaica HIV/AIDS epidemic update. January–June 2005.
17. McCaw-Binns A, Alexander S, Lindo JLM, Escoffrey C, Spence K, Lewis-Bell K, Lewis G. Surviving pregnancy in Jamaica—changing epidemiology and challenges for the 21st century. [Unpublished paper].
18. Jamaica, Ministry of Health. Report. 2004.
19. Jamaica, Ministry of Health. Monthly Clinic Summary Report. 2004.
20. Jamaica National Family Planning Board; Statistical Institute of Jamaica; Centers for Disease Control and Prevention. Jamaica Reproductive Health Survey (RHS) 2002–2003.
21. Jamaica, Ministry of Health. Adolescent Contraceptive Survey. 2001.
22. United Nations Population Fund; United Nations Children's Fund. Meeting adolescent development and participation rights in Jamaica: the findings of five research studies on adolescents in Jamaica. 2002.
23. Eldemire D. Ageing in Jamaica. 2002.
24. Jamaica, Ministry of Health. Annual report. 2004.
25. Jamaica, Ministry of Health. Family health report. 2005.
26. Jamaica, Ministry of Health. Annual tuberculosis reports. 2003–2004.
27. Jamaica, Ministry of Health. Leprosy. Annual reports. 2003–2004.
28. University of the West Indies, Tropical Metabolism Research Institute, Sickle Cell Unit. Report. 2006.
29. Global Fund to Fight AIDS, Tuberculosis, and Malaria. Grant Performance Report (JAM-304-G01-H). February 2006.
30. Jamaica, Ministry of Health. Report of National Knowledge, Attitudes, Behaviour & Practices (KABP) Survey, 2004. May–August 2004.
31. Jamaica, Ministry of Health, National HIV/STI Programme. November 2004.
32. Jamaica, Ministry of Health. The Jamaica Road Map to Scaling Up Universal Access to HIV Prevention, Care, and Treatment Support Services. Draft document. April 2006.
33. Wedderburn M, Bourne D. Report on HIV/AIDS second generation surveillance: behavioural surveillance survey among female sex workers. Jamaica; August 2005. Page 8.
34. Jamaica, Ministry of Health. National KABP Survey. 2004.
35. Jamaica, Ministry of Health. Report. 2002.
36. Blake G, Hanchard B, Gibson T, Wolff C, Samuels E, Waugh N, Simpson D. Gynaecologic cancer incidence, Kingston and St Andrew, Jamaica, 1973–1997, and gynaecologic cancer mortality, Jamaica, 1999. West Indian Med J. 2003; 52(4): 273–7.
37. Impact Assessment of Decentralization and Delegation Initiatives. Draft Report. In: Jamaica Human Development Report 2005. May 2003.
38. Pan American Health Organization. Review of the Water Quality Monitoring Programme of the Ministry of Health in Jamaica. 2004.
39. Pan American Health Organization. Report on the Regional Evaluation of Solid Waste Management in Latin America and the Caribbean. 2002.
40. Jamaica, Statistical Institute of Jamaica. Jamaica's Environment 2001. Environment Statistics and State of the Environment Report. STATIN; February 2002.
41. United States Agency for International Development. Report on the environmental audits for sustainable tourism, 1997–2005.
42. Kozyr E. The negative effects of tourism on the ecology of Jamaica. Caribbean Studies, University of York; 2000.
43. Steffen R, Collard F, Tornieporth N, Campbell-Forrester S, Ashley D, Thompson S, et al. Epidemiology, etiology, and impact of traveler's diarrhea in Jamaica. JAMA. 1999; 281:811.
44. Lewis M. Evaluation of Ministry of Health 2001–2005 Strategic Plan. Final report. 2005.

MEXICO

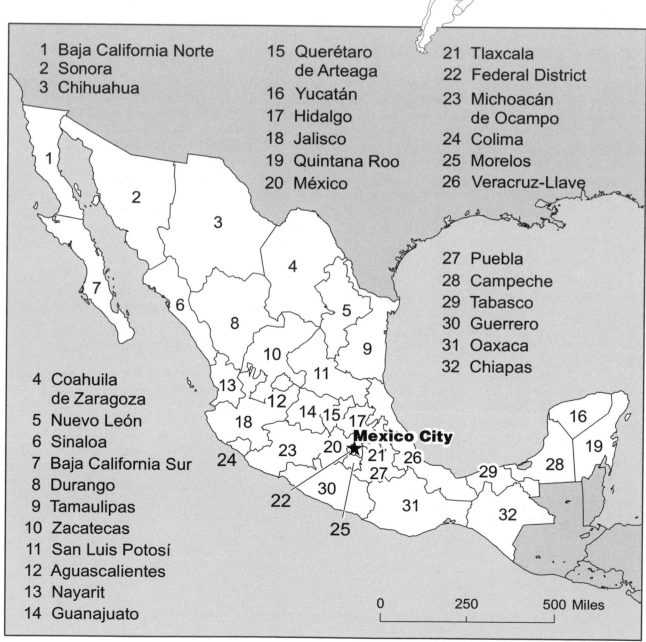

1 Baja California Norte
2 Sonora
3 Chihuahua

15 Querétaro
   de Arteaga
16 Yucatán
17 Hidalgo
18 Jalisco
19 Quintana Roo
20 México

21 Tlaxcala
22 Federal District
23 Michoacán
   de Ocampo
24 Colima
25 Morelos
26 Veracruz-Llave

27 Puebla
28 Campeche
29 Tabasco
30 Guerrero
31 Oaxaca
32 Chiapas

4 Coahuila
   de Zaragoza
5 Nuevo León
6 Sinaloa
7 Baja California Sur
8 Durango
9 Tamaulipas
10 Zacatecas
11 San Luis Potosí
12 Aguascalientes
13 Nayarit
14 Guanajuato

Mexico City

0   250   500 Miles

T he United States of Mexico is a representative and democratic republic consisting of 32 federal entities: 31 states and the Federal District (Mexico City, capital of the country). The federal and state governments are hierarchically equal and abide by principles of autonomy and association.

GENERAL CONTEXT AND HEALTH DETERMINANTS

The federal and state governments change every six years, and municipal governments change every three years. Between 2001 and 2006, the country was governed by a different political party for the first time in seven decades. In July of 2006, presidential elections were held that resulted in a virtual tie between the two parties. The slight difference in favor of one of the parties prolonged by more than two months the decision of the Electoral Tribunal of the Judicial Branch of the Federation (TRIFE) in declaring an official winner, amid political crisis and massive protests.

Social, Political, and Economic Determinants

The Mexican economy grew 4.2% in 2004 and 3.0% in 2005, while the per capita gross domestic product (GDP) grew 1.6% between 2004 and 2005 and inflation remained stable. The per capita GDP went from US$ 5,110 in 2000 to US$ 6,230 in 2003 (1). Remittances sent to Mexico have grown annually by more than 20% since 2002, and in 2005 they surpassed US$ 20 billion. In 2004, remittances accounted for approximately 70% of foreign income from oil and 87% from the maquilador sector (2). Remittances constitute a strong source of income and economic activity with important repercussions for populations living in the country's interior. The economically active population has maintained high levels of employment since 2001, between 95% and 96%. In the first quarter of 2006, employment was maintained at around 96.3%, with no difference between men and women (3). Six states in northern Mexico that border the United States of America (U.S.A.) receive close to 29% of the direct foreign investment, constitute 23% of the national GDP, and represent 17% of the population (4). In 2004, the Federal District and the State of México supplied more than 30% of the national GDP, while states such as Chiapas, Oaxaca, Campeche, and Yucatán collectively accounted for 6% of the national GDP (5).

The three categories defined by the Technical Committee on Poverty Measurement (CTMP) are: food poverty (households with insufficient income to satisfy basic food needs); capacity poverty (households that cannot satisfy their basic food, health, and educational needs); and patrimony poverty (households that cannot satisfy their basic food, health, education, clothing, shoes, housing, and public transportation needs). The National Household Income and Expenditure Survey (ENIGH 2000) found that 24.2% of the population lived with food poverty (42.4% rural and 12.6% urban); that 31.9% lived with capacity poverty (50.0% rural and 20.2% urban); and 53.7% lived with patrimony poverty (69.3% rural and 43.8% urban) (6). The 2004 ENIGH showed a reduction in levels of poverty: food poverty included 17.3% of the population (27.6% rural and 11.0% urban); capacity poverty was 24.6% (35.7% rural and 17.8% urban); and patrimony poverty was 47.0% (56.9% rural and 41% urban). In absolute terms, this signifies a reduction in food poverty between 2000 and 2004 of 5.6 million people, largely in rural areas. This reduction is considered a positive trend, but it is not sufficient to achieve the Millennium Development Goal (MDG 1) of reducing by half between 1990 and 2015 the percentage of persons living in extreme poverty. The main government program to fight poverty and improve human development is the Opportunities Program, where mothers receive monetary support to improve the nutrition, health, and education of their families. In 2005, the program had 5 million households enrolled, selected based on household socioeconomic characteristics (7).

In 2002, the poorest 10% of the population received 1.4% of the national income, while the richest 10% received 40.5% (8). The levels of poverty in Mexico continue to be high for a high-income country; Mexico has been a member of the Organization for Economic Cooperation and Development (OECD) since 1994, which includes the 30 most industrialized countries of the world, in which the Mexican economy ranks 9th (9).

Over the last 15 years, Mexico has improved its place on the Human Development Index (HDI), and in 2005 was categorized as one of the countries with high human development and ranked 53rd with a score of 0.814 (10). However, while estimating the HDI in terms of subnational units and municipalities, significant differences in development are seen. The Report on Human Development in Mexico 2004 (11) ranked 14 states with an HDI greater than 0.800 (high human development), and the 18 remaining states showed midlevel human development. The range varied from 0.883 in the Federal District to 0.707 in the State of Chiapas. The same report grouped the Mexican states into five regions, and the highest value (0.873) in human development belonged to the Northeast Region, which is composed of the states of Coahuila, Chihuahua, Durango, Nueva León, and Tamaulipas (four of them share a border with the U.S.A.). The other extreme was found in the states of Campeche, Chiapas, Guerrero, Oaxaca, Quintana Roo, Veracruz, and Yucatán (HDI 0.742), located in the south of the country. When this index is measured at the municipal level, the differences are even more strongly demarcated, going from 0.38 in the municipality of Metlatónoc in the State of Guerrero to 0.91 in the Benito Juárez area of the Federal District (11).

The marginalization index of the National Population Council (CONAPO) (12) uses data on population size, education level, and housing and income characteristics that together measure the difficulties in technological development, as well as the social exclusion of population groups who do not benefit from certain benefits or goods. The 2000 CONAPO report showed that the states of Chiapas, Guerrero, Hidalgo, Oaxaca, and Veracruz were highly marginalized, and Chiapas, located on the border with Guatemala, had the highest level of marginalization in the country. In Chiapas, 23% of the population older than 15 years is illiterate, 50% of the state's population did not complete primary education, 25% of the houses did not have piped water, and 40% had dirt floors (12). Nine federal states were considered to be highly marginalized; six had midlevels of marginalization; eight had low marginalization; and four had very low marginalization. The marginalization index at the municipal level shows even greater variation. Of the 2,444 municipalities, 1,292 were highly or very highly marginalized and also included historically defined territorial patterns and a concentrated indigenous population. The gaps, the inequities, and the differences in opportunity among the population groups are characteristic of Mexico in the context of a multicultural, multiethnic, and multilingual nation.

In 1992 the Mexican Constitution recognized the country as being multicultural, although this has not had any important legal repercussions. After the armed uprising of the National Liberation Zapatista Army (EZLN) in 1994, recognition for indigenous communities and the established autonomous groups in the south has advanced. The fights for water, land access, and employment are important to the indigenous peoples, as are political and religious conflicts and the use and abuse of natural resources in their territories, some of which have been privatized (13). High levels of corruption exist in the political, judicial, and police systems. A lack of security, attacks, kidnappings, and assassinations have continued despite the efforts of government forces, which have not been able to stop organized crime and the drug-trafficking cartels that operate in the country and that caused 1,500 deaths during 2005 (14).

Universal literacy has been reached among youth between 15 and 24 years of age, and the rate of enrollment at primary school for children between 6 and 11 years reached 99.4% in 2004. In 2000, 90.5% of women aged 15 and older knew how to read and write, and 70.5% of the population older than 15 years had completed primary school (15). The average level of education was 7.7 completed grades (7.8 among males and 7.3 among females); the states with the highest levels of education were the Federal District (9.7) and Nuevo León (8.9), and the lowest were Chiapas (5.6), Oaxaca (5.8), and Guerrero (6.3), which have the largest indigenous population in the country. Efforts are focused on those federal entities with the largest levels of marginalization but that also have percentages of primary school enrollment greater than 97%. Among vulnerable populations, such as indigenous populations, rural communities, and migrants, these indicators show the historical gaps in access to education; for example, 40% of the indigenous population older than 15 years has not completed primary school.

Environmental problems remain a challenge. The proportion of lands covered by forests or jungles dropped from 36.6% to 33.4% between 1993 and 2002, with a negative impact on the conservation of natural resources and water and on prevention of natural disasters. As a positive indicator, the proportion of lands protected as natural areas grew from 5.5% in 1995 to 9.1% in 2002 (16).

Demographics, Mortality, and Morbidity

In 2006, Mexico's population was estimated to be 107,525,207, with 24% living in rural areas. The total fertility rate was 2.07 (2.6 in Oaxaca and 1.8 in the Federal District), with a growth rate of 0.99%. In 2006, it was estimated that 1,942,914 children were born. The specific fertility rate per 100 women between 15 and 19 years was estimated to be 4.9, with extremes in the State of Guerrero (7.1) and the Federal District (1.3). The general mortality rate was 4.5 per 1,000 population (5.0 in men and 4.0 in women). In 2006, approximately 479,000 people died. By 2010 the total fertility rate is expected to drop to 1.97, with a growth rate of 0.88% (17), and the population will reach 111.6 million. Life expectancy at birth in 1995 was 70 years for men and 75 for women, and in 2006 it is estimated to be 74 years for men and 78 years for women (18).

The adolescent population doubled in absolute numbers over the past 30 years; the population of those 15–29 years was 30.2 million in 2004 (28.7% of the total population) and continues to grow (19). Half of adolescent youths (49.9%) live in seven of the 32 federal entities (20). In 2005, the school-aged population (youth less than 14 years) was 30% of the total, and by 2010 will drop to 26.7%. By comparison, the population of productive age (15–59 years) will grow from 62.3% to 64.5% for the same period, and the population of adults older than 60 years will grow from 7.7% to 8.8% (18).

It is estimated that between 2005 and 2025, due to the sustained decrease in the fertility rate, the population replacement

FIGURE 1. Population structure, by age and sex, Mexico, 2005.

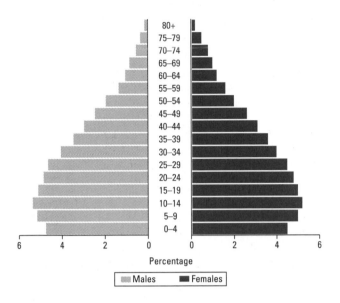

Males   Females

rate will be maintained (each couple has the number of children to replace them on the population pyramid), and by 2025 it will decline to 1.85 children per woman. These results are congruent with the population policies oriented to satisfy the demands for contraceptives, and it is estimated that by 2006 more than 74% of women of reproductive age will be using some method of contraception. Consequently, the demographic transition will change the population pyramid, with more persons of productive age and older persons. (See Figure 1 for the country's population structure in 2005).

Between 2005 and 2025, Mexico will experience a "demographic bonus," where a beneficial relationship will exist in the ratio between the population of productive age (15–59) and the dependent population (children less than 14 years and those older than 60). Given the smaller burden of the dependent population on Mexican families, it is considered that this period will represent an opportunity that will favor development policies, a generation of employment, the formation of social and human capital, and, above all, an opportunity to reduce disparities (21). This period will also be characterized by an increase in the demand for middle- and high-level education, access to health services and social security, as well as housing needs. The dependency rate (relationship between the population less than 15 years and those older than 64 years to the population between 15 and 64 years, expressed as a percentage) was estimated to be 61.9% in 2004 (22).

In 2000, the healthy life expectancy (HALE), taking into consideration the extremes among the states, was 55.2 to 63.1 years for men and 61.0 to 67.3 years for women. This indicator measures the years of life a person can live without disability. The five leading causes of loss of healthy years are perinatal injuries, road traffic injuries, diabetes, violence, and cardiopathies.

A significant migration of Mexicans to the U.S.A. has occurred historically and continues. In 2002, it was estimated that 9,503,928 U.S. residents were born in Mexico (23). It is also estimated that 24 million persons of Mexican origin (born in Mexico or children of Mexicans) reside in the U.S.A., representing 11.6% of the total population (24). The net international migration is −0.38% annually, predominantly in men, and it is expected to remain constant until 2010. The states with the highest emigration of Mexicans to the U.S.A. are: Jalisco (18%), Michoacán (12%), Guanajuato (8%), and Zacatecas (8%). A total of 162 municipalities are considered to have high levels of migration, of which 30 are located in Oaxaca, 28 in Michoacán, and 25 in Jalisco.

In 1980, the leading causes of death were infectious intestinal diseases and pneumonia and influenza, which together represented 18.3% of the total deaths reported. The same causes in 2004 represented only 3.9% (25). Table 1 shows the 10 specific leading causes of death for 2004, with diabetes as the leading cause of death, which represented about 13% of the total number of deaths and a specific mortality rate of 59.0 per 100,000 population. There are no significant changes among the leading causes of death in the last 5 years, although the burden of death due to diabetes continues to rise, representing 10.7% of all deaths and with a rate of 46.3 per 100,000 population in 2000. Underreporting of death was estimated to be 0.8% for the 2000–2005 period (26).

Communicable diseases, maternal conditions, perinatal conditions, and nutritional conditions were the four largest groups of mortality causes, representing 26% of deaths in 1990, compared to 13.4% in 2004; noncommunicable diseases caused 57.8% of deaths in 1990 and 73.8% in 2004; external causes represented 13.9% in 1990 and 10.8% in 2004; and ill-defined causes accounted for 2.3% in 1990 and 2% in 2004 (25). Table 2 shows the causes of mortality according to PAHO's 6/67 list for 2003 (27).

HEALTH OF POPULATION GROUPS

Children under 5 Years Old

Infant mortality was 36.2 per 1,000 live births in 1990, 23.3 in 2000, and 19.7 in 2004. If this trend is maintained, Mexico will achieve the MDG goal of reducing infant mortality by two-thirds by 2015. The infant mortality rates show inequalities among the states: in 2004, the extremes were found in Chiapas (26.3 per 1,000 live births) and the Federal District (14.4 per 1,000 live births) (22). Seventy percent of infant deaths were due to perinatal conditions or congenital malformations, with a decrease in infectious causes such as diarrhea and respiratory infections (28). Acute lower respiratory infections represented the leading cause of death among children 1 to 4 years (10.3% of the total) with a rate of 8.4 per 100,000 population. The fourth cause of death was motor-vehicle accidents (29). Mortality among children less than 5 years dropped from 44.2 per 1,000 live births in 1990 to 24.0

TABLE 1. Ten leading causes of general mortality, Mexico, 2004 compared to rate in 2000.

ICD-10 code	Description	Deaths	%	Rate[a]	Rate in 2000
A00–Y98	Total	472,273	100.0	448.3	433.0
E10–E14	Diabetes mellitus	62,201	13.2	59.0	46.3
I20–I25	Ischemic heart disease	50,461	10.7	47.9	43.5
I60–I69	Cerebrovascular disease	26,975	5.7	25.6	25.2
K70, K72.1, K73, K74, K76	Cirrhosis and other chronic liver disease	26,867	5.7	25.5	25.2
J40–J44, J67	Chronic obstructive pulmonary disease	18,806	4.0	17.9	15.8
P00–P96	Certain conditions arising during the perinatal period	16,501	3.5	15.7	19.3
	Motor vehicle traffic accidents	14,312	3.0	13.6	13.7
J10–J18, J20–J22	Acute lower respiratory infections	14,215	3.0	13.5	14.3
I10–I15	Hypertensive diseases	12,203	2.6	11.6	9.7
N00–N19	Nephritis and nephrosis	10,774	2.3	10.2	9.7

[a]Rate per 100,000 population.
Source: General Directorate of Information of the Mexican Secretariat of Health.

TABLE 2. Causes of death, according to PAHO's 6/67 list, Mexico, 2003.

Group of 6/67 causes	ICD-10 code	Total	Standardized rate[a]
All causes	A00–Y89	470,692	630.4
Signs, symptoms, and ill-defined conditions	R00–R99	9,941	12.6
Communicable diseases	A00–B99, G00–G03, J00–J22	33,289	48.4
Tumors	C00–D48	62,891	82.9
Circulatory system illnesses	I00–I99	107,570	143.6
Certain illnesses originating in the perinatal period	P00–P96	17,081	35.7
External causes	V01–Y89	51,712	35.7
All other	Rest of D50–Q99	188,208	256.7

[a]Rate per 100,000 population.

per 1,000 live births in 2004. If this trend continues, Mexico will achieve the fourth MDG by 2015. However, the work is more difficult given that the sustained decline over the past decade is due to the infectious disease control strategies. For example, 30% of the deaths in children 5 years and younger in 1990 were due to diarrhea and acute respiratory infections, which in 2004 accounted for 15% (28).

Between 1990 and 2003, the rate of acute diarrheal disease in children less than 5 years dropped almost 84% (from 155.1 to 24.9 per 100,000 population), while in the case of acute respiratory infections, the reduction was slightly greater than 70% (from 142.9 to 42.0 per 100,000 population). The 2000 National Health Survey showed the prevalence of diarrhea (at least one episode of diarrhea in the last 2 weeks) in children less than 5 years to be 11.5%, and the 2006 survey showed an increase to 12.9%. At the national level the variation goes from 5.9% in Zacatecas to 21.1% in Chiapas (30). The same survey in 2006 found that 92% of children less than 1 year had been breast-fed some period of time

and that exclusive breast-feeding among infants less than 6 months old was 20%.

Children 5–9 Years Old

In 2004, the mortality rate for children aged 5–9 years was 3.4 per 100,000 population. The leading causes of death were accidents, followed by malignant tumors, congenital malformations, deformities and chromosomal anomalies, cerebral palsy, violence and homicides, other infectious diseases, and malnutrition (31). The leading causes of morbidity were infections of the respiratory system, intestines, and urinary tract; otitis media (middle ear infection); gastrointestinal amebiasis; chickenpox; parasitosis; asthma; and tonsillitis (32).

Adolescents 10–14 and 15–19 Years Old

In the 10- to 14-year-old age group, the leading cause of death in 2004 was motor-vehicle accidents (14.6% of the total number of deaths), with an age-specific rate of 4.64 per 100,000 population. Among this age group, the number of suicides has risen, with suicides being the 10th leading cause of death in 2000 with a rate of 0.98 per 100,000 population and the 8th leading cause in 2004 with a rate of 1.33 per 100,000 population (*33*). Traffic accidents involving a motor vehicle were the leading cause of death for adolescents aged 15–19 years, representing 20% of all deaths and a rate of 13.9 per 100,000. In second place were homicides, with 10.6% of all deaths and with a rate of 7.2 per 100,000. For the combined age group of 10–19 years, the mortality rate for traffic accidents involving a motor vehicle grew from 8.62 per 100,000 population in 2000 to 9.24 per 100,000 population in 2004. Among the same group in 2004, homicides and suicides represented the third and fourth leading causes of death, respectively, with mortality rates of 4.22 and 3.12 per 100,000 population. In 2000, the mortality rate due to homicides among youth 10–19 years was 5.41 per 100,000 population and 2.69 for suicides. The male: female ratio for this age group in 2004 for homicides was 4:1, and for suicides was 2.5:1 (*33*).

Between 2000 and 2004, the average age at sexual debut was 15.4 years: 13.8 years in rural areas and 16.7 years in urban areas. In 2000, 372,000 pregnancies were registered among mothers between 10 and 19 years (17.2% of the total number of births), and 10% ended in abortion. The specific fertility rate for this age group was 70.1 per 1,000 women. According to the 2006 National Health Survey, 29.6% of adolescents between 16 and 19 years reported having had sexual relations, and 63.5% of adolescent males reported using a condom while only 38% of adolescent females reported that their partner used a condom.

Adults 20–59 Years Old

In 1990, the maternal mortality rate was 89 per 100,000 live births; 72.6 in 2000; 62.4 in 2004; and 63.3 in 2005. Over the last 5 years the maternal mortality rate has not continued its downward trend but has been relatively stable, which is not enough to achieve the goal of 22.3 per 100,000 live births by 2015, which is the 5th MDG (*34*). Approximately 75% of all maternal mortality was concentrated in 12 federal entities. In 2004, the state with the highest maternal mortality rate was Guerrero, with 116.4 per 100,000 live births, and the lowest was Nuevo León with 13.1 per 100,000 live births (*22*). In 2003, the Secretariat of Health (SSA), through the General Directorate of Information, began a review to improve underreporting and identified areas with the highest maternal mortality, linked to areas historically known for having poor indigenous populations with little access to health services. In these regions, close to 20% of births are overseen by traditional birth attendants. In the areas of greatest economic development, maternal deaths are largely due to indirect causes and preexisting health conditions of the mother, while in the southern states many of the maternal causes are preventable, such as hemorrhages and toxemias. In 2004, 25% of maternal deaths were due to hemor-

rhages, 30% to hypertension, 6% to complications related to abortion, and 12% to other complications during birth (*28*). The average age of maternal mortality was 29 years. Only 33% of the maternal deaths occurred in women with some type of insurance, largely social security. Approximately 87% of births occur in a health institution, and 10% still occur at home (*35*). According to data from the National Commission on Indigenous Peoples (CNPI), maternal mortality is three times higher in the regions of Tarahumara, Huichola, and Cora than in the rest of the country and is largely linked to high levels of malnutrition.

The 2006 National Health and Nutrition Survey found anemia in 20.6% of pregnant women, compared to 15.5% among nonpregnant women, a situation that has improved since the 1999 survey, which found values of 26.2% and 20.0%, respectively.

According to CONAPO, about 600,000 births are registered annually for women between the ages of 20 and 24 and about 300,000 in adolescents between 15 and 19 years of age, resulting in 45% of all births occurring in women between 15 and 24 years of age. Twenty-two percent of maternal deaths are found in women 20–24 years, and 13% of maternal deaths are found in females 15–19 years (*36*).

Older Adults 60 Years Old and Older

The average annual increase in the number of older adults (60 years and older) is about 270,000 persons. The principal causes of death in 2000 were cardiovascular disease for both sexes (30% of the deaths in men and 33.8% in women); the second leading cause of death among men was malignant neoplasms (14.6%) and in women it was diabetes mellitus (15.7%). In men, diabetes mellitus was the third leading cause of death (11.6%) and malignant neoplasms was third for women (13.4%). Digestive diseases were the fourth cause of death for both sexes (10.2% and 7.7% for men and women, respectively). The fifth cause of death was respiratory infections (7.7% in men and 5.9% in women). Table 3 shows the 10 leading causes of death for adults older than 65 years during 2004, as well as their rates during 2000, for comparison.

The Family

Between 20% and 22% of households are headed by women (*37*). The number of domestic units headed by women is 4.6 million, up from 2.8 million in 1990. One important fact to consider about female-headed households is that half are low income, which often contributes to the incorporation of minors in economic activities. Female heads of household frequently are the only adult in the household, which requires them to assume the role of provider as well as the responsibilities of caring for and raising children and other domestic responsibilities, which leaves them overworked. Female heads of household are generally widows (35.9%), separated (24.7%), or divorced (18.4%). This type of household is generally composed of 3.6 people and in half the

TABLE 3. Leading causes of mortality in people 65 years and older, Mexico, 2004 compared to the rate in 2000.

ICD-10 code	Description	Deaths	%	Rate[a]	Rate 2000
A00–Y98	Total	249,267	100.0	4,595.1	4,619.1
I20–I25	Ischemic heart disease	37,509	15.0	691.5	686.9
E10–E14	Diabetes mellitus	37,380	15.0	689.1	587.1
I60–I69	Cerebrovascular disease	20,327	8.2	374.7	404.5
J40–J44, J67	Chronic obstructive pulmonary disease	16,514	6.6	304.4	295.2
I10–I15	Hypertensive disease	9,521	3.8	175.5	156.7
K70, K72.1, K73, K74, K76	Cirrhosis and other chronic liver diseases	8,966	3.6	165.3	164.6
J10–J18, J20–J22	Acute lower respiratory infections	8,161	3.3	150.4	161.5
N00–N19	Nephritis and nephrosis	6,323	2.5	116.6	120.5
E40–E46	Protein energy malnutrition	6,136	2.5	113.1	133.6
C33–C34	Malignant tumor, lungs, trachea	4,653	1.9	85.8	87.8

[a]Rate per 100,000 population.

Source: General Directorate of Information of the Mexican Secretariat of Health.

cases a minor below 15 years of age is present. Single-person households have increased significantly in recent decades and represent almost 1.5 million households (*38*).

The most recent national survey revealed that 25% of women have suffered some form of abuse (*39*). In Guadalajara, the prevalence of violence against women reached 57% in the urban area and 44% in the rural area. The rate of mortality due to homicide against women in 2002 was 2.5 per 100,000 women (*40*).

Workers

Adolescents form an important part of the economically active population. In 2000, working males below 19 years of age represented 44% of the total number of men; in the case of females, 24%. The rate of participation in the labor force varied according to age; however, 8% of all adolescents 12 to 14 years are already in the workforce.

The Mexican Institute for Social Security (IMSS) provides services to 370,000 people annually due to workplace accidents (*41*). The risk of workplace accidents has improved, considering that between 2000 and 2005 the rate dropped from 2.9% to 2.3%. In the same way, permanent disabilities have dropped to 6.8%, and fatal workplace accidents to 3.1% (*42*).

Persons with Disabilities

The population and housing census in 2000 identified 2.2 million persons living with some type of disability, largely related to reduced movement, blindness or visual impairments, mental disabilities, and lastly auditory and language problems. Slightly fewer than half of the total number of disabled people are older adults. The principal causes of disability are previous illness, followed by advanced age, congenital problems, and injuries or accidents (*15*).

Ethnic Groups

In absolute terms, Mexico has the largest indigenous population in the Americas, estimated in 2006 to be 13,528,579 persons, which represents 12.6% of the total population. Mexico defines the indigenous population as persons older than 5 years of age who speak an indigenous language, the population 0 to 4 years of age who live in households whose head is an indigenous language speaker (ILS), and the population who self-describe as indigenous (*15*).

In Mexico, 62 indigenous languages exist, with 30 dialectical variations. One-quarter of the indigenous people speak Náhuat, followed by Maya, Otomí, Tzeltal, Tzotzil, among others. However, 17 of the 62 indigenous languages have a diminishing number of speakers, and reproduction problems leave them with fewer than 500 ILS. The Mexican states with the greatest proportion of indigenous population are: Yucatán (60%), Oaxaca (49%), Quintana Roo (40%), and Chiapas (29%), all of which are located in the southern part of the country.

According to CONAPO estimates, infant mortality in the indigenous population was 34.4 per 1,000 live births in 2000 and 26.8 per 1,000 live births in 2006. The risk of dying due to pregnancy, birth, and peripartum causes is three times higher in indigenous women (*43*). The illiteracy rate among indigenous peoples is 44%, while the national level is 10% (*44*). The prevalence of childhood malnutrition is 58.3% in indigenous children, and iron deficiency among pregnant indigenous women is 60% (*44*). In Oaxaca, the number of physicians per 1,000 indigenous population is 0.13, compared to the state average of 0.94, and a national average of 1.38 physicians per 1,000 population.

The indigenous population is predominantly found in rural areas. Sixty-five percent reside in localities with fewer than 2,500 persons where the historical factors of poverty, marginalization, and social exclusion persist. Of the 871 municipalities considered indigenous, 259 (29.7%) qualify as being very highly marginalized and 363 (41.7%) are highly marginalized (*45*). In 2000, 36% of indigenous housing did not have piped water and 16.9% did not have electricity, while 43.7% had dirt floors and 62.4% cooked with firewood (*15*).

Despite the development of a health information system, it has not been possible to incorporate ethnic variables into the registries. However, gaps and vulnerabilities in matters of health among the indigenous population are recognized, in which communicable diseases, severe malnutrition, the presence of preventable diseases, as well as problems such as alcoholism, accidents, and violence persist (*46*).

Border Populations

The border between the U.S.A. and Mexico is 3,152 kilometers long. Migration to the United States has historically been attractive to the Mexican population, as well as Central Americans, generating a complex social situation on the northern and southern borders. In 2005, 516 migrants died trying to cross the northern border, the greatest number registered in the last 10 years (*47*). A mix of chronic and infectious diseases, including tuberculosis, hepatitis, and HIV/AIDS, are found in this population, with higher incidences than the national averages (*48*). The increase in the number of injection drug users (IDU) among younger users, particularly women, is worrisome and carries with it a higher risk of sexually transmitted infections (*49*).

The southern border is 1,138 kilometers and is shared with Guatemala and Belize. Chiapas is the state that shares historical, cultural, ethnic, and environmental links with the border region of Guatemala. It is estimated that the annual number of illegal migrants who cross the border is 120,000 persons, complicating epidemiological surveillance with the possibility of introducing a new agent of disease or resistant forms of known diseases.

HEALTH CONDITIONS AND PROBLEMS

COMMUNICABLE DISEASES

Vector-borne Diseases

More than 99% of the cases of **malaria** are caused by *Plasmodium vivax*, and only a few, registered in the border states of Tabasco and Chiapas, are due to *P. falciparum*. The principal vectors are *Anopheles pseudopunctipennis* and *An. albimanus*. In 2005, 2,967 cases were reported, representing a reduction of 13% from 2004 (3,406 cases) and down 60% from 2000 (7,390 cases). In 2005, 97% of the transmission was concentrated in the states of Oaxaca (1,432), Chiapas (852), Sinaloa (208), Chihuahua (181), Durango (114), and Tabasco (97). DDT use has been discontinued and the insecticide is no longer being produced; household spraying with insecticides has also been eliminated, as community participation has increased to control vector breeding grounds.

In the 26 federal entities (629 municipalities and 43 million inhabitants), risk factors for the transmission of **dengue** persist.

In 2005, 17,487 cases of classic dengue were registered, with a rate of 16.43 per 100,000 population, a 10-fold increase over 2000, when 1,714 cases were recorded. In 2002, the predominant serotype was DENV-2 (dengue virus type 2), and in 2005, for the first time in 5 years, outbreaks of more than one serotype were registered, which increased the cases of hemorrhagic dengue from 67 in 2000 to 4,418 in 2005. Fatalities have remained at less than 1%. In the last 2 years, four serotypes have been found, which is largely due to the reintroduction of the DENV-1 and DENV-4 dengue virus strains from Central America.

Ecologically favorable conditions for proliferation of the triatomine vectors for **Chagas' disease** exist, and 30 species have been described, among which 10 are epidemiologically important. In 2000, 100 cases were registered, 17 acute and 83 chronic, and in 2005, 361 cases were registered, 14 acute and 347 chronic (17 with cardiopathy, 1 with megacolon, and 329 undetermined).

The transmission of **leishmaniasis** has been linked to five possible species—*Lutzomia olmeca, L. cruciata, L. diabolica, L. shannoni*, and *L. longipalpis*—which vary in importance based on geographic location and endemic area, the species of the transmitting parasite, and the clinical type of illness with which it has been associated. The localized cutaneous form is found most frequently (99%); disseminated cutaneous and mucocutaneous leishmaniasis are responsive to treatment in most cases. The visceral form has been reported annually in the State of Chiapas since 1990 and occasionally in other states. In 2000, 797 cases were reported; in 2005, 868 new cases were reported, for an increase of 9% (*50*).

Trachoma continues to be endemic in five indigenous municipalities of Los Altos-Chiapas. Since 2001, the SSA and other state, national, and civil society organizations have given special emphasis to the Program for Surveillance, Prevention and Control of Trachoma, which has established strategies such as the active search for cases, house by house, social mobilization, and health education, which have permitted the certification process of the elimination of trachoma to begin. The municipality of Oxchuc is the most affected, with more than 50% of the total cases, but the highest prevalence of active trachoma is in the municipality of Tenejapa, with 79 cases.

Vaccine-preventable Diseases

As a result of vaccination campaigns, poliomyelitis, diphtheria, and neonatal tetanus remain eliminated. The last case of diphtheria was found in 1991, and the last case of poliomyelitis was found in 1990. Other illnesses such as measles, whopping cough, mumps, and rubella are also under control. The vaccination schedule consists of 11 immunobiologics: BCG (antituberculosis) at birth; OPV (oral antipoliomyelitis) at 2, 4, and 6 months; pentavalent (DPT-HB-Hib) at 2, 4, and 6 months; MMR (measles, mumps, and rubella) at 12 months. Since 2004, a dosage of flu vaccine for children 6 and 24 months old has been incorporated. For adolescents, a second dose of MR (measles and rubella), as well as TD (tetanus and diphtheria toxoid), is given, and for adults 65 years and older, an annual influenza vaccine is given. Since 2000, the coverage of the basic vaccination schedule for children less than 1 year has been maintained at greater than 95%, and in children aged 1–4, coverage is greater than 96%. The vaccination coverage has been achieved through a combination of two strategies: constant vaccination promotion and intensive phases during the national health weeks, which are conducted three times a year.

Mexico maintains active surveillance of acute flaccid paralysis, and between 2000 and 2005 identified on average 420 cases annually. The last case of autochthonous or native measles was reported in 1996, but in 2000 the first reintroduction of the virus occurred with 30 cases registered in four states. During 2001 and 2002, no cases were confirmed, but in 2003, 44 cases of measles were reported, followed by 64 in 2004, and 6 in 2005. The isolated viral genotypes in this outbreak indicated that the virus came from other continents.

In 2000, 11,751 cases of **rubella** were identified, which dropped to 38 cases in 2005. There were five cases of congenital rubella reported in 2000, and in 2005 only one case was identified. Mumps dropped from 27,911 cases in 2000 to 8,425 in 2004 (reduction of 30%). Both diseases were reduced significantly due to the introduction of the triple viral vaccine (MMR) in 1998 as part of the national vaccination schedule.

In 2000, 53 cases of **whooping cough** were reported, 137 in 2004, and 349 in 2005. Tetanus cases dropped from 103 in 2000 to 71 in 2005. In 2000, 119 cases of meningeal tuberculosis were identified, 147 in 2004, and 199 in 2005.

After the incorporation of the vaccination against *Haemophilus influenzae* type b in 1999, the number of cases dropped from 131 in 2000, to 56 in 2004, and to 39 in 2005. After introduction of the vaccine against **hepatitis B** in 1997, the number of reported cases dropped from 835 in 2000 to 687 in 2004; all national blood banks screen blood for hepatitis B.

Intestinal Infectious Diseases

Between 2000 and 2004, the most common food-borne illnesses were paratyphoid (with an average annual incidence of 93 cases per 100,000 population) and **shigellosis** (which dropped from 36.51 cases per 100,000 population in 2000 to 21.19 cases in 2004). The incidence of other intestinal infections also dropped with 5,203 cases per 100,000 in 2000 and 4,535 per 100,000 population in 2004.

Chronic Communicable Diseases

The number of reported case of **respiratory tuberculos**is has been stable, with an average of 12,372 annual cases over the period 2000 to 2004. The cumulative annual incidence of all forms of tuberculosis between 2000 and 2004 was 15 per 100,000 population, with some 16,000 cases reported per year and more than 3,000 deaths annually. The greatest areas of risk are the states of Baja California, Chiapas, Nuevo León, Tamaulipas, and Veracruz,

where more than 40% of the national cases are found. The pulmonary form of the illness was found in 80% of the deaths reported for the period 2000–2004. The incidence of meningeal tuberculosis was 0.12 per 100,000 population in 2000, and 0.14 in 2004. The treatment strategy of direct observation (DOTS) is utilized in more than 80% of diagnosed cases. The association of tuberculosis with other types of health conditions such as diabetes, malnutrition, alcoholism, and HIV/AIDS increased from 2000 to 2004.

Leprosy does not constitute a public health problem in most Mexican states. In 2000, the incidence was 0.42 per 100,000 population, and 0.24 in 2004 when 252 new cases in 26 states were detected, but with 77% of the cases concentrated in the states of Colima, Guanajuato, Guerrero, Jalisco, Michoacán, Nayarit, Nuevo León, Sinaloa, and Tamaulipas.

Acute Respiratory Infections

Doctor's visits for acute respiratory illnesses dropped from 29,427 per 100,000 population in 2000 to 24,581 in 2004. The cumulative incidence of pneumonia and bronchitis dropped from 204 to 172 per 100,000 population during the same period, and the incidence of influenza dropped dramatically from 0.57 to 0.06 per 100,000 population. Ninety percent of the cases were found in people younger than 44 years, and children aged 5 to 14 years were the most-affected age group. The mortality rate from respiratory illnesses, including pneumonia and influenza, in children less than 5 dropped from 51.6 deaths per 100,000 in 2000 to 35.3 per 100,000 in 2004.

HIV/AIDS and Other Sexually Transmitted Infections

The HIV/AIDS epidemic began in Mexico in 1983 and grew exponentially until 1994, when it stabilized. Up until November 2005, the cumulative number of AIDS cases was 98,933, with a male:female ratio of 5:1. The 2006 estimates indicate 182,000 persons living with HIV/AIDS, of which close to 45,000 are women (male:female ratio of 3:1). In the population aged 15–49, the prevalence is estimated to be 0.3%. However, among specific at-risk groups the prevalence varies: 15% among men who have sex with men, 3.5% in female sex workers, 20% in male sex workers, 6% in intravenous drug users, and 4% in prisoners (*51*). Between 1985 and 2005, 741 cases of AIDS were found in adolescents between the ages of 12 and 17 years (*52*).

An increase in the growth of the epidemic has been seen in the northern border states, due to the increase in the population of intravenous drug users, as much among men as among women (*53*). The situation has become more serious due to the convergence of mobile populations, particularly indigenous groups. In 2004, 4,723 deaths due to HIV/AIDS were registered, representing the 16th leading cause of death in the population as a whole, with a mortality rate of 4.5 per 100,000 population, and the 7th cause of death nationally in the population 15–64 years (*54*). The highest rate of mortality due to AIDS in 2004 was found in the

State of Baja California (9.8 per 100,000 population) and the lowest was in Querétaro (1.7 per 100,000 population). Mortality in Mexico began to drop after access to treatment with antiretrovirals (ARVs) began in 1997 through social security. In 1999, the SSA began giving access to ARVs to the uninsured population, achieving universal access to all registered HIV/AIDS patients in 2003, covering 25,082 persons. The 2005 estimates confirm that more than 30,000 persons living with HIV/AIDS are receiving free treatment through the Mexican health system (*51*). Among other prevention activities, an anti-homophobia campaign began in 2005 through national radio spots. This campaign, supported by UNAIDS, seeks to reduce the stigma and discrimination suffered by gay men, which limits their access to health services and their adherence to therapy. Only 5.4% of pregnant women are tested for HIV (*55*), and the prevention of vertical transmission is not widespread.

In 2004, 10,403 cases of the human papillomavirus were recorded, which represents a rate of 9.8 per 100,000 population, with the highest rate in the State of Nayarit (60.4 per 100,000 population). Five hundred ninety-five cases of gonorrhea were registered, 990 cases of syphilis, 48 cases of congenital syphilis, and 245 cases of soft chancre (*56*).

Zoonoses

Mexico is free of **bovine spongiform encephalopathy**; however, surveillance remains active throughout the country. From 1996 to 2005, a total of 9,903 animals were tested. A restrictive policy is maintained with countries affected by this disease, with a control on importations through a required animal health form. The country has been free of **foot-and-mouth disease** since 1954. A Binational Commission with the U.S.A. oversees a high-security laboratory for the surveillance and prevention of this and other diseases. From 2003 to 2005, more than 1,134 samples were examined through the disease monitoring and surveillance process.

Between 2000 and 2005, 20 deaths from human rabies were identified, 2 of which were transmitted from dog bites, with the rest from wild animals. In 2000, 244 rabid dogs were reported; in 2004, only 42 cases of rabies were identified. The canine antirabies vaccine increased from 13.7 million doses in 2000 to more than 16 million in 2005.

The incidence of brucellosis was stable over the period 2000 to 2004, with an incidence of 2.18 to 2.98 human cases per 100,000 population. The states with the highest number of notifications were Coahuila, Nuevo León, Sinaloa, and Zacatecas, and the principal sources of infections were contaminated milk and milk products, largely from goats. The number of cases of teniasis has dropped and the incidence of this illness in 2004 was 0.37 per 100,000 population, while cysticercosis in humans has remained stable, with an incidence that same year of 0.39 per 100,000 population; for both diseases, most cases were found in the southern states.

Approximately 6.5 million people each year are infected by some infectious agent or parasite (*57*), and it is estimated that two-thirds of them are due to food-borne diseases, which results in more than 4 million cases.

Different species of scorpions are found throughout the country. The lethal species are found principally in the states in the central part of the country and the Pacific coast. In 2000, 208,444 scorpion stings were reported, which represents an incidence of 209.3 cases per 100,000 population, and in 2005 247,976 cases were reported, with a rate of 232.9. This increase is due to improvement in case notification (*58*).

In November 2002, the first case of **West Nile virus** (WNV) was confirmed in Mexico, when seropositive horses were found in the two northern border states of Tamaulipas and Coahuila. Since then, epidemiological surveillance has been strengthened and resulted in confirmation of the presence of WNV in 30 states and 141 municipalities in 2004. During 2005, the presence of WNV was found in 28 states and 135 municipalities; 236 suspected cases were studied in humans, but all were negative. Positive blood tests were reported for 931 horses and 152 birds (*59*).

NONCOMMUNICABLE DISEASES

Metabolic and Nutritional Diseases

Chronic malnutrition in children less than 5 years dropped from 17.7% in 1999 to 12.7% in 2006; moderate malnutrition dropped from 7.5% to 5%; and emaciation dropped from 2% to 1.6%. For the same period, the prevalence of low-height (for age) in children 5 to 11 years dropped from 16.1% to 10.4% for boys and 16.0% to 9.5% for girls. However, overweight and obesity among children aged 5 to 11 years increased from 18.6% in 1999 (20.2% in girls and 17.0% in boys) to 26% in 2006 (26.8% in girls and 25.9% in boys). By 2006, one of three adolescents was considered **overweight** or obese, and 37.4% of women over 20 years of age were overweight and 34.5% were obese (for a total of 71.9%). Among men older than 20 years, 42.5% were overweight and another 24.2% were obese (*30*). In the population 20–49 years, according to health and nutrition surveys from 1988, 1999, and 2006, the prevalence of overweight and obesity was 34.5%, 61.0%, and 69.3%, respectively. The increase is considered a result of changes in food consumption and lifestyle that are causing serious health problems.

The 2006 National Health and Nutrition Survey estimated that 23.7% of preschoolers, 16.6% of school-aged children, and 11.5% of adolescents have **anemia.**

The prevalence of diabetes is estimated to be 7.5% nationally in persons older than 20 years: 2.8 million Mexicans have been diagnosed as diabetics, and close to 820,000 persons are believed to be diabetic without knowing it (*60*). There is a greater prevalence among women aged 50 and older. The prevalence of diabetes increases with age, and it is estimated that one quarter of

70- to 77-year-olds are diabetic. There is a greater prevalence of diabetes in the northern states. Diabetes is the leading cause of death among women and the second leading cause among men, consuming a significant portion of resources for health.

Cardiovascular Diseases

The incidence of cardiovascular diseases increased from 2000 to 2004, largely caused by arterial hypertension, which increased from 401 to 529 per 100,000 population, with a total of 558,139 new cases in 2004. The incidence of ischemic heart diseases grew from 60 per 100,000 population in 2000 to 62 per 100,000 population in 2004. The group most affected was those 65 years and older. Mortality due to heart disease grew over this period, largely caused by circulatory system diseases and ischemic heart diseases. The mortality rate in 2000 from circulatory system diseases was 96.6 per 100,000 population, while in 2004 it was 102.1, and the mortality rate due to ischemic heart disease increased from 43.5 to 48 per 100,000 population. The federal entities most affected were Sonora, Chihuahua, Nuevo León, and the Federal District.

Malignant Neoplasms

In 2000, the mortality rate from neoplasms of all types was 57.1 per 100,000 population, which grew in 2004 to 61.0 per 100,000. Mortality was higher among men than women throughout this period. The tumors with the highest rates of mortality during this period were found in the trachea, bronchial tubes and lungs, stomach, uterus, prostate, and breast (61).

In 2002, the observed rate of cervical-uterine cancer was 20 per 100,000 for women 25 years and older. Despite the decrease in this rate, this type of cancer remains the leading cause of death for this age group. Women who live in indigenous areas have a 30% greater probability of dying from this cause. The mortality rate from breast cancer in 2002 was 17.74 per 100,000 women 25 years and older, and it constitutes the second leading cause of death for this age group (35).

OTHER HEALTH PROBLEMS OR ISSUES

Disasters

Due to its geographical location, as well as its size, Mexico faces natural phenomena such as hurricanes on both the Atlantic and Pacific sides, volcanic activity, earthquakes, cold fronts and heat waves, intense rains, floods, landslides, and forest fires. PAHO's Emergency and Disaster Prevention Program, with information received from Mexican health authorities during 2000–2005, recorded 57 events classified as disasters. Of those events, 72% were classified as natural, and 28% were classified as man-made. The natural disasters included: 14 floods, 7 hurricanes, 8 tropical storms, 4 heat waves, 3 droughts, 2 earthquakes, 2 volcanic eruptions, and 1 landslide. Man-made disasters were: 11

traffic accidents involving transport of dangerous substances, 3 accidents involving miscellaneous explosives and environmental fires caused by man, and 2 industrial accidents. The total number of persons affected by these events was 3,396,106, with 303,800 homes lost and 1,655 injured persons. From 2000–2005, 885 deaths were reported.

In January 2003, an earthquake measuring 7.6 on the Richter scale occurred in Colima that left more than 2,000 homes unsafe, according to experts. These earthquakes are frequent due to the interaction between the Rivera and Cocos plates (62). September 2005 marked the 20th anniversary of the Mexico City earthquake that killed more than 10,000 persons, despite the valiant efforts of the health system. Multiple academic and public efforts were carried out, showing the city's achievements in civil protection. In 2005 alone, the estimated number of hurricanes exceeded the national average of seven tropical storms, with eight total (seven on the Atlantic and one on the Pacific). This was considered one of the most intense years of hurricane activity, affecting the southern states as well as those close to the Gulf of Mexico. Hurricanes Stan and Wilma, among other natural disasters, brought economic loss, displacement of the population, collapse of physical infrastructure, risks of vector-borne diseases, impact on tourism, and damage to agriculture and livestock, which particularly affected the indigenous communities in the Gulf region.

Violence

Discrimination and violence against women persist in Mexico, even resulting in death. Many cases of death among women are unresolved in the judicial system and remain unpunished. Between 1993 and May of 2006, 430 homicides of women in the city of Juarez were documented, with more than 600 disappearances (63). Before being killed, these women were kidnapped, beaten, and raped. Migrant and indigenous girls and adolescents are victims of physical, social, and mental abuse. The need for greater efforts to preserve the rights of women and achieve gender equity in education, salary, and political participation is recognized as necessary to achieve MDG 3.

Addictions

In 2003, the Youth Tobacco Survey indicated that about half of students (51.1%) have experimented or tried cigarettes at some time. One in five students is an actual smoker, with no statistical differences between males (19.6%) and females (19.1%). Among nonsmokers, the rate of susceptibility to start smoking is 25.2%. In secondary schools, the most frequently used drugs are inhalables (4%), followed by marijuana (2.8%), tranquilizers (2.8%), and cocaine (2.5%). Among those between the ages of 12 and 17, 15.1% of males and 5% of females consume alcohol at least once a week (1). It is estimated that 32 million people between the ages of 12 and 65 years consume alcohol, with a per capita annual consumption of 2.8 liters, and an average of 4.5 liters among men between the ages of 18 and 65 years, with growing consumption

The Demographic Bonus: Associated Challenges

With about 100 million inhabitants, Mexico ranks today as the 11th most populated country on the planet and is expected to maintain that position for several decades more. It is estimated that between 2005 and 2025, due to the sustained decrease in the fertility rate, the population replacement rate will be maintained (each couple has the number of children needed to replace them in the population pyramid), but will decline to 1.85 children per women by 2025. Consequently, the demographic transition will change the population pyramid, which will have more individuals of productive age and older adults. Between 2005 and 2025, Mexico will experience a "demographic bonus," where a beneficial relationship will exist between the working age population (15–59) and the dependent population (children under 15 and adults over 60). Given the lesser burden of the dependent population on Mexican families, this period will be an opportunity to favor development policies, job creation, and the formation of social and human capital and, above all, to reduce disparities. However, the benefits of the "demographic bonus" are not automatic. To capitalize on them, Mexico needs to educate young generations in order to develop a better-qualified workforce, invest in or attract investments that generate more and better jobs, and provide a minimum of economic security for older adults. The period will also be marked by an increase in demand for health services and social security, as well as housing. The challenge of providing assistance for the elderly is large since the number of older adults in Mexico (60 years and over) is growing by an average of about 270,000 people each year.

among women (64). The 2006 National Health and Nutrition Survey showed that tobacco use among adolescents between 10 and 19 years old was 7.6%. In 16- to 19-year-olds, it was 25.9% among males and 9.5% among females (tobacco use is defined as smoking more than 100 cigarettes in the course of one's life). Adult males smoke three times more than females, and an increase in the proportion of smokers has been seen since the 2000 Health Survey. Smokers in the 20- to 29-year-old age group increased from 8.4% to 10.7% and in the 50- to 59-year-old age group increased from 9.4% to 10.1% (30).

Environmental Pollution

Nitrogenated products such as fertilizers are used in 5% of agricultural lands, and pesticides are used in 0.14% of lands. The rate of incidence of pesticide poisoning among industrial and rural workers over the period 2000–2003 increased from 0.3 to 0.4 per 10,000 workers.

The Program to Improve Air Quality of the Metropolitan Area of the Valley of Mexico (PROAIRE) 2002–2010 notes that the atmospheric contaminants of greatest importance for public health are ozone (O_3) and particulate matter less than 10 micrometers (PM10). The concentrations of O_3 that were recorded in the Metropolitan Area of the Valley of Mexico (ZMVM) show a 42% decrease over the period 1990–2004, although in 2004, concentrations that exceeded the normal limits for health protection were reported in 6 of 10 days. The lead concentrations in particulates have decreased 94% since 1990, resulting in acceptable levels according to the norm since 1993 (65).

Mexico has a maritime coast of more than 5,000 kilometers and has more than 250 beaches. The result of bacterial quality surveillance in 2005 shows that 17% of the beaches are not safe for recreational use. One-third of the territory is formed by forest or jungle, and 700,000 hectares are deforested each year, resulting, along with fires and change in use of the soil, in only 55% of original jungles being protected (66).

Oral Health

The results of the National Cavity and Dental Fluorosis Survey (1997–2001), with a sample size of 123,293 schoolchildren, show a rate of DMFT (decayed, missing, or filled teeth) of less than 3 for those 12 years of age. The most common dental problems were caries (76%), filled teeth (20%), and lost teeth (1.6%). The prevalence of dental caries for 12-year-olds was 58%. The Epidemiological Surveillance of Oral Pathologies System (SIVEPAB) is working to help people be informed in a trustworthy and convenient way about their different oral health problems including the use of dental fluorosis.

RESPONSE OF THE HEALTH SECTOR

Health Policies and Plans

The 2001–2006 National Development Plan is the principal planning instrument for the federal government. The 2001–2006 National Health Program (PNS) is derived from the National Development Plan and is based on four main principles: 1) good health is one of the development goals and is necessary to achieve true equality in opportunity; 2) health, along with education, is the central component of human capital; 3) health has a strategic potential that should be considered as a social objective and therefore health policies should be complemented with healthy policies; and 4) health protection is a value shared by all societies, all ideological systems, and all political organizations. Good health is a value that can strengthen the social fabric. The challenges the PNS proposes are to achieve equity, technical quality, and quality treatment and to establish a system of financial protection for health (43).

National health authorities have not developed a specific policy for cost containment and have focused sector resources on strengthening prevention programs, whose objective is to improve the quality of life of the population, such as the Even Start in Life (Arranque Parejo en la Vida) Program. The objective of this program is to provide care to boys and girls less than 2 years of age as well as women during pregnancy, childbirth, and postpartum periods, with the goal of combating maternal, neonatal, and infant mortality. The "Care for Pregnant Women" Program (AME) strengthens care to women during pregnancy, birth, and postpartum.

The provision of health services by the SSA was decentralized in two stages: the first during the 1980s and the second during the 1990s. Both processes came about as a response to the perception that the system was bureaucratic and centralized by design. Furthermore, they were developed because health policies resulted in an inefficient assignment of resources to the states and difficult coordination between providers of health services and the uninsured population. The decentralization resulted in a clearer division of responsibilities between federal and state authorities. The federal authorities are responsible for establishing the objectives for health care, defining a legal framework for general system functioning, and ensuring coordination, planning, and follow-up on results. The State Secretariats of Health (SESA) have ample operational flexibility and are responsible for determining the organization and operation of health services for the uninsured population. Coordination between the federal and state authorities is carried out through the National Health Council (CNS), which is made up of the secretaries of health of each state and is presided over by the federal secretary. The CNS has an important role in strengthening and achieving better coordination among the SESA (67).

The IMSS also decentralized its operations, and the reforms tended to transfer the daily administrative decisions to the health service providers, although administration and control of the system remain with the central authorities. The IMSS is divided into 35 delegations clustered into four regions, which are responsible for the strategic planning and control of activities (68).

The health system in Mexico is basically focused on two general laws carried out continuously by the state: the General Law of Health and the Social Security Law. The General Law of Health was reformed on January 1, 2004, to create the System for Social Protection in Health (SPSS) which offers access to health services to all uninsured Mexicans. Also in 2004, an agreement with the tobacco industry was signed to support the SPSS through the Catastrophic Expense Fund. In 2002, the Federal Commission for the Protection Against Health Risks (COFEPRIS) was formed, which unified and homogenized health policy in this area with technical, administrative, and operational autonomy for the regulation, control, and development of sanitary practices in health establishments; availability of organs, tissues, human cells, and their components; availability of blood, medications, toxic or dangerous substances, narcotics, psychotropic drugs, biotech products, primary and additive materials, and establishments dedicated to processing or storing them; sources of ionizing radiation for medical use; harmful effects on human health from environmental factors; international health; and, in general, the required health conditions that cover the processes, products, methods, installations, services, or activities related to the materials described above (69).

Health Strategies and Programs

The 2001–2006 National Health Program includes different efforts 1) to develop conditions and interventions to affect health determinants in an effective way, 2) to achieve better levels of health and well-being of the population, and 3) to support the incorporation of health into national development plans and programs. These goals are translated into 10 priorities that reflect the principal health strategies. They are (43): 1) link health with social and economic development; 2) reduce health risks that affect the poor; 3) combat emerging problems through explicit definition of priorities; 4) launch a crusade for quality in health services; 5) offer financial protection in matters of health to the entire population; 6) construct a cooperative federalism in the area of health; 7) strengthen the oversight role of the Secretariat of Health; 8) advance toward an Integrated Model of Health Care (MIDAS); 9) expand people's participation and freedom of choice in primary health care; and 10) strengthen the investment in human resources, research, and health infrastructure.

The General Law of Health was approved on January 1, 2004, which provided the legal basis for the national System of Social Protection in Health (SPSS). The SPSS, rooted in Popular Insurance ("Seguro Popular") as its fundamental operating mechanism, offers financial protection to those without social health insurance, incorporating it into a scheme with criteria for public insurance.

Popular Insurance coverage reached 1.6 million families in 2004. It is estimated that coverage grew in 2005 to 3.6 million families throughout the 32 states, or more than 12 million people. Within Popular Insurance, 40% of the affiliated families belong to the Opportunities Program, 75% are families headed by women, and 93% are exempt from paying. Popular Insurance provides 154 interventions or services based on the International Classification of Diseases (ICD). For 2005, SPSS had an initial budget of 8,595.7 million pesos (roughly US$ 771 million), 86.5% greater in real terms than in the 2004 budget.

The System of Popular Social Security (SISSP), implemented by the National Council for Social Protection, began in February 2006 (70) and guarantees medical care services, pensions and retirement, and housing to the poorest and is considered a mechanism of equity to fight marginalization. The SISSP functions as an interagency body headed by the President of the Republic. This new system of social security offers beneficiaries a Retirement Savings System, through the Opportunities Program; subsidies for housing, authorized by the National Development Commission; and medical care provided by Popular Insurance.

Organization of the Health System

The Mexican Health System is characterized by its fragmentation in financing as well as in access to health care services. This lack of institutional integration is the source of inequalities in the benefits the population receives, since the various providers receive different levels of payment and provide different levels of care at various levels of quality.

The public sector is characterized by the presence of various insurers and service providers integrated in a vertical fashion that care for different population types, maintain very little contact among them, and differ in the type of financing and organization of the provision of care; the latter is the cause of inefficiencies in the spending of public funds. Furthermore, the system includes a broad, lucrative private health care services sector; persons with the ability to pay can make use of services by paying for the services they receive (43).

In 2005, the social security institutions covered 55 million salaried workers in the formal sector, representing a decrease of 2.56% from 2000, due to a variation in the unemployment rate from 2.2% in 2000 to 3.75% in 2005. The IMSS is the largest insurer, with 44.5 million insured, followed by the Insurance and Social Service Institute for State Workers (ISSSTE), with 10.6 million. This is followed by Petróleos Mexicanos (PEMEX) with 700,000 insured persons and the Armed Forces, the Secretariat of the Navy, and various other insurers for state workers with 600,000. Additionally, the IMSS offers family health insurance for persons with the ability to pay who wish to purchase it through an annual quota payment.

Informal workers, the rural uninsured population, and the unemployed accounted for 45 million people in 2005. They received care from the SSA and the SESA, which oversee public hospitals and clinics. There are huge differences between the states in terms of their availability of per capita resources to provide health services, and there are access problems for those in rural areas.

Furthermore, private nonprofit institutions exist, such as the Mexican Red Cross and numerous nongovernmental organizations (NGOs), which provide medical care with little emphasis on primary health care but play an important role in issues such as HIV/AIDS and the sexual and reproductive health rights of women.

Public Health Services

The principal strategy to address health, education, and nutrition problems in rural areas is the Opportunities Program, which includes comprehensive interventions to improve the health and nutrition of the family, with a special emphasis on vulnerable groups, and provides a special package of health services free of cost (71).

In a parallel way, the National Programs of Health, Environment, and Development conduct lines of work that converge in the promotion of sustainable development with healthier environments and the development of action plans that help overcome the risks and inequalities in this area.

Since 1999, the Mexican Toxicology Network (RETOMEX), which serves as the national registry for poisonings and epidemiological surveillance of environmental health risks, has functioned with the technical collaboration of PAHO/WHO. Better collaboration among national and state entities is required for its full consolidation.

Mexico has been active in various food markets around the globe, particularly with the United States and Canada, within the framework of the Free Trade Agreement (FTA). Efforts over recent years have been aimed at strengthening established norms and the interaction between the health and agriculture sectors to comprehensively address food safety requirements from primary production, through importation/exportation, to consumption, recognizing the need to increase production of clean food to satisfy consumer needs and to take advantage of the opportunities of the international market within the framework of commercial agreements signed by the country.

In the area of food safety, health norms tend to prioritize activity that contributes to the prevention and control of food-borne illnesses, including the production of safe foods. Given this, various federal agencies, state governments, and municipalities, as well as civil society organizations, work together to carry out various programs and activities largely focused on nutritional deficiencies and deficits in four principal areas: food production, promotion of better eating habits, nutritional surveillance, and the complementary provision of food and micronutrients for specific population groups. However, better collaboration between the developed programs and activities is needed by the institutions and the subnational governments; duplication and holes exist that need to be corrected to achieve greater efficiency and impact.

The MDG of reducing the number of homes without water by 50% has been achieved: access to piped water in homes or within the property increased from 75.4% in 1990 to 89.5% in 2004, but significant disparities exist among the states (70.5% in Guerrero and 98.7% in Veracruz, Aguascalientes), and, in rural areas, coverage reaches only 70.5% (72). Approximately 89.4% of the population has sewage and sanitation services, but important variations exist: in Guerrero only 64.7% have these services, while 99.6% in the Federal District have them. Ninety-five percent of the population have electricity and 14.5% have dirt floors in their homes. The latter value reaches 40% in Chiapas, Oaxaca, and Guerrero (22).

In the case of preparedness for disasters, it was estimated that in 2006 there would be 30 hurricanes, five of which could be very intense. For this reason, 27,000 shelters were built and 30,000 guardsmen were made available at the national level. High levels of citizen participation demonstrate the maturity of the population and their civil protection institutions. All these phenomena are constantly monitored by the national system for civil protection. When the municipalities are affected by some sort of natural disaster that exceeds their response capability, the Natural Disaster Fund (FONDEM) is activated to address unforeseen effects (73).

In 2003, the National Committee for Health Security was created as the highest national entity to carry out prevention activities in epidemiological emergencies and disasters, including: those of a hospital-based nature; those resulting from bioterrorism; and those produced by natural disasters, infectious disease outbreaks, or outbreaks due to some other agent (74). The Directorate of Epidemiological Emergencies and Disasters of the SSA coordinates with all the institutions that participate in the response and mitigation of natural disasters (National System of Civil Protection, Social Security, Mexican Red Cross, United Nations agencies, bodies of the National Defense, and nongovernmental organizations).

The SSA, through the National Committee for Health Security, has established a national preparedness plan and response for pandemic influenza, whose principal objective is to maximally reduce the negative health impact on the population. The prevention plan ensures coordination between the different institutions of the country and at the state and jurisdictional levels, ensuring protection to health personnel so they can respond quickly and effectively. Given the eventuality of a pandemic, the epidemiological surveillance systems and the public health laboratory network are being strengthened; identification of priority population groups where vaccinations and antiviral medications would be concentrated is being conducted so that the purchase and strategic storage of medications and goods will be available. The plan is coordinated with the work plans of the other countries in the Region (75).

Individual Care Services

The National Health System provides three levels of personal health services. The first level carries out activities that are focused on health promotion, prevention of disease, and ambulatory care to the ill and is largely provided by general physicians and nurses, with the support of the community. The principal characteristic of the second level of care is ambulatory care and hospitalization, as well as emergency care. This level requires the basic specialties in general hospitals or in specialty hospitals and provides imaging diagnostics and laboratory services. The level of care provided at the tertiary level is specialized, of increasing complexity, and known for clinical and basic research activities. The 12 National Institutes of Health fall into this category.

More than 4,000 hospitals exist in Mexico (or 1 hospital per 100,000 population) (76, 77) and 1,047 belong to the public sector (86.8% are general and 13.2% are specialty).

In 2004, 19,695 health units existed, of which 80.8% belonged to the SSA, IMMS, and Opportunities Program, and 19.2% were used by those with private insurance. Of the health units, 94.31% provided outpatient care and 5.69% hospitalization (78).

The number of outpatient visits by the uninsured and insured populations in authorized public institutions increased from 231 million visits in 2000 to 250 million in 2004. Of the visits, 54.18% were for the insured population and 45.82% were for the uninsured, with the greatest number of visits by the IMSS (41.19%); followed by the SSA (38.56%); the ISSSTE (9.26%); and the IMSS-Opportunities, PEMEX, SEDENA, and SEMAR (the remaining 10.99%).

In 2004, 37.7 million specialty consultations were approved in the National System. The Federal District is the area with the greatest number of consultations of this type, with Tlaxcala and Baja California Sur in last place. Emergency consultations increased by 1.2% (25.5 million) in 2004, and dental visits increased by 6.3% (12.7 million) compared to 2000 (79).

In 2004, 3 million surgeries were performed, 2.7% more than in 2003. The number of births was around 1 million, which was similar in 2002. In 2004, hospital discharges and patient days were 4,719 and 20,613, respectively.

In 2004, 77,705 hospital beds were counted, and 54,113 health units, 2,626 surgical units, and 2,085 clinical laboratories and 1,888 radiology centers were found (80). The greatest percentage of hospital beds was found in the public sector in the SESA hospitals, followed by the IMSS, with a smaller percentage in PEMEX. At the state level, Durango had the greatest availability of counted beds for the population receiving care through the SSA, and the least availability was found in Baja California Sur with less than one bed per 2,000 population. The Federal District had the greatest availability of counted and total beds, and the fewest were found in the state of México (28, 77).

In 2004, the Even Start in Life Program achieved 11 million family planning visits, 69.3% for the uninsured population and 28.37% for the insured population. These visits allowed more than 10,352 patients to continue using their family planning methods and 2.2 million users were able to begin (78).

In 2004, a total of 257,039,893 studies were conducted, including clinical laboratory (87.82%), radiological (7.68%), other studies (2.83%), and anatomical pathology (1.67%) (81). In 2004, the Centers for Rehabilitation and Special Education (CREE) authorized 2.5 million rehabilitation therapy sessions, 1,101,312 consultations, and 32,463 functional interventions (such as prosthesis).

Blood banks are linked through a network headed by the National Blood Transfusion Center, which includes 31 state centers and, in total, covers 598 blood banks, which receive 1.3 million donations annually. Ninety-six percent were replacement donations and 4% were altruistic donations, which was an increase of 3.87% over 2003 (*82*). In 2005, HIV/AIDS transmission was eliminated from all blood transfusion processes.

The Umbilical Cord Blood Bank was established in 2003 and is in charge of securing, processing, studying, storing, selecting, and releasing hematopoietic progenitor cells for allogeneic and/or autologous transplants obtained from umbilical cord blood.

Medical, ambulatory, hospital and emergency, and specialized services have grown in number, material resources, and financing with a positive direct impact on the quantity of services provided, such as visits, studies, donations, number of immunizations, and facilities for federal entities. Programs aimed at prevention, detection, and timely treatment, specifically for vulnerable groups also have been created.

The practice of traditional medicine has been legal in Mexico since 2005 and is defined as: "the joining of systems of health care that have their roots in the profound knowledge of health and disease of the different indigenous and rural populations that has accumulated through their history, based on an interpretation of the world, health, and illness of pre-Hispanic indigenous origin that has incorporated elements emerging from other cultures, such as old Spanish medicine, African medicine, and institutional Western medicine" (*83*). A high number of practitioners such as birth attendants, healers, bonesetters, and herbalists are used, as well as a variety of cultivated flowers. Traditional medicine has social recognition that has become a fundamental resource for the health of millions of people. Dependence on oral tradition, the plundering of natural areas in which practitioners obtain a large part of their resources, bio-pirating, and the exploitation of traditional knowledge are problems that affect the practice and development of traditional medicine. In Puebla, Chiapas, and Oaxaca, hospital based care is being oriented toward a mixed approach, combining allopathic and traditional medicine while incorporating an intercultural focus on health care.

Health Promotion

In 2004, in 29 of the federal entities 466 civil organizations, such as "Avales Ciudadanos" ("Endorsing Citizens"), worked to improve the quality of care in the delivery of health services. The "Avales Ciudadanos" are civil society organizations that, with a commitment to serve, receive training and endorse (or not) the results of indicators of proper conduct in health centers and hospitals (*84*). The program's objective is to incorporate the population into the process of evaluating the quality of health services through their active participation in certifying or endorsing the processes and results of monitoring the indicators of proper conduct in medical settings, which will contribute to providing society with a sense of transparency and trustworthiness (*85*).

The SSA coordinates health promotion campaigns, which rely on mobilization at the municipal level. A total of 1,794 municipalities participated in 2004 in this mobilization and became part of a national network and 30 state networks.

Health Supplies

The federal and state governments and social security allot funds for the acquisition of pharmaceuticals for public sector patients that are included in the basic table established by the General Health Council. The list includes 776 generic medications that have been determined to be effective, safe, high-quality, and accessible. The supply of these products is dominated by national companies and represents 80% of public acquisitions; the volume of sales in the private market represents 20%; in the public market the IMSS and the ISSSTE represent 80.3% and 14.2%, respectively, of the public acquisition of pharmaceuticals, while the federal and state systems represent 5.4%. The public sector is allowed to acquire only medications that are included on the list of bioequivalent interchangeable generics (*86*).

A regulatory framework and drug registry have been established to ensure that the producers comply with norms for effectiveness, safety, and quality. Two types of generic drugs exist: 1) interchangeable generics, which include products where the "substitutability" or possibility of substitution is demonstrated by a collection of clinical studies, and 2) "copycat products," which include medications that lack the safety and effectiveness tests.

With the goal of stimulating the market for interchangeable generics, the General Health Council began requiring in 2002 that all public health institutions purchase interchangeable generics, when available in the Mexican market, instead of "copycat products." Since this decision was made, the number of interchangeable generics has increased from 963 to 2,606 products.

Human Resources

Mexico has 78 medical schools, of which 54 form part of the Mexican Association of Faculties and Schools of Medicine (AMFEM). In 2003, the National Association of Universities and Institutions of Higher Learning (ANUIES) registered 36 postgraduate programs in public health (*87*). Between 2000 and 2002 the number of admissions into nursing programs increased by 21.1% and into medical school by 26.3%.

The human resources of physicians and nurses are largely hired as salaried employees in public institutions, which does not lead to efficiency. On the other hand, a large proportion of physicians maintain private practices and are paid out-of-pocket.

Human resources in health that work in the public sector are distributed as follows: 143,605 physicians, of which 85% have direct patient contact, and of those 45% provide services to the public and 55% work in social security. Nurses number 192,828, with 43% providing care to the population at large and 57% to those in social security (88).

During the last 10 years the number of professionals and technical health staff contracted by public institutions has increased; the number of physicians went from 0.3 per 1,000 population in 1993 to 1.20 in 1997 and to 1.14 in 2002 (89), lower than the Latin American average, which in 2000 was 1.79 per 1,000 population.

The distribution of human resources is unequal across the states. In the Federal District, human resources surpass 2.5 per 1,000 population, while the states of San Luís Potosí, Chihuahua, Michoacán, Oaxaca, Guanajuato, Baja California Sur, Puebla, Chiapas, and México do not even reach 1.0 per 1,000 population. Nationally, almost 45% of doctors are specialists, but there are states where more than 50% are specialists. The SSA is the institution with the largest number of contracted physicians (56,113), followed by the IMSS (55,842), the ISSSTE (15,574), and the IMSS-Opportunities (5,541). Public and private higher learning institutions rarely coordinate or plan their training policies, including content and practices for training, and therefore there is significant variation among their graduates (90). Nurses exceed 190,000: the IMSS contracts the greatest number (79,715), followed by the SSA (74,475), the ISSSTE (19,899), and the IMSS-Opportunities (6,847) (91).

Women outnumber men in the health services workforce. The medical profession is witnessing growth in the number of women, who in 1970 represented 19% of graduating physicians, but by 1999 represented half of graduates. However, there are still twice as many male physicians as women. Nursing is almost completely dominated by women (95%). Sixty-four percent of nurses have some technical training, 34% hold a bachelors degree, and 2% have some level of postgraduate training (92).

Research and Technological Development in Health

The call by the National Council on Science and Technology (CONACYT) during the second half of 2005 lists the following specific priorities for health research: breast cancer, development of health systems, arterial hypertension, emerging infectious diseases (tuberculosis and HIV/AIDS), chronic renal insufficiency, and obesity (93).

The percentage of researchers belonging to the National System of Researchers (SNI) grew in all the National Health Institutes, decentralized hospitals of the SSA, and in the IMSS. In 2004, the National Institutes of Neurology and Neurosurgery, Respiratory Illnesses and Cardiology excelled in their performance.

Advancement has been made in telemedicine, and 1,025 health centers now have access to electronic content and the Internet (2005). Eighteen medical centers in the states of Puebla, Guerrero, Nuevo León, and Oaxaca have the professional equipment to conduct telemedicine, and in 8 federal entities telemedicine services and tele-education are offered (94).

The National Center of Excellence in Technology (CENETEC) has developed the Information Bank of Health Technology (BITS), which provides technological information in terms of efficacy, safety, cost-effectiveness, and norms to facilitate decision making in the purchasing and use of medical equipment (95).

Health Sector Expenditures and Financing

Health services are financed by different sources. Social security is financed through worker-employer quotas and the services to the population at large through two large funds: those generated by the federal government and those that are provided by federal entities. Private financing largely comes from out-of-pocket expenditures or through private insurance (96). In Mexico it is estimated that only 4% of the population has private insurance and that half of that insurance is covered by employers who have the ability to deduct the cost of the premiums through their taxable income. The buyers of private insurance largely come from the high-income segments of the population.

The health sector is characterized by its relatively low public expenditure, below the Latin American average of 7% of the GDP, equivalent to 76,455.9 million pesos in 2005 (US$ 6.863 million). Nonetheless, health expenditures in recent years increased from 5.6% of the GDP in 2000 to 6.3% in 2004, for a 13% increase (28).

Of the total public expenditure, 37.2% was spent in institutions that cover the uninsured population, through the SSA, the Institutes of Health, and the federal entities, which receive resources from the Contribution Fund to Health Services (FASSA); the remaining 62.8% was distributed to institutions that provide care to the insured population, such as the Secretariat of National Defense (SEDENA), PEMEX, IMSS, and ISSSTE, as well as the Secretariat of the Navy.

Technical Cooperation and External Financing

In 2000, Mexico joined with 189 other countries in signing the Millennium Declaration, which carries a commitment to generate and strengthen regional and local programs and activities to eradicate poverty and hunger, improve education, provide gender equity, provide environmental sustainability, improve health, and strengthen global relationships for development (34).

In the area of technical cooperation, five areas of work (which contain 18 priorities and 45 lines of action) have been defined for the next five years. This proposal of strategic areas of work was established based on the reality identified through the Country Cooperation Strategy (CCS) exercise.

The World Bank is conducting the Health Quality, Equity and Development Program with an original budget of US$ 350 million (97). With this program, equity in access to health services in underserved urban areas is promoted; it helps increase access and quality of health services for indigenous populations and persons with lower levels of overall well-being; it supports institutional development; and it develops innovative models of care and preventive care for vulnerable populations.

References

1. México, Instituto Nacional de Estadística Geográfica e Informática. Producto nacional bruto per cápita, países seleccionados, 2005. Available at: http://www.inegi.gob.mx/est/contenidos/espanol/rutinas/ept.asp?t=inte12&c=5110.

2. México, Consejo Nacional de Población. En base a la información del Banco de México. Available at: http://www.banxico.org.mx.

3. México, Instituto Nacional de Estadística Geográfica e Informática. Encuesta Nacional de Ocupación y Empleo. Available at: www.inegi.gob.mx.

4. México, Comisión para Asuntos de la Frontera Norte. Programa de Desarrollo Regional 2001–2006. Available at: http://fronteranorte.presidencia.gob.mx.

5. México, Instituto Nacional de Estadística Geográfica e Informática. Sistema de Cuentas Nacionales de México. Available at: www.inegi.gob.mx.

6. México, Secretaría de Desarrollo Social; agosto 2002. Available at: http://www.sedesol.gob.mx/ofsec/prensa/index.htm.

7. México, Secretaría de Desarrollo Social. Available at: www.oportunidades.gob.mx.

8. Székely M. Veinte años de desigualdad en México. In: Cuadernos de Desarrollo Humano. Secretaría de Desarrollo Social; 2005.

9. Organization for Economic Cooperation and Development. OECD Factbook 2006. Economic, environmental and social statistics. OECD; 2006.

10. Programa de las Naciones Unidas para el Desarrollo. Índice de desarrollo humano 2005. Available at: http://hdr.undp.org/reports/global/2005/espanol/.

11. Programa de las Naciones Unidas para el Desarrollo. Informe sobre el desarrollo humano. México; 2004.

12. México, Consejo Nacional de Población. Índice de marginación; 2000. Available at: http://www.conapo.gob.mx.

13. Naciones Unidas, Oficina del Alto Comisionado para los Derechos Humanos en México. Diagnóstico de la situación de los derechos humanos en México; 2003.

14. Cervallos D. El narcotráfico se ensaña y acalla. Tierra Viva América Latina; 10 de febrero de 2006. Available at: http://www.ipsterraviva.net/LA/viewstory.asp?idnews=413.

15. México, Instituto Nacional de Estadística Geográfica e Informática. XII Censo General de Población y Vivienda, México, DF; 2000.

16. México, Instituto Nacional de Estadística Geográfica e Informática. Cartografía de usos de suelo y vegetación. Serie II y III. Available at: www.inegi.gob.mx.

17. México, Secretaría de Salud. Estadísticas. Available at: http://www.ssa.gob.mx/htdocs/estadisticas.

18. México, Consejo Nacional de Población. Proyecciones de la población de México 2000–2050. Primera edición. CONAPO; 2002.

19. México, Consejo Nacional de Población. 11 de julio, Día Mundial de la Población. México, DF; 2004.

20. México, Secretaría de Salud. Programa de Acción: programa de atención a la salud de la adolescencia; 2002.

21. México, Consejo Nacional de Población. Informe de ejecución del Programa de Acción de la Conferencia Internacional sobre la Población y el Desarrollo. 1994–2003. México, DF: CONAPO; 2004.

22. Organización Panamericana de la Salud. Indicadores básicos de salud 2004. En base al XII Censo General de Población y Vivienda 2000. OPS; SSA.

23. United States of America, Embassy in Mexico. The foreign-born population in the United States; March 1997. Available at: http://www.usembassy-mexico.gov/ecensus.pdf.

24. United States of America, Census Bureau. Data profiles; 2002.

25. México, Secretaría de Salud, Dirección General de Información.

26. Organización Panamericana de la Salud. Indicadores básicos. Washington, DC: OPS; 2005.

27. Organización Panamericana de la Salud. Estadísticas de salud de las Américas; 2006.

28. México, Secretaría de Salud. Salud: México 2004. Informe para la rendición de cuentas. México, DF: SSA; 2005. Available at: www.salud.gob.mx.

29. México, Secretaría de Salud, Dirección General de Información. Tablas de mortalidad; 2004.

30. México, Secretaría de Salud, Instituto Nacional de Salud Pública. Encuesta Nacional de Salud y Nutrición 2006. Cuernavaca; 2006.

31. México, Instituto Nacional de Estadística Geográfica e Informática. Estadísticas de mortalidad. Porcentaje de defunciones de 5 a 14 años por sexo y principales causas 1990–2004. Available at: http://www.inegi.gob.mx/est/contenidos/espanol/rutinas/.

32. México, Secretaría de Salud, Dirección General Adjunta de Epidemiología. Anuarios de morbilidad 2004. Available at: http://www.dgepi.salud.gob.mx/infoepi/index.htm.

33. México, Secretaría de Salud, Dirección General de Información. Lista 165. [Cálculos a partir de cubos de mortalidad de la Organización Panamericana de la Salud-México]. Available at: http://dgis.salud.gob.mx/cubos/.

34. México, Gobierno de la República. Los objetivos de desarrollo del milenio en México. Informe de avance; 2005.

35. México, Secretaría de Salud. Salud: México 2002. Información para la rendición de cuentas. México, DF: SSA; 2003.

36. Magally S. Pide CONAPO revisar programas de salud reproductiva. Alta mortalidad materna entre mujeres jóvenes. CIMAC Noticias. México, DF; 28 de marzo de 2005. Avail-

able at: http://www.cimacnoticias.com/noticias/05mar/05032801.html.

37. México, Consejo Nacional de Población. El impacto de la transición demográfica en los hogares y las familias. Available at: http://www.conapo.gob.mx/prensa/carpetas/carpeta 2002_11.htm.

38. México, Consejo Nacional de Población. 4 de cada 10 de los hogares son vulnerables. Available at: http://www.conapo.gob.mx/prensa/carpetas/carpeta/ marzo 03 2002_11.htm.

39. México, Secretaría de Salud, Programa de Mujer y Salud. Violencia familiar. México, DF; 2002.

40. México, Secretaría de Salud. Encuesta Nacional sobre Violencia contra las Mujeres 2003. México, DF; 2003.

41. Organización Internacional de Trabajo. Perfil nacional de seguridad y salud en el trabajo. [Unpublished document]; 2006.

42. México, Secretaría del Trabajo y Previsión Social, Dirección General de Seguridad y Salud en el Trabajo.

43. México, Secretaría de Salud. Programa Nacional de Salud 2001–2006.

44. Programa Nacional de los Pueblos Indígenas, 2001–2006. Available at: http://indigenas.presidencia.gob.mx.

45. México, Consejo Nacional de Población. Concepto y dimensiones de la marginación. In: Índices de marginación 2000. CONAPO; 2000: 11.

46. México, Secretaría de Salud, Programa de Acción.

47. Radio Nuevitas. Noticias internacionales. Available at: http://www.radionuevitas.co.cu/nuevas_noticias/Internacionales_150406_03.asp.

48. Comisión para Asuntos de la Frontera Norte. XI Salud. Frontera Saludable 2001–2006. Available at: http://fronteranorte.presidencia.gob.mx.

49. México, Centro Nacional para la Prevención y el Control del VIH/SIDA; Consejo Nacional contra las Adicciones. El consumo de drogas inyectadas y la epidemia de VIH/SIDA en México. CENSIDA; CONADIC; 2003.

50. México, Secretaría de Salud, Centro Nacional de Vigilancia Epidemiológica; 2004.

51. México, Centro Nacional para la Prevención y el Control del VIH/SIDA; Secretaría de Salud. El SIDA en cifras 2005. Available at: http://www.salud.gob.mx/conasida/.

52. México, Secretaría de Salud, Dirección General de Epidemiología. Registro nacional de casos de SIDA. Datos al 31 de diciembre del 2005.

53. México, Centro Nacional para la Prevención y el Control del VIH/SIDA; Secretaría de Salud. Dos décadas de la epidemia de SIDA en México. Available at: http://www.salud.gob.mx/conasida/.

54. México, Secretaría de Salud, Dirección General de Información en Salud. Principales causas de mortalidad 2004. SSA; SINAIS.

55. México, CONASIDA, Comité de Monitoreo y Evaluación. Boletín del grupo de información sectorial de VIH/SIDA; diciembre 2004.

56. México, Secretaría de Salud, Dirección General de Epidemiología.

57. México, Secretaría de Salud, Sistema Nacional de Vigilancia Epidemiológica; 2003.

58. México, Secretaría de Salud, Centro Nacional de Vigilancia Epidemiológica; 2004.

59. México, Secretaría de Salud, Dirección General Adjunta de Epidemiología; 2000 y 2005.

60. México, Instituto Nacional de Salud Pública; Secretaría de Salud. Encuesta Nacional de Salud 2000. Vol. 2. La salud en los adultos. 2003.

61. México, Secretaría de Salud. Registro histopatológico de neoplasias malignas. Compendio de cáncer; 2003.

62. México, Secretaría de Gobernación. El sismo de Tecomán, Colima.

63. México, Mujeres de Juárez. Available at: http://www.mujeresdejuarez.org.

64. México, Instituto Nacional de Salud Pública; Secretaría de Salud. Encuesta Nacional de Adicciones (ENA) 2002.

65. México, Secretaría del Medio Ambiente del GDF, Sistema de Monitoreo Atmosférico. Informe del estado de la calidad del aire y tendencias 2004.

66. Organización para la Cooperación y el Desarrollo Económico. Informe anual 2004.

67. México, Secretaría de Salud, Consejo Nacional de Salud. Available at: http://www.salud.gob.mx/unidades/cns/.

68. México, Instituto Mexicano del Seguro Social. Available at: http://www.imss.gob.mx.

69. México, Secretaría de Salud, Comisión Federal para la Protección contra Riesgos Sanitarios. Available at: http://www.cofepris.gob.mx/mj/mj.htm.

70. Comunicado de prensa No. 2006-103 del 22 de febrero de 2006. Available at: http://www.salud.gob.mx/.

71. México, Secretaría de Desarrollo Social. Programa Institucional Oportunidades 2002–2006. México, DF; 2003.

72. México, Instituto Nacional de Estadística Geográfica e Informática. Censo General de Población y Vivienda 1990 y 2000.

73. México, Sistema Nacional de Protección Social. Available at: http://www.proteccioncivil.gob.mx.

74. Diario Oficial de la Federación. Acuerdo por el que se crea el Comité Nacional para la Seguridad en Salud; 22 de septiembre de 2003.

75. México, Secretaría de Salud. Plan nacional de preparación y respuesta ante una pandemia de influenza, 2006. Available at: http://www.dgepi.salud.gob.mx/pandemia/anexoa.pdf.

76. México, Secretaría de Salud. Programa Nacional de Salud; 2004.

77. México, Secretaría de Salud. Observatorio del Desempeño Hospitalario; 2004.

78. Quinto Informe de Gobierno del Presidente de los Estados Unidos Mexicanos Vicente Fox Quesada; 1 de septiembre de 2005. Available at: http://quinto.informe.fox.presidencia.gob.mx/.

79. México, Instituto Nacional de Estadística Geográfica e Informática. Consultas externas otorgadas en instituciones del Sistema Nacional de Salud según tipo de consulta, 1995 a 2005. Available at: http://www.inegi.gob.mx/est/contenidos/espanol/rutinas/ept.asp?t=msal26&c=6074.

80. México, Instituto Nacional de Estadística Geográfica e Informática. Recursos materiales seleccionados en instituciones del Sistema Nacional de Salud, 1995 a 2005. Available at: http://www.inegi.gob.mx/est/contenidos/espanol/rutinas/ept.asp?t=msal26&c=6069.

81. México, Sistema Nacional de Información en Salud. Available at: http://sinais.salud.gob.mx.

82. México, Secretaría de Salud. Datos sobre donaciones de sangre. Available at: http://www.ssa.gob.mx/unidades/cnts.

83. México, Secretaría de Salud, Dirección de Medicina Tradicional y Desarrollo Intercultural.

84. México, Secretaría de Salud. Quinto informe de labores.

85. Hospital General de México. Información sobre el aval ciudadano. Available at: http://hgm.salud.gob.mx/Aval_Ciud/pdf/acta_avalciu.pdf.

86. Organización para la Cooperación y el Desarrollo Económico. Estudios sobre los sistemas de salud en México.

87. México, Asociación Nacional de Universidades e Instituciones de Educación Superior. Anuario estadístico 2003. Población escolar de posgrado. Available at: http://www.anuies.mx/servicios/e_educacion/docs/pep_peeiep03.pdf.

88. México, Observatorio de Recursos Humanos para la Salud. Available at: http://dgces.salud.gob.mx/observatorio/index Inv.html.

89. México, Secretaría de Salud. Boletín de información estadística: recursos y servicios, 2002.

90. Ruiz JA, Molina J, Nigenda G. Médicos y mercado de trabajo en México. In: Calidoscopio de la Salud. México, DF: Fundación Mexicana para la Salud; 2003.

91. México, Instituto Nacional de Estadística Geográfica e Informática; Secretaría de Salud. Encuesta de unidades médicas privadas con servicios de hospitalización; 2002.

92. Ramírez MA, Méndez O, Nigenda G, Vargas MM. Recursos humanos en los servicios de salud: una perspectiva de género. Fundación Mexicana para la Salud; 2002. Available at: http://www.funsalud.org.mx/casesalud/sintesis,%20etc/Recursos%20humanos.pdf.

93. México, Consejo Nacional de Ciencia y Tecnología. Available at: http://www.conacyt.mx/fondos/ssaimss/2005-02/resultados_pertinencia-2.htm.

94. México, Instituto Nacional de Salud Pública. Elevar calidad de los servicios, prioridad de la reforma en salud. México, DF: Secretaría de Salud; 6 de marzo de 2006; Sección: Prensa. Available at: http://www.insp.mx/Portal/Noticias/Marzo06/noticia080306.html.

95. México, Secretaría de Salud, Centro Nacional de Excelencia Tecnológica en Salud. Available at: http://www.salud.gob.mx:8080/JSPCenetec/web_consulta/html/institucion/terminos.html.

96. México, Secretaría de Salud. Manual del Sistema de Cuentas Nacionales y Estatales de Salud en México. 2004.

97. Banco Mundial. Available at: http://www.bancomundial.org.mx/bancomundial/SitioBM.nsf/vwCatProy/DC4D960500400A07306256E7E0068CB59?OpenDocument&pag=2.3&nivel=2.

485

MONTSERRAT

Saint Peter

Saint George

Plymouth

Saint Anthony

Barbuda

Saint Kitts and Nevis

Antigua

Montserrat

Guadeloupe

Dominica

0   2.5   5 Miles

M

ontserrat, one of the Leeward Islands in the Eastern Caribbean, lies roughly 40 km southwest of Antigua. Montserrat is an island of volcanic origin; its topography is dominated by three mountainous regions—Silver Hills, Center Hills, and Soufriere Hills—surrounded by a small coastal lowland belt.

GENERAL CONTEXT AND HEALTH DETERMINANTS

The island's vegetation ranges from lush tropical forest at higher elevations to dry grasslands in some coastal areas. The terrain has hot springs, ravines, black sand beaches, and one white sand beach in the north. The country is well watered with several natural springs. The climate is tropical, usually tempered by sea breezes. Yearly rainfall averages 1,475 mm, with most rain falling in the second half of the year. June to November is the hurricane season.

Montserrat is a British overseas territory with its own system of government. The Executive Council consists of a Chief Minister, three other elected Ministers, a Governor who represents the Queen, an Attorney General, and a Finance Secretary. There also is an 11-seat Legislative Council, 9 of whose members are popularly elected.

Most residents are of African descent. The dominant religious denominations were Anglican (21.8%), Methodist (17%), Pentecostal (14.1%), Roman Catholic (11.6%), and Seventh Day Adventist (10.6%), and the remainder were Church of God, Hindu, Rastafarian, and unspecified. Standard English is the official language but a Montserrat Creole English is most widely spoken on a daily basis.

Montserrat's Geralds Airport provides regular inter-island services to and from V.C. Bird International airport in Antigua, a connecting hub to other destinations. The unit of currency is the Eastern Caribbean dollar (EC$) pegged at EC$ 2.70 to US$ 1.

Montserrat's Soufriere Hills Volcano became active on July 18, 1995. The volcano's subsequent eruptive activity in the late 1990s and the more recent ventings of ash and pyroclastic flows have been at the center of life for the island's residents. More than half of the 12,000 inhabitants left the island after the eruption in 2000.

In early August 2005, a new lava dome grew in the Soufriere volcanic crater, following a period of vigorous ash emission and explosions that began in June of that year. This was the first lava extrusion in two years following the giant collapse of the previous dome in July of 2003. The 1998–2002 Sustainable Development Plan indicated that, based on public consultations and a policy discussion, the future of Montserrat is dependent upon developing the north of the island.

The loss of Plymouth and the other major urban and agricultural areas in Montserrat's south was a key factor affecting the territory's economy. The evacuation associated with the volcano was one of the primary causes of the loss of assets. There is a one in four chance of continued magmatic activity for the next 30 years. Under these conditions, the area north of Lawyers Mountain line is safe from all but the most severe volcanic activity and so is suitable for all forms of development. Continued damage assessment was carried out to determine the true losses from volcanic activities. In the reporting period, sections of the north were developed and this area continued to absorb substantial levels of development without long-term damage to the environment.

The volcanic crisis had a particularly dramatic impact on the private sector. Not only did large inward investors leave the island, but assets were destroyed and local markets which supported small and medium enterprises became fragmented. Many businesses fell into debt and key subsectors that had been targeted for development before the crisis, such as tourism, information technology, and export oriented light manufacturing, were decimated (1).

The Soufriere Hills Volcano continued to have intermittent eruptions, sometimes depositing large amounts of ash in inhabited areas, resulting in disruption in the schools and people's livelihood.

Social, Political, and Economic Determinants

The volcanic crisis has been an ongoing source of vulnerability, dependency, and poverty in Montserrat. In response to the 1998–2002 Sustainable Development Plan's objective seeking protection through social welfare, the Government of Montserrat undertook the development of a comprehensive and integrated welfare system that would provide a safety net for vulnerable groups, thus responding to their immediate needs. The Plan superseded the crisis food voucher payments that were part of the public assistance program before the eruption. Instead, a means tested social welfare system that has been in place since 2000 provides a basic allowance for food. In addition, since 2001 the Government has provided a rental subsidy for vulnerable government housing tenants. The main beneficiaries of this program were the elderly and the mentally and physically disabled, who had no other means of support.

Since the Soufriere Hills Volcano eruption, tourism dwindled to mostly one-day visits from Antigua and Nevis. Data show the number of arrivals of day-trippers and overnight guests increased by 11% in 2000, compared to 1999; there also was a subsequent increase of 9% in 2001. In 2002, there were 12,400 visitor arrivals, representing a 10% decrease from the 13,700 recorded in 2001. This drop was largely attributable to the extension of the Volcano Exclusion Zone, which made many villas and the Vue Pointe Hotel inaccessible.

In 2004, the GDP at factor cost was US$ 35.0 million, compared to US$ 30.6 million in 2001. GDP at market prices for 2004 was US$ 41.0 million, compared to US$ 34.7 million in 2001. The rate of inflation for 2002 was 3.5%.

The majority of persons who participated in a 2002 poverty assessment survey agreed that there was poverty in Montserrat, even if it affected only a few persons (2). Several groups were identified as possibly at risk—single households headed by women who had no support, the elderly (especially without family support), the mentally challenged who are unable to look after themselves, teenage girls needing help, and potentially disaffected male youths who either underachieve at school or leave school without finishing.

The above-mentioned survey established a ranking for people facing difficulties on the island—definitely not making it (scrunting), possibly not making it (scraping through), barely making it (down but not out), making out (but stretched), and making it (doing okay). The matrix illustrated the unique circumstances in Montserrat, highlighting the multidimensional nature of the losses due to the volcanic eruption and its aftermath, particularly the loss of support networks (social capital) that people had relied on in the past to help them through difficult times (2). According to the 2001 census, 2,029 persons were economically active (1,154 males and 875 females). Unemployment stood at 13%, with 169 males unemployed compared to 100 females.

The Montserrat school system includes both public and private schools. In 2005, there were three nursery schools, two government run primary schools, two privately run primary schools, and one public secondary school.

One new day care center opened and another was expanded in 2002, which made it possible for more children to access early childhood education at minimal cost. Access to primary education also increased in 2002 with the addition of a fourth grade in one primary school; in 2005, two additional grades were included. The Government constructed Montserrat Community College in 2004.

Of the 2,082 households recorded in the 2001 census, 1,759 had access to publicly supplied water piped into the home; 210 had publicly supplied water piped to the yard; 72 relied on public standpipes; 10 had water piped by a private provider; 3 used public wells (tanks); and the remainder used other means. Of the total households, 1,521 had a water closet linked to a cesspit, 296 had water closets linked to a sewer, 135 had pit latrines, 77 had no toilet facilities, and 53 relied on other means.

Demographics, Mortality, and Morbidity

The mid-year population in 2005 was estimated at 4,785. The population growth rate for 2003 and 2004 was 2.4% and 2.5%, respectively.

The 2001 Population and Housing Census estimated the resident population at 4,465; 2,405 (53.9%) were males and 2,060 (46.1%) were females. This figure represented a 42% decline from the 1991 census (total population, 10,639, 49.7% male and 50.3% female). This pattern of alternating population growth and decline has been characteristic of Montserrat since censuses began to be conducted. Figure 1 shows the population structure by age and sex, in 1990 and in 2001.

According to the 2001 census, the population under 15 years old accounted for 19.3% (869) of the population that year; the age group 15–64 years old comprised 65.0% (2910); women of childbearing age (15–49 years old) comprised 23.0% (997). There were 82.0% nationals and 18.0% non-nationals. Since the volcanic eruption, Montserrat's population has concentrated in the north of the island.

Chronic noncommunicable diseases that are influenced by lifestyle choices dominated the morbidity and mortality profiles. Hypertension, diabetes, chronic respiratory diseases, and malignant neoplasms were among the leading causes of death.

In 1999–2003, there were 204 deaths from defined causes. The five leading causes were diseases of the circulatory system, 32.3% (84); malignant neoplasms, 16.3% (42); diabetes mellitus, 15.8% (41); diseases of the respiratory system, 8.5% (22); and mental and behavioral disorders, 5.8% (15). Of deaths from all causes (260), more men (139) than women (121) died. There was one maternal death in 2001 due to complications in pregnancy. In 2004–2005 there were 71 deaths from defined causes. The five leading causes were diabetes mellitus, 17.4% (20); cardiac arrest, 15.7% (18); hypertensive diseases, 14.8% (17); cerebrovascular accident, 7.0% (8); and ischemic heart disease, 7.0% (8). Of deaths from all causes (115), more males (65) than females (50) died.

Immigrants to the country mainly came from CARICOM countries (Dominica, Guyana, and Saint Kitts and Nevis top the list), the United States of America, and the United Kingdom.

HEALTH OF POPULATION GROUPS

Children under 5 Years Old

In 2000–2005, there were 252 live births. There were no deaths in this age group. The number of low-birthweight babies (under 2,500 g) ranged from 1 in 2000 to 10 in 2005. There were six stillbirths in the reporting period. Child health clinics are held weekly at all health centers; there was 100% registration of children under 5 in the clinics.

FIGURE 1. Population structure, by age and sex, Montserrat, 1990 and 2001.

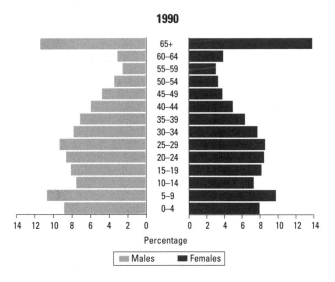

1990

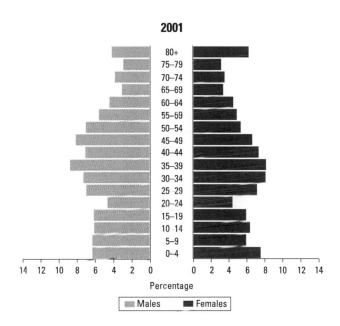

2001

checks, and laboratory tests for hemoglobin. In 2002, 176 students aged 5 to 15 years from five schools were examined (90 males and 86 females). Of them, 78 (44.3%) had normal physical findings and 98 (55.7%) had abnormal findings, with dental caries being the main abnormal physical finding. Other findings included anemia (4), underweight (8), and overweight (18). The male to female ratio of underweight students was 1:3 (3).

Adolescents 10–14 and 15–19 Years Old

There were no deaths among 10–14-year-olds and four deaths among 15–19-year-olds. The causes of death were diseases of the circulatory system (1) and external causes (3). There were 35 births to women under 19 years old in 2000–2005, including four in the age group under 16 years old. There was one reported case of HIV infection in the 15–19-year-old age group.

Adults 20–59 Years Old

There were 16 new adult cases of HIV infection and one AIDS death reported. Family planning clinics were held weekly, offering the contraceptive pill, injectable contraceptives, condoms, and the intrauterine contraceptive device (IUCD). In 2000–2003, the health centers recorded 604 family planning acceptors. Most births occurred at the hospital and were attended by trained health professionals. According to monthly reports from district clinics, 71.4% of infants were exclusively breast-fed at 6 weeks, while 25.7% were exclusively breast-fed up to 5 months. In 2001, 53 pregnant women were registered at district clinics, of whom 9 had mild to moderate anemia. The majority of babies (112) delivered during 2004 and 2005 were born to women between 30 and 34 years old (31), followed by mothers in the 20–24-year-old age group (24). In those same years, 27 mothers delivered by cesarean section, most cesarean sections were performed on mothers 30–34 years.

Older Adults 60 Years Old and Older

In 2001 and 2002, the age dependency ratio was .54; the male to female ratio was 1:1. There was an increasing prevalence of dementia and its complications, and many elderly persons received psychological services geared for older adults.

In those same years, the population older than 60 years old represented approximately 16% of the population. There were 149 persons over age 85 in 2002 and 165 in 2004. Many of the elderly are cared for in their homes by relatives and friends. There were 125 elderly in government institutions in 2003. There were 99 deaths in the age group 65 years and older in 2004 and 2005. The main causes of death were cardiac arrest (18), diabetes mellitus (16), hypertensive diseases (12), ischemic heart diseases (6), and cerebrovascular accidents (5). Of the 1,132 hospital admissions in 2004–2005, 302 (27.0%) were in the age group 65 and older. The elderly represented the majority of persons receiving financial assistance and/or social welfare.

Children 5–9 Years Old

There were no deaths in this age group. In 2000, there were 287 children 5–9 years old; school health data indicated that 119 children in this age group were examined by a medical officer and a family nurse practitioner. There were no reported cases of protein energy malnutrition, but obesity was present. The physical examination of schoolchildren is conducted between April and May each year for specific age groups from the nursery, primary, and secondary schools. The required immunizations due at these ages are administered and immunization records are updated. The physical examination includes height, weight, vision, dental

According to the 2001 census, the average household size was 2.1 persons. Of the 2,082 households, 1,391 were headed by a male and 691 by a female, compared to 1997 when female headed households were greater in number (4).

In 2005, 287 households (on and off the island) received social welfare financial assistance, at an average monthly cost of US$ 39,600. Foster care allowance was issued to 13 children to provide assistance with their living expenses, for a monthly cost of US$ 1,444. One-time grants were approved for 250 persons to provide food packages, home requirements, school supplies, funeral expenses, and medical costs. Total cost of one-off grants was approximately US$ 101,800.

HEALTH CONDITIONS AND PROBLEMS

COMMUNICABLE DISEASES

Vector-borne Diseases

The Breteau index for *Aedes aegypti* was above 5%, which indicated that outbreaks of **dengue** were likely. There were no cases of **malaria**, **yellow fever**, **Chagas' disease**, **schistosomiasis**, or **plague** reported in the reviewed period.

Vaccine-preventable Diseases

There were no cases of **pertussis, rubella, tetanus, neonatal tetanus**, or **diphtheria** during 2001–2005. Vaccination against diphtheria, measles, mumps, pertussis, polio, rubella, and tetanus was maintained at levels of over 95% during the period. The following vaccines are part of the national immunization program: oral polio, diphtheria, pertussis, tetanus, *Haemophilus influenzae* type b, hepatitis B, and MMR.

For 2005, the vaccination coverage of antigens was—MMR (children 12 to 23 months), 100%; for infants (under 12 months), the vaccination coverage for the 3rd doses of DPT/HepB/Hib was 98% and coverage for OPV was 98%.

HIV/AIDS and Other Sexually Transmitted Infections

There were 19 persons (8 males and 11 females) who tested positive for HIV infection in 1999–2005, including two prenatal patients, one voluntary blood donor, and five job seekers who returned to their home countries. Health records prior to 1999 were lost during the evacuation. The majority of the reported cases fell within the age group 20–49 (89.5%); one was age 18 years old and the other, age 50 years.

In 1999–2003, 520 blood donors were tested, and 15 tested positive for hepatitis B.

NONCOMMUNICABLE DISEASES

An audit on quality of care for hypertension and diabetes was conducted in 2001/2002. A total of 137 patients were examined, representing attendance at four public clinics. Of these, 78 (57%)

were females. Of 200 male hospitalizations in 2000, the leading causes of hospitalization were injuries (18%), hypertension/heart-related diseases (15%), diseases of the digestive system (14%), and diabetes/hypercholesterolemia (12%). Of the 189 female hospitalizations, the leading causes were diabetes mellitus (15%), hypertension/heart-related diseases (13%), diseases of the genitourinary system (12%), and diseases of the digestive system (9%).

Cardiovascular Diseases

There were 55 deaths due to this cause group, broken down as cardiac arrest (18), hypertensive diseases (17), ischemic heart diseases and cerebrovascular diseases (8 each), and heart failure and all other diseases of the circulatory system (2 each).

Malignant Neoplasms

Between 2004 and 2005 there were 14 deaths due to malignant neoplasms. The leading cancer sites were the prostate (5), colon (2), breast (2), pancreas and uterus (1 each), and other sites (3).

OTHER HEALTH PROBLEMS OR ISSUES

Mental Health

In 2005, 80% of the clients were schizophrenic, 5% were diagnosed with bipolar disorder, and 15% with other mental illnesses such as drug induced psychoses, alcoholism, organic psychosis, and senile dementia. There were 100 clients registered on the mental health register; 70% were males and 30% females.

Oral Health

A total of 176 children were examined through the school dental health program in 2002. Of these, 75 students (43%) had no dental caries; 48 (27%) had 1–3 or more, 29 (17%) had 4–5 or more, and 24 (14%) had 6 or more.

RESPONSE OF THE HEALTH SECTOR

Health Policies and Plans

The Ministry of Health is charged with ensuring that health services available to the residents of Montserrat are accessible, of good quality, and affordable, and that they promote community participation.

Montserrat's 2003–2007 Sustainable Development Plan encompasses six strategic objectives: to promote the retention of the territory's current population and to encourage the return of Montserratians living abroad; to promote prudent economic management, sustained growth, a diversified economy, and the generation of employment opportunities; to promote human development and well-being and enhance the quality of life for all people on the island; to ensure good governance by strengthening public administration and promoting civil society; to improve and expand external relationships as a way to facilitate Montserrat's integration into the regional and global environment; and to ensure that Montserrat's development is environmentally sustainable and includes appropriate strategies for disaster mitigation. The specific objectives for the health sector under the Plan are to develop appropriate health strategies, including a national health development plan; review regulations and policies governing the operations of the health sector; strengthen the institutional management of the sector; adequately provide for medical and nursing training; adequately provide for specialist services; develop policies for the prevention of HIV/AIDS; strengthen health promotion; strengthen actions and measures that inhibit social, environmental, and behavioral patterns and practices that increase the risk of disease among the population; ensure that adequate procedures and programs are in place to control or eradicate all common communicable diseases through a high coverage immunization program and raising public awareness for the promotion of healthier lifestyles; ensure a comprehensive solid waste management policy aimed at ensuring efficient and effective storage, collection, and disposal of waste on the island; and initiate a national health insurance scheme to ensure appropriate access to all. At the heart of the health sector's objectives is the delivery of adequate, affordable, and accessible health and welfare services to the people of Montserrat. A survey of Montserratians living in the United Kingdom found that the provision of adequate and quality health care service is an essential requirement to encourage Montserratians to return home.

The Ministry of Health's 2005–2008 Corporate Plan details the strategic direction for the implementation of health and community services policies of the Government of Montserrat. The Corporate Plan was developed from the government's Sustainable Development Plan and from feedback from Government agencies, other stakeholders, and from various departments. The strategies in the Corporate Plan form the basis for Annual Business Plans.

Organization of the Health System

Public health and community service functions fall under the responsibility of the Ministry of Education, Health, and Community Services. The Ministry is functionally devided into Headquarters, the Department of Health, and the Department of Community Services. Headquarters is charged with planning and policy analysis to support and strengthen the health system, as well as reviewing any legislation under the Ministry's responsibility. The Department of Health is responsible for providing and administering primary and secondary health care services in the country and assisting Montserratians who wish to access tertiary care elsewhere in the Caribbean. The Department of Community Services is responsible for looking after the well-being of persons in Montserrat by providing policy advice to the Government and protection and care to those in need.

The health care delivery system is organized into primary and secondary health care services. Primary health care is usually provided at the first point of contact in the community, such as at the territory's four clinics (St. Johns, Cudjoe Head, Salem, and St. Peters) and through environmental health, dental, nutrition, and health promotion activities. Secondary care is provided at the 30-bed Glendon Hospital, and includes inpatient and outpatient care, surgery, orthopedics, obstetrics, and gynecology. Access to tertiary care, defined as highly specialized technical inpatient medical care, is offered through referrals to overseas institutions.

Public Health Services

The vector control program emphasized the control of the *Aedes aegypti* mosquito. Bimonthly surveillance was conducted on a bimonthly basis at sea and air ports of entry.

The Montserrat Water Authority is responsible for the distribution of potable water, and the Environmental Health Department, under the Ministry of Health, is responsible for the monitoring of the water supply. The population was reliably supplied with safe water from springs located in the inhabited area. Despite periodic exposure to the volcano's ash fallout, these sources continued to produce good quality water; the water was regularly put through regular laboratory analysis at the Caribbean Environmental Health Institute (CEHI).

Sewage disposal continued to pose a challenge; new technologies were introduced and the public's perception and acceptance of them were low. The most pervasive disposal system was through septic tanks with soakaways. Given the soil structure in Montserrat, it was difficult to attain an acceptable percolation rate for the safe disposal of effluent. Two sewage treatment plants and a proposed maturation pond for the new housing developments are expected to overcome existing challenges. Solid waste management has improved slowly. The operations of the landfill site and a waste reduction strategy saw little success. Health promotion and prevention activities continued to be the main strategies for changing behaviors in the population that would result in a cleaner environment.

Island-wide, air quality remained adequate, helped by prevailing winds and low emissions from sources such as automobiles. However, ash emissions from the volcano continued to affect mainly the population in the south of the island. Dust monitoring was suspended by the Montserrat Volcano Observatory due to equipment failure. Volcanic ashes such as sulphur dioxide and hydrogen chloride were monitored daily. Residents were provided with ash masks and were advised to wear them during ash fallouts or when cleaning areas affected by ash.

Food control efforts centered around monitoring, targeting sanitation, food quality, and building alliances with such agencies as the Consumer Association. Through an increase in the frequency of inspection of food establishments and by networking with stakeholders, particularly the public, the Ministry of Health's Department of Health made significant strides in providing safer food for consumption. There were no confirmed cases of outbreaks of food poisoning, although there appeared to be an increase in the number of ciguatera poisonings associated with various species of fish.

The goal of the food and nutrition policy and program is to improve the food and nutritional health status of the population by improving household food security; protecting consumers through improved food quality and safety; caring for socioeconomically deprived and nutritionally vulnerable groups; promoting proper diet and healthy lifestyles; preventing and managing micronutrient deficiencies; assessing, analyzing, and monitoring food and nutrition situations; and incorporating nutrition objectives and sectoral and national development policies and plans.

Individual Care Services

The Government continuously embarked on programs to improve the standard of health care in both the primary and secondary levels. In 2002, the St. Johns health center was expanded to include consulting rooms, office accommodation, ancillary areas for both doctors and medical staff, and a mental health day care center. St. Peters health center was also upgraded. These improvements ensured a better environment in which to provide basic health services in the various communities. In 2002, US$ 2.1 million was spent to develop the health services. This enhanced the ability to attract specialist surgeons and to expand the types of service procedures available on the island, thereby decreasing the need to fly patients abroad for care.

The operating theatre at Glendon Hospital was completed and fully equipped at a cost of US$ 555,000. A new modern mortuary was completed at Glendon Hospital in 2004. During 2000–2003, 98 patients were transferred from Glendon Hospital to a health care facility overseas for management or specialized care. Patients went to Antigua (80), Guadeloupe (13), the United Kingdom (1), Trinidad (2), and one each to Jamaica and the United States of America. Most transfers (34) occurred in 2001.

One blood bank operates from the hospital laboratory. In 2000, the laboratory achieved a satisfactory level of operation, with all departments fully operational, including the bacteriology department. That year, the laboratory performed 106,475 hematology, biochemistry, bacteriology, rapid plasma regain (RPR), HIV, and hepatitis tests.

Three institutions provide care and housing for the elderly—Margetson Memorial Home, Hill View Home, and the Golden Years Home; in 2004–2005 there were 98 residents. The mental health unit is responsible for enhancing and strengthening the psychiatric/mental health services. To that end, the following initiatives were undertaken: the mental health act was revised; a mental health policy was developed; the mental health committee was reactivated; prioritizing the housing needs of the mentally challenged was prioritized; educational programs for the public

were developed; and an area for establishing a secure facility for providing acute care was identified. There is presently no mental institution in Montserrat; mentally challenged clients are managed in the community. They continue to live in various communities and access care through visits to the mental health clinic and participation in group and occupational therapy. If required, persons are hospitalized at the General Hospital.

A dental health plan prepared in 2003 is designed to develop and implement quality assurance programs for dental care delivery; to revive and review prevention and dental health programs in schools; to improve the Government's dental care program; to develop ongoing training for staff; to establish a data entry and retrieval system of dental records; and to review the policy dealing with accessibility of treatment by the general public.

Health Promotion

The Health Promotion Unit was staffed by a health educator. In 2005 an intersectoral health promotion team was formed, which included the participation of representatives from NGOs and the private sector from within and outside the health sector. The team was conformed to comment on health activities and projects and to help avoid duplication on health efforts. In addition, it advised on health promotion issues and drafted a newspaper column, "Health Corner," covering a variety of health issues and providing health tips, updates, and general health information. The team also collaborated with the HIV/AIDS coordinator, participated in the follow-up of a cervical cancer prevention and care program, disseminated the strategies of the Caribbean Health Promotion Charter to colleagues and others, and taught the health promotion component in a nurses training program.

Human Resources

Continuous education for health workers in the reporting period included participation in seminars or courses on special blood banking; laboratory management and quality management; occupational safety and health; health informatics; anesthesia; psychiatric nursing; public health; nursing education; gerontology; diagnostic radiography; mass casualty; stress management; breast-feeding; use of the fetal monitor; infection control; and a nursing care plan.

Health Supplies

There are no locally produced drugs, reagents, or biologicals in Montserrat. All items are imported through the Organization of Eastern Caribbean States/Pharmaceutical Procurement Service, which audits procurements on an annual basis. The blood bank depended on voluntary/replacement donors to replenish its blood supply. There were no accreditation committees or regulating agencies in place.

Life under the Volcano

After the Soufriere Hills Volcano erupted in 2000, three-quarters of the population left Montserrat. Those who remained and lived in the city of Plymouth and other urban areas in the south, or who farmed the productive agricultural lands in that zone, were forced to pull up stakes, abandoning homes, businesses, and farms and relocating to the north, away from the devastation and continuing volcanic threats. The dislocation of the population sent aftershocks into the economy. Tourism dried up, as many villas and the main hotel were trapped in the volcano exclusion zone. Agricultural and commercial assets were destroyed, crippling the private sector. According to the Government's 2003–2007 Sustainable Development Plan, retaining the territory's current population and encouraging those who have left to return is key to rebuilding Montserrat. To offset the loss of social support networks, the Government has developed a comprehensive welfare system as a safety net for vulnerable groups. It provides a basic allowance for food for the needy and a rental subsidy for vulnerable government housing tenants, mainly elderly and physically or mentally disabled persons.

Health Research and Technology

In October 2000, in an effort to determine the effect, if any, of volcanic ash on lung function, a consultant and his team from the United Kingdom conducted an ash exposure survey on 400 local residents.

Health Sector Expenditures and Financing

In 2003, recurrent expenditures in health amounted to US$ 3.9 million, increasing to US$ 4.3 million in 2004, and to US$ 4.6 million in 2005. Revenue collection from Glendon Hospital in 2003–2005 included US$ 10,000 from the x-ray department; US$ 45,000 from the laboratory; US$ 48,000 for cold body storage; US$ 15,000 for casualties; US$ 34,000 for medicine and materials; US$ 22,000 for surgery; US$ 1,000 for anesthesia; US$ 1,000 for operating theatre use; US$ 13,000 for wards; and US$ 3,000 for electrocardiograms (5). Actual and expected expenditures for the health and social welfare sector in 2003–2005 totaled US$ 3.2 million.

Technical Cooperation and External Financing

Globalization had both a positive and negative effect on Montserrat's development. Montserrat, as one of the founding members of CARICOM and the OECS, continued to play a part in regional affairs and dealt with the challenges that face small island states. The European Union made provisions for a deeper partnership between overseas territories and the European member states. The 1957 Treaty of Rome defined special arrangements for the association of the community with the Overseas Territories, setting up the European Development Fund and providing measures dealing with the right of establishment and trade. Financing was critical for the success of the Sustainable Development Plan and, in turn, for Montserrat to be able to achieve its broad developmental objectives. The funds available determined the pace and success of Montserrat's development. Much of the infrastructure that was lost to the volcano had to be replaced at considerable cost. While considerable resources were expended to replace it, much work remained to be done. The loss of two-thirds of the population led to a decrease in tax receipts and other revenue sources for the Government. This lower revenue, combined with an increase in expenditures, led to a large and unsustainable budget deficit. This deficit required financing by donors. In 2003–2005, ongoing and planned funding was expected from the Caribbean Development Bank (CDB), the United Kingdom's Department for International Development, the European Development Fund (EDF), the Republic of Ireland, the Pan American Health Organization and other regional institutions, private sources, and others (6).

References

1. Montserrat, Ministry of Finance, Development Unit. Montserrat Sustainable Development Plan. Montserrat Social and Economic Recovery Programme. A Path to Sustainable Development 1998–2002. 1998.
2. Montserrat, Ministry of Finance, Development Unit. Making Ends Meet. Participatory Poverty and Hardship Assessment of Montserrat (PPA). July 2000. Final Report. 2001.
3. Montserrat, Ministry of Health, Primary Health Care. School Health Report 2002.
4. Government of Montserrat. Montserrat Social Survey 1997.
5. Montserrat, Medical Records, Statistical Reports 1999–2003.
6. Montserrat, Ministry of Finance, Development Unit. Montserrat Sustainable Development Plan 2003–2007.

NETHERLANDS ANTILLES

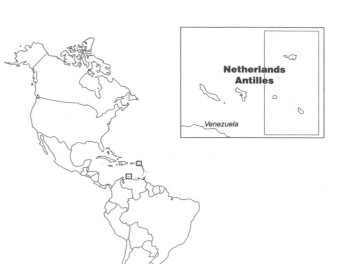

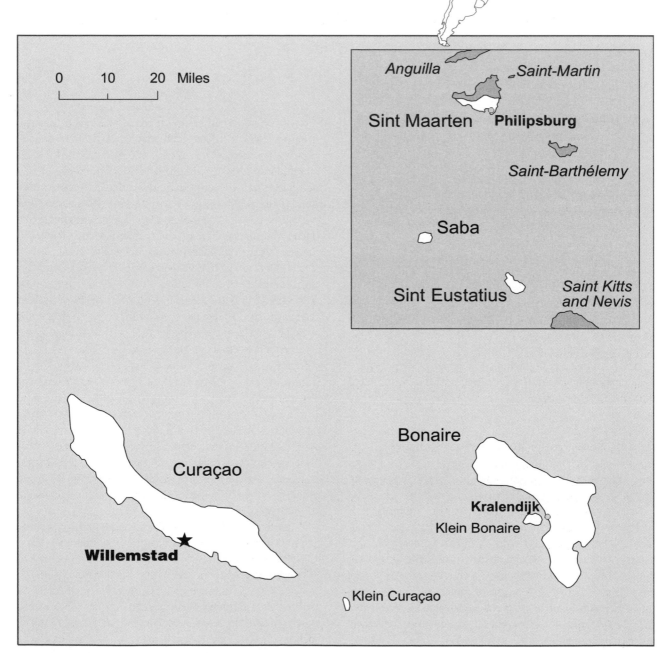

0   10   20   Miles

Anguilla

Saint-Martin

Sint Maarten   **Philipsburg**

Saint-Barthélemy

Saba

Sint Eustatius

Saint Kitts and Nevis

Bonaire

Curaçao

Kralendijk

Klein Bonaire

Willemstad

Klein Curaçao

The Netherlands Antilles are an autonomous territory of the Kingdom of the Netherlands. They consist of five islands in the Caribbean archipelago: the southern Leeward Islands of Bonaire and Curaçao, and the northern Windward Islands of Saba, Sint Eustatius, and Sint Maarten (the southern part of an island shared with France, whose northern part is known as Saint-Martin). The Leeward Islands are separated from the Windward Islands by 900 km. The Netherlands Antilles enjoy a mild tropical climate with an annual average temperature of 27–28° C. The islands are generally hilly with volcanic interiors. Bonaire and Curaçao have a more arid climate than the three Windward Islands, which are lusher and greener.

GENERAL CONTEXT AND HEALTH DETERMINANTS

Social, Political, and Economic Determinants

The Netherlands Antilles possess self-determination on all internal matters and defer to the Kingdom of the Netherlands regarding issues of defense, foreign policy, and some judicial functions.

A Governor who serves a six-year term represents the monarch of the Kingdom of the Netherlands. The Netherlands Antilles' central government is a parliamentary democracy whose seat is located in the capital (and largest city) of Willemstad on Curaçao. The office of the Governor is also based in Willemstad. Each island also has its own local government consisting of an Island Council and a Legislative Assembly. The Island Council is the local equivalent of the central-level parliament and thus each island's highest political body. Its executive council is known as the *Bestuurscollege*, and it is composed of commissioners overseeing the various government services, including the health of the population. Each of the island *Bestuurscolleges* is headed by a Lieutenant Governor. The islands are divided into administrative zones and neighborhoods.

Between 2000 and 2005, referendums were held on each of the islands to determine their future status. This process—which continues as of this writing—has, in effect, initiated the breakup of the Netherlands Antilles. The voting results have led to a series of negotiations and agreements in which Curaçao and Sint Maarten are slated to become separate autonomous entities and Bonaire, Saba, and Sint Eustastius are slated to merge with the Netherlands. Discussions by the Government of the Kingdom of the Netherlands and the island governments on structural and functional changes as regards governance and service provision are ongoing.

The Netherlands Antilles cover a combined area of 800 km². Saba is the smallest island, with a land area of 13 km², and Curaçao is the largest, with a land area of 444 km². In 2004, Bonaire was the least densely populated island, with 37 persons per km², and Sint Maarten was the most densely populated, with 1,030 persons per km².

The population is 85% mixed Black, with the remaining 15% being of White, Amerindian, and Asian background. The overall literacy rate for the population aged 15 and older was 96% in 2001. According to data from the latest (2001) census, 72% of the population is Roman Catholic, another 20% holds membership in other Christian denominations, 1% is Jewish, 5% reports no religion, and the remaining 2% practices another religion or did not specify religious affiliation.

Though Dutch is the official language of the Netherlands Antilles, English is the most commonly spoken language on the Windward Islands of Saba, Sint Eustatius, and Sint Maarten, and Papiamentu—a mixture of Portuguese, Spanish, English, and Dutch words—is the more predominant language spoken on the Leeward Islands of Bonaire and Curaçao. Of the combined Netherlands Antilles population in 2001, 65% primarily spoke Papiamentu, 16% primarily spoke English, 7% primarily spoke Dutch, 6% primarily spoke Spanish, 2% primarily spoke Creole, 2% spoke other languages, and the remaining 2% did not specify primary language.

The 2005 gross domestic product (GDP) per capita was US$ 17,888, with tourism and the services industry making up 84% of GDP. The external debt of the Netherlands Antilles was US$ 2.68 billion in 2004, while the purchasing power parity GDP in the same year was estimated at US$ 2.8 billion. GDP grew almost 8% between 2001 and 2004. Fifteen percent of GDP in 2005 was industry (petroleum refining on Curaçao, petroleum transshipment facilities on Curaçao and Bonaire, and light manufacturing on Curaçao), and 1% was agriculture (aloes, sorghum, peanuts, vegetables, and tropical fruit). The currency of the Netherlands Antilles is the Netherlands Antillean guilder (ANG), with a fixed exchange rate of 1.78 ANG = US$ 1 in 2005.

Tourism and related activities provide the largest source of employment in the Netherlands Antilles. In 2005, the three largest islands of Curaçao, Sint Maarten, and Bonaire had 222,000, 462,000, and 68,000 stay-over tourists, respectively. In that same year, tour ships docked 931 times at these three islands to deliver a total of 1.8 million day tourists.

In 2005, the estimated unemployment rate for the Netherlands Antilles as a whole was 16.3%, with the highest rate being found on Curaçao. Unemployment rates for women were consistently higher than those for men on all of the islands, and employment rates for youth were typically two to three times higher than the overall rates.

During the 2000–2005 period, various different trends and patterns in unemployment rates were noted for the three islands with 98% of the Netherlands Antilles' total population. On Curaçao, where nearly three-quarters of the total population resided during this period, the unemployment rate for the economically active population increased from 14.2% in 2000 to 18.2% in 2005. On Sint Maarten, the island with almost one-fifth of the total population, the unemployment rate remained unchanged at 13.4% during the period, whereas on Bonaire, where only 6% of the population resides, the unemployment rate for the economically active population rose from 5.5% in 2000 to 8.9% in 2005.

A poverty assessment survey conducted during the 2004–2005 period revealed that the percentage of households with a very low monthly income equivalent to approximately US$ 280 (adjusted for household size) ranged from 5% on Saba to 16% on Curaçao, with an overall average of 14% for the five Netherlands Antilles islands. Additionally, an overall average of 32% of households reported that their income was insufficient to cover all necessary expenses, with figures ranging from 27% on Bonaire to 50% on Saba.

The survey found that income inequality was lowest on Saba, the island with the highest median household income, and Bonaire. On Saba and Bonaire, the 20% of households with the highest income levels had an income six times higher than that found among the poorest 20% of households. The highest income inequality, coupled with the lowest median household income, was found on Curaçao, where the 20% of households with the highest income had an income 14 times higher than that found among the poorest 20% of households.

The 2001 census showed that 22% of the population aged 15 or older did not have an income (26% women and 19% men). Twenty-eight percent of female-headed households were living in poverty.

In 2002, secondary school enrollment was 78%. That same year, the average length of schooling for adults from both sexes was approximately 14 years. In 2001, adult literacy was reported to be 96.3%, with men and women having nearly identical rates.

Demographics, Mortality, and Morbidity

The Netherlands Antilles Central Bureau for Statistics estimated the 2005 population to have grown to 185,513 from the census-enumerated population of 175,652 in 2001, at which time 53% of the population was female and 47% was male. With an estimated 73.2% of the total population (135,822 inhabitants), Curaçao has the largest population of the five islands, followed by Sint Maarten with 18.9% (35,035), Bonaire with 5.7% (10,638), Sint Eustatius with 1.4% (2,584), and Saba with 0.8% (1,434).

Figure 1 show the population structure, by age and sex, for the Netherlands Antilles for 1990 and 2005.

The 2001 population of 175,652 was nearly 14,000 persons less than the population enumerated in the previous 1992 census. The population decline on Sint Maarten and Curaçao more than compensated for the population growth experienced on the other three islands. Of the 2001 total population, 7.5% was in the 0–4-year-old age group, 24.0% was in the 5–9-year-old age group, 55.3% was in the 20–59-year-old age group, and 13.2% was aged 60 years or older.

Between the 1992 and 2001 censuses, the overall population had grown older, with a 13% decrease in the population segment aged 19 and under and a 25% decrease in the 20–39-year-old age group. Groups older than 40 years of age increased in numbers over the same time period.

In 2001, one out of every four persons living on the islands was born outside of the Netherlands Antilles. Curaçao had the lowest percentage of foreign-born persons (17%), and Sint Maarten had the largest percentage (63%).

The Dominican Republic was the country of origin with the largest percentage (18.7%) of those who reported being foreign-born and represented approximately 5% of the total population of the Netherlands Antilles. Smaller proportions of the resident population born elsewhere included those born in the Netherlands (15.2% of all foreign-born residents), Aruba (7.0%), Haiti (6.9%), Colombia (5.6%), Suriname (5.2%), Jamaica (4.4%), Dominica (3.9%), Venezuela (3.2%), Guyana (2.8%), and the United States (2.5%).

In 2001, one in five inhabitants indicated that he or she had intentions of migrating from the Netherlands Antilles, and half of the total population was undecided about whether they would choose to migrate. During the 1998–2002 period, approximately 15% of Curaçao's population migrated to other countries due to faltering economic conditions, resulting in a major drain of the population's better-educated and trained segments. The majority of those who migrated were in the 20–35-year-old age group, with a median age at the time of migration of 24 years. However, since 2001, this out-migration trend has slowed and by 2005 was showing signs of reversing itself.

FIGURE 1. Population structure, by age and sex, Netherlands Antilles, 1990 and 2005.

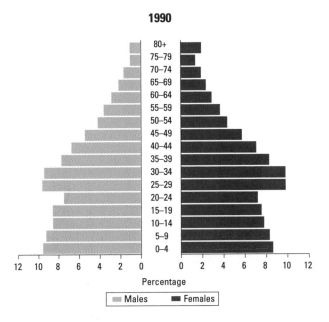

1990

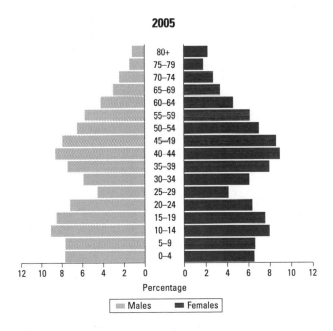

2005

At the time of the 2001 census, 29% of the population aged 30–59 years old reported not having a partner and another 11% reported not living with their partner. For those reporting cohabitation, the average age of the male partner was more than three years older than his female partner.

The overall average size of households was approximately three persons. Larger average sizes of households were found on Bonaire and Curaçao, with the largest share of single-person households being found on Saba, Sint Eustatius, and Sint Maarten. Census data showed a decrease in the fertility rate from 2.4 children per woman in 1992 to 2.2 in 2001. There was also a corresponding increase in mean age of the mother at first birth from 24.5 years in 1992 to 25.5 years in 2001. More than one in every five households in 2001 were single-headed households with children under 18 years of age; of these, 94% were headed by a female. Nearly 90% of the single-headed households were headed by a parent.

For the 2002–2004 period, life expectancy at birth for males was 70.6 years, and for females it was 79.0 years. The difference of more than eight years in life expectancy between males and females was at least partially attributable to differences in lifestyle and risk behaviors. For example, men in the 20–30-year-old age group were disproportionately at a higher risk for death due to accidents and violence than women in this same age group.

For the 1998–2000 period, the mean annual crude mortality rate for Curaçao was 7.5 deaths per 1,000 population, compared to a 1988 crude mortality rate of 6.5 deaths per 1,000 population.

In 2000, chronic noncommunicable diseases were among the leading causes of mortality. In this year, approximately one-third of these deaths were caused by pulmonary, cardiovascular, and cerebrovascular diseases. Malignant neoplasms, diabetes mellitus, and acute respiratory infections were also among the leading 10 causes of death. Neoplasms contributed to approximately one-fourth of all deaths; the most frequently occurring sites for neoplasms were the prostate and the digestive and respiratory tracts. The leading causes of death and corresponding mortality rates for Curaçao during the 1998–2000 period are presented in Table 1.

In the 2001 census, 5.1% of the population reported having a diagnosis of high blood pressure, 3.5% reported having a diagnosis of diabetes, 2.8% reported having a diagnosis of asthma or chronic bronchitis, and 1.7% reported having heart problems.

TABLE 1. Leading causes of mortality and associated mortality rates per 100,000 population, Curaçao, 1998–2000.

Rank	Cause	Mean annual crude mortality rate per 100,000 population
1	Pulmonary and other cardiovascular diseases	90
2	Cerebrovascular diseases	70
3	Ischemic heart diseases	60
4	Malignant neoplasms of the prostate	30
5	Diabetes mellitus	30
6	Acute respiratory infections	30
7	Malignant neoplasms of the digestive tract, excluding the stomach and colon	30
8	Malignant neoplasms of the respiratory tract	20

The prevalence rates of high blood pressure, diabetes, and heart problems increased with age, whereas the prevalence of asthma or chronic bronchitis decreased with age. For each age group after age 14, females were 1.7 times more likely to report having high blood pressure and 1.4 times more likely to report having diabetes than males.

For young adult males, the leading cause of death was homicide and intentional injury. AIDS was in the top three causes of death for both males and females in the 25–44-year-old age group. Adults over the age of 60, females, and individuals with incomes below the poverty line reported a higher frequency of chronic health problems and lower use of preventive health services.

In 2001, 15% of men aged 15–29 and 30% of men aged 30–44 reported smoking tobacco. Among women, 6% in the first age group and 13% in the second age group reported smoking. Overall prevalence of tobacco smoking for the total population was 13%.

HEALTH OF POPULATION GROUPS

Children under 5 Years Old

The estimated infant mortality rate in 2005 was 4 per 1,000 live births, a reduction from the 1990 rate of 7 per 1,000 live births. According to the Netherlands Antilles Central Bureau for Statistics, in 2005 there were 13,378 children aged 0–4, making up 7.2% of the total population. Over the past decade, there has been a steady decline in the annual number of births. In 1998, 3,111 live births were registered, compared to 2,357 in 2004. This decline has been attributed to a reduction in the number of females of reproductive age and to a reduction in the total fertility rate from 2.6 in 1990 to 2.0 in 2000.

The annual number of deaths during the 1998–2000 period for the 1–4-year-old age group was low. On Curaçao, there was an average of four deaths a year among this age group during this period, with accidents and sepsis being the leading mortality causes.

Age Group 5–14 Years Old

External causes are the principal mortality cause for this age group. During the 1998–2000 period, approximately 30% of the deaths among those in this age group were caused by traffic accidents.

According to data from the 2001 census, boys aged 5–14 years old suffered from a higher burden of chronic disease than girls in the same age group, with asthma/bronchitis being the most frequently occurring condition.

Age Group 15–24 Years Old

From age 16, a marked increase in the mortality rate has been shown among males, while for their female counterparts the mortality rate has remained stable. Homicide is the leading cause of death in this age group, followed by traffic accidents. On Curaçao, 40 males and no females in this age group died as a result of homicide during the 1998–2000 period. Youth between the ages of 18 and 25 are three times more likely to be involved in a serious traffic accident than older drivers.

Among the population aged 15–24, females are more frequently hospitalized than males, primarily for pregnancies and deliveries. According to 2001 census data, approximately 10% of all children in the Netherlands Antilles were born to adolescent mothers. The primary reason for hospitalization of males in this age group was due to fractures. Asthma/bronchitis was the most frequently occurring chronic disease.

According to a 2002–2003 study conducted by the Youth Directorate of the Netherlands Antilles, 18% of all youth were facing serious social problems (e.g., drug and alcohol use, parents' gambling addictions, lack of parental guidance and/or involvement, family conflicts) and another 14% were at risk for developing these same social problems. Youth-related risk factors included peer pressure and tolerance toward and/or early exposure to negative social behavior. One-third of the girls in the same study said they knew a victim of sexual abuse, and 21% of the boys reported that they had had sex with an unwilling partner.

In a 2002–2003 public school survey carried out on Curaçao among students aged 13–18, 43% of the boys and 28% of the girls reported being sexually active, with 51% of the boys and 25% of the girls reporting always using a condom.

Adults 25–59 Years Old

During the 1998–2000 period among the 25–44-year-old age group, mortality rates due to traffic accidents and homicides were higher for males than females. Among external causes for death, the third major cause among those in this age group was suicide. Among females in the 25–44-year-old age group and the 45–59-year-old age group, the leading cause of mortality is malignant neoplasms of the breast. The principal cause of death for males aged 45–59 is ischemic heart diseases. For both females and males in the 25–45-year-old age group, AIDS is among the top three leading causes of mortality. In this age group, females are also more frequently hospitalized than males, with the leading reasons for hospitalization being pregnancy and delivery.

In 2002, the leading reasons for hospitalization of males were fractures and other injuries. In the 25–44-year-old age group, migraines and chronic headaches, psychological problems, and dizziness were the most commonly treated chronic conditions, and for those over age 45, hypertension and diabetes were the most common of these conditions.

In the 2001 census, 11% of the population between the ages of 45 and 64 reported having a diagnosis of hypertension and 8% reported having a diagnosis of diabetes, with more women than men reporting these conditions.

Older Adults 60 Years Old and Older

The overall population in the 2001 census was older in comparison with the overall population in the 1992 census. The older age groups increased in both numbers and percentage during this period. The number of hospital admissions was the highest among the elderly. The primary reasons for hospital admissions in this age group were eye diseases, diseases of the kidney and urinary tract, and malignant neoplasms.

The Family

Approximately 85%–90% of all deliveries in the Netherlands Antilles took place in hospitals during the 2001–2005 period. During the 1998–2000 period, 17 late fetal deaths per 1,000 deliveries were reported.

The average number of deaths among children aged 0–12 months remained stable at around 10 deaths per year during the 1998–2003 period. Major causes of death for children under age 1 were respiratory conditions and congenital deformations. During the 1998–2000 period, Curaçao reported a perinatal mortality rate of 23.5 per 1,000 deliveries.

In 1996 and 1997, Curaçao registered 130 and 150 maternal deaths, respectively. In 1998, the number of maternal deaths on Curaçao dropped to 43, then increased to 47 in 2000.

Persons with Disabilities

According to 2001 census data, the number of persons with disabilities (including visual, hearing, physical, mental, and other types of impairments) represented 8.5% of the population. Disabilities disproportionately impacted those over 60 years of age. Among the non-institutionalized persons with disabilities, the most frequently reported disability was visual impairment, followed by limited ability to perform activities of daily living and hearing impairment.

HEALTH CONDITIONS AND PROBLEMS

COMMUNICABLE DISEASES

Vector-borne Diseases

Dengue is endemic on the island of Curaçao. During the past 10 years, all four dengue serotypes have been identified. During the 2001–2005 period, dengue virus types 1 and 3 predominated; type 4 had not been seen since 2000. Circulation patterns of the various serotypes have been associated with patterns of high tourist traffic from neighboring countries, such as Venezuela and Panama. The annual number of laboratory-confirmed dengue cases between 2001 and 2005 was 85, 280, 26, 163, and 132, respectively. Two dengue outbreaks were recorded during the review period, during December 2001–February 2002, with 231 cases,

and during December 2004–February 2005, with 121 cases. During the 2001–2003 period, there were no cases of **dengue hemorrhagic fever**. However, during the 2004–2005 period, five cases were reported.

Vaccine-preventable Diseases

In 2004, overall vaccine coverage in the Netherlands Antilles was 88% for DPT, Hib, and OPV/IPV. Reported MMR vaccine coverage on the individual islands ranged from 75% on Sint Maarten to 95% on Bonaire and Curaçao. Reported individual island coverage for DPT, OPV/IPV, and Hib vaccines ranged from 72% on Sint Maarten to 100% on Saba. Hepatitis B vaccine coverage was 71% on Sint Maarten and 95% on Bonaire.

Chronic Communicable Diseases

In the Netherlands Antilles, the estimated **tuberculosis** incidence rate was 9 per 100,000 population for the 2001–2004 period, a reduction from the estimated 1990 rate of 11 per 100,000 population. The last TB case was reported on Bonaire in 1999. Sint Maarten reported one to four TB cases annually over the 2001–2005 period. The majority of the TB cases in the Netherlands Antilles were recorded on Curaçao. During the 2001–2005 period, a mean of 10 new TB cases were reported annually on this island. INH-resistant strains were isolated in 2004. The mean age at time of TB diagnosis was 40 to 50 years, with close to two-thirds of these cases being among males. An estimated one-half of the annual cases on Curaçao are imported cases. HIV infection and drug addiction are common comorbidities in TB cases.

Hansen's disease remains at a low endemic level in the Netherlands Antilles. Between 2001 and 2004, a total of 11 cases were recorded on Curaçao and one on Bonaire. One of the cases was originally from Guyana. The annual number of new leprosy cases remained between two and four during this period.

Intestinal Infectious Diseases

The most frequently isolated gastrointestinal pathogens were *Campylobacter* and *salmonella*. Between 2001 and 2005, a cumulative number of 331 cases of **Campylobacter jejune infection** were laboratory-confirmed and a total of 559 *salmonella* infections were laboratory-confirmed. *Shigella* infection was also common during this period, with a cumulative number of 168 isolated cases. *Yersinia* and *E. coli* infections were rare, with one isolated case each during the 2001–2005 period. Around one-third of the campylobacteriosis cases, almost half of the salmonellosis cases, and half of the shigellosis cases were found in children under 5 years old.

HIV/AIDS and Other Sexually Transmitted Diseases

The registration system for HIV infection is limited in scope, capturing HIV cases in voluntary testing at Sint Elisabeth Hospital and the Analytic Diagnostic Center, the leading laboratory in the Netherlands Antilles. Between 1985 and 2005, a cumulative number of 1,623 HIV-positive cases were registered, with 56.9% being males and 43.1% being females. The majority of these cases are from Curaçao (65.5%) and Sint Maarten (31.8%). Of the registered HIV-positive persons, 65.7% were in the 15–24-year-old age group. The main mode of HIV transmission is through sexual contact. As a result of the prevention of mother-to-child transmission program, vertical HIV transmission is very low. Intravenous drug use is rare in the Netherlands Antilles, and a very strict blood donor policy and screening of all donated blood have contributed to a high blood safety level.

NONCOMMUNICABLE DISEASES

Metabolic and Nutritional Diseases

In 1996, 63% of the adult population on Curaçao was over-weight (body mass index > 25 and < 30) or obese (body mass index ≥ 30), with the highest prevalences of **overweight** and **obesity** occurring in females in the 45–64-year-old age group and among women of lower socioeconomic status. In a 2002 health study conducted on all of the Netherlands Antilles islands except Curaçao, over 70% of the adult population was found to be overweight or obese. Women on the five different islands were 32%–93% more likely to be obese than men, depending on the island. In 2002, one out of every four adults in the Netherlands Antilles reported exercising regularly.

Malignant Neoplasms

Based on preliminary tabulations from the Cancer Registry for the Netherlands Antilles (located at the Pathology Laboratory on Curaçao), the five leading sites of new cancer cases (excluding non-melanoma skin cancer) for men during the 1999–2003 period were prostate (40% of all male cases), colon/rectum (10%), lung (8%), stomach (4%), and oral cavity/pharynx (3%). For women, the five leading sites of new cases (excluding non-melanoma skin cancer) were breast (36% of all female cases), colon/rectum (13%), corpus uteri (8%), cervix uteri (6%), and stomach (3%). Ovarian cancer followed stomach cancer closely for women, also at 3%. Non-melanoma skin cancer represented 14% of all cancers for men and 13% for women. A total of 1,646 new cases of male cancers and 1,198 of female cancers were registered during the 1999–2003 period.

OTHER HEALTH PROBLEMS OR ISSUES

Disasters

Bonaire and Curaçao are south of the Caribbean hurricane belt and are rarely threatened by hurricanes. However, Saba, Sint Eustatius, and Sint Maarten are regularly subjected to hurricanes. In August of 2000, Hurricane Debby passed through all three islands, causing minimum damage. In July 2005, the center of Hurricane Emily moved through the southeastern Caribbean islands and passed about 180 km north of Bonaire and Curaçao. In the wake of Hurricane Emily, heavy rains caused flooding in the St. Peter basin on Sint Maarten, resulting in two deaths. The estimated damage was US$ 700,000.

RESPONSE OF THE HEALTH SECTOR

Health Policies and Plans

Between 1998 and 2000, the Netherlands Antilles central government implemented a reform plan entitled the "Governing Accord on the Program for Economic and Financial Recovery." The plan called for urgent action to revive the economy, create jobs, reduce poverty, improve social conditions and public finances, and develop a comprehensive program to reduce unemployment, drug use, and crime among young people through both preventive and law enforcement measures. Strengthening public administration at the central level and on each of the islands was an overarching priority.

As a result of this reform process, the Netherlands Antilles central government identified four core government responsibilities: general policy development, legislation, international affairs, and law enforcement and control.

Under these reforms, health care experienced cuts in expenditures and in administrative personnel. The plan led to the restructuring of the Department of Public Health and Environmental Hygiene in 2001. From 1977 to 2001, the Ministry of Public Health and Environment oversaw the Department of Public Health and Environmental Hygiene, the Inspectorate of Pharmaceutical Affairs, the Psychiatric Hospital, and the National Laboratory. As part of the reform process, the central government dissolved the Ministry of Public Health and Environment and replaced it with a new Ministry of Public Health and Social Development. The legislation for this change was ratified on 4 January 2002. The new Ministry of Public Health and Social Development was reorganized to include a Directorate of Public Health, a Directorate of Social Development, a Support Bureau, and an Inspectorate of Public Health. This latter includes separate divisions overseeing health care, health protection, and pharmaceutical affairs.

Organization of the Health System

The activities of the Directorate of Public Health are administered by the Director of Public Health. By legislative decree, the areas of responsibilities under this Directorate include population health; personal health care; veterinary health; the environment; epidemiological surveillance; monitoring of health status, mortality data, and selected diseases; and research for policy-

A New Future for Public Health Services

The Netherlands Antilles are facing a diversity of major public health problems ranging from dengue and obesity epidemics to high rates of traffic accidents. The newly created Ministry of Health and Social Development, through the Directorate of Public Health, oversees disease surveillance and health status monitoring systems; the resulting data provides input for policy formulation and the development of effective responses to these challenges. In addition to the provision of basic health services throughout the five islands, the Ministry of Health and Social Development also provides a variety of specialized medical services, which are principally located on the most populated island of Curaçao. However, the Ministry currently is in a state of flux. With the break-up of the Netherlands Antilles initiated by earlier referendums on the islands, public infrastructure for the delivery of preventive and curative health services in these newly autonomous territories will require transformation and adaptation to the inevitable uncertainties that lie ahead.

making. The tasks assigned to meet these responsibilities include conducting research and surveillance, the development of partnerships with other governmental and nongovernmental organizations, promotion of international collaboration, policy and regulations formation, implementation of cost-cutting measures, and the promotion of equitable access to health care and of health services' effectiveness and efficiency.

Due to the results of voter referendums held at the beginning of the decade signaling the breakup of the Netherland Antilles, discussions continue between government authorities at all levels on how best to minimize the impact on local populations of major structural and functional changes to health care, public health services, and other public services.

Several different health insurance systems exist in the Netherlands Antilles. The government-sponsored Social Insurance/Security Bank (SVB), which is located on all five islands and is headquartered on Curaçao, provides health insurance coverage for employees of nongovernmental organizations and the private sector. Pro-Pauper Insurance is health coverage provided by the individual local island governments for the unemployed, the population living in poverty, and the retired who lack insurance. Civil Servant Health Insurance is provided by the island territorial governments for government civil servants. Private health insurance is purchased by the population earning an annual salary which exceeds the maximum salary enabling eligibility for SVB insurance.

Health care insurance coverage reported in the 2001 census included SVB (36% of the population covered), Pro-Pauper Insurance (16%), other government-subsidized insurance (15%), private insurance (11%), coverage by employer (7%), and other (3%). Eleven percent of the population reported being uninsured. This segment was disproportionately distributed among the islands and ranged from 3% of Bonaire's population to 30% of Sint Maarten's population.

Public Health Services

Based on the 2001 census, in the three most populated islands of San Maarten, Curaçao, and Bonaire, 89%–98% of household dwellings relied on water supplied by desalination plants, whereas 94% and 97% of the household dwellings on Sint Eustatius and Sint Maarten, respectively, relied on water from cisterns or groundwater. Curaçao and Sint Maarten have wastewater plants, while the other islands rely heavily on septic tanks.

Pesticide contamination is not an issue in the Netherlands Antilles due to low agricultural production. Oil spills in the port areas remain a public health concern.

Individual Care Services

In October 2001, there were a total of 1,343 hospital beds in the Netherlands Antilles. Of these, 729 were located in medical centers and general hospitals. The remainder of the beds were designated for specified needs in specialized institutions: 200 were in the Psychiatric Hospital, 160 were in a chronic care facility, 117 were for handicapped children, 75 were for drug rehabilitation, 45 were in a surgical clinic, and 17 were in a maternity clinic. In October 2001, a disproportionate 88% of these hospital beds and medical services were located on Curaçao, where 73% of the population resides. As of this same date, there were 44 pharmacies and 11 geriatric homes with 700 beds evenly distributed throughout the five islands.

Sint Elisabeth Hospital in Curaçao is the largest of all the islands' hospitals and is supported by a private foundation owned by the Catholic Church; more than 80% of its income is provided directly or indirectly by the government. Among other services, it has a decompression unit to assist scuba divers suffering from decompression sickness. Various private clinics on Curaçao provide satisfactory to excellent medical services. In Bonaire, the 35-bed San Francisco Hospital also provides decompression facilities for divers in addition to an air ambulance service to transport patients to Curaçao and Aruba. The Sint Maarten Medical Center, with 79 beds, provides for general surgery. Complex cases are sent to Curaçao. The 20-bed Queen Beatrix Medical Center on Sint Eustatius and the 14-bed Saba Clinic on Saba are both well-equipped first aid facilities. Surgery cases are transported to Sint Maarten. The Saba Marine Park also has a decompression chamber.

Human Resources

As of October 2001, there were 333 physicians practicing on the five islands. The distribution of the 138 general practitioners was reasonably proportionate throughout the islands, as was the distribution of the 216 paramedics, the 47 pharmacists, and the 9 midwives. However, out of the 143 specialized physicians practicing in the Netherlands Antilles, a disproportionate 88% were practicing on Curaçao. Likewise, out of the 60 practicing dentists, 88% were located on Curaçao; out of 676 registered nurses, 87% were on Curaçao; out of 467 practical nurses, 93% were on Curaçao; and out of 41 operating assistants and 14 anesthetist assistants, 85% and 86%, respectively, were based on Curaçao.

Technical Cooperation and External Financing

Leading international collaboration partners with the Ministry of Public Health and Social Development include various entities of the Pan American Health Organization and World Health Organization, such as the Caribbean Epidemiology Center and the International Agency for Cancer Research.

Bibliography

Arnell F. To be or not to be safe. A study on the determinants that influence the sexual behavior and condom use of the secondary school students of Curaçao [Thesis]. Health Science, Department of Health Education and Promotion, Curaçao Medical and Public Health Service, Epidemiology and Research Unit. September 2002–August 2003.

Boas GM. Rapport Quick Scan Kosten Gezondheidszorg, 2003.

Curaçao Medical and Public Health Service, Epidemiology and Research Unit. Isolated gastrointestinal pathogens per year, 2007.

Deloitte and Touche. Quick scan of poverty alleviation programs Curaçao and Bonaire. Final report. Netherlands Antilles and Aruba. Version 1. 27 October 2005.

Directie Jeugd-en jongerenontwikkeling. Indicatoren voor probleemgedrag bij jongeren op de Nederlandse Antillen. Jeugdmonitor 2002/2003.

Fuchs G, Grievink L, O'Niel J, van Sonderen E, Gerstenbluth I, Alberts JF. St. Maarten health study; methodology and main results. Curaçao: Foundation for Promotion of International Cooperation and Research in Healthcare (ISOG); 2002.

Gemeentelijke Gezondheidsdienst (GGD). Tandheelkundig onderzoek Curaçao, 2001.

Grievink L, Fuchs G, O'Niel J, van Sonderen E, Gerstenbluth I, Alberts JF. The Bonaire health study; methodology and main results. 2002. Curaçao: Foundation for Promotion of International Cooperation and Research in Healthcare (ISOG); 2002.

Grievink L, Fuchs G, O'Niel J, van Sonderen E, Gerstenbluth I, Alberts JF. The Saba health study; methodology and main results. Curaçao: Foundation for Promotion of International Cooperation and Research in Healthcare (ISOG); 2002.

Grievink L, Fuchs G, O'Niel J, van Sonderen E, Gerstenbluth I, Alberts JF. The St. Eustatius health study; methodology and main results. Curaçao: Foundation for Promotion of International Cooperation and Research in Healthcare (ISOG); 2002.

Halabi Y. Tuberculosis [PowerPoint presentation], 2007. Epidemiology and Research Unit, Curaçao Medical and Public Health Service.

Nederlandse Antillen, Centraal Bureau voor de Statistiek. Huishoudens in de Nederlandse Antillen. Publicatiereeks Census 2001.

Nederlandse Antillen, Centraal Bureau voor de Statistiek. Huishoudens met zorgbehoevende kinderen. Publicatiereeks Census 2001.

Nederlandse Antillen, Centraal Bureau voor de Statistiek. Modus Statistisch Magazine, Jaargang 7 (1).

Netherlands Antilles, Bonaire Strategic Plan for HIV/AIDS Prevention 2002–2006.

Netherlands Antilles, Central Bureau of Statistics. Demography of the Netherlands Antilles: an analysis of demographic variables (Census 2001 publications). CBS; 2005.

Netherlands Antilles, Central Bureau of Statistics. Fourth Population and Housing Census. Netherlands Antilles 2001. Extended analysis of health and disability. April 2004.

Netherlands Antilles, Central Bureau of Statistics. Statistical yearbook. Netherlands Antilles 2005. Willemstad (Curaçao): CBS; 2006.

Netherlands Antilles, Curaçao. National Strategic Prevention Plan HIV/AIDS/STDs 2003–2008.

Netherlands Antilles, Department of Preventive Health, Section Policy, Epidemiology and Prevention. St. Maarten's Strategisch HIV/AIDS Plan 2001–2005.

Netherlands Antilles, Ministry of Public Health and Social Development, Directorate of Public Health. National Health Plan. Health sector reform conceptual framework [PowerPoint presentation], 2007.

Netherlands Antilles, Ministry of Public Health and Social Development, Directorate of Public Health. [PowerPoint presentation]. Valencia, September 2007.

Netherlands Antilles. (2002) National General Law for the execution of articles 13, 15, 16 and 17 of the Lands Ordinance of the Organization of the National Government, regulating the organization and tasks of the Directorate of Public Health and the Directorate of Social Development of the Ministry of Health and Social Development. 4 January 2002.

O'Niel J, Gerstenbluth I, Aberts T, Heuvel van de W. Project Ontwikkeling gehandicaptenbeleid Nederlandse Antillen. Hoofdrapport, 2004.

Pan American Health Organization/Caribbean Epidemiology Center. International evaluation of the Expanded Program of Immunization, Netherlands Antilles. 21 February–7 March 2005.

Pan American Health Organization. Netherlands Antilles. In: Health in the Americas 2002. Washington, DC: PAHO; 2002.

United States Embassy in Netherlands Antilles. Available from: http://travel.state.gov/travel/cis_pa_tw/cis/cis_981.htm.

United States of America, Bureau of Western Hemisphere Affairs. Background note: Netherlands Antilles. September 2006. Available from: http://www.state.gov/r/pa/ei/bgn/22528.htm.

United States of America, Centers for Disease Control and Prevention. Traveler's health. Available from: http://www.cdc.gov/travel.

United States of America, Central Intelligence Agency. World factbook. Netherlands Antilles. Available from: https://www.cia.gov/cia/publications/factbook/geos/nt.html.

Wijk van N, Gerstenbluth I. Statistisch overzicht van de gezondheidszorg Curaçao 1996–2000.

World Health Organization. International travel and health. Geneva: WHO; 2007. Available from: http://www.who.int/ith.

NICARAGUA

0   25   50 Miles

Honduras

Nueva
Segovia

Jinotega

North Atlantic
Autonomous
Region

Madriz

Estelí

Matagalpa

South Atlantic
Autonomous
Region

Chinan-
dega

León

Boaco

Managua

Chontales

Managua

1

2

Carazo

Rivas

Río San Juan

1 Masaya
2 Granada

Costa Rica

N icaragua has a surface area of 120,339.54 km^2 (*1*) and an estimated population (2005) of 5,142,098 inhabitants, 59% of whom reside in urban areas (*2*). The average population density is 42.7 inhabitants per km^2. The population is distributed unevenly among three geographical regions: the Pacific region (15.2% of the total land area, 54% of the population), the Central region (28.4% of the land area, 32% of the population), and the Atlantic region (56.4% of the land area, 14% of the population).

GENERAL CONTEXT AND HEALTH DETERMINANTS

The country is divided into 15 departments and two autonomous regions, which comprise 153 municipalities, most of which are rural or semiurban. While Spanish is the principal language, the nation is multiethnic and pluricultural, with mestizos making up the majority of the population. The indigenous peoples native to the Pacific and Central regions and the northern part of the country (Cacaoperas, Chorotegas, Nahuas, and Xiu), and the indigenous and Afro-descendant communities of the Atlantic region, consisting of Miskitos, Mayagnas, Garífunas, Ramas, Sumus, and Creoles (the latter also referred to simply as "Blacks"), make up close to 10% of the population (*3*).

Social, Political, and Economic Determinants

The political scenario over the last 15 years has been marked by problems of governance (*4*). A structural adjustment program launched in 1988 to reduce economic imbalances has been assessed as satisfactory (*5*); however, it has not received adequate support in the form of compensatory social measures and, consequently, it has generated widespread dissatisfaction and prompted frequent conflicts, expressed through strikes in key sectors of the economy (*6*), with negative effects for the population (*7, 8*). Government corruption during the 1997–2002 period (*9*) hindered economic development and governance, leading the current government to step up efforts to combat corruption and ensure transparency in the public sector. The fraudulent declaration of bankruptcy by several commercial banks, followed by government support measures, increased the country's internal debt and exacerbated an already unfavorable economic situation, further compromising fiscal sustainability in the last five-year period (*10*). The agricultural sector continued to account for the largest share of gross domestic product (GDP), followed by the manufacturing sector (whose share of exports has grown) (*11*)

and the commerce and services sector. The tourism sector is gaining importance in the country's overall economic development strategy, and a regulatory scheme is being developed for its management and strengthening (*12*). The positive economic growth observed since 1994 (3.9%, on average, between 1996 and 2003, 5.1% in 2004, and 4.0% in 2005) is the result of better macroeconomic performance and an increased flow of external resources, including family remittances and foreign direct investment. These factors, as well as the additional increase in public expenditure devoted to poverty reduction efforts, however, have not translated into better living conditions for the majority of the population (*13*). In 2004, GDP per capita was US$ 754 (*10*).

In 2004, the Heavily Indebted Poor Countries (HIPC) initiative reached a culmination point, leading to cancellation of 80% of Nicaragua's foreign debt. The doubling of prices for petroleum and its byproducts between 1999 and 2004 (9.0% of GDP) created imbalances in the national budget and in the balance of payments, notwithstanding the adoption of compensatory measures (*10*). Nicaragua remained highly dependent on external aid (10.3% of GDP in 2004) to maintain exchange stability, stimulate public investment, and pay off the public debt. The international environment continued to affect the Nicaraguan economy adversely, with diminishing terms of trade for its products owing to higher petroleum prices, an unfavorable balance of trade (more imports than exports), and increased public expenditure. The reduction of interest payments on the foreign debt, an increase in family remittances from abroad (12.2% of GDP in 2005) (*11*), and tourism helped to offset the trade deficit (*10*). In some areas of the Atlantic coastal region, drug trafficking was a factor in illegal foreign currency income (*14*).

In 2001, close to 2.3 million Nicaraguans (45.8% of the population) were poor; of this group, 15.1% lived in extreme poverty, with a higher proportion of poverty in rural areas (4.4 times more extreme poverty in rural areas than in urban ones) and in the Atlantic coastal region, where 12 out of 19 municipalities were extremely poor. Data from the Fourth Living Standards

Survey, conducted in 2005, seem to indicate a rise in levels of poverty (*15*).

The employment situation is critical. Although unemployment has shown a downward trend, there continue to be high levels of informal employment. While the minimum wage increased between 8% and 10% in 2004, the annual inflation rate that year was 9.8%. Workers' real wages declined despite the adoption of compensatory measures. The lowest monthly wage, in the agricultural sector, was only US$ 41.50, and the highest, in the banking sector, was US$ 98.00, neither of which is enough to cover the cost of a basic basket of goods and services in urban areas, estimated at US$ 157.40 in December 2004. In 2004, the economically active population was estimated at 2,117,600 persons. According to official figures, of this group, 93.5% were employed (69% fully employed and 31% underemployed), and 6.5% were openly unemployed (*16*). There are obvious gender inequalities in the labor sector: in 2000, women's net rate of participation in the labor market was lower than that of men (38.6% versus 53.8%); female unemployment was higher than male unemployment (7% and 5.3%, respectively) (*17*); and women's rate of employment in the informal sector was higher and their wages were lower. Case studies on women's working conditions reveal lower wages, less job security, longer working days, and higher rates of temporary work and home-based subcontracting, all of which illustrates the disadvantaged situation of women (*18*). Employment in the maquiladora assembly industry increased; there were 59 companies operating under the duty-free regime, accounting for a total of 61,090 jobs.

In terms of the Human Development Index, in 2005 Nicaragua ranked 112th and was classified as a country with medium human development (*19*). However, development is unequal and there are enormous socioeconomic inequities associated with geographic location, sex, residence in an indigenous area, access to services, and income level. By way of illustration, the lowest income quintile received only 5.6% of national income, whereas the highest income group received 49.2%.

Indigenous peoples are concentrated in the lowest income quintile. Poverty is overwhelmingly rural: 7 of every 10 people in rural areas are poor and 3 of every 10 children are undernourished. The most frequent violations of women's rights are domestic and sexual violence. In the case of children, child labor and lack of adequate access to health services, educational opportunities, and food are the most common human rights violations.

The Reinforced Strategy for Economic Growth and Poverty Reduction (ERCERP), implemented during 2001–2003, rested on three pillars: broad-based economic growth and structural reform, investment in human capital, and protection of vulnerable groups (*20*). In 2003, the Government recognized that prevailing conditions (political climate, fiscal measures, international environment, and anti-corruption efforts) were not suitable for the application of this strategy (*21*), and it put forward a proposal for a National Development Plan (second-generation ERCERP) that

redefines expenditure on poverty and orients public investment towards enhancing the competitiveness of the private sector (rapid generation of employment and development of exports) (*10*). The productive strategy seeks to encourage the formation of production conglomerates (principally coffee, meat, dairy products, shrimp, forestry products, tourism, and light industry). Spending on poverty reduction (12.3% of GDP in 2004) is still financed out of external cooperation resources (6.2% external financing and 2.7% external debt relief under the HIPC initiative), with insufficient allocation of internal resources for that purpose (only 3.4%).

The Government views free trade treaties—with the Dominican Republic, Central America, and the United States of America (Central America–Dominican Republic–United States Free Trade Agreement [DR-CAFTA]); with Mexico and the Dominican Republic (already signed); and with Canada, Chile, Taiwan, and the European Union (under negotiation)—as concrete opportunities to stimulate development and expand Nicaragua's participation in the international market.

The country has embraced the Millennium Development Goals (MDGs) and has incorporated them into its National Development Plan (*22*). However, assessments indicate that most of the Goals (particularly those related to reduction of hunger and improvement of maternal and child health) (*23*) are not being met, nor are the mid-term targets (*24*), and that in order to achieve them it will be essential to increase public investment, address the needs of excluded groups (*25*), encourage citizen participation, and improve communication between local governments and civil society.

A government evaluation revealed high transaction costs, dispersion of resources, lack of linkage with local initiatives, and low impact in the achievement of the MDGs (*26*). A wide gap exists between the estimated available resources and the amount considered necessary to achieve the Goals. A recent study (*27*) projected that to attain the MDGs and national development goals, US$ 5,300 million and US$ 6,400 million would be needed, respectively, in cumulative social investment between 2001 and 2015.

The Nicaraguan Government is currently engaged in a reform process. In the health sector, headway has been made in recent years in the formulation of health policies and of a National Health Plan (2004–2015), and work on a policy on institutional reorganization is currently being intensified, with emphasis on decentralization (*10*).

In 2004, per capita expenditure on education was US$ 79.30. The proportion of the school-aged population not being served decreased from 41.6% (1997–2001) to 36.5% (2002–2004). In 2003, 36.8% of the population aged 3–18 (836,980 children and adolescents) was not attending school; among children in poor households, the proportion was six times higher (*10*). In 2004, the net preschool enrollment rate was only 30.8%; net primary school enrollment was 82.6%, and net secondary enrollment was

40.1%. The illiteracy rate among the population over 10 years old was 18.7%.

Within the framework of agricultural policies that are unable to assure a sustained food supply for the population, poverty and rurality are decisive factors in the high level of food insecurity that affects many municipalities. The main causes of food and nutrition insecurity have been the limited availability of food, limited access to health services and education, and low levels of maternal formal schooling; their effects on the health situation are seen in height and weight deficits, higher maternal and child morbidity and mortality, higher rates of infectious and nutritional diseases, and reduced learning capacity and productivity (28).

Environmental degradation is worsening, as is the deterioration of production and habitat conditions. Nicaragua's great forest potential is being threatened by environmentally unsustainable practices, such as indiscriminate timber harvesting and ongoing expansion of the agricultural frontier, which have reduced dry forest cover by 85% and rain forest cover by 65% (29).

Social, political, and economic violence in recent decades has led to a rise in crime rates (30). In 1998, surveys of living standards included, for the first time, questions about domestic violence, which revealed that one in three Nicaraguan women had been a victim of abuse (31).

A high degree of population dispersion poses a challenge for the country's development and, in particular, access to health services. There are a total of 7,099 communities in the country, of which only 0.5% have more than 15,000 inhabitants, 2% have between 2,500 and 15,000, and 97.5% have fewer than 2,500. Under the social protection policy espoused by the Ministry of the Family, which emphasizes solidarity for development, various programs targeting vulnerable groups have been implemented, providing assistance to 366,349 children, adolescents, and adults in high-risk situations (3.8% of the total population).

With regard to the risk of emergencies and natural disasters, the country is exposed to hurricanes, earthquakes, volcanic eruptions, floods, landslides, and droughts. From 1931 to the present, earthquakes and hurricanes have claimed 14,897 lives. In recent years, hurricanes, floods, and serious food emergencies have occurred, mainly in the Atlantic region (32).

Imbalances created by unregulated economic development have increased the risk of technological disasters. The combination of poverty and environmental degradation in vast areas of the country has spawned high-risk enclaves in a country already recognized for its vulnerability to natural disasters. In several areas, water courses have been modified substantially and vulnerability to flooding has increased markedly, compounding soil deterioration and reducing the possibilities for sustainable production.

Demographics, Mortality, and Morbidity

During the 1995–2005 period, the annual rate of population growth decreased to 1.7%, which represents a significant change with respect to the previous inter-census period (3.5%) (2). Population growth rates remained high in the North Atlantic Autonomous Region and in Nueva Segovia (4.9% and 3.4%, respectively). In 2001, the total fertility rate was estimated at 3.2 children per woman (7.2 in Jinotega and 5.2 in the North Atlantic Autonomous Region) and the crude birth rate at 26.9 per 1,000 population (15). Major disparities between urban and rural areas persist. In the current population structure (Figure 1), the expansion of the segment aged 10–30 years is apparent. Urban dwellers make up 59% of the total population. A comparison of the population pyramid from 1980 with the 2005 pyramid reveals a broadening of the base (population under 20 years of age), a phenomenon associated with declining population growth rates. That expansion will be even more evident after the adjustments resulting from the last census (2005)—which showed the population to be almost 10% smaller than estimated—are incorporated. During the period 2000–2005, life expectancy at birth was estimated at 69.5 years (70.4 years for women and 65.7 for men) (33), an increase of 1.5 years over the previous five-year period for both sexes.

Emigration and internal migration continue to be important demographic phenomena. Approximately 4% of the population has emigrated to another country, the most popular destinations being Costa Rica (45%) and the United States (39%) (34). Seventy-six percent of Nicaraguan emigrants lived in urban areas, 61% of this group have emigrated within the last 10 years, and 90% are working in the destination country. The quest for better opportunities has led to growing internal migration. The areas attracting the largest numbers of internal migrants during the 1990–2001 period were Managua, the North Atlantic Autonomous Region, and Río San Juan. The departments that lost the largest proportions of population were Matagalpa and Chontales. Internal migrants, the majority of whom are women who work in domestic service and the informal sector, tend to cluster around Managua and in urban areas in general. Internal migration by men is associated with agricultural production. Nicaraguan emigrants to Costa Rica have an irregular migration status and work in situations characterized by job instability, low wages, labor subcontracting, and lack of legal protection.

The crude death rate has shown a downward trend (5.6 per 1,000 population over the five-year period 1995–2000 and 5.2 per 1,000 population over the five-year period 2000–2005) (33). Mortality by age group in 2004 was 49.5 per 100,000 population in the group aged 1–4, 25.9 per 100,000 among those aged 5–14, 99 per 100,000 among those aged 15–34, 253 per 100,000 among those aged 35–49, and 1,759 per 100,000 in the group aged 50 and older (35). According to data from 2004, the mortality rate was 3.19 per 1,000 population among men and 2.35 per 1,000 population among women (36). Male mortality exceeded female mortality in all age groups. The population aged 50 and older accounted for the largest proportion of deaths (58%), and the population under 1 year of age accounted for the smallest (14.6%).

FIGURE 1. Population structure, by age and sex, Nicaragua, 1980 and 2005.

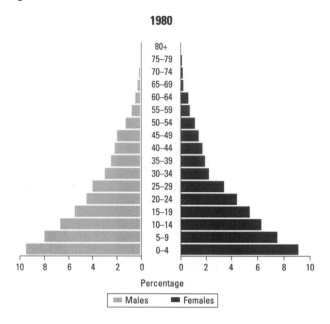

1980

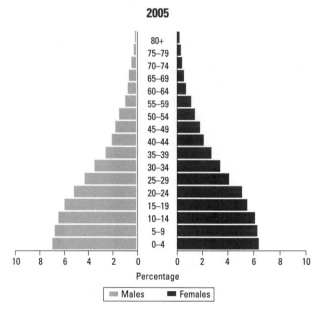

2005

Source: Based on estimates from the National Statistics and Census Institute (INEC); figures do not reflect adjustments from the last census (2005) due to data unavailability.

The North Atlantic Autonomous Region and the South Atlantic Autonomous Region were the departments with the highest death rates.

The most recent five-year period saw a rise in the proportion of deaths due to diseases of the circulatory system and cancer

(malignant neoplasms). Between 1996 and 2004, diseases of the circulatory system remained the leading cause of death, accounting for 23.1% in 1996 and 26.0% in 2004, followed by external causes, which remained in second place (14% in 1996; 13% in 2004), and by cancer, which continued to rank third, although the proportion of cancer deaths increased markedly over the period (from 9.7% to 12.0%). Deaths from communicable diseases decreased from 9.3% to 8.0%, and deaths from disorders originating in the perinatal period fell from 7.7% to 6.0%, those two groups of causes ranking fourth and fifth, respectively, as causes of death (*35*). As can be seen in Table 1, the three leading causes of death in 2004 were ischemic heart diseases (11.1%), cerebrovascular diseases (6.9%), and diabetes mellitus (6.1%).

The coverage by the information systems of the Ministry of Health, the Vital Records Bureau, and the National Vital Statistics System is incomplete. Under-registration of deaths and births is estimated at 50% and 40%, respectively, with especially large gaps in data from the country's most geographically isolated regions. The statistics compiled by the Ministry of Health reflect demand by the population that has access to its services (approximately 60%–65% of the total population) (*13*). The morbidity and mortality figures cited in the following section on population groups were calculated by the Ministry of Health using as denominators the population estimates of the National Statistics and Census Institute, based on the previous census. As the new census conducted in 2005 found the population to be smaller than had been estimated, these figures may change in the near future (the final census data are not yet available). In view of the level of underreporting inherent in the Ministry of Health statistics, infant mortality rates were obtained using data from Demographic and Health Surveys conducted in 1998 and 2001.

HEALTH OF POPULATION GROUPS

Children under 5 Years Old

Children under 1 year old made up an estimated 2.7% of the population in 2003. The infant mortality rate (estimated for a five-year period) dropped from 40 per 1,000 live births in 1998 to 31 per 1,000 in 2001 (Figure 2). The leading causes of death among children under 1 year of age were respiratory conditions of the newborn, sepsis of the newborn, asphyxia, pneumonia, congenital malformations, and intestinal infectious diseases. The rates were higher among males (39 per 1,000 live births versus 32 per 1,000 among females; these data are derived from an analysis of infant death rates for the last 10 years), among children born to mothers over the age of 40 (45 per 1,000 live births), among children born to mothers with more than seven children (59 per 1,000 live births), among children born within two years of the mother's previous birth (60 per 1,000 live births), among low-birthweight babies (36 per 1,000), and among children whose mothers received no care during the pre-

TABLE 1. Leading causes of death, Nicaragua, 1990 and 2004.

Causes	1990 (%)	2004 (%)
Ischemic heart diseases	4.1	11.1
Cerebrovascular diseases	5.7	6.9
Diabetes mellitus	1.5	6.1
Cirrhosis and other diseases of liver	1.4	4.6
Respiratory disorders specific to the perinatal period	4.9	4.3
Diseases of the urinary system	3.0	4.1
Hypertensive diseases	1.1	3.1
Influenza and pneumonia	7.5	3.0
Assault (homicide by firearm and/or sharp object)	1.3	2.9
Ill-defined causes	2.1	1.7
Other causes	67.4	52.2
Total	100	100

Source: Dirección de Estadísticas y Sistemas de Información, Ministerio de Salud de Nicaragua.

FIGURE 2. Infant mortality trends, Nicaragua, 1997–2004.

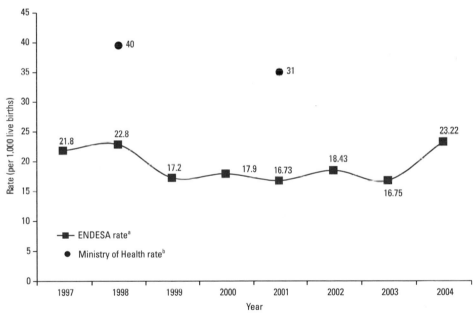

[a]Nicaraguan Demographic and Health Survey (ENDESA) data are from surveys conducted in 1998 and 2001.
[b]Ministry of Health (MINSA) figures are estimated to be underreported by 40%–50%.

natal period or during childbirth (66 per 1,000) (*37*). Infant mortality was also higher among children born to mothers with no formal education (54 per 1,000), mothers in the lowest income quintile of the population (49.6 per 1,000), mothers living in rural areas (43 per 1,000), and in the Atlantic region (48 per 1,000). As can be seen in Figure 3, close to 70% of infant deaths were concentrated in 50% of the population. The Lorenz curve, both for infant mortality and for maternal mortality (Figures 3

and 5), illustrates the uneven distribution of infant and maternal deaths in the population.

Children 1–4 years old accounted for 10.6% of the population in 2003. Mortality in this group was 10 per 1,000 live births, and was higher among children born to mothers over 40 years of age (18 per 1,000), children born to mothers with more than seven children (16 per 1,000), children born within two years of the mother's previous birth (15 per 1,000), children born to

FIGURE 3. Lorenz curve for infant mortality, Nicaragua, 2001.

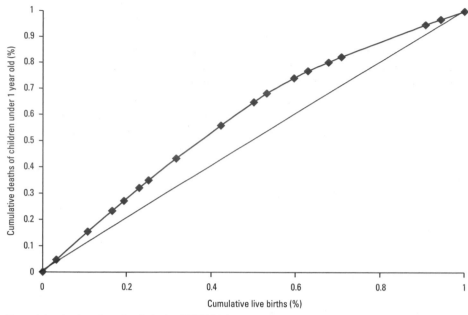

Source: Infant deaths estimated on the basis of ENDESA infant mortality figures for 2001; the number of live births was obtained from National Statistics and Census Institute (INEC) estimates of population and birth rates for 2001.

mothers who had received no care during the prenatal period or during childbirth (31 per 1,000), children born to mothers with no formal education (19 per 1,000), and children in rural areas (13 per 1,000), in the Central and Atlantic regions (13 and 12 per 1,000, respectively), in the departments of Jinotega and Madriz, and in the North Atlantic Autonomous Region (*37*). Pneumonia and intestinal infectious diseases were the leading causes of death (*13*).

In summary, estimated child mortality for the last five-year period was 40 per 1,000 live births (*37*). As Figure 2 shows, infant mortality declined between the 1998 and 2001 Demographic and Health Surveys; however, the rates calculated on the basis of Ministry of Health sources indicate a fluctuating pattern, which is partially a reflection of under-registration of deaths. The infant mortality rate was higher among male children (48 per 1,000 live births), among children born to mothers over the age of 40 (62 per 1,000 live births), among children born to mothers with more than seven children (74 per 1,000), among children born within two years of the mother's previous birth (74 per 1,000), among children born to mothers who had received no care during the prenatal period or during childbirth (95 per 1,000), among children born to mothers with no formal education (72 per 1,000), and in rural areas (55 per 1,000), in the lowest income quintile (64.3 per 1,000), in the Central and Atlantic regions (50 and 59 per 1,000, respectively), in the departments of Jinotega and Madriz, and in the North Atlantic and South Atlantic Autonomous Regions (64.3 per 1,000) (*37*).

In 2001, half of children under 5 years of age (48% of those under 1 year and 51% of those aged 1–4 years) had been ill in the month preceding the last survey of quality of life; the most frequent causes were respiratory problems (16% and 20%, respectively, in the two age groups), diarrheal diseases (28% and 24%), chronic diseases (0.2% and 1.6%), and other problems, including accidents and injuries (4.6% and 5%). Among children under 3 years of age, 94.5% had been breast-fed at some time, but of those children, 26.7% had received some other type of food before breast-feeding was initiated. Only 12% of children under 6 months of age were being exclusively breast-fed, and the median duration of breast-feeding was 17 months (*37*).

Children 5–9 Years Old and Adolescents 10–14 and 15–19 Years Old

In 2003, children aged 5–9 made up 13% of the population. The leading causes of death in this group were transport accidents, pneumonia, leukemia, meningitis, malnutrition, and accidental drowning. The group aged 10–14 made up 12.5% of the population and the group aged 15–19, 11.7%. There is little analysis of the information on these age groups, and the data compiled generally cover the age range from 5 to 14 years. In 2001, 31% (31.5% of males and 30.5% of females) were reported to have been ill in the month preceding the last quality of life survey: 18% due to respiratory problems, 2% due to diarrhea, 3% due to chronic problems, and 8% due to other causes, including accidents and injuries. The main causes of death among adolescent boys were homicide, transport accidents, and suicide, while among adolescent girls the leading causes were problems related to pregnancy and childbirth, homicide, and suicide. Maternal deaths among adolescent girls accounted for one-third of total maternal mortality (38). The main causes of morbidity in male adolescents were injury, poisoning, other external causes, and sexually transmitted infections, while among female adolescents they were complications of pregnancy, childbirth, and the puerperium; domestic and sexual violence; injury; and poisoning. Adolescents aged 15–19 accounted for an estimated 32% of self-inflicted injuries (intentional self-harm) (39).

A 2005 study found that 11% of Nicaraguan women had become sexually active before the age of 15 (40). The fertility rate among adolescents aged 15–19 decreased from 130 per 1,000 population in 1998 to 119 per 1,000 population in 2001 (41). The proportion of births to adolescent mothers fell from 31.0% of all births in 1997 to 27.7% in 2004 (36). Education is one of the key determinants of adolescent motherhood: 46% of adolescent girls without formal schooling had children or were pregnant, whereas among adolescents with a university education the figure was 5% (36). The proportion of pregnant adolescent girls receiving prenatal care was 85.7% (37). An estimated 12.1% of adolescents aged 15–17 have children (42), and 19.8% of young women aged 15–19 reported having unmet family planning needs (37). Knowledge among adolescents about how to prevent sexually transmitted infections was insufficient, even though 91% had heard of AIDS and 24% of syphilis (43).

Adults 20–59 Years Old

In 2001, one-third of the adult population (32% in the segment aged 25–34, 44% in the segment aged 35–49, and 60% among those aged 50 and older) reported having been ill in the month preceding the last quality of life survey: 16% due to respiratory problems and 22% due to other problems, including accidents, injuries, and chronic disorders. The proportion of women reporting illness was higher than that of men; there is also more information available on the health of women.

The total fertility rate fell from 3.6 children per woman in 1998 to 3.2 in 2001 (37). The gap between desired fertility and actual fertility rate was significantly wider in the lowest income strata (5.5 actual versus 3.8 desired) than in the highest income strata (1.7 actual versus 2.5 desired). An estimated 66% of women of childbearing age have used some method of family planning. Among women currently living with a male partner, 88% have used a family planning method, generally a modern one: contraceptive pills (59%), injections (38%), female sterilization or IUD (25% each), condom (23%), or the lactational amenorrhea method (16%) (37). Sixty-six percent of pregnant women received prenatal care, 34.4% of them beginning in the first trimester (23.7% in Río San Juan) (36). The proportion of

births occurring in health care facilities increased slowly, due in large part to increased access and participation by the private sector in urban areas; in 2004, the proportion was 51.6% (30.6% in Río San Juan, 31.3% in Chontales, 37.5% in Boaco, 40.6% in the North Atlantic Autonomous Region, and 41.1% in the South Atlantic Autonomous Region, the area with the least road infrastructure and the highest degrees of poverty). Among women who did not give birth in a health care facility, 72% received no postpartum care (37). Nevertheless, the percentages of women receiving institutional care during the puerperium have improved, rising from 20% in 1994 to 46.8% in 1997 and 50% in 2000, but then increasing only slightly between then and 2004 (50.7%).

Between 1992 and 2005, maternal mortality fluctuated, reaching its highest levels in 1996, 1997, and 1999. The rate has declined over the last five years, dropping to 87.3 per 100,000 live births in 2004 (35) (Figure 4). Like infant mortality, maternal mortality has shown a variable pattern, trending downward during the period under study.

Postpartum hemorrhage remained the leading cause of maternal mortality, accounting for 48%, followed by puerperal sepsis (15%) and eclampsia (14%); these causes were associated with high fertility, short birth spacing, and limited coverage and quality of services providing prenatal care, attendance at birth, and care for complications. Although maternal mortality has declined for the country as a whole, rates remained high in rural areas (e.g., Jinotega, 214.9); in the autonomous Atlantic regions, which have large ethnic communities (Autonomous North Atlantic Region, 184.7; South Atlantic Autonomous Region, 180.6); and in areas where access to health care facilities is limited, educational levels are low, and poverty rates are high. Figure 5 shows that 50% of the population accounted for 80% of maternal deaths.

Older Adults 60 Years Old and Older

Older adults accounted for 5.0% of the population in 2000, with women outnumbering men (male-female ratio = 1:1.2). In 2000, the aging index, which is the ratio of the population over 60 years of age to the population under 15 years of age, was 11 older adults per every 100 children under 15. It is estimated that around 60% of older adults are heads of household; of these, 76% of them are men and 24% are women; 42.2% of older adults are economically active, 94% are employed, and 6% are openly unemployed. In general, they are self-employed or they work in some capacity for their families. No differences were found between men and women, although in Managua the percentage of older women who worked was higher than that of men (15). According to the last quality of life survey conducted in 2001, 75% of the population over the age of 65 years (79.9% of women and 70.0% of men) reported having been ill in the month preceding the survey, 45% due to chronic diseases, 17% due to respiratory problems, 1% due to diarrheal diseases, and 12% due to other problems.

FIGURE 4. Maternal mortality rates, Nicaragua, 1992–2004.

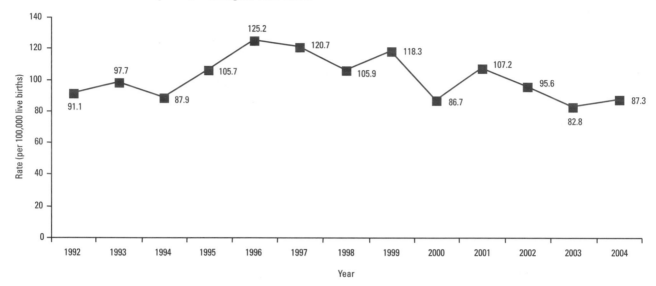

Source: Department of Statistics and Information Systems, Ministry of Health of Nicaragua.

The Family

The 2005 census counted 1,044,476 households with an average of 4.9 people per household. According to data from the eighth population census and the fourth housing census, both conducted in 2005, 94.7% of dwellings are inhabited by one household; 4.1%, by two households; and 1.2%, by three or more households (2). The proportion of families headed by males has remained stable: 71.9% in 1993, 72.3% in 1998, and 71.1% in 2001, although in urban areas a higher proportion of households are headed by women, most of them widowed or separated (15). The proportions of female single parents participating in productive and reproductive work were 47.3% and 87.8%, respectively. The new comprehensive health care model focuses on the health of the family and the community in a framework of health promotion and disease prevention. Morbidity and mortality data on family health are included in the analysis of the health of the various age groups.

Workers

The number of workers in the country was estimated at 1,973,100 in 2004. Most of them (82.4%) received health care from public facilities operated by the Ministry of Health, which do not keep specific statistics on occupational accidents and diseases. For the 17.6% of workers covered by the social security system, reporting of occupational accidents and diseases is mandatory. Employers are also required to report work-related accidents and diseases to the Ministry of Labor, but the inspections conducted by the Ministry to monitor compliance with this

requirement only cover 6.4% of the working population. A study carried out in León on working conditions in the informal sector (44) found that the main obstacles to the achievement of health goals are poverty; lack of coverage of basic health services; the growing proportion of households headed by women—who carry out the double function of earning wages to sustain their families and performing unpaid domestic labor; low and unstable incomes; performance of work that is not socially valued; and exposure to multiple risks, many of them environmental, including exploitation and mistreatment in the workplace.

Official surveys conducted on child labor indicate that the number of children aged 5–17 participating in the labor market fell from 314,012 in 2000 to 266,000 in 2005 (45). Of that number, 90% were working at the time of the survey (76% in the informal sector). The male-female ratio was 2.8:1. Of these active child workers, 74% were male and 26% female, and 11% were between 5 and 9 years of age. Although under current legislation children under age 14 are not allowed to work, eight out of 10 adolescent workers began working before their 14th birthday. Two-thirds worked as unskilled laborers, and more than half did not attend school for work-related reasons. An estimated 20% of children aged 7–17 are illiterate; this percentage is three times higher in rural areas. Approximately one-third of working adolescents reported having suffered work-related injuries. There are no official statistics on sexual exploitation of children; however, specialized agencies serving children agree that sexual exploitation of children for commercial purposes and the trafficking of minors are a reality of growing concern, especially in border, tourist, and industrial cities of the Central American countries

FIGURE 5. Lorenz curve for maternal mortality, Nicaragua, 2001.

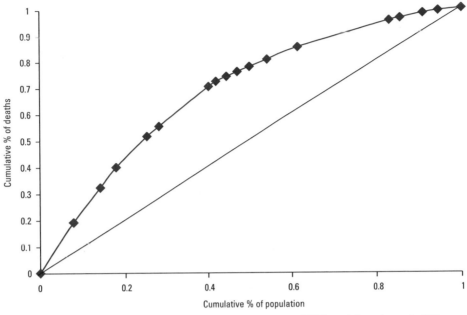

Source: Maternal mortality figures are obtained from Ministry of Health data and INEC population estimates for 2001.

(*46, 47*). In August 2001, the Government of Nicaragua approved a public policy against the commercial sexual exploitation of children and adolescents.

Trafficking of women and forced prostitution are recognized problems in Nicaragua. According to the Nicaraguan Center for Human Rights, there are some 1,200 sex workers in Managua, 40% of whom are girls under 18. A study conducted among 300 girl prostitutes found that 56% became sexually active at 12 or 13 years of age, 28% had been raped, and 50% had sex with more than five clients per day (*48*).

Persons with Disabilities

According to the results of a 2003 survey, the prevalence of disabilities in the population over 6 years of age was estimated at 10.3% (11.3% among females and 9.1% among males, 10.5% among urban dwellers and 10.1% among rural dwellers) (*49*). The prevalence of disability increases with age, the percentages ranging from 3.7% among children aged 6–9 to 85.3% among adults over age 80. The prevalence of impairments affecting the ability to perform certain activities was estimated at 58.0% for comprehension and communication, 75.2% for mobility, 22.6% for self-care, 26.6% for ability to relate to others, 49.9% for household activities, 30.2% for work or school activities, and 53.9% for participation in society. With regard to causes, disabilities are associated mainly with chronic diseases (67%); birth defects and injuries (9%); falls, injuries, and other accidents (9.5%); infec-

tious diseases (4%); occupational diseases (3.4%); motor vehicle accidents (2.3%); war (2.2%); and assault (1.8%). Fifteen percent of people with disabilities had suffered physical or psychological violence, and 14% had suffered some kind of accident during the last year.

Ethnic Groups

The areas with the highest proportions of indigenous populations have the worst health disparities in the country. In 2005, the maternal mortality ratio in the North Atlantic Autonomous Region was 2.1 times higher than the national average and the perinatal mortality rate was 1.6 times higher (*36*). The percentages of indigenous populations living in areas at high risk for natural disasters are estimated at 100% for the Ramas, 90% for Mayagnas, and 61.6% for Miskitos, compared to the national average of 31.8%. Indigenous communities reported less access to family planning services, prenatal care, and care during childbirth. For example, 29.3% of Miskito mothers received no prenatal care (versus 12.3% for the country as a whole), and 57.4% did not give birth in a health care facility (compared to 27.7% for the country as a whole) (*50*). More than a third (33.7%) of Miskito children and 100% of Ramas children suffered from chronic malnutrition (19.6% for the country as a whole); 12.8% of Miskito children suffered from overall malnutrition (8.9% for the country). Miskito communities consume the equivalent of only 70% of the average per capita food intake in Nicaragua and 49.8% cannot afford a basic food basket (34% for the country as a whole) (*50*). The higher incidence of *Plasmodium falciparum* malaria and of tuberculosis was found in the indigenous Atlantic regions. More than 90% of all *P. falciparum* malaria cases in 2001 were concentrated in 24 municipalities with indigenous populations.

Border Populations

Residents in the Río Coco area along the northern border with Honduras and the Río San Juan region along the southern border with Costa Rica face situations of isolation and lack of access to health services. Nicaraguan women who emigrate to Costa Rica exhibit a less favorable maternal and child health profile than their Costa Rican counterparts: they have a lower educational level, they use contraceptives less, and they have less access to health services in general and to preventive services in particular. On the positive side, Nicaraguan female emigrants have lower rates of tobacco use (6% have smoked at some time versus 14% of Costa Rican women) and fewer cesarean births (13% versus 20%), and a higher proportion of them have been vaccinated against tetanus in the last 10 years (83% versus 73%) (*51*).

HEALTH CONDITIONS AND PROBLEMS

COMMUNICABLE DISEASES

Vector-borne Diseases

Much of the information presented in this section is based on Ministry of Health national surveillance data (*52*).

In the last 10 years, the number of **malaria** cases has declined significantly, the annual parasite incidence (API) having dropped from 1.72 per 1,000 population (71,380 cases) in 1995 to 0.11 per 1,000 (6,373 cases) in 2005. Over the 2001–2005 review period, eight comprehensive local health systems (SILAIS) recorded high rates of malaria transmission: those of the North Atlantic Autonomous Region, the South Atlantic Autonomous Region, Río San Juan, Chontales, Matagalpa, Jinotega, Chinandega, and Nueva Segovia. Approximately 36 high-risk municipalities accounted for 93% of the total morbidity burden for the country. In 2004, reported morbidity was 10.7 per 10,000 population, with high rates in the North Atlantic Autonomous Region, the South Atlantic Autonomous Region, Matagalpa, Jinotega, and Chinandega. Around 83% of the cases were caused by *Plasmodium vivax* and 17% by *P. falciparum*; less than 1% were mixed infections. *Anopheles albimanus*, the main vector in Nicaragua, is found in all of the country's 17 departments and regions. Limited foci of transmission exist for *A. pseudopunctipennis* in the Pacific region (Chinandega and Managua). By age group, the highest rates occurred among children 1–4 years old (21.4 per 10,000) and those 5–14 years old (14 per 10,000). The male population was most affected (accounting for 70% of cases). Ninety-five percent of the *P. falciparum*

cases were concentrated in the North Atlantic and South Atlantic Autonomous Regions. In 2005, the malaria mortality rate was 0.13 per 100,000 population. Eight deaths were registered in 2002, seven in 2003, one in 2004, and six in 2005. Malaria morbidity and mortality have shown a slow but steady downward trend, and the goal proposed by the World Health Organization (WHO) of halving malaria mortality by 2010 and reducing the malaria morbidity burden by 2015 is considered to be feasible, provided the control strategies applied to date are consolidated. These strategies have strengthened the capacity for early diagnosis and timely treatment, as well as detection of epidemics, control of breeding sites, human resources development focusing on vector behavior, and malaria stratification to the "malarious household" level (i.e., households with at least one malaria-positive individual).

In the last five years, **dengue** has shown an endemic-epidemic pattern, with outbreaks associated with the introduction of a new serotype in a specific area of the country. Between 2002 and 2005, all of the 17 departments and regions reported dengue cases. Circulation of serotypes 1, 2, and 4 was confirmed by the national reference laboratory, but it is serotype 2 that has had the greatest impact in terms of morbidity and mortality. The reported dengue morbidity rate in 2003 was 4.7 per 10,000 population for classical dengue and 0.4 per 10,000 for hemorrhagic dengue, decreasing in 2005 to 3.2 per 10,000 and 0.3 per 10,000, respectively. In 2004, the areas most heavily affected by the classical form were the departments of Masaya and Madriz and the North Atlantic Autonomous Region, and those most heavily affected by the hemorrhagic form were Masaya and Granada. The population aged 5–14 had the highest morbidity (4.5 per 10,000 population), followed by the group aged 15–49 (3.0 per 10,000); 54% of the cases occurred among women and 46% among men. In 2005, overall dengue mortality was 0.2 per 100,000 population (six deaths). The case fatality rate for hemorrhagic dengue was 3% (*53*).

Three forms of **leishmaniasis** have been identified in Nicaragua: cutaneous (99% of cases) and atypical cutaneous (0.57%), caused by *Leishmania chagas*; mucocutaneous (0.4%), caused by *Leishmania (V.) braziliensis* and *Leishmania (V.) panamensis*; and visceral (0.03% of cases). Thirty-one species of *Lutzomyia* have been identified, two of which are vectors of cutaneous and mucocutaneous leishmaniasis—*Lu. panamensis* and *Lu. ylephiletor*—and one is a vector of cutaneous and visceral leishmaniasis—*Lu. longipalpis*. Leishmaniasis in its various clinical forms has shown an upward trend, the number of cases rising from 959 in 1995 to 3,312 in 2005. In 2004, the incidence of leishmaniasis was 3.5 per 10,000 population (*54*). The highest incidence was recorded among the group 1–4 years of age (10.5 per 10,000 population), followed by the group aged 5–14 (8 per 10,000) and by the group aged 15–49 (4.2 per 10,000). Women accounted for 52% of the reported cases and men for 48%. Sixty percent of the cases occurred in Jinotega; 22% in Matagalpa; 9% in Chontales; and the remaining 9% in Río San Juan, the North Atlantic Autonomous Region, and the South Atlantic Autonomous

Region. The geographic distribution of the disease is related to the opening up of new agricultural lands in jungle areas (in the case of the cutaneous and mucocutaneous forms) and to unplanned urbanization (in the case of the visceral form) (55).

The main vectors of **Chagas' disease** were investigated by means of entomological surveys conducted during the 1998–1999 period, which found *Triatoma dimidiata*, *Rhodnius prolixus*, and *Triatoma ryckmani* in Diriamba, San Fernando, and Chinandega; *Triatoma nitida* in San Rafael and Jinotega; and *Panstrongylus geniculatus* in El Rama, San Carlos, and San Miguelito. *R. pallescens*, detected in Río San Juan, was not reported until 2002. The disease is significantly underreported, which makes it difficult to determine its true magnitude. Seroprevalence studies of 150,000 blood donors during the 1990s found rates of 0.3% in Managua and 11% in the northern portion of the country (mainly Madriz, Nueva Segovia, and Matagalpa). In 2000, a serologic survey of schoolchildren aged 7–14 in all 15 departments (56) found an overall seroprevalence of 3.6%. Another serologic survey, carried out in 2003 among children under 15 years of age in communities with a known presence of *R. prolixus*, revealed a seroprevalence of 10.8% in Madriz, 4.3% in Nueva Segovia, 1.8% in Chinandega and Jinotega, and 0.2% in Masaya. In the municipality of Esquipulas, in communities infested with *T. dimidiata*, seroprevalences of 1% among children under 15 and 1.7% among pregnant women were reported.

Vaccine-preventable Diseases

There have been no reported cases of **poliomyelitis** since 1981, none of **diphtheria** since 1987, and none of **measles** since 1994. A national vaccination campaign targeting the population aged 6–39 was carried out against **rubella** and congenital rubella syndrome in 2005, and coverage of 100% was achieved. Between 2001 and 2005, 38 cases of non-neonatal **tetanus** were reported (mostly among adults), 11 cases of **whooping cough** (10 of them in the South Atlantic Autonomous Region in 2002), and 3 cases of neonatal tetanus (the last one in 2005). Nicaragua has taken advantage of Vaccination Week in the Americas to reach vulnerable populations and children who had never been vaccinated, thus improving immunization coverage in all municipalities.

Intestinal Infectious Diseases

Mortality due to intestinal infectious diseases decreased from 1.9% in 2002 to 1.4% in 2004 (57). Reported morbidity from acute diarrheal diseases remained virtually unchanged (372 per 10,000 population in 2000 and 358 per 10,000 in 2004), with the Caribbean regions reporting rates 2.2 times higher than the national average. The departments with the highest rates were those with the lowest rates of drinking water services coverage. The last 12 cases of cholera were reported in 2000. In 2005, the prevalence of geohelminth infection was found to be 49.3% (58) among 8-year-old children in urban and rural areas of four departments (Chinandega, Chontales, Estelí, and Granada). Intense infection

was reported in rural and periurban schools in Chinandega and Chontales (between 2.0% and 4.5% of the children examined).

Chronic Communicable Diseases

Tuberculosis is endemic in Nicaragua, but has shown a downward trend over the past decade. The incidence of all forms of tuberculosis for the country as a whole fell from 88 per 100,000 population in 1987 to 39 per 100,000 population in 2004 (although very high rates persist in the North Atlantic Autonomous Region, where the incidence is 110.3 per 100,000, and in the South Atlantic Autonomous Region, where the incidence is 58.8 per 100,000). Between 2003 and 2004, case detection decreased by 2.7%. In 2004, 2,220 cases were detected, of which 60% were sputum-positive pulmonary cases, 20% were sputum-negative pulmonary cases, 15% were extrapulmonary forms of tuberculosis, and 5% were relapsed cases (with higher percentages in the North Atlantic Autonomous Region and the South Atlantic Autonomous Region). The 15–34-year-old age group accounted for 49.2% of the sputum-positive cases in 2004. More than half (55%) of the new sputum-positive cases occurred among males. The tuberculosis death rate in 2003 was 1.4 per 100,000 population. In 2003, analysis of a cohort of patients who had received Directly Observed Treatment, Short Course (DOTS) and who were subsequently retreated revealed a mortality rate of 4.6% (79 of the 1,699 patients died). The highest incidence rates, sputum-positive rates, and relapse rates occurred in the North Atlantic Autonomous Region. Between 1987 and 2005, a total of 52 patients with tuberculosis and HIV infection were reported. The SILAIS of Chinandega reported a total of 11 coinfection cases (21.1%) and the SILAIS of Managua, 19 (36.5%). Tuberculosis-HIV coinfection is most frequent in the population aged 20–30.

During the 2001–2005 review period, five new cases of **leprosy** were diagnosed each year; all were from the departments of Managua and Chinandega.

Acute Respiratory Infections

Diseases of the respiratory system were the leading cause of morbidity reported by interviewees in the 2001 Demographic and Health Survey who reported having been ill in the 30 days prior to the survey (38.2%) (37). The incidence of acute respiratory infections for all ages decreased from 2,513 per 10,000 population in 1999 to 2,338 per 10,000 population in 2004 (36). In 2005, the South Atlantic Autonomous Region and Matagalpa had the highest rates. **Influenza** and **pneumonia** accounted for 3.7% of deaths in 2002, a figure which decreased to 3.2% in 2004 (57).

HIV/AIDS and Other Sexually Transmitted Infections

The prevalence of HIV infection in the general population remained low (< 1%). The annual incidence of HIV infection increased from 2.52 per 100,000 population in 2000 to 7.66 per 100,000 population in 2005, with a rapid rise in the rate observed. Prevalence of over 9% was reported among men who have sex with men (*59*). Among HIV-positive heterosexuals, the proportion of infected women rose from 31% in 2000 to 37% in 2005 (*60*). As of December 2005, 2,031 cases of HIV/AIDS had been reported, 72% among males and 28% among females, with 0.68% occurring among persons under 15 years of age. During 2005, 420 HIV-positive cases were reported (323 carriers and 97 cases). Of those 97 cases, 46 remained alive and 51 had died from the infection (*61*). The male-female ratio in 2005 was 2.4:1. The largest number of cases was recorded in Managua, Chinandega, and León. HIV/AIDS is significantly underreported. The prevalence of AIDS in the population aged 15–49 was estimated at 0.2% in 2005 (*62*). Sexual transmission is the predominant form of HIV transmission, accounting for 92.0% of cases (74.0% heterosexual transmission and 26.0% transmission between men who have sex with men), followed by perinatal transmission (3.0%), injection of intravenous drugs (3.0%), and blood transfusion (0.2%). Data on transmission are incomplete in 2.2% of cases.

Other sexually transmitted infections are found most frequently in the population aged 20–24 (30% of cases). In 2005, 3,517 cases were reported, mainly of **gonorrhea**, **condyloma**, and **acquired syphilis**. The male-female ratio for all cases of sexually transmitted infections was 1:1; however, women had a higher frequency of condyloma and men of gonorrhea. The Atlantic region, Chinandega, and Managua had the highest incidence rates (*61*).

Several studies have identified early initiation of sexual activity and deficient knowledge, attitudes, and practices with regard to sexuality as risk factors for sexually transmitted infections; 60% of those interviewed in a 2001 survey stated that condoms are not effective in preventing HIV/AIDS, 86% reported that they did not use condoms with their regular sexual partner, and only 15% said they used condoms as a contraceptive method (*63*). Sixty percent of male respondents and 65% of female respondents did not believe that they were at any risk of contracting HIV/AIDS (*64*), and 20.4% of female respondents did not know how to avoid becoming infected with HIV/AIDS (*37*).

There were 19% of men in Managua and 24% in the Caribbean region (which comprises the North Atlantic Autonomous Region and South Atlantic Autonomous Region, and the Río San Juan area along the Caribbean coast) who reported having experienced at least one sexually transmitted infection, in most cases gonorrhea. Although those interviewed had basic knowledge about sexually transmitted infections, it was evident that many myths and widespread misinformation continue to exist with regard to these infections and to condom use (*63*).

Zoonoses

The incidence of urban canine **rabies** declined sharply, with only two cases being reported during the 2001–2005 period under review. No cases of human rabies have been reported since 2000 (*65*). In some municipalities (Sauce, Bluefields, Jinotega, León, Achuapa), **leptospirosis** remained endemic during 2001–2005, with 318 cases but no deaths. The proportion of laboratory-confirmed cases increased (29%), and overall incidence of the disease rose from 0.33 per 100,000 population in 2000 to 1.65 per 100,000 population in 2005 (*66*).

NONCOMMUNICABLE DISEASES

Metabolic and Nutritional Diseases

Child **malnutrition** remained severe in 2001; 20% of children under 5 years of age suffered from chronic malnutrition and 6.3% from severe chronic malnutrition (*37*) (14.3% in the North Atlantic Autonomous Region, 12.1% in Jinotega, 11.8% in Madriz, and 10.7% in Matagalpa). An estimated 9% of infants were born with low birthweight, and around 4% of women of childbearing age had nutritional problems. Among children under 5 in the poorest quintile, the proportions suffering from chronic and overall malnutrition were 35.2% and 16%, respectively; these are significantly higher percentages than among children in the highest income quintile (4.4% and 2.7%, respectively). This disparity is due to food insecurity, which affects rural areas in particular. Deficits in early stimulation and adequate nutrition increased children's vulnerability, which was also affected by the mother's educational level and the number of young children in the household. According to the second national height census conducted among first-grade schoolchildren in 2005, 27.2% of children aged 6–9 suffered from chronic malnutrition, and 6.5% exhibited severe stunting. The prevalence was higher among males in rural areas, and it increased with age. The departments with the highest rates were Madriz, Jinotega, Matagalpa, Nueva Segovia, and the North Atlantic Autonomous Region. In 46.3% of municipalities, the prevalence of growth retardation was higher than the national average; the most affected municipalities were Las Sabanas, San José de Cusmapa, San Juan de Río Coco, Telpaneca, Totogalpa, and San Lucas, in the department of Madriz; Rancho Grande, Tuma-La Dalia, and San Ramón, in the department of Matagalpa; and El Tortuguero in the South Atlantic Autonomous Region. The prevalence of **vitamin A deficiency** has shown a clear decline, dropping from 31.3% in 1993 to 25.9% in 2003 and 17.0% in 2004. Only 13.4% of the population was found to have urinary excretion of **iodine** below 10 μg/dL, indicating that iodine deficiency is no longer a public health problem at the national level. With regard to **fluoride**, 50% of the population overall has intake levels below the values recommended by WHO; exceptions are the populations of Managua, Moyogalpa, Tisma, and La Cruz de Río Grande.

In 2003, the prevalence of **diabetes** was 8.1% (*67*) (8.3% among women and 7.9% among men), with higher figures in older age groups (2.8% among those aged 20–39, 17% among those aged 40–64, and 22% among those over 65). In 2005, mortality from diabetes mellitus was 18.9 per 100,000 population (compared to 8.9 per 100,000 in 1992), and the majority of the deaths occurred in the over-50 age group. In the population aged 60 and over, more women than men died from diabetes (245.2 per 100,000 population versus 193.6 per 100,000 population) (68).

Cardiovascular Diseases

Between 1996 and 2004, the proportion of deaths from diseases of the circulatory system showed an upward trend, rising from 23% to 26% (68). These diseases continued to be the leading cause of death, with rates of 76.9 per 100,000 population in 1996 and 71.4 per 100,000 population in 2004. The death rates in 2004 were higher among men (74.7 per 100,000) than among women (68.1 per 100,000). The main reported causes were: **acute myocardial infarction** (43%), **stroke** (27%), and **hypertensive disease** (12%). Men accounted for 52% of the deaths, with more than half dying from acute myocardial infarction (56%). Among women, the leading cause was stroke, which accounted for 52.4% of female deaths. According to a 2003 study, the prevalence of hypertension was 25% (25.4% among women and 24.7% among men), and prevalence rose with age (13.5% among those aged 20–39 and 61.8% among those over 65 years of age); newly detected cases made up 9.8% of those figures (23.4% in the population over 65 years of age). The most frequent risk factor was overweight, present in 65.6% of cases (71.4% among women and 59% among men); 80.8% of those with hypertension between the ages of 40 and 64 were overweight, and obesity was a factor in 28.3% of cases. The prevalence of hypercholesterolemia was 19.7% (21.1% among women and 18.1% among men; 31.9% were between the ages of 40 and 64) (69).

Malignant Neoplasms

The proportion of mortality due to malignant neoplasms has increased (7.6% in 1990, 9.7% in 1996, 10.5% in 1999, 11.7% in 2002, and 12% in 2004). Cancer remained the third leading cause of death over the last five years. The specific death rate from this cause rose from 31.2 per 100,000 population in 2000 to 35.2 per 100,000 population in 2004. By site, stomach cancer accounted for 12.5% of all cancer deaths, cervical cancer for 10.5%, and breast cancer for 4.9%. In 2004, cancer mortality was higher among women (38.4 per 100,000) than among men (30.4 per 100,000). Cervical cancer was the leading cause of cancer death among women, and, together with breast cancer, accounted for 18% of all reported deaths from cancer (70). The prevalence of detected cervical cancer was 13.7 per 100,000 women over the age of 15 in 2001; it rose to 13.9 in 2002. The prevalence of breast cancer was 5.2 in 2001, rising to 5.8 per 100,000 women over the age of 15 in 2002 and affecting mainly women over 50. During the period 2000–2005, cervical cancer was the leading cause of morbidity among patients treated at the National Radiotherapy Center, followed by breast cancer (17.2% of cases) and cancer of the digestive and hematopoietic systems (7.3% of cases each) (71). Access to diagnostic and treatment services is limited.

In 2002, the estimated incidence of malignant neoplasms among men was 12.2 per 100,000 for lung cancer and 24.1 per 100,000 for stomach cancer. Among women, the estimated incidence of malignant neoplasms was 47.2 per 100,000 for cervical cancer, 23.9 per 100,000 for breast cancer, 17.6 per 100,000 for stomach cancer, and 5.5 per 100,000 for lung cancer.

OTHER HEALTH PROBLEMS OR ISSUES

Disasters

Since Hurricane Mitch (1998), some 13 natural phenomena have occurred (heavy rains, floods, earthquakes, droughts, and other hurricanes), creating disaster situations and exacerbating existing environmental vulnerabilities. In 2004, a massive landslide in the area around Musún Mountain, caused by intense rainfall, claimed 125,000 victims, approximately 4,800 of whom lost their homes. At the other extreme, drought affected mainly the Atlantic region, further worsening food insecurity. The immediate consequences of these disasters were overburdening of health services, increased incidence of diarrheal diseases owing to contamination of water supplies, and higher rates of respiratory and vector-borne diseases. The most affected population groups were children, the elderly, and pregnant women.

Violence and Other External Causes

The contribution of injuries to total mortality has remained about the same in recent years: 14% in 1996 and 13% in 2004. However, a steady rise in violent injury, rape, and suicide was noted. It is estimated that 30% of women between 15 and 49 years of age have at some time been physically abused by their partners (72). A 2004 study conducted in five Nicaraguan hospitals (73) revealed that injuries accounted for 18% of all emergency room visits; 35% were for falls, 23% for assault by bodily force, 12% for transport accidents, 12% for stabbings, 3% for poisoning, 2% for burns, and 1% for firearm injuries. Burns (36%), poisonings (33%), and firearm injuries (31%) accounted for the highest rates of hospitalization, and firearm injuries (17%), poisoning (14%), and traffic accidents (12%) accounted for the highest case fatality rates. The injuries causing the most premature deaths were those resulting from traffic accidents (2% case fatality), the main causes of which were alcohol consumption (9% of drivers) and failure to use a helmet, seatbelt, or child car seat (only 0.9% of traffic accident victims were wearing a seatbelt). Accidents involving bicycles (33%) and cars and trucks (18%) also produced significant numbers of injuries. The burden placed on hospitals was very heavy, in terms of both inpatient and outpatient care, raising health care costs (74). Almost half of burn injuries involved children under 10 years of age and were associated with contact with hot liquids, food preparation, use of household appliances, burning of waste, housing conditions (in many cases precarious, with a single room serving as kitchen, living room, and workplace), not wearing shoes, and family negligence. Burns occurring outside the home were associated with unsafe handling of explosives and, in occupational settings, with unsafe practices in welding and use of electricity (75).

Mental Health

Demand for care in mental health facilities in 2004, expressed as rates of care provided per 100,000 population, was 145 in outpatient facilities, 19 in psychiatric hospitals, 3.4 in day treatment facilities, and 0.34 in community-based hospital psychiatric units (76). Of the population receiving care in outpatient mental health facilities, 60% were female and 40% were male. By age groupings, 8% were children and adolescents. The leading diagnoses in psychiatric hospitals were schizophrenia (36%), mood disorders (21%), and substance abuse (17%). In community-based psychiatric units, neuroses (70%) and substance abuse (13%) were the most common diagnoses, while in outpatient care facilities, neurotic disorders (44%) and schizophrenia (12%) were the most frequently diagnosed conditions. Attempted suicide has shown a rising trend, as have suicide deaths. More than half of all self-inflicted injuries occurred in the 15–24 age group; 22% were associated with alcohol use and 84% with pesticides use, particularly phosphine, as a means of intentional self-poisoning (39). Suicide and attempted suicide among pregnant young women are important causes of maternal morbidity and mortality.

Grisi siknis ("crazy sickness"), a culture-bound syndrome associated with various manifestations of mental illness, occurs in the Atlantic coastal regions. The disease is currently under study, and no conclusive data are available as of yet. Outbreaks of the illness—marked by aggressive behavior, hallucinations, and convulsions—occur sporadically and have gained notoriety over the last five years as cases have been reported in one or more community almost every year. In 1999, cases were reported in Bilwi (North Atlantic Autonomous Region) and in Raiti (Jinotega). In early 2004, the communities of San Juan de la Bodega, Florida, Bulkian, Leymus, Tusku Tara, Santa Fe, and Santa Isabel, in the municipality of Waspam, and Wawa Bar, in the jurisdiction of Puerto Cabezas (North Atlantic Autonomous Region), were affected. It has been suggested that this ailment may be a sequela of war or that it may be linked to the exacerbation of famine in the North Atlantic areas. In 2004, in one of the most studied outbreaks, a total of 100 cases were reported in Walakistan, a community of 1,200 inhabitants (hence, 8% of the population was affected); half of those cases showed severe symptoms, which were treated with traditional medicine techniques.

Addictions

According to a 2005 survey, 78.7% of men and 43.8% of women in Nicaragua have consumed alcohol at some time in their lives; of those numbers, 21.9% reported having consumed alcohol in the year preceding the survey (77). Between 1992 and 1996, hospital-based epidemiological surveillance systems found the following lifetime prevalence of use figures: tobacco (36.5%), alcohol (42%), tranquilizers (16%), marijuana (6%), cocaine (1%), crack (0.5%), and inhalants (1%) (78). During the same period, the prevalence figures found in detection centers doubled for tobacco and alcohol, remained about the same for tranquilizers, and increased by 5–15 times for other drugs.

Environmental Pollution

In 2005, 1,332 cases of acute pesticide poisoning were reported (rate of 2.43 per 10,000 population), with 153 deaths (mortality of 2.79 per 100,000 population and case fatality rate of 11.5%) (79), but these figures only hint at the magnitude of the problem. In 2001, a national study estimated underreporting of cases at 98%, yearly incidence at 2.3%, and the annual number of cases at 67,868 (80). Several studies have found cases of delayed polyneuropathy in agricultural workers exposed to methamidophos, chlorpyrifos, and malathion (81–85); fertility problems linked to exposure to dibromochloropropane; and chronic effects of exposure to paraquat (86). In Managua, lead poisoning rates of 50 per 1,000 were reported in children living near small battery repair shops (87). In rural water systems in some municipalities in the northern and central parts of the country, arsenic concentrations exceeded permissible levels (88). The accepted standards are < 0.01 mg/l for drinking water and < 0.05 mg/l for safe water. Concentrations of over 0.05 mg/l were found in 8% of samples from Nueva Segovia and in 5.4% from Madriz. Previous studies carried out in Valle de Sébaco, Matagalpa, found levels so high that rural wells had to be closed. Arsenic poisoning cases have been reported in several communities, as have significant chronic effects in the exposed populations.

Oral Health

The development of oral health in the country has been described as "emergent," and a National Salt Fluoridation Program is being implemented (89). The prevalence of dental caries among children aged 6–15 years was 85% in 1999 (90). A 2005 study carried out in indigenous communities of the Atlantic region indicated that the caries rate in temporary teeth was higher among males. Children aged 6–12 years had the highest average amount of bacterial plaque, followed by children under 5 years of age. All dental caries indicators showed a straight-line increase with age (91).

Occupational Accidents and Diseases

The level of undercounting of occupational accidents by the Nicaraguan Social Security Institute (INSS) was 93%–98% in the primary and tertiary sectors of the economy and 64% in the secondary sector (92), and the Ministry of Labor reports 30% fewer cases than the INSS. The number of reported occupational accidents decreased from 14,864 in 2001 to 12,902 in 2004, for an accident rate of 4.8% in 2004, the majority of these events

TABLE 2. Principal health challenges and priority areas for action, Nicaragua, 2004–2015.

Health sector challenges	Problems

• Channel investment to the health sector
• Increase health care coverage
• Shift the sector's focus and activities toward a health promotion and disease prevention approach
• Stimulate social participation in health promotion and protection issues
• Create sectoral coordination mechanisms
• Implement decentralization
• Improve managerial capacity
• Develop human resources
• Implement a new services delivery model
• Seek new sources and mechanisms
	Group 1:
	  • Maternal mortality
	  • Infant mortality
	  • Malnutrition
	Group 2:
	  • Diarrheal and acute respiratory diseases
	  • Vector-borne diseases (malaria, dengue, tuberculosis, Chagas' disease, leishmaniasis)
	  • HIV/AIDS and other sexually transmitted infections
	Group 3:
	  • Disability
	  • Mental health
	  • Violence and injuries
	  • Occupational accidents and diseases
	Group 4:
	  • Noncommunicable diseases (diabetes, hypertension, cervical cancer)

Source: National Health Plan (2004–2015).

concentrated in the secondary sector. In that year, the most frequent occupational injuries were bruises (41%) and puncture wounds (25%). According to the Ministry of Labor, between 2000 and 2005, 183 fatal accidents were reported, yielding an average of 37 deaths per year; 25% of them occurred in the manufacturing sector and 20% in the construction sector (*93*). The case fatality rate for occupational accidents remained at 0.35% during the period (*93*).

Occupational diseases are also highly underreported. In 2004, the INSS reported 235 cases. The most frequent specific pathologies were functional dysphonia (31%), hypoacusia (19%), and carpal tunnel syndrome (8%). In addition, eight cases of byssinosis (2%), three of silicosis (1%), and three of asbestosis (1%) were reported (*94*). Chronic diseases related to exposure to dibromochloropropane and an epidemic of chronic kidney failure were reported among agricultural workers in the western part of the country. A high prevalence of disability due to decompression syndrome has been noted in Miskito divers along the Atlantic coast. A study undertaken by PAHO, the University of the Autonomous Regions of the Nicaraguan Caribbean Coast, and the Institute of Traditional Medicine and Community Development in September 2005 found that there were between 2,500 and 3,000 active divers in 2000, based on data from the International Labor Organization. By 2005, according to the divers' union SIBURAAN, the number of divers in the two autonomous regions had risen to 6,000. Based on information provided by 15% of the divers' families, it is estimated that 1,000 people are currently suffering permanent disability as a result of decompression syndrome. Of a sample of divers interviewed, 19.5% reported some sequela of decompression syndrome.

RESPONSE OF THE HEALTH SECTOR

Health Policies and Plans

The National Health Policy (2004–2015) (*95*) establishes the following general policy objectives: expansion of the coverage and improvement of the quality of health services, strengthening of the primary health care strategy, promotion of good governance in the health sector, consolidation of the national health system, strengthening of managerial capacity, development of human resources, and implementation of innovative strategies in the autonomous regions of the Atlantic coast and in border municipalities.

The National Health Plan (2004–2015) (*95*) is the fundamental tool for carrying out recently formulated national policies. Its aim is to ensure the right to equitable and universal access to a set of basic health services designed to increase the population's life expectancy and quality of life. The plan seeks to promote the adoption of healthy habits and practices of individuals, families, and communities, to expand social participation, to improve user satisfaction, and to enhance equity in the financing of health care, prioritizing vulnerable groups (extremely poor, rural, ethnic, and indigenous populations). To implement the plan, it is necessary to increase the response capacity of the health sector and ensure the sustainability of activities. Table 2 summarizes the main health problems and challenges in Nicaragua.

An evaluation of the health policies implemented between 1997 and 2002 (*96*) found that while health indicators had improved for the country as whole, these advances had not extended to the areas with the least access to health services or to the lowest income households. The financial risk to individuals associated with health care has increased as the share of private spending in total health financing, the percentage of people paying out-of-pocket for care, and the amounts paid have grown. The lowest income strata have been hardest hit by these conditions. No significant change in user satisfaction was found during the six-year period under consideration.

The issue of medicinal drugs in Nicaragua is critical. A national policy formulated in 1996 promotes access to essential drugs and use of generics, and strategies are being developed to expand access to essential and low-cost generic drugs and reduce prices. Regulation policies are also being formulated. However, the restrictions imposed by free trade treaties and customs union agreements have negatively impacted policies on access to drugs.

Performance of the essential public health functions (EPHF) was measured in Nicaragua in 2001 (97), and the country received a total score of 0.49 (on a scale of 0 to 1, with 0 being the lowest score and 1 the highest). The lowest scores were in the areas of public health research (0.15), ensuring and improving the quality of health services (0.17), and evaluation and promotion of equitable access to necessary health services (0.29). The most recent EPHF assessment was carried out in Managua (98), which received a total score of 0.53, the lowest scores being in the areas of public health regulation and enforcement (0.21), health research (0.24), and quality of services (0.25).

The health sector is currently engaged in a process of decentralization. The 17 SILAIS (one per department or region) are the providers and managers of health care at the subnational level. They organize and coordinate units at the primary and secondary levels, carrying out functions that include enforcement of the regulatory framework, public health surveillance, management of resources and establishments, oversight of the provision of care, and promotion of social participation in health. The statute governing the North Atlantic and South Atlantic Autonomous Regions gives them responsibility for participating in the formulation and execution of development plans and programs, administering health programs, and implementing their own economic, social, and cultural projects. The Ministry of Health and the Regional Councils of the two autonomous regions have entered into a collaboration agreement aimed at strengthening the Regional Councils and respective local governments for the transfer of resources, competencies, and responsibilities for the health of their respective populations. The North Atlantic Autonomous Region has its own health model and has made the greatest headway in this regard.

Close to 40% of Nicaraguans lack access to health services, and the 60% that do have access to services often find the care to be of poor quality. Among Afro-descendent and indigenous populations (Creoles/Blacks, Miskitos, and Mayagnas), the proportion lacking access to health services is estimated at more than 75% (99).

The results of a 2001 survey indicate that patients who seek care in health services operated by the Ministry of Health come mainly from urban areas and from the non-poor segment of the population. More than 50% of those participating in the survey said that they did not seek care when they were sick (the proportion is higher in rural areas and among the male population). The main reasons cited for not seeking care were knowledge of the illness (41%), lack of money (18.5%), mildness of the illness (16.4%), distance to the health care center (5%), and poor quality of care (3.6%) (100).

In 2004, the vast majority of workers (92.3%) were not covered by social security. Among rural workers, 93.6% were not affiliated with the INSS, and among urban workers, 78% were not insured. Of the workers who were covered by social security, 36.8% were in the commercial sector, 22.4% in the services sector, 14.6% in the agricultural sector, and 13.4% in the industrial sector.

The National Health Plan has nine objectives: to increase survival and quality of life among women of childbearing age; to increase survival and quality of life among children under 5 years of age; to improve nutrition among children under 5 years of age; to prevent and control diseases in general; to promote knowledge of healthy attitudes and practices among individuals, families, and communities; to reduce the incidence of accidents, disabilities, occupational diseases, and mental disorders; to reduce the incidence of risk factors associated with temporary and permanent disability; to increase survival among older adults; and to promote healthy community environments. Health programs are organized with a view to achieving these objectives, with a priority focus on services for women, children, and adolescents (family planning, prenatal and puerperal care, growth and development monitoring, immunization, integrated management of childhood illness, and sexual and reproductive health). Disease prevention and control programs stress vector-borne diseases, HIV/AIDS, tuberculosis, and, to a lesser extent, chronic diseases, environmental health, toxicology, and occupational health.

The Five-year Plan 2005–2009 identifies three objectives for institutional development: (a) extension of coverage and improvement of the quality of care, especially for populations without access to services or for whom access is difficult, rural populations, deprived populations, and indigenous communities; (b) strengthening of the health services system, including physical rehabilitation and equipping of facilities, functional organization and articulation of networks of services, and improvement of the management of primary and secondary care facilities; and (c) strengthening of governance, complemented by processes of decentralization and deconcentration.

Implementation of this plan presupposes the introduction of a new health care model, the conceptual framework for which has already been defined (101), although discussion of the economic viability of the two options—a comprehensive model versus a targeted model—is ongoing.

Since 2002, changes in the health system have been rooted in General Health Law #423 and its respective regulations, which establish the institutional and functional activities of the Ministry of Health, its governance role, and the principles underlying the comprehensive health care model and the provision of services in the public system (promotion, prevention, recovery, and rehabilitation); the regulations concerning the delivery of services by the private sector and the social security system; the provision of public health services; environmental sanitation; regulation of health products and services; and administrative, safety, and emergency measures.

Organization of the Health System

The system is made up of a public sector and a private sector. The public sector consists of the Ministries of Health, Interior, Defense, and the Environment and Natural Resources; the Nicaraguan Social Security Institute; and other state institutions that carry out health activities. In the context of the Government's overall strategy to reduce poverty, the Ministry of the Family and the Fund for Emergency Social Investment focus on vulnerable population groups. The private sector is subdivided into for-profit and nonprofit subsectors.

The Ministry of Health is the main supplier of health services and is by law the lead institution in the sector. It carries out essential public health activities benefiting the entire population, and it also provides individual health care for the vast majority of the uninsured. The Ministry is currently engaged in a process of institutional reorganization, in the framework of the State reform initiative launched by the national Government several years ago. The new functional organic structure of the Ministry of Health is intended to enhance its regulatory capacity, decentralize administration and reduce bureaucracy, eliminate duplication of functions, improve the linkages between management and services, integrate information systems, strengthen implementation and follow-up of plans, reallocate and target health system financing in order to better meet the needs of priority groups, facilitate the development of a new model of comprehensive care with a preventive focus, and increase the coverage of the services system.

The primary insurer is the INSS, which provides health care to its beneficiaries and their dependents through 49 private health care providers (*Empresas Médicas Previsionales*, or EMPs) from which it purchases services. The INSS does not have its own health care establishments, but it has spurred the development of the private sector by contracting for services with EMPs, many of which operate out of public facilities, affecting the availability of public resources through their use of buildings, resources, indirect subsidies, etc. Disbursements by the INSS are made on the basis of the services purchased from the EMPs under a prepaid health care model.

Information on the private subsector is limited. A total of 203 private health facilities have been identified (*102*), including both for-profit and nonprofit entities. Some are independent, and some are organized into networks (e.g., PROFAMILIA). They are concentrated in Managua and, to a lesser extent, in Chinandega,

Matagalpa, Estelí, and León. The overwhelming majority of private facilities are located in Managua; eight are hospitals, with a total of 250 beds, and the rest are outpatient care clinics.

The Ministry of Health has registered 90 nongovernmental organizations (NGOs) that offer a variety of health services, with differing degrees of specialization. National and international NGOs have the capacity to provide services on a national scale, mainly in conjunction with community-based activities, in some cases covering areas not reached by public services (such as the organization Acción Médica Cristiana in the Atlantic coastal region). The community subsystem is made up of networks of community health workers, midwives, and other volunteers who work in their respective communities. The subsystem includes basic health care centers and maternal health care centers, which play a central role in promoting health, as called for under the new National Health Plan.

Responsibility for the provision of health care is distributed as follows: Ministry of Health, 60%; INSS, 7.7% (including beneficiaries and their spouses and children under age 12); and private institutions, 4%. Civil servants and members of the armed forces have their own health care services.

In 2004, the INSS had 348,200 affiliates (*103*), which, based on a working population of 1,973,100 individuals, made its coverage 17.7%. Adding all family beneficiaries brings the total number of individuals covered by the INSS to 427,139, which is approximately 7.7% of the total population, as noted in the preceding paragraph. However, not all INSS beneficiaries have comprehensive illness and maternity coverage. If the services offered by the Ministry of Health and by the INSS are compared, it is evident that the care provided to the insured and the uninsured populations is very different: the Ministry provided 1.47 medical visits per person, 1.13 prescriptions per visit, and 5.6 hospitalizations per 100 population, whereas the INSS provided 5.18 medical visits per beneficiary, 1.9 prescriptions per visit, and 9.84 hospitalizations per 100 beneficiaries.

Health care for the various ethnic groups (indigenous peoples and Afro-descendant communities) is limited by geographic, cultural, and economic barriers and by marginalization and lack of information. The provision of services to these communities poses serious difficulties for providers and, even more so, for health services users. Care is provided largely by personnel performing their social service who have not been specially trained to work in these areas; most are male and do not speak the local languages of the Atlantic communities, which breeds mistrust among the population, especially women who are thus doubly excluded. At the national level, there is no specific unit that is responsible for the health care for these populations, although the creation of such a unit has been proposed in a draft law on traditional medicine and alternative therapies. Law #28 establishes that knowledge of natural medicine is to be compiled and preserved in a scientific manner and in coordination with the health system.

Public Health Services

Primary health care was adopted as a health policy in 2004, and it is also being incorporated into the new model of comprehensive care, with emphasis on family and community health, and on the implementation of innovative strategies for the Atlantic coastal region. The development of health promotion is still incipient, and intersectoral coordination and citizen participation still need to be strengthened. Nevertheless, there are initiatives to promote healthy schools, healthy workplaces, and healthy municipalities. Some health issues are being addressed through networks (of women, of workers, for children, etc.).

Priority has been given to programs oriented towards the prevention and control of HIV/AIDS and other sexually transmitted diseases; vector-borne diseases; chronic diseases, such as hypertension and diabetes; immunization; and health of women, children, and adolescents. Most of these programs have been launched by the Ministry of Health, with support from community organizations and NGOs. However, budget problems and limited resources in general have resulted in low coverage and in service quality that is far from optimal. In 2004, service production statistics for maternal and child health programs indicated low percentages of coverage with pentavalent vaccine and live polio vaccine (OPV3) among children under 1 year of age (79.4% and 79.8%, respectively), and somewhat better coverage with tuberculosis (BCG) vaccine in the same age group (87.6%) and trivalent measles-mumps-rubella (MMR) vaccine among 1-year-old children (84.3%) (36). The proportion of births attended in health care facilities in 2004 was also low overall (51.6%), and the figures were even lower in the Atlantic coastal area. Prenatal care coverage fell from 75% in 2000 to 66% in 2004 (with only 34.4% initiating prenatal care in the first trimester of pregnancy). The proportion of women receiving postpartum care has remained virtually unchanged over the last five years (50.1% in 2000 and 50.7% in 2004).

Although it was a difficult process, a new health information system has been organized and is now functioning. The system comprises seven integrated subsystems: health regulation, planning, services production, health situation, supply of technical and material resources, human resources, and management of projects and financial resources. The traditional information system has been maintained, although it does not integrate sector information and exhibits technological limitations. The information obtained is used for descriptive purposes and, in some cases, is linked to monitoring and evaluation of services. Nevertheless, there is a clear need for significant enhancement of the country's capacity for information analysis.

The Nicaraguan National Epidemiological Surveillance System is also functioning. This system focuses in particular on communicable diseases and reportable events, such as maternal deaths, compiling epidemiological information collected weekly by the health units of the 17 SILAIS. The great majority of public health reference laboratories (including the bacteriology, virology, parasitology, and food-testing laboratories) are located within the National Diagnostic and Reference Center in Managua. For specific types of laboratory work, the Center collaborates with university centers, such as the one at the Autonomous National University (UNAN) in León (for enteric viruses) and the center at UNAN in Managua (for aquatic resources).

The national drinking water company administers more than 500 electrically powered wells, whose operating and maintenance costs have presented challenges as regards the capacity to ensure continuous delivery of services (104). In 2004, national drinking water coverage was 74.5%. In urban areas, the level was 92.9%, albeit with significant limitations in quantity, continuity, cost, and quality. In rural areas, coverage was 48.6%, with a trend towards deterioration of water systems and lack of support for the management of local drinking water committees (10, 105). More than half (53.3%) of water supply sources were contaminated, especially in rural areas.

Per capita production of solid waste in 2003 was 0.585 kg/person/day, for a total of around 3,000 metric tons daily of household solid waste. Seventy-eight percent of municipalities had solid waste collection services, but only 18% of the waste collected was being disposed of in sanitary landfills (106), and only 35% of the urban population was served by sewerage systems (29). Only five of the 151 municipalities have adequate procedures for the elimination of solid waste, and there is no nationwide program for sorting or recycling of solid waste. Seventy percent of urban waste is not disposed of properly (107), and hospital waste also is not managed properly (108).

The main source of air pollution in Managua is vehicle emissions. Levels of ozone and particulates exceeding the WHO air quality guidelines have been found. The vehicle fleet numbered 102,024 units in 1999, and it is estimated to be growing at a yearly rate of 5%–10%. In rural areas, the use of firewood for cooking and heating is the main cause of indoor air pollution (29).

The Ministry of Environment and Natural Resources (MARENA) is the lead regulatory agency charged with implementing environmental policy and enforcing environmental laws (109). A National Environmental Information System has been established and is coordinated by an environmental coordinating body and a network of 16 institutions and regional bodies. Fifty-two environmental indicators are currently monitored in 10 key thematic areas (water, natural threats, biodiversity, environmental pollutants, energy, forest resources, mines, fisheries, soil and land use, and tourism) (110).

Nicaragua became a signatory to the Stockholm Convention in 2001 and is currently engaged in a project entitled "Initial Assistance to Enable Nicaragua to Fulfill Its Obligations under the Stockholm Convention on Persistent Organic Pollutants" (Global Environment Fund [GEF]/MARENA), aimed at strengthening national capacity to carry out the obligations arising from the Convention. The DDT/GEF project (Ministry of Health/PAHO) seeks to reduce the use of chemicals for malaria control and includes a component for the elimination of DDT in the country.

The Ministry of Health has a center for information, surveillance, technical advice, and toxicological assistance that offers workers' health programs and incorporates the National Toxicology Center and a toxicology testing department. The Pesticides Program, with national coverage, carries out health promotion and acute pesticide poisoning prevention and control activities.

Activities to alleviate the situation of food and nutrition insecurity in Nicaragua are oriented mainly towards strengthening public policies and formulating a national food and nutrition security agenda, in addition to improving national and local capacity to analyze and address food and nutrition issues and ensure food and nutrition security at the local level. This entails the identification and assignment of priority to the most vulnerable municipalities, sensitization, municipal and community organization and strengthening, introduction of food and nutrition security issues on the agendas of local governments, ongoing training for municipal stakeholders and sectors (including the respective communities), and strengthening of the capacity of health workers at the local level for the prevention and treatment of the main forms of malnutrition, especially among women and children. With regard to public policy, the Technical Commission for Food and Nutrition Security has been reactivated with the participation of Government agencies, NGOs, universities, and representatives of civil society, as well as international cooperation agencies. Thus far, a national policy on food and nutrition security, a national law on breast-feeding, and technical standards for micronutrient fortification of foods (e.g., iodized salt, iron-enriched wheat flour) have been adopted.

Regulatory schemes have been put in place for disaster prevention and response (111, 112), and corresponding sectoral regulations (113, 114) and methodological guidelines for the health sector have been issued (115, 116). The National Disaster Prevention System comprises the National Committee for Disaster Prevention, Mitigation, and Response; national Government agencies and institutions; and committees at the departmental, municipal, and autonomous region levels. In recent years, the country has made significant strides in the establishment of an intersectoral network for emergency preparedness and alert and for mitigation and timely response. The Ministry of Health has designated disaster focal points in the SILAIS, developed local health emergency plans and hospital emergency plans, drawn up lists of essential inputs for various types of disasters, trained personnel, and carried out intersectoral coordination.

Individual Care Services

The network of services operated by the Ministry of Health includes 1,039 outpatient care units and 32 hospitals. In Managua, there are 16 departmental hospitals, in addition to specialized hospitals in the fields of pediatrics, obstetrics/gynecology, surgery, and ophthalmology. The hospitals in León and Managua serve as teaching hospitals. The most recent survey of health facilities conducted by the Ministry of Health (in 2001) identified 203 private establishments, including 5 hospitals, 99 clinics and polyclinics, 41 EMPs, 49 clinics associated with NGOs, and 9 maternity clinics. At the primary care level, health promotion, disease prevention, and basic recovery services are offered in 97% of facilities (82% in health posts and 18% in health centers). Outpatient care services provide care through preventive programs, outpatient visits, and emergency visits, while hospitals provide emergency and inpatient care. The secondary level comprises departmental hospitals and national referral hospitals, and the tertiary level, national centers for cardiology, radiotherapy, ophthalmology, dermatology, psychiatry, and laboratory services (the National Diagnostic and Reference Center, an agency of the Ministry of Health). In 2004, 1.8 outpatient visits, 1.2 medical consultations, and 0.07 dental visits per person were provided (36). With regard to hospital services, the number of beds available per 10,000 population was reported to be 8.9, with an occupancy rate of 68%; the duration of the average hospital stay was four days.

Laboratory, radiology, and ultrasound equipment is insufficient at the secondary and tertiary levels, in spite of recent investments. Existing equipment and facilities tend to wear out and/or reach the end of their useful life, with insufficient money available to maintain and/or replace them, even in the private sector. In 2004, there were 20 blood banks affiliated with the Ministry of Health and four with the Red Cross, distributed throughout the country (at least one in each department). That same year, 33 transfusions centers were operated by the Ministry of Health, 10 by private services, and one by the Red Cross. These centers perform screening tests to detect HIV, hepatitis B surface antigen (HBsAg), hepatitis C virus, syphilis, and Chagas' disease. The Transfusion Security Law, enacted in 1999, promotes voluntary donation. In 2004, 48,713 donations were collected; 55% were from replacement donors, and 45% were from volunteer donors.

There is a national program, a hospital, and a network of services and therapeutic activities offered by NGOs for children with disabilities, although a much larger volume of resources is needed to be able to provide adequate assistance for the more than 600,000 persons with disabilities currently estimated to be living in the country.

Nicaragua has no gerontology services as such, and 90% of older adults are not covered by social security. A scant 0.4% of this group has private insurance coverage. The Ministry of Health recognizes that it is not equipped to provide appropriate care for older adults, especially in the areas of medications and rehabilitation for chronic conditions, without negatively impacting other disease control and hospital services. The social security system promotes care for chronic conditions and offers some programs for retirees, but they are mainly recreational programs (13). The Ministry of the Family has a specific program for seniors that includes technical advisory services for public and private centers; health care; recreational, cultural, and occupational activities; and awareness-raising among the general population.

A network of dental services exists at the primary care level (125 services distributed across 77% of the country's municipalities), but these basic services are only reaching 50% of the population, and have limited capabilities due to deterioration of equipment and insufficient availability of supplies and materials (*117*).

Although the country still has no specific policies or legislation on mental health, there are some plans in effect and interventions have been designed for disaster situations. A national program for integration of services exists within the Ministry of Health, and there is one psychiatric hospital in operation (with the equivalent of 2.98 beds per 100,000 population), five day-treatment facilities, and three community-based psychiatric hospital units (supplying 0.3 beds per 100,000 population). However, the INSS does not cover psychiatric disorders, and the supply of drugs is insufficient. In addition, there is tremendous inequality in access to mental health services for ethnic minorities, as is clearly evidenced by the fact that in the entire Atlantic coastal region (comprising both the North Atlantic Autonomous Region and the South Atlantic Autonomous Region) there is a single psychiatrist for a total population of 620,640 (*76*).

The UNAN Center for Research on Health, Work, and the Environment, based in León, offers occupational health services and provides specialized training in occupational health for technicians and professionals (graduates, with master's degrees and clinical residencies). Several large companies also have occupational health services, and the INSS has an Occupational Risks Management Department.

Health Promotion

Relatively little progress has been made with respect to an intersectoral approach to determinants of health, as evidenced by the scant attention accorded to such determinants in the five-year health plan. However, citizen participation in public affairs has acquired the standing of a constitutional right. The National Health Council, an entity organized under the Ministry of Health to stimulate dialogue and joint collaboration between the public and private sectors, has been strengthened, as have municipal health councils, and in the North Atlantic and South Atlantic Autonomous Regions, Regional Health Councils exist as part of the legislative branch of government. At the local level, community development committees function as self-management bodies for local development projects (drinking water supply, construction of latrines, energy, etc.).

With a view to improving occupational health, the Ministry of Health has promoted (as have other Central American countries) the use of a "toolbox for creating healthy working environments." The Ministry of Labor designed the National Strategic Plan of Action for Occupational Health and Safety with the support of the National Council on Occupational Health and Safety, but the Ministry needs to increase its institutional resources in order to expand coverage. The workers' health network has been consoli-

dated and is currently functioning as a commission of the National Council on Occupational Health and Safety with ongoing participation by the various Ministries concerned (Health, Labor, Education), INSS, universities, and labor unions.

In the area of child health, in 2005 a network for the development of healthy environments for children was formed, involving more than 20 organizations (Government ministries, universities, private sector, and unions), which carried out a situation assessment of child vulnerability, presented a policy proposal, and designed various educational materials.

Health Supplies

The 22 laboratories that manufacture drugs as third-tier producers are nominally national firms, but they import the entirety of their raw materials. There are also 83 drug importers and distributors, three of which account for 93% of total imports (US$ 113 million in 2004). Between 1993 and 2002, the number of registered pharmaceutical products increased 600% (from 2,061 products to 12,546). The proportion of generic drugs increased from 13% in 1993 to 26% in 2001. There are only 51 registered pharmacists, and not all units in the network of services have pharmacists on staff. The Ministry of Health suffers from a significant shortage of medical inputs for the various diagnostic and treatment services, which affects surgical services in particular.

The health units of the Ministry of Health at the primary care level have an inventory of 1,681 pieces of equipment, of which 75% are in good operating condition. Sixty-one percent of health posts have refrigerators, 28% have ice chests, and 82% have thermal containers for vaccines. As for the availability of telecommunications, only two-thirds of health centers with beds, half of health centers without beds, and one-fourth of health posts are equipped with radio and telephone services. Two-thirds of health centers with beds and just 3% of health posts have emergency transport means (*13*).

Human Resources

In 2004, there were 3.8 doctors, 3.1 nurses, and 0.5 dentists per 10,000 population (*36*). It was estimated that there were 0.9 psychiatrists, 2.1 psychologists, 0.57 social workers, and 0.07 occupational therapists per 100,000 population (*76*). In 2005, of all Ministry of Health human resources, 60% were assigned to direct care and 40% to services management (administration, instruction, and executive management). The average age of the country's health workers is 40, and 63% have held their jobs for more than 10 years. Health workers are concentrated in the capital and in the Pacific region, and are less abundant in the Atlantic region and the rest of the country. In the Atlantic region, nurses provide 88% of outpatient care and 74% of health personnel are women (93% of nurses, 86% of nursing auxiliaries, 76% of laboratory technicians, 52% of physicians, 37% of hygienists, and 21% of vector control technicians) (*118*). Training of health personnel is carried out in nursing schools and in seven public and private universities. The principles that should guide training for the health professions are currently being defined. The Ministry of Health is promoting a process of continuing education for health personnel.

Despite staff reduction policies implemented since 1990 (which resulted in a decrease of 18% between 1990 and 2003), the Ministry of Health remains the main employer of health professionals. Little information is available on the health workforce in the private sector. The latest survey of health facilities yielded above-average numbers of professionals in the private sector in comparison with Ministry of Health personnel in the fields of pediatrics, gynecology and obstetrics, and technical and administrative services.

A deficient salary policy for the health sector in the last two decades has meant low wages, and health workers have resorted to collective bargaining in order to improve their incomes, negotiating 15 incentives since the 1980s. This modality does not solve the problem, however, and generates distortions, since the incentives represent more than half of earnings, while the base wage makes up scarcely one-third of the total earned. This situation gives rise to constant grievances and prolonged strikes. A draft law on health occupations, with a new salary policy, is currently being drawn up.

Research and Technological Development in Health

The Department of Health Research and Education is responsible for formulating a national research plan and coordinating with training institutions and bioethics committees. Progress has been made in developing a research regulatory scheme and in drafting specific standards. The Ministry of Health, together with the academic community, has begun to put together a health research agenda.

Researchers are trained in the schools of public health in Managua and León. Most research is conducted without oversight by a bioethics committee (except in León and except for some larger-scale studies). Most of the results are published only as gray literature—i.e., they are never formally published and their distribution is limited—which restricts their application and follow-up. No regulatory policies are currently in place for the incorporation of new technologies or for technology assessment and development, nor is there a policy or strategy on information management. The main source of access to information is the National Health Library, which is linked to a network of documentation centers and virtual libraries.

Health Sector Expenditures and Financing

Health financing comes from a three-part mixture of the public sector (35.8%), the private sector (52.8%), and external cooperation (11.4%) (*119*). The amount available from public sources and

from external cooperation has tended to decline, while private funding has increased, driving up household spending. Between 2001 and 2003, expenditure for preventive and public health services made up 9.3%, 8.2%, and 7.3% of total health spending, reflecting a downward trend in this type of expenditure as a proportion of the overall health budget. Medical inputs account for the largest percentage of health spending (43.8%), followed by curative services (33%). By category of expenditure, the largest budget item in the private sector was materials and supplies (30%, mainly for drugs), and in the public sector, it was personal services (22.7%). The following example is illustrative: 1% of the total health budget went to mental health, and of that amount, 91% was expenditure for the psychiatric hospital. Reported spending for the research and training component was 7.3%.

During the period 1999–2005, the gap between available financing and the amount needed to ensure drug coverage for 80% of the population was estimated at 66% (*119*). In 2001, public spending on drugs totaled US$ 6 million (*120*); external cooperation contributed US$ 6.8 million, and the private sector spent US$ 60 million. Drugs accounted for three-fourths of total household spending on health. Access to essential drugs is limited for 45% of the population (especially vulnerable groups, such as hospitalized patients and some patients with chronic diseases) (*121*). A comparative study of prices for one product from the basic drugs list found that the cost in the private market was 4 to 10 times higher (*122*).

Health sector financing has risen since 1995. Per capita spending on health increased from US$ 53.80 in 2001 to US$ 59.40 in 2003. Health expenditure as a percentage of GDP rose from 2.4% in 1997 to 3.1% in 2004, and health spending as a percentage of total public expenditure went from 11.0% to 12.3%. Private sector spending climbed steadily, tripling between 1995 and 2001, which resulted in higher expenditure on the part of households. The latter constituted the main source of financing in 2003, accounting for nearly half of the total (46.8%). During the period 2001–2003, the specific per capita expenditure of households ranged from US$ 27.70 to US$ 29.10. The population continued to use out-of-pocket spending as a compensatory mechanism for obtaining needed services in a context of limited supply of services by the public sector and the gap between population growth and the response of the health sector to needs, especially with regard to supply of drugs and laboratory exams. The Ministry of Health is the second largest source of funding in the sector. Between 2001 and 2003, it accounted for one-third of total sector financing (32.1% in 2001, 34.8% in 2002, and 38.2% in 2003). This increase was associated with the allocation of the interim debt relief fund, fiscal funds, and external funds. Specific per capita spending by the Ministry of Health rose from US$ 17.30 in 2001 to US$ 22.70 in 2003 and US$ 24.90 in 2004. The various levels of the INSS together constituted the third leading source of funding, contributing an average of 16% of total health financing during the period 2001–2003 (16.1% in 2001, 14.7% in 2002, and 15.1%

in 2003), although there has been a downward trend in the number of active INSS beneficiaries. Other sources accounted for 8.9% in 2001, 5.1% in 2002, and 8.2% in 2003. The in-kind contributions of community organizations are not reflected in health accounts, but the existence of 6,324 midwives, 12,748 community health workers, 6,926 health volunteers, 2,841 health promoters, and 339 community leaders is recognized. In terms of infrastructure, 4,369 basic health care centers and 30 maternity health care centers were reported (13).

Technical Cooperation and External Financing

An effort to coordinate, harmonize, and align external cooperation has been under way since the late 1990s with the aim of increasing its effectiveness and impact. Nicaragua is one of four developing nations among the partner countries of the Organization for Economic Cooperation and Development in which the Joint Country Learning Assessment (JCLA) initiative is being implemented with a view to enhancing the harmonization of aid. The Ministry of Health launched its organizational efforts to establish coordination mechanisms to ensure more efficient use of international cooperation resources in 1997, and in 1998 a legal instrument was adopted—Resolution 74-98, creating and implementing rules and procedures for the administration and channeling of such resources. In 1998, the Interagency Modernization Support Commission was formed to serve as a mechanism for consultation between the Ministry of Health and cooperation agencies. This was the starting point for the creation, in August 2001, of the Interagency Health Sector Support Commission as a forum for dialogue, consultation, and coordination between the Ministry of Health and cooperation partners. This process has made it possible to define a sector-wide approach for the health sector, with cooperation modalities such as direct budget support (a method for disbursing cooperation funds aimed at reducing costs and aligning aid with the national budget system and with the national priorities identified in the National Development Plan 2005–2009), creation of the National Health Fund (FONSALUD), and sectoral coordination tables.

The sector-wide approach aims to increase the efficiency of the health sector, reduce transaction costs, and increase the effectiveness of the health system. Key stakeholders in this process are the Ministry of Health, the Ministry of Finance and Public Credit, the Technical Secretariat of the Office of the President, and the Ministry of Foreign Affairs, together with development partners. The objective is to coordinate interventions in support of the five-year plan and harmonize national procedures for budget management, procurement, joint missions, and common indicators. The sector-wide approach also establishes a broad array of financing modalities, ranging from the common fund for budget support (FONSALUD) to specific projects.

During the period 1997–2004, the health sector received US$ 324.6 million, or an average of US$ 46.4 million per year. Al-

though the external cooperation contribution fluctuated, declining between 1995 and 2001 and then increasing in 2003 as a reflection of the poverty reduction strategy (19.2% in 1995, 7.7% in 2001, and 10.0% in 2003), it continued to be important for the development of the sector. In 2004, health cooperation totaled US$ 51.3 million (US$ 10 million less than in 2003) (123). That year, the country had 39 agreements and projects under way, 33% of them aimed at strengthening SILAIS, 26% for institutional development of the Ministry of Health, 24% for strengthening medical infrastructure and equipment, and 17% for health programs (124).

Nicaragua's multilateral cooperation partners include the World Bank, the Inter-American Development Bank (IDB), and various agencies of the United Nations system: PAHO/WHO, the United Nations Development Program, the International Atomic Energy Agency, the United Nations Population Fund (UNFPA), and the United Nations Children's Fund (UNICEF). In 2004, the IDB contributed 29.2% of all external financing and the World Bank, 5%, mainly for the health sector modernization program. The United Nations agencies together accounted for 22% of total cooperation (PAHO/WHO, 4.1%; UNFPA, 4.3%; and UNICEF, 12%). The principal bilateral agencies working in the health sector were those of Austria, Canada, Finland, Germany, Ireland, Italy, Japan, Luxembourg, the Netherlands, Spain, Sweden, the United Kingdom, and the United States. In 2004, the largest donors were Japan (6.9%, for rehabilitation and equipping of health centers), Sweden (5%, for strengthening of SILAIS), Luxembourg (4.5%), and the Netherlands (3.5%, for the sector-wide approach). Since 2005, a portion of international health cooperation has been received in the form of direct budget support allocated to FONSALUD. The Global Fund to Fight AIDS, Tuberculosis, and Malaria increased its contribution from 0.4% in 2003 to 8.2% in 2004, providing specific support for these three program areas. The Norwegian Development Fund contributed 4.1% towards modernization of the health sector. The contribution of the European Union in 2004 was 2.6%.

The nongovernmental sector is represented by numerous institutions sponsored by national and international donors that provide cooperation for specific projects. In 2003, the Ministry of Health received support from more than 30 international NGOs, among them Save the Children, CARE (Cooperative for Assistance and Relief Everywhere), Catholic Relief Services, the International Red Cross, Doctors of the World, and Doctors without Borders (125). A wide range of national NGOs exists, two of the most notable ones being the Federación Red Nica-Salud (NicaHealth Network Federation), an important partner for the implementation of initiatives supported by the Global Fund to Fight AIDS, Tuberculosis, and Malaria in the country, and PROFAMILIA, an organization dedicated to the promotion of reproductive health.

According to the most recent report of the Ministry of Foreign Affairs, in 2005 there were 220 international NGOs registered in the country, 70% of which had a signed framework agreement,

A Call to Protect the Health of Women, Children, and Adolescents

In 2003, maternal deaths among adolescent girls accounted for one-third of total maternal mortality. The main causes of morbidity among female adolescents were complications of pregnancy, childbirth, and the puerperium; domestic and sexual violence; injury; and poisoning. Adolescents aged 15–19 accounted for an estimated 32% of self-inflicted injuries (intentional self-harm).

One of the objectives of the National Health Plan is to increase the survival rate and the quality of life among women of childbearing age. Health programs are organized with a view to achieving this objective, with a priority focus on services for women, children, and adolescents (family planning, prenatal and postnatal care, growth and development monitoring, immunization, integrated management of childhood illness, and sexual and reproductive health). Most of these programs have been undertaken by the Ministry of Health with support from community organizations and NGOs.

16% were inactive, and 14% were active but without a framework agreement. The largest proportions of organizations were from the United States (30%), Spain (14%), and Italy (10%); the rest, in descending order by proportion, were from Germany, Switzerland, Canada, France, Finland, Norway, Denmark, Sweden, the United Kingdom, Belgium, Austria, and the Netherlands. The number of civil society organizations in Nicaragua is estimated at between 300 and 400 (*126*).

References

1. Nicaragua, Instituto Nicaragüense de Estudios Territoriales. Managua; 2006.

2. Nicaragua, Instituto Nacional de Estadísticas y Censos. VIII Censo de Población y IV de Vivienda, 2005. Cifras oficiales. Managua: INEC; 2006.

3. National Geographic; Tierras Nativas; Universidad de las Regiones Autónomas de la Costa Caribe Nicaragüense. Mapa de las regiones indígenas en Nicaragua. Managua; 2003. Actualización de la Asociación Pro Desarrollo Infantil y OPS/OMS; 2004.

4. Delgado R. La gobernabilidad democrática en Nicaragua: principales desafíos. Revista Probidad, edición 24; septiembre de 2003. Available at: http://www.revistaprobidad.info/024/015.pdf.

5. World Bank. Country assistance strategy for the Republic of Nicaragua. World Bank; 2002: 24–26. Available at: http://wbln0018.worldbank.org/LAC.

6. Fajardo R. El caso de Nicaragua. In: Las organizaciones sindicales centroamericanas como actores del sistema de relaciones laborales. Organización Internacional del Trabajo; 2003: 405–527. Available at: http://www.ilo.org/public/english/dialogue/actrav/publ/orgsindca/nicaragua.pdf.

7. Martínez M. Daños colaterales de huelga médica. El Nuevo Diario; 24 de mayo de 2006, Managua. Edición 9257. Available at: http://www.elnuevodiario.com.ni/2006/05/24/nacionales/20175.

8. EFECOM. Nicaragua casi paralizada por huelgas en los diferentes sectores. Agencia Efe; 6 de febrero de 2006, Managua. Available at: http://www.finanzas.com/id.8970865/noticias/noticia.htm.

9. Transparencia Internacional. Informe global de la corrupción 2004. Informes de países. Londres: TI; 2004: 291–294. Available at: http://www.transparency.org/publications/gcr/download_gcr/download_gcr_2004.

10. Nicaragua, Secretaría Técnica de la Presidencia. Informe política social y económica 2004. Managua; 2005.

11. Banco Central de Nicaragua. Informe anual 2005. Managua; 2006.

12. Instituto Nicaragüense de Turismo. Plan nacional de desarrollo turístico. Managua: Gobierno de Nicaragua; INTUR; 2005.

13. Nicaragua, Ministerio de Salud. Análisis de situación de salud. Propuesta plan nacional de salud. Managua: MINSA; 2003.

14. Regiones Autónomas del Atlántico Norte y Sur. Análisis de situación de salud, propuesta de plan de salud de las regiones autónomas de la costa atlántica de Nicaragua. Managua; julio 2004.

15. Nicaragua, Instituto Nacional de Estadísticas y Censos. Encuesta Nacional de Medición de Nivel de Vida, 2005. Unpublished.

16. Nicaragua, Sistema Nacional de Seguimiento a Indicadores de Desarrollo. [Labor statistics]. Managua: SINASID; 2004. Available at: http://www.secep.gob.ni/sinasid/.

17. Trejos JD. Características y evolución reciente del mercado de trabajo de Nicaragua. [Report prepared for the Interna-

tional Labor Organization]. San José: Proyecto NIC Empleo; 2003.

18. Programa de las Naciones Unidas para el Desarrollo; Fondo de Desarrollo de las Naciones Unidas para la Mujer; Agencia Sueca de Desarrollo Internacional. Perfil de género en la economía del Istmo Centroamericana. UNIFEM; ASDI; 2006.

19. United Nations Development Program. Human Development Report. UNDP; 2005.

20. Gobierno de Nicaragua. Estrategia reforzada de crecimiento económico y reducción de pobreza. Managua; 2001.

21. Gobierno de Nicaragua. Segundo informe de avance de la estrategia reforzada de crecimiento económico y reducción de pobreza; 2003.

22. Nicaragua, Secretaría de Técnica de la Presidencia. Propuesta del plan nacional de desarrollo. Managua; 2004.

23. Nicaragua, Secretaría Técnica de la Presidencia; Naciones Unidas. Primer informe de avance hacia los ODM, Nicaragua. SECEP; NNUU; 2003.

24. Nicaragua, Ministerio de Salud. Evaluación de indicadores intermedios ERCERP. Managua: OPS; MINSA; 2003.

25. Nicaragua, Secretaría Técnica de la Presidencia; Naciones Unidas. Primer foro nacional ODM Nicaragua. SECEP; NNUU; 2005.

26. Gómez M. Los ODM y la cooperación externa en Nicaragua. [Intervention of Nicaraguan Vice Minister for External Cooperation at first national MDG-Nicaragua forum]; 2005.

27. Nicaragua, Secretaría Técnica de la Presidencia; Naciones Unidas. Escenarios de inversión social para alcanzar los ODM. Managua: SECEP; NNUU; 2004.

28. Gobierno de Nicaragua. Política nacional de seguridad alimentaria y nutricional. Managua; 2001.

29. Nicaragua, Ministerio del Ambiente y los Recursos Naturales. Estado del ambiente en Nicaragua, 2003. II Informe GEO. Managua: MARENA; 2004.

30. Programa de las Naciones Unidas para el Desarrollo. El desarrollo humano en Nicaragua. Equidad para superar la vulnerabilidad, 2000. Managua: PNUD; 2001.

31. Nicaragua, Instituto Nacional de Estadísticas y Censos. Encuesta de Medición de Nivel de Vida, 1998. Managua: INEC; 1999.

32. Programa de las Naciones Unidas para el Desarrollo. Informe de desarrollo humano 2005. Las regiones autónomas de la costa caribe: ¿Nicaragua asume su diversidad? PNUD; 2005.

33. Nicaragua, Instituto Nicaragüense de Estadísticas y Censos. Estimaciones de población 1950–2050. Managua: INEC; 1999.

34. Organización Internacional para las Migraciones, Sistema de Información Estadística sobre las Migraciones en Mesoamérica. Boletín: Movimientos internacionales en mesoamérica. Volumen 10. Nicaragua: un país de emigrantes. Encuesta de Hogares para la Medición del Empleo Urbano-Rural 2004. OIM/SIEMMES. Available at: www.siemmes.iom.int.

35. Nicaragua, Ministerio de Salud, Dirección de Estadísticas y Sistemas de Información. [Statistics]. Managua: MINSA; 2006.

36. Nicaragua, Ministerio de Salud. Indicadores básicos de salud, 2005. Managua: MINSA; 2005.

37. Nicaragua, Instituto Nacional de Estadísticas y Censos. Encuesta Nicaragüense de Demografía y Salud (ENDESA) 2001. Managua: INEC; 2002.

38. Nicaragua, Ministerio de Salud, Programa de Atención Integral a la Mujer, Niñez y Adolescencia.

39. Nicaragua, Ministerio de Salud. Boletín epidemiológico. Semana N° 39, año 2004. Managua: MINSA; 2004.

40. Organización Panamericana de la Salud, Organización Mundial de la Salud. Estudio de metanálisis de promoción de la salud sexual y reproductiva y prevención del VIH/SIDA en los adolescentes. OPS/OMS; 2005.

41. Nicaragua, Instituto Nacional de Estadísticas y Censos. Encuesta Nicaragüense de Demografía y Salud (ENDESA) 1998; Encuesta Nicaragüense de Demografía y Salud (ENDESA) 2001; Encuesta sobre Salud Familiar 1992–1993.

42. Nicaragua, Comisión Nacional de Promoción y Defensa de los Derechos del Niño y de la Niña.

43. Nicaragua, Instituto Nacional de Estadísticas y Censos. Encuesta de Juventud (ENJOVEN) 2004. Managua: INEC.

44. Centro de Investigación, Salud, Trabajo y Ambiente. Mercado laboral en León: sector informal y sus repercusiones en la salud. León: Universidad Nacional de Autónoma de Nicaragua; 2006.

45. Nicaragua, Ministerio del Trabajo; Organización Internacional del Trabajo. Encuesta Nacional sobre Trabajo Infantil (ENTIA) 2000 y 2005. Managua: MINTRAB: 2000; 2005.

46. Cerda A. Firman acuerdo binacional contra explotación sexual infantil. La Prensa; 20 de junio de 2006. Available at: http://www-ni.laprensa.com.ni/archivo/2006/junio/20/noticias/nacionales/125232.shtml.

47. ECPAT International; Casa Alianza. Proyecto de fortalecimiento de la protección de niñas, niños y adolescentes ante la explotación sexual comercial en Centroamérica. Available at: http://www.ecpat.net/eng/ecpat_inter/projects/central_america_project/publications/panfleto%20nicaragua%20corregido1.doc.

48. Organización Mundial contra la Tortura. Violencia contra la mujer en Nicaragua. Informe redactado para el Comité para la Eliminación de la Discriminación contra la Mujer. OMCT; 2001: 18.

49. Nicaragua, Instituto Nacional de Estadísticas y Censos; Ministerio de Salud. Encuesta Nacional de Discapacidad (ENDIS) 2003. Managua: INEC; MINSA; 2004.

50. Organización Panamericana de la Salud, Organización Mundial de la Salud. Análisis de la variable etnia en ENDESA y EMNV 2001. Managua: OPS; 2004.

51. Centro Centroamericano de Población. Migrantes nicaragüenses en Costa Rica: volumen, características y salud reproductiva. Universidad de Costa Rica; 2001.

52. Nicaragua, Ministerio de Salud, Dirección de Epidemiología Aplicada, Enfermedades de Transmisión Vectorial y Sistema de Vigilancia Epidemiológica Nacional.

53. Nicaragua, Ministerio de Salud. Informe del programa nacional de dengue. Managua: MINSA; 2006.

54. Sistema Nicaragüense de Vigilancia Epidemiológica Nacional. Enfermedades de Notificación Obligatoria (ENO), 2004.

55. Nicaragua, Ministerio de Salud. Informe del programa de leishmaniasis. Managua: MINSA; 2006.

56. Nicaragua, Ministerio de Salud. II Encuesta Serológica en Escolares, 2000. Managua: MINSA; OPS.

57. Nicaragua, Ministerio de Salud. Indicadores básicos de salud 2003 y 2005. Managua: MINSA; 2003 y 2005.

58. Nicaragua, Ministerio de Salud. Estudio de geohelmintosis en escolares rurales, 2005. MINSA; OPS; UNICEF.

59. Joint United Nations Program on HIV/AIDS. AIDS Epidemic Update. Geneva: UNAIDS; WHO; 2005: 63.

60. Nicaragua, Comisión Nicaragüense de SIDA. Plan estratégico nacional de ITS/VIH/SIDA, 2006–2010. CONISIDA; 2006.

61. Nicaragua, Ministerio de Salud. Programa Nacional de ITS/VIH/SIDA. Informe anual de vigilancia epidemiológica de ITS/VIH/SIDA, 2005. Managua: MINSA; 2006.

62. Joint United Nations Program on HIV/AIDS. [Estimates for Nicaragua]. UNAIDS; 2005.

63. United States of America, Johns Hopkins University. [Survey conducted by Center for Communication Programs/Bloomberg School of Public Health]. 2001.

64. Nicaragua, Ministerio de Salud. Encuesta de Conocimientos, Actitudes y Prácticas: participación de hombres en programas de salud sexual y reproductiva. MINSA; Organización Panamericana de la Salud; Fondo de Población de las Naciones Unidas; Cooperación Técnica Alemana; 2004.

65. Nicaragua, Ministerio de Salud. Informe anual del programa de zoonosis. Managua: MINSA; 2005.

66. Nicaragua, Ministerio de Salud, Departamento de Zoonosis. Informe de leptospirosis comparativo 2000–2006. Managua: MINSA; 2006.

67. Nicaragua, Ministerio de Salud. Encuesta de Diabetes e Hipertensión y sus Factores de Riesgo, Iniciativa Centroamericana para la Diabetes (CAMDI) 2003. MINSA; OPS.

68. Nicaragua, Ministerio de Salud, Dirección de Estadísticas y Sistemas de Información. Estadísticas de mortalidad. Managua: MINSA; 2006.

69. Nicaragua, Ministerio de Salud; Organización Panamericana de Salud; Centros para el Control y la Prevención de Enfermedades. Resultados finales de la encuesta de diabetes e hipertensión y sus factores de riesgo, CAMDI, 2003. MINSA; OPS; CDC; 2005.

70. Nicaragua, Ministerio de Salud. Estadísticas de mortalidad. Managua: MINSA; 2005.

71. Nicaragua, Ministerio de Salud. Informe del Centro Nacional de Radioterapia. Managua: MINSA; 2006.

72. Nicaragua, Instituto Nacional de Estadísticas y Censos. Encuesta Nicaragüense de Demografía y Salud (ENDESA) 1998. Managua: INEC; 1999.

73. Nicaragua, Ministerio de Salud. Violencia y otras lesiones en cinco hospitales de Nicaragua. MINSA; CDC; OPS; 2004.

74. Nicaragua, Ministerio de Salud. Boletín epidemiológico. Semana Nº 51, año 2001. MINSA; 2001.

75. Nicaragua, Ministerio de Salud. Boletín epidemiológico. Semana Nº 48, año 2001. MINSA; 2001.

76. Organización Panamericana de la Salud, Organización Mundial de la Salud, Instrumento de Evaluación para Sistemas de Salud Mental. Informe sobre los sistemas de salud mental en Nicaragua, El Salvador y Guatemala. IESM/OMS; 2006: 11–28.

77. Pan American Health Organization. Multicentric study of gender, alcohol, culture, and harm. PAHO; 2005.

78. Nicaragua, Consejo Nacional de Lucha contra las Drogas. [Compilation from various information sources]; 2005.

79. Nicaragua, Ministerio de Salud. Boletín epidemiológico. Semana Nº 52, año 2005. Managua: MINSA; diciembre 2005.

80. Nicaragua, Ministerio de Salud; Organización Panamericana de la Salud. Incidencia de intoxicaciones agudas por plaguicidas y estimación del subregistro en Nicaragua. Proyecto Plagasalud. Managua: OPS/OMS; DANIDA; 2002.

81. Miranda J, McConnell R, Wesseling C, Cuadra R, Delgado E, Torres E, et al. Muscular strength and vibration thresholds during two years after acute poisoning with organophosphate insecticides. Occup Environ Med 2004 Jan; 61(1):e4.

82. McConnell R, Keifer M, Rosenstock L. Elevated quantitative vibrotactile threshold among workers previously poisoned with methamidophos and other organophosphate pesticides. Am J Ind Med 1994 Mar; 25(3):325–34.

83. Rosenstock L, Keifer M, Daniell WE, McConnell R, Claypoole K. Chronic central nervous system effects of acute organophosphate pesticide intoxication. The Pesticide Health Effects Study Group. Lancet 1991 Jul 27; 338(8761):223–7.

84. McConnell R, Delgado-Tellez E, Cuadra R, Torres E, Keifer M, Almendarez J, et al. Organophosphate neuropathy due to methamidophos: biochemical and neurophysiological markers. Arch Toxicol 1999 Aug; 73(6):296–300.

85. Miranda J, Lundberg I, McConnell R, Delgado E, Cuadra R, Torres E, et al. Onset of grip- and pinch-strength impairment after acute poisonings with organophosphate insecticides. Int J Occup Environ Health 2002 Jan–Mar; 8(1):19–26.

86. Castro-Gutierrez N, McConnell R, Andersson K, Pacheco-Anton F, Hogstedt C. Respiratory symptoms, spirometry and chronic occupational paraquat exposure. Scand J Work Environ Health 1997 Dec; 23(6):421–7.

87. Nicaragua, Ministerio de Salud; Centro de Información, Vigilancia, Asesoramiento y Asistencia Toxicológica. Estudio de incidencia de intoxicaciones por plomo en niños. Managua: MINSA; CIVATOX; 2004.

88. Organización Panamericana de la Salud, Organización Mundial de la Salud; Fondo de la Infancia de las Naciones Unidas Evaluación rápida de la calidad del agua de bebida. OPS/OMS; UNICEF: Managua; 2005.

89. Organización Panamericana de la Salud, Organización Mundial de la Salud. Salud oral. Available at: http://www.paho. org/Spanish/GOV/CD/doc259.pdf. [Document CD40/20 presented to PAHO 40th Directing Council in September 1997].

90. Nicaragua, Ministerio de Salud. Estudio epidemiológico de salud bucal en niños de 6, 7, 8, 12 y 15 años de escuelas y colegios públicos de Nicaragua. Managua: MINSA; 1999.

91. Organización Panamericana de la Salud, Organización Mundial de la Salud. Informe final. Project 15. Interprogrammatic Oral Health Activity, Health Canada. Modelos de atención para mejorar la salud bucal de las poblaciones indígenas y vulnerables en la frontera entre Honduras y Nicaragua.

92. Organización Internacional del Trabajo. Perfil nacional sobre salud y seguridad en el trabajo en Nicaragua. OIT; 2004.

93. Nicaragua, Ministerio del Trabajo. Estadísticas de accidentabilidad laboral 2000–2005. Managua; 2006.

94. Instituto Nicaragüense de Seguridad Social. Anuario estadístico. INSS; 2004.

95. Nicaragua, Ministerio de Salud. Política Nacional de Salud, 2004–2015. MINSA; 2004.

96. Sanigest Internacional. Evaluación de las políticas nacionales de salud durante el periodo 1997–2002. Managua: SANIGEST; 2004.

97. Nicaragua, Ministerio de Salud; Organización Panamericana de la Salud. Medición del desempeño de las funciones esenciales de salud pública ejercidas por la autoridad sanitaria de Nicaragua. Resultados del taller de aplicación del instrumento. Managua: MINSA; OPS; 2001.

98. Nicaragua, Ministerio de Salud; Organización Panamericana de la Salud. Informe final medición del desempeño de las funciones esenciales de la salud pública en el SILAIS. Managua; 2006.

99. Organización Panamericana de la Salud, Organización Mundial de la Salud. Proyecto inequidad en salud, etnicidad, Nicaragua. Managua: OPS/OMS; 2004.

100. Nicaragua, Instituto Nacional de Estadísticas y Censos. Encuesta de Medición de Nivel de Vida (EMNV) 2001.

101. Nicaragua, Ministerio de Salud. Marco conceptual del Modelo de Atención Integral en Salud (MAIS). Managua: MINSA; 2005.

102. Nicaragua, Ministerio de Salud. Encuesta de establecimientos de Nicaragua. Managua: MINSA; 2002.

103. Instituto Nicaragüense de Seguridad Social. Memoria institucional 2004. Managua: INSS; 2005.

104. Nicaragua, Ministerio de Salud; Empresa Nicaragüense de Acueductos y Alcantarillados; Instituto Nicaragüense de Acueductos y Alcantarillados; Organización Panamericana de la Salud; Agencia Suiza para el Desarrollo y Cooperación; Banco Interamericano de Desarrollo; Banco Mundial; Fondo de las Naciones Unidas para la Infancia. Análisis sectorial de agua potable y saneamiento en Nicaragua. Managua; 2004.

105. Empresa Nicaragüense de Acueductos y Alcantarillados. Informe 2004. Managua: ENACAL; 2004.

106. Organización Panamericana de la Salud, Centro Panamericano de Ingeniería Sanitaria y Ciencias del Ambiente. Evaluación regional de los servicios de manejo de los residuos sólidos municipales. Informe analítico de Nicaragua. OPS; CEPIS; 2003.

107. Instituto Nicaragüense de Fomento Municipal, Sistema de Información de Servicios Municipales. Managua: SISEM/INIFOM; 2006.

108. Nicaragua, Ministerio del Ambiente y los Recursos Naturales. Estado del ambiente en Nicaragua 2003. II Informe Geo. Managua: MARENA; 2004.

109. Nicaragua. Ley 217: Ley General del Medio Ambiente y los Recursos Naturales. Managua; 1997.

110. Nicaragua, Ministerio del Ambiente. Indicadores ambientales de Nicaragua. Volumen I. Managua; 2004.

111. Nicaragua. Ley 337: Ley creadora del Sistema Nacional para la Prevención, Mitigación y Atención de Desastres. Managua; 2000.

112. Nicaragua. Decreto 98-2000. Reglamento de la Ley 337: Ley Creadora del Sistema Nacional para la Prevención, Mitigación y Atención de Desastres. Managua; 2000.

113. Nicaragua. Decreto 98-2000. Reglamento de asignación de funciones del Sistema Nacional para la Prevención, Mitigación y Atención de Desastres a las Instituciones del Estado. Managua; 2000.

114. Nicaragua. Decreto 118-2001. Reformas e incorporaciones al Reglamento de la Ley 290: Ley de Organización, Competencia y Procedimientos del Poder Ejecutivo. Managua; 2002.

115. Nicaragua, Ministerio de Salud. Guía para la elaboración de planes de emergencias hospitalarios para situaciones de desastres. Primera edición. Managua: MINSA; OPS/OMS; 2005.

116. Nicaragua, Ministerio de Salud. Guía metodológica para la elaboración del plan de emergencia sanitaria local. Segunda edición. Managua: MINSA; OPS/OMS; 2002.

117. Nicaragua, Ministerio de Salud. Informe del programa de salud oral. Managua: MINSA; 2006.

118. Nicaragua, Ministerio de Salud, Dirección de Recursos Humanos. Cálculos del Centro de Inteligencia Sanitaria/Organización Panamericana de Salud. MINSA; 2006.

119. Nicaragua, Ministerio de Salud, Dirección de Insumos Médicos; 2005.

120. Nicaragua, Ministerio de Salud, Dirección de Insumos Médicos; 2000.

121. Nicaragua, Ministerio de Salud. Cuentas Nacionales en Salud 2002. Managua: MINSA; 2003.

122. Nicaragua, Comisión Nacional de Medicamentos. Comparación de precios.

123. Nicaragua, Ministerio de Salud. Cuentas Nacionales en Salud; 2005.

124. Nicaragua, Ministerio de Salud. Informe de cooperación externa de MINSA en 2005. Managua; 2006.

125. Nicaragua, Ministerio de Salud. Informe de cooperación externa de MINSA en 2004. Managua; 2005.

126. Braunschweig T, Stöckli B. La perspectiva de la sociedad civil respecto a su participación en el seguimiento de ERP: evaluación de limitaciones y potenciales en Nicaragua. Berna (Suiza): Alliance Sud; 2006.

PANAMA

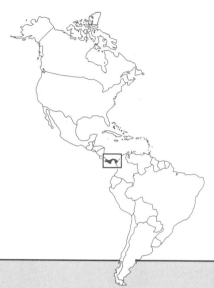

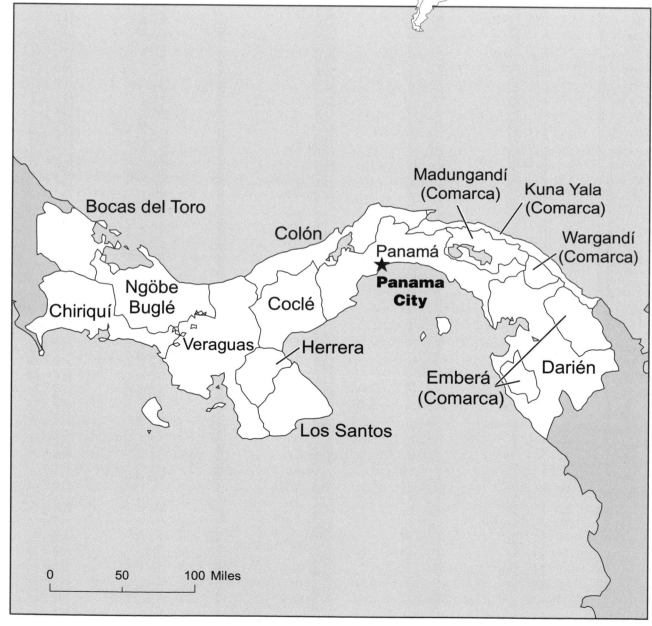

Bocas del Toro

Madungandí
(Comarca)

Kuna Yala
(Comarca)

Colón

Wargandí
(Comarca)

Panamá

**Panama
City**

Ngöbe
Buglé

Chiriquí

Coclé

Veraguas

Herrera

Emberá
(Comarca)

Darién

Los Santos

0   50   100 Miles

P anama has an area of 75,517 km^2, which is distributed into nine provinces, five indigenous territories called comarcas (three of which are at the provincial level), 75 districts
or municipalities, and 621 mayoral jurisdictions or *corregimientos* (two of which are
indigenous) (*1*).

GENERAL CONTEXT AND HEALTH DETERMINANTS

Social, Political, and Economic Determinants

Panama has been classified as an upper middle-income country (*2*). Its economy has experienced sustained growth (with the long-term growth rate close to 5% a year and 2% per capita over the last 15 years). Its nominal gross domestic product (GDP) in 2005 was US$ 15.46 billion and its per capita GDP was US$ 4,318 (*3*) (growth of 6.4% and 2.0% respectively compared to 2004). Productive activity is strongly concentrated in the services sector (76.3% of GDP), with little linkage to the rest of the economy, while manufacturing and construction together contribute 12.0% and the primary sector of agriculture and mining contributes 8.1% (*4*). Despite the relative economic boom, in 2005, the registered public debt, excluding the debt contracted with government sources such as the Social Security Fund (CSS) and with public financial institutions, was US$ 10.23 billion, equivalent to 66.2% of GDP. Of this, 25.9% (US$ 2.65 billion) was internal debt and 74.1% (US$ 7.57 billion), external debt (*3, 4*).

The country's political and economic situation is influenced by its recent past, whose most salient aspects are the return to democratic life (1990) (*5, 6*), the pullout from the Canal zone, and the transfer of administration of the Canal to Panama in 1999 (*7*). A study on the opinions of Panamanians found that they considered the following problems to be important: the national issue (the Panama Canal), the political issue (democracy), and the economic situation (the impoverishment of the population) (*8*), which continue to be present in the country's political and economic life. The 2003 Standard of Living Survey (ENV 2003) confirmed the public's views that unemployment was the most pressing problem (*9*). Almost two-thirds (61.4%) of households identified the job shortage as the main reason for deterioration in the standard of living and poverty among the population. Also, with regard to community life, heads of households mentioned the lack of infrastructure (30%), the lack of access to basic services (26%), and the lack of security (12%) as problems that needed urgent attention (*9*). Consistent with this reading of the political and social context, the national dialogue among different sectors (*10, 11*) has included among policies and objectives poverty reduction, economic reforms, and sustainable growth.

A new president was elected for the period 2004–2009, also obtaining a majority in the legislature (52% of the seats) and in the municipal governments (69% of mayorships). The new government's program (*12*), expressed in its economic and social policies (*13*) and its objectives and goals (*14*), seeks sustainable economic development with social inclusion, by building up the competitiveness of national production, creating and maintaining a climate that favors investments, promoting social participation, strengthening the capacity of individuals and communities, and developing social investment programs that guarantee equitable access to basic services, particularly for the most vulnerable groups.

In 2005, the economically active population (EAP) numbered 1,407,458 people (with a participation rate of 63.5% of the population 15 years of age and older); 90.2% of the EAP was employed, 43% of them in informal activities. The open unemployment rate was 7.2% (*15*) ENV 2003 (*9*) found that the Panamanian labor market reflects a lack of gender equity with respect to job opportunities, with women having higher unemployment rates than men (15.1% and 8.0%, respectively). Almost one half (44%) of the unemployed are between the ages of 15 and 24. Unemployment is fundamentally a problem in urban areas, where the rate is 12.4% and 75% of the country's unemployed are found, while underemployment is typical of rural and indigenous areas. The unemployment rate among the poor is 11.7% (extreme and non-extreme poor together) and 10.3% in the non-poor population. The problem is more serious in urban areas (17.6% and 11.4%, respectively).

The average monthly wage for non-indigenous workers 15 years of age and over in 2005 nationally was US$ 322.30 (US$ 326.30 for men and US$ 314.90 for women), and differed by sector: domestic services, US$ 115.50; agriculture, US$ 136.50; fisheries, US$ 241.70; manufacturing, US$ 311.90; construction, US$ 350.60; public administration, US$ 434.50; teaching, US$ 506; and financial institutions, US$ 551.70 (*15*). Average per capita annual income exhibited extreme contrasts among provinces, such as between the indigenous Comarca Ngöbe Buglé, with US$ 370.50 (males US$ 513 and females US$ 228), and the Province of Panama, with US$ 3,138 (males US$ 3,977 and females US$ 2,299) (*15*). An analysis of per capita income by deciles performed using ENV 2003 showed a national average of US$ 2,482 a year, with US$ 81 in the first decile and US$ 10,943 in the tenth. Accordingly, the poorest 20% of the population obtains just 1.9% of total income while the wealthiest 20% obtains 61.2%. In that year, the Gini coefficient for income distribution was 0.58 (9). General inflation measured by the consumer price index for Panama City and the district of San Miguelito was 3.3%, and inflation in the cost of the basic food basket was 4.8% in 2005 (3), both of which are relatively high for Panama, where the rate had been below 1.0% in the previous five years. The total monthly cost of the basic food basket (2,305 calories per person per day for a household with 3.84 members) in December 2005 was US$ 207.32 (16).

In this context, ENV 2003 found that nearly four out of every 10 people lived in poverty (36.8% of the population, with total consumption of US$ 953 per person per year) and 16.6% (508,700 people with total consumption of US$ 534 per person per year) lived in extreme poverty (17). From 1997 to 2002 (18), poverty was reduced by just 0.5%. In urban zones it grew to affect one out of every five people (in 2003, general poverty, 20.0% and extreme poverty, 4.4%) and in indigenous rural zones it deepened, affecting 98.4% of the population, with nine out of 10 people living in extreme poverty.

Children under 6 years are the most affected by poverty. About one out of every three lived in extreme poverty (29.2% of children from 0 to 5 years), and more than half lived in abject poverty (54.1% of children from 0 to 5 years). Among the young population from 15 to 24 years of age, the incidence of poverty was 36.7% and of extreme poverty 16.2%. As for households, one out of every four (25.9%, 196,232 families) lived in general poverty, more than two-thirds of which (66.8%) are rural families. One family out of every ten (9.6%, 72,498 families) lived in extreme poverty (84% in the rural area, including indigenous areas) (9). As for the districts, 68% (51/75) presented high levels of poverty with low levels of inequality and are home to 20% of the population and 56% of the country's poor. Overall they have a low population density (17.4 people per km²) and a high percentage of rural population (74%). Of the districts, 27% (20/75) presented low levels of poverty with low levels of inequality and are home to 62% of the population and 38% of the country's poor. Overall they had the highest population density (141 people per km²) and a lower percentage of rural population (38%) (19).

Distribution of per capita consumption in 2003 was very unequal, with a Gini coefficient of 0.47. The scant consumption in the poorest population quintile (average annual consumption of US$ 371 per person, 4.0% of total national consumption) implied that for each dollar consumed by a person in the wealthiest quintile (average annual consumption of US$ 4,803 per person, 51.9% of total national consumption), a person from the lowest quintile consumed just 8 cents. In other words, people who are better off consumed 13 times more than the poor (17).

In terms of the human development index, Panama was classified as high (20), at 0.804 (it ranks 56th out of 177 countries)

and its human poverty index was 7.7% (ranking 9th out of 103 developing countries). The distribution of this development potential, measured by Panama's potential human development index (IDHP) in 2002, indicated that for all urban areas, human development was 0.753 while for the rural areas it was 0.46 (21). An analysis of the gaps between provinces for each component of the IDHP revealed that life expectancy was the indicator with the greatest progress and lowest disparity, where the province with the least progress (Comarca Emberá, 0.657) presented an average that is equivalent to 76.4% of the figure for the province with the highest life expectancy (Panama, 0.860). In education, there was a significant gap in progress between the province with the poorest results (Comarca Ngöbe Buglé, 0.396), with the equivalent of 51.8%, and the province with the highest level (Panama, 0.764). The decent level of living aspect (which includes indicators for income, employment, housing, and basic services) presents the most critical situation, since it made the least relative progress and exhibited the widest disparity. The province with the lowest figure (Comarca Emberá, 0.108) represents just 17.9% of the province with the highest figure (Panama, 0.605) (22).

On the economic, social, and cultural levels, the situation is disadvantageous for women. In spite of having better levels of education (total schooling: men 8.6 years, women 9 years), women earn lower wages for their work (urban employees with incomes above the minimum wage: men 68.4%, women 59.7%). In addition, their participation in politics is limited (political positions: men 89.6%, women 10.4%) (23). The standard of living index on the national level is 0.551 for men and 0.521 for women, but in the case of rural and indigenous women, inequality has reached alarming levels (Ngöbe Buglé: men 0.135, women 0.072; Kuna Yala: men 0.185, women 0.065).

As for public education, the country has made significant progress. In 2003, the literacy rate for the population 15 years of age and over was 93.1% (24). The illiteracy that exists is largely due to the high rates that are prevalent among people 40 years of age and older who live in poverty. National primary education coverage was 94.2%. Coverage continued to be low, however, for preschool (50.0%), secondary (70.2%), and higher education (23.9%). The gender parity index indicated that 94 girls in urban areas attend primary school for every 100 boys, while the disparity was greater in indigenous zones, with 86 girls for every 100 boys. This inequality in access to primary education among indigenous girls increased on the secondary level, where just 68 girls attend for every 100 boys. The gaps in access to higher education were even wider in regards to levels of socioeconomic status: the population in the four lowest consumption deciles had net coverage rates of under 10% for youths between the ages of 18 and 24, while in the highest decile coverage was 57.1%.

The national average years of schooling for the population 25 to 39 years of age was 8.6 grades, but there was a large difference between the population in the first quintile, with 4.1 grades, and the fifth quintile with 12.1 grades. The indigenous population, which is mainly poor, had just 2.9 grades (9).

In 2004, public spending on education was US$ 607 million, distributed among the preschool and primary, secondary, and postsecondary levels as follows: US$ 393.98, US$ 724.67, and US$ 1,181.37 per student, respectively. Spending on preschool, primary, and secondary education has been progressive (concentration coefficients of −0.219, −0.275, and −0.029 respectively) in contrast to higher education (concentration coefficient of 0.3858). Educational assistance in the form of grants benefited 6% of the student population. Most of the government's grants in 2003 were for secondary (58%), primary (35%), and postsecondary (7%) education, but fewer than one third (30%) of the beneficiaries were poor. In the case of higher education, 100% of the grants were for the non-poor (9).

As for the diet of Panamanian families, apparent daily energy consumption was 6,832 kcal per family (non-poor 6,529 kcal and poor 7,475 kcal) and 1,608 kcal per person (non-poor 1,697 and poor 1,326 kcal), while among the rural indigenous population and persons living in extreme poverty the figures were significantly lower (1,200 kcal and 1,144 kcal, respectively). The energy consumed came from proteins (11.8%), carbohydrates (59.7%), fats (27.9%), and alcohol (0.5%). The energy contribution of proteins, fats, and carbohydrates varied from 9.5%, 15.3%, and 76.4%, respectively, in indigenous areas to 13.1%, 33.5%, and 52.5% in Panama City (25).

In the main urban centers, levels of pollution are not critical. The Specialized Analysis Institute of the University of Panama began a program to monitor air quality in Panama City in 1996. The city's topography, its proximity to the sea, and the prevailing winds prevent smog from building up. It is estimated that 90% of urban emissions come from the transportation sector and the rest from fixed sources. To date there is no program to control vehicle emissions (26). In the highlands where fruit, vegetables, and coffee are grown, air pollution comes from the intensive use of pesticides. In 2000, 320,953 kg of powdered pesticides were used in agricultural activities (2,769.5 km²) (26). It is estimated that on average the country uses four times more pesticides each year than the average world consumption estimated by the World Health Organization (0.6 kg/person) (27).

As for natural resources, protected areas cover 30% of the country (26). The loss of forest cover between 1992 and 2000 is calculated to have been 3,305.69 km² (28); 27% of the soil has been classified as degraded. Most rivers close to urban centers present a significant degree of pollution, owing to discharges of semi-treated or raw sewage. The situation is particularly critical in Panama City, where the population (900,000 people) and industries in the metropolitan area generate about 280,000 m³ of liquid waste a day, which is dumped untreated into the rivers that cross the city and directly into Panama Bay, through a system of sanitary sewers that only covers 70% of the city.

In comparison with other Central American countries, historically Panama has suffered fewer emergencies and disasters; however, its environmental vulnerability is high due to the degradation of ecosystems as a consequence of human activity. Recurrent flooding affects the provinces of Bocas del Toro, Colón, Panama, and Darién.

Panama's risk of epidemics is unique due to factors that derive from its development, including the airport, which moves close to 2.5 million travelers a year, and the 14,000 ships that sail through the Panama Canal. The ecoenvironmental profile (wetlands) favors the presence of resting places for migratory birds and of insects and rodents that play a very important role in the transmission of diseases.

Demographics, Mortality, and Morbidity

The population in 2005 was estimated to be 3,228,186 (29), with slightly more males (51%). Population density was 42.3 people per km², with extremes ranging from 1.7 in the district of Sambú (Comarca Emberá) to 6,630.1 in the district of San Miguelito, province of Panama (1). The urban population accounted for 59.5% of the country's inhabitants (with an increase in absolute numbers of 623,697 people since 1990) (30), 73% of whom lived in the metropolitan area. At the other extreme, indigenous peoples accounted for about 10% of the total population and are composed of a number of clearly defined ethnic groups: Wargandi, Madungani, Kuna Yala, Emberá and Wounaan, Ngöbe Buglé, Teribe, and Bokota (31). The Ngöbe Buglé represented 64.5% of the country's indigenous population.

Panama is undergoing a rapid process of demographic transition, which is expressed in a downward trend in the population growth rate (from 2.08% in 1990 to 1.7% in 2006), the total fertility rate (from 2.87 children per woman in 1991–1995 to a projected 2.62 in 2006–2010), and the gross mortality rate (from 5.26 deaths per 1,000 population in 1991–1995 to a projected 5.11 in 2006–2010) (32).

As a result of these changes, life expectancy at birth has risen from 72.9 years (estimated for 1991–1995) to 75.6 years for the period 2006–2010. The average life span for the male population rose from 70.2 to 75.6 years in the same periods, while for females it increased from 75.7 to 78.2 years. Estimates for 2006 indicate that children under 15 years made up 30.1% of the population and people 65 years and over made up 6.0% (Figure 1). The average age was estimated to be 26.2 years (29).

Nonetheless, there are varying demographic scenarios, probably associated with the different levels of development in the provinces. Thus, life expectancy at birth presents unequal distribution among the population quartiles defined by the HDI. Los Santos and Herrera, the most highly developed provinces, had

FIGURE 1. Population structure, by age and sex, Panama, 1980 and 2006.

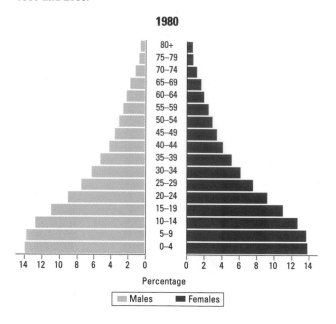

1980

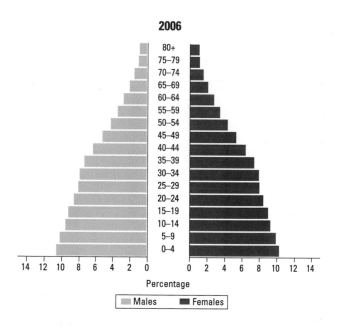

2006

longer life expectancies with 72.4 years and 76.7 years, respectively, while in the indigenous territories life expectancy ranges from 64 to 66 years. Similarly, the average number of live births for females 15 to 49 years of age in the country during 2003 was 2.8, with the figure for the non-poor being 2.3 and for the extreme poor 4.3 (9).

In 2004 (33), 13,475 deaths were reported, for a gross rate of 4.2 deaths per 1,000 population. Underreporting that year was calcu-

lated at about 16% for general mortality. Three out of every five deaths took place in health care institutions, and nine out of every 10 were certified by a physician; deaths reported in the group of unclassified symptoms and signs amounted to just 2.9%.

The leading causes of death per 100,000 population were: diseases of the circulatory system (119), malignant tumors (72.7), external causes (43.6), diseases of the respiratory system (40.1), and certain infectious and parasitic diseases (31.7).

On the national level, the main causes of death include cerebrovascular diseases (which rank first with 44.7 per 100,000 population), diabetes mellitus (third place with 24.4), HIV/AIDS (sixth place with 14), pneumonia (seventh place with 13.6), land transportation accidents (ninth place with 12.8), homicides (11th place with 10.2), prostate cancer (14th place with 8.2), diarrhea and gastroenteritis of presumed infectious origin (20th place with 6.1), hypertension (22nd place with 5.7), respiratory tuberculosis (23rd place with 5.5), cervical cancer (24th place with 4.4), and breast cancer (25th place with 4.2) (33).

The main causes of mortality vary by province. In Comarca Ngöbe Buglé (the poorest with the lowest IDHP), diarrhea and gastroenteritis of presumed infectious origin rank first (with a rate of 48.1 deaths per 100,000 population), followed by accidents, self-inflicted wounds, acts of aggression, and other violence (38.0); tuberculosis (34.1); malnutrition (17.1); and pneumonia (13.2), while in the province of Panama (where the metropolitan area is located) the leading causes are malignant tumors (79.7 per 100,000 population), ischemic heart disease (51.6), cerebrovascular diseases (47.5), accidents, self-inflicted wounds, acts of aggression, and other violence (40.3), and diabetes mellitus (26.5) (33).

The causes of mortality have shifted significantly over the years (Tables 1 and 2). For example, changes in the leading causes of death show that malignant tumors, which were responsible for 51.6 deaths per 100,000 population in 1980 (males 53.7 and females 49.4), were responsible for 72.7 deaths per 100,000 in 2004 (males 75.5 and females 69.7). Cerebrovascular diseases, with 28.4 deaths per 100,000 population in 1980 (males 30.8 and females 25.8), caused 44.7 deaths per 100,000 population in 2004 (males 46.4 and females 42.9). Accidents, self-inflicted wounds, acts of aggression, and other violence, with 53.4 deaths per 100,000 population in 1980 (males 83.2 and females 22.7), caused 43.5 deaths per 100,000 population in 2004 (males 71.5 and females 15.0). Diabetes mellitus, with 8 deaths per 100,000 population in 1980 (males 6.9 and females 9.1), caused 24.4 deaths per 100,000 population in 2004 (males 19.9 and females 29.0).

Out of all deaths reported in 2004, 6.9% corresponded to children under 1 year; 2.4% to children from 1 to 4 years; 0.8% to children from 5 to 9 years; 2.3% to adolescents (10 to 14 years, 0.8%, 15 to 19 years, 1.46%); 25.1% to adults from 20 to 59 years; and 62.1% to adults 60 years and over.

TABLE 1. Number of deaths and mortality rate by the five leading causes of death[a], by sex, Panama, 1980, 1985, 1990, 1995, and 2000–2004.

Year	Tumors (malignant neoplasms)		Cerebrovascular diseases		Ischemic heart disease[b]		Accidents, self-inflicted wounds, acts of aggression		Diabetes mellitus	
	Number	Rate[c]	Number	Rate[c]	Number	Rate[c]	Number	Rate[c]	Number	Rate[c]
Total										
1980	1,000	51.6	550	28.4	908	46.8	1,035	53.4	155	8.0
1985	1,105	50.7	822	37.7	960	44.0	1,072	49.2	215	9.9
1990	1,398	57.8	964	39.9	1,096	45.3	1,232	51.0	266	11.0
1995	1,601	60.9	1,124	42.7	1,157	44.0	1,571	59.7	403	15.3
2000	1,938	67.9	1,201	42.1	1,147	40.2	1,337	46.8	623	21.8
2001	1,929	64.2	1,367	45.5	1,215	40.4	1,348	44.9	698	23.2
2002	2,009	65.7	1,310	42.8	1,223	40.0	1,434	46.9	795	26.0
2003	2,239	71.8	1,391	44.6	1,319	42.3	1,492	47.9	784	25.2
2004	2,305	72.7	1,417	44.7	1,390	43.8	1,381	43.5	774	24.4
Males										
1980	528	53.7	303	30.8	539	54.8	818	83.2	68	6.9
1985	568	51.1	417	37.5	559	50.3	843	75.8	98	8.8
1990	773	62.8	511	41.5	618	50.2	1,009	82.0	106	8.6
1995	915	68.8	611	45.9	674	50.7	1,282	96.4	171	12.9
2000	1,087	75.4	603	41.9	663	46.0	1,114	77.3	260	18.0
2001	1,058	69.8	705	46.5	722	47.6	1,130	74.5	314	20.7
2002	1,136	73.5	684	44.3	701	45.4	1,175	76.1	324	21.0
2003	1,239	78.8	750	47.7	769	48.9	1,228	78.1	343	21.8
2004	1,209	75.5	743	46.4	817	51.0	1,145	71.5	319	19.9
Females										
1980	472	49.4	247	25.8	369	38.6	217	22.7	87	9.1
1985	537	50.2	405	37.9	401	37.5	229	21.4	117	10.9
1990	625	52.6	453	38.1	478	40.2	223	18.8	160	13.5
1995	686	52.7	513	39.4	483	37.1	289	22.2	232	17.8
2000	851	60.1	598	42.3	484	34.2	223	15.8	363	25.7
2001	871	58.6	662	44.5	493	33.1	218	14.7	384	25.8
2002	873	57.6	620	41.3	522	34.4	259	17.1	471	31.1
2003	1,000	64.8	641	41.5	550	35.6	264	17.1	441	28.6
2004	1,096	69.7	674	42.9	573	36.5	236	15.0	455	29.0

[a]Based on the mortality list of 93 groups of causes in the International Classification of Diseases (9th Revision) and the list of 80 groups of causes in the International Statistical Classification of Diseases and Related Health Problems (10th Revision).

[b]The group of ischemic heart diseases includes acute myocardial infarction.

[c]Per 100,000 population, based on the estimated total population, by sex, as of 1 July of the respective year.

HEALTH OF POPULATION GROUPS

Children under 5 Years Old

Children under 1 year old (69,662) were estimated to make up 2.2% of the Panamanian population in 2005. In 2004, 62,743 births were registered (34). Estimates for the level of registration of live births suggest that 5.2% were omitted in the period 1996–2000 (29). It was calculated that there would be 34.1% omissions in reporting infant deaths in 1996–2000, which would double the level of underreporting in the total population

(1996–2000, 18.6%), which rose to 78.5% in the indigenous territories (33). According to official calculations for 2004, the mortality rate was expected to be 19.15 per 1,000 live births, with a declining trend (from 28.6 per 1,000 in 1990); in fact, the rate reported in that year was 14.9 per 1,000 live births and the difference between the two rates is 4.25 per 1,000.

The leading cause of infant mortality reported in 2004 was certain conditions originating in the perinatal period (5.53 per 1,000 live births), representing 37.2% of all deaths among children under 1 year. Congenital malformations, deformations, and

TABLE 2. Number of deaths and mortality rate by selected causes of death[a], by sex, Panama, 1980, 1985, 1990, 1995, and 2000–2004.

Year	Other heart diseases		Chronic lower respiratory diseases[b]		HIV		Pneumonia		Certain conditions originating in the perinatal period	
	Number	Rate[c]	Number	Rate[c]	Number	Rate[c]	Number	Rate[c]	Number	Rate[c]
Total										
1980	234	12.1	171	8.8	...	...	313	16.1	490	25.3
1985	320	14.7	228	10.5	4	0.2	275	12.6	572	26.2
1990	374	15.5	148	6.1	63	2.6	299	12.4	550	22.7
1995	401	15.2	196	7.4	294	11.2	258	9.8	500	19.0
2000	441	15.4	494	17.3	484	16.9	293	10.3	463	16.2
2001	455	15.1	555	18.5	473	15.7	371	12.4	441	14.7
2002	454	14.8	537	17.5	473	15.5	361	11.8	359	11.7
2003	510	16.4	534	17.1	424	13.6	377	12.1	338	10.8
2004	632	19.9	568	17.9	444	14.0	431	13.6	347	10.9
Males										
1980	124	12.6	87	8.9	...	...	161	16.4	273	27.8
1985	192	17.3	113	10.2	3	0.3	158	14.2	312	28.1
1990	191	15.5	89	7.2	56	4.6	160	13.0	306	24.9
1995	207	15.6	111	8.3	239	18.0	154	11.6	292	22.0
2000	239	16.6	282	19.6	362	25.1	155	10.8	257	17.8
2001	246	16.2	315	20.8	360	23.7	223	14.7	247	16.3
2002	259	16.8	290	18.8	338	21.9	190	12.3	210	13.6
2003	289	18.4	306	19.5	315	20.0	205	13.0	196	12.5
2004	363	22.7	328	20.5	328	20.5	223	13.9	204	12.7
Females										
1980	110	11.5	84	8.8	...	...	152	15.9	217	22.7
1985	128	12.0	115	10.8	1	0.1	117	10.9	260	24.3
1990	183	15.4	59	5.0	7	0.6	139	11.7	244	20.5
1995	194	14.9	85	6.5	55	4.2	104	8.0	208	16.0
2000	202	14.3	212	15.0	122	8.6	138	9.8	206	14.6
2001	209	14.1	240	16.1	113	7.6	148	10.0	194	13.0
2002	195	12.9	247	16.3	135	8.9	171	11.3	149	9.8
2003	221	14.3	228	14.8	109	7.1	172	11.1	142	9.2
2004	269	17.1	240	15.3	116	7.4	208	13.2	143	9.1

[a]Based on the mortality list of 93 groups of causes in the International Classification of Diseases (9th Revision) and the list of 80 groups of causes in the International Statistical Classification of Diseases and Related Health Problems (10th Revision).

[b]Until 1995, chronic lower respiratory diseases corresponded to chronic and unspecified bronchitis and to emphysema and asthma.

[c]Per 100,000 population, based on the estimated total population, by sex, as of 1 July of the respective year.

chromosome abnormalities (4.36 per 1,000 live births) represented 29.4%; pneumonia (1.03 per 1,000 live births), 6.9%; diarrhea and gastroenteritis of presumed infectious origin (0.73 per 1,000 live births), 4.9%; and accidents, acts of aggression, and other violence (0.46 per 1,000 live births), 3.1% (33).

An analysis of the trends in causes of death in the structure of infant mortality showed that in the 1960s and 1970s, infectious-contagious diseases prevailed (vaccine-preventable diseases, diarrhea, and respiratory diseases), with about 60% of deaths, while in the 1980s and 1990s as part of a transition process there was an in-

crease in endogenous causes, with 76.3% and 84.7% of deaths, respectively. In 2004, endogenous causes accounted for 67% of deaths; pneumonia, diarrhea, and gastroenteritis of presumed infectious origin persisted (12%), and external causes appeared among the five leading causes of death in this age group, with 6% (35). Figure 2 shows the trend in infant mortality rates from 1990 to 2015.

In a sample of 28,747 newborns in 2005 (36), 9.8% were premature and 3.6% presented some difficulty at birth (respiratory distress syndrome was the most frequent for 23.4%, followed by infections for 12.2%, and hyperbilirubinemia for 11.8%).

FIGURE 2. Infant mortality, Panama, 1990, 2000, 2003, 2004, and Millennium Development Goal for 2015.

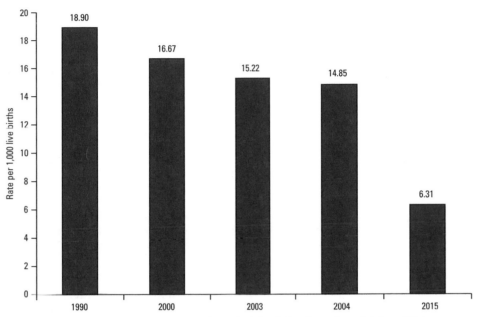

Source: Panamá. Contraloría General de la República. Dirección de Estadística v Censo. Segundo Informe Objetivos de Desarrollo del Milenio, septiembre 2005.

Coverage of check-ups for children under 1 year old was 67.7% of the population of that age estimated for that year, with an average of 3.1 check-ups per child (the national standard calls for nine check-ups for children under 1). The highest coverage was in the regions of Kuna Yala (115.0%) and Darién (109.8%) and the lowest was in Panamá Este (44.6%).

The probability of surviving infancy is uneven and depends on the socioeconomic situation (concentration index of 0.21). The lowest income quintile was the focus of 32% of deaths among children under 1 and the highest income quintile, 12%. Panamanian children have, on average, three times the risk of dying before they reach their first birthday if they belong to the 20% of the poorest population than if they belong to the wealthiest quintile. A breakdown of infant mortality into its components shows that the neonatal mortality rate (under 28 days) was 8.4 per 1,000 live births, or 56% of reported deaths among neonates, while post-neonatal deaths (28 days to 11 months) amounted to 6.5 per 1,000 live births and accounted for the remaining 44%. Between 1980 and 2003, neonatal mortality tended to decline, with rates that ranged from 8.1 to 13.3 deaths per 1,000 live births. In that period there was a percentage drop of 32.5%, which means that the risk of death among neonates was 1.5 times greater in 1980 than in 2003. Post-neonatal mortality in the same period ranged from 9.7 to 5.3 deaths per 1,000 live births, with a downward trend (reduction of 25%). The risk of dying in the post-neonatal period was 1.3 times higher in 1980 than in 2003 (35).

As for the Millennium Development Goals (MDGs), current projections indicate that if the trend in infant mortality continues, the goal will be attained in about 2026.

In 2005, the group of children under 5 years accounted for 10.6% of the total population. Coverage of growth and development check-ups nationwide in this age group in 2004 was 56.2%, with the highest coverage in the Kuna Yala (127.1%) and Darién (109.8%) regions and the lowest in Bocas del Toro (36.6%). The average was 2.5 per child (the standard calls for three check-ups between 12 and 23 months, followed by two check-ups a year until age 5).

The rate for diarrhea in children under 5 years has risen steadily, from 16,046.5 per 100,000 population in 1987 to 22,938 per 100,000 in 2004, mainly due to increases in the 1-to-4 age group, where the figure has doubled, from 11,605.6 per 100,000 population, to 20,357 per 100,000 in 2004.

The mortality rate in children under 5 was 19.95 per 1,000 live births. The proportion of deaths in this age group, including children under 1 year of age, accounted for 9.28% of deaths in the country.

Children 5–9 Years Old

Schoolchildren make up 10.3% of the population (325,887), and 48.9% of them are girls. The mortality rate was 3.25 per 100,000 population, and the volume of deaths in this age group accounted for 0.8% of deaths in the country.

Adolescents 10–14 and 15–19 Years Old

In 2005, the population in these age groups numbered 608,299 (18.8% of the total population). The coverage of health check-ups for adolescents between the ages of 10 to 14 and 15 to 19 years was 20.9% and 7.8%, respectively, for the country as a whole. The main causes of death in this group were external causes (accidents, suicides, homicides, and other violence) and malignant tumors, which ranked second. Deaths in this age group represented 2.3% of all deaths in Panama (33).

In the area of sexual and reproductive health, about one out of every three students (36.4%) said that they had had sexual relations. The average declared age for the first sexual relationship was 14 years (males 13 years and females 15 years); 45.7% of students who were sexually active did not use any contraceptive method in their most recent sexual relationship. One out of every four used condoms, and 11.9% reported using birth control pills. Some 4% of girls reported that they had been pregnant at least once, and 69.4% of those girls said they had interrupted the pregnancy. The average age at which the girls became pregnant was 15 (35). According to ENV 2003 (9), 17% of girls between the ages of 15 and 19 reported that they were pregnant at the time of the survey, a situation that appears to be more prevalent among the non-poor (25% were pregnant compared to 12% for the poor). The value of this indicator does not vary significantly by geographic zone. The specific fertility rate among adolescents (girls 15 to 19 years of age) in 2004 was 0.0849 per 1,000 population, which accounts for 7.9% of total births in this age group. In 2004, the mortality rate in the 10-to-19-year group was 9.44 per 100,000 population.

Adults 20–59 Years Old

In 2005, this group contained an estimated 1,667,330 people (51.7% of the total population), with 851,266 being women of fertile age (15 to 49 years of age). In a sample of 31,823 reported pregnancies (36), 83.5% of the women received prenatal check-ups; 61.0% began in the 20th week of pregnancy and 7.7% after 30 weeks, with an average of five check-ups during pregnancy. Pregnancies ended in spontaneous delivery in 75.2% of women and delivery by cesarean section in 21.5%; 8.4% of women in the puerperium were discharged with a contraceptive method. During pregnancy, delivery, and the puerperium, 18.5% of women presented some kind of problem, with the most frequent being premature rupture of membranes (8.7% of all pregnancies), followed by hemorrhaging (4.0%) and gestational hypertension (3.8%).

The mortality rate among the population between 20 and 59 years was 40.76 per 100,000 population in 2004; the deaths reported in this age group accounted for 25.1% of all deaths in the country. The main causes of death were external causes, malignant tumors, HIV, and ischemic heart disease. In the 25-to-34-year and the 35-to-44-year groups, HIV was the second cause of

death and accounted for 51.8% of deaths from external causes and caused 1.4 times more deaths than tumors (33).

The estimated maternal mortality rate in 2003 was 70 per 100,000 live births, with differences in rural and urban rates (Figure 3). Maternal deaths accounted for 0.8% of deaths in women and 5.2% of deaths in women of fertile age. In 2003, the main specific causes of maternal mortality were hemorrhage (26.8%), indirect obstetrical causes (24.4%), gestational hypertension (17.1%), abortion (12.2%), sepsis (9.7%), and other direct obstetrical causes (9.7%). Death occurred during adolescence in 17% of cases, while the age distribution of women who died was similar to the distribution of deaths among the five-year groups between the ages of 15 and 39 years. The analysis of maternal deaths reported in 2001–2005 showed that 29% took place in third-level care establishments, 28% at home, 21% in second-level establishments, and 7% in first-level establishments. The percentage of women who die without receiving timely medical care could be 40%, if the deaths reported by forensic medicine institutions are considered (15%).

Older Adults 60 Years Old and Older

This age group is estimated to represent 8.6% of the total population at present. ENV 2003 found that 53% were women. Sixty-one percent of the adult population lives in urban zones, while 35% lives in rural areas and 4% in indigenous areas. One fourth of older adults are poor. Health insurance coverage extends to 71% of older adults (non-poor 80%, non-extreme poor 39%, and extreme poor 23%). Two thirds of them receive health benefits from the Social Security Fund, and 5% are served by private health insurance systems in addition to the services offered by the Fund (9). Based on population projections for 2050, the group of older adults will grow to 22.3%, which will mean increased demand related to chronic noncommunicable diseases and psychosocial problems (37).

In 2003, the general mortality rate among the population 60 years and older was 259.24 per 10,000 population; the risk of death is higher among males. Malignant tumors, cerebrovascular diseases, ischemic heart disease, diabetes mellitus, and chronic lower respiratory diseases were the main causes of death among the elderly (33).

The Family

The National Population and Housing Census 2000 estimated that the country had a total of 681,928 households, 12.6% of which were single person, 50.7% were nuclear families (parents and children), 30.2% were extended families (including a relative), and 6.4% were compound (one or more nuclear families with other relatives and non-relatives). ENV 2003 determined that the average size of households was four people (5.8 people in poor households and 3.4 people in non-poor ones); the indigenous population has the largest families among the poor (almost

FIGURE 3. Maternal mortality, by rural and urban areas, Panama, 1990, 2000, 2003, and Millennium Development Goal target for 2015.

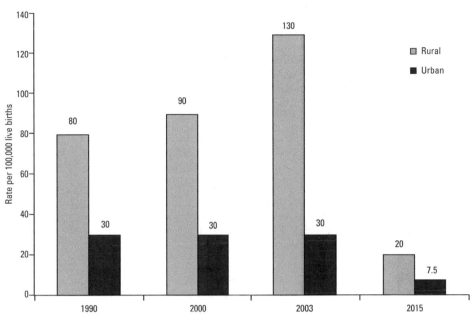

Source: Panamá. Contraloría General de la República. Dirección de Estadística y Censo. Segundo Informe Objetivos de Desarrollo del Milenio, septiembre 2005.

8 per household). Women headed 27.0% of households; 7.6% of heads of households were young, with a larger percentage of men (11.7%) than women (3.5%) (*22*).

In 2005, 26.4% of people over the age of 15 were married, 29.5% lived in stable unions, 31.4% were single, and 12.6% were separated, divorced, or widowed. The divorce-to-marriage ratio has remained stable over the last five years (23.8 in 2001, 22.6 in 2005). Average age at marriage was 31 for men and 28 for women. Based on the IDHP 2004 report, young people described their families and family relations as average to highly positive (25.0%), while 20.6% described them as negative, attributed to poor quality family relations (*22*).

Workers

According to the Social Security Fund (CSS) (*1*), 45,136 people received benefits in 2004, 67.7% for illness and maternity, and 25.7% for occupational risks. A total of 20,113 (44.6%) benefits were for temporary disability, 9,757 for labor accidents, 1,119 for accidents traveling to and from work, and 312 for occupational diseases. In 2003, of the total number of people receiving benefits under the occupational risks program (12,003), 25.0% were agroindustrial workers, 21.5% worked in the services sector, 20.2% worked in manufacturing, and 11.2% worked in construction. The main causes of accidents are related to the mishandling of materials (46% of cases) and improper use of manual tools (24%) (*38*).

Persons with Disabilities

The last census (2000) reported 52,197 people with disabilities (1.8% of the country's population), which affected 29,236 males and 22,961 females; 31,258 lived in urban areas and 20,939 in rural ones. Significant underreporting is believed to exist. The Ministry of Education, in coordination with the Ministry of Health, launched a national education inclusiveness program (2005) involving a pilot project in 65 schools around the country intended to create positive attitudes in the community, particularly the school community, for the inclusion of children with disabilities (*39*).

There are no precise figures on social security coverage for persons with disabilities, but the scant information available indicates that it is low, particularly for rehabilitation services. According to information provided by the National Secretariat for Social Integration of Persons with Disabilities, all rehabilitation services are concentrated in the capital, which greatly limits access to those services for people living in the provinces.

Ethnic Groups

There are seven different indigenous peoples (*40*) who belong to the following linguist groups: Ngöbé, Buglé, Kuna, Emberá, Wounaan, Naso (Teribe), and Bri-bri, with a population that represented 10% of the national total in 2005 (*41*); 51% of them live in the different territories covering more than 20% of the country (*21*).

In 2000, the largest ethnic group, the Ngöbé, made up 59.3% of the country's indigenous people (40), followed by the Kunas (21.6%). The smaller groups include the Teribes, the Bri-Bri, and the Bokotas (which accounted for 1.1%, 0.9%, and 0.4% of the total, respectively) (42). The indigenous and non-indigenous populations have contrasting economic subsistence and market models. The quest for development opportunities has led to a change in how indigenous people take part in the labor field, since from a family economy—in primary agriculture—they have been pushed, in some cases, to sell their labor, generally under the worst possible labor conditions (43). Of every 100 indigenous persons, 98 are poor and 86 of them live in extreme poverty.

In demographic terms, indigenous groups have high population growth rates. In the period between 1990 and 2000, annual growth was 3.8%, higher than the rate for the Panamanian population in 1960–1970 (31). Among indigenous peoples, the average fertility rate was 6.6 children per woman, in contrast with 2.9 for non-indigenous women. Life expectancy shows a difference of almost nine years between non-indigenous and indigenous males (72 years compared to 63.2 years, according to the 2000 census) and of almost 12 years between women (non-indigenous 77.3 years, indigenous 65.4 years). The percentage of young population is high (45.8% are under 14 years of age) (31).

Displaced Persons

The border zone with Colombia, which covers the province of Darién and Comarca Kuna Yala, has been receiving displaced people fleeing the military conflict in Colombia for a number of years. At the end of 2002, the United Nations High Commission for Refugees reported 989 Colombians displaced inside Panama, 91% of whom lived in the province of Darién. The conditions under which basic services, health care, education, housing, water and sanitation, and employment are available in the border region are difficult for people who were born there and are even more so for displaced persons and refugees (44).

HEALTH CONDITIONS AND PROBLEMS

COMMUNICABLE DISEASES

Vector-borne Diseases

Autochthonous transmission of **dengue** has been reported in Panama since 1993. Since then, according to the records of the epidemiological surveillance system, the annual variations in cases can be grouped into three categories: years of endemic transmission (1994, 1996, and 2002), with about 800 cases a year; epidemic years (1995, 1997, 1998, 1999, 2001, and 2005), with an average of 2,500 cases a year; and low-transmission years (1993,

2000, 2003, and 2004), with an average of 350 cases a year. The total number of cases notified since reporting began is 21,830, 6,980 (31.9%) of which were notified in the last four years (2002–2005). The dengue-1 and dengue-2 serotypes have predominated, although in earlier years, the four serotypes circulated. Morbidity from dengue has been from classical dengue in all years, with just 31 cases (0.2%) of hemorrhagic dengue; however, 17 (68%) of the cases of hemorrhagic dengue were notified in the last five years, which indicates that the risk of hemorrhagic dengue is on the rise. There were very few deaths from hemorrhagic dengue and dengue shock syndrome—just five in the entire period—with a cumulative death rate of 16%. The largest dengue epidemic reported since the start of transmission in Panama in 1993 occurred in 2005, when a total of 5,489 cases was reported for a rate of 170 cases per 100,000 population; 99.8% of those cases were classical dengue.

Infestation by the mosquito *Aedes aegypti* now affects all parts of the country. The hardest hit areas in the last two years have been San Miguelito with a Breteau index in 2005 of 7.0, Kuna Yala with 4.7, Panamá Oeste with 4.4, and Panamá Metro with 3.7. The indexes are even more serious given that these regions comprise zones with the greatest hygienic-sanitary complexity.

There are 221,000 people living in zones classified as having moderate risk of **malaria** and 107,000 people live in zones at high risk. Morbidity caused by malaria increased steadily between 2000 and 2005, with 3,668 cases per 100,000 population in 2005. In the same period, transmission intensity increased from an annual parasite index per 1,000 of 0.33 in 2001 to 1.2 in 2005. Also the index for *Plasmodium falciparum* rose from 0.01 in 2001 to 0.25 in 2005. The annual index for blood tests per 1,000 was 4.9 in 2001, 5.3 in 2004, and 5.7 in 2005, with positive blood slide indexes of 0.6%, 3.0%, and 1.8%, respectively. Of the 3,668 cases reported in 2005, Comarca Ngöbe Buglé presented 21.0%, followed by Veraguas with 20.1%, Bocas del Toro with 16.0%, and Darién with 12.0%. Darién and Panamá Este notified 83.0% of the 764 cases caused by *P. falciparum* in the country. The mortality rate from malaria continues to be low, at 0.16 deaths per 100,000 population in 2003. *In vitro* studies performed in 2003 by the Gorgas Memorial Institute for Health Studies (ICGES) showed that strains of *P. falciparum* presented mutations associated with resistance to chloroquine, sulfadoxine, and pyrimethamine. The presence of *P. malariae* has not been detected since 1972.

Ever since it was diagnosed in Panama for the first time in 1931, **Chagas' disease** has maintained its presence in the country, although there have been no reports of major outbreaks of the disease in recent years. Between 1974 and 2006 (epidemiological week no. 20) 522 cases were reported, 67.6% of which were notified between 1974 and 1984. The most important endemic zone for the disease is La Chorrera district, province of Panama. In a serological survey performed in 2003 of a sample of

DOTS Strategy: Progress in Controlling Tuberculosis

In 2005, 1,565 cases of tuberculosis were reported (48.5 per 100,000 population). Males were more frequently affected, with a male-to-female ratio of 1.2:1. The search for cases among individuals with respiratory symptoms has been stepped up, leading to an increase in tuberculosis reporting in recent years, from 8,011 in 2000 to 15,195 in 2005. The Directly Observed Treatment Short-course (DOTS) is the internationally recommended strategy being applied gradually to improve the detection and examination of individuals with respiratory symptoms. The population covered by DOTS grew from 51% in 2000 to 90% in 2004.

school-aged children, seroprevalence of 2.9% was obtained. Screening during 2003 at the blood bank of the regional hospital in that area (Nicolás Solano Hospital) showed a seroprevalence of 0.9% among volunteer donors.

The main vectors were *Rhodnius pallescens*, which continue to be wild, frequently visiting houses but not living there. The main endemic zones lie in the provinces of Panama, Colón, and Darién. *Triatoma dimidiata, T. dispar,* and *Panstrongylus geniculatus* are other important vectors in transmission. Indexes for the infestation of housing by *T. dimidiata* range from 16.4% in Gualaca (province of Chiriquí) to 3.2% in La Chorrera (province of Panama).

Studies of natural infection in insects caught in the vicinity of homes in La Chorrera identified the presence of *Trypanosoma cruzi* and *T. rangeli* in 30% to 60% of the specimens. Tests with the pyrethroids deltametrine and lambdacyhalotrine demonstrated that the strains of *R. pallescens* in the La Chorrera and Chilibre areas in the province of Panama were susceptible to these insecticides.

In 2003, 1,602 cases of **leishmaniasis** were reported, with an incidence of 51.3 cases per 100,000 population. The most affected provinces were Bocas del Toro (534.5 per 100,000 population), Coclé (143.5), and Darién (91.2), which together had 58% of all cases. In the period 1993–2003, the behavior of this disease fluctuated, with a total of 22,634 cases, for an annual average of 2,058 cases and a monthly average of 172 cases. During 2005, 1,590 cases were reported, 36.6% in children under 5 and 35.5% in people between the ages of 15 and 64 years; 51.2% of the cases were in males.

Vaccine-preventable Diseases

The country has not reported **poliomyelitis** since 1972. In 1974, it reported the last case of jungle **yellow fever.** There have been no cases of **diphtheria** since 1981, and none of **measles** since December 1994. The last case of congenital **rubella** was reported in 1999, and no cases of **meningitis** caused by *Haemophilus influenzae* type b were reported in 2005. Epidemiological surveillance for vaccine-preventable diseases is performed

through negative weekly notification throughout the country's entire network of health services.

In 2005, national vaccination coverage in children under 1 year was: BCG 100%, hepatitis B for newborns 78.5%, polio 94%, DPT and Hib 94.2%, and MMR 99%. National coverage with the pentavalent vaccine (DPT+HB+Hib) averaged 86.5%. Vaccinations against yellow fever have been carried out annually since 1991 in the health regions of Panamá Este, Darién, and Comarca Kuna Yala, with a total population of 160,997 people. In the 1991–2004 period, a total of 226,329 doses were given. In 2006, the government included new vaccines in the immunization program, including those against rotavirus for children under 6 months and against influenza for children 7 to 18 months, adults over 65 years of age, and health care workers.

Intestinal Infectious Diseases

In 2003, 1,073 cases of **food poisoning,** 189,914 of **diarrhea,** 35 of **salmonellosis,** 345 of **infectious hepatitis,** and 5,639 of **amebiasis** were reported. There have been no cases of **cholera** since 1994. In that year, 14 outbreaks of waterborne diseases were investigated, with 630 cases and one death. The etiological agent was identified in 25% of the outbreaks. The Panama City metropolitan region had the highest rate in the country, which was double the national average, followed by Chiriquí, Los Santos, and Panamá Este, with 51, 49.6, and 46.6 cases per 100,000 population, respectively. Since 1995, when the PAHO-proposed guide for surveillance of foodborne diseases was adopted, 147 outbreaks of foodborne diseases have been reported (3,253 cases and eight deaths). In the period 2001–2003, the food poisoning rate ranged from 59.8 to 34.4 cases per 100,000 population (*35*).

The cases of diarrhea reported in 2003 represented a national incidence of 6,075 cases per 100,000 population. The province with the highest incidence of diarrhea was Bocas del Toro (11,449.4 cases per 100,000 population), followed by Chiriquí (7,916.2 per 100,000 population) and the areas of San Miguelito (7,594 cases per 100,000 population), the metropolitan area (7,438.3 per 100,000 population), and Panamá Este (6,066.8 per 100,000 population).

Chronic Communicable Diseases

Tuberculosis has been on the rise. In 2005, 1,565 cases were reported (48.5 per 100,000 population). The areas at greatest risk are the provinces of Kuna Yala (210 per 100,000 population), Ngöbe Buglé (152.6), Bocas del Toro (107), and Colón (97.7). Males are more frequently affected, with a male-to-female ratio of 1.2:1 (49.9 per 100,000 population for men and 40.8 per 100,000 for women). The disease's pattern differs among the Kuna Yala, Ngöbé Buglé, Bocas del Toro, and San Miguelito regions, where rates are higher among women (in this last region, the risk for women was three times higher).

The Directly Observed Treatment Short-course (DOTS) strategy is being applied gradually to improve the detection and examination of respiratory symptoms, which rose from 8,011 in 2000 to 15,195 in 2005, with a higher rate of detection of new tuberculosis cases, which increased from 1,123 in 2000 (rate of 39.2 per 100,000 population) to 1,565 in 2005 (rate of 48.5 per 100,000). The population covered by DOTS grew from 51% in 2000 to 90% in 2004. In that last year, of the 860 reported cases of bacilliferous tuberculosis, 557 patients were discharged as cured (64.8%) and 116 completed the treatment, that is, in total, a successful outcome of 78.3%. The percentage of patients who abandoned treatment was 10.5%; transfers and those awaiting evaluation, 7.7%; deaths, 2.3%; and those with failed treatment, 1.2%. From the start of the epidemic in 1984 to 2005, HIV/tuberculosis coinfections totaled 1,655 cases. In 2003, 9.6% of tuberculosis cases were associated with AIDS (137/1,427).

Acute Respiratory Infections

It is compulsory to report clinically identified influenza. Annual outbreaks occur associated with the increase in rainfall in May to October. The accumulated incidence in 1995–2004 grew from 6,250 to 9,822 cases per 100,000 population. In 1999, there was an epidemic that affected a national total of 46,262 per 100,000 population.

HIV/AIDS and Other Sexually Transmitted Infections

The number of people infected with HIV is estimated as 18,000 to 22,000 people between the ages of 15 and 49. From 1984 to 2005, 7,111 cases of AIDS were notified, with a national prevalence of 0.9%. Cases have been reported in 88% of the districts (66 out of 75). Since the start of the epidemic, males have been most heavily affected with 75.6% of AIDS cases and the highest seroprevalence rates are found in men who have sex with men (17%). The male-to-female ratio nationwide has declined gradually, from 17:1 at the start of the epidemic to 3:1 in 2006; however the ratio is just 1.6:1 in people between the ages of 15 and 24 years (*45*). There have been 203 cases of vertical transmission reported, and more than four out of every five cases (81.7%) were reported from 1999–2006. Higher frequencies are notified for the following age groups: 25 to 29 years (13.3%), 30 to 34 (19.2%), 35 to 39 (16.5%), and 40 to 44 (13.2%). Of reported cases, the mode of transmission was as follows: 67.4% (4,792), sexual transmission; 3.7% (262), vertical transmission (perinatal); 2.0% (139), blood transmission; and 27.0% (1,918), unknown transmission method. The concentration index for inequality in the distribution of new cases of AIDS during 2002, according to data aggregated at the provincial level, was 0.41. Panamanians in the poorest quintile accounted for 6% of the new cases of AIDS, while 47% were found in the highest income quintile. The relative risk between the wealthiest and poorest quintiles was 7.6. No national studies have been conducted to provide useful information on the behavior of the population at risk or the consistent use of condoms as a means of prevention of sexually transmitted infections/HIV. Antiretroviral treatment is administered to 70.5% of people with reported cases of HIV (*46*).

According to the Department of Epidemiology of the Ministry of Health, in 2005 the rates of sexually transmitted infections were as follows: **vulvovaginitis** (962.4 per 100,000 population), **inflammatory pelvic disease** (315.2), **papillomavirus** (150.6), **gonorrhea** (41.1), **nonspecific urethritis** (23.6), **acquired syphilis** (13.3), **genital herpes** (12.8), **white canker** (1.0), **congenital syphilis** (0.1), and **venereal lymphogranuloma** (0.1).

Zoonoses

The last cases of urban **rabies** were reported in 1973; subsequently two human cases were reported in 1994, caused by bat bites, and in 1995 there was a case in a Colombian child who had been bitten by a wild cat. The most recent notification of wild rabies was in 2002, with two cases of human rabies caused by hematophagus bats.

As for enzootic **Venezuelan equine encephalitis** (VEE), ever since enzootic subtype ID was identified in Panama in 1968, frequent endemic-enzootic outbreaks of the disease have occurred, and the virus has been isolated in vector mosquitoes, host or reservoir rodents, horses, and humans. Reports indicate that the virus was isolated in 39 human cases between 1991 and 2005. The largest outbreak took place in the Darién region in 2001, with 11 pediatric cases diagnosed in the laboratory, one of which was a girl under 5 who died.

Among emerging viral zoonoses, **hantavirus** was reported in Panama in December 1999. Up to 2006 (epidemiological week no. 28), there were 83 cases of hantavirus cardiopulmonary syndrome, with 15 deaths, for a lethality rate of 18.8%. The seroprevalence study conducted in the affected communities revealed seropositivity of 12.9% (40/311), an average age of 31.5 years, and a range of 1 to 79 years, with no differences by sex or age. Two new hantavirus serotypes have been identified, one of which is associated with the rodent *Oligoryzomys fulvescens* (pygmy rice rat), that has infected humans, and the other with the rodent *Zygodontomys brevicauda* (cane rat or grey mouse).

In the fight against this set of diseases, emphasis has been placed on vaccinating dogs against rabies; controlling the sources of hantavirus, VEE, Chagas' disease, and leishmaniasis; and maintaining surveillance to prevent the introduction of the West Nile virus.

Noncommunicable Diseases

Metabolic and Nutritional Diseases

The prevalence of total **malnutrition** (weight for age) in children under 5 years was 6.8% (non-poor 2.1%, non-extreme poor 4.6%, extreme poor 16.3%), and rose to 21.5% in children aged 5 years in rural indigenous zones. In this age group, 22.1% were at risk of malnutrition (non-poor 16.7%, extreme poor 31.6%), while at the other extreme, **overweight** affected 4.1% (non-poor 6.3%, non-extreme poor 3.5%, extreme poor 1.1%). About 9.2% of children under 5 were at risk of being overweight (non-poor 13.1%, extreme poor 3.8%) (25). The 1997 Standard of Living Survey contained similar figures for total malnutrition (18). The prevalence of moderate/severe chronic malnutrition (height/age) in this same group was 20.6% (non-poor 10.2%, non-extreme poor 19.1%, extreme poor 39.6%), and was 56.6% among children under 5 years in indigenous rural zones. In comparison with the data from 1997, chronic malnutrition increased by six percentage points (18). Acute malnutrition (weight/height) affected 1.3% (non-poor 0.8%, non-extreme poor 1.5%, extreme poor 2.0%). The risk of malnutrition among children under 5 was 9.2% (non-poor 8.9%, extreme poor 9.9%) (25). There was a slight increase in acute malnutrition, which was 1.0% countrywide in 1997 (18).

Among the adolescents evaluated for body mass index, 4.5% had low weight (non-poor 5.1%, poor 3.8%), 6.9% were overweight (non-poor 10.1%, poor 2.9%), and 12.1% were at risk of being overweight (non-poor 13.0%, poor 11.1%) (25). ENV 2003 found that 33.6% of the population was overweight, without distinction by sex, and 18.3% were obese (females 21.8%, males 14.4%). In combination, these conditions affect 56.4% of the urban population, 43.8% of the rural indigenous and non-indigenous population, and 36.8% of the population in indigenous areas. When the prevalence of excess weight and obesity is compared by economic level, these conditions affect 56.8% of the non-poor, 39.7% of the poor, and 35.0% of people living in extreme poverty (25).

With regard to nutrition during pregnancy, in the second and third trimesters, 21.6% of pregnant women presented low weight (non-poor 10.0%, non-extreme poor 17.4%, extreme poor 39.9%), rising to 38.2% of pregnant women in rural indigenous zones; and 39.3% were overweight (non-poor 50.6%, non-extreme poor 40.7%, extreme poor 23.3%) (25). In 2005 (47), 9.3% of newborns had low birthweight, which is less than the 13.1% found in ENV 2003 (non-poor 10.7%, non-extreme poor 12.3%, extreme poor 21.6%). For indigenous newborns the figure was one in four (24.6%) (9). Eighteen percent of babies were fed nothing other than breast milk until the age of 6 months (15% in

urban zones, 22.4% in rural ones), for 13% among the non-poor, 20% among the poor, and 26% among the extreme poor (25).

As for micronutrients, the analysis by socioeconomic level showed that the indigenous rural group and the group living in extreme poverty presented lower levels of apparent consumption of calcium (national average 307 mg, indigenous rural 126 mg), iron (national average 7.3 mg, indigenous rural 5.2 mg), and vitamin A (national average 376 mg, indigenous rural 111 mg) (25). Iron-deficiency **anemia** affected more than one-third of children under 5 and pregnant women and women of fertile age, and so since 1998 the Ministry of Health (MINSA) has been carrying out a preventive iron supplement program for preschool and school-aged children and pregnant women. In evaluations performed in 2005, it was found that the prevalence of iron-deficiency anemia in schoolchildren who had received supplements since grade one was just 1.8%. The National Vitamin A Survey 1999 indicates that 10% of children between 12 and 59 months presented blood retinol levels below 20 μg (24% in indigenous children and 7% in nonindigenous ones). In 2002, Panama was certified as free from iodine-deficiency disorders thanks to universal iodization of salt. In 2004, the National Secretariat for Coordination and Monitoring of the Nutrition Plan (SENAPAN), which reports to the Office of the President, was established to optimize nutritional interventions.

Among metabolic diseases, **diabetes mellitus** has increased. The rates in 2000 and 2005 were 134.5 and 170.1 per 100,000 population, respectively. In 2005, distribution by province indicated that Los Santos, Panamá Oeste, and San Miguelito presented rates of 648.3, 483.5, and 259.6 per 100,000 population, respectively.

Diabetes is the fourth leading cause of death, and rose progressively from 11 per 100,000 population in 1990 to 24.4 per 100,000 in 2004. In the latter year, there was a predominance of cases in women (29 per 100,000 population) compared to men (19.9 per 100,000).

Cardiovascular Diseases

As for **arterial hypertension,** the records point to an increase: from 529.4 per 100,000 population in 2000 the rate climbed to 905.9 per 100,000 in 2005. Diseases of the circulatory system represent the leading cause of death in almost all provinces. Ministry of Health records for **ischemic heart disease** reported a rate of 40.2 per 100,000 population in 2000 and 43.8 per 100,000 in 2004. In the latter year, males were more affected, with 51.0% of cases compared to 36.5% for women. **Cerebrovascular disease** rose from 42.1 per 100,000 population in 2000 to 44.7 per 100,000 in 2004.

Malignant Neoplasms

Medical records presented a predominance of **prostate cancer** in men, with a rate of 25.6 per 100,000 population in 1990 which rose to 66.5 per 100,000 in 2004. In women, cancer of the cervix predominated, but dropped from 81.2 per 100,000 population in

1990 to 47.2 per 100,000 in 2004, while breast cancer rose from 22.6 per 100,000 population in 1990 to 39.4 per 100,000 in 2004.

OTHER HEALTH PROBLEMS OR ISSUES

Disasters

In 2005, floods in the Tocumen area caused more than 20 deaths and numerous injuries. The situation was similar when the Sixaola River flooded. General seismic activity is moderate, but the country can still be affected by earthquakes. In 1991, an earthquake in Bocas del Toro caused several deaths and many injuries. Major seismic movements have been recorded recently in the high part of Chiriquí Province.

Violence and Other External Causes

Surveys indicate that 24.6% of Panamanians consider insecurity to be the worst problem in their municipality; 8% said they had been victims of a crime (58.8% unarmed robbery with no physical threats, 18.5% robbery with aggression, 11.0% robbery in the home, 6.2% physical aggression without robbery, and 4.0% rape), but 48.6% of them did not report the crime (8). Official figures (48) show that during 2003, 63,988 people (26.5%) were arrested for crimes against life and bodily security; against property, 21.5%; and against modesty and sexual freedom, 2.6%. The highest crime rate is among the following age groups: under 18 (13.0%), from 18 to 20 (10.6%), and from 20 to 24 (22.5%). The national detention rate was 20.3 per 1,000 population; for Panama City it was 26.9, and for the city of Colón it was 75.5.

In 2003, 36,176 traffic accidents were reported (97.1 accidents per 1,000 registered vehicles), which injured 11,161 people (2.5% seriously) and caused 421 deaths; 56.7% of the injured and 53.9% of the deaths were in the 15-to-39-year age group. The national rate was 13 deaths per 100,000 population. The province of Panama with 76.5%, Colón with 7.2%, and Chiriquí with 6.8% reported the largest number of accidents. In 2003, traffic accidents occurred about every 15 minutes and caused one death every 20 hours; 62% of those deaths occurred on weekends (Friday to Sunday), and 48.5% were on Saturday and Sunday; 39.4% of the victims were pedestrians, 30.2% drivers, 29.9% passengers, and 0.5% horseback riders (49).

In 2004 external causes (accidents, suicides, homicides, and other types of violence) ranked as the third cause of death, with 1,035 victims (33), and affected men (55.3 per 100,000 population) more than women (11.8 per 100,000 population) (50). In this context, domestic violence is growing in epidemiological, economic, and social importance. Statistics from a Ministry of Health report show that the number of victims of domestic violence or other forms of abuse treated in the public health care system remained stable between 2002 and 2004: 2,462 cases in 2002, 2,371 in 2003, and 2,476 in 2004. Distribution by sex in 2004 was: women, 78.9%; men, 20.5%; and unspecified, 0.6% (50).

Mental Health

Ministry of Health statistics on mental health are limited. In 2004, the main reasons for outpatient consultations for mental health services were stress-related neurotic and somatoform disorders (33%), followed by affective disorders (23%). In Panama's 103 outpatient mental health establishments, 93,239 consultations took place with an estimated five contacts per user. In the National Mental Health Institute, the main diagnoses on discharge were schizophrenia (33%) and affective disorders (26%) (51). Psychiatric beds are distributed as follows: 41% in the National Mental Health Institute (psychiatric hospital) and 59% in psychiatric services in general hospitals. The country has made a major effort to reform and modernize the psychiatric services. The National Psychiatric Hospital reduced the number of beds considerably (63% in the last five years), to become the National Mental Health Institute. Psychiatric services have been developed in general hospitals and mental health teams have been decentralized in almost all the provinces. Estimates indicate that about 3% of the general health care budget is allocated to mental health, and 44% is used by the National Mental Health Institute (51).

Addictions

Different studies indicate that alcohol is the drug that is most widely used by the general population and that men are more apt to consume illegal drugs, while women are more likely to take minor tranquilizers. As for the consumption of hazardous substances, the Global Youth Tobacco Survey (52) showed that one out of every three students between the ages of 13 and 15 (31.6%) had smoked at some point in their lives. The prevalence of tobacco use in the last 30 days was 18.3% (cigarettes, 12.5%); 13.2% said they had never smoked, but would probably start next year. In 2003, the Environmental Tobacco Smoke Surveillance Study (53) revealed that gas-phase nicotine levels in Panama City can be considered low or moderate; however, exposure to tobacco smoke was detected in places where smoking is prohibited, such as airports and hospitals, and the level of exposure in bars and restaurants was classified as high or very high.

RESPONSE OF THE HEALTH SECTOR

Health Policies and Plans

The health sector has two main players—the Ministry of Health and the Social Security Fund (CSS)—which formulate, implement, monitor, and evaluate their own plans and projects, but do not have a unified planning system; there is, therefore, no sector plan. During the last three governments, ministerial planning documents that contain government guidelines were prepared and made into ministerial policies. The current government prepared the document "Health Policies and Strategies, 2005–2009," which reflects the main areas where MINSA proposes to work: strengthening the National Health Authority; the primary health care model; environmental sustainability and protection; increase in social participation; modernization of administrative management; the development and strengthening of human resources in health; and promotion of applied research. The document directly mentions gender equity and human rights, but they are included in a general, not explicit, fashion.

The right of health care access in Panama is enshrined in Articles 109 and 110 of the Constitution, which require the state to guarantee all Panamanians comprehensive, preventive, curative, and rehabilitative services, regardless of their social status or political, ethnic, or religious group. The framework health act (the health code) has been in effect, unamended, for 45 years and is considered obsolete. With regard to the Social Security Code, despite the fact that social security reform (2006) was proposed and discussed, it only touched on social insurance, without resolving the separation of functions of the National Health Authority or unifying the system.

In relation to essential public health functions, function 7 (on evaluation and promotion of equitable access to necessary health services) and function 5 (on policy development and institutional capacity for planning and management of public health) received the best evaluations (with 0.87 and 0.81 points, respectively). Conversely, function 11 (on reducing the impact of emergencies and disasters on health) and function 9 (on ensuring the quality of individual and public health services) received the lowest evaluations (0.32 and 0.29 points, respectively). The score obtained by function 9 reflects the gradual erosion of the steering role that typically comes about when administrative fragmentation results in segmented plans and programs that, in turn, lead to a decrease in the quality of services offered to poorer groups. The remaining functions scored in the higher middle range, with the exception of function 1 (health situation monitoring and analysis), which received almost 0.80 points, placing it in the upper range.

Panama was the second country in the Region to sign and ratify the WHO Framework Convention on Tobacco Control, which has already begun to be implemented and which represents important progress in the fight against smoking. Specific rules have now been developed that restrict the sale and public use of tobacco and its byproducts, which are contained in Law 17 of 2005. Executive Decree No. 17 of 11 March 2005 was issued subsequently, regulating the law and establishing measures in effect for "smoking prevention and the reduction of tobacco use and exposure to tobacco smoke."

The process of health sector reform goes back to the 1990s and its main guidelines were unification of the system, comprehensiveness of service, equity, universal access, and better efficiency, but sustained changes were not achieved. The process was limited to one health region (San Miguel Arcángel) in the Panama City metropolitan area.

Health Strategies and Programs

At the end of 2005, Law 51 was passed, thus reforming the social security statute. An overview of the changes introduced by this new law makes it clear that the main focus was on disability, old age, and life insurance, improving the medium-term sustainability of the program through actions to raise the contribution ceiling and the pensionable age. The ceiling for general health and maternity insurance did not increase, which leaves the problem of the program's financial deficit unaddressed.

As part of the current government's strategy to combat poverty, a social protection system has been implemented that basically seeks to create the capacity to enable 25,000 families to rise out of absolute poverty through conditional cash transfers. The system has not been evaluated yet.

Organization of the Health System

The health system is fragmented and divided into two subsectors: the public (MINSA and CSS) and the private. The public sector institutions are highly centralized and vertically structured and do not involve community participation in the co-management of services; the care model is predominantly curative; and risk and harm prevention programs are targeted to the more prevalent health problems with the greatest negative effects on the population. MINSA has begun a process of deconcentrating some administrative functions and partial management of expenditures, although the processes of budgetary planning, allocation, and management continue to be concentrated at the central level.

As for the degree of segmentation of the population, the CSS had nominal coverage of 2,003,108 beneficiaries in 2004, 33.8% of whom were active contributors, 7.6% pensioners, and 58.6% dependents, while 35.0% were the responsibility of MINSA. Private sector participation is indeterminate but nominally low, given that there are no major private insurers. Cross-subsidies exist, however, since the public system is open and has no mechanisms for identifying selective demand for social security beneficiaries, and MINSA is the only supplier available in some parts of the country.

The CSS is the institution responsible for insuring all public and private sector workers under general health and maternity insurance, occupational accidents and diseases insurance (ATEP), and disability, old age, and death insurance. The types of membership are established in a CSS law: compulsory membership applies to workers in the formal public and private sectors and independent workers who provide services to the government or formally to private enterprise; voluntary membership applies to people who are not subject to the compulsory regime and underage workers who receive the same benefits as workers of legal age. Similarly, this law defines groups of beneficiaries: beneficiaries are spouses or permanent companions and dependents up to age 25 (provided there is no voluntary emancipation, and they are enrolled in the country's formal education system); lifetime beneficiaries are disabled dependents or parents over 60 years of age. The ATEP is applicable to CSS members, which means that only about 30% of the population is covered (formal and affiliated sectors). At present, however, coverage is limited only to care in the case of illness or accident, and financial compensation is limited to temporary or permanent disabilities and does not cover systematic occupational health activities. The CSS has no plan setting out the services covered, waiting periods, or differences in plans between contributors and beneficiaries, which means that the costs of care are growing and will lead to a crisis in general health and maternity insurance, which is forecast to occur in 2011. In the private sector, the coverage plans are varied and subject to the individual's ability to pay, since they operate on the basis of reimbursement.

The regulatory function in public health is the responsibility of the Ministry of Health's Directorate General of Public Health (DIGESA), which is also the focus of a large part of the ministry's functions, such as acting as the National Health Authority. Its structure is divided into the health surveillance and regulatory areas, with the National Directorate of Pharmacy and Drugs reporting to it. Functions overlap in various areas; for example, environmental surveillance and waste management are also the responsibility of the National Environmental Authority (ANAM).

Public Health Services

The Ministry of Health and the Social Security Fund implement programs for vulnerable groups through classical primary care activities centered on age groups, specialties, or pathological processes, such as programs for mental health, sexual and reproductive health, environmental protection, children, adolescents, adults, persons with disabilities, and maternal health, among others. Although all of these programs form part of the health offerings provided by the Ministry and are free of charge to the entire population through different delivery mechanisms, they are not well coordinated and do not constitute a comprehensive system of primary health care.

Services are driven by demand. Another method used for rural and indigenous populations that live in remote areas, with little or no access to regular health services, is traveling care provided by contracted agencies, health fairs organized by the health regions (FOGI), and health caravans organized directly by the Ministry, which provide second level care, including outpatient surgeries. In all cases, the services are limited to those included in the Ministry of Health's basic plan, known as the Comprehensive Health Services Package (PAISS), and do not receive systematic support from the CSS. ENV 2003 indicated that the 17.5% of people with health problems who did not seek care gave financial reasons (11.6% did not have the money to pay for transportation to the place where the care was being offered, and 5.9% said that the health services were expensive). Economic barriers had more impact in rural (26.1%)

and indigenous zones (40.0%), and obviously among the poorer population (28.6% of the poor and 36.1% of the extreme poor), which underlines the need to extend coverage (9).

The ministries of Health and of Social Development and other government agencies and civil society organizations are making efforts to address the problems of accidents, suicides, and violence, using different tools: the Equality Plan for Panamanian Women 2000–2006, Law No. 4 on equal opportunities for women, the National Plan to Combat Domestic Violence and Promote Civic Coexistence (which includes the problem of street gangs), Law No. 16 on the commercial exploitation of sex and human trafficking, and the Protocol to the Convention on the Elimination of All Forms of Discrimination against Women.

An estimated 90.2% of the population has access to potable water (57.2% in indigenous communities, 85.7% in rural areas, and 96.3% in urban ones). Nationwide, 33% of the population obtains water from pipes that are not on their properties. In relation to the quality of drinking water service, 72.2% of households with residential connections receive water uninterruptedly. There are differences between poor and non-poor: in urban areas, just 56.6% of poor households and 45.4% of households in extreme poverty receive water 24 hours a day (9). In general, total annual water consumption is 408.46 hm^3/year and average per capita consumption is 444 liters a day (26).

As for access to adequate sanitation, just 54.3% of the population has sewer connections or septic tanks. In urban areas, 75.4% has access to this service (82.1% for the non-poor and 48.3% for the poor); in rural zones, 67% use pit toilets or latrines. Among the indigenous population, 61% has no sewage disposal system of any kind (9).

The waste generated in the country amounts to 1,463.53 tons a day (26). The percentage of urban housing whose solid waste is collected by the municipality is 86.8%, but 28.5% of poor urban households burn or dump their trash. In rural zones, one-fifth of households have trash collection, 56.0% of households burn their trash, 9.2% bury it, and the rest dump it wherever they can (9). The districts of Panama, Colón, and San Miguelito generate the largest amounts of trash, most of which is deposited in the sanitary landfill at Cerro Patacón. Nationally there is a shortage of sanitary landfills, which means that most waste is disposed of in dumps with little or no sanitary or environmental control. These dumps are often the source of lixiviates that contaminate surface and groundwater and attract the poor who pick through the garbage for usable items (54).

The National Civil Protection System (SINAPROC) is the government agency responsible for emergency preparedness and disaster prevention and for mitigating the consequences and providing a rapid response to victims.

As for the preparations for an influenza pandemic, since 1977, virological surveillance has detected activity by influenza viruses A (H3N2), A (H1N1), and B. This surveillance has detected new strains, some of which have been incorporated into the vaccine antigens. A national intersectoral committee has been established that has prepared a comprehensive plan to deal with an influenza pandemic.

Individual Care Services

For individual care services, MINSA has 14 health regions and, correspondingly, the CSS has the same number of regional directorates. Health care is delivered through the MINSA and CSS service networks, which are composed of provider establishments organized into different levels of complexity and treatment capacity. Panama has three levels of hierarchy and three levels of care. The hierarchical levels are the central and regulatory level (MINSA), the regional and coordination level (health regions), and the local level, which is purely operational. From the standpoint of complexity, there is the primary care level, which includes seven different types of centers classified in accordance with their treatment capability, ranging from community centers that have a traveling health promoter and community volunteers, to the so-called basic polyclinics or health centers with beds. The secondary level of care consists of six institutional subtypes, ranging from specialized polyclinics that have basic specialties, to the main regional hospitals. Last, a tertiary level includes national specialized hospitals (supraregional) and national centers with medical subspecialties. To coordinate the continuity of care by level, MINSA and the CSS created a master referral and counterreferral system (SURCO) in 2003 that is still not fully operative, which means there are no defined entry levels, and levels are duplicated inside the same institution. In 2003, MINSA and the CSS had 846 total establishments, with the following distribution: 39 hospitals, 36 polyclinics, one polycenter, 151 health centers without beds, 31 health centers with beds, 10 local primary care units (ULAPS), nine health promotion centers (CPS), 116 health subcenters, 151 health posts, and two sociosanitary facilities classified as hospitals. However, despite the large number of institutions, there is irregular distribution and integration of diagnostic and/or emergency support, with a higher concentration of resources in the main urban centers to the detriment of the rural and indigenous regions. The third level is overused owing to the shortage of MINSA second tier units.

The country has no unified network of emergency services; however, there are rules that make it compulsory for all institutions, including private ones, to provide first aid at no cost. Panama City has a unified system of ambulances administered by the CSS, which are free of charge for the general public. In the rest of the country, emergencies are the responsibility of different operating units depending on treatment capabilities, but there are no unified operational protocols for emergency management and referral.

With regard to blood supplies and diagnostic aids, there is no network but rather a scattered succession of collection and transfusion centers and a medium-complexity blood bank. The main sources of blood for transfusions in the country are not considered secure, since they continue to be replacement donors and paid donors. Voluntary donations do not amount to 3% of the total collected and do not involve more than 0.5% of the population. The situation with clinical laboratories is similar. Each hospital has one laboratory which generally lumps services together indiscriminately into a single area. The country does not have a legally established reference laboratory, although the ICGES has been acting in that capacity. A quality guarantee program began in 2006, which includes private and public sector institutions, represented in the National College of Laboratory Technicians (CONALAC).

The National Comprehensive Health Office for the Disabled has been operating since October 2004, and the National Physical Medicine and Rehabilitation Institute has been offering physiotherapy, occupational and language therapy, and medical and dental services since 1985. The CSS offers rehabilitation programs for children and adults in different hospitals and in some polyclinics. There are no precise data on social security coverage for people with disabilities, but it is estimated to be low, particularly in rehabilitation. According to SENADIS, all rehabilitation services are concentrated in the country's capital, which means there is no comprehensive rehabilitation network. The network of orthotics and prosthetics workshops and other technical aids currently consists of five small workshops, three of them private, and one that works exclusively for the CSS. They are concentrated in the capital, are not coordinated, and provide low coverage of technical aid requirements in general.

With regard to care for the indigenous population, the number of health care facilities and their distribution in the indigenous territories in 2000 pointed clearly to the lack of specialized personnel to serve this group. Most of the facilities were health posts that were managed by the community and visited by a nurse at intervals, which indicates the insecure conditions affecting these people. Comarca Kuna Yala has hospitals, health centers, and subcenters but there are not enough staff, as reflected in the percentage of medical coverage, which is the worst of all the provinces (2,701 people per physician) (40). In 2002, the population in Comarca Kuna Yala presented the following coverage for maternal and child services: prenatal check-ups, 121.8%; puerperal check-ups, 66.9%; tetanus vaccinations in women of fertile age, 50.8%; and growth and development checks in children under 5 years, 73.3%. In Comarca Ngöbe Buglé, coverage was: prenatal check-ups, 68.9%; puerperal check-ups, 74.7%; tetanus vaccinations in women of fertile age, 25.0%; and growth and development checks in children under 5 years, 62.5%. No data are available for Comarca Emberá (55).

Health Promotion

To boost community participation in health, health committees and rural water supply system management boards have been established by law. Other forms of participation have also been promoted, such as involvement by community leaders and groups and by volunteer groups such as health promoters and the so-called health guardians. However, community participation has not developed as a mechanism for social control or participation in decision-making, and continues to have a welfarist connotation. The national government has recently made commitments to allow community groups and interested sectors to participate in health programs for adolescents, older adults, diabetics, persons with hypertension, and persons with HIV, among others. During the period under study, MINSA has been preparing a National Health Promotion Plan that also envisages cooperation by the local level.

Human Resources

To operate the network of public services on the national level, the health system has 4,321 physicians (13.63 physicians per 10,000 population), 3,665 nurses (11.55 nurses per 10,000 population), and 923 dentists (2.91 professionals per 10,000 population) however, the number of resources per 10,000 population is up to 10 times lower in the indigenous territories than in the rest of the country (Comarca Ngöbe Buglé 0.62 physicians per 10,000 population, and province of Panama, 17.96 physicians per 10,000 population). This situation continues despite financial incentives (bonus of 40% of the base salary) to get professionals to move to these areas. Almost two-thirds (61.8%) of children who had problems with diarrhea and respiratory infections were treated by competent personnel (in 57.3% of the cases by a physician, 2.7% by a nurse or nursing assistant, and 1.8% by a health promoter). The figure ranges from 69.8% in urban areas (69.4% by a physician and 0.4% by a nurse) to 35% in indigenous areas (14.5% by a physician, 12.5% by a nurse, and 7.7% by a health promoter). Two-thirds (65.3%) of indigenous children with respiratory problems, diarrhea, or both were not taken to a health facility and were treated by family members (58%) or by a traditional indigenous doctor or healer (4.7%). From the standpoint of social service, just over half of poor children (52%) who suffered from diarrhea or respiratory infections were treated by appropriate personnel in contrast to 75% of non-poor children. Most children who received care from competent personnel were treated in public health institutions (82%) and more than half of them (53%) came from poor families. On the other hand, 87% of the non-poor were treated in private institutions (9). As for care during delivery, 95.4% were assisted by trained personnel (88.9% of the time by a physician), and 95.1% were assisted in health care institutions. There are significant differences in assistance during delivery between urban and indigenous zones: in Comarca Ngöbe Buglé, for example, out of a total of 904 reported births, 10.2% were attended by qualified personnel, and of them just 38.0% were attended by a physician.

At the end of 2005, certification of technical and professional health workers began with the regulations to Law 43 of 2004, which created councils and interagency certification and recertification procedures for health professionals. These processes were interrupted in mid-2006 when MINSA repealed the regulations through Executive Decree 329, so that at present the country has no mechanisms for certification or recertification of its technical and/or professional staff. An administrative career path is being implemented, but does not yet cover 100% of sector employees and lacks transparent mechanisms for performance evaluation.

Health Supplies

As for the regulation, sale, and distribution of complementary supplies such as medications and medical-surgical equipment and materials, Law 1 of 2003 and Law 54 of 2005, which regulate supplies and medications, respectively, have been promulgated and are being implemented. Through this legislation, the country has a list of essential medications and mechanisms for updating it; protocols for imports and a single registration process for medications and for medical-surgical equipment; clear rules on bioequivalency and the interchangeability of generic medicines; and an early system of post-marketing technosurveillance and pharmacosurveillance.

Research and Technological Development in Health

The area of health research is the responsibility of the Gorgas Memorial Institute for Health Studies (ICGES). The overlapping of functions leads to scattering of resources and limited coordination among the entities that work in this area. In 2000, the Ministry of Health prepared guidelines and policies in the fields of ethics and bioethics, and in 2005 regulations were introduced on conducting research on human subjects.

Health Sector Expenditures and Financing

Although there are no systematic records of expenditures in the health sector and only general estimates are available, there is a consensus that the Panamanian government spends close to US$ 363 per person a year on health-related services. All the resources in the public system are used to subsidize the supply of health services through the public network. In the public system, close to 70% of funds are used to pay personnel and close to 2% for maintenance and investments in infrastructure, which means that less than 30% is used to purchase and provide medications and other supplies. According to data provided by the National Directorate of Welfare Services, the distribution of spending in the CSS is similar. There are no official figures on spending on research, but it is estimated to account for 0.5% of the total.

The funds come from the Ministry of Economic Affairs and Finance, from employees and employers in the case of the CSS, from out-of-pocket spending, and to a lesser extent, from international cooperation. With regard to the origin and allocation of funds, Panama spent over US$ 1.1 billion, or 8.4% of its GDP, which is one of the highest figures in the region. It is estimated that US$ 360 million (31%) came from direct contributions by users, either in the form of out-of-pocket payments for care or for medications, prostheses, etc. or as payments to private health insurers. The remainder (close to US$ 794 million) was financed to similar extents by the Social Security System (US$ 363 million) and the Ministry of Health (US$ 431 million). Panama does not receive more than 1% in nonreimbursable cooperation. The Office of the Comptroller General is responsible for scrutinizing the use of resources, which is done prior to their execution.

ENV 2003 showed that on average, national household spending on health for children under 5 in the month before the survey was US$ 9.50 (US$ 11.60 in urban areas, US$ 6.90 in rural ones); health spending by level of poverty indicates that the non-poor spent US$ 14.10, while the poor spent US$ 6.80 (extreme poor US$ 6.50).

More than three-quarters of the money spent was used to buy medications and to defray the cost of doctors' visits and laboratory tests (53.9%, 23.0%, and 11.0%, respectively). The cost levels maintain a fairly homogenous structure in the different geographic areas, with the exception of the indigenous area, where a larger proportion of spending went to pay for doctors' visits (38%), medications (32%), and laboratory tests (25%). A cost analysis by poverty level shows that people who live in extreme poverty spend more on health services: 44.0% (25.1% for doctors' visits, 17.5% for laboratory tests, and 1.4% for consultations with healers), while the non-poor spent 30.5% (24.1% for doctors' visits, 6% for laboratory tests, and 0.4% for consultations with healers). Medications account for 41.2% of spending by the non-poor and 59.6% by the poor (9).

The suprarcgional hospitals and specialized national institutes are administered as foundations (*patronatos*) chaired by the Minister of Health or his delegate, with autonomy to legislate and control the entity, and whose legal representative is a manager appointed by the minister of health and paid by the public treasury to run the institution.

Another control mechanism recently incorporated by MINSA is the so-called management agreements that contain commitments (prior to receiving the budget) made by the 14 health regions and the four national hospitals to attain specific goals. This accountability tool is in its second year and facing its first evaluation; it is therefore too early to discuss the results.

Technical Cooperation and External Financing

Arranging and negotiating international cooperation is the responsibility of the Ministry of Economic Affairs and Finance, in close cooperation with the Ministry of External Relations and the International Cooperation Coordination Office of the Office of the President. Also, each ministry has a liaison office for international cooperation. Significant funding comes from reimbursable loans from bilateral and multilateral banks, such as those made for the channeling and treatment of liquid waste in neighborhoods that still dump that sewage into Panama Bay (US$ 50 million) and the Multiphase Program for the Institutional Transformation of the Health Sector (US$ 50 million), that the Ministry of Health participates in. The latter program has three subcomponents: to strengthen MINSA's role as lead agency (US$ 5.8 million); to extend coverage to areas that are not served, by contracting external organizations and establishing a comprehensive health services plan, PAISS (US$ 28 million); and to transform health services to boost their productivity (US$ 10 million).

The United Nations system agencies have a strong presence in response to the incentive plans established by the Government. Currently, the Pan American Health Organization/World Health Organization, United Nations Development Program, United Nations Children's Fund, United Nations Educational, Scientific and Cultural Organization, United Nations High Commission for Refugees, the World Food Program, the United Nations Joint Program on HIV/AIDS, and the United Nations Organization for Food and Agriculture have offices and accredited representatives in the country, who participate actively in implementing the Government's plan, particularly in activities related to the Millennium Development Goals, the exercise of individual freedoms, and access to opportunities.

References

1. Panama, Contraloría General de la República, Dirección de Estadística y Censo. Panamá en cifras: años 2000–2004. Panama City; 2005.

2. World Bank. World development indicators 2005. Washington, DC: International Bank for Reconstruction and Development/World Bank; 2005.

3. Panama, Ministerio de Economía y Finanzas. Informe económico anual, 2005. Panama City; 2006.

4. Panama, Ministerio de Economía y Finanzas, Dirección de Análisis y Políticas Económicas. Estadísticas económicas, 2005. Panama City; 2006.

5. Gandásegui M. Democracia y movimientos sociales en Panamá en el centenario de la República. Revista Tareas. 2003; 115:5–30.

6. Brown H. Hacia la consolidación del sistema de partidos políticos panameños. Revista Tareas. 2002; 111:5–26.

7. Gandásegui M. La transferencia del Canal de Panamá. Revista Tareas. 2000; 105:5–34.

8. Pérez O; Gandásegui M, Seligson M, editores. La cultura política de la democracia en Panamá, 2004. Percepciones de la población en torno al sistema político. Nashville, Tenn.: Vanderbilt University; 2004.

9. Panama, Ministerio de Economía y Finanzas, Dirección de Políticas Sociales. Pobreza y desigualdad en Panamá. La equidad: un reto impostergable. Panama City; 2006.

10. United Nations Development Program. Visión nacional 2020. Panama City; 1999.

11. International Labor Organization. Programa InFocus sobre fortalecimiento del diálogo social. Diálogo social en Panamá: el camino hacia la democracia. Geneva; 2002.

12. Patria Nueva. Programa de gobierno 2004–2009. Panama City; 2004.

13. Panama, Presidencia de la República. Visión estratégica de desarrollo económico y de empleo hacia el 2009. Panama City; 2005.

14. Panama, Ministerio de la Presidencia, Secretaría de Metas Presidenciales. Objetivos y metas del gobierno de Patria Nueva 2005–2009. Panama City; 2005.

15. Panama, Contraloría General de la República, Dirección de Estadística y Censo. Encuesta de Hogares 2005. Cifras definitivas. Panama City; 2005.

16. Panama, Ministerio de Economía y Finanzas. Canasta básica, diciembre 2005–enero 2006. Panama City; 2006.

17. Panama, Ministerio de Economía y Finanzas, Dirección de Políticas Sociales. La pobreza en Panamá. Encuesta de Niveles de Vida, 2003. Principales resultados (edición revisada). Panama City; 2005.

18. Panama, Ministerio de Economía y Finanzas, Dirección de Políticas Sociales. Encuesta de Niveles de Vida, 1997. Panama City; 2003.

19. Inter-American Development Bank. Pobreza y desigualdad a nivel de áreas menores en Panamá. Serie de estudios económicos y sectoriales. Washington, DC; 2005.

20. United Nations Development Program. Human development report 2005. International cooperation at a crossroads: aid, trade, and security in an unequal world. New York: UNDP; 2005.

21. United Nations Development Program. National report on human development: Panama 2002. Panama City; 2002.

22. United Nations Development Program. National report on human development: Panama: 2004. Panama City; 2004.

23. United Nations Development Fund for Women; United Nations Development Program; Universidad de Panamá, Facultad de Economía. Economía y género en Panamá: visibilizando la participación de las mujeres. Panama City; 2005.

24. Panama, Ministerio de Economía y Finanzas, Dirección de Políticas Sociales. Pobreza y desigualdad en Panamá. La equidad: un reto impostergable. Panama City; 2006.

25. Panama, Ministerio de Economía y Finanzas, Dirección de Políticas Sociales. Situación nutricional, patrón de consumo a alimentos de la población panameña. Segunda Encuesta de Niveles de Vida 2003. Panama City; 2006.

26. Panama, Autoridad Nacional del Ambiente. Informe del estado del ambiente. GEO Panamá 2004. Panama City; 2004.

27. Pan American Health Organization/World Health Organization. Plaguicidas en el Istmo Centroamericano (PLAGSALUD). Situación epidemiológica de las intoxicaciones por plaguicidas en el istmo centroamericano. San José: OPS/OMS; 2002.

28. Panama, Autoridad Nacional del Ambiente. Informe final de la cobertura boscosa y uso del suelo de la República de Panamá, 1992–2000. Panama City; 2003.

29. Panama, Contraloría General de la República, Dirección de Estadística y Censo. Situación demográfica. Estimaciones y proyecciones de la población total del país: años 1950–2050. Boletín Nº 7. Panama City; 2002.

30. Economic Commission for Latin America and the Caribbean. Statistical yearbook for Latin America and the Caribbean, 2004. Official document LC/G.2264-P/B. Santiago de Chile; 2005.

31. Economic Commission for Latin America and the Caribbean, Latin America and the Caribbean Demographic Center. Los pueblos indígenas en Panamá: diagnóstico sociodemográfico a partir del censo del 2000. Santiago de Chile; 2005.

32. Panama, Contraloría General de la República, Dirección de Estadística y Censo. Estimaciones y proyecciones de la población total en la República de Panamá, por provincia y comarca indígena, según sexo y edad: período 1990–2030. Boletín N° 8. Panama City; 2005.

33. Panama, Contraloría General de la República, Dirección de Estadística y Censo. Estadística panameña: situación demográfica. Estadísticas vitales: volumen III. Defunciones, año 2004. Panama City; 2005.

34. Panama, Contraloría General de la República, Dirección de Estadística y Censo. Estadística panameña. Estadísticas vitales: volumen II. Nacimientos vivos y defunciones fetales, año 2004. Panama City; 2005.

35. Panama, Ministerio de Salud. Situación de salud de Panamá. Documento marco. Panama City; 2005.

36. Panama, Ministerio de Salud, Jefatura Nacional de Registros Médicos y Estadísticas de Salud. Reporte del Sistema de Información Perinatal (SIP). MINSA; julio 2006.

37. Panama, Gabinete Social. Política nacional a favor de las personas mayores en Panamá. Edificar una sociedad para todas las edades. Panama City; 2004.

38. Panama, Contraloría General de la República, Dirección de Estadística y Censo. Situación social. Seguridad social 2003. Panama City; 2004.

39. Panama, Ministerio de Salud; Pan American Health Organization/World Health Organization. Discapacidad en Panamá. Panama City; 2005.

40. World Bank. Perfil de los pueblos indígenas de Panamá. Panama City; 2002.

41. Panama, Contraloría General de la República, Dirección de Estadística y Censo. Informes metodológicos y resultados de los censos de: 1911, 1920 a 2000.

42. Panama, Contraloría General de la República, Dirección de Estadística y Censo. Censos 1990 y 2000. Resultados finales, total país. Panama City; 2001.

43. World Bank, Latin American and the Caribbean Regional Office. Poverty in indigenous populations in Panama: a study using LSMS Data. LCSHD paper series. Washington, DC; 2000.

44. Pan American Health Organization/World Health Organization; Panama, Ministerio de Salud. Análisis del contexto general de la región de Darién y su situación de salud. Panama City; 2004.

45. United Nations Population Fund. Desafíos de Panamá en materia de población y desarrollo, salud sexual y reproductiva y equidad de género. 2005.

46. Asociación Viviendo Positivamente. Proyecto Acción sida en Centroamérica (PASCA). Sondeo de opinión de la atención integral en salud y los derechos humanos de las personas viviendo con VIH/SIDA. Panama City; 2006.

47. Panama, Contraloría General de la República, Dirección de Estadística y Censo. Estadísticas vitales. Cifras preliminares. Año 2005. Panama City; 2006.

48. Panama, Contraloría General de la República, Dirección de Estadística y Censo. Estadística panameña: situación política, administrativa y justicia. Estadística de detenciones y penitenciarias. Año 2003. Panama City; 2004.

49. Panama, Contraloría General de la República, Dirección de Estadística y Censo. Estadística panameña. Accidentes de tránsito. Año 2003. Panama City; 2004.

50. Panama, Ministerio de Salud, Dirección Nacional de Políticas de Salud, Departamento de Análisis de Situación y Tendencias de Salud. Estadísticas de salud, 2004. Panama City; 2005.

51. Pan American Health Organization/World Health Organization. Informe sobre el sistema de salud en Panamá, 2004. Panama City; 2006.

52. Panama, Ministerio de Salud. Encuesta Mundial de Consumo de Tabaco en Jóvenes. Panama City; 2002.

53. Panama, Ministerio de Salud, Dirección Nacional de Políticas del Sector Salud. Estudio de vigilancia del humo ambiental de tabaco. Panama City; 2004.

54. Organización Panamericana de la Salud. Evaluación 2000 de los residuos sólidos. OPS; 2003.

55. Panama, Ministerio de Salud; Organización Panamericana de la Salud/Organización Mundial de la Salud. Indicadores básicos por provincias y comarcas indígenas. Panama City; 2004.

PARAGUAY

Bolivia

Alto
Paraguay

Boquerón

1 Cordillera
2 Caaguazú
3 Alto Paraná
4 Central
5 Guairá

Brazil

Amambay

Concepción

Presidente Hayes

San
Pedro

Canindeyú

Asunción

6 Paraguarí
7 Caazapá
8 Ñeembucú
9 Misiones
10 Itapúa

Argentina

1

2

4

3

5

6

7

8

9

10

0   50   100 Miles

araguay has a total land area of 406,752 km² and borders Argentina, Bolivia, and Brazil. The Paraguay River divides the country into two clearly differentiated natural regions: the western side, or Chaco, with three departments, and the eastern region which, divided into 14 departments, includes the capital (Asunción) and the main cities and population centers, roads, and networks of basic services.

GENERAL CONTEXT AND HEALTH DETERMINANTS

Social, Political, and Economic Determinants

After 35 years of dictatorship, the country has seen almost two decades of incipient democracy, but has not achieved the rule of law. Presidential and parliamentary elections were held in 2003; they were considered democratic by the international observers. In the 2002 municipal elections, 44.6% of the poorest population quintile voted, as compared to 57.9% of the wealthiest quintile. Of those who went to the polls, 39.3% of individuals from the poorest quintile went on their own initiative, as compared to 87.6% of the wealthiest (1). A high proportion of poor people are taken to the polls by political workers. According to the report by Transparencia Paraguay (2), the civil service is deficient in transparency, integrity, and efficiency, despite significant attempts at improvement.

Decentralization has not been effectively implemented. The principal problems observed in terms of decentralization and local government are: the lack of political agreement about the meaning and implications of decentralization, limited autonomy and capacity for decision making and management on the part of the municipalities, and lack of clarity regarding the governments' territorial authorities.

There are significant deficiencies in terms of the protection of individual rights and the administration of justice. In the country's principal prison, 79.8% of the inmates have not yet been sentenced (3). Certain factors weaken the judicial and political system, for example: complaints of police abuse, inefficiency of the security system, "legal flexibility" by means of decrees and regulations that leave laws partially effective, lack of clarity about the order of precedence of laws, and uncertainty and unpredictability of legal rulings. There are limitations on the constitutional and legal guarantee of ownership and uncertainty about property rights due to the absence of a consistent, reliable registration system (3). There is also a perception of corruption on the part of the system's operators and dysfunctions in the stability of legal norms and judicial decisions.

A deep economic recession began in 1997. At the end of 2003 the per capita GDP was 30.0% below that of 1991. In 2002 and 2003, the domestic currency lost 54.0% of its value (4), and inflation rose to 14.6% in 2002 after several years of single-digit variations; in 2003, an additional 9.3% increase (5) in the overall price level further decreased the citizens' buying power. The economic crisis, marked by stagnation of GDP growth rates, along with persistent demographic growth, set the stage for increased unemployment and underemployment, and structural poverty. Expansion of social spending is limited by the decline of productivity, tax evasion, and the regressive tax structure.

The country has a significant social deficit with respect to the Millennium Development Goals (MDGs) and discouraging prospects for meeting its goals. Poverty levels rose from 30.3% in 1995 to 33.7% in 1999 and 41.4% in 2003, and levels of extreme poverty or indigence rose from 13.9% to 15.5% and to 20.1%, respectively. In 2003, 2,346,000 people were considered poor and half of those were considered indigent (6).

The highest proportion of poverty continues to be found in the countryside: 43.4% as compared to 39.8% in urban areas. However, as a result of ongoing urban development, in 2003 some 1,269,000 poor people were located in the cities as compared to 1,077,000 in the countryside. Growing poverty brings women and children to the labor market; they add the hours of paid work to the hours of their domestic work. Women have fewer job opportunities and lower income levels, and the differences between poor women and women who are not poor become increasingly apparent. Unemployment among poor women is twice that of unemployment among women who are not poor; more than 20.0% of women who are not poor have access to higher levels of education, as compared to just 3.0% of poor women (6). Women owned just 7.4% of the lots enumerated in the 2001 Census of Communities (7).

Impoverishment of children, adolescents, and indigenous populations is noted. Half of the population under 18 years old is poor, as compared to 41.4% of the total population (8). Poverty leads to child labor, with consequent negative effects for the present and for overcoming poverty in the future (9). Unemployment rates are higher among young people than among adults; their access to land in the rural sector is increasingly limited (6). In the indigenous population, a sign of the extreme poverty is the lack of land ownership (45% do not own land), and the majority live in huts without basic services. Just 3% of the indigenous population has access to drinking water, 1.1% to basic sanitation, and 9.7% to electricity (10).

The Paraguayan government has three initiatives for addressing poverty;[1] all three include the perspective of gender and excluded groups such as the indigenous populations, but significant progress has not been made in their implementation.

The gross preschool enrollment jumped from 27% in 1990 to 81% in 2001; the gross enrollment in the first and second cycles of basic education remained around 100%, and the gross enrollment in the third cycle increased from 27% to 53%. The gross enrollment rate for secondary education was 22% in 1990 and 44% in 2001 (11). The national illiteracy rate was 9.7% in 1992 and 7.1% in 2002, but the principal gap is found between the national figure and the figure for the indigenous population, which has an illiteracy rate of 51%. The average years of schooling for the population 15 years old and older were 7.1 in 2002, with no difference between the sexes, slightly higher than the average for 1992 (6.4 years); the indigenous peoples attend school for an average of just 2.2 years. There continues to be a marked difference in years of schooling between urban and rural areas, albeit with a decrease of the gap: from 8.1 to 8.4 years, respectively, in the censuses of 1992 and 2002 for the urban area and 4.5 and 5.3 years, respectively, for the rural area (10, 12).

Despite the implementation of educational reform with a gender perspective, there are teaching practices and formal and informal regulatory frameworks at the institutions that reinforce the traditional roles assigned to females and males. The higher educational level among women has not had positive effects on the labor market or on women's participation in politics (from 5.5% in the Chamber of Senators and 4.2% in the Chamber of Deputies in 1989 to 11% and 10%, respectively, in 2005). In social/labor spheres, just 42% of working age women are in the job market, as opposed to 75% of men, with a growing trend toward unpaid work (6).

With regard to environmental sustainability, there is continual loss and degradation of the ecosystems as a result of the competent entities' low institutional capacity, non-compliance with the law, institutional weakness of the Department of the Environment (SEAM), an agrarian policy that does not focus on sustainability, lack of planning for the rational use of water resources, little decentralization of environmental management, meager budget, and deficient management of the system of protected areas in a context of unplanned expansion and uncontrolled extraction of natural resources. Citizens have limited knowledge about their rights, in particular about collective environmental rights.

In 2004, Law No. 2,524 "on prohibition, in the eastern region, of transformation and conversion of land areas with forest coverage" became effective. In 2005, the National Environmental Plan (PAN) of Paraguay was approved. Also, the 2004–2009 National Strategy and Action Plan for Preservation of Paraguay's Biodiversity was passed (6).

Paraguay has part of one of the world's largest aquifers and two of Latin America's biggest rivers, but geographic, cultural, and socioeconomic factors make the country vulnerable to drought, floods, tornados, and man-made disasters. Floods are due mainly to periods of rising of the Paraguay River and its tributaries, affecting the populations in poor districts or shantytowns on the river banks. In Chaco, drought is a chronic disaster.

Demographics, Mortality, and Morbidity

The annual average growth rate was 2.2% between 1992 and 2002; the total population in 2002 was 5,163,198 (12), with a significant proportion living in rural areas (43.3%), 49.6% women, and a sex ratio of 101.7 (94.4 in urban areas and 112.1 in rural areas). As Table 1 shows, the age structure shows a young population: those under 15 years old represent 37.1%, a situation that is higher in rural areas (41.3%) than in the urban areas (33.9%). The population 65 years old and older represents 4.9% of the total population.

The indigenous population totaled 89,169 in 2002 (10), representing 1.7% of the country's total population (but 31% of the population of Chaco); 90.1% lived in rural areas. Some 20 ethnic groups in five linguistic families were identified, the most numerous being the Guaraní, with six ethnic groups and a 3.7% growth rate (much higher than that of the total population). Because of the high fertility rate, the structure of the indigenous population is younger than that of the total population, with a slight predominance of males (51.7%), which is more accentuated in certain ethnic groups. Some 47.1% of the indigenous population is under 15 years old and just 2.6% is 65 years old and older.

Population density is low, with a very unequal distribution: 12.7 inhabitants/km^2 nationwide, 31.5 inhabitants/km^2 in the eastern region, and 0.5 inhabitants/km^2 in Chaco, a region which, despite representing 60% of the country's land area, has just 2.6% of the total population. The capital, Asunción, and the Central Department have 36.3% of the population in less than 1% of the territory (for a density of 4,377 inhabitants/km^2 in the capital and 552.9 inhabitants/km^2 in the Central Department).

Urban growth was a consequence of significant trends in migration from small urban centers outside the metropolitan Asunción area and from rural areas, with women being the principal demographic component of both the migrations and urban resi-

TABLE 1. Population distribution, by age group and sex, Paraguay, 2007.

Age group	Total	%	Women	%	Men	%
Under 1	148,519	2.4	72,752	2.4	72,767	2.5
1–4	584,687	9.6	286,884	9.5	297,803	9.6
Under 5	**733,206**	**12.0**	**359,836**	**11.9**	**373,570**	**12.1**
5–9	714,131	11.7	350,716	11.6	363,415	11.8
10–14	690,550	11.3	339,363	11.2	351,187	11.4
15–19	657,891	10.8	323,976	10.7	333,915	10.8
10–19	**1,348,441**	**22.0**	**663,339**	**21.0**	**685,105**	**22.1**
20–59	2,887,303	47.2	1,425,870	47.1	1,461,434	47.2
60+	436,560	7.1	226,037	7.5	210,523	6.8
Total	6,119,642	100	3,025,598	100	3,094,044	100

Source: Paraguay, Ministerio de Salud Pública y Bienestar Social, Departmento de Bioestadísticas. Estimates according to data from the Bureau of the Census, Statistics, and Surveys (DGEEC).

TABLE 2. Demographic indicators by five-year periods, Paraguay, 1995–2015.

		1995–2000	2000–2005	2005–2010	2010–2015
Crude birth rate (per 1,000 population)	Total	29.3	26.9	24.8	22.78
	Urban	…	25.1	22.9	…
	Rural	…	29.3	27.3	…
Crude mortality rate (per 1,000 population)	Total	6	5.7	5.6	5.53
Infant mortality rate (per 1,000 live births)	Total	39.2	35.5	32.0	28.80
Life expectancy at birth (in years)	Total	69.4	70.8	71.8	72.76
	Men	67.2	68.7	69.7	70.70
	Women	71.7	72.9	73.9	74.92
Global fertility rate (children per woman)	Total	3.9	3.5	3.1	2.76
	Urban	…	2.9	2.6	…
	Rural	…	4.5	3.9	…

Source: Paraguay, Dirección General de Estadísticas, Encuestas y Censos. Data and estimates.

dence (100 women to 94 men). The 1997–2002 period saw a reduction in the intensity of internal migration in relation to 1987–1992. The foreign population as part of the total has declined: 4.6% in 1992 and 3.4% in 2002, with 47.1% from Brazil, 36.5% from Argentina, and 16.4% from other countries. The Brazilian migration is predominantly rural and the Argentine migration is predominantly urban.

The total fertility rate fell 22% in urban areas and 34% in rural areas in the 1995–1998 and 2001–2004 periods (*13*). In the same periods, the fertility rate of adolescents 15–19 years old fell 26%, from 90 to 67 births per 1,000 women. The most significant decline was observed in women 20–29 years old, which strongly affects the total fertility rate, because the majority of births occur in this group. The specific rate for women 20–24 years old dropped from 206 to 150 births per 1,000 women and from 204 to 142 births per 1,000 for women 25–29 years old (*13*). Indigenous women have an average of 6.3 children, much higher than the national average (*10*). Other general demographic information is found in Table 2.

The most recent mortality data available are for 2003 (*14*). It is estimated that, between 2001 and 2003, deaths were underreported by approximately 40%. Of the deaths reported (18,400 in 2001, 18,934 in 2002, and 19,779 in 2003), 50% occurred while under medical care in 2001 and 2002 and 53% in 2003. Ill-defined causes ranged from 18.1% to 21.4% in the same years. Among the deaths while under medical care, this percentage ranged from 3.0 to 4.5. The 10 leading causes of death for the years 2001 to 2003 are shown in Table 3.

Analyzing the deaths while under medical care and with defined cause, and using the 6/67 list, Figure 1 shows the proportional distribution of the six major groups of causes for 2003 and Figure 2 shows the urban/rural differences and differences by sex.

HEALTH OF POPULATION GROUPS

There are many limitations in Paraguay's health data. Most of the data come from the Ministry of Public Health and Social Welfare, and many of the data at other institutions in the sector are not reported or the Ministry does not have knowledge of them. Morbidity data from the services (outpatient consultation, hospitalization) are characterized by low coverage, poor quality, low

TABLE 3. Ten leading causes of death, Paraguay, cumulative 2001–2003.

	TOTAL		
Total deaths	57,113		
Total deaths with defined causes	45,554		
% deaths with defined causes	79.8		
Total population	16,700,718		
Causes	Total	%	Rate per 100,000
Cerebrovascular disease	4,837	10.6	29
Ischemic heart disease	3,660	8	21.9
Diabetes mellitus	3,340	7.3	20
Certain disorders originating in the perinatal period	2,539	5.6	15.2
Influenza and pneumonia	2,186	4.8	13.1
Assaults (homicides)	2,064	4.5	12.4
Cardiac insufficiency	1,950	4.3	11.7
Land transport accidents	1,367	3	8.2
Hypertensive disease	1,058	2.3	6.3
Malignant neoplasm of the uterus	1,019	2.2	6.1
Other	21,534	47.3	128.9
Total	45,554	100	272.8
	MEN		
Total deaths	31,773		
Total deaths with defined causes	25,726		
% deaths with defined causes	81.0		
Total male population	8,450,014		
Causes	Total	%	Rate per 100,000
Cerebrovascular disease	2,312	9	27.4
Ischemic heart disease	2,164	8.4	25.6
Assaults (homicides)	1,890	7.3	22.4
Certain disorders originating in the perinatal period	1,421	5.5	16.8
Diabetes mellitus	1,400	5.4	16.6
Influenza and pneumonia	1,177	4.6	13.9
Land transport accidents	1,085	4.2	12.8
Cardiac insufficiency	1,014	3.9	12
Neoplasm of the trachea, bronchial tubes, and lungs	726	2.8	8.6
Malignant neoplasm of the prostate	607	2.4	7.2
Other	11,930	46.4	141.2
Total	25,726	100	304.4
	WOMEN		
Total deaths	25,335		
Total deaths with defined causes	19,823		
% deaths with defined causes	78.2		
Total female population	8,250,704		
Causes	Total	%	Rate per 100,000
Cerebrovascular disease	2,524	12.7	30.6
Diabetes mellitus	1,940	9.8	23.5
Ischemic heart disease	1,496	7.5	18.1
Certain disorders originating in the perinatal period	1,116	5.6	13.5
Malignant neoplasm of the uterus	1,019	5.1	12.4
Influenza and pneumonia	1,009	5.1	12.2
Cardiac insufficiency	936	4.7	11.3
Malignant neoplasm of the breast	569	2.9	6.9
Hypertensive disease	563	2.8	6.8
Conditions of pregnancy, birth, and puerperium	447	2.3	5.4
Other	8,204	41.4	99.4
Total	19,823	100	240.3

Sources: Paraguay, Ministerio de Salud Pública y Bienestar Social, Dirección General de Planificación y Evaluación, Departamento de Bioestadística. Pan American Health Organization. List of Causes.

FIGURE 1. Proportional distribution of reported deaths while under medical care, with defined causes, according to the six major groups of causes, Paraguay, 2003.

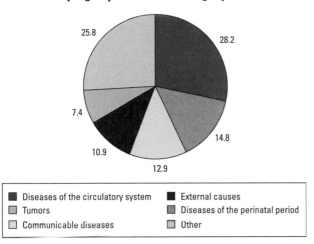

25.8

28.2

7.4

14.8

10.9

12.9

- ■ Diseases of the circulatory system
- ■ External causes
- ▤ Tumors
- ▤ Diseases of the perinatal period
- ☐ Communicable diseases
- ☐ Other

Source: Paraguay, Ministerio de Salud Pública y Bienestar Social, Departamento de Bioestadísticas.

availability, and very low reliability. Moreover, the data available on the programs vary according to their service coverage and their capacity to suspect, diagnose, and report. Mortality data suffer from the difficulties mentioned above, and are particularly deficient for infant deaths, which are about 70% underreported and with respect to which the certification is of poor quality. There are also difficulties with the use of denominators, such as in the analysis of infant or maternal mortality, given the underreporting of births. Consequently, information for this age group must be viewed with caution.

Children under 5 Years Old

For 2003, a total of 151,281 births per year were estimated; of these, 86,739 live births were reported, with 43% underreporting (high even compared with 1992, when the estimate was 49.4%).

MDG 4 (reduce mortality in children under 5 years old by two thirds before 2015) is significantly behind schedule, and progress cannot be adequately measured (*15*). Reported infant mortality

FIGURE 2. Proportional distribution of reported deaths, by area and sex, Paraguay, 2003.

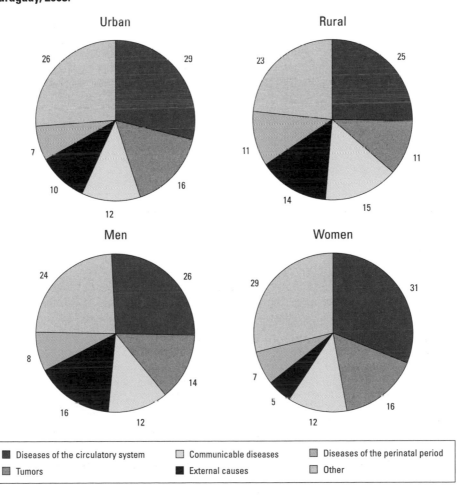

Urban

26   29

7

10   16

12

Rural

23   25

11   11

14   15

Men

24   26

8

16   14

12

Women

29   31

7

5   16

12

- ■ Diseases of the circulatory system
- ☐ Communicable diseases
- ▤ Diseases of the perinatal period
- ▤ Tumors
- ■ External causes
- ☐ Other

FIGURE 3. Trends in estimated infant mortality rates by five-year periods, Paraguay, 1990–2015, and reported infant mortality rates from 1990–2003.

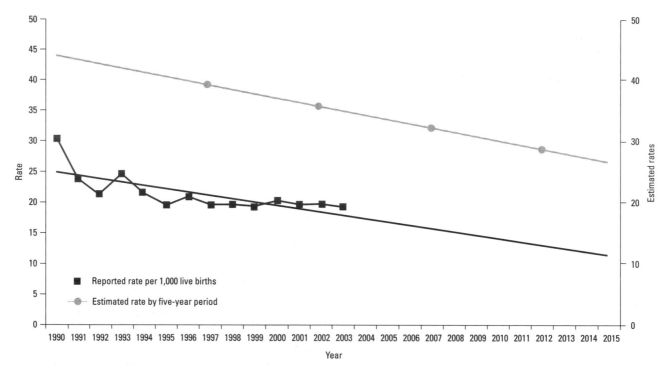

Sources: Estimates from Paraguay, Secretaría Técnica de Planificación, Dirección General de Estadísticas, Encuestas y Censos.
Reported infant deaths and certified live births from Paraguay, Ministerio de Salud Pública y Bienestar Social, Departmento de Bioestadística.

has not changed significantly since 1991, remaining around 20 per 1,000. Estimated infant mortality based on the national censuses shows a rate of decline of just 10% per five-year period, which makes achieving, or at least approaching, the goal impossible, as Figure 3 shows.

For infant deaths reported between 1999 and 2003, 60% occurred in the neonatal period and, of these, 38.5% were due to birth injuries; of the deaths that occurred in the post-neonatal period, 16.2% were due to pneumonia and influenza, and 15.8% to diarrhea.

In the population 1–4 years old, in 2003, the leading causes of morbidity were mild respiratory infections, diarrhea without dehydration, moderate respiratory infections, anemia, and parasitosis (14). Reported mortality in the population 1–4 years old dropped from 78.4 per 100,000 in 1998 to 67.4 per 100,000 in 2003. In this population, the principal causes of death while under medical care and with defined cause were communicable diseases (48%), especially pneumonia, diarrhea, septicemia, and external causes (12.4%) (14).

Children 5 to 9 Years Old

The most common causes of morbidity in this group were mild respiratory infections, parasitosis, anemia, and trauma from

external causes. The mortality rate reported in the population 5–9 years old for 2003 was 24.2 per 100,000. Some 32.7% of those reported deaths were from infectious diseases (acute respiratory infections and septicemia), and 29.1% were from external causes (accidents) (14).

Adolescents 10–14 and 15–19 Years Old

The illiterate adolescent population numbers 42,694 (4.2% are 10–14 years old and 2.6% are 15–19 years old). Adolescents from homes above the poverty line have, on average, two more years of schooling than those who come from poor homes, and 55% of the adolescent population is in school. Entry to the tertiary level is the most difficult time for remaining in the educational system: the poorest of the adolescent population barely finishes basic education, while those with more resources are assured of moving on to higher education (12).

Paraguayan women begin childbearing at a young age. Some 10.9% of adolescents 15–19 years old said they had had one or more pregnancies. Of adolescents 15–19 years old, 36% had had sexual relations. One of every three women who reported sexual experience had her first relations before the age of 16. With regard to the use of contraceptives, of all women with sexual experience, 56.3% used contraceptives the first time. Among women 15–24

FIGURE 4. Reported maternal mortality rate, Paraguay, 1990–2003, and trend to 2015.

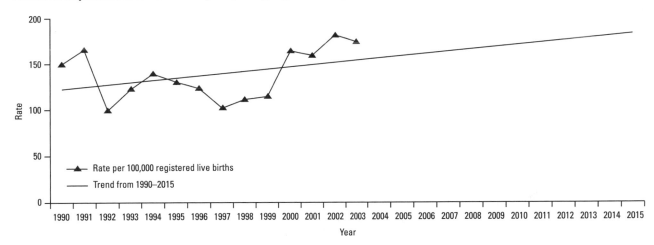

Source: Paraguay, Ministerio de Salud Pública y Bienestar Social, Dirección General de Planificación y Evaluación, Departamento de Bioestadística.

years old, 39.5% used contraceptives in their first marital experience and 57.6% used them in their first premarital experience (61.6% for urban women and 47% in rural areas). Of women with 12 or more years of education, 66.6% use contraceptives the first time, as compared to 38.4% of women with no education or just a fifth-grade education (*13*).

In a study of a population of students 12–18 years old, 66% had already consumed alcohol. The second most used drug among Paraguayan students is the cigarette; the average starting age is 14 for females and 13.8 for males. For marijuana, the average starting age is 15 (*16*). According to the Global Youth Tobacco Survey, 36.8% of youths 13–15 years old in Asunción smoked, 33.6% in Alto Paraná and Itapúa, 30.0% in Amambay and Caaguazú, and 26.0% in the Central Department. Prevalence is higher than in the general population and there are no significant differences between the sexes: adolescent girls smoke as much as boys (*17*).

The specific mortality rate by age was 32 per 100,000 for the population 10–14 years old and 74 per 100,000 for the population 15–19 years old in 2003. In the former group, 57.6% of the reported deaths occurred while under medical care and had a defined cause. Of these, 41.5% were from external causes (78% in males; 59% from accidents; 18% from suicide) and 18.6% from communicable diseases (septicemia and acute respiratory infections). For those 15–19 years old, in 50% of the deaths while under medical care and with a defined cause, 53.5% were from external causes (77.2% in males; 50% from accidents; 10.5% from suicides) and 11% from communicable diseases (*14*).

Adults 20–59 Years Old

The maternal mortality rate reported in Paraguay in 1999 was 114.4 per 100,000 live births, with a 23.8% reduction in relation to 1990, 20% being adolescents. Surveillance of maternal deaths was initiated in 2000 and, given the better record keeping, the

rates rose, to 174.1 per 100,000 live births in 2003 (*14*). Performance with regards to the MDG 5 (of reducing maternal mortality by three-fourths between 1990 and 2015) can be seen in Figure 4 and, judging by the pattern, it is impossible for Paraguay to achieve the goal by 2015.

There are significant differences in maternal mortality rates from region to region, and that is related to the quality and timeliness of care as well as the greater or lesser underreporting of deaths. The causes of maternal deaths are related to barriers in access to health services, with 46% due to a delay in arrival at the service and 23% due to the services' deficient decision making; the remaining 31% die at home without care (*18*). The principal biological causes of maternal death (hemorrhage, abortion, toxemia, and septicemia) continue to be avoidable. According to 2004 figures, in 94.2% of births, the mothers received prenatal care at least once and 68.6% did so during the first trimester; there are still differences among regions. The percentage of institutional births increased from 56.3% in 1998 to 74.1% in 2004. Some 10% of births are attended at home by technicians or individuals with degrees in obstetrics, and 15.8% by traditional birth attendants (*13*).

The mortality rate for the group 20–59 years old was 210.9 per 100,000 population between 2001 and 2003, while for defined causes it was 177.8 per 100,000. Assaults/homicides are the principal specific cause of death, followed by cerebrovascular disease and ischemic heart disease, for both sexes. For women, uterine cancer is the leading cause of death, and complications in pregnancy, childbirth, and the puerperium are the third leading specific cause of death.

Older Adults 60 Years Old and Older

A high percentage of the population of older adults is illiterate (26.4%). The incidence of poverty among people 60 years old and older is lower than that observed for those 10–59 years old, in both urban and rural areas. Coverage of the retirement and pension systems is low (just 14% of people 60 years old and older receive social security), with significant differences between urban and rural areas (almost 20% in urban areas and 6.8% in rural areas) (19).

Some 11,273 deaths were reported in this group (2,966.8 per 100,000) in 2003. Of the 5,119 deaths that occurred while under medical care and from a defined cause, 41.5% were from diseases of the circulatory system (62% pulmonary circulatory disease and 25% ischemic heart disease), with no significant differences between the sexes, and 16.7% were from malignant neoplasms (of the trachea, bronchial tubes, and lungs, and of the prostate in men; and of the digestive system, breast, and cervix in women) (14).

Workers

Some 76.4% of the population is of working age (10 years old and older, according to Paraguay's definition) and of these, 63.4% constitute the economically active population; this percentage is slightly higher in rural areas (64.9%) than urban areas (62.4%). The population 10–14 years old has a high rate of economic participation at the national level and is included in the labor market with an activity rate of 20.8%, with male participation (28.6%) being higher than female participation (12.8%). There are high levels of participation of the population 15–29 years old, with an activity rate of 53%, and more participation by men than women. Men and women work in the tertiary sector in a proportion of 39.8% and 79.2%, respectively, while 36.6% of men and 79.2% of women work in the primary sector (20).

From 2001 to 2005, the annual average of on-the-job accidents was 1,000, with variations from 900 to 1,200. The most common injuries from these accidents are fractures of the legs or arms. The causes range from lack of protective equipment to inexperience or inattention. Of all sectors, the commercial sector generates the most on-the-job accidents, and this is due to the transport of merchandise (almost exclusively traffic accidents). The commercial sector is followed by the lumber industry, the construction industry, and the bottling industry. Bottling plants keep very good records of all their on-the-job accidents (21).

The problems related to the sexual exploitation of children are significant. There is evidence that human trafficking is a situation that affects Paraguay, but there is no up-to-date information. Children who do not have birth certificates are more vulnerable and exposed to all types of exploitation. The majority of the adolescent victims of sexual exploitation are 16–18 years old, and commercial sexual activity starts among children 12 and 13 years old, but also occurs in girls as young as 8 (22).

There is a legislative and regulatory framework for matters related to childhood. Paraguay has ratified International Labor Organization Convention 182 on the worst forms of child labor, and ratified the state's commitment to safeguard the moral and physical health of minors and adolescents in labor matters through Law No. 1,657/2001. In 2005, Decree 4,951, which establishes the regulations for that law, was promulgated, with a list of activities considered dangerous child labor. The challenge is the full implementation of the Code on Childhood and Adolescence and of the National System for Comprehensive Protection of Childhood and Adolescence envisaged by the Code.

Ethnic Groups

In a study of 18 indigenous communities (23), seroprevalence for Chagas' disease ranged between 11% and 78%. With regard to hantavirus infection, in a sample of 957 persons from 18 communities, prevalence was 15%. In the same study, in 1,801 blood sera of indigenous people, 0.2% was positive for hepatitis B, while 7% was positive for syphilis. Of 1,720 indigenous people, 10% were obese; of 1,159 individuals, 5.4% were found to have diabetes mellitus and 7.2% were found to have altered fasting glycemia. The serious health deficiencies in these communities, especially among women and children, are associated with poverty, environmental risks, the scarcity of water, and the devastation of fauna and flora.

Displaced Persons

Displacement of communities due to lack of food and water has resulted in a drastic decrease in the number of their members, and they exhibit high prevalence of gastrointestinal and respiratory diseases and a high risk of vector-borne diseases such as Chagas' disease and hantavirus. These groups have the highest incidence rates of tuberculosis in the country.

HEALTH CONDITIONS AND PROBLEMS

COMMUNICABLE DISEASES

Vector-borne Diseases

Subsequent to the 1999–2000 **malaria** epidemic, with 16,799 cases, ongoing surveillance and control activities have achieved a 97% reduction in the number of cases per year, with 376 cases in 2005. *Plasmodium vivax* accounts for 99.8% to 99.9% (24, 25). No malaria deaths have been reported. In the rural areas of three endemic departments in the east-central zone (Alto Paraná, Caaguazú, and Canindeyú), 75% of cases are found.

Subsequent to the **dengue** epidemic in 2000, caused by dengue-1, which affected the entire country (but mainly Asunción, the Central Department, and the Brazilian border), every year saw small outbreaks or sporadic cases, with circulation of dengue-1, dengue-2, and dengue-3 in different parts of the country, especially in the metropolitan area and on the Brazilian border. Between February and May of 2006 there was an outbreak in Asunción and the Central Department, with 1,937 suspected cases and 1,213 confirmed cases (814 confirmed by laboratory test and 29 by epidemiological link). The *Aedes aegypti* mosquito is widely distributed throughout the country and the vector density is consistently high.

The first national serologic survey for prevalence of **Chagas' disease** in children 1–5 years old was carried out in 2001. Some 11,654 samples from children were analyzed and 57 were found to be infected. The samples were taken in 632 localities from 110 of the country's 227 municipalities. Of the total of seropositive children, three had seronegative mothers. The prevalence of seropositivity for *Trypanosoma cruzi* in blood banks ranged from 3.8% to 4.7% between 1996 and 2000 and from 2.8% to 4.5% between 2001 and 2005 (*26*). Control of transmission by transfusion achieved very high coverage.

The principal endemic zones for **American tegumentary leishmaniasis** are in the north, center, and east of the eastern region, where areas of tropical rain forests are still found. However, the first periurban outbreak of the disease was reported in early 2004 in a district of the Central Department. The transmission pattern is undergoing changes related to the loss of the original forest. Between 1999 and 2003 there was an increase in reported cases of American tegumentary leishmaniasis, from 409 to 1,133; 73% occurred in the departments of San Pedro, Alto Paraná, and Canindeyú; and 22.3% were of mucous forms.

With respect to **visceral leishmaniasis**, the number of cases has increased significantly in recent years. After just one reported case in 1995 and one in 2000, cases have been reported annually since 2002, and are increasing, reaching 23 in 2004, 16 in 2005, and 110 up to June of 2006; 90% of the cases come from the Central Department and the capital.

From 1995 to December 2005, 203 **hantavirus** infections were reported (positive IgG and IgM serology), of which 118 developed hantavirus pulmonary syndrome, with a mortality rate of 24%. Up to 2005, the cases were limited to the western region of the country which is considered endemic. But, starting in June of that year, cases were diagnosed in two departments of the country's eastern region (*27*).

Vaccine-preventable Diseases

Paraguay has been free from circulation of the **measles** virus since 1998. Between 2003 and 2005, the annual average of eruptive febrile diseases was 518 cases, and measles was ruled out in all of them (*28*). Between 1977 and 1995, the measles vaccine was given at 9 and 15 months of age and starting in 1995, at 1 year (*29*). In 2002 the triple virus vaccine (MMR) was introduced into the regular series and, in 2003, there was a mass vaccination of 93% of the population 1–4 years old with double viral (MR) vaccine. The average coverage increased from 78% between 1995 and 1999 to 90% between 2000 and 2005. In 2003 an outbreak of **rubella** was identified, with 11 laboratory-confirmed cases. To eliminate rubella and congenital rubella syndrome and consolidate measles eradication, 99.7% of the population 5–39 years old (63% of the country's population) was vaccinated with MR in 2005 (*30*).

The last case of **poliomyelitis** was reported in 1985; the rate of acute flaccid paralysis ranged from 0.5 to 1.6 per 100,000 children under 15 years old between 1999 and 2005. The average coverage with oral polio vaccine (OPV) in the 1996–2000 period was 77%, and it increased to 87% for 2001–2005. In 2003, 93% of children under 5 years old were vaccinated with OPV.

No cases of **diphtheria** were reported between 1995 and 2000; in 2001 one case was found; and from 2002 to 2003 there was an outbreak of 50 laboratory-confirmed cases. The outbreak extended to six districts in two regions. The incidence in the general population was 0.9 per 100,000; attack rates were higher in 1–4-year-olds and 5–14-year-olds. Of the confirmed cases, 68% had no history of vaccination or had an incomplete series. The mortality rate was 15%. There were four confirmed cases in 2004 and none in 2005. The outbreaks were controlled with vaccination of individuals up to 49 years old in areas with cases and areas with low coverage, and with prophylaxis for contacted persons.

The average incidence of **neonatal tetanus** in the 1996–2000 period was 7 per 100,000 live births (12 cases), and in the 2001–2005 period, 0.4 per 100,000 live births (7 cases). Cumulative vaccination coverage in women of reproductive age with tetanus-diphtheria toxoid was 78% in the 2001–2005 period; despite that, there are still cases of neonatal tetanus, so the vaccination strategy was focused on women of reproductive age in high-risk areas.

In 2001 it was determined that 60% of the invasive diseases in children under 1 year old were due to *Haemophilus influenzae* type b (*31*). In 2002 the combined (Hib+DPT+Hep B) vaccine was introduced for this group and, with an average coverage of 87% from 2003–2005, it was noted that in 2005 just 3% of meningitis cases in children under 2 years old were due to Hib. In 2005, surveillance for **whooping cough** was implemented and *Bordetella pertussis* was isolated in 11 cases in children under 1 year old, not old enough for completion of the primary vaccination series (*31*).

With the introduction of the combined MMR and pentavalent vaccines, the cost of the program increased considerably; Law No. 2,310, which guarantees funds for the annual purchase of vaccines, was approved in 2003. That year, surveillance of adverse events from vaccines was implemented.

Intestinal Infectious Diseases

Diarrhea is the second most common reason for outpatient visits at the Ministry of Public Health and Social Welfare services, mainly in children under 5 years old (69% of reported cases). From 2001 to 2005, approximately 49,000 cases were reported on average, a slight increase in comparison with the previous period (42,000 for 1996–1999). Diarrhea with dehydration represents approximately 10% of the total. Studies on the etiology and pattern of the enteropathogens are still insufficient. The **intestinal parasitoses** are the third most common reason for consultation, right after diarrhea. Intestinal infectious diseases are the fourth leading cause of death in children under 1 year old and the second leading cause of death in children 1–4 years old (*14*).

Chronic Communicable Diseases

With respect to **tuberculosis** (*32*), Paraguay does not have national studies of prevalence and annual risk of tubercular infection. The World Health Organization estimated, for 2004, a rate of 71 cases per 100,000 for all forms of tuberculosis (*33*). Detection of cases of all forms of tuberculosis has been fairly regular from 1995–2004; detection of pulmonary cases with positive bacilloscopy showed a slight increase, which may be attributed to increased detection activity in 2003 and 2004. In 2004, 2,300 new cases were reported, 54% of the estimated cases (rate of 38 per 100,000). Of these, 2,097 were pulmonary (91%); and of these, 57% had a positive bacilloscopy. Of the 203 cases of extrapulmonary tuberculosis (9% of the total), 36 (18%) were tuberculous meningitis. The Chaco region has the highest reporting rate, and the highest number of cases is reported in the metropolitan area. The mortality rate is high (4.7 per 100,000) and is associated with delayed diagnosis (*33*).

In 2000, the National Control Program for Tuberculosis adopted the Directly Observed Treatment, Short-course (DOTS) strategy in two demonstration areas and, for 2004, it reports that 27% of the country's population lives in DOTS areas. Analysis of the 2004 cohort of new positive bacilloscopy (BK+) cases (744 cases) in non-DOTS areas shows a 71.4% treatment success rate, 1.5% unconfirmed transfers, 14.2% abandonment, 0.1% failure, and 5.5% deaths. In DOTS areas, of 361 BK+ cases, the treatment success rate was 84.8% and the abandonment rate was 6.1%. The percentage of deaths remains high (5.8%).

The rate of primary resistance to a single drug is 6.9%; the rate of primary multidrug resistance (MDR) is 2.1% (*34*). The rate of secondary resistance to a single drug is 13.7%,[2] and the rate of secondary MDR is 4%. The high percentage of primary MDR may be related to self-administered treatment that includes rifampicin.

The goal of eliminating **leprosy** as a public health problem was achieved between 2001 and 2003, with prevalence rates of 0.92 to 0.97 per 10,000 (*35*). However, the rate climbed to 1.2 per 10,000 in 2004, and 14 of the 18 health regions still have a prevalence higher than 1 per 10,000. The rate of detection of new cases per 100,000 population increased from 8.0 in 2000 to 9.2 in 2003, the highest in the previous 10 years.

The coverage of polychemotherapy in 2003 was 94.4% (*36*). In a representative sample of 591 patients, it was found that 84%

had had the disability evaluation, 71.1% of the patients were multibacillary, and 4.5% were under 15 years old. The rate of detection of new cases with disabilities (grade 1, 2, and 3) was 25.5% in 2000 and 20.5% in 2003. The lag between the onset of symptoms and diagnosis was 60.9 months in 2003 as compared to 34.6 months in 2000 (*36*).

Limited access to health services and the opportunity for diagnosis result in a significant proportion of new cases with disabilities and a high hidden prevalence. The percentage of new multibacillary cases remains between 70% and 80%, which would also be a sign of delayed detection. Care for lepers is mostly outside the Ministry of Health services in specialized services included in the National Program's patient care department. Just 7.8% of the Ministry's services deliver polychemotherapy.

Acute Respiratory Infections

Acute respiratory infections continue to be the leading cause of consultations involving children under 5 years old. In the demand for Ministry of Health services for 2001, in the group of children under 5 years old, consultations for respiratory infections accounted for 63%. Of all consultations in children under 1 year old, 71% were for respiratory infections; 59% were among children 1–4 years old. Between 2001 and 2003, influenza and pneumonia was the third leading cause of death in children under 1 year old, the leading cause of death in children 1–4 years old, the second leading cause of death in children 5–9 years old, and the fifth leading cause of death in people 60 years old and older, responsible for 57,166 years of potential life lost (*14*).

HIV/AIDS and Other Sexually Transmitted Infections

The epidemic remains concentrated, and it was estimated in October 2004 that 16,000 to 18,000 people 15–49 years old were living with HIV. This estimate, compared to the number reported for the same age group on the same date, indicates underreporting of 80%. The prevalence of HIV/AIDS in pregnant women increased from 0.2% in 2000 to 0.8% in 2002, and in sex workers, from 0.6% in 2000 to 2.6% in 2002,[3] which could be an indication of a significant expansion and possible dispersion of the epidemic. Even with this level of underreporting, the progression of the epidemic in the female population[4] and in young people 15–24 years old is worthy of special attention; equally telling is the increasingly frequent reporting of cases outside the metropolitan area. The prevalence of HIV in blood donors ranged from 0.16% to 0.34% in the 1999–2004 period (*26*).

---

[2]The analysis of secondary resistance to a single drug was conducted with an insufficient sample.

[3]Prevalence was obtained by seroepidemiological surveys on HIV/AIDS infection in pregnant women and sex workers, conducted by the National Program for the Control of HIV/AIDS and STIs (PRONASIDA) in 2000 and 2002. In both studies the sample size was inadequate.

[4]In 1992, for every infected woman, there were 28 infected men, and in 2004, for every infected woman there were 2.8 men infected with HIV/AIDS.

The prevalence rate of condom use among women remains low: 10.5% in 2004 as compared to 1.9% in 1990. Among young women 15–24 years old, the prevalence rate of condom use in the last sexual encounter in the prior three months was 31.8% in 2004, higher than the 15.7% reported in 1996. But, in this same group, just 2.2% of the women had knowledge of all methods of HIV/AIDS prevention (13).

In 2005, the National Program for the Control of HIV/AIDS and STIs provided free antiretroviral therapy (ART) to 588 adults and 92 children (19% was based on the estimate of persons who need ART). There is no medication for prophylaxis of opportunistic diseases. Decentralization of care and distribution of ART for persons living with HIV/AIDS to the Ministry of Public Health and Social Welfare health services in border areas with Brazil and Argentina have been initiated. Prevention of the vertical transmission of HIV was initiated in 2005 with the distribution of rapid HIV diagnostic tests in the MSPyBS maternal-child hospitals in 17 of the country's 18 health regions.

The prevalence of **syphilis** in pregnant women ranged from 5.3% to 6.2% in the 2000–2004 period. The incidence of congenital syphilis for the same period increased from 1.1% to 4.9%.[5] The prevalence of syphilis in blood donors in the 1999–2004 period ranged from 0.2% to 0.3% (26).

Zoonoses

Subsequent to the annual average of more than 300 cases of canine **rabies** in the late 1990s and the mass vaccination and change of control strategy in 1999, sporadic but persistent cases and foci were reported between 2000 and 2005. Human rabies, associated with canine rabies, remains a problem. Seven cases were reported between 2000 and 2004 (37).

About 100 cases a year of bovine rabies, more closely related to wild rabies, were reported between 1998 and 2003, while 51 cases were reported in 2004 (38). Given the constant and ongoing occurrence of cases in bovines, the veterinary service advises the annual administration of bovine rabies vaccine in areas with a high occurrence of cases.

In 1997 the country received certification as a country free of **foot-and-mouth disease** with vaccination, granted by the World Organization for Animal Health (OIE), a condition maintained and recognized during 1998 and 1999 (39). In view of the achievement of the eradication goals, vaccination was eliminated in July 1999, but in 2000 vaccination was reinstated in the border areas because of the reintroduction of the disease in the department of Canindeyú. No cases of foot-and-mouth disease were reported in 2004 and 2005. The control measures, such as mandatory vaccination, epidemiological follow-up, monitoring, and quarantine on the border, were maintained.

---

[5]Data is furnished by the Ministry of Public Health and Social Welfare's Department of Biostatistics based on the records of outpatient prenatal services, the coverage of which is limited and not uniformly distributed throughout the country.

NONCOMMUNICABLE DISEASES

Metabolic and Nutritional Diseases

Some 6% of newborns had low birthweight (<2,500 grams), without significant changes between 1999 and 2003 (14). The average duration of exclusive breast-feeding in children 0–5 months old is 22%, and 27.6% were mainly breast-fed (breast-milk, water, or other liquids, excluding other types of milk) (13).

Nationwide, 5% of children under 5 years old suffer from acute **undernutrition**, defined as more than two standard deviations (SDs) below the mean, and up to 6.3% in rural areas. It is estimated that 20.5% of children suffer mild undernutrition or are at risk for undernutrition (–1 SD) (rural areas, 23.6% and urban areas, 17.1%). Of children under 5 years old nationwide, 10.9% suffered from chronic undernutrition, defined as height-for-age –2 SD from the mean (14% in rural areas and 7.4% in urban areas) (40).

In 2002, 3,646 children under 5 years old were evaluated at health services of 12 health regions, and global undernutrition was found in 8.3%, chronic undernutrition in 15.9%, overweight in 14.2%, and obesity in 8%. In 2004, an anthropometric evaluation found 5.9% global undernutrition, 14.4% at risk for undernutrition, and 9.3% obesity in the same age group. In pregnant women, 32.5% were found to be underweight, 18.6% overweight, and 19.6% obese (41).

Diabetes was the third leading cause of death between 2001 and 2003, the second leading cause of death for women and the fifth for men.

Cardiovascular Diseases

In the 2001–2003 period, diseases of the circulatory system were the leading cause of death, accounting for 28% of all deaths reported with defined causes, in comparison to the 33% average for the 1996–1999 period. Among these, the male-female ratio was 1.1 and it was 3.8 to 5.6 times higher in urban areas, which is an indication, in addition to underreporting, of the poor quality and low coverage of care in rural areas. Among the specific causes of death, cerebrovascular accident was the leading cause for both sexes, 10.6% of all deaths with a defined cause and a rate of 29 per 100,000 (27.4 per 100,000 men and 30.6 per 100,000 women); ischemic heart disease was the second leading cause of death for both sexes (8% and 21.9 per 100,000) and for men (8.4% and 25.6 per 100,000), and the third leading cause of death for women (7.5% and 23.5 per 100,000) (14).

In a non-random, multicentric, predominantly urban study on the prevalence of **coronary risk** factors in 14 cities in different regions of the country (much of Chaco was excluded) (42), 8% were found to have diabetes (with regional variations between 5% and 12%), of which 33% were unaware of their status; 26% were found to have dyslipidemia, of which 57% were unaware of their status; 23% were found to be active smokers (with variations between 15.8% and 31% of residents), 15% were found to be former smokers; 21% were obese and 38% were overweight; 44% had sedentarism (with variations between 35.5% and 58%); and 35% had hypertension (with regional variations between 23.1% and 42.6%). **Hypertension** was found in 31.5% of women and 38.9% of men. Some 31% were aware that they were hypertensive and 85% had had their pressure taken at least once; 27% were medicated and, of these, just 37% had their pressure under control.

In a study of schoolchildren 8–18 years old in Asunción (*43*), 47% mentioned a family history of diabetes, 14% were overweight, and 19% were obese.

Malignant Neoplasms

Malignant neoplasms are the second leading cause of death, accounting for 14%–15% of deaths reported with a defined cause and occurring while under medical care between 2001 and 2003. Among total deaths, no significant differences were noted between men and women, but there were significant differences between urban and rural areas, with a value 5.3–6.7 times higher in urban areas, suggesting significant underreporting, very low health care coverage, and poor quality of death certification. Among deaths from tumors with a defined cause and occurring while under medical care, the leading cause of death in women was uterine cancer, followed by breast cancer and cancer of the digestive organs and peritoneum, excluding the stomach and colon. In men, the leading cause of death was cancer of the trachea, bronchial tubes, and lung, followed by cancer of the digestive organs and peritoneum, excluding stomach and colon (second leading cause), and prostate cancer (third leading cause) (*14*).

Considering all deaths reported and excluding those with ill-defined causes, aggregated for the 2001–2003 period, and analyzing the specific causes of death, uterine cancer is the fifth leading cause of death in women (10th overall), with a rate of 12.4 per 100,000; unfortunately, half of the cases reported do not have a site identified, but among those that do, the ratio of cervical cancer to uterine cancer was 12:5. Breast cancer is the second most common cancer in women.

OTHER HEALTH PROBLEMS OR ISSUES

Disasters

In August 2004, a massive fire destroyed Asuncion's Ycuá Bolaños Shopping Center, putting the lives of some 1,500 people in jeopardy. Given the magnitude of the event, a State of Emergency and a State of Health Emergency were declared. In the prehospital response, numerous rescue workers from different organizations were mobilized. Thirty-three health facilities treated 304 people injured in the fire. A total of 357 people died, and 204 children were orphaned. More than two years of psychological follow-up were provided to the families of the victims. The situation led to greater awareness among the population and heightened vigilance by government authorities, and some attempts

were made to improve conditions in public areas to prevent similar events from occurring.

In 2002, PAHO warned (*44*) of the increase of potential risks of chemical emergencies and disasters due to mishandling of hazardous products deposited in vulnerable places. In July 2003, a fire broke out in downtown Asunción's Cotton and Tobacco Inspection Warehouse, where tons of pesticides, fungicides, herbicides, and insecticides were stored. Firefighters were exposed to hazardous chemicals for at least four hours before safety measures were instituted. The population living near the site of the disaster had to be evacuated. At least 735 people were treated in the health services.

In 2002, the intense drought in western Paraguay, with its consequent food shortages and contaminated water, seriously damaged the national economy and the health of the population. At least 17 people died from drinking the contaminated water (*45*). In September 2005, an emergency was declared in Paraguay's Chaco region. The drought caused at least five deaths, attributable to the use of water unfit for human consumption. The State channeled resources to more than 20,000 indigenous people and 14,000 families in the disaster area.

Violence and Other External Causes

Between 2003 and 2005, traffic accidents represented an important cause of hospitalization and death, especially in the young population. During those years, the Medical Emergency Center in Asunción saw 21,560 people, 20% of all care for injuries from external causes. Of these, 4,225 patients needed to be admitted. Of all deaths from injuries due to external causes at that institution, in 2004 and 2005, 41% were the result of traffic accidents. In 2005, when there was a 23% increase in comparison to 2004, approximately 72% of traffic accident victims were young: 17% were 0 to 14 years old, 55% were 15 to 34 years old, and 28% were 34 years old and older (*46*).

According to the National Demographic and Sexual Reproductive Health Survey 2004 (*13*), violence against women is as follows: 33.0% verbal, 19.0% physical, and 8.0% sexual. Law No. 1,600/00 of 2000 recognizes domestic violence as a social problem and made it easier for women to file complaints. However, progress has not been made in terms of the institutional framework and the training of human resources to address the problem.

External causes accounted for 11% of deaths with a defined cause and occurring while under medical care in 2003, compared to 9.5% the previous year. The male/female ratio was 4:3, similar to previous years; the urban/rural ratio was 3:5 (*14*).

Considering all the deaths reported and excluding those with ill-defined causes, aggregated for the 2001–2003 period, and analyzing the specific causes of death, homicide is the sixth leading cause of death for both sexes (rate of 12.4 per 100,000) and the third leading cause of death in males (22.4 per 100,000), seventh in urban areas, and third in rural areas; land transportation accidents are the eighth leading cause (8.2 per 100,000), and seventh for males (12.8 per 100,000) (*14*).

The National Observatory of Violence was established in 2002, joining several institutions and sectors together under the coordination of the Ministry of Public Health and Social Welfare. Violence is monitored from the perspective of the different institutions. Special emphasis has been placed on monitoring traffic violence, including measuring the impact of policies in Asunción.

Mental Health

Care is based in the Psychiatric Hospital; efforts have been made to direct care to the community, with limited success. Resources are scarce and centralized. There are 26 outpatient mental health services. Of these, 8% are exclusively for children and adolescents. These services treat 263 users per 100,000 population. Women represent 53% of all users, and 40% of all consultations involve patients 20 years old or younger. There are no data on the proportion of users who are children and adolescents.

The principal diagnoses of persons seen at outpatient services were schizophrenia and related disorders (21%) and affective disorders (20%). The information on the diagnosis is based on the number of patient consultations, not the number of users. The average number of consultations per user is 2.8. Some 15% of the outpatient services provide follow-up in the community, while 12% have mobile teams. Some of these services offer psychosocial treatment (*47*).

Mortality from suicide is moving in the direction of younger age groups: in 1999 the highest incidence rate was found in the 50–59 year-old group (6.6 per 100,000); in 2000 the highest rate was found in the 40–49-year-old group (4.6); and in 2001 the highest rate was found in those over 60 years old (5.6); but in 2002 and 2003 the rate was higher in the 20–29-year-old group (5.6 and 4.9, respectively) (*14*).

Environmental Pollution

From July 2000 to May 2004, of a total of 2,570 diagnoses of poisoning, 352 (13.7%) were caused by pesticides, with annual increases of 30% to 53%. Of those, 47.1% were caused by organophosphates, 28.7% by rodenticides and carbamates, and 10.5% by piretroides. Some 87.5% of patients poisoned by pesticides were under 45 years old; those 16–30 years old (50.3%) and those younger than 15 years old (24.1%) were affected most. The reports for 2000 to 2003 on a total of 269 patients showed that poisonings affected primary and secondary level students (22.6%), followed by domestic cases (18.2%) and farmers (11.5%) (*48*). Up until 2006 there was clear underreporting of cases of acute and chronic pesticide poisoning, but in 2004 surveillance of pesticide poisoning was initiated in some of the departments outside the metropolitan Asunción area, with training of health professionals, farmers, and others involved in handling pesticides. Data are still limited in coverage and quality, but the

increased capture of acute pesticide poisoning cases outside the metropolitan Asunción area, from less than 30 per year up to 2003 to 270 cases in 2004, is an important step forward. There is no information about any eco-toxicological studies that may evaluate the situation of pollution or accumulation of pesticides in the soil or in land or aquatic animals.

RESPONSE OF THE HEALTH SECTOR

Health Policies and Plans

Article 68 of the National Constitution of 1992 addresses the right to health and provides that the state shall protect and promote health as a fundamental right of individuals and in the community's interest. The 2005–2008 National Health Policy is based on: a) health reform; b) health promotion; c) social protection in health with joint financing and insurance; d) environmental health and basic sanitation; and e) development of human resources and ongoing education. With certain exceptions, the greatest difficulty for the governing entity is in complying with the policies and plans that are formulated, associated with the frequent changes in the leadership levels.

Law 1,032 of 1996 (*49*) established the guidelines for decentralization, but in practice, little progress has been made. There was a pilot experiment in 1998, with the participation of 23 municipalities which signed decentralization agreements, but just 10 are implementing this mode of operation. The experiments are isolated agreements and there is no comprehensive official assessment of their effect on decentralized operation. Despite the existence of legal frameworks that support social participation in health, through regional and local councils, its implementation has been scarce and controversial, since it includes the management of financial resources in its actions.

Table 4 presents an overview of the legal framework of the health system. It is evident that there are limits on rule-making and on the implementation of laws.

Health Strategies and Programs

The care delivered by the network of services is not comprehensive, is highly fragmented, lacks coordination among the various levels, and suffers from a dearth of decision making at the first level. Some 18.4% of the population has medical insurance (27% in the urban areas and 7% in the rural areas) through the Institute of Public Welfare (IPS) or another type of insurance (individual, employment, family, military, police, local, and abroad), while 81.6% have no medical insurance. Some 48.8% of those seeking services in 2003 did so at a public establishment, while in 2004 the percentage increased to 55.1%. In contrast, consultations at private hospitals or offices declined from 30.8% in 2003 to 27% in 2004; the rest of those who were ill or injured sought

TABLE 4. Legal framework of the National Health System, Paraguay.

Legal framework	Remarks
National Constitution of the Republic of Paraguay, 1992	
Law No. 836/60	Organic Law of the MSPyBS. Amended by Decree 4674/99, with regard to the organization chart.
Sanitary Code, 1980	Update has not been approved at this time.
Law No. 1,032 of 1996	Creation of the National Health System. Regulations not issued.
Decree 19,996/1998	Establishes the regulations for local health decentralization.
Decree 20,553/1998	Establishes the regulations for the Superintendency of Health.

outpatient services at pharmacies, with traditional healers, and others. Mechanisms have not been established to guarantee equal access to services and actions have not been implemented for evaluation of quality and user satisfaction.

Organization of the Health System

Law 1,032/96 establishes the regulations for the National Health System; it has both public and private components, and health services are delivered through four subsectors: public, private non-profit, private for-profit, and mixed. There is much segmentation of providers and a lack of coordination among the various subsectors, without clear separation of functions. The Ministry of Public Health and Social Welfare performs governance, delivery, and financing functions. The IPS and the private sector perform insurance, delivery, and financing functions, but the three are autonomous and there is no coordination among them.

Public Health Services

In 2005, the National Health Authority conducted a wide-ranging interinstitutional analysis aimed at establishing strategies that would make a process of primary health care renewal possible.

At the Ministry of Public Health and Social Welfare, the prevention and control of disease is principally the responsibility of the General Directorates of Health Surveillance (DGVS) and Health Programs (DGPS). The former includes the Directorate of Communicable Diseases, with responsibility for surveillance, prevention, and control programs for priority problems, the Directorate of Noncommunicable Diseases, established in 1999 and operational since 2003, the National Vector Control Service (SENEPA), with re-

sponsibility for surveillance, prevention, and control of vector-borne diseases, and the Central Laboratory for Public Health.

In 2005 a strategic plan was drawn up for the elimination of malaria as a public health problem, including diagnosis and treatment in the health services in and including the local governments in the environmental regulation process. Since 2005, the Integrated Management Strategy for the prevention and control of dengue has been included, strengthening actions in border areas, which are considered more vulnerable. The vector control program achieved, between 1999 and 2006, 100% nationwide coverage for spraying of endemic areas, with its own funds. Concurrently, in the departments in which action was taken, surveillance of the vector was initiated through sampling, with an active community (rural leaders and schools) and institutional base.

In addition to the specific actions by the National Cardiovascular Prevention Institute of the Ministry of Public Health and Social Welfare, in 2005 the country joined the CARMEN Network and set up an interinstitutional and intersectorial team for an integrated approach to the principal risk factors for chronic diseases.

The DGPS is responsible for the comprehensive child care programs, programs for the care of adolescents and women, sexual and reproductive health, mental health, and the National Institute for Food and Nutrition (INAN).

Responsibility for health information and analysis is shared by the Department of Planning and Evaluation (DGPE) and the DGVS. The DGPE includes the Department of Biostatistics, which is responsible for vital statistics in coordination with the Vital Records Office and the General Directorate of Statistics, Surveys, and Censuses, and for the records of services delivered by the Ministry's health establishments. The DGVS is responsible for the surveillance of health events. Both directorates are responsible for analyzing the data to support decision-making at the national level. However, the deficiency of infrastructure and human resources trained for analysis at all levels is recognized. The data flow from the local to the regional level and from the regional to the national level without processing or analysis; they are poor in quality and untimely; occasionally the data are collected from other institutions or sectors at each level. The surveillance data are published every four months in an epidemiological bulletin and on a weekly basis in a weekly bulletin; neither is of high quality. The pamphlet of basic health indicators was published from 1998 to 2004, but no analytic documents are produced on a regular basis and there is no systematized mechanism for health situation analysis. The Ministry of Public Health and Social Welfare does not perform regular monitoring of the MDGs. The current Health Code (dating back to 1980) establishes mandatory reporting of communicable diseases by the medical care services, be they public, private, or social security, although in practice the coverage of reporting is limited. Since the late 1990s, the Central Laboratory for Public Health has experienced strong growth at the central level in its surveillance support function. By 2006 it had an expanded diagnostic capacity, quality control, relationships with several international reference laboratories, and participation in regional and subregional networks. For surveillance of certain problems it has networks involving private laboratories and reference hospital laboratories in and outside of the Ministry of Public Health and Social Welfare, in the capital, and in some regions. Its principal limitations are not having a national network of public health laboratories and the lack of a surveillance budget.

Three entities are considered the country's most important providers of drinking water and sewer system services, with four distinct types of operation: Sanitary Services of Paraguay (ESSAP), with specific services for population centers with more than 10,000 residents; the Sanitation Boards, supported by the National Environmental Sanitation Service (SENASA), and with services for population centers with less than 10,000 residents; and the private operators (water carriers) and community operators (neighborhood committees).

In 2000, Law 1,614/00 (50) established the bases and principles for delivery of drinking water and sanitary sewer services and created the Sanitary Services Regulatory Entity (ERSSAN) to regulate and supervise the quality and efficiency of the services, protect the community's interests, and control and verify the correct application of current provisions. Decree 18,880/2002 established the regulations for that law and empowered the Ministry of Public Works and Communications (MOPC) to develop public policies, including financing. The MOPC does not have a structure for carrying out that function, and governance of the sector is in limbo.

Despite the progress in recent years, there is low coverage of water and basic sanitation, with an enormous urban/rural gap, especially for the indigenous population. From 1992 to 2002, the percentage of the total population with access to water through a residential connection increased from 29.8% to 63.4% (84.4% of the urban population and 35.5% of the rural population) (12). The highest percentages of coverage through a residential connection are in Asunción (8), with 97.2%, and in the Central Department, with 86.4%. Of the 46.4% of households with a residential connection, 60% belong to households of the wealthiest population quintile and just 30.3% belong to the poorest 20%. The increased coverage has not been accompanied by improved water quality, and in many of the small communities and rural areas, drinking water is disinfected irregularly or not at all.

Sanitary sewer coverage is low and little progress has been made: it increased from 7.2% in 1992 to 9.4% in 2002 (12), concentrated in the urban sector (16% coverage). Asunción has the most sewer coverage in the country with 70.5%, but in 10 departments the coverage is less than 5%. Some 49.2% of all homes eliminate their excreta through a septic tank: 62.5% of all homes in the urban areas and 30.0% in the rural areas. Common latrines are used by 35.5% of all households while 2.8% use another sys-

tem and 1.1% do not have a bathroom. In urban areas, 15.2% use common latrines and in rural areas, 64.8% (8).

With respect to solid waste management, the 1992 National Constitution and various laws establish the legal, administrative, tax, and penal framework. However, this legislation contains a great deal of overlap and significant gaps in relation to the sector. There is no policy or law on solid waste with high enough legislative status for the sector (51). The SEAM is the principal authority for enforcement in all matters related to the environment, and in particular, in the area of solid waste. The Ministry of Public Health and Social Welfare is the authority when human health may be affected by the improper handling of solid waste. Solid waste management services are the only basic services that are truly decentralized; municipalities are responsible for them through direct municipal administration, privatization, outsourcing, and operation of municipal and private services concomitantly in the same city. In 2006, 66% of service delivery was in the hands of the public sector, 30% in the private sector, and in 4% there was a combination of both modalities (51).

The average rate of urban solid waste generation is about 1.0 kg/person/day, fluctuating between 0.5 and 1.8 kg/person/day, which is approximately 3,700 tons/day in the urban population centers (51). Some 33.6% of the solid waste generated in the country is collected (55.6% in the urban areas and 2.5% in the rural areas); 54.5% of the country's total population (35.9% in urban areas and 80.1% in rural areas) burns garbage (12). Final disposal of 72% of the waste is in an open-air dump, while 28% is disposed of in a controlled manner (13), mainly in the metropolitan area dump.

In relation to environmental control, it bears mentioning that agriculture and livestock generate about 27.2% of the GDP (52) and 33% of the working population carried out primary activities in 2004. More than 55% of exports are of agricultural products and a significant part of the national industry is based on the processing of just those products. The demand for chemical products for pest control has led to the use of products apparently brought in as contraband, according to accusations in the press in 2003 (53). The country has legislation through the Ministry of Public Health and Social Welfare, the Ministry of Agriculture and Livestock (MAG), the SEAM, and the Ministry of Industry and Commerce. But intersectorial coordination is weak and the institutions do not have sufficient resources to enforce the legislation. Also, there are few provisions on the matter at the municipal and departmental levels, lack of knowledge, little enforcement effort by the local and regional governments, and scant compliance with these provisions (53).

The country does not produce chemical substances, although it packages and mixes them. The distribution of pesticides in any type of packaging at the retail level and the final disposition thereof are not always in keeping with the international regulations for marketing these chemicals. The mechanisms for control of the distribution, sale, and use of pesticides are not effective enough (53).

With regard to food protection and control, the National Institute for Food and Nutrition, an institution under the Ministry of Public Health and Social Welfare, is the governing body for food and nutrition, the taking of actions for the control and prevention of iodine deficiency, and standardization of fortification with iron, folic acid, B1, B2, B3, and fluorine. It performs food and nutrition surveillance for the population in need of services (those under 5 years old and pregnant women) and promotes the implementation of nutrition guidelines. It is also responsible for control of food registration and laboratory determinations on micronutrients and foods.

The National Institute for Technology and Standardization (INTN) supports consumers, industry, commerce, and the services with assistance in research, development, standardization, certification, and metrology, in order to guarantee the quality of food. It also develops national technical guidelines for international standardization, certifies food products using product testing and analysis services, and provides technical assistance aimed at the transfer of technical knowledge.

In 2004, the National Animal Health Service was restructured to provide greater coverage, efficiency, and reliability of the services delivered (Law 2,426/04) and to address OIE quality standards, evaluation of third parties, and rapid response in the case of emerging diseases (54). Also in 2005, the system of health records of cattle owners was strengthened, and the system for traceability of the bovine species was instituted (55). The sanitary control of the slaughtering of cattle for local consumption is still weak, very often taking place in establishments that are not properly equipped and that lack ongoing veterinary inspection.

The Program for Food and Nutritional Assistance is a national program implemented in 2005 by the Ministry of Public Health and Social Welfare with the goal of delivering promotion, prevention, and food assistance and nutritional recovery services to children under 5 years old with global undernutrition and at risk, and to low-weight pregnant women, through best nutrition practices and access to nutritional supplementation.

Paraguay made progress in institutionalizing disaster preparation, prevention, and mitigation in 2005 and 2006 in relation to previous years. Law 2,615/2005 created the National Ministry of Emergency (SNE) under the Presidency of the Republic, giving higher status and priority to the issue of disaster prevention and mitigation in Paraguay; it created the National Disaster Fund, and transferred all the employees, assets, credits, and obligations of the National Emergency Committee to the SNE. In 2004, the Ministry of Public Health and Social Welfare initiated the National Program for Health in Emergencies and Disasters, under the Vice Ministry of Health.

Faced with the threat of avian influenza, in 2005 the Ministry of Agriculture and Livestock initiated epidemiological surveillance of bird flu in zoos, associated with the program for surveillance of Newcastle disease. The veterinary service's capacity to diagnose and classify viruses is still lacking. A program of education and decentralization of the veterinary service to zone offices was initiated, along with an alliance with the Paraguayan poultry production chain to control the transit of fowl and their products, implement biosafety measures with farm personnel, and support epidemiological surveillance.

Individual Care Services

In 2004, the Ministry of Public Health and Social Welfare had 670 health posts, 50 dispensaries, 130 health centers, 23 district hospitals, 17 regional hospitals, 18 specialized hospitals, and 7 specialized centers (14, 56). Despite having a wide network, there are distribution problems. Many of these installations do not have the human resources necessary for their operation, and there are serious limitations on adequate supply. The network has grown because of political decisions and not in order to structure a network of services in keeping with the population's needs. The great functional weakness of the first level of care distorts the operation of the network of services, which focuses on hospital care.

The IPS has one general and specialized one hospital, 10 regional hospitals, five outlying clinics, and 60 first level units. It has cooperative agreements with other institutions that deliver services and train human resources in health. It covers the member and his or her descendants up to the age of 18, as well as the relatives in the ascending line, if the member is responsible for them. Police and Military Health cover less than 1% of the population. The most complicated care is delivered at the Police Clinic of Asunción, with 80 beds. The National University of Asunción has a teaching hospital attached to the School of Medicine, caring mainly for low-income sectors.

The private nonprofit subsector has 30 first level establishments. The private for-profit subsector consists of prepaid companies and insurance companies, hospitals, and clinics (153 establishments), clinics, centers, and institutes (425 establishments), physician offices (474 establishments), 342 laboratories, 15 emergency services, and 1,965 pharmacies.

The country has 49 blood bank services or hemotherapy centers, public and private (23 under the MSPyBS, 6 under the IPS, and 20 in the rest of the system). The current system for acquisition of blood is the so-called "by replacement" system. The Ministry of Public Health and Social Welfare network of ambulances consists of 196 ambulances throughout the country, of which 28 are not operating.

Health Promotion

Some of the pillars of the 2005–2008 National Health Policy are health promotion, intersectorial action, and social participation, including joint intersectorial work with community participation. Another is proposing the strengthening of the initiatives of Municipalities, Communities, Healthy Borders, and Health Promoting Schools, their operation in networks, and the creation of a National Intersectorial Committee for Health Promotion, with

Natural and Man-made Disasters: the System's Response

In August 2004, a massive fire destroyed Asuncion's Ycuá Bolaños Shopping Center, putting the lives of some 1,500 people in jeopardy. Given the magnitude of the event, a State of Emergency and a State of Health Emergency were declared. In the prehospital response, numerous rescue workers from different organizations were mobilized. Thirty-three health facilities treated 304 people injured in the fire. A total of 357 people died, and 204 children were orphaned. More than two years of psychological follow-up were provided to the families of the victims. The situation led to greater awareness among the population and heightened vigilance by government authorities, and some attempts were made to improve conditions in public areas to prevent similar events from occurring. In July 2003, a fire broke out in downtown Asunción's Cotton and Tobacco Inspection Warehouse, where tons of pesticides, fungicides, herbicides, and insecticides were stored. Firefighters were exposed to hazardous chemicals for at least four hours before safety measures were instituted. The population living near the site of the disaster had to be evacuated. At least 735 people were treated in the health services. In 2002, the intense drought in western Paraguay, with its consequent food shortages and contaminated water, seriously damaged the national economy and the health of the population. At least 17 people died from drinking the contaminated water. In September 2005, an emergency was declared in Paraguay's Chaco region. The drought caused at least five deaths, attributable to the use of water unfit for human consumption. The State channeled resources to more than 20,000 indigenous people and 14,000 families in the disaster area.

Paraguay made progress in institutionalizing disaster preparedness, prevention, and mitigation in 2005–2006 in relation to earlier years. Law 2,615/2005 created the National Emergency Secretariat (SNE) under the Office of the President of the Republic, raising the profile, and hence the priority, of disaster prevention and mitigation in the country; the law also created the National Disaster Fund, transferring all the staff, goods, credits, and obligations of the National Emergency Committee to SNE. In 2004 the Ministry of Public Health and Social Welfare launched the National Emergency and Disaster Health Program under the Vice-Ministry of Health.

technical groups for management and support of specific areas. The Network of Healthy Municipalities has bylaws and an organizational structure, with a management committee named in the Assembly. However, it lacks financing and mechanisms for self-support, is little known, and still unconsolidated. The implementation of the Healthy Schools initiative can be considered a result of the healthy municipalities movement. There are 22 schools in the network in the department of Misiones and 10 more schools in Paraguay, and they have the potential to become the element that sustains the healthy initiatives in the community.

Human Resources

A human resources policy is in place, but there are still structural problems, such as the existence of personnel training models not in line with the services' requirements, insufficient staff trained in public health, and the incipient development of processes for management and regulation of professional practices. The year 2005 saw the initiation of a process of coordination of health careers for the target personnel in order to improve the position and salary structure.

The rate of Ministry of Public Health and Social Welfare doctors per 10,000 residents increased from 5.6% in 2002 (57) to 6.3% in 2005 (58), ranging from 19.6% in Asunción to 1.2% in Caazapá

(59). The rate of professional nurses in 2003 was 2.2 per 10,000 residents (57), and 2.8 in 2005 (58), ranging from 7.2% in Asunción to 1% in Caazapá (59). As for the distribution of Ministry of Public Health and Social Welfare health personnel, by occupational category, 40% are administrative, 26% auxiliary, 23% administrative professionals, and 11% technicians; 56% of the personnel are permanent and 44% are contracted. These indicators clearly show problems of inequity in access to and quality of care.

The medical residency programs do not have an adequate system for planning and quality control. Work is being done to unify the selection and admission of residents and to standardize curriculum content. There is an excess of doctors being trained, with the opening of five private universities that generate an annual cohort of more than 300 doctors, of which just 60% will be accepted in residency programs. It is estimated that approximately 40% of physicians in the health institutions are general physicians.

Health Supplies

Since 2001 there has been a National Drug Policy focusing on prescriptions. The principal developments have been: the implementation of a national system for the registration of drugs and pharmaceutical establishments; the implementation of actions for oversight of the establishments, resulting in the closing of those that fail to comply with the standards for manufacture or dispensing; and the implementation of a program for quality control of drugs. As of 2006 (*60*), Paraguay had 172 authorized production laboratories, 1,529 authorized external pharmacies in the capital and 2,034 outside the metropolitan Asunción area, 13,400 records of pharmaceutical specialties, 137 distributors, and 127 importers of drugs. There are 113 authorized packagers. From 2003 to 2005, 174 products were analyzed and of these, 5% were not in compliance. In the same period, there was intervention with 23 pharmacies and 27 non-pharmaceutical businesses, and there were 31 inspections of production laboratories, packagers, and distributors.

Paraguay does not produce vaccines or human hyperimmune sera; these are obtained through the PAHO Revolving Fund for Vaccine Procurement. In 2005, the National Vaccine Regulatory Authority was established under the General Directorate of Health Surveillance. This entity registers and releases batches of immunobiologicals at the public and private level.

Since 1988, the Health Sciences Research Institute of the National University of Asunción has been producing ELISA diagnostic kits for canine visceral leishmaniasis, Chagas' disease, and toxoplasmosis; the latter two are exported to other countries.

In 2004 the Ministry of Public Health and Social Welfare took a census of the hospital equipment and furnishings in the 18 health regions and in the specialized and pediatric hospitals of the capital and the metropolitan area. There are serious deficiencies in maintenance, inasmuch as this is not included in the regular structure of operating costs. A plan for maintenance and control of the efficient use of biomedical technology has been initiated in six health regions, involving the checking of 4,464 items of hospital equipment and furnishings and the detection of equipment that is underutilized due to lack of supplies, reagents, replacement parts, or human resources.

Research and Technological Development in Health

The existing entities include the National Council for Science and Technology (CONACYT); the National Secretariat of Technology, under the National Institute for Technology and Standardization; a System of Science, Technology, and Innovation, with the legal force; CONACYT as a governing body for policies on science and technology; and a National Fund of Science and Technology (FONACYT), whose goal is to finance the related activities. In 1998, the National Accreditation Agency (ONA) was created as part of CONACYT. However, there is an absence of clarity in policies, coordination, prioritization, and regarding mechanisms for accessing funds.

Health Sector Expenditures and Financing

The General Budget of the Nation has three types of sources of income: funds from the Public Treasury (FF10—tax revenues, royalties, contributions of state-owned companies, and other revenue); public credit funds (FF20—loans received by the state to finance public investment expenses); and institutional funds (FF30—generated by the institutions and administered by the receiving entity, and the donations received by the government). The status of total expenditures on health between 2002 and 2004, and their impact on the national GDP, are shown in Table 5.

Per capita public expenditures on health have averaged, for the period under analysis, US$ 25, and private expenditures have averaged US$ 48. Of the private expenditures, approximately 88% to 90% are expenditures by households; the rest correspond to the prepaid drug companies authorized to do business by the Superintendency of Health (*61*).

During the 2002–2004 period, personnel services accounted for the highest proportion of the structure of total public sector health expenditures (between 59.4% and 61.2%), followed by drugs (between 18.4% and 22.2%) and investments (between 5.6% and 7.5%). Public funding increased from 29.7% of the total in 2002 to 33.1% in 2004 (*61*).

Technical Cooperation and External Financing

In 2003, Paraguay received, in the areas of health and population, total non-reimbursable cooperation in the amount of US$ 17,121,548, of which 80.7% represents multilateral cooperation (PAHO/WHO; the United Nations Population Fund, UNFPA; European Union, EU; and the United States Agency for International Development, USAID), and 19.3% represents bilateral cooperation (Canadian International Cooperation Agency, CIDA, and the Japanese International Cooperation Agency, JICA) (*62*); these funds represented 18.1% of the Ministry of Public Health and Social Welfare's budget. For 2004, the country received US$ 20,390,540, of which 73.9% was contributions from multilateral cooperation (Food and Agriculture Organization of the United Nations, FAO; PAHO/WHO; UNFPA; UNICEF; EU; and USAID) and 26.1% was from bilateral cooperation (CIDA and JICA), representing 20% of the Ministry of Public Health and Social Welfare's budget for that year. In 2005, Paraguay received US$ 15,087,795, of which 88.1% was from bilateral cooperation (Brazil, France, the United States, and Taiwan) and the rest was from multilateral cooperation (FAO and PAHO) (*63*), representing 15.9% of the Ministry of Public Health and Social Welfare's budget.

With regard to poverty reduction (*64*), Paraguay received, for 2003, a total of US$ 34,130,488, of which 42.5% was from multilateral cooperation (EU; the Organization of American States, OAS; the Inter-American Institute for Cooperation on Agriculture, IICA); and 57.5% was from bilateral cooperation (CIDA; Spanish Agency for International Cooperation, AECI; and Taiwan). For 2004, this amount increased to US$ 46,112,151, of which 60.5% was from multilateral cooperation (IICA, OAS, United Nations Development Program, EU, and PAHO/WHO), and 39.5% was from bilateral cooperation (CIDA, AECI, and Tai-

TABLE 5. Macroindicators of health expenditures, Paraguay, 2002–2004.

Item	2002	2003	2004
Expenditures of Central Administration (millions of Guaranis)	7,332,412	8,071,525	8,716,322
Total public expenditures (millions of Guaranis)	14,292,510	15,546,136	16,564,956
Total health expenditures (millions of Guaranis)	2,431,032	2,494,813	2,693,917
GDP (millions of Guaranis)	31,976,903	38,805,548	42,102,405
Total health expenditures/GDP (%)	7.8	6.6	6.5
Ministry of Public Health expenditures/GDP (%)	1.3	1.1	1.1
Institute of Public Welfare (IPS) expenditures/GDP (%)	1.0	1.1	1.3
Public expenditures on health/GDP (%)	2.6	2.2	2.3
Private expenditures on health/GDP (%)	5.2	4.4	4.3
Public expenditures on health/total public expenditures	5.8	5.9	6.7
Ministry of Public Health expenditures/ Expenditures of Central Administration (%)	5.8	5.1	5.4
Out-of-pocket expenditures/GDP (%)	4.5	3.7	3.6

Sources: Public Sector: Presupuesto obligado. SICO. Ministerio de Hacienda. Instituto de Previsión Social.
Private Sector: Dirección General de Estadísticas, Encuestas y Censos; Ministerio de Salud Pública y Bienestar Social; Banco Central de Paraguay.
Prepared by: Comité Interinstitucional de Cuentas de Salud. March 2006.

wan). Up until 2006, residuals were used from an Inter-American Development Bank loan for Reinforcement of Primary Care, reformulated to support Strengthening of the Health System, in the amount of US$ 21,587,201.

References

1. Paraguay, Secretaría Técnica de Planificación de la Presidencia, Dirección General de Estadísticas, Encuestas y Censos. Condiciones de vida de la población paraguaya según la encuesta de 2002. Fernando de la Mora; 2002. P. 38.
2. Transparencia Paraguay. Índice de transparencia, integridad y eficiencia: medición de la administración pública basada en elementos objetivos. Asunción; 2005.
3. United Nations Development Program. Informe nacional de desarrollo humano: Paraguay 2003. Asunción: UNDP; 2003.
4. Paraguay, Banco Central del Paraguay. Cuentas nacionales N° 40. Asunción; 2004.
5. Paraguay, Banco Central del Paraguay. Informe económico, abril 2005. Asunción; 2005.
6. United Nations. Common country assessment, Paraguay. 2005.
7. International Labor Organization. Políticas de empleo para superar la pobreza. Santiago de Chile; 2003.
8. Paraguay, Secretaría Técnica de Planificación de la Presidencia, Dirección General de Estadísticas, Encuestas y Censos. Encuesta Permanente de Hogares (EPH). Principales resultados 2003; 2004.
9. International Labor Organization, International Program to Eliminate Child Labor; United Nations Children's Fund. Seguimiento de indicadores sobre la niñez trabajadora de Paraguay. Asunción; 2003.
10. Paraguay, Secretaría Técnica de Planificación de la Presidencia, Dirección General de Estadísticas, Encuestas y Censos. II Censo Nacional Indígena de Población y Viviendas 2002. Pueblos Indígenas del Paraguay. Resultados finales. Fernando de la Mora; 2002.
11. Paraguay, Ministerio de Educación y Cultura, Dirección General de Planificación Educativa y Cultural. Análisis cuantitativo de la evolución educativa, 1990–2001. Asunción; 2004.
12. Paraguay, Secretaría Técnica de Planificación de la Presidencia, Dirección General de Estadísticas, Encuestas y Censos. Censo Nacional de Población y Viviendas 2002. Resultados finales. Fernando de la Mora; 2004.
13. Paraguay, Centro Paraguayo de Estudios de Población. Encuesta Nacional de Demografía y Salud Sexual y Reproductiva 2004. Asunción; 2005.
14. Paraguay, Ministerio de Salud Pública y Bienestar Social, Dirección de Planificación y Evaluación, Departamento de Bioestadística; 2006.
15. United Nations Development Program. Objetivos de desarrollo del milenio: informe del Paraguay 2005. Asunción; 2005. Available from: http://www.undp.org.py/rc/ODMPY2005.pdf.
16. Paraguay, Observatorio Paraguayo de Drogas. Plan nacional antidrogas 2001–2005. Secretaría Nacional Antidrogas; 2001.
17. World Health Organization; Centers for Disease Control and Prevention. Global Youth Tobacco Survey, 2003. (No. for Paraguay: 7,916).
18. Paraguay, Ministerio de Salud Pública y Bienestar Social, Dirección General de Programas de Salud. Comisión Nacional

Vigilancia Epidemiológica de la Salud Materna y Neonatal. Informe interno. Asunción; 2005.

19. Paraguay, Secretaría Técnica de Planificación de la Presidencia, Dirección General de Estadísticas, Encuestas y Censos. Características socio-demográficas de los adultos mayores en Paraguay. Asunción; 2005.

20. Paraguay, Secretaría Técnica de Planificación de la Presidencia, Dirección General de Estadísticas, Encuestas y Censos. Indicadores del mercado laboral en Paraguay EPH 2004. Asunción; 2005.

21. Paraguay, Instituto de Previsión Social. Información preliminar. [Information for the insured]. Asunción; 2006.

22. Petit JM. Relato especial sobre la venta de niños, la prostitución infantil y la utilización de niños en la pornografía. United Nations, Commission on Human Rights and Economic and Social Council; 2004.

23. Paraguay, Universidad Nacional de Asunción, Instituto de Investigación en Ciencias de la Salud. Situación de salud de la comunidad indígena del Chaco paraguayo, 2000. Informe técnico. Asunción; 2003.

24. Paraguay, Ministerio de Salud Pública y Bienestar Social, Dirección General de Vigilancia de la Salud, Servicio Nacional de Erradicación del Paludismo. Informes técnicos internos. Asunción; 2006.

25. Pan American Health Organization. Malaria in Paraguay: time series epidemiological data from 1998 to 2004. Available from: http://www.paho.org/english/AD/DPC/CD/mal-2005par.ppt.

26. Paraguay, Ministerio de Salud Pública y Bienestar Social, Centro Nacional de Transfusión Sanguínea. Unpublished. Asunción; 2006.

27. Paraguay, Ministerio de Salud Pública y Bienestar Social, Dirección General de Vigilancia de la Salud. Informe técnico. Asunción; 2006.

28. Pan American Health Organization; Ministerio de Salud Pública y Bienestar Social, Dirección General de Vigilancia de la Salud, Programa Ampliado de Inmunizaciones. Sistema de Vigilancia para la Eliminación del Sarampión. Asunción; 2006.

29. Paraguay, Ministerio de Salud Pública y Bienestar Social, Dirección General de Vigilancia de la Salud. Normas para el Programa Ampliado de Inmunizaciones. Asunción; 1996.

30. Paraguay, Ministerio de Salud Pública y Bienestar Social, Dirección General de Vigilancia de la Salud. Sistema información campaña de vacunación para la eliminación de rubella y CRS. Asunción; 2005.

31. Paraguay, Ministerio de Salud Pública y Bienestar Social, Dirección General de Vigilancia de la Salud, Programa Ampliado de Inmunizaciones, Laboratorio Central de Salud Pública. Informes técnicos varios. Asunción; 2006.

32. Paraguay, Ministerio de Salud Pública y Bienestar Social, Dirección General de Vigilancia de la Salud, Programa Nacional de Control de la Tuberculosis. Informes técnicos varios. Asunción; 2006.

33. World Health Organization. Global tuberculosis control: surveillance, planning, financing. WHO Report 2006. Geneva: WHO; 2006.

34. Pan American Health Organization; Ministerio de Salud Pública y Bienestar Social, Dirección General de Vigilancia de la Salud, Programa Nacional de Control de la Tuberculosis. Estudio sobre multidrogorresistencia. Washington, DC; 2003.

35. Paraguay, Ministerio de Salud Pública y Bienestar Social, Dirección General de Vigilancia de la Salud, Programa Nacional Control Lepra. Documentos internos. Asunción; 2005.

36. Pan American Health Organization; Ministerio de Salud Pública y Bienestar Social, Dirección General de Vigilancia de la Salud. Leprosy Elimination Monitoring (LEM). Asunción; 2003.

37. Paraguay, Ministerio de Salud Pública y Bienestar Social, Dirección General de Vigilancia de la Salud, Centro Antirrábico Nacional. Informes técnicos. Asunción; 2006.

38. World Organization for Animal Health. Handistatus II. Situación zoosanitaria plurianual.

39. Pan American Health Organization, Pan American Foot-and-Mouth Disease Center. Situación de los programas de erradicación de la fiebre aftosa: América del Sur; 1999–2003.

40. Paraguay, Secretaría Técnica de Planificación de la Presidencia, Dirección General Estadísticas, Encuestas y Censos. Encuesta Integrada de Hogares, 2000/2001. Fernando de la Mora; 2001.

41. Paraguay, Ministerio de Salud Pública y Bienestar Social, Dirección General de Programas de Salud, Instituto Nacional de Alimentación y Nutrición. Sistema de vigilancia alimentaria y nutricional. Asunción; 2005.

42. Sociedad Suramericana de Cardiología. Estudio de factores de riesgo coronario en Sudamérica (Argentina, Bolivia, Chile, Ecuador, Paraguay, Peru, Venezuela); 2005.

43. Paraguay, Ministerio de Salud Pública y Bienestar Social, Dirección General de Vigilancia de la Salud, Programa Nacional de Diabetes. Factores de riesgo para diabetes tipo 2 en niños y adolescentes. Asunción; 2001.

44. Pan American Health Organization. Health in the Americas. Washington, DC: PAHO; 2002. (Scientific publication 587; 2 vol).

45. Paraguay, Red Cross. Información del llamamiento internacional; 2002.

46. Paraguay, Ministerio de Salud Pública y Bienestar Social, Observatorio Nacional de Violencia y Lesiones de Causa Externa. Centro de Emergencias Médicas. Informe técnico. Asunción; 2006.

47. World Health Organization. Instrumento de evaluación para sistemas de salud mental. Preliminary report. Geneva: WHO; 2005.

48. Paraguay, Ministerio de Salud Pública y Bienestar Social, Centro Nacional de Toxicología. En: Plan de Acción Nacional de Salud Ambiental Infantil 2004–2008. OPS/OMS; 2004.

49. Paraguay. Ley N° 1.032/96 que crea el Sistema Nacional de Salud. Asunción; 1996.

50. Paraguay, Secretaría Técnica de Planificación de la Presidencia. Evaluación regional de los servicios de manejo de residuos sólidos municipales: informe de Paraguay. PAHO/WHO; 2004.

51. Paraguay. Ley N° 1.614/00: Ley General del Marco Regulatorio y Tarifario del Servicio Público de Provisión de Agua Potable y Alcantarillado Sanitario del Paraguay. Asunción; 2000.

52. FAOSTAT. Informe del servicio de estadísticas y análisis socioeconómicos; World Bank. World Development Indicators 2005.

53. Paraguay, Ministerio de Salud Pública y Bienestar Social. Plan de Acción Nacional de Salud Ambiental Infantil 2004–2008. PAHO/WHO; 2004.

54. Paraguay, Ministerio de Agricultura y Ganadería, Servicio Nacional de Calidad y Salud Animal. Informe sobre la situación del Programa de Erradicación de la Fiebre Aftosa en el país. Asunción; 2005.

55. Paraguay, Asociación Rural del Paraguay. Sistema de trazabilidad del Paraguay: reglamento. Asunción; 2005. Available from: http://www.arp.org.py.

56. Paraguay, Ministerio de Salud Pública y Bienestar Social, Dirección General de Vigilancia de la Salud, Dirección de Control de Profesiones y Establecimientos de Salud. Documento interno. Asunción; 2005.

57. Paraguay, Ministerio de Salud Pública y Bienestar Social, Dirección General de Recursos Humanos. Documento interno. Asunción; 2002.

58. Paraguay, Ministerio de Salud Pública y Bienestar Social, Dirección General de Recursos Humanos. Base de datos. Asunción; 2005.

59. Paraguay, Ministerio de Salud Pública y Bienestar Social, Dirección General de Recursos Humanos. Censo integral de funcionarios MSPBS, 2003. Asunción; 2004.

60. Paraguay, Ministerio de Salud Pública y Bienestar Social, Dirección General de Vigilancia Sanitaria. Documento interno. Asunción; 2006.

61. Paraguay, Comité Interinstitucional de Cuentas Nacionales. Informe preliminar. Asunción; 2006.

62. Paraguay, Secretaría Técnica de Planificación de la Presidencia. Cooperación técnica internacional no reembolsable. Ejecución acumulada a diciembre 2003. Asunción; 2004.

63. Paraguay, Secretaría Técnica de Planificación de la Presidencia. Cooperación técnica internacional no reembolsable. Informe preliminar. Datos parciales. Asunción; 2006.

64. Paraguay, Secretaría Técnica de Planificación de la Presidencia. Cooperación técnica internacional no reembolsable. Ejecución acumulada a junio 2004. Asunción; 2004.

PERU

1 Tumbes
2 Loreto
3 Amazonas
4 Piura
5 Lambayeque
6 Cajamarca
7 San Martín
8 La Libertad
9 Ancash
10 Huánuco
11 Ucayali
12 Pasco
13 Junín
14 Lima
15 Constitutional Province of El Callao
16 Madre de Dios
17 Huancavelica
18 Ayacucho
19 Apurímac
20 Ica
21 Cusco
22 Arequipa
23 Puno
24 Moquegua
25 Tacna

Colombia

Ecuador

Brazil

Lima

Bolivia

Chile

0   100   200 Miles

I n 2005, the Republic of Peru had a population of 27,219,264 inhabitants. The country has a land area of 1,285,215 km², distributed over three major geographic regions: the coast, the Andean highlands, and the Amazon jungle. It is politically divided into 25 departments (including the Constitutional Province of El Callao) and encompasses 194 provinces and 1,829 districts.

GENERAL CONTEXT AND HEALTH DETERMINANTS

Social, Political, and Economic Determinants

Peru strengthened its democratic process during 2000–2005, maintaining its economic stability and substantially increasing the country's fiscal revenue: its international reserves rose from US$ 8.8 billion to US$ 13.8 billion, while the country's fiscal deficit decreased from 3.2% of the gross domestic product (GDP) to 1.0% during that same period. One transcendental aspect of Peru's situation is the vast inequality in living conditions and welfare among population groups, among regions, and between rural and urban areas. In general, nearly all welfare indicators show that rural areas, indigenous populations, females, the jungle region, and the central and southern highlands are at a disadvantage.

Since 2002, the GDP has grown by more than 4.0%, and it reached 6.7% in 2005. This increase has raised the per capita GDP to more than US$ 2,000 per year (Figure 1). In 2005, Peru ranked 50 among the 180 member countries of the International Monetary Fund (in terms of the size of its economy, measured by GDP according to purchasing power parity) and was 97 in terms of per capita GDP (US$ 5,983) (1), placing it in the category of "middle income" countries.

Very careful financial management in Peru has resulted in continually low inflation rates (3.7% in 2000, 0.1% in 2001, 2.0% in 2002, 2.5% in 2003, 3.5% in 2004, and 1.5% in 2005). In addition, in spite of low levels of confidence in Government (below 10% in mid-2005), private and foreign investment continued to grow (from 14.9% of the GDP in 2002 to 15.7% in 2005) (2); foreign investment largely went to the primary sector of the economy, particularly mining, which, in conjunction with construction, has been one of the largest growth areas of the economy. However, this sound economic performance with its perceptible macroeconomic results has not necessarily translated into improved living conditions for the majority of the population in terms reducing poverty, inequality, and exclusion. From 1997 onward, in a sustained fashion, external public debt has accounted for more than 30% of the GDP with a slight trend toward growth, and interest on the debt has totaled 2.0% of the GDP.

Income is highly concentrated in Peru: while the 20% of the population with the highest income received 47.5% of national income, the 20% of the population with the lowest income received only 6%. The unequal distribution of income, expressed as a ratio between the highest and lowest quintiles, rose from 4.9 to 7.9 between 1997 and 2000 (3). The Gini index for income distribution by population deciles was 0.51 for 2003 (4); that same year, the monthly average national household income was 387.8 *nuevos soles*, ranging from 628.6 in metropolitan Lima to 138.4 in Huánuco.

Total poverty increased from de 48.4% in 2000 to 52.0% in 2004 and was greater in rural areas (73.6%). The percentage of people living in extreme poverty rose from 15.0% to 20.7% during that same period and was 42.5% in rural areas. In departments such as Huancavelica, poverty was 88.5% and extreme poverty 74.1% (4). These levels of poverty are similar to those recorded at the beginning of the 1990s.

The unemployment rate remained steady in urban areas at around 7.5% between 2001 and 2004. Unemployment increased during that same period in metropolitan Lima from 7.8% to 10.5%; underemployment also rose from 41.7% to 42.8% (5). A major labor phenomenon in Peru is the large proportion of the economically active population (55.0%) that works in the informal sector of the economy and that therefore has no access to social security, does not receive a steady income, and has no provisions for retirement. Both unemployment and underemployment are greater among women. In 2004, unemployment affected 9.4% of men and 12.0% of women, and underemployment 35.9% of men and 52.5% of women (5). One reason that unemployment and underemployment have remained high in spite of the sustained economic growth over the last five years is that growth has primarily occurred in sectors such as mining, which generate few employment posts.

In 2002, the National Agreement—which draws together the country's main political parties, churches, and business and worker organizations, as well as the Consultation Committee for the Fight against Poverty—defined 31 governmental policies that included goals related to the Millennium Development Goals (MDGs), regardless of whether direct reference was made to them. These objectives included reduction of poverty, promotion

FIGURE 1. Per capita gross domestic product, Peru, 1982–2004.

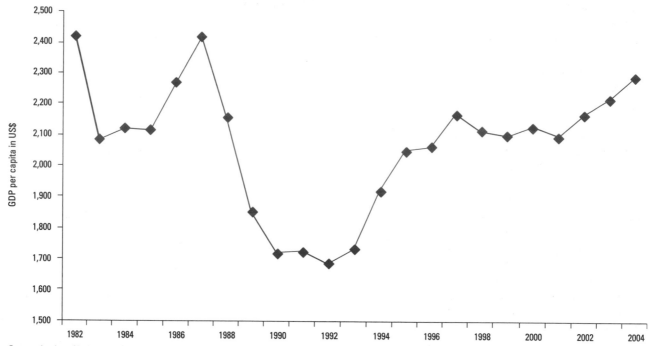

Source: Instituto Nacional de Estadística e Informática, Dirección Nacional de Cuentas Nacionales. Preliminary data for 2002 and 2003. 2004 data estimated by Instituto Cuánto.

of equal opportunities without discrimination, universal access to free quality public education, universal access to health services and social security, promotion of safe food and nutrition, sustainable development and environmental management, and development in infrastructure and housing. These are governmental policies, which the signing organizations have committed themselves to carrying out, and each has goals for the next 10 years.

In 2004, the Research Center of the Universidad del Pacífico in Lima created a model to predict fulfillment of the MDGs in Peru. According to this model, growth policies, redistribution policies, and specific social policies must be merged to meet the MDGs. With an annual average economic growth rate of 5%, fulfillment of the goals would require annual transfers of resources of close to 1.4% of the GDP (0.75% through income redistribution and 0.65% for specific social policies). The primary specific sectoral policies are to increase access to drinking water and basic sanitation services, coverage of health services for mothers and children under 5, investment in public complementary child feeding programs, the educational levels of mothers, the number of births in which care is provided by qualified health professionals, the number of prenatal exams by qualified health professionals, and the quality of the infrastructure and care received at health facilities. This would make it possible to meet all the objectives associated with the first five MDGs, with the exception of the prevalence of caloric deficit. That goal will not be reached even

with annual sustained economic growth rates of 7% because of its vast scope (32.5% during 2003–2004) (6).

In 2004, the illiteracy rate was 11.6%, with a wide gap between men and women (5.8% and 17.2%, respectively) as well as in poor areas with a high percentage of campesino and Quechua-speaking populations, such as Apurímac, Ayacucho, Cusco, and Huancavelica, where these percentages exceed 6% for men and 25% for women. Preschool attendance for children between 3 and 5 years old was 50%; primary school attendance among children between 6 and 11 years old was 90.5%, and secondary school attendance among 12- to 17-year-olds was to 67.6% (68.3% for men and 66.8% for women). The average number of years of study for the population 15 years and older was 9.1 years: 10.2 in urban areas and 6.5 in rural areas, and 9.3 among men and 8.9 among women (7). This is compounded by quality issues in state education establishments, which seriously limit the possibilities of the country's development and particularly that of the poorest populations (8). Investment in the education sector totals 16% of public spending.

Air quality is deficient in the metropolitan areas of Lima, Callao, and Arequipa and in the industrial urban centers of Chimbote, Ilo, and Cerro de Pasco, due to industrial development without adequate pollution control and the increase and poor maintenance of automobiles in circulation. Measurements taken in Lima and Callao in 2000 found an annual average concentration of total suspended particles greater than 200 $\mu g/m^3$; in addition, annual average concentrations of nitrogen dioxide, sulfur dioxide, and lead, measured in the center of Lima, surpassed WHO-recommended levels (*9*).

Peru is exposed to such natural disasters as earthquakes, volcanic activity, landslides, floods, droughts, tsunamis, and the El Niño phenomenon. It is also subject to accidents caused by humans, particularly fires and chemical spills.

Demographics, Mortality, and Morbidity

The population of Peru was 27,219,264 inhabitants in 2005 (*10*), and it is estimated to reach 30 million by 2010 (*11*). The Peruvian population has almost doubled over the last 30 years, even though the total growth rate has decreased from 23.8 per 1,000 inhabitants during 1980–1985 to 14.9 during 2000–2005. This has been the result of the reduction in the total fertility rate from 4.7 to 2.8 children per woman during this same period. During the 2000–2005 period, the birth rate was 23.3, and the mortality rate was 6.2 per 1,000 population. The decrease in overall and child mortality contributed to increased life expectancy at birth from 61.6 to 69.8 years during 1980–2005. During the 2000–2005 period, life expectancy at birth was 67.3 for men and 72.4 for women (*11*).

Between the censuses of 1993 and 2005, the percentage of people under 15 years of age decreased from 37.0% to 31.1%, even though the absolute numbers rose from 8,155,376 to 8,455,390. Those over the age of 65 went from 4.6% to 6.2% (1,026,119 to 1,693,657) (Figure 2).

Migration, both internal and external, is a major demographic phenomenon in the country and the result of industrialization, deteriorated living conditions in rural areas, and, during the 1980s, the internal war and the profound economic crisis that produced hyperinflation. The departments that traditionally lose population are located in the southern highlands (Huancavelica, Ayacucho, Apurímac, Cusco, and Puno); they are the poorest and have the highest percentage of rural population. In 2001, 37.6% of the population living in Lima were immigrants: 36.2% from Tacna, 28.4% from Arequipa (located on the coast and more industrialized), 38.2% from Madre de Dios, and 32.9% from Ucayali (both located in the Amazon jungle) (*12*). In terms of international migration, it is estimated that 141,000 people left Peru between 1975 and 1985 and that 370,000 left between 1990 and 1995. The improved economic situation and defeat of subversive groups at the beginning of the 1990s are reversing this trend, and it is estimated that the exodus of Peruvians dropped to 50,000 between 2000 and 2005 (*11*).

In 2005, 72.6% of the Peruvian population lived in urban areas. During 2000–2005, mortality and birth rates and the total fertility rate were higher in rural areas (7.9, 31.0, and 4.6 per 1,000, respectively) than in urban areas (5.5, 20.3, and 2.4) (*11*). While the reproductive growth rate is higher in rural areas than in urban areas (23.1 compared to 14.9 per 1,000 population), there is less total population growth (9.8 compared to 16.9) be-

FIGURE 2. Population structure, by age and sex, Peru, 1981, 1993, and 2005.

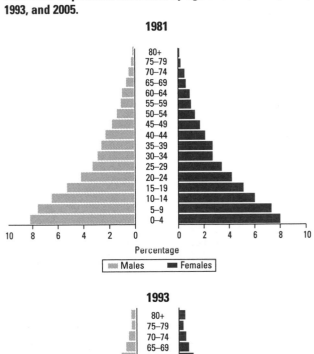

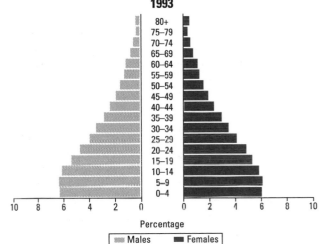

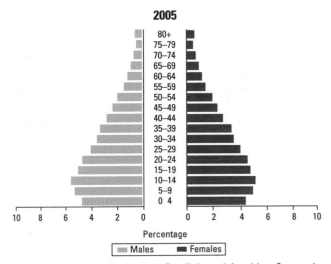

Source: Peru, Instituto Nacional de Estadística e Informática, Censos de Población y Vivienda.

TABLE 1. Leading causes of mortality, Peru, 2004.

	Causes of mortality (PAHO List 6/67)	Mortality rate per 100,000 population
1	Acute respiratory infections	68.0
2	Ischemic heart diseases	25.7
3	Cerebrovascular diseases	24.3
4	Septicemia, except for neonatal	21.5
5	Cirrhosis and certain other chronic liver diseases	21.4
6	Hypertensive diseases	16.9
7	Malignant stomach tumors	15.6
8	Respiratory disorders originating in the perinatal period	14.7
9	Tuberculosis	13.2
10	Diabetes mellitus	12.3

Source: Adapted from Peru, Ministerio de Salud, mortality database.

TABLE 2. Selected sociodemographic characteristics and mortality, Southern Highlands departments, Lima, and Callao, Peru.

	Peru	Southern Highlands	Lima and Callao
Poverty (%)	52.0	70.0	35.7
Rural population (%)	27.8	56.2	0.4
Quechua or Aymara as native language (%)	19.5	71.2	10.1
Public drinking water (%)	64.4	42.3	82.4
Elimination of excreta via a public system (%)	50.9	23.2	80.2
Population under 15 years of age (%)	31.1	36.3	26.0
Total percentage of the population	100.0	14.7	32.1
Mortality rate[a]	6.2	11.2	4.5
Mortality rate for communicable diseases[a]	124.6	228.9	91.3
Mortality rate for certain diseases originating in the perinatal period[a]	34.4	61.1	16.8
Mortality rate due to external causes[a]	66.1	158.2	30.5

[a]Rate per 100,000 population.
Source: Adapted from Peru, Ministerio de Salud, mortality database.

cause of internal migration. The percentage of the population under 15 years of age is greater in rural areas than in urban areas (39.9% and 29.4%), while the reverse is true for those over 64 years of age (4.7% and 5.4%, respectively).

During 2000–2005 there was a 7-year difference in life expectancy at birth between the urban and rural populations (73.2 and 66.9, respectively), due to higher mortality rates, particularly child mortality, in rural areas (24.2 per 100,000 urban and 49.2 per 100,000 rural).

With regard to the leading causes of death, it should be mentioned that there is a serious problem in the Peruvian health information system with regard to low coverage of death records (55% in 2004, of which 88% were certified by physicians). Between 1990 and 2000, there was a significant reduction in mortality[1] from communicable diseases, from 236.2 to 124.6 per

100,000; likewise mortality from certain diseases originating in the perinatal period decreased from 53.8 to 34.4, while deaths from neoplasms or tumors increased from 96.2 to 108.4, as did deaths from external causes (from 59.0 to 66.1). While chronic diseases predominated among the main causes of death in 2004, acute respiratory infections were the leading cause, and certain other communicable diseases had high mortality rates (Table 1).

Analysis of mortality by sex shows that acute respiratory infections were the leading cause of death for both males and females (71.3 and 64.7). Ischemic heart diseases had a higher mortality rate among men than women (29.7 and 21.7), as did cirrhosis and other chronic diseases of the liver (27.5 and 15.1), tuberculosis (17.1 and 9.2), and overland transportation accidents (15.1 and 5.5). Malignant uterine tumors (cervix, uterus, unspecified part) were the sixth leading cause of death among women (15.6 per 100,000), and malignant prostate tumors were the fourteenth leading cause of death among men (12.4 per 100,000).

Mortality profiles in Peru are very heterogeneous; departments in the southern highlands—with a high proportion of

---

[1]Mortality rates for groups and subgroups from PAHO List 6/67 were obtained by using the estimation procedures described in *Health Statistics from the Americas. 1992 Edition.*

TABLE 3. Leading causes of death, Southern Highlands, Peru, 2000.

	Causes of mortality (List 6/67 PAHO)	Mortality rate per 100,000 population
1	Acute respiratory infections	147.9
2	Cirrhosis and certain other chronic liver diseases	51.0
3	Cardiac insufficiency	46.5
4	Nutritional deficiencies and anemia	44.8
5	Appendicitis, hernia of the abdominal cavity, and intestinal obstruction	44.2
6	Cerebrovascular diseases	41.3
7	Respiratory disorders originating during the perinatal period	31.3
8	Septicemia, except for neonatal	26.2
9	Land transportation accidents	25.9
10	Malignant stomach tumors	25.0

Source: Adapted from Peru, Ministerio de Salud, mortality database.

TABLE 4. Leading Causes of Mortality in Lima and Callao, Peru, 2000.

	Causes of mortality (List 6/67 PAHO)	Mortality rate per 100,000 population
1	Acute respiratory infections	41.0
2	Ischemic heart diseases	21.1
3	Cerebrovascular diseases	20.2
4	Tuberculosis	18.1
5	Malignant neoplasms of stomach	14.5
6	Hypertensive diseases	12.6
7	Diabetes mellitus	12.4
8	Cirrhosis and certain other chronic liver diseases	12.2
9	Septicemia, except for neonatal	11.8
10	Overland transportation accidents	10.1

Source: Adapted from Peru, Ministerio de Salud, mortality database.

people of Quechua or Aymara origin and high levels of poverty and rural areas, such as Apurímac, Ayacucho, Cusco, Huancavelica, and Puno—have higher mortality rates from communicable diseases, certain diseases originating in the perinatal period, and external causes compared with Lima and Callao—areas with greater industrial development, lower poverty rates, and better access to basic services (Table 2).

In 2000, the leading causes of death in Lima and Callao were chronic diseases, while in the southern highlands they were communicable diseases, nutritional deficiencies, and problems related to accessing health services (Tables 3 and 4). Acute respiratory infections were the leading cause of death in the southern highlands as well as in Lima and Callao, but to very different extents. The risk of dying from this cause was 3.6 times greater in the southern highlands. Transportation accidents in the southern highlands, the ninth leading cause of death, were generally due to the fall or overturn of interprovincial transportation vehicles carrying passengers, which occurs because of the poor state of roadways and of the vehicles.

It also bears mentioning that 20% of the poorest population accounted for 50% of deaths from nutritional deficiencies and anemia (Gini of 0.43); 40% of deaths from intestinal infectious diseases (Gini of 0.38), and 62% from appendicitis, abdominal hernias, and intestinal obstruction with no mention of hernia (Gini of 0.57) as a result of unstable living conditions and limited access to quality health services.

HEALTH OF POPULATION GROUPS

Children under 5 Years Old

In 2005, children under 5 years old constituted 9.45% of the population (2,572,220). Chronic malnutrition is still high among this group, and there was no significant change between 1996 (25.8%) (13) and 2004 (24.1%), with a marked difference between urban and rural areas (10.1% and 39.0%, respectively) (14). In 2000, acute malnutrition affected 0.9% of children under 5 years old, although it was 3.0% in Ayacucho (15).

Infant mortality decreased from 33 per 1,000 live births in 2000 to 23 in 2005 (14,15), although there were broad differences among departments, from 84 in Cusco to 17 in metropolitan Lima (14), and a Gini index of 0.20 (Figure 3). There are also differences according to the mother's level of education (an indicator of the family's socioeconomic situation); in 2000, infant

FIGURE 3. Infant mortality, Peru, 2000.

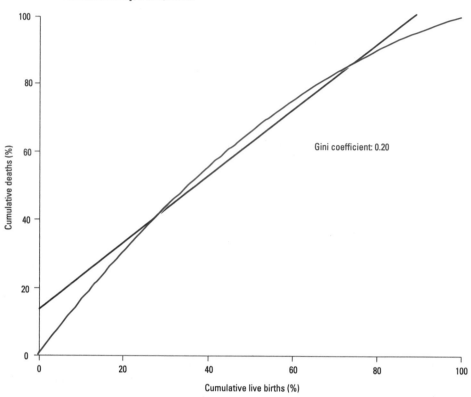

Gini coefficient: 0.20

Source: Peru, Instituto Nacional de Estadística e Informática; United Nations Development Program. *Human Development Report.* Peru 2002.

mortality among children of women with no schooling was 73, and 20 among those with higher education (*14*).

The child mortality rate decreased from 47 to 31 per 1,000 live births between 2000 and 2005 (*14,15*), but there were also vast differences among departments (108 in Cusco and 23 in metropolitan Lima) (*15*). The reduction in infant and child mortality was primarily due to the decrease in deaths from communicable diseases, from 2,467.5 per 100,000 children under 1 year in 1990 to 712.2 in 2004 (*16*). In 2004, the leading causes of death among children under 1 year old were respiratory diseases specific to the perinatal period (669.8 per 100,000 children under 1 year old); acute respiratory infections (448.3); delayed fetal growth, fetal malnutrition, short gestation, and low birthweight (402.1); and bacterial sepsis in newborns (287.0). The leading cause, respiratory diseases specific to the perinatal period, is related to low coverage of birthing care in health facilities and lack of immediate attention for the newborn, including resuscitation of children who are not responsive at birth (*17*); the third leading cause has its roots in maternal malnutrition (25.4% prevalence of anemia among women between 15 and 49 years of age) (*15*).

Exclusive breast-feeding is one of the main strategies that the Ministry of Health has been promoting in recent years. Accord-

ing to available data (*14*), 97.9% of children under 5 years old have been breast-fed at some point: 87.4% during the first day of life, although 27.4% received some type of feeding before breast-feeding. Exclusive breast-feeding in children under 6 months of age was 63.9%, and the average duration was 3.9 months.

Children 5–9 Years Old

Children between 5 and 9 years of age represent 10.6% of the Peruvian population. In 2004, the mortality rate for this group was 11.3 per 100,000; the leading causes of death were acute respiratory infections (12.2 per 100,000), undefined events (10.3), land transportation accidents (8.6), leukemia (6.3), and septicemia (5.8) (*16*).

Adolescents 10–14 Years Old and 15–19 Years Old

Adolescents 10 to 19 years old represent 21.2% of the total population. Among those between 10 and 14 years of age, external causes were the leading causes of death in 2004 (21.1 per 100,000), followed by communicable diseases (11.5). Death is greater in males than in females for acute respiratory infections (5.4 and 4.1, respectively), leukemia (4.3 and 3.0), land transportation accidents (6.2 and 1.2), and drowning and accidental submersion (2.8 and 1.0) (16).

Among adolescents between 15 and 19 years of age, the mortality rate due to external causes was double that of communicable diseases and triple that of neoplasms (35.4, 15.1, and 11.7, respectively) in 2004. The five leading causes of death among males were undefined events (14.5), land transportation accidents (8.9), tuberculosis (6.5), acute respiratory infections (6.3), and accidental firing of firearms (5.4); among females, the leading causes were undefined events (5.3), acute respiratory infections (3.9), leukemia (2.9), accidental poisoning by (and exposure to) harmful substances (2.5), and land transportation accidents (2.4). Complications of pregnancy, birth, and puerperium (2.3) were the sixth leading cause of death among females in this age group (16).

In 2004, 12.7% of adolescent women were already mothers or were pregnant, a very similar situation to that in 2000 (13.0%), with a much higher percentage in rural areas than in urban areas (20.3% and 9.5%, respectively) and much higher among adolescents in the lowest income quintile (27.0%) than in the highest income quintile (3.3%) (14).

Adults 20–59 Years Old

This group makes up 50.1% of the Peruvian population (approximately 13.5 million people). The total fertility rate dropped from 2.9 children per woman during 1997–2000 to 2.4 during 2001–2004; during the latter period, the figures were 3.6 in rural areas and 2.0 in urban areas (14). The highest fertility rates were among women between 25 and 29 years of age (115 births per 1,000 women) and between 20 and 24 (113). The interval between pregnancies increased from 37 to 43 months between 2000 and 2004; the interval was lower for uneducated women (27 months) and higher for women with higher education (52 months). The age of initial procreation was higher in urban areas (23.3 years) than in rural areas (20.2) and higher still in metropolitan Lima (24.2).

In 2004, 98.5% of all women between 15 and 49 years of age in domestic partnerships had knowledge of some modern contraceptive method, but only 44.7% used any, which represented a slight decrease from 2000 (50.4%); in contrast, the use of traditional methods increased from 17.5% to 22.0% (14).

Maternal mortality decreased from 265 per 100,000 live births in 1996 to 185 in 2000 (13,15); however, during the latter year it exceeded 300 per 100,000 live births in departments such as Puno (361), Huancavelica (302), and Ayacucho (301), and it was less than 100 in Arequipa (96), Tacna (87), Lima (52), and Ica (48) (18). The leading causes of maternal death were postpartum hemorrhaging (33.4%), eclampsia (11.6%), complications of labor and delivery (10.7%), and abortion (6.2%).

In 2004, mortality from external causes was four times higher among men than women (101.8 and 24.2 per 100,000) and from communicable diseases it was twice as high (80.3 and 39.1), while death from neoplasms was higher among women (83.8 and 57.3). The leading causes of death among adult men were cirrhosis and other chronic liver diseases (25.8), HIV/AIDS (24.9), acute respiratory infections (20.7), tuberculosis (19.7), and overland transportation accidents (18.2). Among women, the leading causes were malignant tumors of the uterus (17.9), acute respiratory infections (12.9), malignant breast tumors (11.5), cerebrovascular diseases (11.2), and tuberculosis (9.7) (16).

Older Adults 60 Years Old and Older

Of the total Peruvian population, 8.8% are 60 years old or older; in 2004, acute respiratory infections were the leading cause of death among men and women (555.1 and 530.1 per 100,000, respectively) in this group, and ischemic heart diseases ranked second (309.0 and 226.8). Among men, cerebrovascular diseases (237.5), cirrhosis and other chronic liver diseases (197.0), and hypertensive diseases (180.6) held third, fourth, and fifth places, while for women these were hypertensive diseases (181.1), septicemia (137.3), and malignant stomach tumors (130.1) (16).

The Family

In 2004, 57.8% of the total of families in the country were nuclear families, 23.6% were extended, 6.2% were blended, 7.6% were single person, and 4.8% were homes with no core structure. Women headed 21.1% of families, with a higher percentage in urban areas (23.9%) than in rural areas (16.0%) and a higher percentage in nonpoor homes (24.1%) than in poor ones (17.3%). The majority of single-parent families were headed by women (78.7%). Poverty levels in single-parent families were similar for men (39.2%) and women (39.8%), even though there was a significant difference in rural areas (59.9% and 67.0%) (7).

Workers

Between 1996 and 2001, the percentage of children and adolescents between 6 and 17 years old who worked increased from 20.8% to 28.6% (19, 20). In 2001, of the total of children between 6 and 17 years of age who worked, 54.0% were male, and 42.4% were between 6 and 11 years old. Working children between 6 and 13 years of age were concentrated in nontechnical activities and family businesses and received little or no remuneration. Among adolescents between 14 and 17 years old, 48.7% worked as manual laborers, 11.6% as vendors in kiosks and markets, 8.6% in domestic labor, and 7.0% were weavers, spinners, or mechanical assistants; 70% of working adolescents lived in rural areas. The Ministry of Labor and Employment Promotion developed the National Plan for Children and Adolescents; its goal is to eliminate the worst forms of child labor, including, among others, in small-scale mining (in which 50,000 children and adolescents work), garbage picking, small-scale brick making, domestic labor in outside homes, gathering of coca leaves, and working in bars.

The main health problems facing workers were the lack of protection at work and low coverage for occupational health services. In 2003, social security covered 50.2% of all workers (66.3% from the formal sector, and 10.6% from micro-businesses—with up to five employees) (21). There is little information about work accidents and occupational illnesses, but according to social security reports, in 2002, there were 16,914 work accidents, 60% of them in Lima. The highest mortality from work accidents occurred in the mining industry, with 68 per 100,000 mining workers; it is followed by construction (58), transportation (37), and industry (14) (22).

Persons with Disabilities

There is little information about this population group, and available data differ a great deal. The 1993 Population Census found that people with some form of disability represented 1.3% of the total population. That same year, another study stated that 13.1% of the population had some form of handicap, 31.3% some disability, and 45.4% some impairment (23). The percentage of people with disabilities is higher in urban areas than in rural areas (36.3% and 16.4%, respectively). The primary disabilities included the side effects of poliomyelitis and the loss, or loss of use of, lower or upper extremities (28%); blindness (21%); deafness (14%); mental retardation (12%); mental disorders (10%); and muteness (7%). In 2005, according to the preliminary results of the Continuous Survey of the Population Census, 8.7% of the population had some form of disability, whether it was visual, verbal, auditory, motor, or cognitive; this percentage was greater in metropolitan Lima (10.9%) than in rural areas (8.0%) and other urban areas (7.6%) (24).

HEALTH CONDITIONS AND PROBLEMS

COMMUNICABLE DISEASES

Vector-borne Diseases

It is estimated that 13 million people live in areas at risk of **malaria** transmission (1.2 million in high-risk areas); in 2005, a total of 87,699 malaria cases were reported, a significant decrease from the 247,229 cases reported in 1998, although the El Niño phenomenon of 1997 and 1998 must be taken into consideration. Reported cases came from the Amazon jungle and the northern coast; the former is a very wet and rainy area nearly all year long, and the latter is a desert area, but with rice plantations that require large amounts of water, making them suitable places for the vector to reproduce. Seventeen percent of malaria cases were caused by *Plasmodium falciparum*. Mortality is low in Peru, and four deaths were reported in 2005.

In terms of **dengue**, there are 10 million people living in cities infested with *Aedes aegypti*; these cities are located on the northern coast and in the jungle. There are four dengue virus serotypes in Peru. There was an outbreak in 2001 on the northern coast, and 23,329 cases were reported, of which 250 were **hemorrhagic dengue**. In 2005, a total of 7,360 cases were reported, 926 of them confirmed; the same year there was an outbreak for the first time in the northern zone of the city of Lima (with 813 cases), which lasted from March to April. During that outbreak, serotype 3 was isolated, and entomological surveys found the vector in most of the districts in northern Lima and in two southern districts.

It was estimated that 1.5 million people live in areas at risk for the transmission of **Chagas' disease**, in the departments of Ica, Arequipa, Moquegua, and Tacna. Prevalence in blood banks in these areas was 0.8% in 2003. In the city of Arequipa, which has a population of approximately 1 million inhabitants, where the vector exists and the disease is transmitted, a plan is being implemented to eliminate *Triatoma infestans*, using funds from the Arequipa regional government and with international cooperation.

Leishmaniasis is widespread in the mountain and jungle areas of the country. In Peru, there are two clinical forms of leishmaniasis, cutaneous and the mucocutaneous; the latter is found only in the Amazon jungle. In 2005, a total of 7,127 cases were reported, 95.3% of which were cutaneous, and 4.7% of which were mucocutaneous; 70% of the reported cases originated in Amazonas, Madre de Dios, Cajamarca, and Cusco.

Between 2001 and 2005, there were 226 reported cases of **yellow fever** (30, 42, 12, 67, and 75, respectively). A massive universal vaccination campaign was initiated in 2004 in endemic departments and in those from which workers traveled to the jungle during seasonal harvest and planting; 90% coverage was achieved.

Vaccine-preventable Diseases

Morbidity and mortality from vaccine preventable diseases remained low during 2001–2005, due to high vaccination coverage obtained, in spite of the reduction between 2000 and 2004 in coverage for DPT3 (diphtheria, pertussis, tetanus) (from 98% to 91%), OPV3 (oral polio vaccine) (from 93% to 91%), BCG (bacillus Calmette–Guérin) (from 93% to 92%), and measles vaccine (from 97% to 86%) (25). In 2004, there were 1,580 reported cases of **whooping cough**, and 4 cases of **neonatal tetanus**; the last case of **measles** was confirmed in 2000. Peru has remained free of acute **poliomyelitis**, and neonatal tetanus has been eliminated as a public health problem. In 2004, in spite of high national coverage, there were still departments without optimal coverage. For example, Ucayali had coverage of 70.2% for DPT3, 69.4% for OPV3, and 86.2% for the measles vaccine.

The General Law on Vaccines was enacted in June 2003 and it states that vaccination activities are mandatory and that funds allocated for this purpose should be flexible. Peru has made the pentavalent vaccine universal for children under 1 year old; this vaccine has been part of the vaccine scheme since 2004. There is also a proposal to include boosters with the DPT and measles-rubella vaccines in the vaccine scheme. An intense **rubella** outbreak occurred during 2005–2006 with more than 5,000 cases, as well as the presence of **congenital rubella syndrome** (CRS). In 2006, a massive vaccination campaign was initiated among men and women to eliminate rubella and congenital rubella syndrome.

Intestinal Infectious Diseases

There was a 15% rate of prevalence of **diarrhea** in children under 5 during the 2 weeks before the demographic and family health survey in 2000 as well as in 2004 (*14,15*). Although intestinal infectious diseases are not a leading cause of death at the national level (49.8 per 100,000 children under 5), they are in several departments in the Amazon jungle, such as Madre de Dios (202.6), Ucayali (153.7), and Amazonas (144.1), and in the poorest departments such as Puno (113.9) and Huancavelica (89.8); in Lima and Callao, rates are 11.5 and 9.8, respectively (*16*).

Chronic Communicable Diseases

In 2005, 30,226 new cases of **tuberculosis (TB)** were identified (109.7 per 100,000 inhabitants), representing a decrease from 2000 when 34,280 cases were identified (133.6 per 100,000 inhabitants). In 2005, 668 patients were diagnosed with TB/HIV coinfection (2.4 per 100,000 inhabitants); that same year the rate of relapse was 11.6%, and the percentage of failure to respond to first-line drugs was 2.8%.

Between 2001 and 2005, 8,561 cases of multidrug resistant tuberculosis (MDR TB) were diagnosed and treated. As of 2004, the cure rate was less than 40%, so beginning in 2005, new rules were established for caring for these patients, which incorporate a highly efficient drug regimen. This measure is expected to raise the cure rate to 85% in 2007, and, beginning in 2008, to reduce the annual MDR TB rate by 5%. During the last quarter of 2005, the third National Survey on Resistance of *Mycobacterium tuberculosis* was carried out; the second survey was completed in 1999 and found MDR TB in 3.0% of new cases and in 12.3% of people who had been treated previously.

In 2002, the prevalence of **leprosy** was 0.03 per 10,000 population. Eighty-three new cases were reported between 2003 and 2005 (34, 20, and 29, respectively). Of the 29 cases reported in 2005, 20 were multibacillary and 9 were paucibacillary; 2 were in children under 15, and 12 were in females. All cases originated in the jungle (Loreto and Ucayali).

Acute Respiratory Infections

These infections are one of the leading causes of morbidity and are the leading cause of death. In 2004, 17.0% of children under 5 had some episode of this disease during the 2 weeks before the survey; the percentage was higher among children in the poorest quintile (22%) than among those in the wealthiest (15%) (*14*). That same year, the mortality rate for the entire population was 68.0 per 100,000 population, but it was 7 times higher among

children under 1 year old (483.3) and 11 times higher among people over 64 years old (722.2). The highest mortality rates were observed in the poorest departments, such as Ucayali (298.4), Apurímac (290.4), and Puno (278.9), while rates were 82.5 in Lima and 69.3 in Tacna.

HIV/AIDS and Other Sexually Transmitted Infections

As of December 2005, a total of 18,117 cases of AIDS had been reported in Peru. It is estimated that there are 70,000 people with HIV, and 7,000 of them have progressed to the AIDS phase. The average age of the reported cases was 31 years. The ratio of men to women with AIDS has continuously and progressively declined from 13.3:1 in 1990 to 2.8:1 in 2005. In 97% of the cases, AIDS was transmitted sexually; transmission was vertical in 2% of the cases, and parenteral in 1% (*26*). In 2002, HIV seroprevalence among carriers between 15 and 24 years of age was 0.21% (*27*) and, depending on the study, HIV prevalence among men who have sex with other men varied from 11% to 18%. A population sample study was carried out in 2002 of those between 18 and 29 years of age, in 24 cities with more than 50,000 inhabitants, with the exceptions of Lima and Callao. The primary findings showed an HIV prevalence rate of 0.4% among men and 0.1% among women. Twelve percent of the men had had sex with other men. Twenty-four percent of men used a condom during their last casual sexual relation with a woman, and 32% did so during their last same-sex encounter. The prevalence of **syphilis** was similar among men and women (1.1%), and the prevalence of **chlamydia** was higher among women (4.0% and 6.8%, respectively), as was **gonorrhea** (0.3% and 0.8%) (*28*).

Peru obtained funding in 2003 from the Global Fund to Fight AIDS, Tuberculosis, and Malaria for the project Strengthening the Prevention and Control of AIDS and Tuberculosis in Peru. The majority of the funding for the HIV/AIDS component of the project was allocated to provide antiretroviral treatment. Before the project, fewer than 2,000 people received this treatment (the majority of them through social security). As of December 2005, treatment had been provided to 7,075 people. Starting in 2006, the Ministry of Health (MINSA) financed the purchase of antiretroviral treatments for people not affiliated with social security.

Zoonoses

There are active pockets of the **plague** in extremely poor areas, like the departments of Cajamarca, Piura, and Lambayeque. Two cases were reported in 2004, and five in 2005. Elimination of these pockets will depend on constructing and maintaining small-scale silos to store agricultural harvests and on improving housing and living conditions among the rural population, with the support of local governments.

Anthrax is endemic in several areas along Peru's coast, and its presence in humans is associated with handling infected animals. During 2003–2005, 136 cases were reported in the departments of Lima (65), Ica (43), Piura (18), and Tacna (10).

Human **brucellosis** is generally caused by consuming unpasteurized cheeses contaminated with *Brucella melitensis*. There were 5,397 cases diagnosed during 2002–2005 (2,450 in 2002, 1,358 in 2003, 1,108 in 2004, and 481 in 2005); the cities of Lima and Callao had the most cases. There is still no mechanism for learning the true magnitude of the problem nor how to control it, which must include the participation of goat ranchers, the milk industry, and consumers.

Since 2001, there had been no reported cases of human **rabies** transmitted by dog bites until 2005, when a human death was reported from this disease in the Department of Puno. There is a declining trend in canine rabies: in 2004, there were 24 cases, and in 2005, there were 22. The National Rabies Control Program bases this success on community education and information about the risk of contracting rabies, on timely and universally available access to preventative drugs before and after exposure, and to improved coverage of canine vaccination programs stemming from intensive vaccination campaigns from 25.5% in 2002 to 49.1% in 2004. On the other hand, outbreaks of wild rabies transmitted by vampire bats have been reported in indigenous communities in Amazonia: eight cases in 2004 (Amazonas) and seven in 2005 (four in Amazonas and three in Loreto).

Peru has made progress in controlling **foot-and-mouth disease** with the objective of eliminating it. Since October 2000, there had been no incidence of this disease, until 2004, when there was an outbreak caused by the type O virus. The outbreak was brought under control and the World Organization for Animal Health has certified 10 departments in southern Peru as being free of this disease. This will facilitate free trade of South American camelids and other agricultural products important to the rural economy and society.

NONCOMMUNICABLE DISEASES

Metabolic and Nutritional Diseases

The highest mortality rates from anemia and nutritional deficiency, in both the general population and among children under 5 years old, are in the country's poorest departments such as Huancavelica (72.5 per 100,000 inhabitants, and 168.8 per 100,000 children under 5, respectively), Huanuco (22.2 and 114.8), Ucayali (53.8 and 156.8), Puno (40.8 and 69.9), and Apurímac (31.9 and 45.2), while Lima had the lowest rates (4.9 and 9.4, respectively).

In 2004, 32.5% of the Peruvian population suffered from caloric deficit (28.6% of the urban population and 39.7% of the rural population). The poorest departments also had the highest percentages of people suffering from caloric deficit—for example, Huancavelica (63.5%), Huanuco (48.3%), and Puno (44.3%) (7).

In 2000, the percentage of children under 5 suffering from acute **malnutrition** was 0.9%, with the highest rate among children between 12 and 15 months of age (1.9%). That same year,

chronic malnutrition affected 25.4% of children under 5, and this rate was more than 30% after 16 months of age. The latter type of malnutrition affected boys and girls equally, although there was a significant difference according to area of residence: higher in rural areas (40.2%) than in urban areas (13.4%). Since this problem is associated with poverty, departments such as Huancavelica, Cusco, and Apurímac, where more than 70% of the population lives in poverty, had prevalence rates much higher than the national average (53.4%, 43.2%, and 43.0%, respectively) (15); the correlation coefficient between chronic malnutrition and poverty is 0.92 (Figure 4).

In 2000, the prevalence of iron-deficient **anemia** among women between 15 and 49 years of age was 31.6%, with 37.0% in rural areas and 29.2% in urban areas. By department, figures ranged from 45.9% in Ayacucho to 16.9% in Lima. Among children under 5 years of age, 49.6% had some form of anemia; the percentage was higher in rural areas than in urban ones (53.4% and 46.6%, respectively); at the same time, anemia affected 70.7% of children under 5 years old in Cusco and 61.5% in Puno (15). To decrease this problem, as well as deficiencies of other micronutrients, a high-level decree was issued in 2005, stating that wheat must contain iron (55 mg/kg), niacin (48 mg/kg), folic acid (1.2 mg/kg), vitamin B1 (5 mg/kg), and vitamin B2 (4 mg/kg).

A policy was begun in 1986 geared toward eliminating **iodine deficiency**, by promoting universal consumption of iodized salt, particularly in the mountains and jungle areas where the deficiency existed. In 1998, it was declared that iodine deficiency as a public health problem was eliminated. Since then, there has been continued monitoring of the consumption of iodized salt. A survey carried out in 2003 (29) found that the consumption of iodized salt at the national level was appropriate for 92.9% of children between 12 and 35 months of age and for 92.8% of women between 15 and 49 years of age; prevalence was lower in Loreto (86.2% and 85.0%, respectively), which is located in the Amazon jungle.

Assessments carried out between 1997 and 2001 by the National Health Institute found high levels of **vitamin A deficiency** in children under 5 years old. At the national level, this deficiency decreased from 19.2% to 13.0% during this period. In 2001, vitamin A deficiency was more prevalent in the southern highlands (22.9%) and the jungle (17.9%), while it was 10.3% in Lima. That same year, 8.7% of women between 15 and 49 years of age were affected by vitamin A deficiency; this rate was somewhat higher in the southern highlands (11.2%) (30). In 1996, the Ministry of Health set up a program for preventative vitamin A supplementation for babies and children between 6 and 59 months of age as well as for improved complementary feeding practices after 6 months of age for children and during gestation, focusing actions on the poorest provinces in Peru.

In 2000, the prevalence of **overweight** in mothers between 15 and 49 years of age was 33.7% and the prevalence of **obesity** was 13.0% (15). Among adults, the prevalence of overweight was up

FIGURE 4. Chronic malnutrition in children under 5 years of age, by levels of poverty, Peru, 2000.

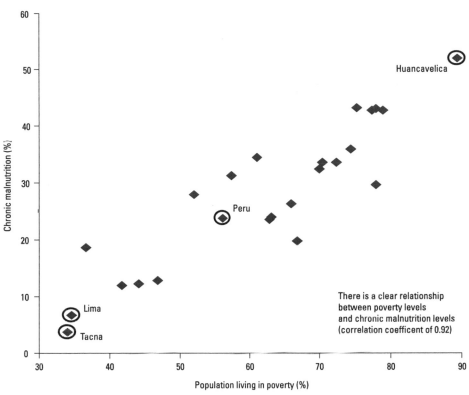

There is a clear relationship between poverty levels and chronic malnutrition levels (correlation coefficent of 0.92)

Source: Perú, Instituto Nacional de Estadística e Informática. Encuesta Demográfica y de Salud Familiar 2000. Encuesta Nacional de Hogares 2001.

to 40%, and up to 20% for obesity (*31, 32, 33*). The prevalence of high cholesterol among adults varied according to the area under study, ranging from 47.2% in the district of Castilla (Piura) to 10.6% in Huaraz (Ancash) (*32*).

In Peru, **diabetes mellitus** was the fifteenth leading cause of death in 2000 and the tenth leading cause in 2004, the same year when it was the sixth leading cause of death for people between 45 and 64 years of age. In 2000, there was a 7.0% rate of prevalence of diabetes mellitus in the city of Lima, 6.7% in Piura, 4.4% in Tarapoto, and 1.3% in Huaraz (*34*). Although there are not many studies on the economic impact of this disease, a study carried out by Cayetano Heredia National Hospital in Lima found that the cost for the initial diagnosis and evaluation of a patient with diabetes mellitus varied between US$ 120 and US$ 200. When the patient had complications because of chronic renal insufficiency, the cost could rise to between US$ 8,000 and US$ 12,000 per year (*34*). In Lima, diabetes mellitus was responsible for 10% of the cases of chronic renal insufficiency (*35*).

Cardiovascular Diseases

In 2004, **ischemic heart disease** was the second leading cause of death in Peru (25.7 per 100,000 inhabitants) and was more

common among men (29.7) than women (21.7). The mortality rate for people between 45 and 64 years of age was 41.4 per 100,000 inhabitants (58.1 for men and 24.9 for women), and it was 352.1 among those over 65 years old (405.3 in men and 306.1 in women in this age group). **Hypertensive diseases** had a mortality rate of 16.9 per 100,000, less than that of ischemic heart disease and **cerebrovascular diseases** (24.3 per 100,000 inhabitants), although arterial hypertension is a problem associated with the other two. Studies carried out between 1997 and 2001 found a prevalence of between 15% and 20% of arterial hypertension in men and around 10% in women among certain select population groups (*31, 32*).

Malignant Neoplasms

In 2004, malignant stomach tumors were the seventh leading cause of death from all causes (PAHO List 6/67), with a mortality rate of 15.6 per 100,000 inhabitants; there was no difference between men and women. After stomach cancer, malignant prostate tumors were the second leading cancer among men (mortality rate of 12.4 per 100,000), even though after the age of 65 it surpassed stomach cancer as a cause of death (228.9 and 205.0, respectively). That same year malignant tumors of the uterus (cervix, uterus, and unspecified part) were the sixth leading cause of death from all causes among women (15.6 per 100,000 women) and the first leading cause of death among women between 25 and 44 years of age (48.6 per 100,000). In spite of the importance of this type of cancer as a cause of morbidity and mortality, the Ministry of Health does not have a program in charge of its prevention and control. However, in 2004, the General Office of Human Health and the Specialized Institute for Neoplastic Diseases drafted the Rules and Procedures Manual for the prevention of cervical cancer to improve coverage for Pap smears and reduce morbidity and mortality levels.

OTHER HEALTH PROBLEMS OR ISSUES

Disasters

In recent decades, there have been three types of natural disasters: floods and the overflow of rivers in the north as a result of the El Niño phenomenon, earthquakes in the south and east, and flooding in the mountains during periods of intense rain. In the north of the country, where there is usually little rain, the El Niño phenomenon appears at irregular intervals, every 2 to 7 years, with increased precipitation and overflowing rivers. This affects agriculture and drinking water and sewage systems and increases the presence of vectors that significantly affect public health, including those that transmit malaria. One of the last two major earthquakes was in Arequipa, Moquegua, and Tacna (on June 23, 2001, a 6.9 magnitude on the Richter scale). There were 83 deaths, 219,420 injuries, and 22,052 homes destroyed. The second was in San Martín (on September 25, 2005, a 7.5 magnitude), but it did not cause major damage because its epicenter was far from urban centers with high concentrations of population (36).

Mental Health

In Lima, in 2002, 56.7% of the adult population thought that the main problem facing Peru was unemployment; poverty, 16.4%; corruption, 5.1%; and violence, 2.8%. This situation created a state of disillusionment (26.6%), bitterness and rage (25.9%), resignation (5.3%), and indifference (3.3%); moreover, 76.9% did not feel protected by the State. High levels of stress affected 49.5% of women and 41.6% of men. In terms of feelings of dissatisfaction, 40.6% related it to economic concerns, 29.5% to their upbringing, and 29.5% to their social relationships (37). Among this same population, the prevalence of lifetime anxiety was 20.3% among men and 30.1% among women and that of any psychiatric disorder was 32.9% for men and 41.5% for women. Among the adults interviewed, 30.3% had thought about killing themselves at one point, and 5.2% had tried it. The main reasons were problems in romantic relationships (45.1%) and economic problems (15.5%). The prevalence of psychotic disorders was 1.0% (0.7% in men and 1.3% in women). Also in 2002, among adolescents in Lima, 1 of every 7 had thoughts of suicide; the

prevalence of depressive disorders was 14.5% for males and 23.3% for females, and 1 of every 12 adolescents showed signs of depression (37).

Addictions

In 2002, the prevalence of alcohol and tobacco consumption at some point during their lives was 94.2% and 68.0%, respectively, for those between 12 and 64 years of age. The annual prevalence of alcohol consumption was 75.1% and was greater among men than women (79.8% and 71.0%); prevalence of tobacco use was 37.5% (53.3% for men and 23.7% for women). Among 12- and 13-year-old children, 36.0% had consumed alcohol during the year prior to the survey (42.6% of males and 28.4% of females) and 4.4% had used tobacco (6.8% of males and 1.6% of females). The average for initial consumption of alcohol was 13.7 years for the 12- to 19-year-old age group, 16.1 for the 20- to 29-year-old age group, and 17.4 for the 30- to 39-year-old age group. This difference shows that initial alcohol consumption has been taking place at a younger age in recent years.

The lifetime prevalence of illegal drug use was 5.8% for marihuana, 2.1% for basic cocaine paste, and 1.8% for cocaine hydrochloride. Among adolescents between 12 and 19 years of age, 5.2% had used marihuana, 1.1% basic cocaine paste, and 2.0% cocaine hydrochloride.

Alcohol dependence among 12- to 64-year-olds was 10.6% (17.8% among males and 4.3% among females), with higher rates among the group between 20 and 30 years of age (14.5%) and among those 31 to 40 years of age (13.4%). Tobacco was the second most common dependency at 4.4% (6.3% among males and 2.2% among females), with a higher rate among those between 20 and 30 years of age (6.8%) and those between 31 and 40 years of age (4.9%) (38).

Environmental Pollution

The National Agricultural Health Service has prohibited the registry, importation, local formulation, distribution, and marketing of the chloride pesticides aldrin, endrin, dieldrin, chlordane, mirex, heptaclor, and toxaphene. In 1991, all use of DDT and its derivatives was prohibited; the Ministry of Health does not use DDT in controlling malaria vectors. In 2003, symptoms of chronic pesticide poisoning were found in 1 of every 6 farmers in the provinces of Huancayo, Jaén, and Tarapoto (39). In addition, there is no program for farmers that would enable them to store and appropriately handle pesticides in rural areas; this has led to several instances of massive poisoning, such as the poisoning of 50 children with parathion (24 of whom died) in the community of Tauccamarca (Cusco) in 1999 and the poisoning and subsequent death of 2 adults and 4 children in the district of Andarapa (Apurímac) in October 2003.

In 2002, an inventory was taken of the sources of the emission of dioxins and furans, and, in the city of Lima, dioxin levels of 21 ng/g were found (normal readings are 0.0072 to 14 ng/g, according to WHO-TEQ). The primary sources of emissions are the incineration of municipal waste and hospital waste, the production of cement and metals, the generation of electricity, motorized vehicles, and paper pulp factories.

Oral Health

In 2001, the last year a national evaluation was carried out, the prevalence of dental caries among students between 6 and 15 years of age was 90.7%, and fluorosis was 35.7%. The DMFT (decayed, missing, filled teeth) index was 5.7, and it fluctuated between 8.3 in Ayacucho and 3.5 in Ancash. The DMFT index was 3.9 among 12-year-old children. Oral diseases were the second leading cause for medical visits to Ministry of Health facilities and represented more than 10% of all visits in 2004. Of the total of dental visits, 20.6% were for tooth extractions, and 18% were for fillings. In spite of the high demand for dental services, only 16% of all health facilities of the Ministry of Health provide these services, and the number of dentists working in them has not increased in recent years (1,681 in 2002 and 1,607 in 2004). However, with Comprehensive Health Insurance, it is hoped that access to basic oral health care will be improved for the poor, for dispersed populations, for children, and for pregnant women, who do not have social protection in health. As part of prevention activities, the National Technical Standard on Salt for Human Consumption has been reformulated and incorporates imported salt and increases the concentration of fluoride. On the coast, more than 80% of the urban population consumes iodized and fluoridated salt, but in the mountains and jungle, this figure is only 60% (40).

RESPONSE OF THE HEALTH SECTOR

Health Policies and Plans

In July 2001, the Peruvian Government called upon political parties and a group of political, religious, and civil society organizations to achieve a national consensus that would act as the basis for the transition and consolidation of democracy, affirmation of national identity, and development of a shared vision for the country's future. Of the 29 government policies approved, the 13th highlights the commitment to universal access to health services and social security, while the 15th is related to the promotion of food safety and nutrition.

The Sectoral Policy Guidelines for 2002–2012 guide the actions of the health sector and define the basis for modernization of the sector. The nine defined guidelines emphasize health promotion, comprehensive health care, universal insurance, financing for the poorest, and modernization of the Ministry of Health. Their strategic objectives include health promotion, prevention of chronic and degenerative diseases, health education, development of Comprehensive Health Insurance, reduction of child and maternal morbidity and mortality, expanded access to and rational use of drugs, and sectoral decentralization.

In 2002, the Basic Decentralization Law (Law No. 27783) was promulgated. It regulates the structure and organization of the State in the national, regional, and local spheres; defines rules that regulate administrative, economic, productive, financial, tax, and fiscal decentralization; assigns responsibilities for the three levels of government and determines the goods and resources for regional and local governments; and regulates government relations at its different levels. In January 2003, regional governments began operating with the functions and responsibilities, as well as budget management, that had been transferred to them.

In 2005, the Ministry of Health began the transfer process from health offices to regional governments[2] by means of an accreditation process carried out by the National Decentralization Council. This process involves the development of capacities in the regions to lead, direct, and manage health services following the transfer of certain responsibilities agreed upon with the National Decentralization Council. Although this process is due to be completed in 2010, extraordinary progress was made between 2004 and 2005, meaning that the goal of transferring responsibilities could be achieved sooner than planned. Several regions (La Libertad, Lambayeque, and Arequipa) have used participatory and consultation processes to establish regional health priorities, policies, and plans.

The Coordinated and Decentralized National Health System was created in 2001 as a mechanism for sectoral articulation among public subsectors (which include the Ministry of Health and the health services of the armed forces and national police) as well as private and social security subsectors. The first evaluation of the Coordinated and Decentralized National Health System was carried out in 2005 and showed that several adjustments were needed; since the Ministry of Health did not take on the leadership role for the Coordinated and Decentralized National Health System, primarily because it has neither the structure nor the competencies needed, it also became clear that the rules governing the agencies that comprise the Coordinated and Decentralized National Health System needed to be harmonized, so that these agencies could interact under the guidance of the Ministry and be compatible to operate as a coordinated system. The major progress observed in the Coordinated and Decentralized National Health System was the decentralization process in which the Ministry of Health played a key role.

The impact of decentralization on the public health sector is still in its initial phases, because the process of transferring functions, competencies, responsibilities, and resources is progressive by stages and by areas, as per the timeline agreed upon by the national government and regional governments. The main changes have been in the provision of public health services, which have been transferred to regional governments, and in the transfer of certain public health and health promotion activities, such as basic sanitation, to local governments.

---

[2]One for each department, with the exception of Lima, where the metropolitan area constitutes one region, and the rest of its provinces another.

As of June 2006, 34 competencies and responsibilities have been transferred to 24 of the 26 regional governments, which have shown that they have the ability to exercise decentralized functions. This makes them responsible for providing all of the health services, including negotiating finances, which are carried out through management contracts and results indicators. Between 2005 and 2006, all regional governments were evaluated using the measurement instrument known as the Essential Public Health Functions, which made it possible to learn about the level of performance for each regional government in terms of the Essential Public Health Functions as well as about existing gaps and needs. The central government will carry out a program to develop capacities based on the results of this evaluation.

Health Strategies and Programs

In 2004, 63.2% of the Peruvian population had no medical insurance (70.1% of the poor and 56.1% of the nonpoor were in this situation) (41). The main restriction on access to health services was economic: 32.1% of the poor with symptoms of diseases or who had accidents and thought medical treatment was necessary did not seek it out for this reason. As a strategy to improve access for the poor, the Comprehensive Health Insurance was created in 2001 from the merger of an insurance program for schoolchildren (created in 1977) and a maternal and child health insurance program (created in 1998). The Comprehensive Health Insurance covers those under 18 years of age, pregnant women, and certain groups of adults living in poverty. According to Comprehensive Health Insurance data, in 2004, there were 8.8 million members (32.0% of the total population). The National Household Survey stated that 20.1% of the entire population was affiliated with this medical insurance. In spite of the discrepancy in these numbers, this strategy has improved the population's access to health services, even though 40% of the population is still excluded from health services in some way, and 10% (2.7 million people) is completely excluded from the health system. Factors such as poverty, living in a rural area, and social and ethnic discrimination explain some of this situation, although internal problems of the health system are also important factors, including deficient provision of essential services in the poorest areas (42). For example, in 2000, preventable death from problems related to low-complexity surgery (mortality from appendicitis, abdominal hernia, and intestinal obstruction without hernia) was 1.7 per 100,000 population in Lima, while in the poorest departments in Peru, like Apurímac and Huancavelica, it was 30 times higher (62.1 and 59.0, respectively) (16).

The trend is to continue progressively toward universal insurance. Comprehensive Health Insurance is the public insurer for the poor and extremely poor, as well as for the population working in the informal sector. The social security system (ESSALUD) would insure the salaried population, leaving complementary plans and insurance open to the private sector for those who prefer them.

After deactivation of the National Health Programs in 2001, in July 2004, the Ministry of Health established 10 national health strategies, which are related to the health priorities and are the areas the Ministry of Health will promote and target in coming years: immunizations, prevention and control of metaxenic diseases and other diseases transmitted by vectors, prevention and control of sexually transmitted infections and HIV/ AIDS, prevention and control of tuberculosis, sexual and reproductive health, prevention and control of noncommunicable injuries, road safety, health of indigenous peoples, healthy food and nutrition, mental health, and a culture of peace.

Organization of the Health System

Peru's health system is segmented and has various actors in both services provision and public insurance, which carry out different but not necessarily complementary functions and with high degrees of overlap. This situation could become more marked with decentralization of the Peruvian government. The health system comprises ESSALUD (medical insurance and insurance for workplace risks and occupational health) which is public in nature and mandatory for salaried workers (in 2004, it covered 17.6% of the total population) (41); the Ministry of Health (with decentralized public national institutions: ophthalmology, cancer, rehabilitation, and pediatrics, among others); regional governments (to which were recently transferred functions and human and financial resources to provide public services) and local governments (to which responsibilities are being transferred in the areas of water and basic sanitation); the health services of the armed forces and the police (which cover approximately 3% of the population); and the nonprofit and for-profit private sector (with 10% coverage), of which the latter is extremely fragmented. Comprehensive Health Insurance is a public insurer and financer, which facilitates free access to basic health care for poor and extremely poor pregnant women and minors under the age of 18. There is also Mandatory Traffic Accident Insurance which covers care for injuries caused by this type of event.

There are also regulatory and research institutions, such as the National Health Institute (public health and health research laboratories), the Human Resources Institute for Health, and the Superintendence for Private Insurance, among others. Public services and those of ESSALUD are organized into geographically distributed care networks and by levels of complexity for the member population. They have general and basic hospitals and health centers and posts, most of which are categorized and regulated and which include a group of volunteer community agents that incorporates health promoters and midwives. The public sector and ESSALUD are based on the conceptual framework and criteria of the primary health care strategy.

To provide care to the poor and disperse populations living in the most distant rural areas of the mountains and the indigenous population in Amazonia, the regional governments and the Ministry of Health have organized mobile care units, supported by Comprehensive Health Insurance, that provide care at regular intervals to this population and offer a package of basic or essential services as well as promotional and community organization actions. This service covers approximately 200,000 people.

Public Health Services

The Ministry of Health established the application of the primary care strategy as one of its national priorities for 2006–2012, and, as a result, has developed a set of actions, including implementation of the Comprehensive Health Care Model, which lists the health services to which a person is entitled to according to his or her life stage, and of the National Sanitary Strategies (as a replacement for the former Health Programs), social participation, development of rules for the organization of networks and categorization of health facilities, cultural adaptation of services, the gender focus, intersectoral action, and elimination of social exclusion in health through progressive implementation of universal insurance. In this context, the Comprehensive Health Care Model has defined and is implementing a set of basic actions according to life cycle or stage (vaccination, complementary feeding, a reproductive health package, and a promotional preventative package for adolescents, older adults, the family, and the community, etc.), which includes promotional, curative, and rehabilitative care for individuals, families, and communities. Collective care is the responsibility of regional and local governments, while individuals are the responsibility of care networks.

National Health Strategies are units for health analysis, surveillance, evaluation, programming, planning, and intelligence and are responsible for overseeing the control of specific high-impact or high-risk problems such as vaccine-preventable diseases, TB, malaria, maternal and child mortality, and the health of indigenous populations, among others.

In 2004, 64.4% of homes received water from the public system. Coverage for this service was greater in nonpoor homes (77.4%) than in poor homes (47.7%). Eighteen percent of all homes, 28.3% of the poor, and 46% of the rural population received water from rivers, streams, springs, or similar sources (7). This deficit was even greater in sewerage services: only 50.9% of homes were connected to the public network; 26.8% had latrines, blind wells, or septic tanks; and 22.3% had no system for excreta disposal. The latter figure was 52% in rural areas. Among indigenous populations in Amazonia, only 11.7% have some type of water supply system, mainly wells and public cisterns. Disinfection of water is practically nonexistent in nearly all these communities, and, in those where it does exist, it is done intermittently. Only 9.7% had some system for elimination of excreta, mainly latrines.

In 2004, only 23.4% of wastewater was treated in some way (primarily in the city of Lima) before final disposal (43), which represents a serious environmental pollution problem. Another major source of water pollution is industrial activity, particularly mining. Monitoring of water quality has found that the majority of hydrographic basins are polluted by metals, including lead, arsenic, and cadmium (44). In some areas, the bioconcentration of metals is several times above the standards for food quality, as in the case of mercury in the fish sold in the public markets of Puerto Maldonado.

Solid waste collection reaches 73.7% of the population, and only 65.7% of this waste (8,532 tons per day) receives some form of final disposal: 14.7% is recycled, 29.8% (2,545 tons per day) is dumped in the environment (rivers and beaches are the main locations), and the rest is placed in landfills. This situation causes serious environmental pollution, which poses major risks to the stability of ecosystems and human health. Only certain hospitals in Lima have waste treatment systems. The Ministry of Health, through the General Office of Environmental Health has set up an environmental and health monitoring system for handling solid wastes at the national level, emphasizing final disposal and coverage of services, and already has a property register of all the systems currently operating. In addition, actions have been implemented to eliminate the clandestine treatment of solid wastes, especially those to be fed to swine and other livestock.

In terms of food safety, caloric availability in 1998 was 2,584 calories per capita per day. Cereals (wheat and rice) were the main source of energy and protein; 30% of wheat used in Peru is imported. Only 7% of all hydrobiological resources extracted are destined for direct human consumption and provide 10% of the total protein consumed by the Peruvian population.

In terms of preparation for a possible influenza pandemic, in October 2005, the Ministry of Health and the Ministry of Agriculture, with the support of PAHO and the Communicable Diseases Commission of the Coordinated and Decentralized National Health Council drafted the National Plan on Preparedness and Response to a Potential Influenza Pandemic; the objective of the plan is to facilitate an effective and coordinated national response to a potential influenza pandemic, providing recommendations to support health services and other institutions in preparing their own contingency plans. The plan includes vaccination against seasonal influenza for vulnerable groups (primarily the elderly and children) and health personnel: chemoprophylaxis with antivirals for 20,000 people for 6 weeks, treatment with antivirals for 100,000 people for 5 days, purchase of 2 million personal protection items, and the purchase of 100 ventilators. The cost of these activities is estimated at US$ 47,185,000 (45).

Individual Care Services

At ESSALUD, individual care services are provided according to a specific organizational schematic for each subsector. In the public sector, it is carried out via care networks comprising facilities of varying complexity, coordinated by levels of care interwoven through a system of references and counter-references; the point of entry into the system is general or comprehensive care practitioners or facilities with a lower level of complexity, and a national standardized clinical history is used, with mandatory content but free format. In public services, the basic health care of the Comprehensive Health Care Model or of the National Health Strategies is prioritized, and the user must pay a regulated and subsidized tariff (except for maternal and child care under Comprehensive Health Insurance).

The Peruvian health system provides nearly all types of routine and most frequently needed medical and technological care, but ESSALUD has greater technological development and routinely carries out kidney, marrow, and liver transplants. In all regions, there are intensive and perinatal care units with varying levels of functionality and equipment. The country has all clinical specialties and highly complex equipment, but they are not equitably distributed because they are concentrated in the main cities of Peru.

The National Center of Public Health Libraries is the regulatory technical body of the National Health Institute, in charge of researching, regulating, developing, and evaluating, from a comprehensive view, research into the development of new technology related to communicable and noncommunicable diseases. This Center is the reference laboratory for the 19 regional public health laboratories of the country.

In 2003, there were 92 blood banks in Peru, with the majority located in Lima, Callao, and the main cities; 93.3% of the blood units collected were through recovery, and only 5.3% were obtained from voluntary donors. More than 96% of the units were tested for the major blood-borne diseases; in 2003, there was a 0.27% prevalence of HIV, 0.62% for hepatitis B surface antigen, 0.55% for hepatitis C virus, 1.58% for syphilis, and 0.84% for *Trypanosoma cruzi*. However, there is no regulation, monitoring, and evaluation system to guarantee the quality of transfused blood, nor are there networks of blood banks or specialized units for their centralized management. In July 2006, the Ministry of Health approved the Policy Guidelines for the National Hemotherapy and Blood Banks Program, with a view toward creating the foundation for the National Network and Regional Networks of Transfusion Services, as well as guaranteeing the quality and safety of blood for transfusion in health facilities.

By law, emergency care must be provided at the closest possible facility regardless of the patient's ability to pay. Except for health care services provided under Comprehensive Health Insurance or the ESSALUD, users generally must pay for drugs, laboratory tests, and in-hospital and ambulatory procedures. In the public sector, there are central state purchases of basic and generic drugs, which are then distributed to health facilities.

Peru's health care provision system has a component for managing the quality of care that includes medical audits; however, in spite of repeated attempts, it has not been possible to accredit facilities. Certification of health personnel is the responsibility of professional associations.

Health Promotion

With implementation of the Local Health Administration Committees, Law on the Coordinated and Decentralized National Health System, law on decentralization, and the Comprehensive Health Care Model, operative and legal foundations have been created to increase citizen participation in the collective promotion of health. Peru is encouraging the community participation of midwives; community workers; hospital volunteers; patient associations; family members of patients; health boards and committees; local and regional participatory health plans; and regional, provincial, and district health councils. At the same time, civil society is developing national health forums that bring together thousands of participants. These efforts consolidated the trend toward greater citizen participation and culminated at the end of 2006 in the National Health Conference.

Special mention should be made of the Local Health Administration Committees, which represent the association of communities with the Ministry of Health and in which organized citizens are delegated the authority to administer the local provision of health services; one-third of primary care facilities are administered in this manner. In the regions of Arequipa, Tacna, and Moquegua all facilities are administered by Local Health Administration Committees.

In addition, major efforts are being carried out for intersectoral actions, above all with the educational sector and the private sector, as was the case with the "*Juntos*" (or "Together") program (subsidy to the poor in exchange for vaccination, breast-feeding, institutional births, and school attendance). In general, Peru has been working toward greater and more sustainable social participation in health and toward improved health status based on rights and duties.

Health Supplies

Peru has a pharmaceutical industry that produces generic and national brands as well as laboratories that import and market most of the drugs the country needs. It is regulated and supervised by the General Office of Medications, Supplies, and Drugs (DIGEMID), which is the health authority on medications, medical devices, and reagents. It is estimated that only about half of the population with a health problem can access drugs prescribed through health services, primarily due to the limited ability of people to pay (with differences between urban and rural areas). Another major problem with regard to medications is the high incidence of forgery and contraband, which has led the Ministry of Health to strengthen the body in charge of controlling medications. In coming years, the effect of intellectual property in negotiations of a Free Trade Agreement could affect access to

---

A Strategy to Improve Access to Health Care by the Poor

The Comprehensive Health Insurance system was created in 2002 as a subsidy for the very poor who do not have health insurance (the population under 18 years of age, pregnant women, and targeted adult groups). The purpose is to reduce the limitations on access to health services represented by the existence of economic barriers and cultural and geographic differences. Some of the system's achievements are:

- It delivered approximately 79.1 million health benefits in just 60 months.
- It focuses efforts on free maternal and child care in rural and marginal urban areas.
- More than 1.2 billion *soles* have been spent on financing health benefits throughout the country.
- Free care has been provided for pregnant women, and by the end of 2006, 1,554,896 deliveries had been assisted by trained personnel.
- More than 2.7 million children up to age 4 and more than 196,000 poor mothers are covered.
- The system covers 7.1 million schoolchildren and youths (from 5 to 17 years old) even if they do not attend school regularly.

---

drugs, particularly if measures are not taken to prevent a substantial increase in prices (46).

There are standards that ensure Good Manufacturing Practices and a mandatory national registry of drugs and medical devices. During 2006, the national list of essential drugs for the public sector was revised, and centralized and joint purchasing for the entire sector was initiated with major savings. However, ESSALUD and the health services of the armed forces have not yet incorporated this mechanism.

The national capacity to produce vaccines is limited to anti rabies vaccines, and the rest are purchased through the PAHO Revolving Fund for Vaccine Procurement. The Ministry of Health provides free vaccines to all public and some private providers.

Peru produces all low-complexity equipment and instruments used in health and medicine. More complex equipment is imported, primarily from the European Economic Community, Japan, the United States, Argentina, Brazil, Chile, and Colombia.

Human Resources

In 2005, there were 23,804 physicians, 21,332 nurses, 8,104 obstetricians, and 3,614 dentists working at the Ministry of Health, ESSALUD, and health provider companies (which jointly provide services to approximately 80% of the population). That same year, the rates per 10,000 population were 11.5 for physicians, 10.3 for nurses, 3.9 for obstetricians, and 1.7 for dentists. However, the distribution of these resources was unequal: Lima had a rate of 18.6 physicians per 10,000 population, which was 3.8 times higher than that of Huancavelica (4.9). In addition, there was a shortage of medical professionals in Ministry of Health facilities in 19 of the 25 departments; for example, the deficit of physicians in Cajamarca was 65% (47). If an equitable distribu-

tion were to be achieved, 24% of physicians, 14% of nurses, 12% of obstetricians, and 22% of dentists would have to be relocated (absolute index of dissimilarity).

The number of medical schools increased from 13 to 28 between 1992 and 2003, and nursing schools went from 34 to 44. Educational opportunities increased the number of medical graduates (from 951 in 1993 to 1,238 in 2003) and nursing graduates (from 1,402 to 1,760 during the same period) (47). In spite of the shortfall of professionals in most departments in Peru, there are few work posts available in health institutions, leading to unemployment and underemployment and migration of graduates (47). Between 1996 and 2004, 2 years after leaving Peru, 13,711 physicians, 7,340 nurses, 2,112 dentists, and 1,110 obstetricians had not returned to the country. This progressive imbalance is compounded by shortcomings in the training of human resources in health. The overcrowding in professional and technical health education has led to a deterioration in educational quality; the health education model is still centered on the hospital and disease and on highly specialized clinical and surgical care, to the detriment of education geared more toward public health (47).

Over the last 5 years, Peru has created an infrastructure to address problems in human resources, such as the Institute for Human Resources Development and the General Office for Human Resources Management, as a direct subsidiary of the highest managerial level of the Ministry of Health; in addition, Peru is carrying out efforts to strengthen leadership capacity by issuing National Human Resources Policies approved by the National Health Council. Also, there are signs that the situation could be beginning to correct itself: the recent development of regulatory mechanisms for educational training, the creation of the National System of Preliminary Study in Health (SINAPRES) for better coordination of universities and health services, and the reorientation of financing, prioritizing only 22 medical specialties, which are better adjusted to the population's needs.

Sectoral reform processes and decentralization require a change in the occupational profiles of the work force. There is a broad supply of training with different sources of financing, administrative forms, and pedagogical concepts, which generates duplications and contradictions. Investment in training exceeded 2 million dollars in 2004. However, the high turnover of trained personnel calls into question the effectiveness of this investment (48).

The imbalance between the unplanned supply of professionals who graduate from universities and the limited capacity of the health system to absorb them can be seen in the number of posts for physicians offered by the Marginal Urban Rural Health Service (SERUMS), which in 2004 had 2,308 vacancies for 7,551 applicants. Those who did not obtain a position provided service of an equivalent nature, i.e. without remuneration.

Changes in contractual relationships of the last decade that made health employment precarious for a high percentage of health employees have begun to reverse. In November 2004, the Ministry of Health incorporated, through appointments, 3,040 physicians, who had been working with contracts. However, even though this change in labor relationship created employment stability for this group of professionals, it widened the gap of inequity in distribution because there were more appointees in departments with a higher number of physicians. This process of appointing hired people is extending to the rest of professional and technical staff. However, it conflicts with the fiscal ceiling set by the Peruvian government and aggravates the labor conflict that has been increasing in recent years: from 6 national strikes in 2003 to 11 in 2004.

Health Sector Expenditures and Financing

In 2000, national health spending was 4.4% of the GDP, and public health spending was 2.8%, while the per capita health cost was US$ 97 (49).

As per the National Health Accounts for Peru, 1995–2000, in 2000, the main sources of financing were households (37.3%) through out-of-pocket expenses, the formal economy via payments of workers and employees into social security in health (35.0%), the government via the public treasury through indebtedness and ordinary resources (24.0%), and other organizations (including international cooperation) (3.7%) (49).

Technical Cooperation and External Financing

In 2004, 12.5% of total international cooperation funds to Peru were for the health sector (US$ 48.6 million dollars, 50.4% were nonreimbursable international cooperation, and the rest was nongovernmental). There is a declining trend toward nonreimbursable official cooperation (in 1994, it was US$ 56.8 million and, in 2004, it was US$ 24.5 million), as well as nongovernmental cooperation (in 1998, it was US$ 58.6 million and, in 2004, it was US$ 24.1 million).

Of the total money provided through international cooperation in 2004, 66.9% (US$ 260.9 million) was aligned with an MDG. Of this quantity, 1.9% was directed toward the reducing infant mortality; 0.3% toward improving maternal health; and 2.9% toward combating HIV/AIDS, malaria, and other diseases (50).

REFERENCES

1. International Monetary Fund. World Economic Outlook Database; 2006.
2. Peru, Banco Central de Reserva del Peru. Reporte de inflación: panorama actual y proyecciones macroeconómicas; 2006.
3. Instituto Cuánto. Anuario estadístico: Peru en números 2005.
4. Peru, Instituto Nacional de Estadística e Informática. La pobreza en el Peru 2003–2004; 2005.
5. Peru, Ministerio de Trabajo y Promoción de Empleo. Informe Estadístico Mensual. Año 9, N° 106; marzo 2005.
6. Programa de las Naciones Unidas para el Desarrollo. Hacia el cumplimiento de los objetivos de desarrollo del milenio en el Peru. Informe 2004.
7. Peru, Instituto Nacional de Estadística e Informática. Condiciones de vida en los departamentos del Peru: 2003–2004; 2005.
8. Peru, Ministerio de Educación. IV Evaluación nacional del rendimiento estudiantil, 2004; 2005.
9. Peru, Ministerio de Salud, Dirección General de Salud Ambiental. Programa Nacional de Vigilancia de la Calidad del Aire 1999–2000; 2001.
10. Peru, Instituto Nacional de Estadística e Informática. Censo de Población y Vivienda 2005; 2006.
11. Peru, Instituto Nacional de Estadística e Informática. Peru: Estimaciones y proyecciones de población 1950–2050. Boletín de Análisis Demográfico N° 35; 2001.
12. Peru, Instituto Nacional de Estadística e Informática. Condiciones de vida en el Peru: evolución 1997–2001. Encuesta Nacional de Hogares (ENAHO); 2002.
13. Peru, Instituto Nacional de Estadística e Informática. Encuesta Demográfica y de Salud Familiar (ENDES) 1996; 1997.
14. Peru, Instituto Nacional de Estadística e Informática. Encuesta Demográfica y de Salud Familiar (ENDES) Continua 2004–2005; 2005.
15. Peru, Instituto Nacional de Estadística e Informática. Encuesta Demográfica y de Salud Familiar (ENDES) 2000; 2001.
16. Peru, Ministerio de Salud. Base de datos de mortalidad 2000–2004.
17. Sistema de las Naciones Unidas en el Peru. Hacia el cumplimiento de los objetivos de desarrollo del milenio en el Peru. Informe 2004; 2004.

18. Watanabe T. Tendencias, niveles y estructura de la mortalidad materna en el Peru, 1992–2000. Instituto Nacional de Estadística e Informática; 2002.

19. Peru. Instituto Nacional de Estadística e Informática. Peru: trabajo infantil y adolescente; 1998.

20. Peru, Instituto Nacional de Estadística e Informática; Organización Internacional del Trabajo. Visión del trabajo infantil y adolescente en el Peru, 2001; 2002.

21. Organización Internacional del Trabajo. Panorama laboral 2004. América Latina y el Caribe; 2004.

22. Peru, Ministerio de Salud, Dirección General de Salud Ambiental. Manual de salud ocupacional. Lima; 2005.

23. Peru, Instituto Nacional de Estadística e Informática. Estudio de prevalencia de deficiencia, discapacidad y minusvalías en el Peru, 1993.

24. Peru, Instituto Nacional de Estadística e Informática. Nota de prensa N° 134, junio 2006.

25. Peru, Ministerio de Salud. Indicadores básicos 2005.

26. Peru, Ministerio de Salud, Dirección General de Epidemiología. Boletín Epidemiológico Mensual; marzo 2006.

27. Peru, Ministerio de Salud, Dirección General de Epidemiología. Vigilancia Centinela VIH, 2002.

28. Universidad Peruana Cayetano Heredia; Universidad de Washington, Seattle; Imperial Collage, Londres. Prevención comunitaria de enfermedades de transmisión sexual (PREVEN); 2003.

29. Miranda M, Calderón M, Riega V, Barboza J, Rojas C. Consumo de sal fortificada con yodo en niños de 12 a 35 meses de edad y mujeres en edad fértil en el Peru. Rev Peru Med Exp Salud Pública 2004;21(2).

30. Peru, Instituto Nacional de Salud, Centro Nacional de Alimentación y Nutrición. Informe nacional de deficiencia de vitamina A en niños menores de 5 años y mujeres en edad fértil 1997–2001; 2002.

31. Seclén S. Prevalencia de diabetes mellitus, hipertensión arterial, hipercolesterolemia y obesidad, como factores de riesgo coronario y cerebrovascular en población adulta de la costa, sierra y selva del Peru. Lima; 1997.

32. Peru, Ministerio de Salud, Dirección General de Epidemiología. Prevalencia de factores de riesgo de enfermedades cardiovasculares y diabetes en familias nucleares de seis ciudades del Peru, 1998–2000.

33. Rosas A, Lama G, Llanos-Zavalaga F, Dunstan J. Prevalencia de obesidad e hipercolesterolemia en trabajadores de una institución estatal de Lima, Peru. Rev Peru Med Exp Salud Pública 2002;19(2):87–92.

34. Seclén S. La diabetes mellitus, problema de salud pública en el Peru. Lima: Universidad Peruana Cayetano Heredia; 2000.

35. Cieza J, Huáman C, Álvarez C, Gómez J, Castillo W. Prevalencia de insuficiencia renal crónica en la ciudad de Lima. 1990. Rev Peruana de Epidemiología 1992;5(1):22–27.

36. Peru, Ministerio de Salud. Plan sectorial de prevención y atención de emergencias y desastres del sector salud; 2004.

37. Peru, Instituto Especializado de Salud Mental. Estudio epidemiológico metropolitano en salud mental 2002. Informe general. Anales de Salud Mental 2002;18(1; 2).

38. Peru, Comisión Nacional para el Desarrollo y Vida sin Drogas. II Encuesta Nacional sobre Prevención y Consumo de Drogas 2002. Informe ejecutivo. Proyecto RLA7AD/PER/99/D77.

39. Red de Acción en Agricultura Alternativa. Diagnóstico de salud y plaguicidas en los corredores económicos de Huancayo, Jaén y Tarapoto; 2003.

40. Peru, Ministerio de Salud. Informe de la Estrategia Sanitaria Nacional de Salud Bucal, 2005.

41. Peru, Instituto Nacional de Estadística e Informática. Condiciones de vida en el Peru: evolución 1997–2004; 2006.

42. Organización Panamericana de la Salud; Agencia Sueca para el Desarrollo Internacional. Exclusión en salud en países de América Latina y el Caribe; 2003.

43. Peru, Superintendencia Nacional de Servicios de Saneamiento. Nota de prensa del 28 de octubre de 2005.

44. Peru, Consejo Nacional del Ambiente. Informe nacional del estado del ambiente 2001; 2002.

45. Peru, Ministerio de Salud. Plan nacional de preparación y respuesta frente una potencial pandemia de influenza; 2005.

46. Peru, Ministerio de Salud. Evaluación de los potenciales efectos sobre el acceso a medicamentos del Tratado de Libre Comercio que se negocia con los Estados Unidos. Lima; 2005.

47. Peru, Ministerio de Salud, Instituto de Desarrollo de Recursos Humanos. Situación y desafío de los recursos humanos en salud. Gobernabilidad y desempeño con desarrollo humano. Primera edición; 2005.

48. Peru, Ministerio de Salud, Instituto de Desarrollo de Recursos Humanos. Observatorio de Recursos Humanos, Peru 2005.

49. Peru, Ministerio de Salud; Organización Panamericana de la Salud. Cuentas Nacionales de Salud: Peru 1995–2000. Lima; 2003.

50. Peru, Agencia Peruana de Cooperación Internacional. Situación y tendencias de la cooperación internacional en el Peru 2004; 2005.

PUERTO RICO

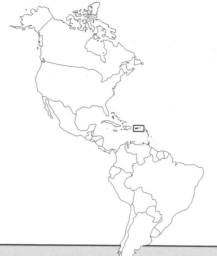

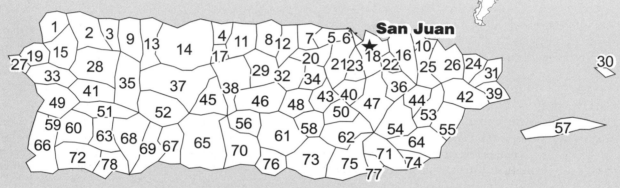

San Juan

1 Aguadilla	21 Bayamón	41 Las Marías	61 Coamo
2 Isabela	22 Trujillo Alto	42 Naguabo	62 Cayey
3 Quebradillas	23 Guaynabo	43 Comerío	63 Sabana Grande
4 Barceloneta	24 Luquillo	44 Juncos	64 Yabucoa
5 Toa Baja	25 Canóvanas	45 Jayuya	65 Ponce
6 Cataño	26 Río Grande	46 Orocovis	66 Cabo Rojo
7 Dorado	27 Rincón	47 Caguas	67 Peñuelas
8 Vega Baja	28 San Sebastián	48 Barranquitas	68 Yauco
9 Camuy	29 Morovis	49 Mayagüez	69 Guayanilla
10 Loíza	30 Culebra	50 Cidra	70 Juana Díaz
11 Manatí	31 Fajardo	51 Maricao	71 Patillas
12 Vega Alta	32 Corozal	53 Las Piedras	72 Lajas
13 Hatillo	33 Añasco	52 Adjuntas	73 Salinas
14 Arecibo	34 Naranjito	56 Villalba	74 Maunabo
15 Moca	35 Lares	57 Vieques	75 Guayama
16 Carolina	36 Gurabo	59 Hormigueros	76 Santa Isabel
17 Florida	37 Utuado	58 Aibonito	77 Arroyo
18 San Juan	38 Ciales	54 San Lorenzo	78 Guánica
19 Aguada	39 Ceiba	55 Humacao	
20 Toa Alta	40 Aguas Buenas	60 San Germán	

0   15   30 Miles

P uerto Rico is an island in the Caribbean Sea's Greater Antilles. In addition to the main island, it includes Vieques, Culebra, and Mona, as well as several islets. It has an area of 9,105 km^2 and is divided into 78 municipalities, each of which is administered by a mayor and a municipal council. The capital, San Juan, is located on the northern coast.

GENERAL CONTEXT AND HEALTH DETERMINANTS

In 1952, Puerto Rico became a commonwealth; it has its own system of government with administrative autonomy for internal affairs. It is governed by a republican system and is divided into three branches: the executive, the legislative, and the judicial.

Social, Political, and Economic Determinants

The educational level among persons 25 years old and older increased between 1990 and 2000, but there are gender differences in school enrollment. In the lowest school grades, males had higher enrollment, primarily in private schools up to grades 9 to 12. After that point, gender differences in enrollment began to reverse, and by the university level, most students were women.

In 2000, three out of every five people had completed some form of higher education, one out of every four (25.4%) had completed a university or high school degree, and 12.2% had attended university without completing it. School attendance increased from 65.5% to 78.3% among those between 16 and 19 years of age.

There have been major changes in the economy. With industrialization, agriculture was outranked as the primary economic sector and, as a result, employment opportunities shifted from rural areas (inland and agricultural areas) to urban and coastal areas. Puerto Rico's development and modernization led to, among other things, increases in the population's income, as well as high rates of unemployment, more families living below the poverty line, minimal changes in income distribution, very expensive housing projects, environmental problems, high crime rates, marked increases in family violence and child abuse, and high teen pregnancy rates.

The gross national product (GNP) was US$ 50.3 billion in 2004, representing a 6% increase compared with 2003. Per capita income was US$ 12,965, and the gross domestic product (GDP) was US$ 78.8 billion, with a real growth rate of 1.9%. The per capita GDP was US$ 17,700. The breakdown of the GDP per sector was as follows: manufacturing (42.1%); insurance, finances, and properties (17.1%); trade (11.6%); services (9.9%); government (9.6%); transportation and other utilities (6.9%); construction and mining (2.4%); and agriculture (0.3%).

In 2004, the workforce comprised 1.4 million people between 16 and 64 years of age, of which 1.2 million (88.6%) were employed. The distribution per sector was as follows: services (28%); government (21%); trade (21%); manufacturing (11%); construction and mining (7%); finances, insurance, and properties (5%); transportation and other utilities (4%); and agriculture (2%). In 2004, the unemployment rate was 11.4%.

The population's rate of participation in the workforce decreased from 47.3% in 1990 to 40.7% in 2000; this reduction was greater for men (from 58.4% to 48.5%) than for women (from 37.2% to 33.7%). In 2000, one out of every five persons in the workforce was unemployed, and unemployment was higher among women. The southern region (Ponce) had the highest unemployment rate (27%), and the Metropolitan Region had the lowest (14.2%).

In 1990–2000, the number of persons living below the poverty line decreased from 2,057,377 to 1,818,687, and the highest percentage corresponded to persons 0–17 years old (66.8% in 1990 and 58.4% in 2000). Of the total population living below the poverty line, women accounted for 53.3%. Poverty levels decreased among older adults from 57.5% to 44.0%. In 2000, 48.2% of the total population and 44.6% of all families lived below the poverty line, and in 68 of the 78 municipalities, 50% of the population lived below the poverty line. The population with the highest concentration of poverty lives in the center of the island.

The country faces serious environmental problems, due partly to its small territory and accelerated urban growth. The Environmental Quality Board, the Department of Natural Resources, the Solid Waste Authority, and the United States Environmental Protection Agency are responsible for regulating and monitoring environmental protection activities.

Water quality varies. According to 2003 reports from the Environmental Quality Board and the Environmental Protection Agency, approximately 40% of Puerto Rico's bodies of water do not meet quality standards. The quality of surface water is generally poor due to discharged sewage and agricultural and industrial waste. In 2002, the United States Geological Survey and the Environmental Quality Board stated that the main pollutants in surface water were fecal bacteria and volatile organic nutrients and compounds. These pollutants come from treatment plants, agricultural activity, septic tanks, and domestic discharges. Pollution of aquifers is serious in some 19 places, preventing their use for human consumption. Water resources also have been affected by indiscriminate urbanization and the removal of vegetation and topsoil, which has played a role in changing watershed processes.

Air quality meets most of the established parameters, even though the Environmental Protection Agency occasionally fines the Electric Energy Authority for higher sulfur emissions than allowed. A determining factor contributing to air pollution is the excessive use of motor vehicles. In 2005, it was calculated that there were approximately one million motor vehicles in circulation.

Demographics, Mortality, and Morbidity

According to the most recent national census, Puerto Rico had a total population of 3,808,610 in 2000, of which 51.9% were women (1,975,033); urban dwellers represented 94% of the population. The male-to-female ratio decreased from 93.9:100 to 92.8:100. Among persons under 15 years old, the male-to-female ratio was 104.9:100; among persons 65 years old and older it was 74.9:100. The average rate of population growth in 1990–2000 was 0.8%, but due to a decreased fertility rate, there was a 23% reduction between 1990 and 2004. The average age of the population increased, meaning that the country had an older age structure. Birth rates have decreased, and life expectancy varied between 76.1 in 2000 and 77.5 in 2004. Figure 1 shows changes in the population structure between 1990 and 2005.

In 2000, population density was 429 persons per km^2, with 25% of the population residing in six municipalities on the country's northeastern coast. Between 2000 and 2003, life expectancy increased from 72.2 to 73.7 for men and from 79.9 to 81.1 for women; the fertility rate decreased to 1.8 children per woman in 2004. This rate is below the population replacement level (2.1 children per woman), which is largely attributed to the use of permanent contraceptive methods. Professional women have children at a later age and tend to have fewer children.

The population under 15 years old decreased from 958,219 (27.2%) in 1990 to 906,368 (23.8%) in 2000, and the number of persons 65 years old and older increased to 84,900. This trend is linked to changes in birth, mortality, and migration rates, as well as to medical advances and changes in eating habits and lifestyles. The average age for both men and women varied from 28.5 in 1990 to 32.1 in 2000.

Migration flows have increased substantially, and everything indicates that this trend will continue. In 2000, the immigrant population comprised 185,218 permanent residents (0.5% of the population), although some studies put this figure as high as 225,000. The population of non-regular foreign residents was estimated at between 100,000 and 120,000 persons. Outmigration mainly involves young people leaving Puerto Rico in search of new opportunities. Adults, on the other hand, return to the island to spend the later years there.

FIGURE 1. Population structure, by age and sex, Puerto Rico, 1990 and 2005.

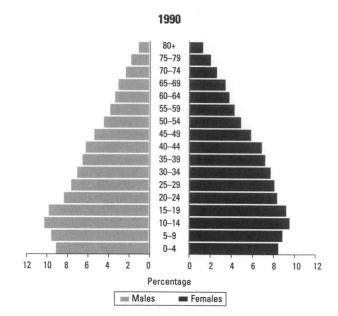

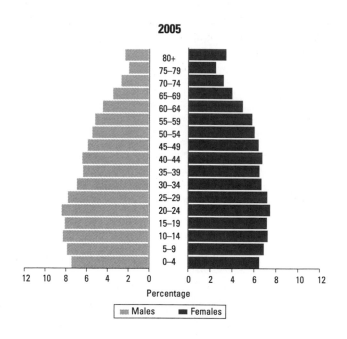

The general mortality rate increased from 7.3 per 1,000 population in 2003 to 7.5 per 1,000 in 2004, but there was a decrease compared with 1995 (8.3). One factor contributing to these changes was the decrease in the number of deaths due to heart disease (from 162.5 per 100,000 population in 1995 to 129.1 in 2004), the equivalent of a 20.6% reduction. Mortality rates due to AIDS decreased 64%, and remained higher among men. In 2004,

TABLE 1. Leading causes of death, Puerto Rico, 2004.

Cause of death	Rank	Number	Percentage	Rate (per 100,000 population)
All causes	—	29,066	100.0	746.1
Heart disease	1	5,031	17.3	129.1
Malignant neoplasms	2	4,829	16.6	124.0
Diabetes mellitus	3	2,569	8.8	66.0
Cerebrovascular diseases	4	1,532	5.3	39.4
Alzheimer's disease	5	1,211	4.2	31.1
Chronic pulmonary disease	6	1,165	4.0	29.9
Hypertensive diseases	7	1,133	3.9	29.1
All accidents	8	1,101	3.8	28.1
Pneumonia and influenza	9	1,030	3.5	26.4
Nephritis and nephrosis	10	832	2.9	21.4
Other causes	—	8,633	29.7	221.6

Source: Departmento de Salud, Annual de Estadísticas Vitales; 2004.

the mortality rate in men was 8.6 per 1,000 population and 6.4 per 1,000 in women.

Eight of the 10 leading causes of death (Table 1) were chronic diseases, accounting for nearly two-thirds of the country's deaths. Heart disease, malignant neoplasms, and diabetes have been the three leading causes of death for many years, accounting for nearly half of all deaths (44%). Even though heart disease remained the leading cause of death, it showed a downward trend, topping malignant neoplasms by approximately 1%. Mortality from AIDS has been largely reduced, and this cause now ranks as the 13th leading cause of death after being among the top ten for much of the 1990s. Mortality from septicemia also has considerably decreased in recent years. Accidents and murders remained among the twelve leading causes in 2001–2005, primarily affecting persons 15–19 years old.

The maternal mortality rate for 1991–2003 was 14.5 per 100,000 live births; in 2004, it was 17.6 per 100,000 (Figure 2), even though

the Department of Health's Division of Mothers, Children, and Adolescents states that cases may have been underreported. The 2002–2003 Descriptive Study on Maternal Mortality in Puerto Rico recorded 22 pregnancy-related deaths, while the Vital Statistics Report recorded only 11.

Data supplied by the Health Insurance Administration show that the primary diagnoses of the population covered by the Commonwealth's health insurance were hypertension (19.6%), diabetes mellitus (14%), and asthma (12%). These diseases represented 46.3% of the demand for service. In terms of morbidity by sex, there was a greater prevalence of hypertension (22.1%), diabetes (15.9%), anxiety (5.1%), asthma (13.2%), and depression (6.5%) among women, while the prevalence of schizophrenia (2.1%) was slightly higher among men. The prevalence of asthma is higher among the younger population, with those under 18 years old and young adults 18–24 years old being the most affected. The prevalence of diabetes is highest among per-

FIGURE 2. Maternal mortality rates, Puerto Rico, 1980–2004.

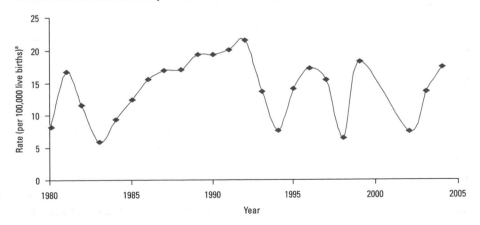

sons 55–64 years old, and hypertension is most prevalent among persons 65–74 years old. The prevalence of heart disease, cerebrovascular events, and congestive heart failure is highest among persons older than 75 years old. The frequency of mental disorders, specifically anxiety, depression, and schizophrenia, increases with age; the highest prevalence is found among 45–54-year-olds, decreasing among persons older than 74 years old. Most medical consultations were for hypertension and diabetes, cardiovascular events, and mental disorders; most emergency room visits were for asthma and diabetes. Coronary disease and cerebrovascular events were the reason for the greatest number of hospital admissions; diabetes was responsible for the highest number of laboratory services.

In 2000–2003, the highest rates of enteric diseases subject to mandatory reporting corresponded to salmonellosis, hepatitis A, shigellosis, campylobacteriosis, and giardiasis. Category II diseases with the highest incidence rates were grippal syndromes and influenza, gastroenteritis, conjunctivitis, and meningitis. Morbidity rates for diseases subject to mandatory reporting have remained at expected levels, except during outbreak years. In 2003, there was an outbreak of conjunctivitis in the entire country with 1,438 cases, and in 2004 there was an outbreak of aseptic meningitis, with a rate of 25.2 per 100,000 population. As of 2005, there had been no reported cases of West Nile virus in humans, even though it was identified in four animals in February 2004.

HEALTH OF POPULATION GROUPS

Children under 5 Years Old

The infant mortality rate decreased from 13.4 per 1,000 live births in 1990 to 8.1 per 1,000 live births in 2004. Neonatal mortality and postneonatal mortality also decreased. Approximately 50% of infant deaths occurred during the first 7 days of life (Figure 3).

In 2004, the five leading causes of infant mortality were short gestation and low birthweight, congenital malformations, respiratory problems originating in the perinatal period, other perinatal conditions and diseases, and circulatory system diseases. The three leading causes of neonatal mortality were short gestation and low birthweight, sepsis, and respiratory problems originating in the perinatal period. The three leading causes of postneonatal mortality were congenital deformations, septicemia, and diseases of the circulatory system.

An evaluation of the distribution of infant and fetal deaths that considered age at death and birthweight, as well as a calculation of excess mortality according to the categories of maternal health, maternal care during pregnancy, and newborn and infant care, determined that the decrease in infant deaths was largely due to technological advances in the neonatal intensive care

rooms, rather than to improvements in the mother's health during pregnancy or to prenatal care. WHO's Perinatal Periods of Risk model was used to evaluate the indicators.

The most important of the variables associated with infant mortality was low birthweight. Seven out of every ten deaths (73.4%) in 2001 occurred in children with low birthweight, and 50% of all infant deaths occurred among children who weighed less than 1.5 kg. Approximately 1 out of every 10 infant deaths were to adolescent mothers.

According to a paired case-control study carried out between 2000 and 2003 by the Department of Health's Division of Mothers, Children, and Adolescents, the number of children with low birthweight increased from 10.8% in 2000 to 11.5% in 2003. The major factors that contributed to this were preeclampsia, a weight increase of fewer than 20 pounds or of more than 30, obesity, vaginal bleeding during the first trimester, having had fewer than eight prenatal visits, and suicide attempts during pregnancy.

Adolescents 10–14 and 15–19 Years Old

According to the 2000 census, there were 619,236 adolescents (17% of the population), of which 49,339 were enrolled in the Commonwealth's Health Plan.

A study by the Mental Health and Anti-Addiction Services Administration carried out in 2000–2002 and involving 426,038 Puerto Rican private- and public-school students from the fifth to twelfth grades showed that the most frequently used drugs, at least once, among adolescents in the fifth and sixth grades were alcohol (34.4%), cigarettes (6.1%), and inhalants (2.7%). Among adolescents between the seventh and ninth grades, the most used drugs were alcohol (43.6%) and cigarettes (15.5%). A total of 6.8% indicated that they had consumed illegal drugs. The drugs most commonly used by adolescents between the tenth and twelfth grades were alcohol (76.2%) and cigarettes (40.4%). A total of 20.6% stated that they had consumed some illegal drug, with marihuana (18.9%) and designer drugs (3.8%) being the most frequently used (1).

It is difficult to estimate the total number of adolescent pregnancies because there is no reliable record of the abortions performed each year. Data available from clinics on pregnancy termination in fiscal years 2002/2003 and 2003/2004 show that of the 14,593 induced abortions, 4,166 (29%) were performed on mothers 15–19 years old. Birth rates among adolescent mothers 10–19 years old have decreased, from 42.9 per 1,000 in 1997 to 31.4 per 1,000 in 2004.

Older Adults 60 Years Old and Older

The proportion of persons older than 60 years old increased from 13.2% in 1990 to 15.4% in 2000. The rate of growth of the population of 60-year-olds has been higher than that of the pop-

FIGURE 3. Infant, neonatal, and postneonatal mortality rates, Puerto Rico, 1990–2004.

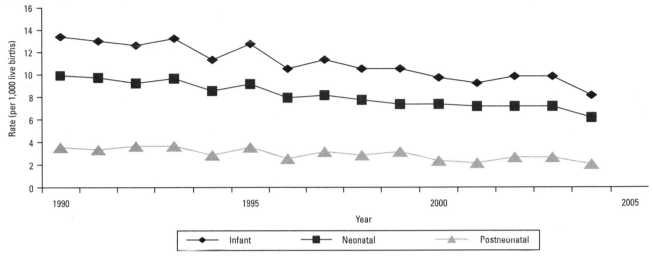

Source: Departmento de Salud, Informe Annual de Estadísticas Vitales, 1990–2004.

ulation as a whole. According to data from the Health Conditions of Older Adults in Puerto Rico, during 2002–2003 the prevalence of hypertension, arthritis, obesity, diabetes, incontinence, and depression was greater among older adults and higher among women than men in this group.

Workers

Musculoskeletal conditions gave rise to most of the cases of occupational diseases in the last decade. In the private sector, injuries due to repetitive motion caused the highest number of workdays lost (35–45 days, on average). In 2001, the public sector reported 31 workdays lost due to repetitive motion. The Government Insurance Fund, the body responsible for providing health care, reported that the injuries responsible for the most number of cases were back contusions and injuries, with figures varying between 12,000 and 15,000 annually.

Persons with Disabilities

The 2000 census included two questions specifically directed to persons with disabilities: one dealing with sensory and physical disabilities and the second with mental disabilities, limitations on activities of daily living, and employability. There were 934,674 persons older than 5 years old who had some disability, representing 26.8% of the total population—6.9% of those 5–15 years old, 26.8% of those 16–64 years old, and 59.1% of persons 65 years old and older had some form of disability.

According to the 2002 Behavioral Risk Factor Surveillance System survey, 14.9% of those interviewed stated that they had some type of limitation. Women reported more limitations (15.8%) than men (13.9%). The most common health problems among people with some form of limitation were back problems (18.2%), followed by emotional problems, depression, and anxiety (13%).

According to data from the 2001 Ongoing Health Study, chronic conditions were the most prevalent among the disabling conditions studied (1,897 per 10,000), followed by physical disabilities (264 per 10,000), mental disorders (253 per 10,000), conditions associated with developmental deficiencies (98 per 10,000), and severe injuries (41 per 10,000).

HEALTH CONDITIONS AND PROBLEMS

COMMUNICABLE DISEASES

Vector-borne Diseases

According to data from the Environmental Health Division and the Epidemiology Program of the Department of Health, during 2001–2005, there were a significant number of suspected cases and deaths due to **dengue**: 5,233 suspected cases and one death in 2001; 2,906 suspected cases and no deaths in 2002; 3,735 suspected cases and one death in 2003; 3,289 suspected cases and one death in 2004; and 5,775 suspected cases in 2005 (no data available on deaths).

Vaccine-preventable Diseases

The incidence of cases due to these diseases decreased notably; the highest number was recorded in people 60 years old and older who had not completed their vaccination series.

In 2001, there were three cases of **rubella**, one of **parotiditis**, and one of **meningitis;** in 2002, there were three cases of **tetanus** (who died), two of **rubella,** two of **mumps**, and two of meningitis. Between 2003 and 2005, one case of **whooping cough**, four cases of tetanus, nine of meningitis, and one of rubella were recorded. There were a significant number of cases of **hepatitis A**: 258 cases in 2001, 242 in 2002, 104 in 2003, 65 in 2004, and 66 in 2005. The number of **hepatitis B** cases was: 297 in 2001, 221 in 2002, 145 in 2003, 88 in 2004, and 63 in 2005. The number of reported cases of **chicken pox** was 2,186 in 2001; 1,141 in 2002; 652 in 2003; 445 in 2004; and 779 in 2005. There were no reported cases of **diphtheria** or **polio**.

Chronic Communicable Diseases

The incidence of **tuberculosis** increased from 121 cases per 100,000 inhabitants in 2001 to 129 cases per 100,000 in 2002. In 2003, the incidence of tuberculosis was 115 per 100,000 inhabitants; in 2004, 123 per 100,000; and in 2005, 113 per 100,000. Incidence was greater among men (70% of cases). Persons 15–44 years old were the most affected.

HIV/AIDS and Other Sexually Transmitted Infections

In 2002, Puerto Rico had the seventh highest incidence rate for AIDS cases in the United States and its territories. In 1990–2002, there were 28,701 accumulated AIDS cases reported. Men were the most affected (76.4% of the cases reported). Most cases were diagnosed among persons 30–39 years old (43.4%), and this distribution was the same for men and women. There were 18,154 reported deaths up to 2004, and from that year forward the number of AIDS deaths decreased. AIDS-related deaths were the 23rd leading cause of death between 2000 and 2004.

Use of intravenous drugs (50.2%) and unprotected heterosexual contact (24.3%) were the most prevalent HIV transmission modes; 16.6% of cases were among men who have sex with other men.

Up to 2002, the number of pediatric AIDS cases rose to 404, with mother-to-child HIV transmission being responsible for exposure in 94.8% of pediatric cases. No cases of pediatric AIDS were reported in 2003–2004.

Chlamydia infection has been the sexually transmitted disease with the highest incidence in recent years, with a rate of 72.1 per 100,000 population in 2003; the greatest number of cases were found in women. **Gonorrhea** has been declining, but this could be the result of underreporting, because in recent years a technique has been used that does not allow for taking cultures from certain areas of the body.

Rates of primary and secondary **syphilis**, which include early latent and late latent syphilis, increased from 6.4 per 100,000 population in 2001 to 7.0 in 2002, decreasing to 5.2 per 100,000 in 2003 and to 4.7 in 2004. In 2005, the rates of primary and secondary syphilis increased to 5.8. The disease affects men more, and the age groups most affected were persons 20–24 years old and 30–34 years old.

Zoonoses

The Surveillance System reported 98 cases of **animal rabies** in 2001, 87 in 2002, 71 in 2003, 61 in 2004, and 71 in 2005. Cases were reported in mongooses, cats, dogs, horses, and cows, in descending order.

NONCOMMUNICABLE DISEASES

Metabolic and Nutritional Diseases

Diabetes has been the third leading cause of death for the last 15 years, with rates steadily increasing in the period. Between 2001 and 2004, the diabetes mortality rate increased 5.6% (from 62.5 per 100,000 population to 66.0 in 2004). In 2004, about 1 of every 10 deaths was caused by diabetes. Diabetes deaths increase with age, and the highest rates were among those over 85 years old. In 2004, the mortality rate due to diabetes was 68.8 per 100,000 in men and 63.3 per 100,000 in women.

Some 19.3% of the population follows some form of diet, and women are more likely to do so. Data for 2002 from the Behavioral Risk Factor Surveillance System (BRFSS) showed that 14.5% of the population reported that they consumed five or more fruits and vegetables per day, 10.2% reported that they consumed little or no fruits and vegetables, and 44.7% reported that they consumed one or two portions.

BRFSS data showed that in 2002 nearly 61.6% of persons interviewed were **overweight**. A report from the Women, Infants, and Children (WIC) Program showed that among children 3–5 years old who participated in the Head Start Program, 7.7% were classified as obese.

Overweight and obesity were also major risk factors among older adults. According to the Puerto Rican Elderly Health Conditions report, 33% of women and 27% of men 60 years old or older had a body mass index (BMI) of 30 or more in 2002–2003. According to BRFSS, 49.2% of older adults stated that they did not exercise at all in their free time in 2001; 46.9% did so in 2002.

Cardiovascular Diseases

Deaths due to cardiovascular diseases were mostly recorded among people 65 years old and older. Considering the distribution of deaths due to heart disease with the aging of the population, it would be expected that the number of cardiovascular deaths would remain equal or increase. Instead deaths due to cardiovascular disease decreased between 1999 and 2004.

Malignant Neoplasms

Malignant neoplasms are getting to be the leading cause of death, after having ranked second in 1999. Neoplasms in diges-

Streamlining the Health System and Reaching Out to Vulnerable Groups

Fueled by the Government's reform processes, Puerto Rico's health system has undergone far-reaching changes designed to improve performance and granting the state government the leadership role for the health sector. To improve access to services and extend their reach, the Government of Puerto Rico has embraced as a priority the development of systems to provide support to vulnerable groups such as women, young people, women who are heads of households, children, and retirees. To this end, it has engaged in various health promotion and protection initiatives. In addition, the Government is carrying out a disease prevention public policy and reformulating the health policy that sets the Department of Health's functions. Administrative Order 179, issued on 15 January 2003, is the most recent mechanism for reorganizing the Department by streamlining its structure, better coordinating related activities, reducing duplication and overlap, bolstering coordination, establishing lines of supervision, and establishing frameworks for activities or intervention.

tive organs were the leading cause of death, accounting for 31.8% of total deaths; followed by prostate neoplasms (10.3%); neoplasms in lymphatic, hematopoietic, and related tissues (9.0%); and breast neoplasms (8.4%). Breast and prostate neoplasms have increased considerably since 1990. The highest numbers for malignant neoplasms were recorded among persons 60 years old and older. Among women, malignant neoplasms of the breast accounted for nearly one-third of malignant neoplasms, followed by colorectal and cervical neoplasms. Among men, prostate, lung, and colorectal neoplasms ranked highest.

OTHER HEALTH PROBLEMS OR ISSUES

Mental Health

Prevalence rates of severe mental disorders in adults and severe emotional disturbance in children and adolescents were estimated using the standards set by the Center for Mental Health Services. At least two of the following criteria (2) must be met for a mental illness to be classified as severe: have a psychiatric diagnosis as defined in the Diagnostic and Statistical Manual of Mental Disorders (DSM-IV-TR) (3); have a score of 5 on the subscales of the Psychiatric Symptoms and Dysfunctional Scales; and have a score of 23 or more on the subscales of the Center for Epidemiological Studies Depression Scale.

In 2000, the prevalence rate of severe mental diseases among the population older than 18 years old was approximately 8.3% (225,470). This estimate coincided with figures from a study on the patterns of use of mental health services (4). The last epidemiological study of the population of children and adolescents 4–17 years old showed that nearly 140,528 children and adolescents meet the criteria for mental disorders in the DSM-IV-TR,

with slight to moderate impediments, and nearly 59,125 meet the criteria for severe emotional disturbance (5).

In fiscal year 2003, some 32,521 children were treated through the Health Reform in the Area of Mental Health and the Mental Health and Anti-Addiction Services Administration. Of these, it is estimated that 50% (16,260) met the criteria for severe emotional disorders (6–9). Some 42,865 (72.5%) of the 59,125 children and adolescents with a severe mental condition and severe disability did not receive mental health care. It was estimated that nearly 51,016 persons 65 years old or older suffer from some defined psychiatric problem and that between 64,000 and 106,000 older persons could have a major mental health problem.

Addictions

According to data from the 2002 Ongoing Health Study, 29.9% of persons older than 17 years old had smoked at some point; 14.7% continued to smoke, with greater prevalence among men (21.3%) than women (9.6%); 62% of regular smokers stated that they intended to quit.

According to the Ongoing Health Study, approximately 16% of those older than 17 years old had consumed five or more drinks per day in 2002. Men tended to have consumed three and a half times more alcohol than women.

Oral Health

BRFSS data for 2002 showed that nearly 75% of the population visited a dentist or dental clinic within the year prior to the interview; 21.7% of the population stated that they had lost six teeth or more due to cavities or periodontal disease. According to PREHCO data, more than 40% of adults older than 60 years had lost most or all of their teeth; 60.4% of the elderly had bridges or dentures, and 93.3% used them.

RESPONSE OF THE HEALTH SECTOR

Health Policies and Plans

The Government's reform processes have brought about major changes in the health system over the last decade. The Government was given the steering role in the health sector, and it has made major efforts to increase access to health services, control costs, and improve user satisfaction, as well as to pay greater attention to health promotion and the prevention and control of diseases.

The Department of Health was reorganized through Administrative Order 179 (15 January 2003) in order to streamline the organizational structure, improve the coordination of related operations, facilitate coordination of activities, establish lines of supervision, and define frameworks for action or intervention.

Between 1994 and 2000, the Government sold most of the health service infrastructure to private investors and contracted out the health insurance of the indigent population. Puerto Rico was divided into 10 health regions, and public health centers were privatized. The 10 health regions were incorporated into the Health Reform (Commonwealth Plan) and beginning in 2002 were restructured into eight regions: North, Northeast, Metro-North, East, Southeast, West, Southwest, and San Juan.

The privatization of health services produced negative effects, including a lack of comprehensive coordination in multiple institutions; competition between general hospitals for patients and for reimbursements by insurers; duplication of services at all levels of service provision; limitation of endovascular neurosurgery services; division of physical and vocational rehabilitation services and limited access to psychiatric services, both in hospitals and in intensive ambulatory care and care in distant facilities; lack of traditional psychiatric rehabilitation services for long-term care patients; lack of comprehensive psychiatric services in general and specialized hospitals; need for telemedicine services for the entire island, which currently operate only in a limited basis in Vieques; and a lack of coordination in the provision of services.

Health Strategies and Programs

In its effort to improve access and expand the provision of services, the Government offers educational opportunities and implements support systems for women, female heads of household, young people, children, and retirees. Various initiatives and projects are being carried out to promote and protect health. In addition, a public policy has been established to prevent diseases, and the Department of Health's health policy, which is part of its steering role, is being recast.

In order to improve health services for the medically indigent population, achieve greater efficiency, and improve price and quality, "controlled competition" was established. Those eligible

for this first stage were persons living up to a 200% level of poverty. Poverty level was calculated as US$ 401 for a one-person family, with US$ 95 added for each additional person. Coverage was provided to families with monthly incomes up to US$ 791 and low deductibles were set. The deductibles would not be applicable for people with a 50% level of medical indigence. Complete coverage is offered through insurers to individuals with a 200% level of medical indigence.

Organization of the Health System

Health services include public facilities, privatized public facilities, and private facilities, all of which are duly accredited by the Department of Health's Deputy Secretariat of Standardization and Accreditation.

The Health Insurance Administration (a public corporation with an independent legal status and separate from any other Government entity, agency, department, or instrument) is responsible for negotiating and contracting quality health insurance for eligible residents regardless of their economic situation. The Administration was charged with ensuring the right to choose among several insurance companies working in the region. It cannot do so, however; as a result of the current situation's complexity, there is only one insurer operating in each region.

The Government, through the Health Insurance Administration, offers health plans such as the Basic Coverage Plan, the Special Coverage Plan, and the Mental Health Coverage Plan, health plans that must provide quality medical and hospital services, regardless of a person's capability to pay for them.

The Basic Coverage Plan includes preventive, surgical, hospitalization, maternity, outpatient, and emergency-room rehabilitation services, as well as diagnostic tests; dental care; sea, air, and land ambulances; drugs; and others.

The Special Coverage Plan offers intensive care services, cardiovascular and neurosurgery procedures; peritoneal dialysis treatments; hemodialysis and related services; intensive neonatal care; malignant neoplasm treatments; diagnostic tests that include tomography and magnetic resonance imagery; and other services. Services are offered through the network of participating providers, who have contractual arrangements with insurers throughout the island. The Plan also includes services for the medically indigent recipients of Medicare, which have been approved by the Medicaid program.

The Mental Health Coverage Plan includes medical exams and the evaluation and treatment of mental illnesses; ambulatory psychiatric and psychological services; partial hospitalization; stabilization, detoxification, and medication; and ambulance services.

The Catastrophic Coverage Plan includes treatment for AIDS, leprosy, and substance abuse, as well as the implantation of pacemakers, valves, and artificial heart equipment. As a rule, insurers prefer to disburse special coverage expenses to retain greater

TABLE 2. Persons treated through the Reform's mental health area, Puerto Rico, 2000–2003.

Year	Number of patients	Number of insured	Percentage of access or use
2000	125,238	1,795,067	7.0
2001	125,511	1,730,623	7.3
2002	146,584	1,623,169	9.0
2003*	136,937	1,521,848	9.0

Source: Administración de Servicios de Salud. Database, March 2004.

control over catastrophic conditions because these services are very expensive.

According to data from the Office of the Insurance Commissioner, 3,154,582 people had some health insurance plan in 2003, but this figure could double because some persons may have enrolled in health insurance plans with more than one insurance company, because of differences in the type of medical insurance, or because of how the information was gathered.

In 2003, 40% of the population was covered under the Commonwealth Medical Plan, 14% received medical care through Medicare, 37% had some form of private insurance, and 8% had no medical plan.

Health reforms in mental health have enabled services to be provided to approximately 1.5 million persons, even though service utilization is extremely low when compared to the magnitude of the country's problem (Table 2).

Public Health Services

The law requires that children be vaccinated before being enrolled in school. Thanks to this requirement, annual coverage levels among the student population (which is currently 726,511 students) is between 80% and 87%, meaning that 8 out of every 10 students have up-to-date vaccinations. The Health Department provides vaccines against influenza, pneumonia, and tetanus/diphtheria for the medically indigent and at-risk populations, which has taken coverage above 90% as a rule. May 2001 marked the beginning of a shortage of the diphtheria, tetanus, and whooping cough (DTaP) vaccine, which caused a decrease in coverage from 94.1% to 31% in 2002.

In 2002, a surveillance system was developed to combat West Nile virus, and work was being carried out on the design and implementation of a health database (DATAWAREHOUSE) that will provide a sophisticated system for capturing events and that includes appropriate and reliable information for strategic planning and for measuring health results.

In 2000, 99% of the population had a home connection to potable water. In 2005, the Aqueducts and Sewer Authority provided services to 1,174,000 residential clients (93.1% of homes). Several communities have established their own potable water

system and, according to the Department of Health's Division of Potable Water, have provided services to some 2% of homes. The Aqueducts and Sewer Authority reported that 678,000 homes (54%) were connected to the sewerage system. Water supply in urban areas is uninterrupted throughout the day; all water systems are disinfected through treatment plants.

Waste is mainly disposed of in landfills, which has created a critical problem. According to data from the Solid Waste Authority, five million tons of waste are generated annually and, of those, nearly 2,600,000 are household waste (1.8 kg per person per day). Most of this waste is processed in municipal dumps; only 15% is recycled.

Individual Care Services

There were 68 hospitals in fiscal year 2001–2002, 12 of which belonged to the public sector, and 56 to the private sector. In terms of distribution, 37% (25) of the hospitals were in the Metropolitan Region; 16% (11), in the Ponce region; 13% (9), in Arecibo, Caguas, and Mayagüez; and only 7% (5) in Bayamón. The Metropolitan Region had the highest proportion of hospitals per population (1 per 40,420), while Bayamón had the lowest, at 1 per 120,144 population.

The distribution of available beds per 1,000 population also varied significantly. The national average was 3.3 beds per 1,000 population, but the Metropolitan Region accounted for 41% of the 12,562 beds, with a rate of 5.0 beds per 1,000 population; Ponce, for 16%, with a rate of 3.3; Caguas, for 12%, with a rate of 2.7; Bayamón, for 13%, with a rate of 2.6; Mayagüez, for 11%, with a rate of 2.5; and Arecibo, for 7.5%, with a rate of 2.0.

Human Resources

According to the registry of health professionals, there were 54,120 active professionals in 2001–2004 (38.8% were concentrated in the Metropolitan Region): 8,225 physicians, 24,777 nurses, 2,779 medical technicians, 2,428 pharmacists, 1,457 dentists, and 14,454 other professionals. Of the total health professionals, 75.2% of physicians and 70.9% of other health professionals worked in the private sector; the rest worked in the public sector or in volunteer work (24.5% and 0.3%, respectively). There were 30.2% working as general practitioners; 11.8% worked in internal medicine; 10.7%, in pediatrics; and 47.3%, in specialties, including obstetrics and gynecology, family medicine, general surgery, and anesthesiology.

Primary centers were staffed by primary medicine physicians, such as family physicians, internists, pediatricians, obstetrician-gynecologists, and general practitioners; they also had the support of other physicians depending on morbidity and mortality patterns in the area. In addition, they may have the support of dentists, optometrists, clinical laboratories, x-rays, and pharmacies.

TABLE 3. Health Plan budget, Puerto Rico, fiscal year 2002–2003.

Source	Amount (US$)	Percentage
Medicaid	189,000,000	14.8
Health Insurance Program for Children	26,000,000	2.0
Municipalities	136,000,000	10.6
General Fund	931,000,000	72.6
Total	1,282,000,000	100.0

Source: Departamento de Salud de Puerto Rico, Administración de Seguros de Salud.

Research and Technological Development in Health

One of the most important aspects of the health system is the investment in the automatization and technological development of health processes and services. Both the public and private sectors have major technological resources at their disposal. In recent years, the Government has invested approximately US$ 300 million to purchase highly sophisticated diagnostic and treatment equipment, as well as the most advanced and secure information and data processing technology, which it has made available to patients. The vast majority of these resources are concentrated at the central level (Metropolitan Region); other health regions scarcely have basic resources such as printers, photocopiers, personal computers, Internet access, and others.

Health Sector Expenditures and Financing

In Puerto Rico, the flow of funds between sources and agents is channeled through public financing, payment of public or private insurance premiums, and user fees or quotas. The flow of funds between agents and providers is channeled via different payment mechanisms, including budgets, fees for services, and training. In 1999–2003, the health sector held one of the most important positions in the country's economy, with spending increasing from US$ 10.1 billion to US$ 12.2 billion. This increase was reflected both in the amount of resources used by the health sector and in the increase of the prices for said resources. The public sector was an extremely important component in the provision and financing of health services. In 1994–1995, financing of the health card amounted to US$ 82.3 million. The health sector represented 16.4% of the GDP for fiscal year 2003. Annual per capita health spending was US$ 3,143 in current prices for fiscal year 2003, which represented an increase of US$ 466 in per capita spending compared with 1999. Table 3 shows the breakdown of the Health Plan budget for fiscal year 2002/2003.

Before the Reform, the Government offered health services through the corresponding agencies (the Health Facilities and Services Administration and the Department of Health). All of these services were considered central government expenses. After the Health Plan, these expenses were considered part of the private sector. The Government paid the insuring company a premium so that people who were members of the Plan would receive a health card and be able to receive medical services and medicines. The premium payment was considered as a transfer payment to individuals, becoming part of their personal income. As a result, people's consumption spending increased for medical services, medicines, and other related expenses. As the Health Plan has been progressively implemented, the Government's consumption spending has decreased and income and spending for personal consumption have increased. Health reforms have resulted in a system that has exceeded 20% of the gross domestic product in health care expenses, even though quality is questionable, and both subscribers and providers are dissatisfied.

References

1. Administración de Servicios de Salud Mental y Contra la Adicción. Universidad Central del Caribe. Programa de Evaluación de Necesidades de Abuso de Sustancias de Puerto Rico. "2002 Household Survey" Puerto Rico; 2003.
2. Plan for Comprehensive Community Mental Health Services for Adults with Severe Mental Illness and Children and Adolescents with Seriously Emotionally Disturbances for Fiscal Year 2004. Puerto Rico: Mental Health and Anti-Addiction Services Administration; 2004.
3. Diagnostic and Statistical Manual of Mental Disorders (DSM-IV-TR). Washington, DC: American Psychiatric Association; 2000.
4. Alegría M, McGuire T, Vera Canino G, Calderón J. Changes in access to mental health care for the poor and the Non-poor with manager care: Results from the Health Reform in Puerto Rico *American Journal of Public Health* 2002;91:1421-1434.
5. Canino G. The prevalence of specific psychiatric disorders and mental health utilization among children in Puerto Rico. *Archives of GeneralPsychiatry* 2003;61:85-93.
6. Lanhey BB, Flagg EW, Bird HR, Schwab-Stone M, Canino G, Dulcan MK, Leaf PJ, Davies M, Brogan D, Bourdon K, Horowitz SM, Narrow WE, Weissman MM, Kandel DB, Jensen PS, Richters JE, Regier DA 1996 ; The NIMH method for epidemiology of the child and adolescent mental disorder (MECA) study : background and methodology. *Journal of the American Academy of Child and Adolescent Psychiatry* 1996; 37.2:855-864.
7. Leaf PJ, Alegría M, Cohen P, Goodman SH, Horowitz SM, Hoven CW, Narrows WE, Vaden Kierman M, Regier D. Mental health service use in the community and schools: results from the four-community MECA study. *Journal of the American Academy of Child and Adolescent Psychiatry* 1996;37.2: 889–897.

8. Ribera JC, Canino GJ, Rubio-Stipec M, Bravo M, Bird HR, Freeman D, Shrout P, Bauermeister J, Alegría M, Woodbury M, Huertas S, Guevarra LM. 1996. The diagnostic interview schedule for children (DISC 2.3): Description, acceptability, prevalences and performance in the MECA study. *Journal of the American Academy of Child and Adolescent Psychiatry* 1996;37.2:195–204.

9. Shaffer D, Fisher P, Dulcan M, Davis D, Piacentini G, Shwab-Stone M, Lanhey B, Bourdon K, Jensen P, Bird H, Canino G, Regier D. The NIMH Diagnostic Interview Schedule For Children (DISC 2.3): Description, acceptability, prevalences and performance in the MECA study. *Journal of the American Academy of Child and Adolescent Psychiatry* 1996;35.7: 865–877.

SAINT KITTS AND NEVIS

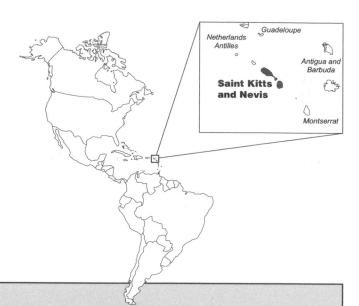

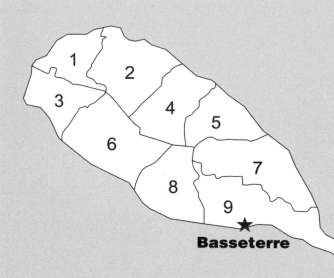

Basseterre

Saint Kitts

1 Saint Paul Capisterre
2 Saint John Capisterre
3 Saint Anne Sandy Point
4 Christ Church Nichola Town
5 Saint Mary Cayon
6 Saint Thomas Middle Island
7 Saint Peter Basseterre
8 Trinity Palmetto Point
9 Saint George Basseterre

Nevis

10 Saint James Windward
11 Saint Thomas Lowland
12 Saint Paul Charlestown
13 Saint John Figtree
14 Saint George Gingerland

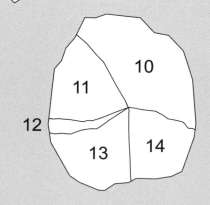

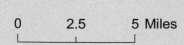

0   2.5   5 Miles

The Federation of Saint Kitts and Nevis lies in the northern section of the Eastern Caribbean's Leeward Islands. Saint Kitts and Nevis are of volcanic origin; they are separated by a 3 km channel at their closest point. Saint Kitts measures 176.12 km²; Nevis, 93.2 km².

GENERAL CONTEXT AND HEALTH DETERMINANTS

Saint Kitts and Nevis attained political independence from Great Britain in 1983. The titular Head of State is the Queen of England, whose local representative is the Governor General. The constitution provides for a federal government based in Basseterre, Saint Kitts, which is responsible for foreign affairs, national security, and justice, as well for the oversight of Saint Kitts' domestic affairs. The constitution provides Nevis with full autonomy through the Nevis Island Administration. The heads of the executive branches of government are the Prime Minister at the federal level and the Premier at the local level in Nevis. Legislative powers are vested in the Federal Parliament and Nevis Island Assembly, each of which has specific jurisdictions.

The political relationship between Saint Kitts and Nevis has always been a point of contention since the 19th century during the British colonial rule, when Nevis (and at that time also Anguilla) was annexed to Saint Kitts for administrative purposes. The constitution envisions a process for the eventual secession of Nevis that includes the holding of a referendum. The most recent of these was in 1998, in which the vote for secession was 61%, short of the required two-thirds.

In the administration of health, some responsibilities are federal and others are local. The Federal Ministry of Health, based in Saint Kitts, administers health in Saint Kitts and handles some integrated functions such as public health surveillance, health professional regulation, disease management programs (such as HIV/AIDS), disease prevention programs (such as the Expanded Program on Immunization), and matters involving international dealings.

Health service delivery functions, such as the financial and budgetary management of health institutions, are administered separately. Personnel administration also is separate, but the nomenclature of posts is virtually the same. As a rule, public service arrangements are identical and each island's Ministry of Health operates within the framework of the same General Orders.

Social, Political, and Economic Determinants

Despite the political divide, there is no social distinction between the people of Saint Kitts and those of Nevis, who freely move, live in, and work in both islands. There is inter-island communication, mostly by a 40-minute ferry between the capitals, and, to a much lesser extent, by plane (5-minute flight). The increase in number of ferryboats from two in 2001 to six in 2005 is an indicator of heightened inter-island movement and commercial activity.

Saint Kitts and Nevis has a small, open economy based on services (73% of GDP in 2004), and secondary activities such as manufacturing and construction. GDP performance was mixed in the years under review.

From 2001 to 2003 GDP growth at constant prices showed negative values, while growth was 5.1% and 6.8% in 2004 and 2005 respectively. The decline registered from 2001 to 2003 was attributed to the negative impact on travel and tourism after the 2001 attacks in the United States. According to data from the Ministry of National Security, United States citizens make up 42% of visitors, and total visitor arrivals declined by one-third from 333,361 in 2001 to 246, 364 in 2002, and 246,787 in 2003.

The sugar industry had historically been the major contributor to economic activity (especially in Saint Kitts). It closed down in 2005 after three centuries of operation and several years of financial losses that led to unsustainable debt. Sugar production at the Saint Kitts Sugar Manufacturing Corporation fell 16.1% between 1983–1993 and 1994–2002, and output declined by 24% between 2002 and 2003. The industry's closure left approximately 1,500 people unemployed, which led to an increased demand for government health and social services. The financial burden of medical services for sugar industry workers, hitherto paid for by the former employer, was immediately transferred to the Ministry of Health and the Ministry Responsible for Social and Community Development and Gender Affairs. Former sugar industry workers, including immigrant workers, are entitled to free community clinic and hospital care until they find employment.

Improved GDP performance in 2004 and 2005 reflects robust performance in the tourism sector, with visitor arrivals estimated at 389,868, a 58% increase over 2003. According to information from the Ministry of Tourism, the number of hotel rooms increased by 14%, from 1,611 in 2003 to 1,825 in 2004.

A survey of living conditions cosponsored by the Caribbean Development Bank and the Government of Saint Kitts and Nevis, which was conducted in 1999–2000, documented an unemployment rate of 5.6% for Saint Kitts and 8.6% for Nevis. The workforce increased 8%, from 21,741 persons in 1999 to 23,361 in 2004. Average wages also increased 28.6% over the same period, from US$ 6,295 to US$ 8,098.

The Saint Kitts and Nevis 2000 Poverty Assessment Survey, sponsored by the Caribbean Development Bank, showed a poverty[1] rate of 30.5% in Saint Kitts and of 32% in Nevis. In Saint Kitts, 56% of the poor were female, 68% were under 25 years, and 57% of the working poor had no secondary education certification. In Nevis, 26% of the poor were female, 58% were under 25 years, and 37% of the working poor had no secondary education certification. Of the population in Saint Kitts, 11% was defined as indigent[2]; in Nevis, 17% of the population was defined as such. Adult education and skills training programs have been developed to improve competitiveness within the new service economy.

According to the 2001 Population and Housing Census, there are 15,680 households in the country, an increase of 23.2% from the previous census in 1991. The average household size in 2001 was three persons, with 79% having installed toilet facilities and 94% having piped water. In Saint Kitts, 20% of the water supply is treated, compared with 90% in Nevis; a project is ongoing to ensure that the entire water supply meets WHO standards.

Every child has access to preschool, primary, secondary, and tertiary education, regardless of income status or national origin. Saint Kitts and Nevis has attained a 98% literacy rate; this achievement is driven by the 1975 Education Act (updated in 2005), which mandates compulsory school attendance from 5 to 16 years. Preschool attendance is actively promoted, and enrollment levels are near 100%. The policy of universal primary and secondary education has resulted in a nearly total transfer rate from primary to secondary school. Enrollment in advanced vocational programs has increased from 60 persons in 2000 to 113 in 2004, consistent with the Government's policy to encourage the acquisition of skills necessary for employment in hospitality, construction, electronic and mechanical technology repair, and handicraft.

There are two Government tertiary institutions, one on each island, which are integrated to provide education and training along academic, technical, and professional streams. Diploma and associate degrees programs are available in various subject

areas, including teacher education and nursing. Average enrollment increased from 450 students in 1995–1999 to 575 in 2000–2004, as more persons availed themselves of quality, low-cost university education at home. The Government has expanded the availability of higher education: along with the primary affiliation with the University of the West Indies, other options include credit transfer arrangements with several United States universities and colleges and study arrangements in Cuba, all handled by Government-supported financing arrangements. Low-cost student loans are available through the Development Bank of Saint Kitts and Nevis: in 2004, 284 loans were issued to students, compared to 156 in 2001. Several countries, including the Republic of China (Taiwan), provide postgraduate scholarships. The human resource investment dividend is emphasized by the return of an unprecedented nine medical doctors and two dentists from study and training in Cuba since 2002.

Demographics, Mortality, and Morbidity

According to the 2001 Population Census, there were 46,325 persons living in the country (22,973 males and 23,352 females), a 12% increase from the figure of 40,618 in the 1991 census; 76% of the population resides in Saint Kitts. The estimated population in 2005 was 48,781 with 36,676 persons in Saint Kitts and 12,105 persons in Nevis. The country's population is relatively young, with persons younger than 20 years old representing 38.6% of the total population, and persons younger than 25 years old representing approximately 50% of the total population (see Figure 1). Life expectancy at birth in 2003 was 70 years (69 for males, 72 for females). The crude birth rate dropped from 17.3 live births per 1,000 population in 2001 to 13.7 in 2005 and the number of births ranged from 803 in 2001 to 654 in 2004. Average total fertility declined from 2.6 children per woman in 1996–2000 to 2.4 in 2001–2005.

Compared to the population distribution in the 1991 census, the population distribution in 2001 shows a relative increase in the proportion of persons aged 35 to 50 years, an age group that makes up a substantial segment of the workforce (see Figure 1). There was migration into Saint Kitts and Nevis from Guyana, the Dominican Republic, and, to a lesser extent, Jamaica attracted by job expansion in the service and construction sectors. Increased job opportunities also encouraged nationals to stay in Saint Kitts and Nevis.

The country's epidemiologic profile is dominated by chronic noncommunicable diseases, with diabetes, hypertension, heart disease, and malignant neoplasms increasingly challenging the organization and financing of services. Drug abuse and injuries also are significant morbidities, especially among adolescents and young adults. Dengue fever is the only endemic disease reported with outbreaks occurring every three to four years. The major morbidities in children are acute viral upper respiratory infections and viral gastroenteritis.

[1]Poverty is defined as a monthly income below that needed to meet the cost of food and other basic needs, or US$ 104 for Saint Kitts and US$ 122 for Nevis.

[2]Indigence is defined as earning less than US$ 64 per month in Saint Kitts and less than US$ 75 per month in Nevis.

FIGURE 1. Population structure, by age and sex, Saint Kitts and Nevis, 1991 and 2001.

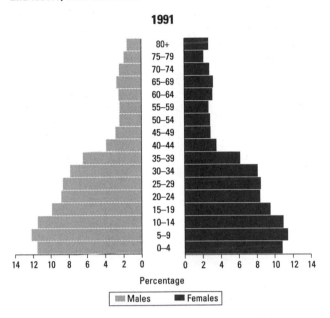

1991

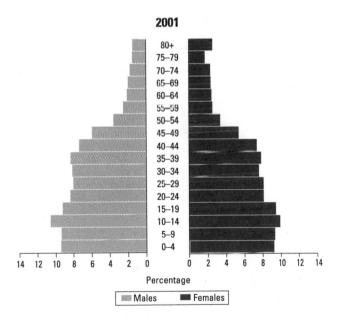

2001

1996–2000 figures, the infant mortality rate has declined from an average of 20.3 to 16.2 per 1,000 live births. Table 1 shows crude mortality rate figures and a breakdown of deaths and mortality rates by age group for 2001–2005. When compared to 1996–2000 figures, the infant mortality rate has declined from an average of 20.3 per 1,000 live births to 16.2.

Table 2 shows the leading causes of death in Saint Kitts and Nevis, as well as their rank order. In 2002–2004, the list was headed by diseases of the circulatory system (cerebrovascular diseases and ischemic heart disease).

The ten leading causes of death in 2002–2004, based on estimated deaths defined by cause, were cerebrovascular diseases (13.2%), ischemic heart disease (11.3%), septicemia (7.1%), influenza and pneumonia (7.0%), cardiac arrest (5.7%), diseases of the urinary system (4.2%), certain conditions originating out of the perinatal period (3.3%), heart failure and complications and ill-defined heart disease (3.1%), malignant neoplasm of prostate (2.4%), and pulmonary heart disease and diseases of pulmonary circulation (2.0%). Both in 1996–1997 and in each year in 2002–2004, cerebrovascular disease ranked either first or second. Diabetes ranked second in 1996–1997, but did not make the top ten disease categories in either 2003 or 2004, and ranked tenth in 2002.

HEALTH OF POPULATION GROUPS

Children under 5 Years Old

The average number of live births in 2001–2005 was 736, a decline of 14% from the 855 figure in 1996–2000. From 2001 to 2005, the number of live births declined by 17%, from 803 to 668 infants. An average of 12 deaths per year occurred in infants under 1 year old, mainly due to conditions originating in the perinatal period, chief among them being respiratory distress syndrome due to immature lungs of premature infants of less than 32 weeks gestation. The incidence of low birthweight (under 2,500 g) remained constant at 10%.

According to information from the 2005 Community Health Report, the immunization schedule includes BCG, polio, DPT, Hib, and hepatitis B, and coverage is virtually 100%.

Growth and development are monitored in community clinics and by private sector pediatricians. Although breast-feeding is actively promoted, exclusive breast-feeding of infants for the first four months of life is hindered by mothers' usually returning to work by the third post-partum month.

Children 1–4 Years Old

In 2001–2005, there were 16 deaths, or 0.9% of total deaths, in this age group, primarily due to complications of congenital anomalies. Acute viral respiratory and viral gastrointestinal infections were the main causes of illness, with 167 and 123 reported cases, respectively; there were no deaths due to these two

During 2001–2005, crude death rates (Table 1) fluctuated between 7 and 9 deaths per 1,000 population. Infant deaths ranged from 17 in 2002 to 9 in 2005, and infant mortality rates in 2001–2005 averaged approximately 16 per 1,000 live births. Neonatal mortality ranged from 6 deaths in 2001 to 15 deaths in 2002; there were 9 deaths in 2005. Late fetal deaths ranged from 6 in 2002 to 15 in 2001; there were 11 in 2005. When compared to

TABLE 1. Total deaths, crude mortality rate, and deaths and mortality rates, by age group, Saint Kitts and Nevis, 2001–2005.

Mortality category	Years				
	2001	2002	2003	2004	2005
Total deaths	375	341	348	395	333
Crude mortality rate (per 1,000 population)	7.6	7.6	8.0	8.6	6.8
Infant deaths	10	17	13	11	9
Infant mortality rate (per 1,000 live births)	12.5	22.4	17.6	17.3	13.5
Neonatal deaths	6	15	11	10	9
Neonatal mortality rate (per 1,000 live births)	7.5	18.5	14.9	15.3	12.0
Maternal deaths	0	0	2	0	0
Late fetal deaths	15	6	15	12	11
Late fetal death rate (per 1,000 live births)	18.7	7.9	20.3	18	16.2
Deaths in 1–4-year-olds	7	5	2	1	1
Deaths in 5–9-year-olds	3	3	0	0	2
Deaths in 10–14-year-olds	2	1	2	2	2
Deaths in 15–19-year-olds	2	4	6	8	1
Deaths in 20–59-year-olds	78	71	70	81	75
Deaths in 60–79-year-olds	132	113	136	142	101
Deaths in persons older than 80 years	141	127	119	150	142

Source: Health Information Unit, Ministry of Health.

TABLE 2. Rank, number of deaths, percentage, and cumulative percentage of leading causes of death, Saint Kitts and Nevis, 2002–2004.

Cause	2002–2004			
	Rank	Number	Percentage	Cumulative percentage
Cerebrovascular diseases	1	135	13.2	13.2
Ischemic heart disease	2	116	11.3	24.5
Septicemia	3	73	7.1	31.6
Influenza and pneumonia	4	72	7.0	38.6
Cardiac arrest	5	58	5.7	44.2
Diseases of the urinary system	6	43	4.2	48.4
Certain conditions originating in the perinatal period	7	34	3.3	51.7
Heart failure and complications and ill-defined heart disease	8	32	3.1	54.8
Malignant neoplasm of prostate	9	25	2.4	57.3
Pulmonary heart disease and diseases of pulmonary circulation	10	21	2.0	59.3

conditions. Nutritional status is measured using height and weight criteria, as established in the Caribbean Food and Nutrition Institute growth chart. According to 2005 data from the Ministry of Health's Nutrition Unit, combined mild, moderate, and severe undernutrition levels remained low, at 2.6%, while the prevalence of obesity remained relatively constant—11% in 2000 and 11.3% in 2005. Fewer than 1% of community clinic clients presented hemoglobin levels under 10 g/dl. Measles, mumps, and rubella are included in the immunization schedule; coverage was 100%.

Children 5–9 Years Old

Children of this group represented 9.4% of the 2001 population. The main causes of morbidity in this age group were acute respiratory infections and gastroenteritis. There were eight deaths in this age group from 2001 to 2005, or 0.4% of the total number of deaths in this time period.

Adolescents 10–14 and 15–19 Years Old

The Adolescent Health Survey conducted in 1998–1999 studied major health challenges such as drug use, physical violence, and sexual violence. These issues were still considered matters of concern in 2005. The study surveyed 341 high school students, equally distributed by sex. Of students surveyed, 4% admitted using cocaine, tobacco, marijuana, heroin, or cigarettes; 46% used alcoholic beverages "once or a few times." Use was confined mainly to 16–19-year-olds, who generally did not regard marijuana and alcohol as drugs. Police data showed that approximately 5%–10% of crimes were committed by juveniles. Gang membership is a growing problem, and the Ministry of National Security has established a "Youth at Risk" program to engage young men and women who may benefit from behavioral-change and skill-development services.

The prevalence of obesity among adolescents is of serious concern. In 2005, a study on adolescent obesity conducted by the Ministry of Health in conjunction with the Caribbean Food and Nutrition Institute found a prevalence rate of 19% among 13–15-year-olds. Daily consumption of fruit was 15% and daily consumption of vegetables, 26%; nutrition knowledge was rated as "very poor." However, most (82%) of the study participants had engaged in physical activity in the week prior to the survey.

Teen motherhood rates also are of great concern; they averaged 18.3% in 1996–2000 and 19.1% in 2001–2005. In the same period, 13 infants were born to girls 10–14 years old.

Adolescents 10–14 and 15–19 years old accounted for 10.3% and 9.4% of the population, respectively. There were nine deaths among 10–14-year-olds and 21 among 15–19-year-olds; 17 of the latter were males. These age groups recorded 0.5% and 1.2% of total deaths, respectively, mostly due to injuries.

Adults and Older Adults

Adults 20–59 years old accounted for 51.4% of the population in 2005, up from 43% in the 1991 census. Persons aged 60–79 years old and persons older than 80 years old represented 8.2% and 2.1% of the 2005 population, respectively, compared to 10.5% and 2.2% in 1991. Chronic noncommunicable diseases were the major causes of illness, with women having higher rates of diabetes and hypertension; female rates were 1.5 times greater than male rates.

In 2001–2005, 20.9% of deaths occurred among persons 20–59 years old, while the age groups 60–79 and older than 80 years accounted for 34.8% and 37.9%, respectively. Between 2002 and 2004, cerebrovascular diseases were the leading cause of death, with a rate of 94.6 per 100,000 population, followed by ischemic heart disease (81.5) and septicemia (51.1). There were two maternal deaths in 2003.

The Family

Data from the 2004 and 2005 Maternity Ward Birth Registers showed marriage rates of 20% in Saint Kitts and 35% in Nevis. According to a 1998 study conducted by the Pan American Health Organization, single women head approximately 50% of households. All family members have access to primary and secondary level health services. Free community clinic services include maternal and child health, dental health, mental health, health maintenance for persons with chronic diseases, care and treatment of acute illness and injuries, and HIV-related volunteer counseling and testing. Seniors also have free access to public sector health

services. Home care and material assistance are provided through outreach programs. Social Security also provides financial assistance to the aged.

Expectant mothers receive care from nurse-midwives and obstetricians, including at high-risk obstetric clinics provided in the community clinics. Almost all deliveries occur in hospital, where early neonatal care is rendered by pediatricians and trained nurses. Hospitals have special care units where sick neonates receive high dependency care, including limited assisted ventilation.

Workers

Occupational health is limited to advocacy and inspections provided by the Labor Department. A robust program of activities is the remit of the Environmental Health Department, but program execution is hindered by the absence of trained personnel. Every worker is required by law to contribute to the Social Security Scheme, which provides injury benefits to members, contingent upon submission of medical certification of illness or injury. Health care for former sugar-industry workers from the Dominican Republic is integrated with that of local workers. New immigrants have the same access to health care as locals. Between 2001 and 2004, the average number of claims for injuries was 459 and the average annual amount paid was US$ 125,000. In the previous four-year period, the average number of claims was 483 and the average annual amount paid was US$ 90,000. Women comprised slightly less than 50% of the workforce in 2004 (48% in 1999) and earned US$ 770 less than did men in 2004. Social Security maternity grants decreased from 582 in 2001 to 449 in 2004, consistent with the declining birth rate.

Persons with Disabilities

Disabled persons receive financial and other material assistance from a variety of sources including service sector organizations, the Social Security Scheme, and the Social Assistance Units (welfare) of the governments. Public sector health services are provided at no charge.

HEALTH CONDITIONS AND PROBLEMS

COMMUNICABLE DISEASES

Vector-borne Diseases

In 2001–2005, there were two reported cases of **malaria**, both imported. There were 144 cases of **dengue fever** reported between 2001 and 2004, with 115 occurring during the 2001 outbreak, and 29 between 2002 and 2004; there were no cases reported in 2005. All reports are followed up by the Community Health Department, using teams of doctors, nurses, and environmental health officers. Mosquito surveillance is actively carried out by vector control officers. The Breteau index dropped from 9 in 2004 to 4 in 2005; heightened surveillance was made possible by increased staff.

Vaccine-preventable Diseases

During 2001–2005, vaccination coverage of administered antigens varied between 95% and 100%. Hib vaccine was introduced in the national immunization schedule in 2000 as a component of the pentavalent vaccine—DPT/HepB/Hib. The immunization schedule includes BCG, polio, DPT, Hib, hepatitis B, and MMR. The vaccination coverage of administered antigens in 2005 is as follows: BCG,100%; MMR,100%; third dose of OPV, 100%; and DPT/HepB/Hib, 100%.

The last case of **polio** was in 1969. There were no reported cases of **measles, rubella, congenital rubella syndrome, diphtheria, pertussis, tetanus,** or **neonatal tetanus.**

Intestinal Infectious Diseases

In 2001–2005, there were 613 cases of gastroenteritis in children under 5 years old and 1,038 in persons 5 years old and older. Clinical and laboratory data suggested a viral cause. There were 45 reported cases of **giardiasis.**

There were no reported cases of **helminthiasis.**

HIV/AIDS and Other Sexually Transmitted Infections

From 1984 to the end of 2004, there were 261 HIV-positive tests reported. The number of annual tests has increased, from fewer than 1,000 in 1988 to 2,836 in 2004. The number of reported HIV-positive cases varied from 9 in 1991 to 34 in 1996; 73 cases were recorded in 2001–2005. The male to female ratio of persons testing positive for HIV has reversed, from 1.5:1 in 1998 to 1:1.6 in 2005. The most affected age group continued to be persons 25 to 44 years old, especially among females. HIV infection among males tended to cluster in the 15-to-24 years old and 45 and older age groups. The age and gender distributions stimulated advocacy interventions targeting youth, especially young women and girls. Highly active antiretroviral therapy (HAART) medications were started in 2005. There were 14 AIDS deaths in 2001–2005, compared to 16 in 1996–2000.

Chronic Communicable Diseases

In 2005 there was one case of **tuberculosis** (not linked to HIV), which was being managed by the Directly Observed Treatment, Short-Course (DOTS) regime.

NONCOMMUNICABLE DISEASES

Diabetes, hypertension, cerebrovascular diseases, and heart diseases accounted for the majority of adult hospital admissions according to data from the main referral center. Diseases of the circulatory system were the leading cause of death with a rate of 315.5 per 100,000 population.

Saint Kitts and Nevis has experienced an epidemiologic profile shift from diseases of nutritional deficiency and poor sanitation prevalent prior to the 1980s, to noncommunicable conditions attributed to lifestyle (nutrition, behavior) choices. The Government considers health promotion to the a key component in the fight against chronic noncommunicable diseases. The Government's initiatives in this regard are discussed in detail in the subsection on "Health Promotion" within the section on Response of the Health Sector.

Metabolic and Nutritional Diseases

In 2000, a chronic disease survey conducted by the University of Newcastle in conjunction with the Ministry of Health reported overweight prevalence rates of 60% in men and 70% in women, and that 54% of adults had at least one chronic illness.

Among adolescents 13–15 years old, 19% were overweight, with a female-to-male ratio of 1.4 to 1. There was a cumulative total of 2,390 registered diabetics and hypertensives attending community clinics, representing approximately 8% of the population 20 years old and older.

Malignant Neoplasms

Malignant neoplasms ranked as the fourth highest cause of death, with a rate of 111.4 per 100,000 population. Of a total of 213 deaths between 2001 and 2005, prostate cancer accounted for the highest number in men (47 out of 119), while in women, the highest number was due to cancer of the breast (20 out of 94). Men are encouraged to undergo regular physical exams and any physician recommended tests and procedures to detect malignant neoplasms. Women are also encouraged to have periodic breast examinations; ultrasonography and biopsy services are available. Cervical cancer screening also is widely available in the community clinics at no charge, as well as from private-sector gynecologists. In collaboration with a private non-profit U.S.-based organization, colorectal screening (colonoscopy) services are provided twice yearly at minimal charge, with low-income persons receiving financial assistance where necessary. The noncommunicable disease component of the National Health Plan envisions a cancer registry and disease specific management protocols.

OTHER HEALTH PROBLEMS OR ISSUES

Violence and Other External Causes

Injuries were the third leading cause of death, with a rate of 118 per 100,000 population. In 2001–2005, the number of cases of assault (without gunshot wounds) and wounding tripled, compared to the previous five-year period. Of the 73 deaths in 2002–2004, 82% occurred in males, and assault accounted for 30%. This trend occurred at a time when drug-related, violent gang activity involving adolescents and young men had increased. Of all deaths, 20% were due to motor vehicle accidents;

there was minimal change in the average number of motor vehicle accidents, injuries, and deaths compared to 1996–2000. A review of external causes of death at Joseph N. France Hospital emergency room showed that injuries due to accidents ranged from 215 in 2004 to 318 in 2005. Assaults and wounding ranged from 310 in 2001 to 518 in 2005. Gunshot wounds ranged from 6 in 2001 to 36 in 2004. Assaults and wounding were up tenfold in 2005, compared with those in 1998–2000, and accidents in general had almost doubled by 2005 when compared to 1998.

Mental Health

The country promotes the community approach to mental health, although the effort has been curtailed due to a shortage of trained personnel in psychiatry, psychology, and occupational therapy. The number of registered patients has not increased from the 1996–2000 average of 224 persons. In 2004 and 2005, an average of 212 persons received service, with approximately equal numbers of males and females. The most common conditions were schizophrenia, depression, and substance abuse.

Asthma

Since 2002, asthma has replaced gastroenteritis as the most frequent admitting diagnosis in children. A clinic is conducted where children and their caretakers receive disease management education and supplies such as spacers and peak flow meters. Bronchodilators and corticosteroids are readily available in the government pharmacies. Hospital admissions confirm the need for an expanded response including the development of management guidelines.

Oral Health

Preventive and treatment services are provided by two public sector clinics (one on each island). Children are the principal focus for preventive work. A sealant program sponsored by the private sector was started in 2005. Outreach efforts are ongoing to promote dental health among adults.

RESPONSE OF THE HEALTH SECTOR

Health Policies and Plans

It is a matter of public policy that all residents have equitable access to quality health care. To this end, the governments of the two islands are committed to ensuring a sustainable package of services designed to meet prevailing health care needs. Services not available locally may be accessed on neighboring islands, either through publicly financed arrangements or through personal funding, including insurance plans. A public health insurance plan is under consideration, but at this writing, there is no public health insurance on either island.

The 2006–2011 National Health Plan began to be developed in the period under review. This multisectoral effort represents a logical, goal-driven approach to meeting specific health sector priorities, including health systems development, human resource development, environmental health, mental health and substance abuse, HIV/AIDS/STIs, chronic noncommunicable diseases/food and nutrition/physical activity, and family health services. These priority areas closely approximate those enunciated in the Caribbean Cooperation in Health, Phase III, a regional approach to addressing common health challenges.

Saint Kitts and Nevis' investment in population health and social development programs has been largely responsible for the country's attainment of many of the UN Millennium Development Goals. For example, the provision of financial aid, skills training, assistance to displaced workers from the sugar industry, and a vibrant school meals program works to eradicate extreme poverty and hunger (goal 1). The country has already attained universal education (goal 2). In terms of the promotion of gender equality and women's empowerment (goal 3) Saint Kitts and Nevis' constitution protects against discrimination based on gender—60% of Permanent Secretary posts, the most senior administrative officer in the Ministry of Health, are occupied by women. The emphasis on free obstetric care in community clinics targets child mortality reduction (MDG 4).

Notwithstanding the gains, there is continuing investment of resources towards quality improvement in immunization, nutrition, maternal and child health, housing, potable water access, environmental sanitation, infrastructure development, and human resource training.

Chronic, incurable, and expensive medical conditions drive Saint Kitts and Nevis' engagement with regional partners and health institutions in re-orienting services around health promotion strategies and collaborative approaches to solving common problems. Through frameworks such as the Caribbean Cooperation in Health (CCH) and the Pan Caribbean Partnership Against HIV/AIDS (PANCAP), Saint Kitts and Nevis strives to address the pressing challenges of diabetes, hypertension, heart disease, malignant neoplasms, drug abuse, HIV/AIDS, and violence.

Among salient health-related legislation in the country are the 1938 Medical Act, the 1946 Quarantine Act, the 1969 Public Health Act, the 1951 Accidents and Occupational Disease Notification Ordinance, the 1956 Mental Health (Lunacy) Act, the 1956 Nurses Registration Act, the 1976 Immunization Act, the 1986 Drug (Prevention and Misuse) Act and the Solid Waste Management Act, the 1989 Litter Abatement Act, the 2000 Pharmacy Bill, and the 2002 Institutions-based Health Services Management Bill.

Public health sector operations are divided into three program areas, which are designed to meet priority areas and deliver essential public health functions. The Ministry of Health, as the administrative health authority, is responsible for policy formulation, finance and budget, regulation of professionals and facilities, human resource management, and health information. The Community Service program provides public health services, including environmental health, mental health, oral health, family health, health maintenance, and health promotion and advocacy. The component dealing with managing health institutions provides primary, secondary, and limited tertiary medical services, as well as care of senior citizens.

Saint Kitts and Nevis' health sector operates under the following strategies: leadership, health promotion, equitable universal access to health, human resource development, and disease management.

Organization of the Health System

The health system of Saint Kitts and Nevis is organized so as to effectively and efficiently respond to meet the health needs of the entire population.

The Ministry of Health administers the public health sector and is accountable for the delivery of quality public and individual health services. Both islands have parallel organizational structures, with each island's Minister leading final policy determination. Permanent Secretaries, as heads of administration, are responsible for matters related to finance, budget, personnel, and procurement. The two Ministers regularly confer with one another to harmonize policies.

The delivery of essential public health functions is integrated and incorporates the federal-based direction of health status monitoring, surveillance, research and information, health promotion, disease prevention, management of chronic diseases, and the regulation of health professionals. There are 17 community clinics, 11 in Saint Kitts and 6 in Nevis. The strategic location of these clinics is such that each household is within three miles of a clinic.

Institutions in Saint Kitts include the country's main referral center, the 150-bed Joseph N. France General Hospital, and two former cottage hospitals that are currently being recast as 24-hour urgent care centers with limited inpatient capacity. The Cardin Home accommodates approximately 100 senior citizens. In Nevis, Alexandra Hospital has 50 beds, to which the 36-bed Flamboyant Home for senior citizens is attached. In recent years, four (two on each island) private senior citizen facilities have been established. There are no private hospitals.

There is no single public-payment mechanism for health services. Public sector health and medical services are either highly subsidized or free to users, and so are universally accessible. Personal and group medical plans are readily available from several private sector vendors; 30% of the workforce is estimated to be covered.

Public Health Services

The National AIDS Program manages the response to HIV/AIDS, with oversight from the National Advisory Council on HIV/AIDS. Activities include prevention of mother-to-child transmission; voluntary counseling and testing, provision of free antiretroviral medications, coordination of clinical care, free distribution of condoms, outreach services for affected persons, plus research, and monitoring and evaluation.

The threat that an avian influenza could spread to humans has been acknowledged. Saint Kitts and Nevis has issued a draft response plan to this effect, following PAHO's template. The main action lines include the strengthening of animal health and human health surveillance systems, capacity building to meet the anticipated surge in demand, and the procurement of medication and vaccine (when available). Public sensitization has commenced with respect to reporting dead birds, and the dissemination of food safety information is ongoing.

Environmental health receives priority consideration. Capacity building activities in human resources are ongoing to fulfill all of the mandates of food safety, vector control, water quality surveillance, sanitation, occupational health, port health, and solid waste collection and disposal.

Individual Care Services

Currently, mental health and substance abuse are managed as a component of family health services, with links to psychiatric wards in hospitals. It is acknowledged that mental health services need to expand in the area of community mental health education, treatment, and support. The community-based approach is the operant strategy, with targeted services designed to promote inclusiveness of mental health patients in society. Efforts are ongoing to recruit and retain professionals in psychiatry, child and adolescent psychology, and occupational therapy.

Health Promotion

The Health Promotion Unit coordinates the response to diabetes, hypertension, cancer, and asthma, utilizing the defining strategies that underpin health promotion. Several studies have underscored the work to de done in reducing the burden from overconsumption of foods high in calories and from lack of physical activity. The Unit coordinates the response to chronic noncommunicable diseases through advocacy, education, and health status monitoring focused on dietary lifestyle change, increased physical activity, and evidence-based case management. An expected outcome is a decline in hospital admissions commensurate with improved community care.

In 2005, protocols for diabetes monitoring were formally disseminated to practitioners; each case record is expected to contain a standard set of data including blood pressure readings; serum levels of lipids and glycosylated hemoglobin; and the findings of cardiac, foot, and eye examinations. Community clinic attendees have free access to anti-coagulants, anti-hypertensive drugs, and blood sugar and lipid lowering medications.

Hospital admissions for diabetes ranged from 131 in 2003 to 109 in 2005, while new clinic enrollments for diabetes ranged from 107 in 2002 to 60 in 2005. Hospital admissions of patients

Fighting Diabetes and Hypertension; Containing Hospital Costs

Diabetes and hypertensive diseases were among the country's leading causes of death between 2002 and 2004 and topped the list of leading causes for hospitalization. The Ministry of Health's Health Promotion Unit coordinates activities to address chronic noncommunicable diseases, including advocacy, education, and health status monitoring that focuses on dietary lifestyle changes.

for symptoms of hypertension ranged from 180 in 2002 to 95 in 2005, while new clinic enrollments for symptoms of hypertension ranged from 170 in 2003 to 126 in 2005.

The Health Promotion Unit also has increased its efforts to combat the high prevalence of obesity or overweight. Activities included use of the national print and electronic media to disseminate nutrition information. Brochures also are readily available in community clinics and schools. Nutrition information billboards are posted in strategic locations around the islands.

Government agencies responsible for adolescent health and gender affairs conduct programs designed to empower and protect adolescents through psychosocial support services in crisis situations, pregnancy prevention, family planning, and the promotion of condom use. Teen mothers are actively encouraged to complete their secondary education and beyond. An emergency contraception policy is being developed.

In 2004, the first patient satisfaction survey was conducted in Saint Kitts' health centers. More than 90% of respondents reported a favorable assessment of the quality of care. Respondents also expressed satisfaction with interpersonal care, information and education, and provider attitudes. The main areas of dissatisfaction related to physical comfort in some centers and regularity of staff availability. These findings have been used to improve the care environment and motivate the staff to achieve higher quality of care standards.

Human Resources

The health sector maintains favorable provider-to-population ratios, except for a few gaps in some specialized skills, particularly in mental health and nursing; health care is readily accessible. Overall, the number of medical doctors per 10,000 population increased from 11 in 2001 to 13 in 2005. On the other hand, the number of nurses decreased from 49 to 32 per 10,000 in the same period; this decrease was a result of retirement and, to a lesser extent, migration. The situation is more acute in public health nursing, where the number of trained nurses entering employment is less than the number retiring. Given that the strengthening of community-based services is a central strategy in health promotion and disease burden reduction, the public

health training of nurses and doctors continues to be emphasized. Priority attention is paid to attracting committed persons into the nursing profession; those with aptitude but who lack the qualifying academic standards for entry into the registered nurse program are trained as nurse attendants and nurse assistants and encouraged to upgrade their qualifications over time.

Health Supplies

All supplies are imported. Medications for the public sector are obtained through the Organization of Eastern Caribbean States Pharmaceutical Procurement Service, a subregional collaboration among the smaller English-speaking Caribbean islands. A similar mechanism for medical equipment is under consideration. Administrative supplies are sourced from the government's central purchasing unit.

Essential drugs are readily available at minimal cost within the public sector pharmacies. Antiretroviral medications are provided free through assistance from an international partner in the fight against HIV/AIDS.

Health Sector Expenditures and Financing

The Government is the leading provider of health care financing. In 2001–2005, the federal government's recurrent health expenditures averaged 8% of total recurrent expenditures. On each island, 60% of the health ministry budget is devoted to operational expenses of hospitals and other institutions. Cost recovery efforts are in place for hospital services, although there are significant fee-exempt service categories such as those targeting schoolchildren and senior citizens. Hospital service fees are nominal, and community-clinic services are free of charge. Given this, expenditure exceeds revenue by a factor of 9 to 1 in health institutions; community health services are totally subsidized by the Government.

Technical Cooperation and External Financing

Saint Kitts and Nevis is a committed partner in regional integration processes. Policies, plans, and programs are consistent with the agreed collaborative frameworks, such as those of the

Caribbean Cooperation in Health, Phases I, II, and III, and the Pan Caribbean Partnership Against HIV/AIDS. Through these arrangements, priority areas are identified and ranked, governance structures are developed, and resources are mobilized for implementing population health programs and other activities, including research, monitoring, and evaluation. Various regional institutions provide technical cooperation in different areas. Among the highlights: the Caribbean Food and Nutrition Institute provides cooperation in monitoring nutrition status and in the conduct of overweight prevalence studies; the Caribbean Epidemiology Center provides assistance in HIV seroprevalence studies; the Caribbean Environmental Health Institute has focused on assessing landfill operations; the Caribbean Health Research Council has provided assistance in producing guidelines on management of diabetes, hypertension, asthma, and HIV monitoring and evaluation; and the Pan American Health Organization participated in the development of the National Health Plan and the mental health policy, in providing training in emergency care and management of mass casualties and in emerging diseases preparedness.

Five priority areas in the National AIDS Program are supported by technical assistance from regional health institutions such as the Pan American Health Organization, the Caribbean Food and Nutrition Institute (CFNI), the Caribbean Epidemiology Center (CAREC), the Caribbean Health Research Council (CHRC), the Caribbean Environmental Health Institute (CEHI), and the Caribbean Regional Drug Testing Laboratory (CRDTL). The program is funded by the central government and various external donors.

In addition, several countries provide financing to complement Government funding of the public health sector. Chief among them is Taiwan (Republic of China), whose grant contributions meet selected capital equipment needs. In addition, the National HIV/AIDS Program benefits from a World Bank loan, and grant support from the Global Fund, UNAIDS, and the United Kingdom's Department of International Development.

SAINT LUCIA

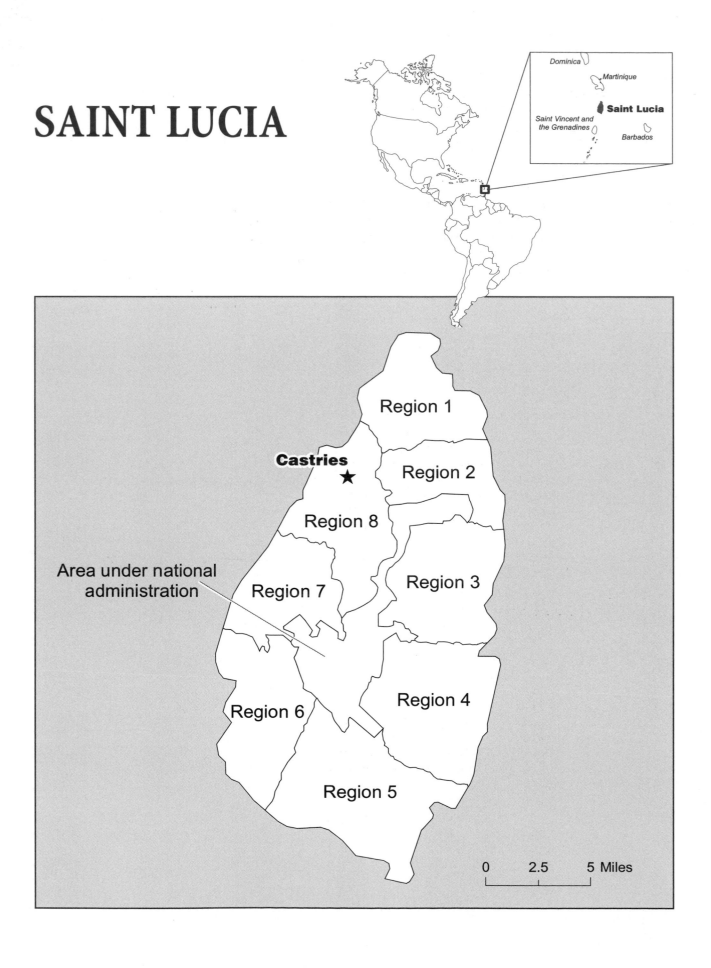

Dominica

Martinique

Saint Vincent and
the Grenadines

Saint Lucia

Barbados

Region 1

Castries

Region 2

Region 8

Area under national
administration

Region 3

Region 7

Region 4

Region 6

Region 5

0   2.5   5 Miles

Saint Lucia is a small, Caribbean island nation with a total land area of 616 km^2 located between the islands of Martinique and St. Vincent and the Grenadines. Castries is the capital city, and the twin pitons in Soufrière represent the island's most impressive landmark.

GENERAL CONTEXT AND HEALTH DETERMINANTS

Social, Political, and Economic Determinants

The country experiences both dry and rainy seasons, the latter spanning from June to November, and is prone to hurricanes that pose a continuous threat to its agriculture and physical infrastructure.

Saint Lucia attained political independence from the United Kingdom in 1979 and now has a democratic system of government based on the Westminster model; parliamentary elections are held every five years. The country is a member of the Commonwealth of Nations, the Organization of Eastern Caribbean States (OECS), and the Caribbean Community (CARICOM).

The official language is English, but a French patois is commonly spoken, particularly among most of the rural population. Roman Catholicism is the dominant religion (practiced by 67% of the population), followed by the Seventh-day Adventist (9%) and the Pentecostal (6%) religions; other religions are practiced by the remaining population (18%).

According to the 2001 population census, 83% of the population is of African descent, 3% is of East Indian descent, 1% is Caucasian, and 12% are of mixed ancestry (1). Most of the population inhabits the coastal areas and less mountainous regions of the north and south, and approximately 41% lives in the district of Castries. The city of Castries is the hub of the country's economic activity and political life.

Saint Lucia experienced an economic recession in 2001 due to a decline in tourism, the principal engine of economic growth, resulting in a growth rate of –3.8%. After 2001, however, the growth rate rose from 0.8% in 2002 to 5.4% in 2005. Gross domestic product (GDP) per capita increased from US$ 2,928 in 2001 to US$ 3,070 in 2005. Tourism accounted for 13.6% of real GDP in 2005, and real growth in the sector was further reflected by a 6.3% expansion of the hotel and restaurant subsectors. During 2005, output of the agriculture sector, with the exception of the livestock subsector, recorded contractions of varying magnitudes—the largest (36.2%) in the banana subsector (2); real output in the sector fell by 22% in 2005, following marginal growth of 1.8% in 2004, and, in keeping with this decline, the contribution of the agriculture sector to real GDP fell to 3.4%. Throughout the period under review, the exchange rate remained constant at ECD$ 2.70.

The 1995 poverty assessment, conducted by the Caribbean Development Bank and based on expenditures on food and non-food items, revealed that 25.1% of the population was poor. In rural areas, 29.6% were poor, compared to 17.4% of those living in urban areas. Poverty was slightly higher among males (25.5%) than females (24.7%).

According to the 2004 core welfare indicators questionnaire survey (CWIQ), the unemployment rate was 18.8%—a slight increase from the 2001 rate of 17%. Data for 2004 indicated a significant gender difference, with a 14% unemployment rate for males compared to a 25% rate for females. Youth unemployment was markedly higher at 39% and that of female youth was especially high at 44%. Lower unemployment among females could prove to be a major constraint to the country's achieving the MDG of gender equality and empowerment of women. The overall rate of underemployment was 8%—6% in urban and 11% in rural areas. Disaggregated by gender, the rates of underemployment were 10% for males and 6% for females (3).

According to the CWIQ, the adult literacy rate in 2004 was 89%, a significant increase over the 54% rate of 1990. Females had a higher literacy rate (90%) than males (87%), and the literacy rate of youth (persons 15–24 years of age) was high at 98.1%—in line with an indicator of the MDG pertaining to attainment of universal primary education. The primary school enrollment rate (children 6–11 years old) was 93%—91% for males and 94% for females; the secondary school enrollment rate was 79%—72% for males and 86% for females. Enrollment rates were similar for urban and rural areas, but secondary school enrollment was lower for the poorest households, especially in rural areas (67%). Although the school dropout rate was low (1% of the school population), females were more likely to be in school than their male counterparts (3).

Safe drinking water is accessible to 98% of the population—to 99% in urban areas and 96.7% in rural areas; among urban households 95% had safe water compared with 88% among rural households. Two-thirds of households had flush toilets or ventilated improved pit latrines, and 95% had access to public waste disposal services.

For the period 1999–2004, 1,048 cases of child abuse were reported to the Division of Human Services and Family Affairs. The most prevalent forms of abuse are child neglect and abandonment (34% of all reported cases), physical abuse (31%), and sexual abuse (29%). For the period 2000–2004, 2,165 cases of domestic violence were reported, but it is known that many cases go unreported. Ministry of Health interventions targeted alleviating the suffering of victims of domestic violence and interrupting the cycle of abuse. The Women's Support Center provided a temporary haven for women and their children in domestic abuse situations.

For the period 2000–2004, 228 deaths due to accidents and homicides were reported; of those deaths, 116 were homicides, most of them (108) in the 20–59-year age group; males accounted for 106 homicides, females for 10. Of the 112 deaths due to accidents, motor vehicle accidents accounted for 106; of those, 81 (76%) were males and 25 females (24%); 96 of the deaths (91%) occurred in the 20–59-year age group, while 10 deaths (9%) occurred in the 15–19-year age group. During this same period, 39 suicides occurred in the 20–59-year age group, 32 of them males (82%) and 7 (18%) females (4).

In 2002, tropical storm Lili forced 125 persons to seek shelter and resulted in an estimated EC$ 20.3 million in damages to the island, and destroyed over half of the banana crop. Another tropical storm in 2003 and Hurricane Ivan in 2004 together accounted for EC$ 9.9 million in damages. No lives were lost, however, as a result of these three disasters (5).

Demographics, Mortality, and Morbidity

The total mid-year population of Saint Lucia was estimated at 162,434 in 2004, reflecting an increase of 1,814 persons (1.1%) over the 2003 figure of 160,620 (6). Females accounted for 51% of the population, with women of childbearing age (15–49 years of age) representing 32.8% of the population. The population is still relatively young, with 28.8% below 15 years of age, while the elderly account for 7.1% of the total population (Figure 1). The dependency ratio in 2005 was 56.3% (7). In 2004, 2,322 births were registered and the crude birth rate was 14.3 live births per 1,000 population, as compared to 2,486 registered births and a crude birth rate of 15.5 in 2003. The number of births in 2004 is the lowest to date, a trend expected to continue as women delay pregnancies and use prescribed contraceptives and other methods of birth control. The decrease in total number of live births was reflected in the steady decline in total fertility rate, from 2.1 children per woman in 2001 to 1.7 in 2004. In 2004 teen births accounted for 18% of total live births, compared to 20% in 1991. Average life expectancy at birth in 2005 was 72.8 years—71.3 years for males and 74.3 years for females (7).

During the period 2000–2004, 4,860 deaths occurred, including 1,046 deaths in 2003 and 1,114 in 2004—a 6.5% increase from one year to the next. The crude death rate was 6.5 in 2003 and 6.9 per 1,000 population in 2004. Leading causes of death for

FIGURE 1. Population distribution, by age and sex, Saint Lucia, 1993 and 2004.

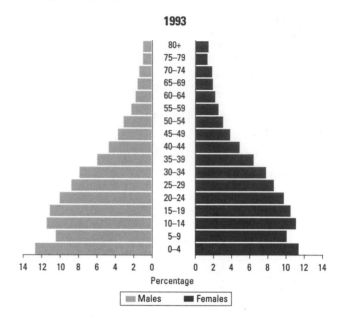

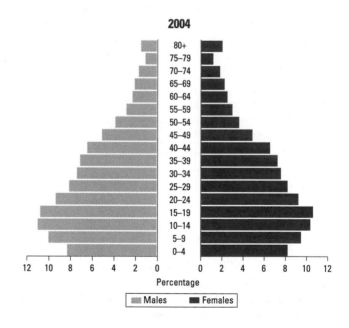

2004 are shown in Table 1 and were consistent throughout the period 2000–2004, although two other disease groups were also noteworthy: conditions originating in the perinatal period showed 92 deaths with a rate of 38.8 deaths per 100,000 population over the three-year period 2000–2002; and hypertensive diseases recorded 83 deaths and comprised 3.3% of total deaths by cause during that same period. The mortality rate of children under 1 year of age was 14.9 per 1,000 live births in 2003 and 19.4 in 2004 (6).

TABLE 1. Number of deaths and rate per 100,000 population for the leading causes of death, Saint Lucia, 2004.

Causes	Rank	No.	Rate
Diabetes mellitus	1	133	81.9
Cerebrovascular diseases	2	116	71.4
Ischemic heart disease	3	61	37.6
Pulmonary heart disease, diseases of pulmonary circulation, and other forms of heart disease	4	51	31.4
Malignant neoplasms of other and unspecified sites	5	45	27.7
Acute respiratory infections	6	43	26.5
Homicides	7	38	23.4
Malignant neoplasms of the digestive organs and peritoneum, except stomach and colon	8	37	22.8
Malignant neoplasm of the prostate	9	36	22.2
Chronic lower respiratory diseases	10	32	19.7

HEALTH OF POPULATION GROUPS

Children under 5 Years Old

In the period 2000–2004, 699 deaths occurred in the 0–4 age group; of those, 601 were due to premature births, 52 were due to slow fetal growth and fetal malnutrition, and 30 deaths were attributed to congenital anomalies.

In 2004, there were 45 infant deaths and an infant mortality rate of 18.5 per 1,000 live births—higher than the 2003 rate of 14.9 and the 2002 rate of 13.5. In 2004, 10.9% of births were low birthweight (< 2,500 g) compared to 9.5% in 2003. Of all births in 2004, 83.7% were of average weight (2,500–4,000 g), compared to 85.1% in 2003. In 2004, 5.4% of infants were overweight (> 4,000 g), and the average birthweight for all babies was 3,155 g—3,218 g for males and 3,081 g for females (6). In 2004, 95% of children in the under 5 year age group participated in three standard development assessment programs—at 6 weeks, 8 months, and 3 years of age. Vaccination coverage was high at over 90% for DPT 1, 2, and 3; BCG; and polio 1, 2, and 3; 7.5% of children under 5 were reported to have had no vaccinations.

Children 5–9 Years Old

During the period 2000–2004, 16 deaths occurred among children 5–9 years of age; 14 were due to accidents and adverse effects, and two to congenital anomalies. Five cases of HIV/AIDS have been reported in this age group since the beginning of the epidemic; of those, two have died (8).

Adolescents 10–14 and 15–19 Years Old

The number of births to mothers under 20 years of age was 443 in 2003 and 444 in 2004. Of those births, 1.8% were to mothers 12–14 years of age in 2004, and 1.4% to mothers in that age group in 2003. In an effort to postpone childbearing and reduce fertility among teens, they have been the target of special programs by the Population Policy Unit, the Ministry of Health, the Ministry of Education, and the Family Planning Unit (6).

During the period 2000–2004, seven deaths occurred among adolescents 10–14 years of age; four were due to land transport accidents, two were suicides, and one was a homicide; males accounted for six of the deaths. In the same period, 24 deaths occurred among 15–19-year-olds; 10 were due to land transport accidents, eight were homicides, and six were due to accidental drowning; males accounted for 22 deaths in this age group. Since the beginning of the HIV/AIDS epidemic, there have been 22 cases: three were 10–14 years of age; 19 were 15–19-years of age; of those 22 cases, five have died—one in the 10–14-year age group, and four in the 15–19-year age group. Among adolescents the preferred measures of preventing HIV/AIDS were condom use (83%) and abstinence (71%); 54% of adolescents indicated that they were sexually active.

Adults 20–59 Years Old

In 2004, there were 2,436 live births; 96% of the respective mothers had prenatal care; births to women in the 20–24-year age group accounted for 25% of all live births.

In 2002–2004, 773 deaths occurred among adults 20–59 years of age. The three leading causes of death were malignant neoplasms, heart disease, and homicides. In the same period, among males aged 20–59 years, the leading causes of mortality were malignant neoplasms (prostate, stomach, lung), homicides, and heart disease. The leading causes of death among females were malignant neoplasms of the breast and cervix, leukemia, diabetes, and heart disease. AIDS accounted for 5% of deaths in this age group, in which 195 AIDS deaths have occurred since the beginning of the epidemic.

Older Adults 60 Years Old and Older

During the period 2002–2004, 2,093 deaths occurred among adults 60 years and older. The leading causes of death were malignant neoplasms (29% of total deaths in this age group), diabetes mellitus (24%), cerebrovascular disease (24%), and heart disease (24%). The leading causes of death among males were malignant neoplasms (365), heart disease (252), and cerebrovascular disease (215). Among females, the leading causes of death were diabetes mellitus (304), cerebrovascular disease (285), and heart disease (248). Since the beginning of the HIV/AIDS epidemic, six persons in this age group have died of AIDS.

A 2002 report on care of the elderly in the country revealed that the main problems facing older persons were abandonment by family, inadequate preparation for retirement, isolation, and poverty. Many older persons were unable to access health and other support services due to geographic location, lack of transportation, and the cost of drugs and medical services (9).

The Family

The mean household size in 2004 was 3.4 persons; urban areas had a household size of 3.3, and rural areas of 3.5. Of those households, 43% were headed by females; and 25% of all female-headed households fell into the poorest quintile, compared to 18% of male-headed households. In addition, female-headed households were less likely to own assets such as land, housing, or vehicles, and half of the females who headed households were unemployed (3). During the period 2001–2004, only 2% of babies were not delivered at a hospital or maternity home (3); approximately 85% of live births were born to women out of wedlock.

Persons with Disabilities

The 2001 census revealed that 9,313 persons (6.2% of the total population) had disabilities; 39.1% of disabilities occurred in persons 65 years and older, and 25.1% in persons 15–64 years of age. The most noted disabilities were locomotor and sight disabilities, accounting for 63.4% of all disabilities.

HEALTH CONDITIONS AND PROBLEMS

COMMUNICABLE DISEASES

Vector-borne Diseases

From 2000 to 2002, five imported cases of **malaria** were reported; no cases were reported in 2003 or 2004. In the 2000–2004 period, 80 cases of **dengue** were confirmed, including an outbreak of 60 cases in 2001; dengue virus types 1, 2, 3, and 4 have been identified in the country.

Vaccine-preventable Diseases

Under the Expanded Program on Immunization (EPI), children under 5 years of age are immunized against **diphtheria, whooping cough, tetanus, Hib, hepatitis B, poliomyelitis, measles, mumps, rubella**, and **tuberculosis**. In 2004, vaccination coverage for polio was 91% and for BCG 99%. Only one case of tetanus has been reported in the past five years, in a two-

year-old male in 2001. The near absence of vaccine-preventable diseases attests to the high immunization coverage over the last 10 years.

Intestinal Infectious Diseases

During the period 2000–2005 no case of **cholera** was reported. During the same period, 36 cases of **salmonella** were reported, and 20 cases of **typhoid fever** were confirmed. Gastroenteritis was the first cause of visits by persons to clinics and the cause of 47% of outpatients seeking medical attention.

Chronic Communicable Diseases

There were 73 reported cases of **tuberculosis** for the period 2000–2004, an increase due in part to improved detection of clinical and laboratory diagnoses; of those cases, 53 were new and 20 were relapses. There was an average of 11 new infections per year and an average of four relapses per year. For the period 2000–2004, 53 cases of leprosy were reported—an increase attributable to successful education and awareness programs in schools and media since 2000.

HIV/AIDS and Other Sexually Transmitted Infections

Between 1985 and 2004, 469 persons tested positive for HIV infection; children under 15 years of age accounted for 10% of cases, and adults aged 15–49 for 77%; 251 (53%) have developed AIDS-related diseases, and 230 (49%) of these have died. Males represent 53% of AIDS deaths among adults 15–49 years old and 64% among the 50+ age group. The male-to-female ratio of AIDS deaths in 1995–1999 was 1.4:1. Unprotected heterosexual sex remains the main mode of transmission.

Zoonoses

No cases of **rabies** have been reported in the country for the past two decades. For the period 2000–2004, 18 cases of leptospirosis were confirmed; all cases investigated suggested a link with rodent infestation in homes and workplaces.

Schistosomiasis was still present in the country, especially in the south, with 30 cases confirmed in the 2000–2005 period.

NONCOMMUNICABLE DISEASES

Nutritional and Metabolic Diseases

Between 1998 and 2002, **diabetes** accounted for 518 deaths, with 62% occurring among females. About 23% of all reported deaths from diabetes were in the 45–64-year age group, and 75% were in the 65 year and older age group.

Cardiovascular Diseases

Deaths by **cardiovascular diseases** (heart disease, cerebrovascular disease, and hypertension) totaled 1,577 (32% of all deaths) for the period 1998–2002, with an average of 315 deaths per year.

Heart disease and cerebrovascular diseases represented 85% of cerebrovascular mortality in the country. In 2001, there were 298 deaths from cardiovascular diseases (30% of all deaths) and, in 2002, there were 296 deaths from cardiovascular diseases (31% of all deaths). Deaths due to cardiac arrest accounted for 16% of all cardiovascular deaths for 1998–2002, ranging from 15% to 23% per year. Ischemic heart disease represented about 10% of all deaths due to cardiovascular diseases for 1998–2002 (10).

Malignant Neoplasms

Between 1998 and 2002, 763 deaths occurred due to malignant neoplasms—an annual average of 153 deaths—and represented about 16% of all deaths. Males accounted for 56% of all deaths due to malignant neoplasms, and among males the three sites most frequently reported for these deaths were prostate (36% of all male deaths due to malignant neoplasms), stomach (11%), and the trachea/bronchus/lung (8%). Among females, the leading sites of malignant neoplasms were breast (17% of all female deaths due to malignant neoplasms), cervix (17%), and leukemia (8.8%). Mortality due to malignant neoplasms was higher for women than for men in the 15–44-year age group, but was similar in the 45–64-year age group. In the 65 year and older age group, mortality from malignant neoplasms was twice as high among men than women, with the exception of colon cancer for which rates were higher among women (10).

OTHER HEALTH PROBLEMS OR ISSUES

Mental Health and Additions

The Golden Hope Hospital, a 162-bed mental institution, had an occupancy rate of 72–74%, with an average length of stay of 50 days and 43 days for 2003 and 2004, respectively. According to hospital records, schizophrenia was the most frequent diagnosis, accounting for approximately 60% of all diagnoses in 2003 and 58% in 2004. In 2005, 62 patients had resided at the hospital for more than one year. The models of care most commonly used were physiotherapy, occupational therapy, and other forms of therapy.

In 2005, the Substance Abuse Advisory Council sent survey questionnaires to primary (5–16-year-olds) and secondary (11–16-year-olds) schools; of the 11 schools that responded, 10 indicated that abuse of drugs—crack, cocaine, and marijuana—was a problem in the communities surrounding their schools. Six of the 11 schools reported that students had been caught with drugs in their possession.

Oral Health

In 1997 a community dental survey was carried out, and the results showed an average of six decayed, missing, and filled teeth among children 12 years old, which is considered high. In 2003–2004, the most common activities carried out by the public health dental program were preventive (education, fluoride treatments, and sealants), restorative (fillings and root canal treatment), and emergency (extractions); the most common procedures performed were periodic examinations and extractions.

RESPONSE OF THE HEALTH SECTOR

Health Policies and Plans

The Ministry of Health completed its National Strategic Plan for Health for the period 2006–2011 (11). The plan envisions: strengthening the organization and management of health and social services; improving and sustaining health gains and residents' well-being; achieving greater equity, cost effectiveness, and efficiency in the allocation and use of health resources; ensuring a cadre of well-trained and motivated staff; developing an effective health information system to support evidence-based planning; implementing a quality improvement system; and improving health infrastructure to support the reform process.

In 2005, a draft protocol for the prevention and management of child abuse was developed that is to provide relevant information to facilitate rapid and effective response to all suspected cases of abuse. Also, the country is a part of a domestic violence and family law reform project of the Organization of Eastern Caribbean States that aims to ensure that laws are responsive to the needs of clients. Some of the relevant bills under review relate to the status of children, child care and protection, and adoption. A draft policy for older persons was completed that prescribes various mechanisms to enhance the quality of life of the elderly. The WHO framework convention on tobacco control was ratified by Saint Lucia in 2005. The Disaster Preparedness and Response Act was enacted in 2000 to provide for more effective disaster and emergency mitigation, preparedness, response, and recovery.

Organization of the Health System

The Ministry of Health focuses on providing maximum quality of life for all the country's citizens. Among other priorities, health policies and plans continue to target poor at-risk populations, children, and older adults and to assure gender equity. The Ministry has two main divisions: an administrative arm headed by a permanent secretary and a technical arm headed by the chief medical officer, who is responsible for the health of the nation. The Ministry of Health is the sole provider of primary and secondary health care services in the public sector. The country seeks to strengthen the health sector within the national, regional, social, political, and economic contexts and to position it as a major driver of social and economic development (12).

Outpatient services are provided at medical clinics at health centers and district hospitals and through the casualty or emergency departments of acute general hospitals. Secondary and specialized services are provided by three institutions: Victoria Hospital, the main hospital, located in the city of Castries and managed by the Ministry of Health; St. Jude's Hospital, located in the south of the island, a quasi-public institution that receives an annual subvention from the Government and many of whose specialists come from overseas and serve on a voluntary basis; and Tapion Hospital, a privately owned facility in the city of Castries. Two specialized institutions operate on the island: the psychiatric facility, Golden Hope Hospital, which offers inpatient and outpatient mental health services; and Turning Point, a drug rehabilitation center.

Most tertiary care services are provided through health facilities abroad, primarily in Martinique, Barbados, and Trinidad and Tobago. The national insurance scheme provides assistance to older persons, the disabled, and the indigent, whether or not they are contributors to the scheme. The cost of care for indigent persons is partially funded by the Ministry of Health, while the rest is funded out-of-pocket; private health insurance covers the insured.

Both the Division of Human Services and Family Affairs and the Division of Gender Relations respond to vulnerable and at-risk groups by implementing appropriate social protection programs. The elderly home refurbishment project aims to refurbish the homes of older persons in difficult circumstances, and the Government has committed to build a new home for older persons. Services to vulnerable children are to be increased through establishment of a transit home for children, foster care, and family intervention programs. The Division has implemented a foster care and recruitment program that promotes public involvement in caring and protecting children in need, and the public assistance program likewise targets helping those in need. The Division of Gender Relations is responsible for implementing gender mainstreaming and has developed a program to combat gender-based violence.

Public Health Services

Primary health care services are provided at 34 health centers, a polyclinic, and two district hospitals. These facilities routinely offer medical and pharmaceutical services, maternal and child health care (antenatal and postnatal care as well as immunization of children), prevention and control of sexually transmitted infections, mental health clinics, and services related to diabetes, hypertension, cancer screening, dental care, and food and nutrition.

In the Ministry of Health, the Bureau of Health Education is responsible for health education and promotion; it focuses on control and reduction of noncommunicable diseases such as cancer, diabetes, hypertension, arthritis, and lupus, and promotes good dietary habits and guidelines for treatment and care of those diseases. Community sensitization meetings are held to foster community participation and disseminate information on vector management.

Programs are executed for disease prevention and control, specifically of tuberculosis, leprosy, HIV/AIDS, and other sexually transmitted infections (STI), dengue fever, measles, and some cancers. Activities include surveillance, management, and treatment of cases, and special clinics for STI. A cancer registry was established in 1995, a national tuberculosis register in 1996, and a national diabetes register in 2001. Since 2000, a national tuberculosis management committee meets monthly and follows up on all cases of the disease. The Expanded Program on Immunization (EPI) has maintained high vaccination coverage for many years, and the incidence of vaccine-preventable diseases is very low. High-risk pregnancies are monitored, and all pregnant mothers are provided with folate and iron supplements and counseling services. Screening programs are offered for cervical, breast, and prostate cancer, although few men are being screened for prostate cancer. Preventive services are free except for contraceptives, yellow fever vaccinations, and vaccinations required for college entry. Nutrition protocols and guidelines have been established to manage HIV/AIDS, and the distribution of antiretroviral drugs, through the Global Fund, has commenced.

The communicable disease surveillance system, which was revised in 2001, bolsters the Caribbean Cooperation in Health initiative and aims to improve surveillance, prioritize response to outbreak-prone communicable diseases including emerging and reemerging infectious diseases, and increase sensitivity, preparedness, timeliness, and laboratory diagnosis; the major changes to the system include expansion of syndromic surveillance, discontinuation of suspected cases of diseases, quarterly-basis reporting of tuberculosis, and systematic and standardized outbreak reporting. Data for this system are collected from sentinel sites at the emergency and accident departments of Victoria Hospital, St. Jude's Hospital, and Gros Islet Polyclinic.

The Environmental Health Department within the Ministry of Health is responsible for the delivery of environmental health services including food and water safety, vector control, and sanitation and for monitoring and regulating the disposal of solid waste. Efforts have focused on surveillance and treatment of mosquito breeding sites; conduct of monitoring exercises for dengue, schistosomiasis, and leptospirosis; and port inspection for *Aedes aegypti* at Marigot, Rodney Bay, and Castries harbors. The Department developed and implemented effective mechanisms and strategies for monitoring and enforcing the quality of potable water; in 2005, 29 municipal distribution systems were monitored weekly. The Food Unit of the Department is responsible for food protection, control, and safety and conducts inspections of food service establishments and wholesalers at least three times a year; in 2004, 1,696 food handling establishments were inspected, and follow-up inspections were carried out in 204 to ensure compliance with guidelines. In 2004–2005, the unit trained some 300 farmers in basic food hygiene principles. The draft food and animal health acts were reviewed and circulated for comments.

Government Targets the Well-being of the Youngest Saint Lucians

Saint Lucia's is a young population—more than one in four inhabitants is younger than 15 years old. Given this age distribution, the Ministry of Health considers the country's children as a priority. Over the past decade, efforts to immunize children under 5 years old against diphtheria, whooping cough, tetanus, *Haemophilus influenzae* type b, hepatitis B, poliomyelitis, measles, mumps, rubella, and tuberculosis have resulted in the near-absence of vaccine-preventable diseases. The Government also has established a transitional home for foster care and family intervention services that will protect at-risk and abused children. Among other initiatives, development and guidance services are now being offered to children under 16 years of age, monthly clinics have begun to serve children with handicaps, and several years ago the ministries of Health and of Education collaborated in setting up a school dental health program. Concern for youths' use of drugs—marijuana, crack, and cocaine mainly—and exposure to HIV/AIDS have prompted an array of national efforts to combat these health threats.

Response to disasters caused by human activity centers on training personnel—firefighters, emergency medical technicians, and first responders; in addition, eight ambulances are available on a fee-for-use basis.

Individual Care Services

In addition to the above-mentioned secondary and specialized hospitals, two district hospitals (in Soufrière and Dennery) provide outpatient, hospitalization, and emergency services, as well as inpatient care for minor medical, surgical, and pediatric problems and maternity care for low-risk deliveries. The psychiatric hospital provides inpatient care and some primary care to outpatients through community psychiatric clinics at the hospital and in seven other locations.

Two public and three private laboratories operate on the island. The one at Victoria Hospital serves as the national reference laboratory and employs the country's only pathologist. Blood collection and transfusion services are done at the blood bank unit of Victoria Hospital; there is also a mobile blood bank unit. Blood donors are interviewed about lifestyle and other risk factors before blood is drawn and tested for HIV, VDRL, hepatitis B and C, HTLV-1 and -2, blood group, and antibody screening.

Among specialty services, one of the Ministry of Health's current areas of concern is mental health. The mental health reform initiative articulates a shift from institutional to community-based mental health care that is expected to result in decentralization of, and increased access to, mental health care. The reform process entails mental health policy and legislative reform; human resource development and training; mental health promotion and illness prevention; and community mental health services. In addition, plans were finalized for construction of a new mental health facility, to be opened in 2007–2008; estimates

of personnel needs and the corresponding job descriptions were prepared.

In support of family planning, the Saint Lucia Planned Parenthood Association targets reduction of the incidence of unwanted pregnancies, particularly among adolescents, through a strengthened family life education program and comprehensive reproductive health care services. The Association provides counseling as well as contraceptive and other reproductive health services in clinical settings.

The National Strategic Plan for Health includes the provision of portable public dental health services, many of which are not currently available on a daily basis, to nine community health centers. In collaboration with the Ministry of Education, a school dental program was launched in 2003. Dental services are provided through a number of health facilities as well as the private sector.

Specialist ear, nose, and throat services were available, but those of speech therapists and audiologists were only periodically offered by short-term volunteers. A team of health professionals conducted monthly clinics for children with multiple handicaps. The Child Development and Guidance Center and the Ministry of Education offered services to children from birth to 16 years; their multidisciplinary team of professionals—a volunteer pediatrician, a physiotherapist employed by the Ministry of Education, visiting speech and language therapists, and visiting occupational therapists—provides comprehensive, ongoing assessment and diagnosis of children with physical, mental, emotional, and behavioral problems.

Human Resources

The most recent assessment of public health professionals in the country is summarized in Table 2. The total health sector human resource cost is estimated at US$ 15.2 million, which represented 70% of the latest total national budget.

The country experienced a shortage of health workers, as many of its nurses and other staff obtained more lucrative positions abroad. Approximately half of all nurses and midwives left the service within a year of graduating. The Nursing Council received 170 requests for transcripts in 2004, suggesting the departure of substantial numbers of trained nurses (*13*). The National Strategic Plan for Health emphasizes the development of measures to retain trained health workers.

In the reporting period, 14 persons participated in the PAHO/ WHO environmental health three-step program, the main objective of which is to enhance the skills of environmental health officers. Two nurses were trained in the care and management of diabetic patients and subsequently assisted in developing protocols for the effective management of diabetics. The Ministry of Health implemented an internship program to ensure the quality of new doctors by affording them the opportunity to apply their skills in a supportive learning environment. In 2004–2005, 37 doctors were trained at a cost of almost US$ 400,000. In 2005, a family case worker was trained in Israel, and two welfare officers were trained in social gerontology in Malta.

Health Supplies

The country obtains drugs through the Eastern Caribbean Drug Services, while all vaccines used in the public sector are procured through the PAHO Revolving Fund. The pharmaceutical procurement service of the Organization of Eastern Caribbean States expanded its medical product portfolio from 470 to 680 items to increase economies of scale by international tendering of a diverse range of essential health care products; the 25% increase in tendered medical supplies included a wide assortment of sutures, which previously consumed a significant portion of the health budgets of OECS countries.

Research and Technological Development in Health

In 2004, the Government conducted a knowledge, attitude, and practice survey (KAPS) of young persons (10–30 years of age) regarding HIV/AIDS in Gros Islet, Vieux Fort, Canaries, and Dennery, as part of a joint effort with the Organization of Petroleum Exporting Countries and UNFPA; the survey revealed the need for a deliberate strategy to arrest and control the HIV/AIDS epidemic among Saint Lucian youth (*14*). In 2004, the above-mentioned core welfare indicators survey included the monitoring of poverty and household welfare, covering a sufficiently large and representative sample to provide reliable welfare indicators for planning and policy formulation. In 2005, a UNICEF-sponsored child vulnerability study provided the Government pertinent findings and recommended priorities for action. That same year, a survey conducted by the Substance Abuse Advisory Council Secretariat to determine the level of drug abuse and drug education activities among the secondary school population found that the drugs most commonly used were marijuana, crack, and cocaine.

TABLE 2. Public sector health professionals, by specialty and population covered per specialty, Saint Lucia, 2002.

Category	No.	Population/ specialty
General practitioners	60	2,669
General surgeons	4	40,036
Anesthetists	5	32,029
Pediatricians	3	53,382
Obstetricians/gynecologists	5	32,029
Psychiatrists	5	32,029
Physicians	8	20,018
Accident and emergency	4	40,036
Epidemiologists	1	160,145
Cardiologists	1	160,145
Dermatologists	1	160,145
Internists	2	80,073
Ophthalmologists	1	160,145
Pathologists	1	160,145
Radiologists	2	80,073
Orthopedic surgeons	3	53,382

Health Sector Expenditures and Financing

Health services are funded from four main sources: the cosolidated fund, out-of-pocket payments, private insurance schemes, and donor contributions. The total annual health budget in 2000–2001 was the highest for the decade, at US$ 20.2 million; in 2001–2002 it was US$ 19.5 million, representing 6.2% of the total national budget; and in 2002–2003 it was US$ 19.3 million, representing 6.7% of the national budget.

In terms of distribution of the total health budget, secondary care services accounted for 53% in 2001–2002 and 54% for 2002–2003; primary care services were the second major portion of the total health budget, accounting for 22% in 2001–2002 and 23% in 2002–2003, and community services consumed about half of the primary care services budget; Golden Hope Hospital accounted for 5% each year of the total budget for 2001–2003; and the Ministry of Health's administration, policy, and planning services accounted for 9% of the total budget in 2001–2002 and 10% in 2002–2003 (*10, 15*).

The National Insurance Scheme made an annual contribution to the consolidated fund to cover inpatient hospital expenses for its members. Health expenditures grew by 40% over the period 2000–2006, from US$ 22.6 million to US$ 31.9 million. This upward trend is a reflection of the demand placed on the public health system by the demographic and epidemiological health profile. As a result, the resources allocated to the public health sector were insufficient to adequately respond to the increasing health needs of the population. The universal health care program was developed as the mechanism to improve national health sector financing; universal health care is scheduled to be implemented in 2006–2007.

Technical Cooperation and External Financing

Given the limited resources of the health system, resource mobilization is a major public sector thrust. The country received technical and financial cooperation from several external agencies and foreign governments. The European Union provided support in the form of loans and grants for the new general hospital, the development of the National Strategic Plan for Health, the integrated child protection and development program, the care of the elderly project, and the Women's Support Center. The Government received partial financing from the Caribbean Development Bank to undertake rehabilitation of primary schools and community health centers. It also secured funding to repair and refurbish 24 health facilities—15 through the Central Bank economic reconstruction project, five through the Basic Needs Trust Fund, and four through the World Bank. The World Bank also provided both loan and grant funding to implement the HIV/AIDS prevention and control project. A grant from the Government of Ireland targeted improvement of HIV/AIDS services, and UNFPA funded a project for HIV/AIDS prevention among youth. PAHO provided cooperation through training, scholarships, and direct technical services. The Government of China began construction of the new mental health facility, and the Government of Cuba contributed to improving the national eye care program, by providing free eye care for Saint Lucians in Cuba and technical assistance for development of an ophthalmology center at Victoria Hospital.

Nongovernment organizations such as the Saint Lucia Blind Welfare Association (SLBWA) and the National Council for Persons with Disabilities are critical in their response to eye health and physical disability problems. The SLBWA, through its link with the Hilton-Perkins International funding agency, provides limited, predominantly home and community-based care to a small number of multidisabled and vision-impaired children.

References

1. Government of Saint Lucia, Department of Statistics. Census of 2001.
2. Government of Saint Lucia. Saint Lucia Economic and Social Review, 2005.
3. Government of Saint Lucia. Core Welfare Indicators Questionnaire Survey. A Pilot Study in Saint Lucia, 2004.
4. Government of Saint Lucia, Ministry of Health, Epidemiology Department.
5. Government of Saint Lucia, National Emergency Management Office.
6. Government of Saint Lucia, Statistics Department. Vital Statistics Report, 2004.
7. Pan American Health Organization. Core Data, 2005.
8. Government of Saint Lucia, National AIDS Program Secretariat.
9. Government of Saint Lucia. Care of the Elderly in Saint Lucia, 2002.
10. Government of Saint Lucia. Report of the Chief Medical Officer, 2001–2002.
11. Government of Saint Lucia. National Strategic Plan for Health, 2006–2011.
12. Government of Saint Lucia. Debate on the Budget, 2006–2007.
13. Saint Lucia Nursing Council, Special Committee on the Migration and Training of Nurses. Final Committee Report, August 2004.
14. Government of Saint Lucia; United Nations Population Fund; Organization of Petroleum Exporting Countries. Knowledge, Attitude, and Practice Survey of Youth regarding HIV/AIDS, 2004.
15. Government of Saint Lucia. Report of the Chief Medical Officer, 2002–2003.

SAINT VINCENT AND THE GRENADINES

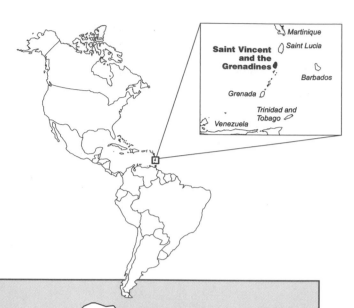

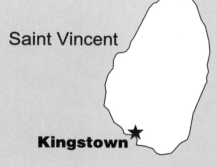

Saint Vincent

★ **Kingstown**

Bequia

Mustique

Canouan

Mayreau

Union Island

Palm Island

Petit Saint Vincent

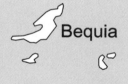

0   10   20   Miles

S aint Vincent and the Grenadines is a multi-island state in the Lesser Antilles; the country's 32 islands, inlets, and cays cover a 345-km^2 land area. The volcanic island of Saint Vincent, which accounts for most of the land area, is where 91% of the country's population lives. La Soufriere Volcano last erupted in 1979. The Grenadines includes seven inhabited islands—Bequia, Canouan, Mayreau, Union Island, Mustique, Palm Island, and Petit Saint Vincent. Sea transport links all the islands; airport facilities are available on Saint Vincent and in Bequia, Canouan, Mustique, and Union Island.

GENERAL CONTEXT AND HEALTH DETERMINANTS

The country has a tropical climate, with temperatures averaging between 72° and 80° F and rainfall averaging 80 inches along the coast and 160 in the central range; the rainy season falls between May and November. Saint Vincent and the Grenadines is susceptible to hurricanes, tropical storms, volcanic eruptions, and earthquakes.

Social, Political, and Economic Determinants

Saint Vincent and the Grenadines gained political independence from Great Britain in 1979 and is governed as a Westminster-style parliamentary democracy. The country is politically stable and free and fair elections are held every five years. The official language is English. The leading religious denominations are Anglican (17.8%), Pentecostal (17.6%), and Methodist (10.9%).

Between 2000 and 2004, Saint Vincent and the Grenadines' GDP grew from US$ 285 million to US $349 million. GDP growth averaged 5.1% per year in 2000–2004, resulting mainly from resilience in the construction, transportation, banking and insurance, electricity and water, communications, and wholesale and retail sectors. The removal of preferential tariffs and quotas on bananas, the country's main export crop, has led to losses in the agricultural sector. The Government has acknowledged the need to develop the services and tourism sectors to offset those losses. There were 77,631 tourist arrivals in 2002, nearly 7,000 more than in 2001.

In 2000–2004, the government annual budget ranged from US$ 150 million to US$ 180 million.

The 1996 Poverty Assessment Report concluded that 37.5% of the population (43,875 persons) was poor[1] and 25.7% (30,069 persons) was classified as indigent poor.[2]

The report also concluded that the country showed high levels of inequality. In 2001, the Government committed itself to address the doubly debilitating conditions of mass poverty and inequality, and established the National Economic and Social Development Council to oversee and guide the poverty reduction strategy. In 2002, the draft Interim Poverty Reduction Strategy Paper, a blueprint for developing policies and programs to address the central elements of poverty reduction in the short, medium, and long terms, was completed.

The overall employment rate[3] declined from 80.2% to 78.9% between 1991 and 2001. Unemployment among males increased from 18.4% in 1991 to 22.1% in 2001; among females, it decreased from 32.1% to 18.6% in the same period. The percentage of the population working in agriculture, construction, and wholesale industries declined from 49.1% of the labor force in 1991 to 41.6% in 2001. This drop was mainly due to a 37% decline in employment in agriculture. Fishing and manufacturing industries declined between 1991 and 2001. In 2001, 52% of the labor force was in the age group 15–43 years old as compared with 60% in 1991.

The unemployment rate in 2001 was 21%. The country's size, limited economic diversification, and extreme vulnerability to hurricanes triggered income insecurity and economic volatility at national and household levels. According to a World Bank document, the impact was particularly felt by the poor and the indigent poor, who were unable to tap savings or were not reached by the government's social protection programs in times of hardship.

The literacy rate in 2001–2005 was estimated at 96% overall, with equal levels for males and females. Saint Vincent and the Grenadines' educational system offers primary, secondary, and tertiary education levels. Since 2003, the Government has granted universal access to secondary education for all children. There

---

[1]Poverty is defined as insufficient diet and a lack of other goods and services necessary for effective functioning in a society.

[2]The indigent poor are persons who are not able to meet their basic food needs.

[3]The overall employment rate is the employed population as a percentage of the economically active population.

are 28 primary and 21 secondary public schools in the country, plus 3 private primary schools and 4 private secondary schools. School enrollment was 96% for the age group 5–9 years old and 94% for 10–14-year-olds. Preschool enrollment was only 33% in 2001. Although there were no full-time tertiary institutions on the island, 5.4% of the population has attained tertiary degrees. There were no observable differences in the number of males and females pursuing university education.

The Central Water and Sewerage Authority distributes potable water to about 90% of the country's population. According to the 2001 census, the water supply for 52.2% of households was publicly supplied into the home; for 17%, publicly supplied water was piped into the yard; for 20.8%, water was privately piped into the dwelling; and for 10%, mainly households on the Grenadines, water came from private catchments.

Food safety continued to be an issue of great concern in the country. Between 2001 and 2005, the number of food establishments increased, but there was no system for registering and licensing them. Food handlers' clinics conducted twice per year at district health centers provided education and information on food safety; attendance is voluntary.

In 2001, 52% of the households used a combination "water closet linked to cesspit" and "water closet linked to sewer," an increase compared with the 32% reported in 1991. Concomitant with this increase, the number of households using pit latrines fell from 62% in 1991 to 44% in 2001. Saint Vincent and the Grenadines has two sanitary landfills, one located at Belle Isle on the island's leeward side and the other at Diamond, on the windward side.

All households in Saint Vincent have their garbage collected once a week; households in the Grenadines have collection twice a week.

Squatting continues to be widespread. Persons who settle in squatting areas usually have no access to potable water or sanitary facilities. The areas where they live also are noted for vermin and rodent infestations, as well as the presence of other disease carrying organisms. Overcrowding, which allows for the easy spread of communicable diseases, is a common feature in these settlements.

Demographics, Mortality, and Morbidity

According to the 2001 Population and Housing Census, Saint Vincent and the Grenadines' total population was 106,253. Of the total population, 30.7% was under 15 years old, compared to 37.2% in 1991. This decline has reduced the dependency ratio, which dropped from 0.8 in 1991 to 0.6 in 2001. There were 29,523 persons 15–29 years old, which accounted for 27.8% of the population in 2001, compared to 29.5% in 1991. The broad age group of 30–44 years old, on the other hand, increased from 16.1% to 21.1% in those same years, while the age group 45–64 years old rose from 10.7% to 13.2%. Persons 65 years old and older represented 7.3% of the total population in 2001, compared to 6.5% in

1991. The census also showed that the female-to-male ratio was 1:1.02. (See Figure 1.)

According to the 2001 census, African descendents accounted for 72.8% of the population, mixed ethnicities for 20%, Caribs for 3.6%, and East Indians for 1.4%. Caribs and other indigenous peoples live predominantly along the country's northeast.

In 2001–2004, there were 3,097 deaths, for an average of 774 deaths per year. In 2001, there were 765 deaths. The five leading causes based on defined causes of death were malignant neoplasms (133), diabetes mellitus (103), cerebrovascular accidents (60), ischemic heart diseases (45), and HIV/AIDS (34). Diabetes, ischemic heart disease, cerebrovascular accidents, hypertensive diseases, and malignant neoplasms were the five noncommunicable diseases that accounted for around 50% of total deaths annually. In 2003 there were 774 deaths. The five leading causes of death were diabetes mellitus (120), malignant neoplasms (119), heart disease (102), hypertension (101), and cerebrovascular accidents (51); together, these causes accounted for 62.4% of total deaths.

Diabetes accounted for 71 female deaths and 49 male deaths; 55 females and 46 males died of hypertension. Nearly equal numbers of males and females died from ischemic heart disease and cerebrovascular disease; economically and socially deprived women were particularly vulnerable to these two diseases.

The leading cause of death in males was malignant neoplasms; in 2001–2003 malignant neoplasms of the prostate was the fifth leading cause of death among males, with 91 deaths. An analysis of mortality data for 2003 showed that there were 69 deaths from malignant neoplasms among males, compared to 49 deaths among females. The most common site for malignant neoplasm in males was the prostate. Cardiac-related conditions have steadily increased in Saint Vincent and the Grenadines over the years; in 2004, 1,205 cases were reported. Chronic obstructive pulmonary diseases were responsible for 23 deaths in males and 5 deaths in females. In 2003, 40 males died from cirrhosis of the liver, alcoholic cardiomyopathy, alcoholic hepatitis, acute pancreatitis, and gastrointestinal hemorrhage; only 16 females died from these diseases that year.

Data from public health care facilities revealed that injuries from poisoning and other consequences of external causes accounted for 827 visits. Males accounted for 468 (57%) visits and females, for 359 (43%). According to an analysis of clinic visits for noncommunicable diseases in 2003, the age group 15–24 recorded the most visits for soft tissue injuries, with 156 (19%), followed by the 25–34 age group with 149 (18%), and the age group 5–14, with 145 (17%).

Injuries and accidents accounted for 124 deaths in 2001–2003, with homicides accounting for 38.7%, drowning for 24.2%, motor vehicle accidents for 21.8%, and suicides for 16.1%. Between 2001 and 2004, motor vehicle accidents increased from 950 to 1,086. In those same years, 134 males were seriously injured, compared to 56 females. In 2003, external causes ranked among the ten leading causes of death in the country for the first time.

FIGURE 1. Population structure, by age and sex, Saint Vincent and the Grenadines, 1990 and 2005.

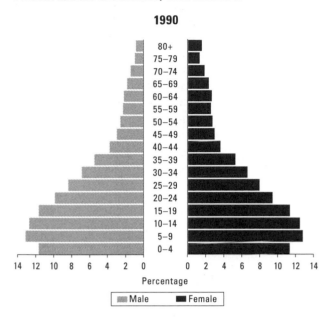

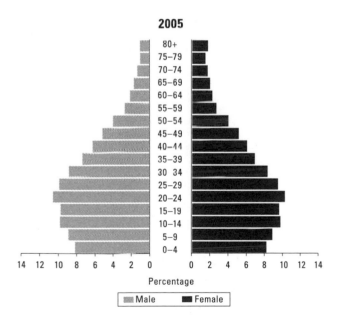

According to clinic data, external causes represented 0.6% of the reason for clinic visits in 1998, increasing to 2.2% in 2003. Police reports indicate that 63 homicides and 4,470 criminal assaults were reported in 2001–2004.

The surveillance system reported 2,500 annual visits for asthma to the emergency room at Kingstown General Hospital in 1998 and 1999, with 45% of these visits from children under 10 years of age. In 2001–2005, asthma continued to be a major reason for clinic visits.

Total life expectancy at birth was 71.6 years in 2005. Life expectancy for males decreased from 69.5 years in 1991 to 68.8 years in 2005; life expectancy for females remained constant at 74.4 years in that same period.

The total fertility rate in 1996–2000 was 2.3 children per woman and 2.2 children per woman by 2005. The fertility rate in 2001 was 2.4; it was 2.1 in 2005. The crude birth rate averaged 19.0 per 1,000 population in 2000–2001, while the crude death rate averaged 6.8.

Infant mortality ranged from 18.5 per 1,000 live births to 17.3 between 2001 and 2004. Three maternal deaths were recorded between 2001 and 2004.

HEALTH OF POPULATION GROUPS

Children under 5 Years Old

There were 4,094 live births between 2001 and 2002; 241 infants were low-birthweight babies (<2,500 g). Perinatal mortality in 1998–2002 registered an annual average of 20 deaths per 1,000 live births. The leading causes of death in this age group were extreme prematurity, birth asphyxia, and respiratory distress syndrome of the newborn. According to data from the maternity unit of Milton Cato Memorial Hospital, in 2002, 34.4% of admissions to the special care nursery were as a result of prematurity. Other leading morbidities seen at the nursery included sepsis, jaundice, and respiratory distress syndrome. According to the communicable disease data for 2001 and 2002, acute respiratory infections in the age group under 1 year old accounted for approximately 11% of total reported cases of acute respiratory infections.

Among the 1–4-year-old age group, poisonings were responsible for 47% (37) of reported accidents in 2002; falls were responsible for 32% (25).

A total of 20,324 child health visits were made at the various health centers. Most visits were for growth monitoring (19,606) followed by immunization (10,073); the remainder were for referrals and other health problems. There were 212 (18% of the total) clinic visits for asthma in the age group 1–4 years old. Visits for child health complications accounted for 214 visits, or 1% of total health visits made—problems included malnutrition, respiratory infections, diarrheal diseases, and injuries. In 2003, immunization coverage for BCG, polio, DPT, hepatitis B, and *Haemophilus influenzae* type b was 100%; coverage for MMR was 90.7%. In 2003, there were two reported cases of *Haemophilus influenzae* meningitis in the age group 1–4 years old; both were females.

Children 5–9 Years Old

The age group 5–9 years old accounted for 10.8% of the total population in 2001. Mortality in this age group is generally low. In 2001, there were 8 deaths: 5 males and 3 females. According to data for 2002, there were 6 deaths, 3 males and 3 females. Causes of death for males were unspecified drowning (1) and exposure to electric current (2). The causes of death in females were malignant neoplasm of the kidney (1) and victims of an avalanche (2).

Health center data showed that in 2002–2004, visual problems, impacted cerumen, dental caries, viral illnesses, and tinea were the most common health problems encountered. Each child is examined upon entering and leaving primary school as a public health requirement.

In 2002, asthma workshops were conducted for 37 primary and secondary schools as well as for preschool teachers.

Adolescents 10–14 and 15–19 Years Old

This age group represented 21.1% of the population in 2001, almost equally distributed among the sexes. In 2001, the Pan American Health Organization conducted a national sample survey on healthy lifestyles among adolescents 10–14 years old and found that 11% of respondents admitted to using inhalants, 85% to using marijuana, 7% to smoking cigarettes, and 3% to using alcohol weekly or daily. Nutritional data from 2002 indicated that 87.8% of youth in this age group met criteria for normal nutrition, 8.6% were obese, and 3.6% were moderately undernourished. The Ministry of Health's National Family Planning Unit reported that of the 8,166 live births in 2000–2003, 1,704 (20%) were to teenage mothers. Disaggregated by age group, the 10–14-year-old cohort accounted for 48 live births, while the 15–19-year-old age group accounted for 1, 606 live births. Of the 782 diagnosed cases of HIV in 1984–2004, 48 (61%) were among persons aged 10–19 years old. Ten new cases were diagnosed in 2002, six in 2003, and five in 2004.

In 2000–2002, there were 10 deaths in the age group 10–14 years old. Causes of death included tuberculosis of the lungs, infantile cerebral palsy, secondary malignant neoplasm of the brain, and septicemia.

Adults 20–59 Years Old

This age group accounted for almost 50% of the population in 2001. Of total births (7,166) in 2000–2003, 91% (6,525) were to women 20–44 years old. Twenty-five percent of these women made their first visit to prenatal clinics prior to the 16th week of gestation. Trained personnel at Milton Cato Memorial Hospital delivered 99% of births. According to 2002 maternal and child health data, of the estimated 4,130 pregnancies in 1996–2002, 4.5% (92) had gestational diabetes and 4.2% (85) had hypertension in pregnancy.

In 2002, 9.2% (184) of women had anemia during pregnancy, 5.1% (102) had pre-eclampsia, 16.5% (341) had pregnancy with abortive outcome, 4.1% (85) were Rh-negative, 10.5% (216) gave birth to premature infants, 7.1% (143) had hypertensive disease during pregnancy, and 24.1% (709) gave birth by cesarean section. That same year, there were 141 low-birthweight babies, representing 11.8% of total births. There were 9,023 visits to prenatal clinics in 2002, excluding those made to private health care providers. That same year, there were 1,264 new family planning acceptors, 55% of them opting for oral contraceptives and 38% for injectables; six persons chose sterilization and two were fitted with intrauterine devices. In 2004, the number of family planning acceptors increased to 10,888. There is little data on the extent of condom use, but it is estimated that in 2004, the Government spent roughly US$ 3,875 on free condom distribution. In 2002, 2,926 Pap smears were done; 7.4% showed abnormal results.

Clinic records show that there were 220 obese persons in 2002, with women accounting for 85% (188 cases). Persons 35–45 years old had the most records of obesity (58%), followed by those aged 25–34 years (26%) and those 45–54 years (22%). Persons aged 55–64 years old accounted for 3,432 visits for hypertension, and persons 45–54, for 1,927.

Older Adults 60 Years Old and Older

This age group represented approximately 7.2% of the population in 2001. Persons 60 years old and older always have accounted for the greatest number of attendances for hypertension, which in 2003 reached 5,774 (48.7% of all attendances). Arthritis ranked as the fourth leading reason for clinic visits for this group in 2003, accounting for 3,632 visits, or 8.9% of total visits. Arthritis has always predominantly affected persons 65 years old and older: in 2003, this group accounted for 2,199 visits (60.5% of all visits for arthritis), with women accounting for 75% of the group's visits. Cardiac problems were the primary reason for clinic visits among those 65 years and older. The age group 70 years old and older recorded the most skin cancers, accounting for 41% of the total number reported in 2003.

The leading problems facing this population group include chronic diseases, loneliness, and abuse. Saint Vincent and the Grenadines has a need for psychosocial support services for the elderly. Care for the elderly is provided through the public and private health care systems through a Government-operated home and a publicly operated program that provides care and support to the elderly in their homes. There are also four privately operated homes for the elderly. Two recently commissioned centers cater to the elderly's daytime needs and allow for older persons to interact socially with one another. There are 161 available beds for the elderly; 106 of them are in the public system.

The Family

Ninety percent of households were located on mainland Saint Vincent. In 2003, the mean household size was 3.5 persons, compared with 3.9 persons in 1991. In 2001, 85.2% of the households lived in undivided private houses (single dwelling units that comprise the entire building). The number of persons living in "combined business and dwelling" structures increased by 26.3% between 1991 and 2001. There were 30,518 households (one or more persons living together) in 2001, compared with 27,002 in 1991, an increase of 13.0%; 12,136 households were headed by females, and 39% of them (4,723) were headed by women not in union. During 2001–2004, 35 children lost one or both parents to HIV/AIDS.

Morbidity data for 2003 made special note of spousal abuse—83 males and 49 females were affected. According to an analysis of clinic visits for noncommunicable diseases in Saint Vincent and the Grenadines in 2003, there were 83 clinic visits due to domestic violence recorded in 2003, with males accounting for 49 (59%) and females accounting for 34 (41%).

Workers

Work-related injuries contribute substantially to the country's morbidity profile; some workplaces are unsafe or provide unhealthy working environments. Occupational conditions fall outside the ambit of the Ministry of Health and the Environment, however.

HEALTH CONDITIONS AND PROBLEMS

COMMUNICABLE DISEASES

Vector-borne Diseases

Dengue fever and **leptospirosis** continued to be endemic in the country. National household and Breteau indices of *Aedes aegypti* breeding were 19.84% and 43.57%, respectively, in 2000; both figures were above internationally accepted levels. The introduction of West Nile virus and the rare Chikungunya virus are of real concern to the country's vector control unit.

Vaccine-preventable Diseases

Saint Vincent and the Grenadines vaccinates against **measles, mumps, rubella, diphtheria, pertussis, tetanus, poliomyelitis, tuberculosis,** and **hepatitis b**. In 2003, the pentavalent vaccine was introduced into the immunization program. Although vaccination against *Haemophilus influenzae* **type B** is not routinely offered in the country, private sector physicians administer it on request. Of the approximately 2,000 to 3,000 annual blood donors, 2% tested positive to hepatitis b in 2001–2003.

Saint Vincent and the Grenadines continued to enjoy a steady supply of vaccines, syringes, and needles, and the country's vaccination coverage has remained between 85% and 100% over the years.

Intestinal Infectious Diseases

There were 1,744 cases of **gastroenteritis** reported in 2002 and 4,122 in 2003, more than a twofold increase. The disease was listed as the second most common communicable disease in 2004 and 2003, accounting for 11.3% and 12.3% of cases, respectively.

Helminthiasis diagnoses in the primary care setting are usually based on clinical suspicion, rather than laboratory confirma-

tion. Of the 4,281 stool samples screened for 2003 and 2004, there were 144 positive samples: 47 cases of *E. coli*, 30 cases of **hookworm**, 2 cases of **trichuris**, 34 cases of **strongyloides**, 2 cases of **ascaris**, and 29 cases of **giardia**. In 2003, there were 60 cases of **foodborne illness** reported from the accident and emergency department. Fifteen cases of foodborne illness were reported in 2004; 13 were confirmed.

Pathology laboratory surveillance reports for 2004 identified three cases of **salmonellosis**, two cases of **shigellosis**, and one case of **campylobacterosis**. In 2003, there were four cases of salmonella, two of shigella, and two of campylobacter.

Chronic Communicable Diseases

There were 65 new cases of **tuberculosis** between 2000 and 2004. Each year in that period, the majority of cases were in males; in 2003, 13 of the 14 cases were in males. Diagnosed cases ranged between 15 and 80 years old. In the same period, there were 14 deaths from tuberculosis. Saint Vincent and the Grenadines has adopted the Directly Observed Treatment, Short-course (DOTS) strategy to reduce the number of tuberculosis cases since the Milton Cato Memorial Hospital began to offer the treatment.

The last case of **leprosy** (Hansen's disease) was reported in 2000.

Acute Respiratory Infections

There were 16,374 cases of acute respiratory infections reported in 2003 and 11,030 in 2004. In this two-year period, acute respiratory infections represented roughly half of all reported communicable diseases, which is a matter of grave concern for the country. In 2004, there were 4,654 cases of acute respiratory infections in children under 5 years old, 40% of the total number of acute respiratory infections in the population; the male-to-female ratio was 1.2:1.

HIV/AIDS

There were 60 cases of HIV infection in 2002 and 81 in 2003. In 2004, there were 108 confirmed new cases of HIV infection—the highest incidence since the first case was reported; males accounted for 64 of the cases (59%). There were 40 cases of AIDS, 26 in males (65%) and 14 in females (35%). There were 57 cases of AIDS in 2003.

Vertical transmission accounted for two cases in 2004; there were no new cases in 2003. A formalized system of care and treatment to persons with HIV/AIDS offering antiretrovirals was put in place in August 2003; the program was bolstered in 2005. In 2004, 14 new clients began antiretroviral treatment, adding to the 22 persons (12 males and 10 females) who had been participating since 2003; as of this writing, there were 25 males and 11 females enrolled in the program. The availability of the care-and-treatment program, as well as voluntary HIV counseling and testing programs, may be responsible for more people volunteering to be tested and for more persons accessing treatment centers for managing their infection.

The 17 fewer AIDS cases between 2003 and 2004 may be attributed to the introduction of antiretrovirals treatment and the bolstering of the national HIV/AIDS program through the project jointly funded by the Global Fund to Fight AIDS, Tuberculosis, and Malaria and by the World Bank.

Zoonoses

There were 53 cases of **leptospirosis** in 2000–2004, most of them in males. The mean age of those affected was 34 years.

NONCOMMUNICABLE DISEASES

Metabolic and Nutritional Diseases

Anemia accounted for 531 clinic visits in 2004, representing 1.4% of all noncommunicable diseases clinic visits. The female-to-male ratio was 4:1: females accounted for 429 visits (80.8%) and males, for 102 (19.2%).

The age group 65 years old and older is the most affected by metabolic and nutritional diseases, accounting for 82 visits for these diseases (15.4%), followed by the 15–24 age group with 79 (14.8%), and the age group 5–14 with 78 (14.6%). In 2003–2004 there were more than 500 annual visits for metabolic nutritional diseases.

Diabetes accounted for 4,070 visits, or 11% of total clinic visits, in 2002; males accounted for 23% and females for 77%.

Obesity accounted for 271 visits in 2004. Most visits were among persons aged 25–44 years, accounting for 120 visits, or 44.2%. Results of the 2004 Food and Agriculture Organization/Caribbean Food and Nutrition Institute study of 143 adolescents and adults aged 11–65 years old showed a widespread use of foods high in fats, salt, and sugar. On the other hand, foods rich in fiber and antioxidants were not consumed widely, especially among the younger age group. The study also pointed out that persons who reported daily consumption of vegetables also were vegetable producers. Estimates of national food availability indicated that there was a trend in an oversupply of per capita energy, increasing from 2,540 kcal/day in 1999 to 2,642 in 2000, and then decreasing slightly to 2,609 in 2001. The corresponding figures for protein and fat were 68.1g and 74.9g, respectively, in 2000 to 66.7 g and 73.0g in 2001.

Cardiovascular Diseases

Hypertension accounted for 29% of all clinic visits in 2000. Visits for hypertension rose slightly in 2002, accounting for 30% of all clinic visits (11,082). Males represented 26% of these visits and females, 74%. The age group 65 years old and older accounted for half of all visits for hypertension, followed by the age group 55–64 years, which accounted for 20%.

Cardiovascular diseases accounted for 1,869 (4.6%) clinic visits and ranked as the fifth leading reason for health visits in 2004. That same year, the age group 65 years old and older—the age group with the highest number of visits for cardiovascular diseases—accounted for 1,273 visits (73.5% of all visits). Records at the Milton Cato Memorial Hospital, the main referral hospital, show that in 2000–2003 there were 1,025 admissions for cardiovascular diseases: 237 for myocardial infarction, 279 for chronic ischemic heart disease, and 509 for hypertensive heart disease.

Malignant Neoplasms

Between 2000 and 2003, there were 554 deaths from malignant neoplasms. The six most common sites were: the prostate, 118 (21%); upper respiratory organs and lungs, 56 (10%); upper gastrointestinal tract, 47 (8.0%); female breast, 39 (7.0%); bowel, 30 (5.4%); and cervix, 23 (4.1%). Cervical cancer is the most common form of malignant neoplasm in females.

OTHER HEALTH PROBLEMS OR CONDITIONS

Mental Health and Addictions

During 2002–2004, there were 1,437 admissions to the mental hospital, 282 of them (19.6%) were new cases. According to a breakdown by diagnosis, drug-induced psychoses was the leading cause of admission, followed by schizophrenia, acute psychoses, mental retardation, and manic depressive disorders. Drug users accounted for 85 admissions (40%).

Oral Health

Oral health services are offered through a network of public and private health care facilities. The government operates ten public health dental health clinics that offer primarily preventive care. In 2002, public dental health clinics cared for 15,921 patients. The frequency of procedures performed by the department were: extractions (52%); preventive care (18%), restorations (18%), and other (12%). There is no school dental health program.

RESPONSE OF THE HEALTH SECTOR

Health Policies and Plans

In developing Saint Vincent and the Grenadines' national health policies and strategies, consideration was given to the country's specific and unique local health conditions; to relatively unchanging societal and policy circumstances, such as economic and political organization; to cultural factors, such as the society's and specific groups' values and commitments; and to external factors that influence the country, such as regional and international agreements.

Caring for the Poor, Caring for the Environment

Squatting—the practice of establishing unregulated settlements on state-owned land—is widespread in Saint Vincent and the Grenadines, and it poses major public health and environmental challenges for the country. An estimated 16,000 squatters—more than one in seven of the country's citizens—survive mostly through subsistence farming. As a rule, in these settlements housing is substandard, and the communities are overcrowded and prone to vermin and rodent infestations, which lead to high rates of communicable diseases. The squatters usually have no access to potable water or sanitary facilities. By far the most promising endeavor is embodied in the Government's Integrated Forest Management and Development Program (IFMDP), an ambitious multisectoral effort involving various ministries. The program aims to encourage squatters to relocate to areas that provide better access to health services and to apply better farming practices.

Health Strategies and Programs

In 2004, the Ministry of Health and the Environment began to prepare the 2006–2011 national strategic health plan which is guided by local, regional, and international policies the Government has suscribed to. First, the Government relies on the principle of primary health care as the main mechanism to improve the population's quality of life. Second, in a regional context, priority areas set in the Caribbean Cooperation in Health Initiative will be adhered to. Thirdly, the results of the analysis of the country's Essential Public Health Functions will guide the direction the health sector will pursue during the period of the plan. In addition, the regional initiative for extending social protection in health will facilitate a greater collaboration with the National Insurance Service as a way to address universal access to programs and services. In 2001, Parliament passed the National Economic and Social Development Council Act; the Council finalized the Interim Poverty Reduction Strategy paper in 2003.

Saint Vincent and the Grenadines became a signatory of the WHO Framework Convention on Tobacco Control in 2004, an international treaty that promotes state parties to enact or amend public health laws to control the burden of disease from tobacco use and prevent the initiation of smoking.

Legislation regulating the work of nurse midwives and nursing assistants was amended to incorporate and expand the role and functions of the family nurse practitioner. In 2002, the draft legislation requiring the use of seatbelts while riding in automobiles and helmets while riding motorcycles was enacted in 2006. The 2004 pharmacy act gives greater autonomy to pharmacists.

Organization of the Health System

The Ministry of Health is the agency within the Executive Branch charged with providing equitable, good quality, sustainable, and comprehensive primary, secondary, and tertiary health care. The Ministry also must offer health promotion, nutrition, and health education services to the population, as well as protect and preserve the environment and the country's natural resources, through a health service delivery process, the conduct of environmental assessments and research, and the efficient management of available resources.

The Minister operates as the political director; the Permanent Secretary is the administrative leader; and the Chief Medical Officer (CMO) is the technical head. Administrative and technical leaders follow public service rules and regulations. A Health Planner sits within the Ministry of Health and the Environment, although administratively this officer functions under the Ministry of Finance and Planning.

To support this structure a senior management committee has been constituted, involving senior administrative and technical personnel at the Ministry. The committee's primary responsibility is policy development and implementation. The Ministry of Health and the Environment provides primary, secondary, and tertiary services through its 14 programs.

Thirty-nine health centers provide services across nine health districts. Shifts in population have affected the numbers of persons to be served in various districts, resulting in a need to redefine district boundaries.

On average, each health center is equipped to provide services to a catchment population of 2,900 persons, and no person is required to travel more than three miles to access care. Primary health care services available include emergency care, medical care, prenatal and postnatal care, midwifery services, child health services (including immunizations and school health), family planning services, and communicable and noncommunicable disease control. Dental health services are delivered at selected centers and mental health services are offered at all health centers on a visiting basis. Each health center is staffed with a full-time district nurse, a nursing assistant, and a community health aide. Other district health teams—including a district medical officer, a pharmacist, a nursing supervisor, a family nurse practitioner, an environmental health officer, a family life educator, a social worker, a nutrition officer, and other visiting staff—provide additional support.

Public Health Services

The Government of Saint Vincent and the Grenadines is firmly committed to a program to prevent and control the spread of HIV/AIDS and to alleviate the socioeconomic impact of the disease on the population. A National Strategic Plan was launched in 2001 and a program that will fall under the Ministry of Health and the Environment was budgeted in 2002 expenditure estimates. An updated Plan to be implemented in 2004–2009 includes the following overarching goals: to reduce the incidence of HIV to 0.1% from the current rate of 0.6%; to decrease the case fatality rate of persons living with HIV/AIDS; and to offer support to people living with HIV/AIDS and their families. The Plan targets the following five priority areas: to strengthen intersectoral management, organizational structures, and institutional capacity; to develop, strengthen, and implement prevention and control programs for HIV/AIDS and other sexually transmitted infections with priority given to youth and high-risk or vulnerable groups; to strengthen care, support, and treatment programs for people living with AIDS and their families; to conduct research; and to upgrade surveillance systems. The agencies implementing the Plan include civil society organizations and ministries other than the Ministry of Health.

The response to natural and manmade disasters is the responsibility of the National Disaster Management Organization (NEMO), which includes community disaster committees that are responsible for the response at the community level. Under a World Bank sponsored project, new headquarters for NEMO were constructed, equipped with necessary infrastructure to house an emergency command center. Strategic sea defenses in vulnerable areas have been constructed. All government sectors have developed national disaster plans.

In 2000–2004, the government funded contraceptive distribution at a cost of US$ 89,630.

An assessment of the school feeding program was conducted in 2004 with assistance from the Caribbean Food and Nutrition Institute. An adolescent health and family life survey was conducted in 2002 and a study on how to communicate behavioral change for preventing HIV was carried out in 2003.

Individual Care Services

The 211-bed Milton Cato Memorial Hospital is the country's only acute-care referral hospital in the public sector that provides specialist care in most major areas. The delivery of care is organized into seven departments: accident and emergency, outpatient services, surgery, medicine, operating theatre, pediatric services,

and obstetrics/gynecology. Five rural hospitals with a combined 58-bed capacity provide a minimum level of secondary care. There also is a 10-bed acute-care private hospital, the Maryfield.

The Government also operates the 186-bed Mental Health Centre, which provides care to patients with acute and chronic psychiatric problems, and the 106-bed Lewis Punnett Home, which caters to an indigent elderly population. Five private institutions with a combined bed capacity of 55 offer resident care for the elderly.

With the installation of a Coulter Haematology Analyzer® in 2002, blood testing has been streamlined in the country, with turnaround times significantly cut down and the capability to conduct new tests expanded. In addition, the installation of a BD FACSCount™ cytometry instrumentation system in 2003 has allowed the laboratory to effectively handle an increased demand for CD4 testing, which has led to the introduction of antiretroviral treatment for HIV/AIDS, as well as to handle greater demand for routine hematology. The laboratory also has benefited from two information programs, the Rapid Automated Biological Identification System (RABIS) and Portable High-throughput Integrated Laboratory Identification System (PHILIS).

Saint Vincent and the Grenadines participated in a project sponsored by the European Union designed to strengthen medical laboratories in the Caribbean, which has led to a better understanding of the quality of laboratory services in the country and has set the course for achieving standardization and accreditation in the future. Since 2001, histology specimens have been analyzed locally by a resident pathologist.

In 2001, an additional plain-film unit was installed at Milton Cato Memorial Hospital's accident and emergency department.

Health Promotion

In 2001–2005, some public schools adopted healthy school policies, including providing only healthy food choices in the school feeding program or through vendors at the school. Teachers received additional training in physical education so they could make it more enjoyable for students. All the new schools built included facilities for physical education or had such a facility nearby. The health and family life curriculum included topics related to the prevention of noncommunicable diseases. Of 1,620 schoolchildren screened, 20 were referred to the ENT specialist.

A program to reduce drug demand began in 2004; it is designed to build human resources to address the issue of drug abuse, strengthen treatment and rehabilitation capability, raise public awareness about drug abuse and its attendant problems, and develop a strong multisectoral response to prevention.

Human Resources

According to 2005 figures from the Nursing Council's register, there were 398 nurses of varying categories registered. The country has access to two schools of nursing: the Government-run School of Nursing and the Kingstown Medical College, which is based in Grenada. In 2003, the School of Nursing strengthened its registered nurse program to accommodate increased enrollment and help offset nurse shortages due to nurses migrating out of Saint Vincent and the Grenadines. Table 1 shows the number and ratio of health professionals in the country.

Health Supplies

The Central Pharmacy and the pharmaceutical services are charged with procuring, preparing, dispensing, and distributing all drugs in the national health system, as well as procuring and distributing through medical stores the medical and other supplies that facilitate the health system's proper functioning.

The bulk of pharmaceuticals are purchased through the Organization of Eastern Caribbean States' Pharmaceutical Procurement Services (formerly the Eastern Caribbean Drug Service). According to the Procurement Services' Regional Formulary and Therapeutics Manual Saint Vincent's Ministry of Health and the Environment can purchase drugs from 76 categories. There are 39 district pharmacies that supply drugs to the public health system. There also are 13 registered private pharmacies and 31 registered pharmacists, 19 of whom are employed by the Ministry.

TABLE 1. Number and ratio of health professionals, by category, Saint Vincent and the Grenadines, 2001–2005.

Health professional category	Number	Ratio per 10,000 population
Physicians	101	9.5
Registered nurses	228	21.5
Nursing assistants	124	11.7
Nursing auxiliaries	115	10.8
Laboratory technicians	13	1.2
Pharmacists	36	3.4
Environmental officers	14	1.3
Psychiatrists	2	0.19
Psychologists	1	0.09
Dentists	13	1.2
Counselors	5	0.5
Nutrition officers	12	1.1
Health educators	7	0.66

Health Sector Expenditures and Financing

The Ministry of Health and the Environment collaborates with other ministries and departments in the pursuit of its health care goals and objectives.

Financing from the Government is based on annual budgetary proposals submitted to the Ministry of Finance and Planning and on a program of work derived from strategic and operational planning processes. According to Government estimates, the total health budget for 2000–2004 ranged from US$ 18.6 million to US$ 21.7 million, representing an annual average of roughly 12% of the national budget.

Information on the cost of medications for noncommunicable diseases in the public health system is provided by the report of the audit of the country's pharmaceutical supply. Medications for diabetes cost US$ 407,154 and medications for hypertension cost US$ 230,032 in 2004; the two combined represented 20% of the annual pharmaceutical budget in the public system. According to information from the Family Nurse Practitioner and asthma initiative coordinator, the most recent medication costs for asthma are for 2002; they totaled US$ 21,283.90.

Technical Cooperation and External Financing

Technical and financial assistance is obtained from international organizations such as the World Health Organization, the World Bank, the Pan American Health Organization, the European Union, the Caribbean Epidemiology Center, and the Organization of Eastern Caribbean States; from individual governments such as the governments of France, Japan, and Taiwan; and from private institutions such as St. Georges University.

Bibliography

OECS Fiscal Issues: St. Vincent and the Grenadines, December 2004.

National Health Plan of Saint Vincent and the Grenadines, Working document, 2006–2010.

Saint Vincent and the Grenadines Population and Housing Census, 2001.

National Family Planning Unit, Ministry of Health and the Environment.

SURINAME

Guyana

Nickerie

Coronie

2

Paramaribo
1
3
4

Marowijne

Para

Brokopondo

*French
Guiana*

Sipaliwini

1 Paramaribo
2 Saramacca
3 Wanica
4 Commewijne

Brazil

0   25   50 Miles

S uriname is located on the northeast coast of South America, and covers 163,820 km². In the north, it borders the Atlantic Ocean; its neighbors to the east, south, and west are French Guiana, Brazil, and Guyana, respectively. The topography encompasses a narrow coastal plain that extends from east to west, consisting mainly of a savanna belt and a highland tropical rainforest.

GENERAL CONTEXT AND HEALTH DETERMINANTS

The land is divided into urban, rural, and interior areas. The urban area, comprising the capital city of Paramaribo, the city of Nieuw Nickerie in the west, and parts of the district of Wanica, covers 0.4% of the country's land surface and is inhabited by 59.4% of the total population. The coastal rural area is inhabited by 29.6% of the population. Both urban and rural areas are located along the coast, covering 10% of the land surface, with a population density of 526.5 inhabitants per km². The remote, heavily rainforested interior to the south, making up the remaining 90% of the country, is home to only 11% of the total population, with a density of 0.2 person per km². The interior's inhabitants are largely Maroons (descendants of runaway slaves) and indigenous tribal settlements of 100 to 4,000 persons, who have little or no basic sanitation, piped water, or electricity.

Social, Political, and Economic Determinants

The Government of Suriname accords high priority to sustainable development, poverty reduction, and improvement of the living conditions of its population within a framework of democracy and the preservation of human rights. Formerly a Dutch colony, Suriname gained independence in 1975. The political system (1) may be characterized as a constitutional democracy. The last elections were held in 2005. The present administration has majority support in the 51-seat National Assembly from a coalition of political parties that represent ethnic groups more than political platforms and ideologies. Below the national level there are 10 District Councils, and at the sub-district level there are 62 Resort Councils.

GDP growth for most of the 2001–2005 period remained high and reached 7.8% in 2004. Mining, agriculture, and manufacturing are the most important sectors in Suriname's economy, with good prospects for the construction and tourism sectors. Bauxite mining and oil extraction continue to account for more than 90% of total foreign exchange earnings while agriculture, forestry, and

fishing accounted for 7.5% of the GDP in 2002. The tourism industry is still in an early stage of development, yet shows encouraging signs of growth: in 2004, there were 137,000 tourist arrivals, compared to 85,000 in 2003.

National statistics indicate that there is a very large informal sector accounting for at least 20% of GDP and composed of remittances from family members living abroad, especially in the Netherlands, and various types of small-scale gold mining and logging operations. The Head of the Judicial Section of the Police Corps indicated in 2000 that narcotics trafficking had become a major challenge and estimated that approximately 26,000 kg of cocaine are shipped to Europe each year, with a street value of slightly over US$ 1 billion. Of this, he estimated that some US$ 300 million stayed in Suriname. The country's location and remote, sparsely populated interior contributed to its desirability as an international transit point for drug trafficking (2).

The country has experienced a significant loss of skilled labor due to emigration. The Netherlands is the country with the highest number of emigrants from Suriname, with 321,000 living there in 2004 (1) and an average migration of 3,300 Surinamese per year to the country (3). The external migration of skilled professionals affects several areas: in the health sector, there is a very high out-migration of nurses.

According to the local definition of poverty, a person or household is considered poor if there are insufficient means to provide for basic human needs, particularly as regards food. Figures for the average poverty lines for the second quarter of 2005 for Paramaribo and Wanica show that the poverty line for a household consisting of one adult would be US$ 135 per month and that of one adult and two children, US$ 281 per month. The General Bureau of Statistics estimates that in 2000, between 60% and 75% of the population lived below this poverty line. Women living in the interior, women without a partner, youth, and older adults are the groups most affected by poverty. Women overall are poorer than men (4), due to persistent gender inequality in the household and in society. A lack of access to employment in the formal sector forces women into informal economic activities, which are often characterized by poor working conditions, health risks, irregular working hours, and low income (5). After the public sector, private sector agriculture is the second largest productive activity of women. The majority of rural families own and work small plots of land, with women and children usually working without pay. Poverty is also common among youth and children below 15 years of age, with 61.6% in this group living in poverty. The prevalence of poverty declines gradually with age, reaching 46.3% in the 45–60-year-old age group. However, of the population over 60 years of age, 52.1% live below the poverty line because the current pension system does not effectively meet the financial needs of retired persons. Although the majority of poor live in urban areas, the sectors living in the most extreme poverty are found in the country's interior (6). However, this latter sector is gradually migrating to Paramaribo; many are women and the majority are poorly educated and possess only minimal job skills (7).

The urban unemployment rate decreased from 14% in 2001 to 8% in 2004 (8). The national unemployment rate is 9.5%, with the unemployment rate for youth ages 15–24 standing at 15.8% for males and 33.4% for females in 2004. While women are disadvantaged by unequal political, social, and economic opportunities, males have poorer school performance and are more frequently involved in negative social and economic activities.

In 2000, the national average school attendance of children was 77.5%, ranging from a high of 80.9% for Paramaribo District to a low of 51.7% for Sipaliwini District in the interior. Low teacher salaries have led to a shortage of trained teachers in the schools, limiting access to a quality education. The overall literacy rate of the population age 15 years and older is 86%; the highest rate (92%) is found among the population aged 15–34. Literacy rates decline with age, dropping to 63% for the population age 65 years old and older. Differences in literacy between sexes increase with age, with an equal gender distribution in the age group 15–24 years, but with a difference of 19.3% higher for males than females at aged 65 and older. Overall literacy is 93% in urban areas (94% for males, 92% for females), 87% in the rural districts (89% for males and 85% for females), and 51% in the interior (66% for males and 44% for females) (9).

Despite institutionalized programs of the Government and initiatives promoted by nongovernmental organizations (NGOs), gender disparities persist. The proportion of seats held by women in National Parliament is 20% (10), and in general there are nearly twice as many men as women holding decision-making positions and other types of high level employment. Women's advancement in the academic world is not reflected in the levels of their participation in the nonpolitical public sector or private enterprise.

Violence against children and women is a major political and public health issue. In the first half of 2005, there were 139 cases of child sexual abuse and 59 cases of cruelty to children reported to police. Children of Creole and Maroon descent represent two-thirds of these cases. There is no formal national registration system for domestic violence. Suriname is both a transit and destination country for human trafficking, especially for the purpose of sexual exploitation such as commercial sex work in the mining camps in the country's interior (1).

Policies and legal frameworks to ensure rights-based, sustainable human development are inadequate, obsolete, or absent, as is the systemic response to violence, particularly against women and children. Also, there are no appropriate measures to ensure equal access to a basic education and health and other social services that would thereby target social investments to those most in need and empower communities with multiple disadvantages. There is also a lack of data collection that would more clearly reveal the disparities and provide the evidence base for policy development and management.

The health sector in Suriname is currently confronted with a series of serious obstacles. These result from macroeconomic problems, the emigration of qualified personnel to other countries, shortages of essential drugs, physical deterioration of health services infrastructure, and health care deficiencies, particularly at the secondary level.

There is inequitable access to water and sanitation services. For every urban dweller without water service, there are two inhabitants in the country's interior without this service. The distribution of sanitation services is even more inequitable: for every one urban dweller without these services, there are four rural dwellers and 17 dwellers in the interior without access to them. The distribution patterns for drinking water quantity and quality are similar. Mercury pollution from small-scale gold mining activities in the interior, excessive pesticide use on agricultural lands in rural coastal areas, and the widespread practice of dumping sewage into street ditches and canals all pose a serious threat to drinking water quality. The only treatment for urban public water supplies consists of aeration and rapid filtration to remove iron and manganese. In the interior, piped drinking water is often sourced from rivers and distributed untreated. The distribution systems are compromised because of poor maintenance, water theft, and leakages, resulting in pump breakdowns, low pressure, intermittent supply, and high potential for contamination.

Surface water quality in urban as well as rural areas is under severe stress due to poor sanitary practices, a high groundwater table, and industrial and mining activities. The aquifer providing water to the population of Paramaribo is expected to be depleted in 15 to 20 years. The situation in the interior is considerably worse than in other regions. Improvements of the water system are under way that are expected to increase water service capacity to approximately 5,680 m^3 per hour, while the demand when the improvements are complete is projected to be 4,430 m^3 per hour.

Littering by the general public contributes to flooding during rainy periods. Polyethylene terephthalate (PET) bottles, household garbage, and even semi-industrial refuse are often thrown into ditches and canals, resulting in massive blockages of sewer and drainage systems.

Demographics, Mortality and Morbidity

According to the 2004 census (*11*), the total population of Suriname was 492,829 (50.3% men and 49.7% women), a small population for the country's geographical size. The ethnic composition is as follows: 27.4% Hindustani, 17.7% Creole, 14.7% Maroon, 14.6% Javanese, 12.5% mixed, 3.7% Amerindian, 1.8% Chinese, 0.6% Caucasian, and 7.2% other/not reported. The principal religions are Christianity (40.7%), Hinduism (19.9%), and Islam (13.5%).

In 1980, the population was 355,240 (*11*). With an absolute growth of 137,589, the population has grown by 38.7% in 24 years. The male-to-female ratio both in 1980 and 2004 was 1:1. In 2004, 10.5% of the population (51,837) was under age 5 and 39% was under age 20. The number of Maroons has more than doubled, from 35,838 in 1972 to 72,553 in 2005. The overall annual growth rate remained at 0.9% (*12*), based on the natural positive growth of the population (6,618 persons in 2001 and 5,773 persons in 2004), with a consistent negative growth migration balance between 2001 and 2004. The population structure of Suriname in 1990 and 2005, by age and sex, is presented in Figure 1.

Ninety-five percent of all births are registered (*9*). The total annual number of births ranged from 9,052 to 10,188 for the 2001–2004 period. Crude birth rates ranged from 19.4 to 22.3 births per 1,000 population annually during that same time. An ongoing problem exists regarding the underreporting of live births due to legal regulations of the Surinamese Civil Code, resulting in less accurate estimates of the infant and perinatal death rates (*13*).

Approximately 85% of all deaths that are registered on the Civil Registry are certified. The total number of registered deaths showed a minor increase from 3,099 in 2001 to 3,319 in 2004.

Crude death rates remained stable at approximately seven deaths per 1,000 population between 2001 and 2004. Life expectancy at birth was 69.7 years in 2005 (66.6 years for males and 73.0 for females). The total fertility rate was an average of 2.0 births per woman in 2004.

Officially registered external migration figures are 2.5 times higher than immigration figures. Immigrants arrived mainly from the Netherlands, China, Guyana, and French Guiana (63%, 13%, 6%, and 4%, respectively, in 2004). As the vast borders of rainforest do not permit reliable controls, there is also a considerable amount of illegal immigration from these countries. Emigration is also underreported. The principal destination country for external migration is the Netherlands; others included the Netherlands Antilles, French Guiana, and the United States (60%, 18%, 12%, and 4%, respectively, in 2004). Internal migration rates have remained fairly stable, with major migration to urban areas.

Table 1 presents the 10 leading causes of mortality in Suriname in rank order for 2004, based on 85% of certified deaths.

Between 2001 and 2004, the largest proportion of deaths occurred between the ages of 65 and 79 years, representing an average of 32% of all deaths. During this time period, the percentage

FIGURE 1. Population structure, by age and sex, Suriname, 1990 and 2005.

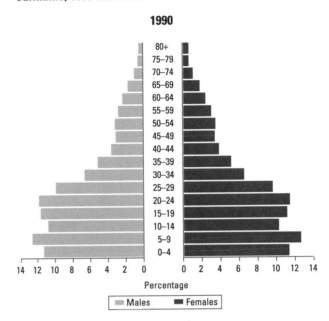

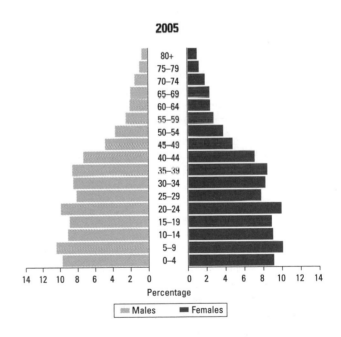

of deaths by gender remained constant at 57% for males and 43% for females (*3*). Until age 25, there is an almost equal percentage of mortality between the sexes. Between 25 and 39 years of age, the number of deaths among males is 2.5 times higher than among females. The principal cause of death for the population aged 1–29 years is external causes; for the 30–39-year-old age group, it is AIDS, and after age 40, it is cardiovascular diseases.

TABLE 1. Number of deaths, proportional mortality, and rates for leading causes of mortality, Suriname, 2004.

Rank	Disease category	Number	% total[a]	Cumulative %	Rate[b]
1	Cerebrovascular diseases	456	15.8	15.8	92.5
2	Certain conditions originating in the perinatal period	244	8.5	24.3	49.5
3	Ischemic heart diseases	209	7.3	31.6	42.4
4	HIV disease	152	5.3	36.8	30.8
5	Diabetes mellitus	133	4.6	41.4	27.0
6	Events of undetermined intent	111	3.9	45.3	22.5
7	Heart failure and complications	67	2.3	47.6	13.6
8	Intentional self-harm (suicide)	65	2.3	49.9	13.2
9	Neoplasms of the uterus	31	1.1	51.0	12.7
10	Neoplasms of the prostate	30	1.0	52.0	12.1

[a]Total deaths defined by cause.
[b]Rate per 100,000 population.

External causes remain the principal cause of mortality among males until age 29, while for females external causes remain the principal cause until age 25. AIDS becomes the principal cause of death among females from the age of 25 to 39. For males in this age group, AIDS is the second leading cause, although the number of deaths caused by AIDS is 2.4 times higher among men. For the group aged 50 years and older, cardiovascular diseases ranked first, followed by malignant neoplasms.

In 2003, 68.1% of all deaths occurred among the 25–44-year-old age group. In 2004, this percentage declined to 53.4%, while for the 45–49-year-old age group, the percentage doubled from 8% in 2003 to 16.5% in 2004.

Among malignant neoplasms, those of the digestive organs ranked highest, accounting for 17.2% of all malignant neoplasms, followed by those of the cervix (9.8%), lung (6.1%), prostate (12.1%), and breast (9.0%). When considering malignant neoplasms of the reproductive organs as a whole, in 2004 these comprised 22.5% of all malignant neoplasms among females and 12.1% among males.

Mortality due to diabetes mellitus accounted for 5% of the 10 leading causes of death in 2004. Forty-eight percent of all deaths due to diabetes mellitus that year occurred among the population of Hindustani descent, and 35% of all deaths due to cardiovascular diseases were among this population group. Thirty-one percent of all cardiovascular deaths were among those of Creole descent, as were 25% of all deaths due to diabetes mellitus. The populations of Creole and Maroon descent accounted for 57% and 21%, respectively, of all HIV/AIDS-related deaths.

HEALTH OF POPULATION GROUPS

Children under 5 Years Old

According to the 2004 census, there were 9,872 children under 1 year of age, making up 2% of the total population. The number of live births was 9,717 in 2001 and 9,062 in 2004. Approximately 90% of all births were attended by skilled health personnel, with the remaining 10% by traditional birth attendants in the interior. Of those births attended by skilled health personnel, about 90% occurred in hospitals and 10% in primary health care facilities. The number of stillbirths increased from 202 in 2001 to 243 in 2004. Most stillbirths are due to conditions originating in the perinatal period (48%), followed by obstetric complications (22%), short gestation and low birthweight (15%), complications of diseases of the mother (9%), and congenital malformations (4%). Although virtually all pregnant women receive some type of prenatal care and 91% of all pregnant women visit the prenatal clinics at least once (9), nearly 20% of these women do not have their first visit until the second trimester of their pregnancy.

The infant mortality rate averaged 19 deaths per 1,000 live births during the 2000–2004 period, but dropped as low as 16 deaths per 1,000 live births in 2001. During the years 1990 to 1994, the infant mortality rate was consistently around 21 deaths per 1,000 live births. The number of deaths in the under-1-year-old group increased from 154 in 2001 to 174 in 2004. Major causes of death in this group were intestinal infections, followed by respiratory diseases and congenital malformations. The perinatal mortality rate increased from 29.2 deaths per 1,000 deliveries in 2001 to 39.3 in 2004. There was also a noticeable increase in the early neonatal mortality rate from 9.2 deaths per 1,000 live births in 2001 to 13.6 in 2004. The late neonatal mortality rate was 1.6 deaths per 1,000 live births in 2001 and 1.1 in 2004. The postneonatal mortality rate was 5.0 deaths per 1,000 live births in 2001 and 4.5 in 2004. Most early neonatal deaths are due to complications of short gestation and low birthweight (47%), followed by intrauterine hypoxia and asphyxia (17%), complications of diseases of the mother (16%), congenital malformations (9%), and obstetric complications (6%). Only 13% of children under 4 months of age are exclusively breast-fed.

The major causes of death in children 1 to 4 years old were gastrointestinal infections, followed by respiratory infections and external causes.

About 13.0% of children under age 5 in Suriname are underweight, and 2.1% are severely underweight. Approximately 10% of children are stunted, and 6.5% are wasted. There are noticeable differences between the prevalence of malnutrition in urban, rural, and interior areas. Children in the interior are the group most at risk for chronic malnutrition. The disparity is mainly related to the geographical inaccessibility of the country's interior; many parts are reachable only via air or water, creating formidable obstacles for the availability and distribution of goods and services. More than half of the children hospitalized due to malnutrition are under age 1. Seventy-five percent of children ages 1–4 who are hospitalized for malnutrition are of Maroon and Creole descent. The majority of hospitalized children, equally boys and girls, are from Paramaribo South, an area known for its socially deprived living conditions and the migration of families from the interior, and from the interior Sipaliwini and Brokopondo districts (14).

The marked differences in living conditions found in the interior and the urban and rural regions are also reflected in child morbidity data. Clinic visits in the interior show that children aged 0–4 are the most frequently returning visitors (61%); the most frequently treated conditions among this age group are respiratory infections (59.9%), diarrhea (23.1%), and malaria (15%).

Malaria is a common cause of school absenteeism and one of the leading causes of mortality in the 0–5-year-old age group. Preventive measures, especially the use of mosquito nets treated with insecticide, continue to be implemented. Insecticide-impregnated mosquito nets are used by 72% of children between the ages of 0 and 4 when sleeping. Poor sanitary conditions and personal hygiene practices, as well as limited access to safe water sources, especially during dry season, are the leading contributors to the high incidence of diarrhea in Suriname's interior. The Suriname Multiple Indicator Cluster Survey (MICS) study conducted in 2000 (9) revealed that only 24.2% of children with diarrhea received oral rehydration therapy. In many cases, medical attendance is sought too late, resulting in preventable deaths.

Children 5–9 Years Old

According to the 2004 census, the population 5 to 9 years of age totaled 49,409 persons, representing 10% of the total population. The principal causes of death in this age group are external causes, cardiovascular diseases, and intestinal infections. All schoolchildren are required to have a vaccination card in order to enter elementary school, usually at the age of 6 years.

Adolescents 10–14 and 15–19 Years Old

According to the 2004 census, the population segment ages 10 to 14 years consisted of 45,143 persons, or 9.1% of the total pop-

ulation. Leading causes of death in this age group are external causes, followed by malignant neoplasms and cardiovascular diseases. In 2002, the average number of decayed, missing, or filled teeth at age 12 was 2.7.

The population aged 15 to 19 years in 2004 was 46,508 persons, or 9.4% of the total population. The leading cause of death in this age group is external causes. From 2002 to 2004, there were three deaths due to HIV/AIDS each year among this group.

The establishment of reproductive health services targeted to adolescents is a priority need. For the 2001–2004 period, an average of 16.7% of the total live births were to mothers between 15 and 17 years of age; 4.3% of all live births were to girls between the ages of 10 and 14. Most of these occurred in the Paramaribo and Wanica districts.

The prevalence of tobacco consumption among the population ages 13 to 15 years was 11% for girls and 20% for boys in 2004 (15).

Adults 20–59 Years Old

According to the 2004 census, the adult population between the ages of 20 and 59 stood at 253,039 persons, representing 51.3% of the total population. Within this broad age group, external causes are the leading cause of death, followed by HIV/AIDS, cardiovascular diseases, and neoplasms. Beginning at age 40, diabetes makes its first appearance on the list of the 10 leading causes of mortality; cardiovascular diseases also grow in importance as external causes descend in the rankings.

Maternal mortality decreased from 15 deaths in 2001 to 8 in 2004. The main causes of maternal death during 2001–2004 were hemorrhage (31%), preeclampsia (29%), and sepsis (17%); in most cases the health facility was lacking the necessary supplies for a timely response to the complication (16). The cesarean section rate for 2001 was 12.7%, and for 2002 it was 13.3%. Abortion is illegal but widely practiced, particularly by women under the age of 24. Estimates of 8,000–10,000 abortions performed annually are based in part on sample surveys among adolescents (17). These outcomes indicate an unmet need in family planning. Abortions are performed upon request and are generally socially tolerated. The illegality yet tolerance for and frequent use of abortion are the result of a lack of official mechanisms and/or structures to regulate abortion practices and further increase the risks for unsafe practices and financial obstacles, particularly among poor women with a higher risk of unwanted pregnancies and more barriers to education (18).

The mortality rate due to external causes was 62 per 100,000 population in 2004. Of all external causes, events of undetermined intent had the highest percentage (23%), followed by intentional self-harm (13%). The 20–49-year-old age group accounted for nearly 55% of all deaths due to these causes (75% males and 25% females).

Older Adults 60 Years Old and Older

According to the 2004 census, the population segment aged 60 and older consisted of 42,060 persons, or 8.5% of the total population. The leading causes of death in this age group are cerebrovascular and cardiovascular diseases, followed by malignant neoplasms, diabetes mellitus, external causes, acute respiratory infections, and chronic lower respiratory infections.

The Family

An estimated 40% of all households consist of three to four members, with 62.2% of children living with both parents, 22% living with their mother only although their father is alive, and 7% living with neither parent although both are alive (9). The family structure in the interior is quite different from that found in urban and rural areas along the coast: less than 50% of children live with both parents, 34% live with their mother, and 12% live with neither parent. Cultural standards and expectations dominate decisions with regard to reproductive health issues in the interior. Generally, contraceptive use in rural areas and the interior is low, because producing children in these regions is highly valued. Contraceptive use among Maroon women is low (between 6% and 17%). On average, Maroon boys become sexually active between the ages of 10 and 13 and girls initiate sexual experiences between the ages of 13 and 15 (19).

The oral contraceptive pill is the most popular method of birth control, with 70% of couples practicing contraception choosing the pill. Past studies have found that around 40% of women with a partner use contraceptives (20). According to the 2000 MICS study, contraceptive use in urban areas was 51%, while in the coastal rural areas it was 45%, and in the interior it was 7.1% (9).

Workers

A rapid assessment of child labor conducted in 2002 by the International Labor Organization (21) indicates that 2% of all children between the ages of 4 and 14 years were economically active. Fifty-four percent of children in this group worked more than 15 hours a week and were involved in activities related to fishing, vending, agriculture, gold digging, construction, and boat transport. Some children, especially females, were involved in domestic work and trade (described in the study as "vending a variety of products"). None of the children interviewed reported being involved in commercial sexual activity, the production or sale of illicit drugs, or any form of human trafficking. However, the study notes sporadic reports by NGOs of children being involved in prostitution and becoming victims of sexual exploitation. There were no specific findings to suggest that children were exposed to violence in their work environment, although health concerns were raised related to their exposure to sand, dust, and mercury vapor and the carrying of heavy loads.

There are an increasing number of non-Surinamese workers in the gold mining and other natural exploitation sectors in the interior, including an estimated 30,000 *garimpeiros* (gold diggers from Brazil). Mercury poisoning and malaria and sylvatic yellow fever transmission, as well as HIV/AIDS and other sexually transmitted infections, are serious health threats for miners and local communities. Additionally, traditional community life has undergone sociocultural disruption due to the commercial sex industry, the gold economy, drug use and related crime, and degradation of the natural environment.

Border Groups

The border population along the eastern border, consisting mainly of Maroons, has frequent interaction with the population living in French Guiana across the Marowijne River. It is not uncommon for groups belonging to the same family to be living on both sides of the border, separated only by the river. Women on the Surinamese side prefer to deliver their children in French Guiana because health care there is perceived to be of higher quality. At the northwestern border with Guyana in Nickerie District, as with the French Guiana–Suriname border, related families often live on both sides of the Corentyne River and often cross over. However, the influx of Guyanese nationals into Suriname is much larger than that of French Guianese nationals.

HEALTH CONDITIONS AND PROBLEMS

COMMUNICABLE DISEASES

Vector-borne Diseases

The two most prominent communicable diseases are **dengue** in the coastal area and **malaria** in the interior. Morbidity data on dengue come principally from hospital surveillance. Suspected cases of dengue are also reported by telephone surveillance. The number of suspected cases decreased from 516 in 2001 (of which 64 cases were confirmed) to 309 suspected cases in 2004 (of which 56 were confirmed). As of 2001, dengue serology studies isolated all 4 subtypes. From 2001 to 2004, most hospitalized suspected cases of dengue were among individuals of Hindustani descent (30%), followed by those of Creole (20%) and Javanese descent (15%). The majority of cases came from the densely populated areas of Paramaribo and Wanica, and from less-populated Saramacca. Incidence was equally distributed among the various age groups. The male-to-female ratio of reported cases of dengue was 1:2.

Malaria is an important public health problem in Suriname's interior, where the natural habitat of the vector, *Anopheles darlingi*, is found. In 2000, 13,216 cases of malaria were reported. After the introduction of new treatment policies in 2004, case numbers declined to 8,560 in 2004 and 9,000 (preliminary estimate) in 2005. Half of the new cases of malaria occurred in children under the age of 15 years. No transmission in the coastal area has been reported. Incidence is highest in the Suriname–French Guiana border area along the Marowijne River. Gold mining activities by Brazilian *garimpeiros* and frequent border-crossings by the population have contributed to the increase of malaria in that area. Gold mining activities have spread to new areas in the interior as well, leading to the emergence of malaria in regions where previous transmission seldom occurred. The incidence rate of malaria per 100,000 population was estimated at 3,500 in 2001 and 1,700 in 2004. The national incidence is most probably higher. There is underreporting due to patients receiving clinical treatment without laboratory confirmation and non-reporting by private physicians and traditional medicine practitioners. The number of hospitalized suspected malaria cases was 436 in 2001, with 50% of the cases being confirmed, and 248 in 2004, with 65% being confirmed. Of these confirmed cases, death occurred in 21 cases, or 9.7% in 2001, and 8 cases, or 4.9% in 2004. The male-to-female ratio of hospitalization was 1:2.1 in 2001 and 1:2.5 in 2004.

Chloroquine-resistant malaria due to *Plasmodium falciparum* is widespread, but quinine resistance has not yet been established. In 2003, Suriname introduced malaria treatment with Coartem, resulting in a less severe course of the disease and a decrease in the mortality rate. For several years now, the use of bed nets has been promoted throughout the interior. They are produced, treated with insecticide, and distributed by local women's groups.

Yellow fever has not been reported in Suriname over the past decades. But in view of the disease's reemergence on the South American continent, vaccination activities for yellow fever have been intensified. The mass yellow fever vaccination campaign that started in 2000 was finalized in 2002. Persons traveling to Brazil and French Guiana are vaccinated for yellow fever regularly, as this is mandatory for these countries. Yellow fever serology tests yielded a negative result for six suspected cases in 2003 and four in 2004.

Vaccine-preventable Diseases

During the review period there were five reported **tetanus** cases (excluding neonatal tetanus): two cases each in 2001 and 2002, and one in 2003. There were no reported cases of **measles**, **diphtheria**, or **congenital rubella syndrome** between 2001 and 2005.

The geographic disparities between the urban, rural, and interior regions are also reflected in the immunization status of children. The frequent movement of migrant groups between the interior and Paramaribo and between Suriname and French Guiana places an additional burden on monitoring the vaccination status of children in these groups.

National coverage increased from 82% for measles, mumps, and rubella vaccine (MMR); 68% for the final dose of diphtheria, pertussis, and tetanus vaccine (DPT3); and 65% for three doses of the live oral poliovirus (OPV3) in 2001 to 86.4% for MMR, 84.9% for DPT3, and 83.5% for OPV3 in 2004. In 2005, Suriname introduced the pentavalent vaccine (diphtheria, pertussis, tetanus, hepatitis B, and *Haemophilus influenzae* type B) in the national vaccination schedule for infants. Routine tetanus vaccination of pregnant women was also initiated in 2005, together with yellow fever vaccination for children ages 12–23 months who live in the country's interior.

Intestinal Infectious Diseases

The number of laboratory-confirmed *salmonella* **infections** was 48 cases in 2001 and 104 in 2004. Of these cases, 7 persons (15%) died in 2001, and 14 persons (13%) died in 2004. Children under age 5 (and especially those under age 1) represent the highest percentage of deaths due to *salmonella* infection. Adults aged 60 and older are the group most frequently hospitalized for diarrheal diseases. Creoles had the highest laboratory-confirmed incidence of *salmonella* infection in 2001 and 2003 among ethnic groups, while Hindustanis had the highest incidence in 2002 and 2004. The number of laboratory-confirmed *shigella* **infections** increased from 91 cases in 2001 to 114 cases in 2003, then dropped to 92 cases in 2004. Of the 398 cases of laboratory-confirmed shigellosis during the 2001–2004 period, 7.3% died. Of those who died, 41% were 60 years old or older and 38% were younger than 5 years.

Between 2001 and 2004, there were 25 foodborne outbreaks. In two of these outbreaks *salmonella* infection was laboratory-confirmed, in another outbreak *shigella* infection was laboratory-confirmed, while in the rest, laboratory analyses were unable to identify the responsible microorganism.

Chronic Communicable Diseases

Between 2001 and 2004, the annual incidence of leprosy averaged 1.1 new cases per 10,000 population. The number of new cases of **tuberculosis** (TB) ranged from 80 to 101 annually between 2001 and 2004, equal to annual incidence rates ranging from 18 to 21 new cases per 100,000 population. Pulmonary or respiratory TB is the most frequent type reported, comprising 84% of all TB cases. The indigenous population experienced the highest TB incidence rate.

HIV/TB coinfection ranged from nine out of 80 new TB cases, or 11% of all new TB cases in 2001, to 17 coinfections out of 101 new TB cases, or 17%, in 2004. By far the highest HIV/TB coinfection rate was among the 25–44-year-old age group. Sixty-six percent of treatment outcomes for TB were successful. The Directly Observed Treatment, Short Course (DOTS) strategy has not yet been adopted.

HIV/AIDS and Other Sexually Transmitted Infections

The first case of HIV/AIDS was reported in Suriname in 1983; by 2004 the cumulative number of reported HIV/AIDS cases was 3,032. Newly reported HIV-positive tested cases increased from 255 in 2001 to 524 in 2004. Since 2003, HIV testing has been included in routine prenatal care.

In 2001, persons who were tested for HIV in the 30–34-year-old age group had the highest count of first-time HIV-positive tests of any five-year age group, with 19 positives. In 2002 and 2004, those who were tested for HIV in the 34–39-year-old age group had the highest count of first-time HIV-positive tests of any five-year age group, with 37 and 41 positives, respectively. In 2003, the highest counts of HIV-positive tests occurred among the 20–24-year-old age group, with 42 positives. In 2004, there were 28 HIV-positive tests among children in the 0–4-year-old age group.

In 2005, the HIV prevalence rate among the population aged 15–49 years was estimated at 1.9% (22). In the same year, 610 persons testing HIV-positive for the first time were reported. The gender distribution of new HIV-positive tested cases has shifted from more males than females prior to 2004 to more females than males since 2004 (18). Of newly reported HIV-positive cases, 60% to 80% are between the ages of 15 and 49 years. Transmission of HIV occurs principally through heterosexual contacts. In 2005, there was one case of HIV-positive transmission through donated blood. Prevention of mother-to-child-transmission services began in 2003. Each year there are approximately 10,000 pregnancies, and in 2005 almost 70% of all pregnant women were screened. Between 2001 and 2004, a total of 2,456 persons with suspected HIV/AIDS cases were hospitalized; of these 1,400 (57%) were confirmed as being HIV-positive.

The increase of HIV-positive cases with a coinfection of *salmonella* also contributes to the overall increase of salmonellosis and the increase of death due to HIV and *salmonella* coinfection.

In 2001, 14% of deaths due to *salmonella* infections occurred among individuals who were HIV-positive; in 2004, 50% of *salmonella* infection-related deaths were among individuals with HIV-positive status. There has also been an annual increase in the number of shigellosis patients with HIV-positive status, but coinfectivity with *shigella* has led to a lower case fatality than *salmonella*-HIV coinfections.

Zoonoses

No cases of **plague** and **human rabies** were reported during the 2001–2005 review period.

The incidence of **leptospirosis** can be linked to the incidence of rainfall, with the majority of cases occurring during the rainy season (May to August) and in the country's most densely populated districts. From 2001 to 2004, the average number of hospitalized suspected leptospirosis cases was 149.5 per year, or 12.5 per month, and the average number of confirmed leptospirosis cases was 13.8 per year, or one per month. The male-to-female ratio for hospitalization for leptospirosis is 1:1.95, with the Hindustani and Creole population groups being the ones most frequently hospitalized for this disease.

Meningitis

During the reporting period, the number of hospitalizations for meningitis was 69 cases in 2001 and 72 cases in 2004. The reported incidence rate was 15.2 new cases of hospitalized meningitis per 100,000 population in 2001 and 14.6 per 100,000 population in 2004. The male-to-female ratio for cases of hospitalizations for meningitis was 1:2.1 in 2001 and 1:2.3 in 2004. Fifty-five percent of all cases of hospitalized meningitis were among children under age 5, with the greatest proportion of these under-5 cases being younger than 1 year of age.

NONCOMMUNICABLE DISEASES

Metabolic and Nutritional Diseases

Counts of hospitalizations for malnutrition were 138 in 2001 and 125 in 2004. Of these cases, six (4.4%) resulted in death in 2001, and 11 (8.8%) died in 2004. Children aged 0–4 years accounted for 96% of hospitalizations. The male-to-female ratio was 1:1. Maroons and Creoles were the ethnic groups most frequently hospitalized for malnutrition, followed by those of Amerindian and mixed descent.

Cardiovascular Diseases

Recent studies show that approximately 50% of all persons aged 60 years or older suffer from a chronic disease. The leading condition is hypertensive diseases, followed by diabetes mellitus and a combination of both conditions.

Diseases of the circulatory system, including cardiovascular, hypertensive, and cerebrovascular diseases, have held their position as the leading cause of mortality for a number of years; during the 2001–2004 period, they accounted for 29% of all deaths in Suriname.

Malignant Neoplasms

The highest mortality rates due to neoplasms were caused by neoplasms of the uterus for females, with a rate of 12.7 deaths per 100,000 females, and neoplasms of the prostate for males, with a rate of 12.1 deaths per 100,000 males.

OTHER HEALTH PROBLEMS OR ISSUES

Disasters

Suriname did not experience any major natural disaster during the 2001–2005 period.

Environmental Pollution

The impact of gold mining activities in Suriname's interior, including persistent mercury contamination of the soil, water, and air, as well as other disturbances to the terrestrial and aquatic ecosystems, are recognized by environment authorities as being substantial and difficult to reverse (23).

RESPONSE OF THE HEALTH SYSTEM

Health Policies and Plans

The health sector occupies a key position in the Suriname Government's overall social program. Article 36 of the national Constitution (24) specifies that health is the right of every citizen and that the Government's role is to promote general health care through systematic improvement of living and work conditions and the provision of information to protect health. Availability of and accessibility to health care for the entire population is therefore of crucial importance.

The first phase (1998–2003) of the project "Support for Health Sector Reform" consisted of a series of studies on health sector supply and demand, with the goal of introducing a sector-wide approach as part of the national macroeconomic development strategy. Based on the results, in May 2004, the Sector Plan for Health Care 2004–2008 was approved by the President's Cabinet of Ministers and implementation began. The second phase embodies the principles of efficiency, equity, and quality and focuses on the improvement of primary health care performance, increased access to medicines, and strengthening of the Ministry of Health. The strategies over the 2004–2008 period are: (1) strengthening primary health care and prevention, (2) improving hospital care efficiency and quality, (3) promoting financial access to health care, (4) controlling health care costs, (5) strengthening health support systems, (6) human resources development, and (7) improving and safeguarding quality throughout the health system.

With its stated goal as being "to achieve an integrated and sustainable health care system of good quality and effectiveness, accessible for everyone, and a continuous improvement of health for the whole population," the Plan serves as a guiding document in the development of the national health system. Within this context, the 2004 census provides crucial data and information for assessing the population health status and providing input for health planning over the four-year period.

Suriname signed the Stockholm Convention on Persistent Organic Pollutants (POPs) in 2002, but had already started banning the use of POPs, particularly polychlorinated biphenyls, as long ago as 1971. At present, there is no national policy to ensure the environmentally sound management of persistent toxic substances and wastes. There is little awareness on the part of the private sector and general public of the dangers posed by the un-safe use and disposal of chemicals, whether household, automotive, or industrial.

Health Strategies and Programs

The Government priority of poverty reduction has been translated into several programs managed by the Ministry of Social Affairs and Housing. One target group is the elderly. Various provisions have been implemented that especially support older adults living in poverty, including a subsidy to long-term living facilities, financial support to the needy to cover the cost of living, free medical services to the poor and near-poor, and monthly payments to those with a free medical service card.

The Ministry of Social Affairs and Housing is the institution responsible for certifying those living in poverty or near-poverty and ensuring that the economically disadvantaged population has access to subsidized health care. Approximately 30% of the population qualifies for government-subsidized health care services that are mostly provided by government hospitals and clinics.

Organization of the Health System

The principal tasks of the Ministry of Health are policy-making, evaluation, coordination, setting of standards and protocols, and quality assurance, with overall responsibility for ensuring the availability, accessibility, and affordability of health care.

The health care system's core institutions are the Ministry of Health's Central Office, the Bureau of Public Health, and the Inspectorate. The Central Office and the Inspectorate function at the level of global health planning and standard-setting, inspection, and monitoring, while the Bureau of Public Health is responsible for program development.

The public providers of primary health care are the Regional Health Services (RGD), a state foundation, and the Medical Mission (MM), an NGO. Both institutions are subsidized by the Government. The RGD provides services to the poor and near-poor in the coastal area through 50 clinics, serving approximately 100,000 patients of generally lower socioeconomic means. The MM provides curative and preventive health services to the interior Maroon and Amerindian population through 50 health centers and health posts, serving around 50,000 patients.

The Government also runs vertical programs targeting special populations or conditions, such as sexually transmitted infections, leprosy, youth dental care, malaria, and immunizations.

The private providers of primary health care are the general practitioners (GPs) and some NGOs permitted by the Government to provide specific health care services, such as the Foundation for Family Planning (*Stichting Lobi*), an affiliate of the International Planned Parenthood Federation specializing in reproductive health issues. Large private-sector firms provide health care for their employees and families through their own clinics. Secondary care is provided through five general hospitals, all located in the coastal area. There are three public and two private hospitals and one psychiatric center. The private Diakonessen Hospital, through an agreement with the MM, provides care to patients from the interior.

Medical specialists provide both outpatient and inpatient care. Private physicians are highly centralized in the capital. Secondary care is likewise centralized, since four of the general hospitals and the psychiatric center are located in the capital and one in the rural coastal district of Nickerie.

The contribution of the private sector is at the level of service provider; the majority of its activities are curative, while the government-subsidized RGD and MM provide both preventive and curative health care services. Private participation in the health system is also through larger companies, which employ their own general practitioners. Others have a list of contracted general practitioners from which the employee may select one. Consultation of GPs is required for referral to a specialist or hospital.

Health care is financed through public and private sources: the Government provides the largest share (44%), followed by households (20%), donors (18%), and companies (2%). Distribution of these payments by level of care is primary health care (34%), secondary care (55%), and other (11%).

Approximately 315,000 persons (64% of the total population) are covered by health insurance; another 177,000 persons (36%) are not insured, or do not know if they are.

The distribution of health insurance coverage includes the State Health Insurance Fund, known as SZF (21%), the Ministry of Social Affairs and Housing (24%), the Medical Mission (6%), company medical plans (10%), private health insurance companies (3%), out-of-pocket (19%), other (1%), and no insurance/not known (16%).

Public Health Services

Control of vaccine-preventable diseases is coordinated by the Bureau of Public Health's National Immunization Program that collaborates with the Epidemiology Unit in case investigations.

The RGD's school health program includes growth development monitoring, visual screening, and vaccination of all primary-level schoolchildren in the coastal area. Cases of suspected health problems or special conditions are referred to a physician. The Bureau of Public Health's health education department provides public health information related to the prevention of communicable diseases and the promotion of breast-feeding practices and healthy lifestyles.

Malaria control activities are supervised by the Malaria Board, which developed a multisectoral Roll Back Malaria strategy supported by international donors. Vector control activities, including spraying and promotion of the use of bed nets treated with insecticide, are carried out by the Bureau of Public Health and MM.

The Ministry of Health's National Health Information System (NHIS) Unit is responsible for official national health data. Most of the health information reaches the NHIS Unit through hospital registrations and reports of the Bureau of Public Health, RGD, MM, and professional health associations.

Communicable diseases surveillance is conducted through weekly hospital and sentinel surveillance, and, occasionally, through physicians and outbreak reporting. Hospital surveillance focuses on dengue, leptospirosis, shigellosis, *salmonella* infection, and malnutrition, while the telephone sentinel system reports on gastroenteritis, rash and fever, upper respiratory tract infections, and sexually transmitted diseases. Serotyping is done at the Ministry of Health's Central Laboratory. Data on malignant neoplasms is provided by the Pathology Laboratory.

The Bureau of Public Health's Epidemiology Unit also requests data for known communicable diseases of public health importance from such institutions as the Dermatology Clinic, the TB Clinic, and the National Blood Bank, and presents this information on a regular basis to the Caribbean Epidemiology Center (CAREC). Currently, there is no noncommunicable diseases surveillance system in the country.

Suriname's environmental institutional framework is based on three entities utilizing intersectoral coordinating mechanisms. The National Environmental Council (*Nationale Milieuraad*) is a policy-making body in the Office of the President. It is charged with developing overall environmental policies for the President's consideration, as well as advising and guiding the National Institute for the Environment and Development in Suriname (*Nationaal Instituut voor Milieu en Ontwikkeling*, or NIMOS) in setting priorities for environmental action. NIMOS functions as the Council's operational arm. NIMOS and the Council work together with the Inter-ministerial Advisory Commission (IMAC), which disseminates environmental information among other key government ministries and sectors with responsibilities and activities in this area.

Regulations to control the quality of the environment have been mandated to NIMOS, while the Bureau of Public Health oversees environmental health quality control activities.

Approximately 73% of the population has access to safe drinking water: 92.6% in urban areas, 66.6% in coastal rural areas, and 20% in the interior (9). Coverage of piped water supply varies significantly by region. Ninety-one percent of the urban population uses drinking water that is piped into their dwelling or yard. In the rural areas, 65% use piped water, whereas in the interior only 18% have access to this type of source. In rural areas, the second-most important source of drinking water is rainwater, while in the interior some 60% of residents use river or stream water and the rest collect rainwater. Drinking water is provided by two state-owned water suppliers. Five private companies provide drinking water to village populations near their operations. The piped water is treated and thus potable.

Addressing Inequities in the Interior

One in ten Surinamese, most of them indigenous peoples and Maroons (descendants of African slaves), live in the country's interior. A lack of electricity, difficulties in transportation, and scanty communications infrastructure make it difficult to supply goods and services to those living in this inaccessible region. Grievous inequities in terms of socio-economic development, health status, and access to health care exist between the inhabitants of the interior and those living on the coast, including:

- only 18% of households in the interior have piped water in their homes, and only 31% have sanitary excreta disposal services;
- women in the interior are among the poorest groups in the country;
- one in five Maroon deaths are HIV/AIDS-related;
- children there are at the highest risk for chronic malnutrition; and
- fewer than half of all children in the interior live with both their parents and one in eight live with neither parent.

The Ministry of Health, working through the Medical Mission, provides curative and preventive health care services free of charge to residents of the interior, operating 57 health centers and health posts serving some 60,000 people.

Eighty-eight percent of households have sanitary excreta disposal facilities (99.1% in urban areas, 98.3% in coastal rural areas, and 30.5% in the interior). The most common facilities in urban and rural areas are flush toilets connected to a septic tank.

Responsibility for sewage management and wastewater disposal is shared by the Ministry of Public Works' Sewer and Drain Division, the Bureau of Public Health's Environmental Control Division, and the Ministry of Regional Development, which provides logistical support.

The Ministry of Public Works is responsible for collecting and disposing of garbage and other wastes. Indiscriminate dumping sites are very common in Paramaribo and throughout the coastal and rural areas. Since 2002, a medical waste incinerator has served the hospitals in Paramaribo, while clinics in the coastal area and the interior use low-cost drum incinerators.

Limited waste recycling activities are carried out. Polyethylene terephthalate (PET) bottles are recycled, and the shredded materials are added to reinforce bricks used in the construction industry.

The Bureau of Public Health has a mandate to control air quality. Its inspection activities focus on small-scale entrepreneurs such as backyard industries and automotive paint and repair shops. However, inspection technicians require more training in these activities. All gasoline sold in Suriname is lead-free. Multinational mining companies in Suriname adhere, for the most part, to dust emission policies and guidelines set at their corporate headquarters.

The Bureau of Public Health is responsible for food protection and control, including quality analysis through its laboratory, as well as the inspection of restaurants, food processing plants, and public and private sanitary systems, including the disposal of solid waste and sewage. A food safety program, focusing on the development of food handling and processing protocols, is being implemented. Food aid programs for children of low resource households are carried out by the Ministry of Social Affairs and Housing and by NGOs in selected elementary schools in the coastal area.

Although the Labor Inspectorate of the Ministry of Labor, Technology, and the Environment performs occupational health inspections, these are limited to registered entities; economic activities in the informal sector are beyond the scope of these inspections. Recent studies indicate that low radioactive waste handling and storage do not pose significant public health problems.

A draft national disaster plan addressing both natural and human-made disasters has been recently prepared; the health sector has not yet developed its own plan.

In 2001, the completion of the National Strategic Plan on HIV/AIDS and the availability of two grants from the Global Fund to Fight AIDS, Tuberculosis, and Malaria significantly enhanced Suriname's capacity to develop a comprehensive response to HIV/AIDS during the review period. The Plan outlines the targets, strategies, and activities for the 2004–2008 period. Specific targets toward achieving the Millennium Development Goals include a 25% reduction in the number of new HIV infections in the 15–24-year-old age group and a 25% reduction in the number of HIV-positive pregnant women. Measures currently being implemented are the expansion of the prevention of mother-to-child transmission program and intensified prevention programs based on the ABC strategy, which promotes abstinence, faithfulness to partner, and the consistent and correct use of condoms.

651

Condom availability was increased as part of the strategy. Through the "3 by 5" initiative of the World Health Organization and Joint United Nations Program on HIV/AIDS, whose goal was to provide antiretroviral therapy to three million people in developing countries by the end of 2005, 486 individuals in Suriname, or 15%–20% of the estimated total HIV-positive population, received much-needed medications and treatment. In December 2005, the "Know Your Status" campaign was launched to raise public awareness regarding the importance of HIV testing.

Individual Care Services

Inpatient and ambulatory services are provided by all five hospitals in a variety of specialty services. The public Academic Hospital, which is also a training institution, employs the majority of medical specialists and offers nearly all types of specialty care, some of which are exclusively available at this facility, such as open heart surgery, laparoscopic surgery, orthodontic surgery, pulmonology, and ophthalmology.

There are two emergency medical care units, one in Paramaribo and one in a remote district in the west. The Military Hospital functions as an ambulatory facility for army personnel and their families.

In addition to the laboratories at each of the five hospitals, there are three private laboratories (MyLab, Health Control, and Medilab). The laboratories also offer decentralized services through sample-taking sites.

The National Blood Bank, supervised by the Red Cross, operates exclusively through voluntary blood donations. With 4,844 registered blood donors, 70% of the national demand for 7,000 blood donors is covered. The National Blood Bank supplies all blood for open heart surgery sessions at Academic Hospital, which are now performed on a regular basis.

The National Blood Bank supplies blood products to the country's five hospitals and the Foundation for Renal Dialysis. All blood donations are screened for HIV, HTLV, hepatitis B and C, malaria, and syphilis. Quality control mechanisms for the screening of blood donations for HTLV and HIV have been established through collaboration with the Bureau of Public Health's National Reference Laboratory, CAREC, and the U.S. Centers for Disease Control and Prevention.

Special programs for persons with disabilities are under the coordination of the Ministry of Social Affairs and Housing. Several NGOs have programs for special target groups, including the blind, individuals with hearing impairments, former leprosy patients, children with combined physical and mental disabilities, and older adults diagnosed with Alzheimer's disease.

The Rehabilitation Center, as a subdivision of the Academic Hospital in Paramaribo, provides services to referral patients for the construction of artificial limbs, and physical, occupational, and speech therapy. With a staff of 14 paramedics and medical professionals, the Center registers approximately 6,000 patient visits each year. In 2004, the Center opened a special children's unit under the care of a specialized physiotherapist. The 25 children of the school for the handicapped (Mytylschool) have daily access to this unit. The majority received treatment for conditions related to cerebral palsy and muscular dystrophy. The adult patients received treatment principally for conditions related to hemiplegia or amputations.

The Youth Dental Service Foundation is available in the coastal area through dental clinics located in primary schools and RGD clinics with a staff of 70 youth dental care professionals. Children access these services through payment of an annual membership fee. The Foundation also offers private services to adults. After the primary school age, dental care is available only through private firm health insurance or out-of-pocket payment.

The Suriname Psychiatric Center is the only institution providing mental health care in the country. With a staff of 430 (including 270 nursing staff, 6 psychiatrists, and 3 psychologists) and a capacity of 300 beds, the Center currently houses 245 patients. There are 15,000 polyclinic visits per year. The Bed, Bath, and Bread Center serves approximately 50 persons, mostly the homeless population with problems related to drug addiction. There is an association for patients with Alzheimer's disease and their families. The NGO Ypsilon provides support to families of those affected by schizophrenia. Since 2001, there has been a national mental health plan.

The Foundation for Family Planning promotes responsible parenthood and offers family planning methods, fertility counseling, basic infertility testing, and cervical cancer screening. In 2003, the Ministry of Health initiated a United Nations Population Fund/European Union-funded reproductive health project utilizing a rights- and gender-based framework, with the objective of achieving the targets set at the International Conference on Population and Development (Cairo, Egypt, 1994) and the Millennium Development Goals related to sexual and reproductive health.

All Surinamese nationals over the age of 60 are entitled to a monthly financial compensation from the Government under the coordination of the Ministry of Social Affairs and Housing. The gerontology unit at the Bureau of Public Health aims at improving care for the elderly at all levels, including institutional and home care.

Health Promotion

During the period under review, a variety of health promotion activities in the areas of environmental, reproductive, and community health; disease prevention and control; and public health education were initiated and implemented by government entities and NGOs with the support of international development partners. NGOs have played an active role in attaining targeted health outcomes. Examples include the Community Health Development Program implemented by ProHealth and the environmental health activities undertaken by the Foundation for a Clean Suriname. The national health-promoting schools committee is a Government-led initiative. The Bureau of Public Health's health education department provides information to the public on the prevention of malaria, dengue, leptospirosis, yellow fever, and other communicable as well as noncommunicable diseases and breast-feeding practices.

In general, there is a growing recognition of the need for intersectoral cooperation. This is best demonstrated in the National Strategic Plan on HIV/AIDS approved by the Government in 2004. Priority areas include coordination; policy formulation; legislation and advocacy; prevention; reduction of stigma and discrimination; treatment, care, and support; and monitoring and evaluation.

Human Resources

The availability of health personnel by category in 2004 is presented in Table 2. General physicians receive training at the University of Suriname's Faculty of Medical Sciences, which has a limited admission of 30 students per year. Registered nurses and nursing assistants are trained at the Central Training Institute for Nurses and Allied Professions (Foundation COVAB). Two hospitals (AZP and St. Vincentius) have internal training courses for nurses. Midwives are trained at one public hospital ('s Lands). The Medical Mission and Youth Dental Services provide internal training for their respective medical and dental assistants. The Skillslab is a training facility for medical and paramedical students.

Registration and certification of physicians, midwives, and pharmacists are regulated and supervised by the Ministry of Health. Physicians are licensed through the Ministry and require permission from the Director of Health for clinical practice. Regional licensing and accreditation are currently under review. There are currently no regulations or statutes for official registration or certification of paramedical professionals.

Health Supplies

The state-owned Drug Supply Company of Suriname (BGVS) is the central purchaser, importer, and producer of drugs and medical supplies for local consumption. Ninety percent of all drugs are imported, and 10% are manufactured internally. BGVS distributes medications on the National Essential Drug List to private and public pharmacies and hospitals and also oversees marketing and quality control. All immunobiologicals and nearly all reagents are imported. All vaccines are obtained through the PAHO Revolving Fund for Vaccine Procurement.

Availability of the medications on the National Essential Drug List is not guaranteed. To compensate for scarcities, hospitals and pharmacies may turn to private importers, resulting in extremely high costs. This negatively affects the accessibility of drugs for those with health insurance through the Ministry of

TABLE 2. Number and ratio of health personnel, by category, per 10,000 population, Suriname, 2004.

Category	Number	Number/ 10,000 population
General practitioners	295	6.0
Family physicians	225	4.6
General practitioners in hospitals	70	1.4
Medical specialists	105	2.1
Total number of physicians	400	8.2
Dentists	42	0.9
Non-university trained nursing personnel	1,745	35.4
Registered nurses	778	15.8
Midwives	57	1.2

Social Affairs and Housing or SZF. Many drugs are also accessed directly through personal connections outside of Suriname, bypassing proper customs and quality inspection, or through private pharmacies.

All drugs must be approved by the Governmental Committee on Drug Registration, while the Pharmaceutical Inspectorate oversees inspection of pharmaceutical manufacturing and pharmacies.

There are one CT scan unit and two CD4 count units in the country.

There are a total of 1,378 beds (excluding 60 psychiatric care beds) in Suriname, or 2.7 beds per 1,000 population. The average bed occupancy rate is 70%. In 2002, the average length of hospitalization was 7.2 days, including the longer hospitalization stays of social security patients.

Research and Technological Development in Health

Research projects are funded by international organizations and conducted by the Ministry of Health or other governmental institutions. Most research is limited to conducting surveys on specific health issues, such as malnutrition and mortality, for which current data are required for policy or project development. Training in new technologies and skills for medical and paramedical personnel is also usually sponsored by international entities.

Publications and research reports regarding health and development issues in Suriname are available through the Ministry of Health and the various agencies funding public health projects, including the Pan American Health Organization/World Health Organization (PAHO/WHO).

Health Sector Expenditures and Financing

In 2002, the gross domestic product (GDP) was US$ 879.9 million. GDP per capita was US$ 1,925. The latest available figures on total health expenditure are from 2000, when it was US$ 78,763,778. Total per capita health expenditure was

US$ 180.33, or 9.42% of GDP. In 2002, public health expenditure was US$ 31.7 million and per capita expenditure was US$ 69.40, or 4.97% of GDP. Public and private health care expenditures are nearly equal, with the Government spending about 44% and the private sector (company cost coverage and household out-of-pocket health expenditures) approximately 42%. The remaining 14% comes from external sources (donors). The contribution of the private sector to health care is significant. Out-of-pocket household expenditures are an area of particular concern.

Of total health expenditure for 2000, 55% went to secondary care (public and private hospitals, medical specialists, hospital laboratory and x-ray services, hospital drugs), 34% went to preventive and primary care (Bureau of Public Health, RHS, Medical Mission, private GPs, etc.), while the remaining 11% went to administration, training, and other areas.

The Community Development Fund, United Nations Development Fund GEF (Global Environment Facility) Small Grants Program, Suriname Conservation Foundation, Cordaid, and other NGOS have played a leading role in financially supporting and implementing poverty reduction initiatives. The National Women's Movement is actively involved in initiatives to improve the well-being and living conditions of women in the interior.

Technical Cooperation and External Financing

The principal international development partners working in the health sector are PAHO; the United Nations Development Program; United Nations Population Fund; United Nations Children's Fund; Global Fund to Fight AIDS, Tuberculosis, and Malaria; Inter-American Development Bank; Islamic Development Bank; International Planned Parenthood Foundation; and the European Union. Bilateral donors include the Netherlands, United States, Japan, France, and Germany. Of these, the Dutch Development Cooperation provides by far the largest amount of funding and covers the broadest scope of health-related activities. There is also strong cooperation between local NGOs and Dutch private institutions for development assistance, such as Cordaid.

References

1. United Nations. Common Country Assessment of Development Challenges in Suriname (draft), June 2006.
2. Inter-American Development Bank. Governance in Suriname, IDB report 1999/2000. In: United Nations Common Country Assessment of Development Challenges in Suriname (draft), June 2006. p. 10.
3. Suriname, Ministry of Home Affairs, General Bureau of Civil Registration. Demographic data Suriname 2003–2004. January 2006.
4. United Nations Development Fund for Women, 2001.
5. United Nations, Convention on the Elimination of All Forms of Discrimination against Women. Third Progress Report.
6. Neri M, Menke J. Sustainable combat against poverty: findings and policy recommendations for Suriname, 2000.
7. James V. A strategy for social development and poverty eradication. Paramaribo: United Nations Development Program; 2000.
8. Suriname, General Bureau of Statistics. Statistical Yearbook 2004. p. 49.
9. Government of Suriname; United Nations Children's Fund. Suriname Multiple Indicator Cluster Survey (MICS) 2000. March 2001.
10. Suriname, National Bureau of Gender, 2000.
11. Suriname, General Bureau of Statistics. Seventh General Population and Housing Census. Volume I. 2005.
12. Suriname, Ministry of Home Affairs, General Bureau of Civil Registration. Demographic data Suriname 1998–1999. December 2000.
13. Surinamese Civil Code. Article 46. Paragraphs 1, 2, 4.
14. Suriname, Bureau voor de Openbare Gezondheidszorg. Epidemiologie data 2004. January 2006.
15. Suriname, Ministry of Health. Global Youth Tabacco Survey. November 2004.
16. Ashok M. Confidential enquiries into maternal deaths in Suriname. [Doctoral thesis].University of Leiden (Netherlands); 2000.
17. Leckie G, Pelser R, Grünberg A, Bishoen S. Reproductive health and rights of adolescents in Suriname. Paramaribo; 1997.
18. Suriname, Ministry of Health; United Nations Population Fund; ProHealth. ICPD+10 Report. 2006. p. 106.
19. Adams B. National Women's Movement. Survey report on Maroon fertility in four selected Maroon villages in the interior of Suriname. 2002. In: Third CEDAW periodic report of States parties (CEDAW/C/SUR/3).
20. Stichting L. Contraceptive prevalence study 1992. In: MICS 2000.
21. Schalkwijk M, van den Berg W. Suriname. The situation of children in mining, agriculture and other worst forms of child labour: a rapid assessment. International Labor Organization, Subregional Office for the Caribbean; 2003. Available from: http://www.ilocarib.org.tt/childlabour/library/rapid_assessment/RASuriname.pdf.
22. Suriname, Ministry of Health. HIV/AIDS/SOA Surveillance Report 1983–2005. MOH; 2005.
23. Greenstone Belt Gold Mining Regional Environmental Assessment. Draft report. National Institute for Environment and Development in Suriname; July 2003.
24. Suriname, 1987 Constitution with Reforms of 1992.

TRINIDAD
AND TOBAGO

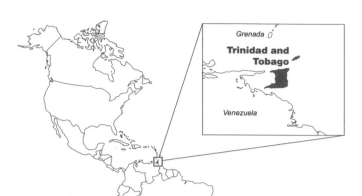

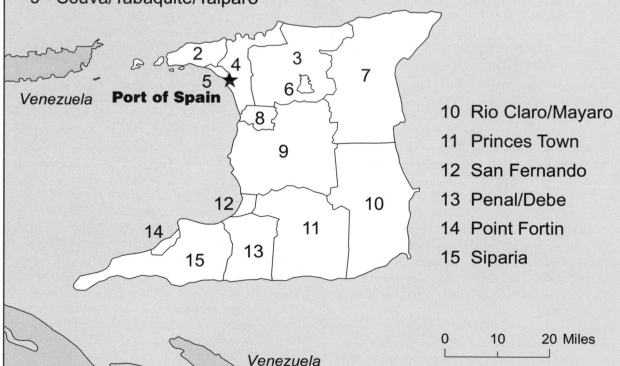

1 Tobago
2 Diego Martin
3 Tunapuna/Piarco
4 San Juan/Laventille
5 Port of Spain
6 Arima
7 Sangre Grande
8 Chaguanas
9 Couva/Tabaquite/Talparo

10 Rio Claro/Mayaro
11 Princes Town
12 San Fernando
13 Penal/Debe
14 Point Fortin
15 Siparia

Venezuela

Port of Spain

Venezuela

0   10   20 Miles

T rinidad and Tobago is the second-largest and southernmost territory of the West Indies. It has a total area of 5,128 km², of which Trinidad covers 4,828 km² and Tobago 300 km². The climate is tropical with a dry and rainy season. The capital city of Port of Spain is located on the northwestern coast of Trinidad. According to the 2000 national census, the population was 1,267,366, which represented a 4% increase over the previous decade. Of this total, 96% reside in Trinidad and 4% in Tobago. The male-female ratio is 1:1, and there is a population density of 246 persons/km².

GENERAL CONTEXT AND HEALTH DETERMINANTS

The twin-island nation gained independence in 1962 and became a republic within the Commonwealth of Nations in 1976 with a parliamentary democracy and an appointed President. Executive power lies with the elected Prime Minister and designated Cabinet with 23 public ministries. Legislative power rests with the Parliament. The bicameral legislature has an elected House of Representatives and an appointed Senate. The local government system consists of 14 corporations made up of two cities, three boroughs, and nine regional corporations principally responsible for maintenance and hygiene of the general environment and public buildings, including solid waste disposal. Tobago has its own political administrative structure under the executive power of the Tobago House of Assembly Act.

Social, Political, and Economic Determinants

In 2005, the Government of Trinidad and Tobago adopted the Vision 2020 National Strategic Plan to strengthen and support initiatives and increased investment in the social sector. The Plan's development priorities center on promoting effective governance, facilitating competitive economic enterprise, and providing sound infrastructure in an environmentally friendly manner. Vision 2020 focuses on human investment and resources development, as evidenced through a sustained increase in national budgetary allocations to the health (30%) and education (32%) sectors for 2005 (1).

The establishment of the CARICOM Caribbean Single Market and Economy in 2006 poses new social challenges that will affect the health and education sectors, due to the resulting rise in the free movement of people, goods, services, and capital between member countries and the need to secure competitive human capital for the global market. Such dynamics also increase the potential risk of disease transmission and require innovative, harmonized, and shared health information and epidemiological surveillance systems and improvements in both the quality and coverage of health services from public and private sources, including coordinated social financing mechanisms.

To achieve the Millennium Development Goals (MDGs) within the context of a stable economy, the Government of Trinidad and Tobago developed, enacted, and implemented plans and policy and legislation reforms and established institutional bodies to expedite achievement of the MDGs. The MDG national assessment report for 2004 indicated that the global partnership for development had increased through anti-dumping and fair trade legislation; access to technology and services had increased; the debt service ratio had declined; and coverage of social assistance programs to vulnerable groups, such as older adults and families living below the poverty line, had increased (2, 3).

The economy has shown robust growth (7% in 2005) with a significant increase in energy exports, a low external debt, and increased external reserves. Core inflation rose on a year-to-year basis, reaching 3% by early 2005 due to rising food costs. Headline inflation has been stationary since 2000 and was approximately 4% in 2004. External current account surplus increased to 14% of GDP in 2004, up from 9% in 2003. Gross national income per capita increased over 2000–2004 by 64%. Real GDP at constant 2000 prices reached 6% in 2005. The dependency ratio was 47% in 2000 and decreased to 41% in 2005. Agricultural production steadily declined over the last decade, with the contribution of the agricultural sector to GDP falling from 2% in 1999 to 0.7% by 2005. This decline is attributed to several factors, such as the closure of the main government-owned sugarcane growing and processing company in 2003 due to a revision of World Trade Organization tariff and trade rules and the removal of European Union sugar subsidies, low wages in the agricultural sector, and the worldwide rise in oil and gas revenues. As a result, the import value of food rose by 31% between 2002 and 2004 (4–7).

The labor force participation rate has remained stable since the 1990s, particularly for males, due to a decrease in the working population group for which qualified laborers and professionals are being imported in the social, productive (such as farm and non-farm enterprises and manufacturing), and construction areas.

Between 1996 and 2000, women's participation in the labor force remained stable at 38%, with a moderate increase in 2002, predominantly in the public services and informal sectors, and at lower clerical and income levels. Women's average income as a percentage of men's in 2000 was lower in all occupational categories, with the smallest disparity being that of clerks (88% for women vs. men) and the largest being that for legislators and senior officer managers (53%). The youth (15–24 years of age) unemployment rate stood at 25.4% in 2001; female unemployment has been consistently higher than male unemployment over the last three decades.

The Ministry of Education's mission statement focuses on a modernization and renewal of the education system with the institutional target of achieving universal primary education by 2015. The objectives of the Ministry's policy are to improve and increase access to educational opportunities at all levels, achieve and sustain quality in schools, provide student support services, and develop well-articulated human resources. Education is compulsory for children up to 12 years of age; the 2004 MDG national assessment report indicated that education coverage goals had been achieved, even though not all segments of the population were fully benefiting from the available opportunities.

In 2000, a policy was established for universal secondary education in Trinidad and Tobago, and during the review period all students completing primary school and taking the Common Entrance Exam for the 221 existing secondary schools were guaranteed placement. Expenditure in public education as a percentage of GDP was 3% in 2003. The annual Education for All (EFA) Global Monitoring Report for 2005 placed Trinidad and Tobago among the countries with a high (97%) EFA development index, a net enrollment rate in primary education of 94%, a gender-specific EFA development index of 96%, and a survival rate to grade 5 of 98%. The national education network has 917 early childhood education centers, 22% of which are public and focus on children ages 3–5. For the 2002–2003 school year, the pupil-teacher ratio was 12:1. There are 483 primary schools for children ages 5–11, yet 50% of students are considered to be at high risk of missing school, due to the schools' geographical location. Following the introduction of universal secondary education, promotion of primary students into secondary level studies increased by 79% for the 2002–2003 school year; female enrollment was 49%, and the pupil-teacher ratio was 19:1. Secondary education focuses on students ages 12–16; among these, those who pass the advanced proficiency examination continue on to an additional final two years of secondary education; in 2003, fe-

male enrollment was 52%, with a pupil-teacher ratio of 20:1. The combined primary, secondary, and tertiary gross enrollment ratio showed a downward trend in the early 1990s due to such socioeconomic factors as structural adjustment, unemployment, and parent migration. The change in the primary and secondary enrollment ratio fluctuated from a negative proportion over 2000–2003 to 28% in primary schools and 1% in secondary schools. With the introduction of universal secondary education in 2000–2001, the declining pattern at the secondary level improved in the advance years of 2002–2003 even though a decline of first entrants was maintained. Females predominated at the secondary and university enrollment levels with a male-female ratio at the latter level of 1:1.5 in 2001.

The estimated literacy rate for 2003 for the population aged 15 and over was 99%, with no significant gender differential. Literacy rates are higher among women of East Indian descent than men of East Indian descent, but lower for women of African descent than men of African descent. Low resource families with children enrolled in public schools receive government subsidies for books, transport, and meals (breakfast and lunch). In 2001, the Government of Trinidad and Tobago initiated the "dollar-to-dollar" program as a way to subsidize tertiary education by matching parents' local tuition fees; the 2005 national budget widened the scope by committing to provide free local first-degree tertiary education for nationals (8–10).

The situation of males poses challenges for achievement of the MDGs due to poor retention in schools and increased mortality from HIV/AIDS, external causes, violence, and crime. The Ministry of Community Development, Culture, and Gender Affairs, in conjunction with an Inter-ministerial Committee and the participation of the National Council of Women in an advisory role, promotes the Government of Trinidad and Tobago policy in support of gender and development. An active movement comprised of nongovernmental and community-based organizations supports the advancement of women in the country together with an ad hoc committee that supports women in the production and trade sectors. The Tobago House of Assembly has also established a Gender Division with a similar advocacy role as that of the various entities working together in Trinidad. The percentage of seats held in Parliament by women increased from 11 to 19 between 2000 and 2004; in 2002, the first female was elected by the Senate to become its President (11).

Key issues related to health are evident in the number of reports on serious criminal and violent events (traffic accidents excluded), ranging from 17,134 in 2000 to 16,387 in 2004 and 11,289 as of August 2005. The National Gender Policy addressing domestic violence is in formulation, together with a central registry for domestic violence data and a national plan of action. A range of nongovernmental organizations (NGOs) is working together to complete these activities, including the National Rape Crisis Society (NRCS), national toll-free hotlines, a network of shelters for women that are largely private, the family court (established in 2004), and 19 community drop-in/information centers, among others. Women and children living with domestic violence and women's intimate partners may access a variety of public services ranging from counseling and alternate job placement to confidential medical services. The NRCS reports rape as the country's principal abuse problem, representing 37% of all cases reported by service users in 2004; those most frequently affected are women of African descent in the 12–17-year-old age group. Females were the group most affected by domestic violence, with a predominance of male perpetrators. Partial data on cases assisted by the NRCS indicate that new cases of child sexual abuse rose from 7% to 10% between 2000 and 2004, while new cases of incest declined from 16% to 8% and crimes and injuries, such as unlawful carnal knowledge (a local term referring to illicit sexual intercourse or contact), narcotic offenses, and attempted suicide, increased. Motor vehicle accidents and fatal collisions increased by 23% and 46%, respectively, over the 2000–2004 period (12–16).

According to the latest (1997–1998) national household survey, within the nine counties there were five defined poverty areas. At the national level, 21% of households in Trinidad and 26% in Tobago were designated as poor. Population groups characterized as poor were those who were uneducated or undereducated, the unemployed or underemployed, unskilled or semiskilled workers, and female-headed households and single-parent households with an average monthly income ranging from US$ 95–160 (at the current exchange of TT$ 6.27 = US$ 1). The root causes identified for these outcomes included lack of educational attainment and intergenerational entrapment by poverty, among others. While there is no significant gender gap identified among the poor, approximately 60% of this group has no qualifications.

One percent of the population is comprised of squatters, of which 26% are poor. Heads of households with no educational qualifications account for 77% of the total poor population. The national MDG assessment of 2004 focuses on the issues of eradication of extreme poverty and hunger and calls for the need to conduct more frequent living conditions surveys, strengthen institutional capacity, carry out poverty eradication programs, set measurable targets, improve data quality, and ensure sustainability of newly created jobs (3, 17).

Population groups such as minors and young adult males and females are predominantly high-risk groups for mortality and morbidity incidence, particularly among those living under the poverty line and those whose behaviors, lifestyles, and social environments increase their exposure to external injuries, crime, violence, HIV/AIDS, and noncommunicable diseases. In 2003, there were 734 socially displaced persons (street children, ex-prisoners, deportees, older adults, substance abusers, those with mental disorders, and those infected with HIV). Males and those who live in the country's two major urban settings (Port of Spain and San Fernando) make up the majority of this group. Between 1997 and 2002, the number of deportees returning to Trinidad

grew. In general, they had left as minors with their families and were now returning to an environment unfamiliar to them and without a support structure. In addition to being socially displaced, they were unemployed and prone to violence and crime. The 2004 Caribbean Epidemiology Center (CAREC) pilot behavioral risk factor survey showed that women experience illness more frequently than men, but also live longer, and persons with lower educational levels seek medical care less often than those with higher levels of education (18).

A 2001 study on overweight, obesity, and skin fold thickness among children of African and East Indian descent, using international standards for overweight and obesity and British (1990) reference curves for body mass index (BMI), showed that those of African descent were taller for their age, but with lower BMI. Obesity was higher among the older Afro-Trinidadian children, particularly among girls. The study concluded that higher BMI was associated with higher BMI in the child's parents, higher reported birthweight, older age of the child's mother, smaller family size, and higher maternal education attainment. The Food and Agriculture Organization estimated the undernourished population at 11.9% for 2001. Food fortification for flour with iron and B complex is mandated and carried out by law, but fortification with calcium is optional. The establishment of "Baby-friendly" initiatives in all the major hospitals and efforts by the National Breast-feeding Committee to improve breast-feeding practices have contributed to the initiation among 95% of mothers of breast-feeding, with the rates of exclusive breast-feeding ranging from 26%–30% for infants under 4 months of age. The 2000 United Nations Children's Fund (UNICEF) Multiple Indicator Cluster Survey estimated that 6% of children under age 5 were underweight, less than 0.5% were severely underweight, and 4% were stunted or showed wasting. In 2002, the Caribbean Nutrition and Food Institute (CFNI) reported a prevalence of 3% overweight among preschool children. Data on food availability indicate that there is an excessive quantity of foods high in energy, proteins, and fats and that the population's ability to access healthy foods in sufficient quantities is affected by income disparities (19–22).

A country assessment of essential public health functions (EPHF) indicated that the national health system identifies outbreaks as they occur but due to weak monitoring practices its predictive capacity is limited. The EPHF exercise also identified the need for regular quality assessments and improved feedback mechanisms for information input utilized for decision-making and policy formulation. Consequently, the institutional response capacity is weak. No official declaration of disease outbreaks occurred during the 2001–2005 review period. Nevertheless, the risk for epidemics remains and is closely monitored at points of entry based on the level of commercial and population movement in and out of the territory (23).

In 2000, 69% of households received water piped into their homes or yards; on the other hand, only 26% of households had a continuous 24-hour water supply seven days a week. Storage of water is therefore commonplace, and 57% of the households had their own water storage tanks. Poor access to potable water is attributed to several factors, including a 40%–50% loss of water in the distribution system, deterioration of assets, and weak institutional and human resources programs. The quality of water delivered meets World Health Organization guidelines for drinking water quality, although this status is challenged by environmental degradation, watershed destruction, and pollution. For sewage disposal, the majority of the population (60%) is served by on-lot septic systems, while 10% is served by central sewage treatment plants, and 30% by pit latrines (24).

Demographics, Mortality, and Morbidity

The population of Trinidad and Tobago is ethnically diverse, with 41% being of East Indian descent, 40% of African, and 19% of other groups, including Chinese, European, and Middle Eastern. Over the last 20 years, the proportion of the population under age 15 declined, while the portion of those 60 years old and older increased. Twenty-one percent of the population falls within the 0–14-year-old age group, 71% in the 15–64 age group, and 8% is 65 years old and older. The country is in a stage of advanced demographic transition, with a low birth rate and decreased fertility rates, resulting in a low population growth rate. Mid-year population estimates indicate a crude birth rate of 14 per 1,000 population and a population growth of 0.3 per 1,000 population for 2000–2005, with a declining trend expected over the next decade. The population structure, by age and sex, for 1990 and 2005 is shown in Figure 1.

The total fertility rate began to decline in the 1970s, and in 2005 was estimated at 1.75 children born per woman, thus placing the country below population replacement level. The decline is principally due to the external migration of nationals in pursuit of better job markets. The net migration rate was –10.87 migrants per 1,000 population for 2005. The life expectancy estimate at birth in 2005 was 71 years for the total population, with 69 for males and 74 for females. Ninety-four percent of households are located in Trinidad, with an average size of 3.7 and a total fertility rate of 1.4 children per woman. Colonial historical roles influence the geographical distribution of ethnic groups, with those of East Indian descent residing predominantly in rural and agriculturally oriented localities, while those of African descent tend to live in urbanized environments, where they principally are employed in the service industries sector and government-related entities (24–26).

General mortality data is available up to 2001, at which time the crude death rate was 8 per 1,000 population. Maternal mortality was 39 per 100,000 live births and infant mortality 19 per 1,000 live births in 2001 (Figure 2). That same year, total deaths increased by 3% in comparison to 2000, with males accounting for 56%; the 50–74-year-old age group accounted for 40% of all

FIGURE 1. Population structure, by age and sex, Trinidad and Tobago, 1990 and 2005.

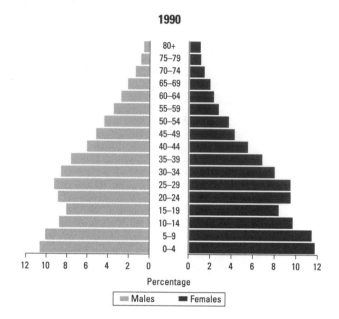

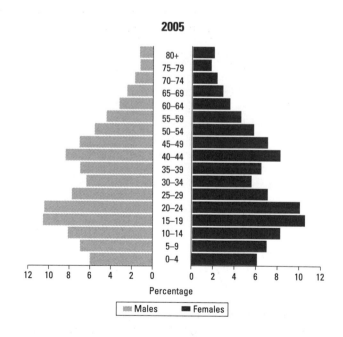

deaths. In 2000, heart diseases, diabetes, malignant neoplasms, and cerebrovascular diseases together accounted for 61% of all deaths (25, 26). The 10 leading causes of mortality for 2001 are presented in Table 1.

Over little more than a decade, mortality rates among infants for conditions originating in the perinatal period more than doubled, from 678 per 100,000 live births for the period 1984–1986 to 1,368

FIGURE 2. Maternal and infant mortality rates, Trinidad and Tobago, 1990–2001.

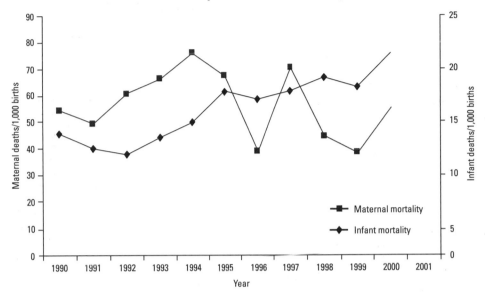

TABLE 1. Leading causes of death, by rank, number of deaths, percentage of total deaths, and cumulative percentage, Trinidad and Tobago, 2001.

Causes of death	Rank	Number	% of total deaths	Cumulative %
Ischemic heart diseases	1	1,631	16.7	16.7
Diabetes mellitus	2	1,340	13.7	30.4
Malignant neoplasms	3	1,211	12.4	42.8
Cerebrovascular diseases	4	972	10.0	52.8
External causes	5	569	5.8	58.6
Human immunodeficiency virus (HIV) disease	6	541	5.5	64.1
Hypertensive diseases	7	406	4.2	68.3
Other heart diseases	8	330	3.4	71.7
Certain conditions originating in the perinatal period	9	224	2.2	73.9
Renal failure	10	173	1.9	75.8

Source: Population and vital statistics report, Central Statistical Office. Ministry of Planning and Development, Government of Trinidad and Tobago.

per 100,000 live births for the 1998–2000 period. This increase is attributed to problems related to the quality of prenatal care and to early detection of high-risk conditions during pregnancy. External injuries accounted for the highest number of deaths in both sexes among the 15–24-year-old age group for the 2000–2005 period. Between 2000 and 2004, mortality rates due to motor vehicle accidents grew from 12 to 19 per 100,000 population. Fatal accidents took place most frequently during weekends and evening hours; in 2004, 87% occurred among the 15–44-year-old age group. Suicide is most prevalent among the population of East Indian descent, with pesticide ingestion being the most frequent mode.

Records from CAREC show that case numbers for some diseases preventable by immunization—chicken pox, meningitis, mumps, rubella, and tetanus (excluding neonatal)—have decreased. Episodes of other diseases or conditions that have also decreased include acute flaccid paralysis, foodborne illnesses, leptospirosis, salmonellosis, scabies, shigellosis, all forms of hepatitis, and viral encephalitis. The diseases that have shown increases are acute hemorrhagic conjunctivitis, dengue in all its forms, gastroenteritis, gonococcal infections, influenza, Hansen's disease, syphilis, and all forms of tuberculosis. During the 2001–2005 period, there were no reports of cases of cholera, ciguatera poisoning, pertussis, human rabies, neonatal tetanus, typhoid fever, and yellow fever (27, 28).

HEALTH OF POPULATION GROUPS

Children under 5 Years Old

There were 383 deaths among children under age 1 in 2000, with leading causes attributed to conditions originating in the perinatal period such as respiratory disorders (intrauterine hypoxia and birth asphyxia) and congenital anomalies. These deaths are related to flaws in the quality of prenatal care provided at all levels of the health system and, consequently, to poor early detection of high-risk conditions. The mortality rate for the 1–4 age group was 8 per 1,000 population in 2000.

Six percent of under-5-year-olds are estimated to be underweight, while 4% were estimated to be stunted or with evidence of wasting. In 2002, exclusive breast-feeding practices were 44%, 33%, and 27% at 1, 2, and 3 months of age, respectively. The Ministry of Health is pursuing a "Baby-friendly" hospital initiative nationwide in order to encourage the establishment of enabling environments for breast-feeding in health facilities and among the population. The number of children ages 1–4 seen at primary health care facilities declined from 4,128 in 2000 to 3,783 in 2003. The five leading hospital discharge diagnoses for the 1–4 age group were diseases of the respiratory system; injury, poisoning, and certain other consequences of external causes; symptoms, signs, and abnormal clinical and laboratory findings; certain infectious and parasitic diseases; and diseases of the digestive system, with a higher prevalence among males. During 2003–2004, 9% of infants were born to HIV-infected mothers.

Children 5–9 Years Old

There were 36 deaths among this age group in 2000, with a slight predominance among males; the major causes were external causes, followed by injury, poisoning, and certain other consequences of external causes; diseases of the nervous system; diseases of the circulatory system; and certain infections and parasitic diseases. Although chronic malnutrition is rare among students in this age group, there are nonetheless pockets of nutritional deficiency, based on reports of protein-energy malnutrition and iron deficiency, together with rising levels of obesity. Violence and early sexual initiation, together with cigarette and drug use, are reported among students and represent challenges to be addressed by the school health services. The Ministry of Health reports that sickle cell, chronic conditions (largely asthma), and external causes and injuries are the major causes of morbidity and mortality among students. A 2004 baseline survey of blood lead levels conducted on 1,761 children in the 5–7 age group on both islands showed levels ranging from

< 1 μg/dL to 29 μg/dL. Only three children in Trinidad met the U.S. criteria for lead poisoning (blood lead level ≥ 20 μg/dL). There were no significant differences by age, sex, ethnicity, or income group (29, 30).

Since 2005, institutional priority has been placed on early detection and resolution of vision and hearing impairments for 100% of children enrolled in primary schools. Of these, 10% received screening during 2005, and 20% failed the first screening.

Adolescents 10–14 and 15–19 Years Old

Mortality rates in 2000 for the age groups 10–14 and 15–19 were 0.49 and 0.87, respectively, per 1,000 estimated mid-year population and were higher among males in both age groups. A 2005 review of services provided to 112 adolescents aged 10–19 nationwide at the country's only public child guidance clinic indicated that depression (33%) was the most prevalent disorder for which treatment was sought, followed by behavioral problems (13%), mental retardation (11%), substance abuse (10%), anxiety (9%), and psychosis (5%). Mental disorders were more prevalent among females than males and among 15–19-year-olds with no difference as to their area of residence; nevertheless, a larger number of cases were children coming from socially and/or economically unstable family environments and residing in underserved areas.

The 2000 Global Youth Tobacco Survey, a school-based study supported by the World Health Organization that collected data from adolescents aged 13–15, showed that 19% of adolescents smoked their first cigarette before they were 10 years of age, with no significant difference between genders; of the representative sample from all secondary schools, 40% of students had smoked cigarettes at least once in their life, which is 5% higher than the number found in a similar prevalence study conducted in 1988. Smoking was more prevalent among males than females and increased in frequency among the older age groups. A similar prevalence pattern was observed among current smokers, with an increase of 11% in 1998 to 14% in 2000. Eighty-four percent of those surveyed reported exposure to tobacco advertisements (31).

The Ministry of Education reported a surge in violent behaviors, including discipline problems, among secondary school students for the 2000–2003 period, with a higher proportion of disruptive behaviors occurring among male students. Pregnancies to mothers ages 13–19 accounted for 15% of live births in 2000. That same year, a representative study related to the sexual health needs of secondary school-age adolescents in Tobago identified the priority concerns driving early initiation of sexual practices as unemployment, drug use, and limited access to educational and developmental opportunities. Other factors, such as poverty, unstable home environments, and seeking multiple sexual partners, further increased their vulnerability to risky behaviors (25, 32, 33).

Adults 20–59 Years Old

Mortality rates are available only for 2000 for this age group; rates range from 2.0 per 1,000 estimated mid-year population among those 20–24 years old to 14.0 among those 55–59 years old, with a higher predominance in both cases among males. The major causes of death were diseases of the circulatory system, followed by neoplasms; certain infections and parasitic diseases; and injury, poisoning, and certain other consequences of external causes. Young males are the population group most affected by deaths due to violence and external causes. The 2004 pilot behavioral risk factor survey by CAREC found that females have a more consistent pattern of health-seeking behaviors than do males; women and older adults were the groups which were the most consistent in monitoring their blood pressure and glucose levels; adults, principally those with higher educational levels, more closely monitored cholesterol levels; only 50% of women in the 35–54 age group reported having had a Pap smear; and more males than females reported always using safety seat belts (18).

Men, youth, and young adults of lower educational levels were the groups that most frequently engaged in physical activities. Males and females were considered slightly obese with an average BMI of 27 for those aged 33–44 and with a normal BMI for those 18–24 years old; the latter younger group consumed fewer fruits and vegetables, with no gender difference observed. Men smoked more than women, particularly those aged 45–54, as well as those of lower education levels; women, however, made more attempts and experienced greater success in their smoking cessation efforts. Marijuana use was not affected by educational levels, with women reporting more frequent use; use of cocaine was insignificant (18, 26).

Older Adults 60 Years Old and Older

By 2000, the size of the population aged 60 and over had increased by 345% over 1985 figures. This age group represented 10% of the total population in 2000, of which 53% were males; among the age group 80 years old and older, females represented 58%, a lesser predominance when compared to the 1985 figure of 63%, thus indicating a gain in life expectancy among older males. This trend in population aging highlights the need for social programs; it is estimated that for 2025, the size of the population 60 years old and older will be larger than that of those under age 18. According to the 2000 census, there were 38 persons over 60 years of age for every 100 children, a situation that will cause a consistent rise in dependency ratios over the next decade. More than two-thirds of older adults receive pension benefits provided by the government; it is estimated that the majority of the population aged 60 and older are inadequately prepared financially for retirement and depend on other sources of income, principally from family members. Older females have lower income levels and fewer employment opportunities than males. Of the total noninstitutional population 65 years old and older, only 9% were represented in the 2001 labor force. The 2000 population census showed that the highest educational attainment for 67% of persons aged 60 or older was at the primary level. In 2001, the mortality rate for the population aged 50 or older was 32 per 1,000 population. Males predominated in the number of deaths, but females 80 years old or older had a higher percentage (79%) of total female deaths registered. The main cause of mortality was heart diseases, followed by diabetes mellitus, malignant neoplasms, cerebrovascular diseases, and diseases of the respiratory system. Public hospital discharge records show no differences by gender but identify the most frequent discharge diagnoses as those related to heart diseases and diseases of the digestive system, followed by injury, poisoning, and cerebrovascular diseases, with the last cause occurring slightly more frequently among females. Based on the 2000 population census data, 40% of persons aged 60–69 years reported having a disability or chronic illness, with a predominance among males; while among those 70–79 years old, the figure was 36%, with males again predominating; and for those aged 80 and older, it was 24%, with a predominance of females (34–37).

The Family

According to the 2000 population census, the average number of persons living in 94% of the households in the country was 2.64 persons, a situation that does not portray households with high occupancy located in marginalized areas. For the same period, the number of marriages decreased by 7% and divorces by 62% when compared with the previous two decades. Sixty-nine percent of households are headed by males; of the 31% of female-headed households, 19% were single mothers. In 2000, 96% of institutional births were assisted by skilled attendants; in 2002, there were 36 births per 1,000 women aged 15–19, a situation that highlights the need to address sexual and reproductive health-related issues in the family environment. The prevalence of contraceptive use, regardless of method, was an estimated 38% in 2000. Domestic violence is a growing public health concern; in 2000, 87% of the victims were females and males were principally the perpetrators. Women and children subjected to abuse of any nature may access a nationwide network of 13 shelters; no similar services currently exist for males. Counseling is offered to the affected women and their intimate partners through NGOs and various public mental health services, or as mandated by the family court system (15, 24). During 2001–2002, there were 17 deaths among adults and 4 among minors associated with domestic violence.

Workers

Over the 2001–2005 period, the National Insurance Board, which provides insurance coverage for more than 50% of the labor force, reported 13,092 workplace-related injury claims, and 2,496 disablement claims. There were 22 deaths due to occupational incidents in 2004 and 57 in 2005. More than 80% of all injuries and disablements recorded occurred to males, while less than 20% occurred to females, although females comprised 39% of the employed for the period under review. Since males predominate in the country's construction and heavy industry labor force, they are more at risk of facing injury or death due to unsafe and/or unhealthy working conditions. For the same period, of the 239 occupational-related registered deaths, only 3% were female. It is estimated that 2%–4% of children aged 5–14 perform some type of labor, with an estimated 1% receiving remuneration in 2000. An International Labor Organization Rapid Assessment Survey conducted in 2002 in Trinidad identified the following areas as those in which children and young workers are engaged: scavenging and agricultural, domestic, and commercial sexual activities (22, 38, 39).

HEALTH CONDITIONS AND PROBLEMS

COMMUNICABLE DISEASES

Vector-borne Diseases

In 2000, 2001, and 2003, the Ministry of Health reported more than 2,000 annual cases of classical **dengue**. In 2002, however, there were 6,000 cases coinciding with the reentry of dengue serotype III. During 2004 and 2005, 400 and 519 cases of classical dengue were reported, respectively. In 2002, there were 218 cases of dengue hemorrhagic fever (DHF) and no cases in 2005. This reduction does not necessarily reflect a trend since all four serotypes of dengue and the *Aedes* mosquito are endemic. There were 45 registered deaths due to DHF during 2000–2002, with a predominance of male deaths in all years. No deaths were registered in 2003–2005 for DHF in the public health system. **Malaria** was declared eradicated in 1965; however, annual reports of imported cases and of a small number of indigenous cases of *P. malariae* in southern Trinidad persist. For the 2001–2005 period, 29 imported cases and 13 indigenous cases were recorded, with no fatalities.

There have been no cases of **yellow fever** since 1979 nor any **lymphatic filariasis** (LF) cases during the 2001–2005 review period. The former is largely due to widespread immunization and the latter to mass chemotherapy in previously affected locations. Ongoing surveillance suggests that there has been successful interruption in transmission of LF, and the country is now pursuing LF-free certification (27, 40).

Vaccine-preventable Diseases

In 2000, hepatitis B and *Haemophilus influenzae* type b (Hib) vaccines were introduced into the national immunization schedule as a part of the pentavalent combination vaccine DPT/HepB/Hib. To extend coverage, vaccines included in the Expanded Pro-

gram on Immunization are administered at public health centers and by private doctors free of charge. National coverage rose from 90% in 2000 to 94% in 2004, and all health personnel, including medical interns, involved in the Program are trained on an annual basis. There have been no outbreaks of vaccine-preventable diseases in the pediatric age group, although one isolated case of **diphtheria** was reported in 2002 (41).

There were no cases of **polio**, **rubella**, or **measles** reported in the country between 2000 and 2005.

Intestinal Infectious Diseases

Gastroenteritis, age unspecified, was the most frequently reported disease to the National Surveillance Unit over the 2000–2005 period. Since 2004, age-specific incidence has shown a discrete drop for the 0–5-year-old age group even though there was no national intervention targeting preschoolers. Changes are attributed to improvements in household safe water sources and health promotion and prevention initiatives, including the "Baby-friendly" hospitals initiative. There are no national-level **helminthes infestation** deworming programs, nor are detailed data by age or sex available, but the National Surveillance Unit registry shows a decrease in the case frequency from 315 in 2000 to 285 in 2005 (42).

Chronic Communicable Diseases

Tuberculosis (TB) shows a higher prevalence of cases among males of African descent and the 25–44-year-old age group, with incidence rates fluctuating over the 2000–2004 period from 16 in 2001 to 18 in 2002 per 100,000 population. In 2004, the annual notification rate was 12 per 100,000 population. TB/HIV comorbidity was 26% in 2004, with an increasing trend when compared to 12% in 1990; other major comorbidities identified with TB are substance abuse (35%) and diabetes (13%). The National Tuberculosis Program reported a 70% cure rate with 15% defaulters and 10% mortality in 2004. **Hansen's disease** (leprosy) prevalence was 0.44 per 100,000 population with a new case detection of 0.24 in 2003. Cases were more prevalent among males than females and showed no ethnic or age group differentiation pattern (28, 43–45).

Acute Respiratory Infections

According to CAREC surveillance reports, over the 2000–2005 period there was an epidemic of acute respiratory infections among the 5-years-and-under age group, with 15 confirmed cases in 2000 and 12,064 cases in 2005. At the same time, suspected **influenza** cases decreased from 41,125 in 2000 to 23,511 in 2005. Surveillance for respiratory diseases increased over the period and continues due to the threat of **SARS** and **avian influenza** outbreaks. Ministry of Health reports for the 2000–2003 period place diseases of the respiratory system among the leading five to 12 hospital discharge diagnoses. The main causes are **asthma**, other acute upper respiratory infections, **pneumonia**, other diseases of the respiratory system, and bronchitis, emphysema, and others.

HIV/AIDS and Other Sexually Transmitted Infections

Over the period 2000–2004, the cumulative number of HIV infections reported in public health facilities since the beginning of the epidemic in 1983 increased by 37%, while the number of new AIDS cases decreased by 34%. Sexual transmission remained the predominant mode of transmission among newly identified cases. The male-to-female ratio for new infections decreased from 1.6:1 in 2000 to 1.2:1 in 2004, with the majority of new infections occurring among females, especially in the 15–49-year age group, which showed an increase over the period of 67% in 2000 and 70% in 2004. AIDS deaths per annum in public facilities declined over the 2000–2004 period, a phenomenon which may be attributed to the provision of antiretroviral therapy free of cost in all public HIV treatment centers. Data from the year 2000 show a slight increase in the number of deaths from 519 in 1999 to 535 in 2000. Sixty-five percent of these deaths occurred among males in the 30–39-year-old age group and predominantly in urban areas (26, 46).

In an effort to raise the population's awareness regarding the importance of knowing individual HIV status, the public health sector scaled up voluntary counseling and testing (VCT) services through the introduction of a National Prevention of Mother-to-Child Transmission (PMTCT) Program for HIV testing of all pregnant women attending public antenatal care clinics; the provision of HIV testing at national clinics for the treatment of sexually transmitted infections (STIs); and the establishment of VCT clinics within selected health centers. As a result, during the 2000–2004 period, samples submitted for HIV testing by public facilities increased by 35%. The improved availability and access to HIV testing by pregnant mothers provided by the PMTCT Program led to an increase in testing from 78% in 2000 to 96% in 2003. The prevalence rate in this group ranged from 19.3 per 1,000 in 2000 to 10.9 per 1,000 in 2003. Access to antiretroviral therapy for HIV-positive mothers is provided free of charge. Follow-up care for all HIV-positive mothers and their infants includes testing of HIV-exposed infants, post-delivery counseling on the importance of breast-feeding avoidance, and the provision of nutritional replacement therapy (baby formula) free of charge for the first six months following birth (47).

Seven HIV treatment centers provide antiretroviral treatment and care for adults, including pregnant women and children; two of the centers are located in Tobago. All HIV-positive individuals have access to diagnostic tests, including CD4 and viral load, and a ready supply of antiretroviral medications. HIV drug resistance testing is not conducted nationally, but there is evidence of resistance to first-line medications at some treatment centers. In 2004, 40% of the newly reported cases of HIV-positive adults and children were receiving treatment and care in public health facil-

ities and 23% were receiving antiretroviral therapy. Ninety-five percent of those receiving treatment and care resided in Trinidad. A 2005 assessment of one of the country's public care and treatment centers highlighted various obstacles to coverage extension. These included a shortage of trained personnel and multidisciplinary teams for in- and outpatient clinics, along with confidentiality issues related to service provision and stigma and discrimination (48–52).

The Queens Park Counseling Center and Clinic is the national health facility for the treatment and care of all conventional STIs through a national network of seven satellite facilities. Over the 2000–2004 period, there was a reduction in the case numbers of **syphilis** (42%), **acute gonorrhea** (42%), **genital warts** (41%), **trichomoniasis** (76%), and **bacterial vaginosis** (53%), while case numbers of **herpes genitalis** increased by 25%. For the same period, there was a higher incidence among females of syphilis, trichomoniasis, and bacterial vaginosis, while males were predominantly affected by acute gonorrhea and genital warts. STI data for Tobago for the 2003–2004 period show a reduction in case numbers for acute gonorrhea (17%) and syphilis (14%), together with an increase in the number of blood specimens testing positive for HIV (88%) (53, 54).

The HIV/AIDS National Strategic Plan for 2004–2008 has targeted various vulnerable and/or high-risk groups for the promotion of healthy sexual attitudes, behaviors, and practices. Specifically, this HIV prevention strategy will focus on young women, youths in or out of school, men who have sex with men, commercial sex workers, the prison population, and substance users (18).

Over the period 2000–2004, the reported cases of HIV show young people in the productive age group to be increasingly affected by the epidemic, with the 25–34-year-old age group recording the highest numbers of new HIV infections per year followed by the 15–24-year old age group (46). Females continue to be increasingly infected with HIV owing to biological factors as well as social factors, including domestic and sexual abuse, economic dependency on men, commercial sex work, and reduced power to negotiate safe sex. Females had the highest incidence of HIV in the 15–24-year-old age group over the 2000–2002 period while males dominated the 24–34 age group. This gender division quickly changed for the period 2003 and 2004 when females in both age groups represented the highest number of new infections of HIV (46).

At the same time that men who have sex with men are being highlighted internationally for their increasing vulnerability to HIV/AIDS, this group continues to face high levels of stigma and discrimination. Drawing from national statistics on sexual exposure among HIV-positive cases, 3%–5% in this group classified themselves as men who have sex with men and 1%–3% identified themselves as men who have sex with both men and women (46).

The current environment of stigma and discrimination inhibits individuals from identifying themselves as men who have sex with men or bisexual, and, as a result, presents obstacles for securing an accurate and reliable assessment of the extent of risky sexual behaviors associated with these groups. Nationally, prevention efforts among men who have sex with men have been minimal.

Since commercial sex work is illegal in Trinidad and Tobago, the activities related to its practice usually are of an underground or covert nature and occur within the context of massage parlors, modeling agencies, tour groups, and night clubs. A study of commercial sex work in the country revealed the range of sex work targeting predominantly young women to include high school and university students and involve street solicitation, escort services, work in locally produced pornographic films, sex tourism involving entertainers and local and foreign female club and casino employees, and commercial sex work among men who have sex with men (49).

Not only do these activities increase the vulnerability of young commercial sex workers to HIV infection, but their human rights are not promoted or protected due to the concealed and unlawful nature of their work.

The prison population in Trinidad and Tobago, as in other countries, continues to face the risk of increased exposure to HIV infection. The Ministry of Health and other national stakeholders have developed a comprehensive health plan to mitigate the spread of various communicable and noncommunicable diseases, including HIV/AIDS, STIs, and TB in national prisons.

According to an NGO Needs Assessment conducted by the National AIDS Coordinating Committee, nongovernmental organizations have been involved in a host of prevention activities at the local and national levels. These activities include school and workplace sensitization on HIV/AIDS prevention and control, condom distribution, and the dissemination of information on STIs and sexual and reproductive health issues. Some of the challenges facing NGOs, however, include lack of training in NGO governance and in human resources, financial, and project management. Monitoring and evaluation skills among NGOs working in HIV/AIDS-related issues are also limited, resulting in difficulty assessing the impact of civil society initiatives (55).

Zoonoses

For 2000–2005, annual reported cases of **leptospirosis** ranged from a high of 161 in 2002 to a low of 102 in 2005. In 2000, there were 29 fatalities, 83% of which occurred in persons over 40 years of age with no deaths reported for the under-15 age group; 76% were males and 24% were females. Similarly, during 2001 there were 16 deaths (9 males and 7 females), with 69% of the fatalities occurring among the over-40 population age group. Since the 1960s, leptospirosis has transitioned from being a disease concentrated in agricultural areas to one that is now common in urban settings. There were no reported cases of rabies for the 2001–2005 period. In 2004, several horses and birds were found to be seropositive for the **West Nile virus**. Since then, all dengue and unspecified fever blood samples are being screened for West Nile virus, with no human cases reported up to the end of 2005 (28).

Noncommunicable Diseases

Metabolic and Nutritional Diseases

Endocrine, nutritional, and metabolic disorders occupy places ranging from 1st to 12th among the most frequent diagnoses at discharge from 80% of hospitals nationwide, with **diabetes** being the first cause during the 2000–2003 period. Mortality data available for 2000 shows rates for endocrine, nutritional, and metabolic diseases at 112 per 100,000 population with higher rates (118) among females than males (108). In 2000, diabetes accounted for 14% of total deaths (26, 56).

Cardiovascular Diseases

The mortality rate in 2000 for diseases of the circulatory system was 279 per 100,000 population, with a higher rate among males (293) than females (264). **Cerebrovascular diseases, hypertension**, and other heart diseases follow ischemic heart diseases, with males accounting for a higher frequency than females in all causes. Despite this, the 2004 CAREC behavioral risk factor study profile showed that both sexes shared various risk factors, such as smoking, sedentary lifestyles, and improper diet (18, 26, 56).

In 2000, hypertension accounted for 4% of total deaths (26, 56). That same year, ischemic heart diseases were the leading hospital discharge diagnosis at 80% of hospitals nationwide; this cause also accounted for the highest proportion of total deaths (17%).

Malignant Neoplasms

The mortality rate of malignant neoplasms per 100,000 population was 99 in 2000, with males accounting for a rate of 104 and females with a rate of 94. According to the National Cancer Registry 2000–2004, at the national level the leading sites of neoplasms overall were prostate, followed by breast, colon and rectum, cervix uteri, and bronchus and lung, while for females they were the breast, followed by cervix uteri, colon and rectum, corpus uteri, and ovary. Over the period 2000–2003, the leading cancers responsible for mortality were those of the prostate (28%), followed by breast (14%), colon and rectum (13%), bronchus and lung (11%), and leukemia (7%). The same site distribution is seen for males and females excepting the breast and with the stomach being the fifth-leading site; 90% of neoplasms of the prostate occurred among the age group 65–85 or older. Among females in the 25–85 and older age group, more than half of all deaths were due to neoplasms of the breast (23%), cervix uteri (11%), colon and rectum (11%), and corpus uteri and ovary (8%) (26, 56, 57).

OTHER HEALTH PROBLEMS OR ISSUES

Disasters

For the period 2000–2005, the Office of Disaster Preparedness and Management reported that localized and island-wide flooding was the main emergency problem, causing disruptions in transportation, agricultural losses, and property damage. In September 2004, landslides related to Hurricane Ivan claimed the lives of three persons in Tobago (12, 16).

Mental Health

There is no community-based national mental health program, but three Regional Health Authorities (RHAs) offer some community-based services through outpatient clinics and primary health care centers where substance abuse services are included. Data on the country's mental health profile is limited, but overall estimates indicate that depression, schizophrenia, suicides, and substance abuse are the most prevalent issues.

Addictions

The Government of Trinidad and Tobago signed and ratified the WHO Framework Convention for Tobacco Control in 2003 and 2004, respectively. Within this context, the Ministry of Health informs all prospective job applicants of its no-smoking policy, has made all publicly funded health organizations and their motor vehicles smoke-free, discourages sponsorship by the tobacco industry of health-related events, and regulates tobacco advertising, including the placement of health warnings on tobacco products. Due to its geographical location and accessible topography, its links to global markets provided through the tourism and maritime industries, and increased local production of cannabis, Trinidad and Tobago is widely viewed as a transshipment point for the international drug trade. The groups most vulnerable to drug use and involvement in narcotics trafficking are out-of-school and unemployed youth, those living below the poverty line, sex workers, and individuals living in unstable family environments. Higher use is reported among males (92%) (32, 58–61).

Environmental Pollution

A five-year study on poisonings (2001–2005) conducted by the Ministry of Health's Occupational Health Unit and based on admission data from five major hospitals shows a total of 2,222 poison-related cases. Of these, 78% were suicide attempts and 21% accidental poisonings, while only 1% were documented as workplace-related events. Four percent of all the reported incidents resulted in deaths. Females accounted for 54% of the poisoning cases. The main poisoning agents were agro-chemical (35%), pharmaceutical (34%), household (21%), and industrial (4%). There is no specific official information available on the status of environmental pollutants, but with the closure of secondary lead-smelting facilities and the removal of lead in gaso-

line in 2004, it is expected that lead exposure levels will decline significantly (62).

Oral Health

A national oral health survey conducted in 2004 with schoolchildren in the 6–8-, 12-, and 15-year-old age groups in 18 primary schools and 19 secondary schools showed significant improvement in the oral health of 12-year-olds when compared to the previous survey conducted 15 years earlier. With the current decayed, missing, and filled teeth (DMFT) index being 0.6, the country surpassed the WHO goal of 3.0 by the year 2000. The oral health of 15-year-olds was good, with a DMFT score of 1.0. However, for the 6–8-year-old age group, it was poor compared to secondary students (DMFT = 2.54). The presence of caries was detected in 62% of the 6–8-year-old age group, 38% of 12-year-olds, and 43% of 15-year-olds. Ongoing research at the University of the West Indies (UWI) School of Dentistry suggests there may be low awareness among parents of the importance of primary teeth and appropriate preventive dental care for young children. Primary school students had higher treatment needs than those in secondary, reflecting a low caries experience among older age groups. Overall, 72% of students aged 6–8 years had some treatment needs, compared with 59% of 12-year-olds and 65% of 15-year-olds. Almost half of the overall sample required fillings, 38% required fissure sealants, and 12% required extractions (63).

RESPONSE OF THE HEALTH SECTOR

Health Policies and Plans

The National Health Services Plan of 1994 remains in force. In the context of the Vision 2020 National Strategic Plan developed for the health sector and discussed earlier, the core principles of affordability, equity, and accessibility will guide ongoing health sector reform activities and help define the future role of health care services. The Health Sector Reform Program (HSRP) has pursued fundamental changes through the strengthening of leadership in the Ministry of Health, development of health systems, and implementation of the Regional Health Authorities Act of 1994. There are currently five RHAs. In order to improve the performance of the essential public health functions, the Ministry of Health is working to strengthen its leadership role and transform itself into an effective policy, planning, and regulatory organization.

Vision 2020 seeks to improve the health status of the population by unifying and enhancing the performance and quality of the health care delivery system and services; strengthening health research systems for evidence-based decision-making, policy formulation, new learning, and development; and creating a client-focused health care environment. Achievement of these goals will depend upon the ability of national authorities to optimize and sustain intersectoral collaboration, which in turn will harmonize the HSRP (64).

In this regard, a pivotal element will be the development of a comprehensive network of new or upgraded primary health care facilities that focus on the promotion of equity, accessibility, community involvement, self-reliance, sustainability, and relevance of services delivery. The HSRP envisaged that a shift would occur from a reliance on secondary level services to primary level and community services, outpatient surgery and care programs, and home care initiatives, with particular emphasis on the primary level management of chronic diseases. However, there is a difference between the building and refurbishment of the primary health care infrastructure and the development of health systems and of skilled human resources to achieve the desired improvements in outcomes of care. Referral protocols require strengthening among the network of providers and with other sectors, such as education and social services.

Trinidad and Tobago's existing legal framework discourages all known forms of discrimination against women, and many provisions are in place based on the Convention on the Elimination of All Forms of Discrimination against Women. These include policies for gender and domestic violence now being implemented, the Married Persons Act, the Status of Children Act, and the Family Law, among others. Women enjoy the same rights as men to enter the labor force, perform public functions at all levels of government, hold political office, and initiate legal action when they feel their rights have been violated. Workplace legislation also is in place to protect women's rights.

The 2004 national plan of action for children addresses maternal and child health, family planning, basic education and literacy, children in special circumstances, and supporting educational goals based on the United Nations' 1990 World Declaration on the Survival, Protection, and Development of Children. All international and regional conventions and accords related to child health have been ratified. To enhance the quality and timeliness of data, the government is taking steps to improve monitoring and response to the priority needs of children. At the same time, the Ministry of Health is finalizing the national school health policy and modernizing the school health program so that clinical and teaching staff will be better able to address hearing, vision, dental, immunization, and psychological needs of all students entering and leaving the educational system. A network of student support services initiated by the Ministry of Education in 2004 seeks to address the concerns identified by guidance officers based on high numbers of events related to attitudinal problems, peer conflicts, learning difficulties, physical and sexual abuse, pregnancy, and substance abuse.

The Mental Health Act of 1975 is currently under review, and the 2000 Mental Health Plan developed by the Ministry of Health was implemented in the national psychiatric hospital and several primary health care centers in three RHAs during the 2001–2005 period.

A research study undertaken in 2002 by the National Drug Council on the impact of drug trafficking on Trinidad and Tobago society underscored the potential capacity of this problem to undermine the political stability of the country and damage the country's international image. The assessment addresses the diversion of national resources to mitigate the negative impact of the drug trade, ongoing practices of bribery and money laundering, and the emergence of a parallel economy outside policymakers' control. The drug trade also contributes to a rise in serious crimes nationwide and aggravates racial tensions and poverty-related issues, thereby introducing a negative dimension into the sociocultural fabric of Trinidad and Tobago society. Stringent controls and intervention measures are being implemented to undermine and discourage the local production of marijuana and all other illicit practices associated with the drug trade.

Organization of the Health System

The health sector is comprised of public and private entities. The foundation of the health sector is the public health system, which includes a network of three tertiary level hospitals, three district hospitals, three specialized long-stay hospitals, and a series of primary health care facilities—3 district health facilities, 67 health centers, and 36 outreach centers—with the district health facility serving as the hub. Persons from other CARICOM islands also come to Trinidad and Tobago seeking tertiary medical care, particularly in the areas of oncology and cardiac surgery. Currently, some publicly funded health institutions outsource some of their health and ancillary services to private providers as a short-term measure to reduce the time spent on waiting lists to receive care in public facilities. The private sector includes private practitioners, hospitals, clinics, pharmacies, biomedical laboratories, and radiological-image diagnostic services; it remains highly unregulated. Several private companies provide health services benefits, with the most common form being that of group medical insurance coverage provided by employers to their employees. In late 2004, a National Health Insurance Steering Committee was established, and a model was prepared and presented to the Cabinet for approval in 2005.

The Regional Health Authorities Act of 1994 defines the Ministry of Health's role as being that of a "purchaser" of health care services and the RHAs being the providers. The Private Hospitals Act, which was amended in 1989, regulates the licensing and oversight of private hospitals. Regulation of health care providers in both the public and private sectors is governed by various health professional acts, including those for the Pharmacy Board, the Medical Board, registration of nurses and midwives, and the dental profession. Dual work practices, which allow many senior public service physicians to work in both the private and public spheres, have resulted in the limitation of their public sector work hours to the detriment of those population segments unable to pay for private sector services. The Ministry of Health has em-

Health Is Critical in the Push to Achieve Developed-nation Status

Trinidad and Tobago's Vision 2020 ushers in comprehensive improvements for the country and its citizens. In preparation for the Plan, Trinidad and Tobago passed fair-trade and anti-dumping legislation, focused on increasing access to technology and services, reduced the debt-service ratio, and boosted social assistance programs for the elderly and the poor. The Plan's health sector goals include improving the performance and quality of health systems and services and promoting patient-centered health care.

barked on a comprehensive Quality Improvement Program as a key strategy for its health sector reform agenda to enhance the country's performance of the essential public health functions. The concepts of total quality management and continuous quality improvement were adopted as strategic management tools to foster effective teamwork, the reengineering of systems and processes, and the improvement of outcomes and efficiency. Accreditation of health institutions is a key element in the Ministry of Health's quality improvement strategy. In July 2002, the Ministry of Health formally issued an accreditation standards manual for the health sector to the heads of health institutions. In order to implement a successful national health insurance system as projected during 2007, all elements in the design and implementation phases, including accreditation of health institutions, will need to be carefully planned. Internal surveys are used to redesign systems and processes to assess and improve services quality, with the intent of achieving a state of readiness for external audits of health facilities in 2007. Infection prevention and control for all health care facilities is a focus of the accreditation standards, and in 2006 the Ministry of Health produced a Manual of Infection Prevention and Control Policies and Guidelines.

Public Health Services

The population-based health services and programs under the responsibility of the Ministry of Health include the Public Health Laboratory, Hansen's Disease Control Program, National Tuberculosis Program, Expanded Program on Immunization, National Surveillance Program, National Population Program, Veterinary Public Health Program, National AIDS Program, National Oncology Program, and School Health Program, among others.

Epidemiology is a weak area in the public health system. The National Surveillance Unit, a centralized service of the Ministry of Health, captures data from the country's primary health care services and hospitals but maintains a passive surveillance system. The National Surveillance Unit depends on the Trinidad Public Health Laboratory and other institutional laboratory facilities for confirmation of outbreak events, but the RHAs and their network of health services are directly responsible for implementing immediate outbreak control measures as needed, with

support from the Ministry of Health. A limited number of trained surveillance nurses and epidemiologists, the latter with both medical and nonmedical specializations, perform these functions and produce monthly reports on the case frequency of specific communicable diseases for which notification is mandatory and surveillance and outbreak control measures are deemed necessary at the RHA level. The system is cumbersome and challenged with partial, untimely reporting, resulting in a passive and poorly informed response capacity. The HSRP envisions decentralizing the system and organizing surveillance units at the RHA level in order to improve quality, data audits, needs assessment, monitoring, and evaluation, as well as to enhance response capacity for surveillance, improve analysis, and ensure the adequate application of strategic information to policy development and planning in the sector.

The Vision 2020 National Strategic Plan articulates environmental policy as "the sustainable use and conservation of the environment for the promotion of social and economic development in order to improve the quality of life of all citizens" (64). Demand on the country's natural resources is increasing at an exponential rate, with increasing exports of natural gas and oil. Increased revenues are fueling the construction of new public buildings, industrial estates, and housing. There is a standing debate between environmentalists and the Government of Trinidad and Tobago over various conservation, pollution, and land use issues. Environmental health services within the Ministry of Health traditionally focus on inspections, registrations, and licensing for food safety, public sanitation, and vector control, with the municipalities sharing responsibilities with the Ministry of Health in the major cities and boroughs. The Pesticide and Toxic Chemicals Board and laboratory are situated within the Ministry of Health. The establishment of the Environmental Management Authority (EMA) in 2000, the passage of legislation protecting the environment, and the implementation of environmental impact assessments have facilitated increased participation by the citizenry in decision-making regarding major new developments that impact not only on the natural environment, but also on human health. Enacted noise pollution rules are in place and enforced under EMA legislation, while water pollution rules are in the introduction phase. The Government of Trinidad and Tobago ratified the Basel Convention on the Control of Transboundary Movements of Hazardous Wastes and Their Disposal and the Stockholm Convention on Persistent Organic Pollutants, and it is currently in the process of ratifying the Rotterdam Convention on the Prior Informed Consent Procedure for Certain Hazardous Chemicals and Pesticides in International Trade. The country's Public Health Ordinance and the Municipal Corporations Act are under review and will be updated in keeping with modern environmental health practices. The Government of Trinidad and Tobago has made a commitment to invest TT$ 1.2 billion over the 2006–2009 period for the purpose of upgrading the quality of water services.

In the absence of a national policy on waste management, the Ministry of Public Utilities and the Environment has overall responsibility for the management of solid and hazardous wastes. Independent contractors employed by local governments collect municipal solid waste, but industrial and hazardous waste treatment and disposal are not adequately supervised. The major landfill sites are operated by the government, and they all would require extensive upgrading in order to be classified as sanitary landfills. A Code of Practice for Biomedical Waste Management was adopted by the Ministry of Health in 2005 and is being implemented in the public health institutions. However, this Code still lacks the necessary supportive legislation to ensure its complete implementation.

The country's energy-based economy benefited from an increase in industrial investments and construction activities beginning in 2003. Between 2001 and 2005, unemployment figures decreased while occupational injuries and deaths increased. There is limited laboratory and testing equipment to monitor occupational health conditions. The Occupational Safety and Health Act (2004) mandates the establishment of an Occupational Safety and Health Authority and an agency responsible for policy development and legislation implementation, to be supported by the Ministries of Labor and Health.

Trinidad, and, to a lesser extent, Tobago, were spared the ravages of hurricanes during the active 2004–2005 seasons. In recognition of the need to strengthen the country's preparedness and emergency response capacity to natural disasters, in 2005 the government replaced the National Emergency Management Agency with an Office of Disaster Preparedness and Management. This office is expected to prepare and introduce new national emergency legislation.

During 2000–2005, the Ministry of Health strengthened its outbreak response capacity with the incorporation of preparedness plans for the West Nile virus, severe acute respiratory syndrome (SARS), and avian influenza A (H5N1). The Ministry of Health adheres to the International Health Regulations and is taking the necessary steps to adequately face the challenges posed by global trade and development—particularly the increased risk of disease transmission—by strengthening institutional response and human resources competencies.

Individual Care Services

Efforts are under way at the RHA level to increase access to and utilization by males of health services in response to the growing prevalence of chronic noncommunicable diseases, as well as to raise awareness among this group regarding common risk factors for these diseases and STI/HIV/AIDS. In 2004, the Ministry of Health approved a new sexual and reproductive health policy that will foster a more comprehensive and gender-based approach to the needs of families and individuals of all ages.

The Ministry of Social Development, Youth, and Sports (MSDYS) holds responsibility for implementing overall policy regarding youth health education and has appointed a national youth council to drive this process. The Ministry of Education provides student support services and counseling in schools nationwide, with individual care being provided on a needs basis; NGOs such as the Family Planning Association of Trinidad and Tobago (FPATT) provide peer counseling services, and a network of youth programs is available through the MSDYS at the community level. To address growing concerns regarding HIV/AIDS stigma and discrimination, the Ministry of Education is implementing the Health and Family Life Education curricula at the primary school level. Sex education and abstinence, values, and morals programs are currently being developed, even though only 7% of schools nationwide have teachers trained in life skills-based HIV education; the Ministry of Health, together with UWI, are training and integrating school health nurses into the system to develop the national program.

A 2004 rapid assessment of the national drug supply system highlighted the need to ensure a constant flow of antiretroviral medications through timely distribution mechanisms which would allow drug delivery directly from suppliers to pharmacies, especially in Tobago. At the same time, there is a need for training of pharmacists to facilitate their increased involvement in the response to HIV/AIDS, particularly as regards encouraging treatment adherence and the provision of first-line counseling to clients. An assessment of STI services identified issues affecting services quality, including the lack of standardized treatment protocols; health, safety, and quality control guidelines; and other quality assurance mechanisms. Clinic services also need to include laboratory facilities for herpes, chlamydia, and HIV testing, to provide continuous training for staff, and to transition from being a strictly vertical STI program into a more holistic, integrated sexual and reproductive health service that facilitates such services as cervical cancer screening and enhances contact-tracing and follow-up of clients (48).

The Ministry of Health is currently implementing a Directly Observed Treatment, Short-course (DOTS) program in two pilot sites, with plans to scale up the program nationwide and thus improve institutional response to tuberculosis.

The Ministry of Health provides institutional care free of cost for all those affected by Hansen's disease.

The National Blood Transfusion Service, with satellite sites at major hospitals, is responsible for screening all blood and blood products and for setting standards for their collection and distribution. All blood donations are obtained on a voluntary basis; screening for HIV is conducted in 100% of all donations.

Intensive care units, including neonatal, are available in the public sector only at the three major hospitals. Individual services include emergency, outpatient, and institutional care for mental health, surgery, oncology, tuberculosis, and substance abuse, together with primary health care preventive and outreach services. General dental services by dental surgeons and dental nurses are provided countrywide free at the point of delivery in primary health care facilities. In 2000, the Emergency Health Service transport system was established and made available free of cost at the point of delivery to persons seeking emergency transfer to a public hospital under the supervision of trained staff. A private emergency health transport system also exists to transfer individuals to private hospitals; however, individuals using these services must pay all expenses out of pocket. Plans are under way to consolidate the Public Health Laboratory; the Chemistry, Food and Drug, Vector Control, and Nutrition and Metabolism Laboratories; and the Queens Park Counseling Center and Clinic into one organization, since the physical infrastructure of these laboratories has deteriorated over time, compromising their ability to render adequate service despite high ongoing maintenance costs. Currently, these facilities operate independently of one another, although some consultants are shared among them. In 2005, the Ministry of Health established a National Laboratory Advisory Committee to oversee the operations of the country's medical laboratory network.

Primary and secondary health care facilities provide health promotion interventions and preventive care and treatment for metabolic diseases, with particular focus on diabetes, hypertension, and cancer. Screening for chronic noncommunicable diseases is available free of cost. The Ministry of Health is currently reformulating its national noncommunicable diseases policy and designing an integrated approach-based program to address common risk factors for the country's major morbidity and mortality causes. Primary health care facilities are now furnished with exercise equipment to encourage increased physical activity, and the RHAs are actively pursuing the implementation of prevention screening in community fairs. The Trinidad and Tobago Diabetes Association has also supported health promotion and education interventions by providing voluntary services at primary health care facilities.

The needs of persons with disabilities are addressed through the Disability Assistance Grant Program, which operates under the purview of the MSDYS. Financial assistance is provided to individuals with medically certified permanent disabilities who are unable to earn an independent livelihood. The Disability Assistance Fund was established in December 2003 to meet the needs of persons with disabilities and/or organizations associated with those who do not qualify for assistance in the existing schemes offered by the Ministry. The main objectives of this program are to support and empower civil society groups that focus on the needs of persons with disabilities and to create the institutional and organizational environment necessary for the easy integration of persons with disabilities into society. Program participants receive assistance to purchase therapeutic aids, devices, and equipment.

There are 9.47 hospital beds per 10,000 population, with only a 0.55 bed ratio in general hospitals; human resources for these services are scarce, with 1 psychiatrist, 0.3 psychologists, 11.4 psychiatric nurses, and 1.64 social workers per 100,000 population. There is only one child guidance clinic unit in the country. The health system offers therapeutic services in psychopharmacology, group and individual psychotherapy, occupational therapy, psychosocial rehabilitation, and behavioral therapy. Current services include training for nurses and mental health assistants and the development of research, even though the information system is inadequate and epidemiological surveillance in mental health is limited. There are several NGOs addressing the consequences of Alzheimer's disease and child autism; there is one center for children with mental retardation and one national mental health association.

The Human Tissue Transplant Act was enacted in 2000, with approval of the accompanying regulations occurring in 2004. A National Unit is being established for the procurement, storage, and distribution of tissues for corneal and kidney transplants; these will be provided free of charge at the point of service together with immunosuppressive drugs for the transplant recipient; during the current phase, kidney transplantation will come from living donors only. Between 1993 and 2003, 17 patients had kidney transplants, and the number of kidney recipients who traveled abroad for transplant operations rose. All public health facilities provide cancer screening services for reproductive organs, but unresolved issues remain regarding response efficiency and quality of care. NGOs such as the FPATT and the Cancer Society of Trinidad and Tobago also provide services. The government is currently planning the construction of a National Oncology Center and establishing a national cancer program, with funding and technical support from the Government of Canada.

Health Promotion

The Ministry of Health, within the framework of the 1993 Caribbean Charter for Health Promotion and the HSRP, adopted health promotion as the principal strategy to improve quality of life and well-being among the population. The strategy addresses individual, social, and environmental risk factors in order to modify individual and collective behaviors that in turn will positively influence health determinants. The process encourages a participatory approach by all stakeholders and the development of policies and strategic plans in the areas of sexual and reproductive health, school health, noncommunicable diseases prevention and control, and HIV/AIDS/STIs, among others. Health promotion programs and efforts to enhance human resources competencies and institutional strengthening are being decentralized to the RHA level, with the purpose of stimulating the creation of healthy settings supported by the basic primary health care principles of accessibility, quality, and equity. The Directorate of Health Promotion and Public Health guides these activities nationwide. A multisectoral National Health Promotion Council was also appointed by the Cabinet in 2001; nevertheless, establishing effective and sustainable mechanisms for intersectoral collaboration between the public and private sectors remains a challenge. In 2000, the Ministry of Health institutionalized the annual observance of Health Promotion Month in April to encourage the participation of community organizations and NGOs and actively advocate for personal responsibility in health by the population, including the adoption of healthy lifestyle practices and a reduction in behavioral risk factors that negatively impact health determinants. The primary health care network is slowly being reoriented, in part through improvements in physical infrastructure that are more conducive to the development of promotional activities and the availability of physical exercise equipment for use by staff and clients. Community health fairs are organized periodically with community organizations, NGOs, and corporate partners that focus on health education activities, voluntary counseling and testing for HIV/AIDS, monitoring common risk factors for noncommunicable diseases, healthy lifestyle counseling, and walks for health. Health promotion activities are reinforced at all levels by sustained, aggressive public awareness campaigns led by the Ministry of Health. A healthy community movement (HCM) initiative is being implemented in three RHA pilot sites with active community participation in the identification of priorities and partnerships with governmental and nongovernmental organizations, including international cooperation agencies. HCM components include local resource mobilization, improving social services' access and quality, developing life skills among vulnerable groups, and strengthening local competencies to enhance intervention planning, implementation, monitoring, and evaluation. The HCM initiative encompasses the development of health-promoting schools; the first phase consists of scaling up school health screening programs and building synergy with similar ongoing programs already existing in the Ministry of Education, as well as through partnerships with NGOs, corporate bodies, civil organizations, and cooperation agencies (65).

Human Resources

While neither the private nor public health sector undertake systematic workforce planning, this activity is conducted to some extent at the unit or departmental levels. Such planning usually occurs in response to the need to fill the requirements of a newly created component within an existing program and does not necessarily form part of a long-term strategy to identify and respond to future health needs. The HSRP, however, has attempted to correct this situation by developing a detailed plan to move human resources from hospitals and health institutions into community services (district health facilities and health centers). This shift supports the Ministry of Health's policy of greater adherence to primary and preventive health care and of encouraging the population at large to assume greater responsibility for individual health by adopting healthy lifestyle practices. There is the need to strengthen the dialogue in strategic human resources planning between the Ministry of Health and other health stakeholders, such as UWI; the National Institute of Higher Education, Research and Technology; and other professional bodies. The public health sector has experienced a chronic shortage of personnel—nurses in particular—since 1996 resulting in the need to contract professionals from abroad. During the review period, nurses and pharmacists were recruited from the Philippines, as were health personnel from Cuba.

Health Supplies

There is only limited medicines production capability. The National Drug Policy, which covers both the public and private sectors, has evolved into an open formulary that is a valuable drug information resource. However, health professionals do not uniformly apply the formulary protocols and guidelines in their daily practice due to infrequent revisions of the formulary and a lack of formal incentives that would encourage better compliance. In addition, there is a Vital, Essential, and Necessary (VEN) list currently purchased by the government on a needs basis when ordered by a public health facility. Purchasing of drugs is through a tendering process based on best value in therapeutic class. Since 1993, the National Insurance Property and Development Company (NIPDEC) has been contracted by the Ministry of Health to procure, store, and distribute pharmaceutical and nonpharmaceutical items on a monthly basis to public health institutions. A Comprehensive Audit Report of the Central RHA in 2000 identified several concerns, including the lack of tracking of drugs once they are dispensed to units outside the pharmacy department (excepting narcotics and other controlled substances) and the over-inflation of orders to NIPDEC in order to receive quantities as close as possible to the required amount by health facilities (66–68).

The Ministry of Health's Chronic Disease Assistance Plan provides prescription drugs free at the point of delivery to patients with specific chronic diseases, using a range of pharmaceuticals that are listed on the drug formulary. Since fiscal year 2005, the program allows universal coverage of the population eligible for benefits once they are diagnosed at a health care institution with any of the following diseases: diabetes, asthma, hypertension, arthritis, glaucoma, cancer of the prostate, mental depression, some cardiac-related diseases, and benign prostatic hyperplasia. The Ministry of Health is upgrading the information system to manage and monitor the program.

Vaccines are acquired through the PAHO Revolving Fund for Vaccine Procurement. In 2003, the Government of Trinidad and Tobago signed a memorandum of understanding with PAHO enabling the country's participation in the Regional Revolving Fund for Strategic Public Health Supplies.

Research and Technological Development in Health

The IISRP includes a plan to develop technology assessment and management capacities and systems, including the accreditation of health care facilities as a way to strengthen health information technology infrastructure and integrated information systems for improved evidence-based planning, policy development, and managerial decision-making. Specialized technology is available in both the public and private sectors. Computerized axial tomography and hemodialysis are available in both sectors, while magnetic resonance imaging is available only in the latter.

The virtual health library was launched in December 2005 as a network of health information sources universally accessible on the Internet and compatible with international databases. The library's goal is to promote universal and equitable access to health, scientific, and technical information and to facilitate the management of essential technologies for achieving equitable access to health information. Developing and strengthening the health research system to facilitate evidence-based decision-making, policy formulation, and new learning and development is one of the seven goals identified by the Vision 2020 Sub-Committee on Health, as well as an essential public health function needed to improve the performance of the public health system. The Ministry of Health plays a major governance role in health research and works in partnership with the Essential National Health Research Council. Established in 1995, the Council holds responsibility for directly developing, or stimulating the development through others, of health research policies and instruments, with special emphasis on research to support equity in health and improve health systems.

Health Sector Expenditures and Financing

There is a need to scale up coverage and increase expenditure; generate and maximize revenue; and improve quality in spending, in terms of efficiency and equity. The source of government health expenditure is general taxation revenues; a health surcharge is deducted from the monthly salaries of all wage earners; however, it is not directed to a fund for health care but to a government consolidated fund.

Total health expenditure as a percentage of GDP was 4% for the 2000–2003 period. General government expenditure on health as a percentage of total expenditure on health decreased over the 2000–2003 period from 40% to 38%, while in the private health sector expenditures increased from 60% in 2000 to 62% in 2003. General government expenditure on health as a percentage of total government expenditure was 6% over this same period. The total per capita expenditure on health at an average US$ exchange rate increased over the 2000–2003 period from US$ 235 to US$ 316; during this same period, governmental per capita expenditure on health at an average US$ exchange rate also increased from US$ 157 in 2000 to US$ 201 in 2003 (69).

Technical Cooperation and External Financing

A variety of United Nations agencies, bilateral agencies, financial institutions, and NGOs partner with the Government of Trinidad and Tobago utilizing a diversity of technical and economic mechanisms to further the development agenda set by the Vision 2020 National Strategic Plan. Two prominent international financial institutions working in the health sector are the Inter-American Development Bank and the World Bank; the first provided a loan for the development of the HSRP until 2006 and the latter for the HIV/AIDS Prevention and Control Program for the period 2004–2008. The European Union provides a grant in support of HIV/AIDS prevention activities and to ensure a well-coordinated implementation of the HIV/AIDS National Strategic Plan for the 2005–2010 period. The International Labor Organization contributes to health with its project on HIV/AIDS in the workplace (55).

References

1. Trinidad and Tobago, Ministry of Finance. Social Sector Investment Programme 2005. Vision 2020: Ensuring Our Future Survival; 2004.
2. Caribbean Commission on Health and Development; 2005.
3. United Nations. United Nations Millennium Development Goals for Trinidad and Tobago. Revised Draft Report; 2004.
4. Central Bank of Trinidad and Tobago. Annual Economic Survey; 2004.
5. Pan American Health Organization, World Health Organization. Health Statistics from the Americas; 2006.
6. Trinidad and Tobago, Ministry of Agriculture, Land and Marine Resources. Agricultural Census; 2004.
7. Trinidad and Tobago, Ministry of Planning and Development, Central Statistical Office. Pocket Digest; 2003, 2004.
8. Trinidad and Tobago, Ministry of Education. Indicators of the Education System of Trinidad and Tobago; 2005.
9. Trinidad and Tobago. Statistical Digest of the Education System; 2005.
10. Trinidad and Tobago. National Policy on Child Care; 2005.
11. Trinidad and Tobago, Office of the Attorney General and Ministry of Legal Affairs. International Convention on the

Elimination of All Forms of Discrimination against Women; 2000.

12. Trinidad and Tobago, Trinidad and Tobago Police Force, Modus Operandi Bureau. Partial Report; August 2005.

13. Rape Crisis Society of Trinidad and Tobago. Annual Reports; 2001–2004.

14. Trinidad and Tobago, Ministry of Gender Affairs. Battered Women Shelter Experience Report; 2001.

15. Pan American Health Organization, World Health Organization. Unabridged Report on the Impact of Domestic Violence on Women's Health and Family Stability in Trinidad and Tobago; 2003.

16. Trinidad and Tobago, Ministry of Planning and Development, Central Statistical Office. Annual Road Traffic Accident Report; 2004.

17. Trinidad and Tobago. Vision 2020. Poverty Alleviation and Social Services Sub-committee. Draft Final Report; 2004.

18. Caribbean Epidemiology Center, Pan American Health Organization, World Health Organization. Pilot Caribbean Behavioral Risk Factor Survey; 2004.

19. Pan American Health Organization, World Health Organization. Trinidad and Tobago Country Cooperation Strategy; 2005.

20. Gulliford MC, Mahabir D, Rocke B, Chinn S, Rona R. Overweight, obesity and skinfold thickness of children of African or Indian descent in Trinidad and Tobago. Int J Epidemiol. 2001; 30(5):989–98.

21. Simmons W. Food fortification in the English-speaking Caribbean.

22. United Nations Children's Fund. Multiple Indicator Cluster Survey. Trinidad and Tobago. Full Report; 2000.

23. Pan American Health Organization, World Health Organization. Public Health in the Americas. Conceptual Renewal Performance Assessment and Bases for Action; 2002.

24. Trinidad and Tobago, Ministry of Planning and Development, Central Statistical Office. 2000 Population and Housing Census. Preliminary Report; 2001.

25. United Nations. Globalis: An Interactive World Map. Available at: http://globalis.gvu.unu.edu. Accessed 11 April 2006.

26. Trinidad and Tobago, Ministry of Planning and Development, Central Statistical Office. Annual Statistical Digest 2001; 2005.

27. Trinidad and Tobago, Ministry of Health, National Surveillance Unit; 2005–2006.

28. Caribbean Epidemiology Center, Pan American Health Organization, World Health Organization. Reported communicable diseases: suspected and confirmed cases. Trinidad and Tobago; 2000–2005.

29. Trinidad and Tobago, Ministry of Social Development. Revised Draft National Plan of Action for Children; 2004.

30. Rajkumar W, Manohar J, Doon R, Siung-Chang A, Chang-Yen I, Monteil M. Blood lead levels in primary school children in Trinidad and Tobago. Sci Total Environ. 2006; 361 (1–3):81–7.

31. Trinidad and Tobago, Ministry of Health. Global Youth Tobacco Survey. Final Report; 2004.

32. Watson G. Analysis of the burden of mental disorders presented by adolescents in Trinidad and Tobago and their relation with family structures and environmental factors among the two main ethnic groups in the population in 2004. Port of Spain; 2005.

33. Family Planning Association of Trinidad and Tobago. Sexual Health Needs of Youth in Tobago; 2000.

34. University of the West Indies. A National Profile on Aging Report with an overview of the Health Care System in Trinidad and Tobago Country Implementation for the Integrated Health Care Response to Rapid Population Aging in Developing Countries; 2005.

35. Simeon D, Ramdath D, Chadee D, Rawlins J. Physical disability, food insecurity and nutritional status of non-institutionalized persons aged 65 and over in Trinidad.

36. Trinidad and Tobago, Ministry of Health, Health Sector Reform Programme, Community Care Development Programme; 2004.

37. Trinidad and Tobago, Ministry of Health, Population Programme Unit. Annual Report; 2004.

38. National Insurance Board of Trinidad and Tobago, Planning and Research Department. Database on employment and injury benefits claims; 2001–2005.

39. International Labor Organization. The Situation of Children in Landfill Sites and Other Worst Forms of Child Labor: A Rapid Assessment; 2002.

40. Trinidad and Tobago, Ministry of Health, Insect Vector Control Division. Statistical database; 2000–2005.

41. Caribbean Epidemiology Center, Pan American Health Organization, World Health Organization. Percentage of children under one year of age fully immunized in Trinidad and Tobago; 2006.

42. Trinidad and Tobago, Ministry of Health. Survey for helminthiasis; 2006.

43. Trinidad and Tobago, Ministry of Health, Hansen's Disease Control Unit. Annual Report; 2002–2003.

44. Caribbean Epidemiology Center, Pan American Health Organization, World Health Organization. Epidemiological Bulletin. Tuberculosis in Trinidad and Tobago; 2002–2003.

45. Trinidad and Tobago, Ministry of Health, National Surveillance Unit. Situational Analysis of National Tuberculosis Programme; 2004.

46. Trinidad and Tobago, Ministry of Health, National Surveillance Unit. HIV/AIDS Morbidity and Mortality Report; 2000–2004.

47. Trinidad and Tobago, Ministry of Health, Prevention of Mother-to-child Transmission of HIV Programme. Annual Reports; 2000–2003.

48. Trinidad and Tobago, National AIDS Coordinating Committee. National HIV/AIDS Strategic Plan 2004–2008.

49. Trinidad and Tobago, Caribbean Association for Feminist Research and Action. Situation Analysis of Commercial Sex Work in Trinidad and Tobago; 2004.

50. Trinidad and Tobago, Ministry of Health. Quarterly Data Report of HIV/AIDS Treatment; 2000–2004.

51. Pan American Health Organization. Assessment and Recommendations on Scaling-up Antiretroviral Therapy in Trinidad and Tobago at the San Fernando and Sangre Grande General Hospitals; 2005.

52. Rapid Assessment on the Antiretroviral Drug Supply System in Trinidad and Tobago; 2005.

53. Trinidad and Tobago, Ministry of Health, Venereal Disease and Yaws Division; Queens Park Counselling Centre and Clinic; Pan American Health Organization. Annual Reports; 2000–2004.

54. Trinidad and Tobago, National AIDS Coordinating Committee. Evaluation for Sexually Transmitted Infections in Trinidad and Tobago; 2005.

55. Trinidad and Tobago, National AIDS Coordinating Committee. Baseline Survey of NGOs, FBOs, CBOs involved in HIV/AIDS. Draft Report; 2006.

56. Pan American Health Organization, World Health Organization. Final Report on Republic of Trinidad and Tobago Ministry of Health. Annual Reports; 1999–2003.

57. Trinidad and Tobago, Ministry of Health, National Cancer Registry of Trinidad and Tobago. Information on cancer in Trinidad and Tobago; 2000–2004.

58. Trinidad and Tobago, Ministry of Health. No Smoking Policy: Public Health Property; 2005.

59. Trinidad and Tobago, Ministry of Health. A Policy for Creating and Maintaining Smoke-free Environment at Head Office, Ministry of Health; 2005.

60. Trinidad and Tobago, National Drug Council. Research Study on the Impact of Drugs on the Society. Available at: http://www.ndctt.com. Accessed 11 April 2006.

61. Trinidad and Tobago, National Alcohol and Drug Abuse Programme. Drug demand reduction research statistics. Available at: http://www.drugtel.org.tt. Accessed 11 April 2006.

62. Trinidad and Tobago, Ministry of Health, Occupational Health Unit. Statistical database.

63. Preliminary Report on the Oral Health Survey of School Children in Trinidad and Tobago; 2004.

64. Trinidad and Tobago, Vision 2020 Sub-committee on Health. Draft Report; 2005.

65. Trinidad and Tobago, Ministry of Health. Report on the Achievements of Health Promotion, Trinidad and Tobago; 2002.

66. Report of the Committee Appointed by the Honorable Minister of Health. Procurement and Distribution of Pharmaceuticals and Related Supplies; 1997.

67. Trinidad and Tobago, Ministry of Health, Central Regional Health Authority. Comprehensive Audit Report; 2000.

68. Trinidad and Tobago, Ministry of Health, Health Sector Reform Programme. Pharmaceutical Services Reform Report; 2003.

69. World Health Organization. World Health Report 2006: Working Together for Health. Geneva: WHO; 2006.

TURKS
AND CAICOS
ISLANDS

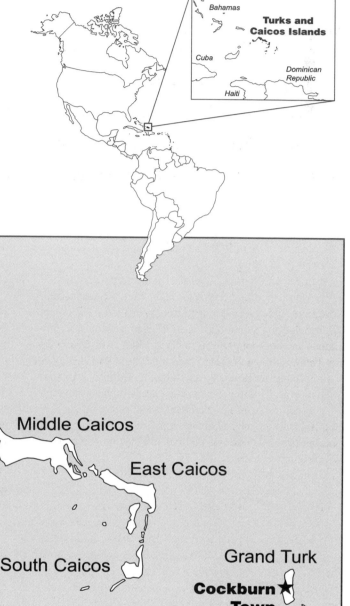

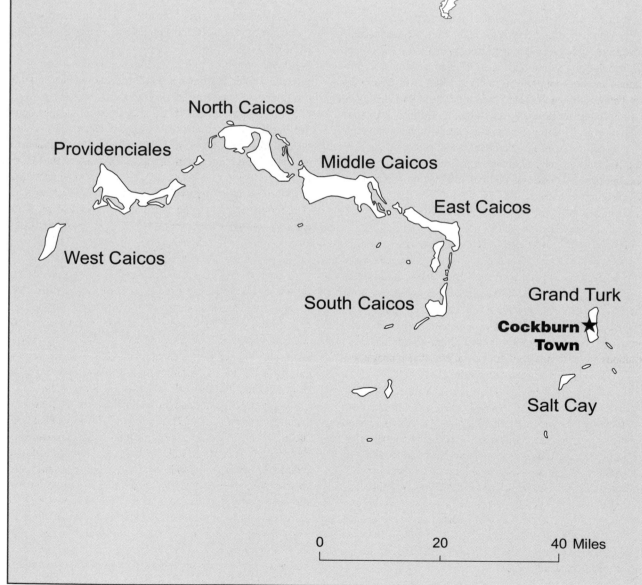

North Caicos

Providenciales

Middle Caicos

West Caicos

East Caicos

South Caicos

Grand Turk

Cockburn
Town ★

Salt Cay

0   20   40 Miles

GENERAL CONTEXT AND HEALTH DETERMINANTS

The total landmass of the territory is 430 km². The archipelago is located to the southeast of the Bahamas and north of Hispaniola. Because of the Turks and Caicos' geographic layout, communication and transportation are important issues. Air transportation between the main islands of Grand Turk, Providenciales, North Caicos, Middle Caicos, South Caicos, and Salt Cay is regular but costly. There is a ferry system between Grand Turk and Salt Cay and between Middle Caicos and North Caicos. Small boats also provide inter-island services. The telecommunication links through telephone and electronic mail greatly facilitate the communication process.

Social, Political, and Economic Determinants

Cockburn Town, on Grand Turk, is the capital and the seat of government. The Governor represents the Queen of England; the Premier, appointed by the Governor, is the head of government. The legislature consists of a unicameral Legislative Council. Government ministries are directed by a minister (political) and a permanent secretary (administrative). Quasi-governmental institutions are often managed through an executive management team led by a general manager or director.

According to the Turks and Caicos Department of Economic Planning and Statistics, the estimated population of the territory in 2005 was 30,602. It was evenly distributed between males and females and mainly concentrated on the island of Providenciales, the commercial and business center, which had 22,296 residents, compared to 13,021 in 2001. Grand Turk had a population of 5,186 in 2005. Parrot Cay, which up to 1999 was uninhabited, had a population of 60 persons in 2005 due to the construction of a luxury hotel, which in turn provided employment and prompted the need for housing and related facilities. Figure 1 shows the population distribution of the Turks and Caicos Islands, by age and sex, for 1990 and 2005.

The term "Belonger status" refers to any person who was born in the Turks and Caicos or who was born outside the islands but has at least one parent who was born in Turks and Caicos. It also includes those who are born outside the islands but are adopted by someone with Belonger status and those granted residency status by the territories' Governor. Belongers accounted for 37.4% of the population in 2005, which represents a 2.6% increase over 2004.

Those who do not meet Belonger requirements (i.e., are not citizens by parentage or birth or through naturalization) are called non-Belongers. The population is comprised mainly of non-Belongers who accounted for approximately 62.6% of the total population in 2005, representing a 17.2% increase over 2004. The growth in the non-Belonger population is due mainly to immigration by non-nationals to the islands for employment purposes. Non-Belongers with illegal immigration status pose a significant challenge for the health system—particularly as regards the prevention and control of communicable diseases—since they usually seek to avoid using government health services for fear of possible deportation.

The five principal activities, which together contributed approximately 75% to the GDP, were hotels and restaurants; construction; transport, storage, and communications; real estate, renting, and other business activities; and financial intermediation. Tourism was the mainstay of economic growth, followed by fishing and offshore financial services. Although tourism is beneficial to the country, it also has brought numerous social challenges related to drug trafficking, substance abuse, and illegal immigration.

Over the last few decades, the archipelago has experienced a rapid economic growth of 9% per annum. This growth has been fuelled by large inflows of foreign capital, labor, and entrepreneurial skills. Following a 7.4% fall in 2002, output of hotels and restaurants surged to 15.5% in 2005 as tourist arrivals increased by about the same rate. Tourists' expenditures are more evident in the value-added growth of restaurant activity, which was 23.7% in 2004 and another 15.0% in 2005. The output of the financial intermediation sector leaped to 24.4% in 2004 and another 18.8% in 2005, reflecting an increased demand for financial services. As businesses and households took advantage of favorable lending terms, loans and advances to clients reached nearly US$ 400 million in 2005.

FIGURE 1. Population structure, by age and sex, Turks and Caicos Islands, 1990 and 2005.

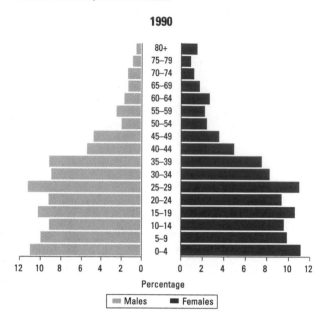

1990

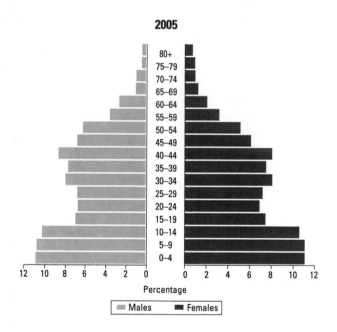

2005

mands on the government to expand both the public health infrastructure and health services, mainly to provide for those who cannot afford private health care services.

Three industries—hotels and restaurants, public administration and defense, and construction—accounted for 41.4% of the employed population. In 2005, 81% of the employed population was in the private sector compared to 11% in the government sector; 8% are self-employed.

There was a decrease in the unemployed labor force from 2004 (9.9%) to 2005 (8.0%). Though still relatively high, the rate was reflective of and consistent with the slight economic upturn that occurred in 2004 (11.4% growth) and 2005 (14%).

The literacy rate in 2001 was estimated at 97.5%. Education for all children of school age is mandatory and free in public schools. In the school year 2005–2006, there were 82% males and 80.3% females, with an overall enrollment of 81.1%. These rates declined from those of the 2004–2005 school year, in which overall primary school enrollment was 83.4% (males 83.8% and female 83.0%). During this time, the gender gap in primary school enrollment rates is apparent, with rates for females being slightly lower than those of their male counterparts. Gender parity in secondary enrollment showed a male-female ratio of 100:97 for the 2005–2006 school year; it had been 100:92 for 2004–2005.

It is important to note that there has been an overall increase in secondary enrollment over the years. In contrast to primary and secondary education, female enrollment in tertiary education surpassed that of men. The gender gap was clearly reversed at the tertiary level when the male-female ratio was 100:206 in 2002 and 100:302 in 2003.

In 2001, most households had private catchments of water (68%) or water piped into their dwellings (22%). In 2001, there were more households with water-closet cesspit/septic tanks (68%) compared to 1999 (56%). Fewer households had pit latrines in 2001 (28%) than in 1999 (34%). However, as the number of households increased during the 1999–2001 period, the percentage of households without sanitation facilities grew (from 1.3% in 1999 to 4% in 2001).

The Turks and Caicos Islands face a variety of environmental inadequacies as regards solid waste disposal, liquid waste management, water quality control, food safety, and institutional hygiene. Solid waste management remains a major challenge on Providenciales, as does pest infestation in areas of the islands where garbage collection systems are poor. The proper inspection of imported food presents difficulties for port health services due to the lack of a port health officer. This situation has led to food inspections being conducted once foodstuffs already have been stored in warehouses or placed on the shelves of retail establishments. In many instances, contaminated or expired food items have been seized from these facilities and destroyed. On occasion, however, this action occurred too late to prevent consumers from purchasing these items. Generally speaking, food handlers

Since 2003, positive per capita GDP growth rates have been recorded. These continued through 2005, when there was a 5.5% growth over 2004 in current market prices and 2.3% in constant (2000) market prices. This was equivalent to US$ 18,636 and US$ 15,683, per capita in current and constant (2000) market prices, respectively. This economic growth placed increasing de-have not received training in proper hygiene and food handling techniques.

Demographics, Mortality, and Morbidity

In 2004–2005, there were more births of females than of males, when compared to other years when this trend was reversed. Census data for 2001 estimated life expectancy at 77.5 years. Of the 318 births which occurred in 2005, about 85% (270) were registered. In 2000–2002, the leading causes of death from defined causes and the corresponding number of deaths were: hypertensive diseases (25); HIV/AIDS (16); accidental drowning and submersion (the majority of deaths were due to illegal immigrants entering on sloops) (11); and diabetes (8). There were 213 deaths from defined causes during the 2001–2005 period. The crude death rate was higher in 2005 for males (2.10) than for females (1.37). There were no maternal deaths during the 2001–2005 period. In 2001, the age-specific fertility rate for the population aged 30–34 was 7.2 births per 1,000 population; the total fertility rate was 3.1 for females of childbearing age (15–45 years).

HEALTH OF POPULATION GROUPS

Children under 5 Years Old

The Primary Health Care Annual Report for 2005 indicated that the majority of infants seen at 3 months were partially breast-fed—that is, mostly being given formula with some breast-feeding. Of the 1,563 children seen in child health services in 2005, 68 were overweight and two were below normal weight.

During the 2001–2005 period, there were 1,255 live births. Thirteen deaths occurred in the age group of 0–4 years. Of these, 7 deaths (5 boys and 2 girls) were under age 1. Asphyxia and slow fetal growth were the major contributors to death. There were two deaths due to HIV/AIDS in the under-1 age group. Intestinal infections and acute respiratory infections accounted for 59% of hospital discharge diagnoses for infants.

There were 6 deaths (3 boys and 3 girls) in the 1–4 age group. Causes of death were HIV/AIDS and external causes. Intestinal and acute respiratory infections and external causes accounted for 47.7% of hospital discharge diagnoses. Of the 371 cases of gastroenteritis that were reported in 2004, 132 were in the under-5-year-old population.

Children 5–9 Years Old

There were seven deaths in this age group in the period 2001–2005. Of the six deaths known by cause, two were from HIV/AIDS, and one each was due to congenital heart diseases, intestinal infectious diseases, drowning, and acute respiratory infections. The most frequent hospital discharge diagnoses were respiratory illness, intestinal infectious diseases, appendicitis, and hernia.

Adolescents 10–14 and 15–19 Years Old

During the 2001–2005 period, there were two adolescent deaths in this age range, both from external causes. The leading hospital discharge diagnoses were external causes, appendicitis, diseases of the nervous system, and asthma. Complications of pregnancy accounted for 8% of all discharges in the 15–19-year-old age group. Of the total number of births in 2002 and 2003, 10.0% and 13.5%, respectively, were to teenagers ages 15–19. Teenagers accounted for 12% and 13% of medical abortions in 2004 and 2005, respectively. The reporting of abortions is not a requirement in the Turks and Caicos Islands, and the only data available on medical abortions reflect those performed in hospitals.

Adults 20–59 Years Old

During the 2001–2005 period, there were 65 deaths in this age group. The leading causes of death were diseases of the circulatory system, injuries and external causes, malignant neoplasms, communicable diseases, and suicide. Data for the 2000–2002 period showed that the leading causes of death were HIV/AIDS (12), hypertensive diseases (6), and accidental drowning and submersion (5).

Diseases of the circulatory system accounted for 30% of all hospital discharge diagnoses. Other causes included endocrine, nutritional, and metabolic diseases; external causes; and complications of pregnancy. Thirty-one abortions occurred in the under-40-year-old age group.

Older Adults 60 Years Old and Older

The 2001 census showed that there were 2,065 persons in this age group, representing 10.4% of the total population. A growth in the elderly population has implications for increased spending on health care and treatment at home and abroad due to chronic diseases. In 2001–2005, there were 125 deaths in this age group. Cardiorespiratory arrest, ischemic heart diseases, diabetes, and malignant neoplasms were the major contributors to mortality.

The principal hospital discharge diagnoses for this age group were hypertension, diabetes mellitus, diseases of pulmonary circulation, cerebrovascular diseases, other diseases of the digestive system, injuries, and acute respiratory infections.

The Family

In 2001, there were 7,254 households, and 30.8% were headed by females. The average income for male-headed households was US$ 30,461, compared to US$ 21,916 for female-headed households.

At the end of 2005, the Social Development Department registered 77 children who had lost either one parent (45 children) or both parents (32 children) to HIV/AIDS. While most were being cared for by extended families, there were several who entered

679

the foster care system and whose upbringing may be negatively impacted by this situation.

In 2005, the Primary Health Care Department of the Ministry of Health reported that most clinic attendees stated that they were unable to breast-feed exclusively due to the necessity of returning to work. Maternal grants (a one-time payment of US$ 400) are provided to all mothers for each live birth when they produce a birth certificate to the National Insurance Board, which provides a variety of social security services to all employed and self-employed persons through compulsory participation. Maternity allowances (60% of average weekly earnings for a 12-week leave period) are awarded to those who have satisfied contribution requirements.

Persons with Disabilities

In 2001, the Population and Housing Census estimated that there were 337 persons living with a disability. Of these, 28.5% had a visual disability, 18.7% a mobility disability, 15.7% a hearing disability, 8.9% mental retardation, 8.3% a speech disability, and 19.9% reported other types of disability.

HEALTH CONDITIONS AND PROBLEMS

COMMUNICABLE DISEASES

Vector-borne Diseases

In the period 2001–2005, there were four imported cases of **malaria**. There was one imported case of **dengue** in 2005.

Vaccine-preventable Diseases

There were no cases of **measles**, **rubella**, **diphtheria**, **pertussis**, **neonatal tetanus**, or **tetanus** during the 2001–2005 review period. Annual mop-up campaigns are conducted in schools and work sites to identify and vaccinate those in the population over age 5 who have missed routine vaccination and previous campaigns. In 2001, the DTP-HB/Hib pentavalent combination vaccine (primary doses) was introduced into the routine child health schedule, with the first of three dosages to be administered at 6 weeks of age. In 2005, the schedule was changed to commence at 2 months. Children were immunized against measles, mumps, and rubella (MMR); diptheria, pertussis/whooping cough, and tetanus (DPT); poliomyelitis (OPV); and tuberculosis (BCG).

The vaccination coverage for administered antigens for the period 2001–2005 was maintained above 90%. For 2005, vaccination coverage for antigens stood as follows: DPT3, hepatitis B, and Hib (95%); OPV3 (97%); and BCG (100%).

Intestinal Infectious Diseases

In 2001–2005, there were 592 cases of **gastroenteritis** in children under 5 years of age and 675 cases in persons over 5 years

old. In the same period, there were 201 confirmed cases of food-borne diseases, the majority caused by *Salmonella*, *Shigella*, and **ciguatera poisoning**.

Chronic Communicable Diseases

In the 2001–2005 period, there were four new cases reported of **Hansen's disease** (leprosy). Of the 21 cases of **tuberculosis** during this period, 7 were coinfected with HIV/AIDS. Between 2003 and 2005, there were 29 cases of **hepatitis B**.

Acute Respiratory Infections

Primary health care data for 2003–2005 showed 4,080 reported cases of acute respiratory infections in children under age 5. Notable increases in these infections normally occur in the months of October through March.

HIV/AIDS and Other Sexually Transmitted Infections

HIV and AIDS remained a challenge for the Turks and Caicos Islands over the 2001–2005 period. The first case was diagnosed in 1985 and up to 2005, there were a total of 732 HIV-positive individuals. The principal mode of transmission is heterosexual. In the period 2004–2005, there were 41 newly reported HIV cases (21 males and 20 females). The majority of these cases were among nonresident work permit applicants, and most of these individuals no longer reside on the islands. The island of Providenciales, which has the largest population, accounted for more than 50% of the HIV-positive cases. Although the data were not disaggregated by sex and age, the trend tended toward more males than females testing positive. Given that the persons living with AIDS were of various nationalities, prevention and care initiatives were challenged to adequately respond to language issues and cultural beliefs, address stigma and discrimination issues, and introduce measures to discourage a general relapse or complacency about minimizing risk behaviors.

The HIV/AIDS surveillance system also faced a number of challenges. Chief among these is a mistrust by some individuals regarding the system's ability to ensure confidentiality given the islands' small population size. This fear resulted in some persons refusing to be tested or in their seeking testing abroad.

There were 21 deaths due to AIDS during the 2000–2003 period and five deaths in 2004–2005. This decrease in case numbers was due to the introduction of an improved treatment and care program and scaled-up access to antiretroviral drugs commencing in January 2003.

The number of reported cases of **syphilis** rose from 13 in 2003 to 35 in 2005. The rise in numbers was attributed to increased detection in persons undergoing testing to acquire work permits.

Other Communicable Diseases

Over a three-year period, **acute hemorrhagic conjunctivitis** contributed substantially to morbidity with 842 cases in 2003,

49 in 2004, and 124 in 2005. The etiology for the outbreak in 2003 was suspected to be a Coxsackie virus but this was unconfirmed. **Influenza-like illness** is one of the most frequently reported health conditions, with 2,809 cases being reported during the 2001–2005 period.

NONCOMMUNICABLE DISEASES

These diseases are managed as part of the primary level of health care services offered at health centers and hospitals. In 2001–2005, the majority of patients were seen for conditions related to **hypertension, diabetes** and related complications, and **malignant neoplasms**. This trend was supported by morbidity data that confirmed hypertension (1,367), diabetes (499), **heart disease** (174), **obesity** (84), and cancer (39) as the leading health problems reported by the health services in 2004.

OTHER HEALTH PROBLEMS OR ISSUES

Mental Health and Addictions

A psychiatrist and mental health nurse provide mental health-related services to the inhabited islands at the primary, secondary, and tertiary levels, and make patient referrals to the Bahamas for care as needed. Data available for 2003 showed that 76 patients were seen, of which 64.5% (49) were males and 35.5% (27) were females. Most of the patients were seen on Grand Turk (27.6%) and Providenciales (21%).

The data also showed that 63% of those seen were in the 20-to-49-year-old age group, while only 9.2% were 19 years of age or younger. The main diagnoses were schizophrenia (28.9%), substance abuse (15.8%), psychosis not specified (7.9%), seizure disorders with psychological problems (7.9%), bipolar affective disorder (6.6%), and adjustment disorder with depressive or anxiety symptoms (6.6%). Visits to mental health clients in the prison population are conducted on a regular basis. Challenges affecting the delivery of mental health services during the 2001–2005 review period included outdated legislation and policies and insufficient human resources to guide services delivery.

Oral Health

Dental health services are provided on all six of the main inhabited islands. There is a school dental program on Providenciales. There were no x-ray machines on the other islands; therefore, no surgical extractions and root canal treatments were carried out.

Similarly, no orthodontic and prosthetic services were offered, as there was no dental laboratory, dental technician, or orthodontist consultant. There was also no dental assistant in the program. As a result, dental nurses are being underutilized, and this adversely affects services delivery.

RESPONSE OF THE HEALTH SECTOR

Health Policies and Plans

The government recognizes health as a basic human right and works to ensure equal access for its residents to health care as needed. The 2005 Five-year Strategic Health Plan takes into consideration the overall vision and mission of the Ministry of Health, provides a framework upon which the Ministry's various departments can develop and implement equitable health programs, and is evaluated and revised on an annual basis.

The 2005 Five-year Strategic Health Plan also serves as the framework to guide and direct the delivery of equitable health services. It includes a restructuring of the Ministry of Health in order to strengthen health planning, systems development, financial management, essential national health research, health promotion, and capacity to regulate public and private health sector activities. Under the Plan, the post of Director of Health Services was created, and the incumbent has overall responsibility for the health status of the country and for developing and directing health policies in the Ministry of Health. The Permanent Secretary chairs the Senior Management Team and is responsible for personnel and fiscal management functions.

Organization of the Health System

The Ministry of Health is responsible for the provision of efficient and effective preventive and curative health care through the health departments. The Ministry's activities are carried out in partnership with the community, the private sector, and overseas providers.

The private health sector is limited mainly to outpatient care and is focused on general practice, although some secondary care services are also offered. The public hospital network consists of Grand Turk Hospital and the Myrtle Rigby Health Complex, located on Providenciales. These are the only two hospitals which offer secondary health care services and some tertiary care services. The Grand Turk Hospital has 21 acute care beds and 10 chronic care beds for geriatric patients. The Myrtle Rigby Health Complex has 10 acute care beds. There is an operating theater in both facilities with full surgical care capabilities to respond to major emergencies and undertake all elective procedures except for those requiring postoperative intensive care, or specialized equipment or personnel not available locally. Both hospitals have maternity units for cases not requiring advanced neonatal care as determined by an antenatal risk assessment. The hospitals provide secondary health care in the areas of internal medicine, pediatrics, general surgery, obstetrics and gynecology, and anesthesiology. Some urological services are provided through collaboration with a private sector urologist. In 2005, there were four private clinics, seven primary health care medical centers, and seven family planning clinics.

Using Research to Assure Health Equity in Turks and Caicos

In an attempt to deliver health services equitably to every resident on the islands, the Government of the Turks and Caicos has crafted the 2005–2009 Five-Year Strategic Health Plan. As part of this plan, the National Epidemiology and Research Unit has been created, whose dual mission is to bolster disease surveillance efforts and respond more effectively to disease outbreaks. To this end, it conducts communicable disease workshops, coordinates efforts with other governmental entities, and informs the development of national health policies.

Public Health Services

The primary health care strategy continued to undergo reorientation to strengthen specific programs geared towards health promotion and management and disease prevention and control. There are primary health care clinics on the six main inhabited islands, and clients are treated regardless of their ability to pay. Primary health care services focus on maternal and child health, dental health, chronic noncommunicable diseases (diabetes and hypertension), communicable diseases, school health programs, safe food handling, and, to a limited extent, nutrition.

In 2005, the seasonal influenza vaccine was introduced among health care workers. The disease surveillance team and the National Epidemiology and Research Unit of the Ministry of Health conducted several workshops geared at completing the development of the national communicable diseases surveillance manual and stepping up the coordination and response to communicable disease outbreaks. Training provided by the Ministry of Health focused on promoting good hygiene practices in the hotel and hospitality industries and contributed to a reduction in the number of foodborne diseases in 2005 compared to previous years.

As regards services for those living with HIV, the government has committed itself to scaling up access to antiretroviral medications by allocating the necessary funds in the national budget for their procurement for all Belongers and non-Belongers with legal status requiring such treatment. These drugs are purchased through the National AIDS Program of the Ministry of Health of the Bahamas based on a contractual arrangement which also allows the Turks and Caicos Islands to benefit from HIV/AIDS laboratory services and staff training in that country. At the end of 2005, some 70 individuals were receiving antiretroviral therapy, and another 12 accessed treatment in the United States through the University of Miami's research program.

In 2005, six sites provided access for the population to prevention-of-mother-to-child-transmission services. Voluntary counseling and testing (VCT) are available at all clinics and public laboratories. HIV testing and counseling are offered on an informed basis as a matter of routine to all women attending prenatal clinics. During 2000–2005, four pregnant women tested positive. Due to the nature of their immigration status, migrant women may not access these services at an early stage out of fear

of being deported. Thirty-five VCT providers were trained in 2005 as part of ongoing efforts to scale up these services and improve their quality. Several additional services are available for persons living with HIV/AIDS. Programs such as Buddy Support and People for Positive Action as well as the Center of Love and Hope (an AIDS hospice) lend support, supervise and monitor drug adherence, and provide information and links to additional community resources. The Social Development Department provides counseling services and welfare grants in addition to foster care services to children orphaned by HIV/AIDS or others needing assistance to meet their basic needs.

During 2001–2005, staff were assigned to implement programs for food safety, water quality, liquid and solid waste management, vector and pest control, institutional hygiene, veterinary public health, occupational health and safety, cemetery management, vaccine-preventable childhood illnesses case investigations, and premises inspection/residential sanitation.

With the increasing volume in air and sea traffic and the persistent threat of hurricanes, the Turks and Caicos Islands are vulnerable to disasters and mass casualties. The health sector, in collaboration with other government and nongovernmental agencies, increased its capacity to manage major emergencies and decrease the impact of disasters. In 2005, staff from health facilities on Grand Turk and Providenciales participated in aircraft simulation exercises. A plan for improvements in the management of disasters was also prepared; it included the conducting of mass casualty training exercises involving first responders from all sectors. During the 2001–2005 review period, the Ministry of Health created an Emergency Preparedness and Response Unit to coordinate disaster responses.

Individual Care Services

The Ministry of Health is responsible for providing affordable and efficient health services to all residents. However, the fee structure for Turks and Caicos nationals (Belongers) is less than that for non-Belongers.

Accessibility to secondary and tertiary care services is difficult in emergency situations due to the geographic dispersion of some of the islands and cays. At present, the government holds the principal market share in providing hospital services to the population even though many individuals travel abroad for diagnostic and hospital care.

The Medical Treatment Abroad Program (MTA) continues to be the single largest recurrent health expenditure line item. Patient travel costs and overseas treatment accounted for approximately 7.3% of the government's recurrent expenditure in the 2004–2005 budget. Treatment may be accessed in the Bahamas and Jamaica, even though the majority of individuals prefer to seek treatment in the United States. In 2005, a total of 456 patients were referred abroad resulting in 730 treatment episodes (patient visits). Of these, 302 had one visit, and the remainder had two or more visits. Twenty-seven cases of cancer were referred abroad for treatment, which accounted for approximately 50% of the total treatment-abroad expenditure. Subsequently, the government introduced a number of strategies to increase the effectiveness of case management for patients referred abroad. These include improvements in monitoring the length of hospital stay and the need for follow-up visits, as well as negotiating for larger discounts for the medical services provided and with third-party administrators for management fees to be placed at fixed rates, as opposed to being based on percentage of savings.

The Visiting Medical Consultant Program continued to be of substantial value for patients in need of subspecialist medical care in the areas of orthopedic surgery, ophthalmology, neurology, dermatology, nephrology, and audiology.

In 2002, a patient satisfaction survey conducted for Grand Turk Hospital showed the quality of services and overall rating to be very high. The Myrtle Rigby Health Complex on Providenciales introduced a system of triaging, in which priority outpatients were given a red card to ensure prompt attention to their health needs. An appointment system also has been set up to reduce the outpatients' waiting time.

Two laboratories are operated by the public sector within the hospital facilities, and there is one privately operated laboratory on Providenciales. Diagnostic services are limited to basic hematology, chemistry, microbiology, and serology. All histopathology and cytology specimens are sent abroad for analysis. Basic radiological, ultrasound, mammography, CT scan, colposcopic, and endoscopic procedures are performed locally. There are two blood banks which operate on a donor-directed or donor-replacement system; both are characterized by a limited blood storage capacity and the unavailability of blood components. The types of surgical procedures that may be performed locally, therefore, are limited by the availability of blood.

There is one dialysis unit on Grand Turk; it is highly dependent upon the blood banks; in 2005 it served 10 chronic renal failure patients. Five of these patients flew three times weekly from Providenciales to Grand Turk for dialysis treatment.

In 2005, the first mobile dental unit on Providenciales was launched at Clement Howell High School. This unit provides preventive and curative services to schoolchildren. There is an ongoing project on the islands of North Caicos and South Caicos in which children are examined and given appointments to dental clinics for conventional and specialized treatments.

Geriatric care services are provided on Grand Turk and South Caicos. The Grand Turk facility houses 14 clients, and the Wellness Center on South Caicos accommodates six in-patients.

Health Promotion

Health promotion activities included such targeted initiatives as the Rapport Youth Peer Education program and the Creole Peer Education program, as well as the development of public service announcements and media campaigns.

Human Resources

In 2005, there were 14 general physicians (7 public and 7 private), 7 dentists (2 public and 5 private), and 16 specialist physicians (14 public and 2 private). Around 80% of the professional staff employed are foreign nationals on contract. Staff turnover is high, since most contracted staff leave the islands after a stay of two or three years.

The rapidly growing population fuels the demand for health care personnel. Government efforts to provide incentives to nationals to return to work in the public sector upon graduation through the granting of scholarships have not reduced the need for international recruitment. At the same time, many trained health care staff have been lost through nonrenewal of their contracts. The constant turnover of professional staff has greatly affected continuity in patient-health care professional relationships and treatment regimens. The Ministry of Health has a small pool of staff upon which it draws for succession planning as a result of this staff turnover. Despite this, a number of health personnel posts remain vacant for long periods of time, thus affecting the delivery of health care services.

In the period 2001–2005, based on per capita needs, there was a shortage of public health nurses and midwives. Nurses are the most vulnerable to migration pressures due to high regional and international demands for their services. Nevertheless, the nursing staff constituted the largest portion of health care workers on the islands. In 2005, the expenditure on human resources represented about 45% of public health sector expenditure. In 2005, the government prepared a Strategic Plan for the Development of Nursing Services as an integral component of the overall strategic plan for human resources development in the health services area.

Health Supplies

Frequent turnover of health professionals has also affected the area of pharmacy, since prescribing habits by physicians tend to be influenced by cultural beliefs and background. This has led some professionals to not prescribe certain drugs even if they form part of the approved national formulary and are widely available. At the same time, the geographic spread of the Turks and Caicos results in long-distance supervision of pharmacists, as there are only two trained pharmacists to cover the entire island population. Pharmaceutical drugs are available in the public sector free of cost for schoolchildren and those over age 55 and for a nominal cost to the rest of the population.

The rotavirus and influenza vaccines were introduced into the Expanded Program on Immunization during the 2001–2005 period.

Research and Technological Development in Health

The National Epidemiology and Research Unit was created in 2005 as part of the restructuring component of the Ministry of Health's Five-year Strategic Health Plan. It is headed by a National Epidemiologist/Chief Medical Officer to enhance disease surveillance and disease outbreak response and to support research activities related to health policies development. In addition, a National Research Committee was created and Ministry of Health staff received training in research ethics. The Ministry continued its consultations with the Caribbean Health Research Council for the establishment of an ethics review board and committee.

Health Sector Expenditures and Financing

Government expenditure (both recurrent and capital) on health services increased in the 2001–2005 period. In 2001–2002, the recurrent expenditure on health was 19% of the total government recurrent expenditure. In the 2003–2004 fiscal year, recurrent expenditure on health was US$ 17,285,202 (per capita expenditure of US$ 790).

In 2005, the Ministry of Health was allocated US$ 19.6 million, which represented 15.9% of the 2005–2006 recurrent expenditure budget. Actual expenditure for the 2005–2006 fiscal year for all health departments (inclusive of environmental health, but excluding the Ministry of Health headquarters) was US$ 27.2 million, with 46.3% and 29.6% of this corresponding to the MTA and human resources, respectively.

The factors contributing to rising health services expenditures included rapid population growth, the introduction of additional secondary and tertiary care services, and increased demands for medical supplies, medications, and staff. The government contin-

ued to provide 100% of the recurrent expenditure for HIV/ AIDS treatment. The increase in expenditure on the MTA was the single most important contributing factor to the general increase in government expenditure on health. In 2001, the MTA expenditure was US$ 6.4 million, with one catastrophic case costing US$ 1.5 million. In 2003, expenditure on primary health care services was estimated at US$ 4 million, while that spent on secondary and tertiary care was US$ 13.5 million. The treatment-at-home program and better enforcement of the MTA policy achieved the objective of reducing the total government expenditure on health services.

The Turks and Caicos' public health services charge user fees in a system in which fees for non-Belongers are much higher than those paid by Belongers. This particularly affects access for non-Belongers to secondary care services. Some categories of users are exempt from these fees: adults over age 55, welfare recipients, the economically indigent, prisoners, schoolchildren of Turks and Caicos nationals under age 18, government employees, and contract workers and their dependents.

Private sector health services are financed by out-of-pocket payments from clients or through private health insurance. In 2005, it was estimated that 20% of the population had private health insurance while the rest of the population was covered by the Ministry of Health or through out-of-pocket expenditure.

Technical Cooperation and External Financing

The Ministry of Health developed various partnerships to improve the delivery of health care services through community participation. These include collaborations with the National Kidney Foundation in the development of a dialysis unit on Providenciales and with the National Cancer Society for the procurement of a mammogram machine and the provision of mammography services at the Myrtle Rigby Health Complex. Other sustained partnerships included those with the Turks and Caicos AIDS Foundation and the Turks and Caicos Cancer Foundation.

The Ministry of Health also continued its collaborations with the Pan American Health Organization and procured the rotavirus and influenza vaccines through the PAHO Revolving Fund. Other key subregional and international partners included the Caribbean Epidemiology Center; Caribbean Community; European Union; Global Fund to Fight AIDS, Tuberculosis, and Malaria; and the Clinton Foundation.

UNITED STATES
OF AMERICA

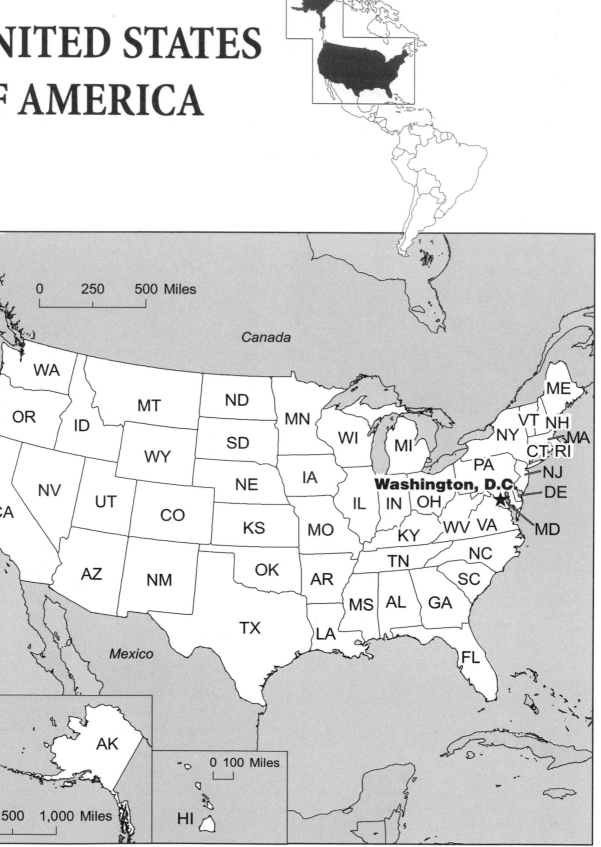

Canada

0   250   500 Miles

WA

OR   ID   MT   ND   MN   ME

WY   SD   WI   MI   VT NH

NV   UT   NE   IA   NY   MA

CA   CO   IL   IN   OH   PA   CT RI

KS   MO   KY   WV VA   NJ

AZ   NM   OK   AR   TN   NC   DE

TX   MS   AL   GA   SC   MD

LA   FL

Washington, D.C

Mexico

AK

0   500   1,000 Miles

0 100 Miles

HI

Throughout the 1990s and early 2000s, the United States experienced economic growth, although inequalities in earnings also widened in those years. Summary health indicators improved, but health differences between population groups persisted. The age structure of the population continued to change during this period, which shifted the population's health needs and the provision of health services.

GENERAL CONTEXT AND HEALTH DETERMINANTS

Macroeconomic, Political, and Social Issues

In 2003, about half the population in the United States lived in large metropolitan areas and only 20% lived in micropolitan areas (smaller urban areas with an urban core of at least 10,000 but less than 50,000) or in rural counties. This distribution is far from static, however. In fiscal year 2003 some 40 million persons (about 14% of the total population) moved, although most did so for only short distances. Non-Hispanic Whites moved less (12%) than either Blacks or Hispanics (around 18%). (See Figure 1 for the country's population structure.)

The country's real gross domestic product (GDP) grew by 37.6% from 1995 to 2005 (Figure 2), despite an eight-month recession in 2001. The percentage of the population living in poverty declined from 13.5% in 1990 to 11.3% in 2000, but increased thereafter, reaching 12.6% in 2005.

Female-headed households with children (a subgroup of all female-headed households) are one of the groups most vulnerable to poverty. The poverty rate for this subgroup followed a trend similar to that of the overall poverty rate during this period, but at a much higher level—36.2% of these families were below the official poverty line in 2005. This "feminization" of poverty has been partially linked to differences in the earnings of employed men and women. In 2005, women with paid work earned considerably less than men—men 15 years old and older earned a median US$ 34,349 per year, whereas women earned only US$ 23,074, or 33% less than men, in part because women tend to be concentrated in lower-paid occupations. In 2005, 20% of working women were in service occupations, while only 13% of men were in these lower-paid jobs; similarly, 22% of working women were in office and administrative support positions compared to 6% of their male counterparts.

Hispanics and Blacks also are among the groups most vulnerable to poverty. Poverty rates for these groups followed trends similar to the overall poverty rate during this period, but at a much higher level; 2005 poverty rates for these groups were 21.8% and 24.9%, respectively.

As the GDP grew in recent decades, so did inequalities in personal income distributions, as measured by the Gini index. Although there have been intervals of stability or decline in the Gini index, such as in 1993–1998, the long-term trend since the mid-1970s has been upward. Over the past 10 years, the Gini index has risen 4.2%, from 0.450 to 0.469.

This widening of the earnings gap has been linked to structural changes in the U.S. labor market, whereby more highly skilled persons in the upper income percentiles experienced real gains in wages, while less-skilled workers experienced real wage losses. This has been explained by an industrial shift towards technical services and retail sales, as well as more frequent use of temporary workers, a proportional drop in union membership, a real-value decline of the minimum wage, and increased global competition and immigration.

In 2005, 16% of the population, or 46.6 million people, had no health insurance coverage, up from 14.2% in 2000. Among those living in poverty, 32% had no health coverage, despite the existence of government health insurance targeting the poor, such as Medicaid. Blacks, Asian/Pacific Islanders, Hispanics, and foreign-born persons had a relatively high risk of lacking health insurance coverage. These groups, except for Asian/Pacific Islanders, also had elevated rates of poverty. The lowest health insurance coverage was in the South and the West, both at around 18%, and in the Midwest and the Northeast with coverage levels between 12% and 14%. Not surprisingly, the regions with the highest poverty rates also had the lowest coverage.

The proportion of children without health insurance declined in the early 2000s, falling from 11.9% in 2000 to 11.2%, or 8.3 million children, in 2005. A decline in health insurance coverage by private insurance was more than offset by an increase in Medicaid coverage; 19% of children in poverty were uninsured.

Demographics, Morbidity, and Mortality

The country's population grew 13% in the 1990s, rising from 249 million people in 1990 to 281 million in 2000 and 296 million in 2005. Some of this growth was due to immigration: in 2000, 11% of the population (about 30 million people) was foreign-born,

FIGURE 1. Population structure, by age and sex, United States of America, 2005.

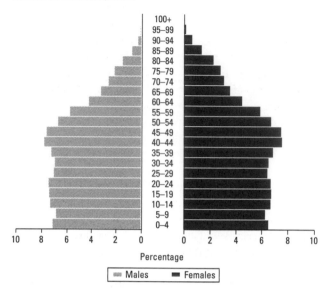

FIGURE 2. Gross domestic product, annual growth (%), United States of America, 1994–2004.

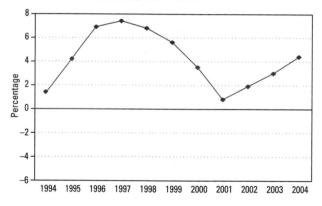

which represents a substantial increase from the 8% figure (almost 20 million persons) in 1990. Many of these immigrants came from Latin America. In fact, throughout the 1990s, the proportion of Hispanics in the country's population changed and increased the population's ethnic makeup. For example, in fiscal year 2004, Mexico had 175,364 immigrants coming to the U.S., ranking it first among the ten countries providing the most immigrants. Also included among the top ten were the Dominican Republic and El Salvador, providing 30,492 and 29,795 immigrants, respectively; other Latin American countries that ranked high included Colombia, Cuba, and Guatemala. The Hispanic population's high fertility rate also contributed to the rapid growth of the Hispanic population in the United States. Hispanic women's fertility rate far exceeds that

of any other ethnic group in the country—in 2004, Hispanic women in the United States had a fertility rate of 97.8 live births per 1,000 women, compared to White non-Hispanic women, who had a rate of 58.4. In 2004, Latinos made up 14.0% of the population, and are now the largest minority group in the country. Of children aged 5–17 years old, 18% spoke a language other than English with their families; for nearly 7 out of every 10 of these children, the language was Spanish.

From 1998 to 2004 the crude birth rates and the fertility rates remained relatively unchanged. Crude birth rates varied between 14.0 live births per 1,000 population and 14.8, and fertility rates fluctuated between 64 and 66 live births per 1,000 women aged 15–44 years. In every ethnic group, women delayed having children until increasingly older ages. From 1998 to 2004, birth rates for teenagers dropped steadily and rates for women in their early 20s generally declined.

Life expectancy continues to improve, with people aged 65 and over comprising 12% of the U.S. population in 2003. In 2003, life expectancy was 77.5 years, compared to 75.8 in 1995. Women's life expectancy was 5.3 years longer than men's in 2003. Although life expectancy for Blacks also improved throughout the past decade, in 2003 they lagged 5.3 years behind Whites. The growth rate of the older population is expected to continue until 2030, when the last Baby Boomers enter the ranks of the older population. The U.S. Census Bureau projects that the population of the oldest, those aged 85 and older, could grow from 4.2 million in 2000 to nearly 20 million by 2050.

The expected growth of the older adult population over the next 50 years will have an extraordinary impact on the U.S. health care system. The supply and demand for health care workers will be particularly affected. On the one hand, the supply of health care providers may decrease, as large numbers of workers retire or reduce their working hours. On the other, older adults consume a disproportionate share of health care services, so demand will grow. The aging of the population also will affect the type of services used and the preparation of the workforce needed to provide those services.

In 2003, the crude death rate in the United States was 841.9 per 100,000 population, a 1.4% decline from the 2000 rate of 854.0 (Figure 3). The age-adjusted death rate (which adjusts for the aging of the U.S. population) declined by 4.2%, dropping from 869.0 in 2000 to 832.7 in 2003. Death rates increased for people aged 40–49 years old. Death rates for persons aged 65–74 years old decreased by 2.6%, the largest decrease of any age group. Death rates also decreased for age groups 55–64, 75–84, and 85 years and over.

In 2003, the leading causes of death for both men and women, in rank order, were diseases of the heart; malignant neoplasms; cerebrovascular disease; chronic lower respiratory diseases; unintentional injuries (accidents); diabetes mellitus; influenza and pneumonia; Alzheimer's disease; nephritis, nephritic syndrome, and nephrosis; and septicemia. The age-adjusted death rate for

FIGURE 3. Estimated mortality, by broad groups of causes and sex, United States of America, 2003.

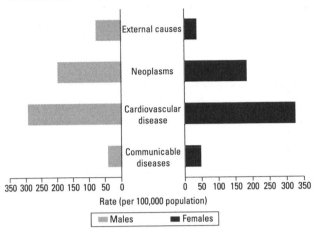

heart disease in women was 33.6% lower than that for men. The rate for cancer was 31.0% lower for women than men, mainly because more males smoked tobacco, the leading cause of lung cancer and other respiratory cancers. Males also were almost twice as likely to die in accidents, more than four times as likely to commit suicide, and more than three times more likely to be a victim of homicide than females. The overall crude death rate for women was considerably lower than that for men throughout the 1990s but was about the same in 2003.

Death rates varied substantially between rural and urban areas, and these differences also varied from one geographical region to another. From 1994–1996 to 2000–2002, overall age-adjusted death rates declined in each geographical region and in each category of urbanization. The overall age-adjusted death rates for the most urbanized, large central metropolitan counties dropped substantially, from 902.5 deaths per 100,000 population to 833.1. Rates in the most rural, non-metropolitan counties declined less, dropping from 945.8 per 100,000 to 914.3. The South, which had the highest age-adjusted death rates in the most rural counties, also had the least decrease in rates in these same counties between 1994–1996 and 2000–2002. In 2000–2002, the South's age-adjusted death rate for large central metropolitan counties settled below the rate of its most rural counties. In the Midwest, the 2000–2002 age-adjusted death rates for the large central metropolitan counties remained higher than the more rural counties.

HEALTH OF POPULATION GROUPS

Children under 5 Years Old

For young children, mortality, morbidity, and access to quality health care are greatly affected by poverty, which explains many of the differences between race and ethnic groups. One-fifth of all children under the age of 6 lived below the poverty threshold in 2005. (In 2005, the official poverty threshold for a family of four was just under US$ 20,000.)

The infant mortality rate dropped throughout the latter part of the 1990s, but rose in 2002. In 1995, infant mortality was 7.57 deaths per 1,000 live births. More recently, the infant mortality rate was relatively stable, fluctuating around 6.84 deaths per 1,000 live births in 2001, 6.95 in 2002, and 6.84 in 2003. The five leading causes of death in infants in 2003 were congenital anomalies (20% of all infant deaths); disorders relating to short gestation and unspecified low birthweight (17%); sudden infant death syndrome (8%); maternal complications of pregnancy (6%); and newborn affected by complications of placenta, cord, and membranes (4%). Non-Hispanic Blacks, who had substantially higher infant mortality rates than any other ethnic or racial group, experienced a decrease in rates, dropping from 14.65 deaths per 1,000 live births in 1995 to 13.60 in 2003. In 2003, as was the case in previous years, infant mortality rates varied widely by state. In general, states in the Southeast had higher rates, while those in the West and Northeast had lower rates.

Neonatal mortality followed a similar pattern. From 1995 to 2001, neonatal mortality rates decreased from 4.92 deaths per 1,000 live births to 4.54; this rate increased in 2002, to 4.67, and was 4.63 in 2003. Non-Hispanic Blacks, again with the highest rate of any ethnic group, dropped from 9.65 per 1,000 live births in 1995 to 9.22 in 1997, and then increased 9.40 in 1998, and 9.57 in 1999. The rate in 2003 was 9.26. For children aged 28 days to 11 months, mortality rates dropped from 2.65 deaths per 1,000 live births in 1995 to 2.27 in 2000. From 2000 to 2003 the rate remained relatively unchanged. American Indians and Alaskan Natives shared the highest postneonatal mortality rates with non-Hispanic Blacks, at 5.00 deaths per 1,000 live births in 1995; in 2003, the rate dropped to 4.18 for American Indians and Alaskan Natives, and 4.34 for Blacks.

Death rates for children 1–4 years old consistently declined throughout the 1990s and early 2000s. In 2003, the death rate in this age group was 31.5 deaths per 100,000 children aged 1–4 years; the highest rate was among Black children, at 46.8 deaths per 100,000. The leading cause of death for these children in 2003 was unintentional injuries, at 10.9 deaths per 100,000 children aged 1–4 years, or 34.6% of all deaths in this age group. More than half of these deaths were related to motor vehicle traffic accidents, many of which could have been prevented—most of the children who died in motor vehicle accidents were not restrained by children's safety seats or seat belts. The second leading cause of death for this age group was congenital malformations, at 3.4 deaths per 100,000, and representing 10.9% of all deaths. Both of these two cause-specific death rates declined substantially throughout the 1990s. The next three leading causes of death for these children were cancer (7.9% of all deaths in 1–4-year-olds), homicide (7.6%), and heart disease (3.7%). The sixth leading cause of death was influenza and pneumonia, representing 3.3% of all the deaths in this age group.

Children 5–9 Years Old

In 2000, children aged 5–9 years old made up a little over 7% of the country's population. Children in this age group had the lowest death rate of any age group, and this rate dropped slightly from 16.4 deaths per 100,000 children aged 5–9 years in 2000 to 14.7 in 2003. The leading cause of death for this group was unintentional injuries, with most deaths due to motor vehicle accidents.

Two of the chronic morbidities seen in these children—asthma and lead poisoning—are more likely to affect children living in poverty. In 2004 about 12% of children of all ages had ever been diagnosed with asthma, with children living in poverty having a slightly higher likelihood of developing asthma (14%). Asthma is believed to be the most common reason for school absenteeism. In 2000, about one million of the country's children under age 6 had high enough lead levels in their blood to adversely affect their development, behavior, and ability to learn; a disproportionate number of them were living in poverty. Problems caused by lead poisoning begin to surface at the time children enter school. Lead-based paint used in older homes was the usual source for the poisoning.

Adolescents 10–14 and 15–19 Years Old

Adolescents living in poverty are at greater risk for poor health. Adolescents who did not live in poverty were 15% more likely to report very good or excellent health than those living in poverty. In 1998, 17% of adolescents came from families living in poverty, and another 20% came from families living in near poverty. Moreover, 40% of all adolescents who lived in families headed by women were living in poverty.

Initiating smoking during adolescence is a good indicator of future smoking rates and smoking-related disease trends. Based on a national survey of adolescents, the percentage of 13–14-year-old eighth graders who had smoked in the previous 30 days dropped from a peak of 19% in 1997 to 9% in 2005. In the same time period, the prevalence of smoking among 17–18-year-old high-school seniors dropped from about 37% to 23%. In 2005, 50% of all 12th-grade students had tried smoking. Rural students smoked more than their urban counterparts.

Under-age alcohol use and most illicit drug use among adolescents declined moderately between 1997 and 2005. In 2005, marijuana was the most commonly reported illicit drug used by adolescents: 38% of 17–18-year-old high-school males and 30% of females reported having smoked marijuana. For 13–14-year-old eighth graders, illicit drug use reported for the 30 days prior to the survey dropped from 13% to 8.5% between 1997 and 2005. Among 17–18-year-old high-school seniors, illicit drug use in the past 30 days dropped from 26% to 23% between 1997 and 2005. Lifetime use of methylenedioxymethamphetamine (MDMA), known as ecstasy on the street, increased between 1997 and 2001 for both groups, however, before beginning to decline. In 1997, 3% of eighth graders had used MDMA, rising to 5% in 2001 be-

fore falling back to 3% in 2005. High-school seniors experienced a similar trend, with rates of MDMA use rising from 7% to 12% between 1997 and 2001, and then falling to 5% in 2005. Adolescent alcohol use is of particular importance because of its association with increased vehicular injuries and fatalities. Use of alcohol among high-school seniors in the 30 days before the survey dropped from 53% to 47% between 1997 and 2005. Likewise, binge drinking (defined as five or more drinks in a row in the last two weeks) by high-school seniors declined from 31% to 28% in the same period. From 1997 to 2005, drug and alcohol use among eighth graders generally followed the same trends, with the prevalence of drug and alcohol use being roughly half that of high school seniors. The exception was in the use of inhalants, which were used by eighth graders at rates twice those of high-school seniors. Rates of inhalant use in the year prior to the survey decreased for both groups between 1995 through 2003. However, in 2003 and 2004 inhalant use increased for both age groups. Alcohol use by eighth graders in the 30 days prior to the survey dropped from close to 25% to 17% between 1997 and 2005; binge drinking in this group dropped slightly, from about 15% to about 11%.

Through the late 1990s through the early 2000s, boys consistently reported using drugs and alcohol at a higher prevalence than girls. In recent years, eighth- and sometimes tenth-grade girls have had higher rates of alcohol and illicit drug use than boys. Boys have higher rates of marijuana use than girls in all grades. Non-Hispanic Whites reportedly used drugs and alcohol at a higher prevalence than Blacks.

Weight issues also plagued adolescents in the United States during the reporting period. Adolescents, along with the rest of the country's population, were increasingly overweight. In 1976–1980, 5% of all 12–19-year-olds were overweight. By 1988–1994, almost 11% were overweight, and by 2003–2004 more than 18% were overweight.

In 2005, nearly one-half (47%) of all high-school students surveyed reported being sexually active: 14% of them reported having had four or more sexual partners and 37% reported not using a condom in their last sexual encounter. Nationwide, almost 8% of high-school students reported that they had had intercourse at least once against their will. Regarding sexually transmitted infections among adolescents, chlamydia and gonorrhea were relatively common and syphilis relatively rare in 2004. Females aged 10–14 and 15–19 years old were estimated to have rates of chlamydia infection close to 132 per 100,000 and 2,762 per 100,000, respectively. Gonorrhea rates among females in these two age groups were 37 per 100,000 and 611 per 100,000, respectively. Males in those two age groups had chlamydia rates of 11 and 458, respectively, and gonorrhea rates of almost 6 and 253, respectively. In 2004, females 15–19 years old had the highest reported rates of both chlamydia and gonorrhea of any sex and age group in the country. Differences in reported STI rates between adolescent females and males were largely attributed to the fact that females are tested and screened more often than males, so detection of sexually transmitted infections is more common among the former. Insufficient funds for services, lack of transportation, and lack of confidentiality made access to STI prevention services more difficult for active adolescents than for older age groups.

From 1997 to 1998, new AIDS cases in 13–19-year-old females dropped by 17%; for males of the same age group they dropped by 22%. By 1999, however, while AIDS cases in adolescent males had declined again, new cases in adolescent females increased by 17%. However, beginning in 2000, the number of new cases for males between ages 13 and 19 began rising at a faster pace than new cases for females. By 2002, the number of new cases was comparable for males and females, and in 2003 males had far more new cases reported than females, at 249 and 209 new AIDS cases, respectively.

In 1991, more than one-quarter of all high-school students reported carrying a weapon. In 2005, nearly 19% of all high school students 14–18 years old reported carrying a gun, knife, or club in the month prior to the survey, and almost 7% reported bringing a weapon to school. With each national survey between 1991 and 1999, fewer high-school students reported carrying a weapon, although there was no change in the rates between 1999 and 2005. Between 1993 and 2003, smaller percentages of high-school students reported carrying a weapon to school in the last 30 days, although there was no difference in this percentage between 2003 and 2005. In addition, in 2005, 43% of male high school students and 28% of female students were involved in a physical fight in the 12 months prior to the survey. Between 1993 and 2003 adolescents also were more frequently the victims of violent crimes than adults. Compared to adults, adolescents reportedly were victimized at rates three times higher for simple assault, two times higher for aggravated assault, two times higher for robbery, and 2.5 times higher for rape and sexual assault. There were more adolescent males who were victims of violent crimes than females.

Adolescent victimization rates increased with age for females, but decreased for males. In 2003, there were reportedly 32 female victims of violent crime per 1,000 females aged 12–15 years and 70 male victims per 1,000 males aged 12–15 years. In 2003, there was an annual rate of 38 female victims per 1,000 females aged 16–19 years and 68 male victims per 1,000 males aged 16–19 years. The overall nonfatal violent victimization rate for youth ages 12–17 decreased by half between 1993 and 2003. Females aged 12–19 years old were more than twice as likely to be victims of reported sexual assault and rape than all other age groups of females.

Many adolescents suffered from depression and many of them were suicidal. In 2005, 17% of all high-school students surveyed reported that they had seriously contemplated suicide. Suicide was reportedly attempted by 8% of all 14–18-year-old high school students in the 12 months prior to the survey. Female high school students were more likely to seriously consider suicide than males.

Adults 20–59 Years Old

This age group makes up most of the country's population. Mortality patterns change drastically from one end to the other of the age range: for example, in 2003, there were 3,250 deaths due to diseases of the circulatory system among 25–34-year-olds, but there were 37,732 deaths due to this cause among 45–54-year-olds. That same year, deaths due to cancer totaled only 3,741 among 25–34-year-olds, but reached 49,843 among 45–54-year-olds. Cause specific death counts for such diseases as Alzheimer's and diabetes followed similar patterns.

Older Adults 60 Years Old and Older

The rapid growth in the proportion of the elderly in the population is challenging health and long-term care service systems, because the elderly require more frequent and more expensive care. In addition to the many distinctive health problems the elderly face, access to health care also complicates the provision of health services for many. Disproportionate numbers of the elderly live in more rural areas where there are greater distances to travel to reach health care facilities and fewer physicians per population.

Older adults suffer from more chronic health problems than other age groups, problems such as heart disease, hypertension, arthritic symptoms, diabetes, and osteoporosis. Women report higher levels of hypertension, asthma, chronic bronchitis, and arthritic symptoms, while men report higher levels of heart disease, cancer, diabetes, and emphysema. The prevalence of some conditions is increasing over time. In 1997–1998, 47% of people older than age 65 reported having hypertension; in 2003–2004, nearly 52% did. During the same period, the percentage reporting diabetes went from 13% to 16%. Roughly half of the elderly showed reduced hip-bone density between 1988 and 1994.

Mental health issues were also particularly important among the elderly—with aging, the incidence of memory impairment due to Alzheimer's disease and other dementias increases. The prevalence of moderate or severe memory impairment is six times as high for people age 85 and older as it is for people age 65–69. In 2002, the proportion of people age 85 and older with moderate or severe memory impairment was 32%, compared to 5% of those age 65–69.

Compared to most other age groups, a disproportionately high percentage of the elderly fall prey to depression, and suicide also is relatively more common among them. In 2002, 16% of women and 10% of men age 65–69 reported depressive symptoms; for those age 85 and older, 22% of women and 15% of men reported such symptoms.

In 1999, approximately 6.6 million Americans aged 65 and older used assistive devices and/or received personal care for a chronic disability. Slightly more than one-half of these persons (3.4 million) relied on help for their long-term care needs from unpaid caregivers, usually family members and friends. The other half either received paid care exclusively while living in their home (314,600), used assistive devices only to maintain independence (1.3 million), or lived in an institution, such as a nursing home or some other type of long-term care facility (1.6 million).

The leading risk factors that contribute to poor health and quality of life among the country's elderly are overweight (in 2003–2004, nearly 30% of those over age 65 were obese and close to three-fourths were overweight), diets deficient in fruits/vegetables and milk products, lack of physical activity (in 2002 only 21% of those over age 65 reported engaging in regular leisure time physical activity), and smoking. The percentage of older Americans who smoke has declined dramatically over the past 37 years.

The leading causes of death for the elderly in 2002–2003 were heart disease (1,632 deaths per 100,000 elderly) and cancer (1,100 per 100,000), which account for more than one-half of all deaths in this group. Additional leading causes of death in this age group were cerebrovascular diseases (stroke; 404 elderly deaths per 100,000 elderly), chronic lower respiratory diseases (301 per 100,000), influenza and pneumonia (155 per 100,000), and diabetes (151 per 100,000). The importance of influenza and pneumonia as a cause of mortality indicates the crucial role vaccines can play in preventing these diseases in this population.

Family Health

According to the Census Bureau's Current Population Survey, in 2000, women heading households with children represented nearly one-quarter of all families in the United States. More than two million of these women were grandmothers who were the primary caregivers for children in their homes, and almost one-fifth of these grandmother-headed families lived in poverty at some time in the 12 months prior to the survey.

Poverty was the most important determinant for family health. Despite attempts by federal, state, and local governments, as well as non-profit organizations, to provide a safety net to protect the health of the most vulnerable families, poor health conditions persisted. Although improvements were seen in child mortality rates, other health indicators often associated with poverty worsened. For example, the proportion of low-birthweight newborns (under 2,500 g) increased from 7.4% in 1996 to 8.1% in 2004. Likewise, the percentage of births with very low birthweight (under 1,500 g) increased from 1.37% to 1.47%. Among mothers 20 years of age and older, low-birthweight rates were highest for those who had not completed high school and lowest for those who had more than a high school education. Non-Hispanic Black mothers, dealing with much higher levels of poverty, were especially vulnerable, with 13.7% of all live births for non-Hispanic Black women having low birthweights in 2004.

Children of families who came off the welfare rolls after the 1996 reforms potentially faced reduced access to health care. The creation of the State Children's Health Insurance Program (SCHIP) in 1997 helped to minimize the number of children who lost health coverage. Poor children (under 100% of the federal poverty guidelines) are largely eligible for Medicaid, and the percentage of poor children who were uninsured fell from 24% to 19% between 1997 and 2005. For near-poor children (between 100% and 200% of the federal poverty guidelines), who are largely eligible for SCHIP, the decline was more significant. The percentage of near-poor children who were uninsured fell from 24% in 1997 to 16% in 2005.

Workers

Occupational risks of death varied by gender and age: men were 10 times more likely to die than women during work, probably partially reflecting the differences in occupation. Workers 35–64 years of age had the highest work-related fatality rate.

From 1980 through 2005 there were 150,799 work-related deaths in the United States. The number of deaths due to injuries at work went from 5,430 in 2000 to 5,702 in 2005. Since 1992, rates have shown corresponding changes, from a high of 5.3 deaths due to injuries at work per 100,000 employed workers to the current rate of 4.0 per 100,000. Leading causes of job-related deaths during this period were motor vehicle accidents, homicides, machine-related accidents, falls, electrocutions, and being struck by falling objects. Risks of death varied by gender and age; males were 12 times more likely to die during work than women, reflecting in part the differences in occupation. Workers 65 years old and older had the highest work-related fatality rate of any age group (11.8 work-related deaths per 100,000 workers 65 years and older, a rate 2.9 times greater than the overall workplace fatality rate for all workers).

In 2005, 60% of women 18 years old and older were either employed or looking for work, and 3.5 million women held more than one job at the same time. In 2005, median weekly earnings were US$ 713 for men 16 years and older vs. US$ 580 for women, approximately 81.3% of male weekly wages. Working women suffered more musculoskeletal disorders such as sprains, strains, carpal tunnel syndrome, and tendonitis than men. In 2004, 34% of all work-related injuries and illnesses suffered by women were musculoskeletal, compared to 30% among men. Women also were the victims of 64% of nonfatal assault injuries at the workplace; most assaults occurred in service occupations.

Persons with Disabilities

Disabilities affected every segment of the population, but those living in poverty are disproportionately affected. According to a Census Bureau survey, 51.2 million people, or 18% of Americans, reported a disability in 2002 and 32.5 million (12%) reported a severe disability. In the adult population, 20% of women and 17% of men reported a disability. Among children under 15 years of age, boys are more likely than girls to report a disability (11% versus 6%, respectively).

From 12% to 23% of children under age 18 have a special health care need—a chronic condition with a functional limitation or other negative consequences. Among the most prevalent conditions in 2002 were asthma (12% of children aged from birth to 17 years), respiratory allergies (12% of children aged from birth to 17 years), learning disabilities (8% of those aged 3–7 years), and attention deficit hyperactivity disorder (7% of those aged 3–17 years). About 12% of children ages 3–21 used special education services in 2003–2004, up from 11.7% in 1999–2000. State and federal government education departments spend US$ 50 billion per year for special education programs for 3–21-year-olds, compared to US$ 27.3 billion spent on regular education.

In 2002, people with severe disabilities were highly likely to have Medicare or Medicaid coverage, to live below the poverty level, to report their health status to be fair or poor, to receive public assistance, and to have a household income below US$ 20,000. The poverty rate for people age 25 to 64 years with no disability was 8%, compared to 11% for those with a non-severe disability, and 26% for those with a severe disability.

Among adults aged 21 to 64 years who had a disability, about 56% had been employed in the one-year period prior to the interview. People with a severe disability reported the lowest employment rate (42%), as compared to those with a non-severe disability (82%) and those with no reported disability (88%).

Disabilities affected every segment of the population, but adults 65 years and older struggled with an inordinate share of disabilities and impairments. According to a survey conducted in 2004, 19.7% reported a chronic disability. About 19% of women aged 65 and older and 14% of men aged 65 and older reported trouble seeing, even when wearing contact lenses or glasses. For women in this age group, 34% reported trouble hearing; for men in this age group, 48% did. Among this elderly population, 13.7% of men and 23.6% of women reported difficulty walking two to three blocks.

Indigenous Peoples and Other Ethnic and Special Groups

Blacks, Latinos, Native Americans, and Asian/Pacific Islanders in the country incur a disproportionate share of mortality, morbidity, disability, and adverse health conditions compared to non-Hispanic Whites. Life expectancy and infant mortality trends show a widening gap between majority and minority ethnic/racial groups, even as these health indicators improved for most groups over the 1990s. These overriding health differences between ethnic and racial populations were strongly related to so-cioeconomic differences and differences in the prevalence of poverty in each group.

The Latino population, the largest and fastest growing minority in the United States, comprised 12.5% of the population in 2000 and included persons of Mexican, Puerto Rican, Cuban, and South and Central American descent, among others. Health disparities within the country's Latino population—age-adjusted death rates were substantially lower for Latinos of Cuban descent than for those of Mexican or Puerto Rican descent—primarily reflected socioeconomic differences. Overall, health indicators for Latinos improved during the 1990s and early 2000s.

African-Americans, who made up more than 12% of the population in 2000, have three times the portion of their population living in poverty than do non-Hispanic Whites; one-third of all Blacks live in poverty. Half of the Black population lives in urban areas often typified by inadequate housing, poorly funded schools, lack of living-wage employment opportunities, and violence. African-American death rates were higher than those for Whites for most leading causes of death. For African-Americans 15–24 years old, homicide was the leading cause of death for males and the second leading cause of death for females. But Blacks had lower age-adjusted death rates for suicide, chronic lower respiratory diseases, Alzheimer's disease, chronic liver disease and cirrhosis, and Parkinson's disease than Whites. Overall, many health indicators improved for Black communities in the 1990s and early 2000s; colorectal, respiratory, and breast cancer death rates dropped, and there were gains in leading health indicators such as infant mortality and overall death rates.

Asian/Pacific Islanders, who speak more than 30 different languages and originate from a variety of very different cultures, represented almost 4% of the country's population in 2000. Overall, they had roughly the same socioeconomic and health status as the majority White population. Some in this group had been in the United States for generations, but others had arrived more recently. Given its diversity, health challenges in this population varied substantially from group to group. Southeast Asian men suffered more lung cancer than the majority male population, and older Filipino men living in California had greater rates of high blood pressure than other California men of the same age. Southeast Asian immigrants are 40 times more likely to have tuberculosis and hepatitis B than the general population.

In 2000, those who reported themselves as only American Indian or Alaskan Native made up 0.9% of the population, accounting for 2.5 million persons, and those reporting as Native American or Alaskan Native plus at least another race represented 0.6% of the population, or 1.6 million persons. This minority resides primarily in urban areas or on reservations, and many receive their health care through clinics and hospitals provided by the federal government's Indian Health Service. The population is very young, partly because many die before reaching old age. This native population was much more likely than the general population to die from diabetes mellitus related to obesity and from liver disease due to alcohol abuse. Accidents and violence (homicides and suicides) are leading causes of death among Native Americans and Alaskan Natives. Alcoholism, which contributed to many of the major causes of death, is a leading health and social problem in this community. Smoking prevalence also is higher among them, increasing risk for smoking-related diseases.

In 2004, nearly 54,000 refugees were admitted into the United States, representing a significant increase from the previous two years of relatively low admissions following the terrorist attacks in 2001 (27,000 in 2002 and 28,000 in 2003). There were two principal groups of refugees admitted in 2004, Somali Bantu from Kenya (totaling about 12,000) and Hmong from Thailand (totaling about 14,000). In addition to these refugees, about 23,000 Cuban entrants were also admitted in 2004. Refugees and entrants often have health problems that need to be addressed as part of their initial resettlement, and federal and state governments provide health care coverage for these new arrivals through Medicaid (if they meet that program's eligibility criteria) or special refugee health coverage available for their first eight months in the country (if they do not meet Medicaid criteria).

HEALTH CONDITIONS AND PROBLEMS

COMMUNICABLE DISEASES

Vector-borne Diseases

Most **malaria** cases reported in the United States were acquired outside of the country. The few that were acquired domestically were due to blood transfusion, congenital transmission, or undetermined mode of transmission. Of the 1,337 cases of malaria reported in 2002, only 5 were domestically acquired: one person acquired malaria from blood transfusion, one from congenital transmission, and three from an undetermined mode of transmission.

In 2004, there were 1,324 cases of malaria reported, representing a 3.6% increase from 2003 (1,278 reported cases). Approximately 50% of the cases reported in the United States in 2004 were due to *Plasmodium falciparum* and 24% of cases were attributed to *Plasmodium vivax*.

In 2005, there were 3,000 cases of **West Nile virus** reported, representing a 15.4% increase from 2004. Of these, 1,294 were West Nile encephalitis or meningitis, 1,607 were West Nile fever, and 99 were unspecified.

In 2004, 19,804 cases of **Lyme disease** were reported, for a national average of 6.7 cases per 100,000 persons. In the 12 states where Lyme disease is most common, the average was 27.4 cases per 100,000 persons.

Most other vector-borne diseases are acquired outside of the country, with the exception of **tularemia** and **arboviral en-**

cephalitis, which are endemic in the United States. **Plague** is extremely rare in the United States, with an average of only 10–15 cases reported each year.

Vaccine-preventable Diseases

Life threatening or debilitating diseases which were once common in the United States, now remain at sustained low levels thanks to the widespread use of vaccines, particularly among children. In 2004, there were no cases of **diphtheria**, **paralytic wild-type polio**, or **congenital rubella syndrome**; there were fewer than 12 cases of **measles** and **tetanus** reported in the country. In March 2005, the U.S. Centers for Disease Control and Prevention announced a major public health milestone, the elimination of rubella virus in the United States.

In 1983, vaccines for seven diseases were available and recommended for routine use in the United States. By the summer of 2006, vaccines for 16 diseases were available and recommended for children and adolescents. Since 2000, pneumococcal conjugate vaccine; meningococcal conjugate vaccine; a comprehensive booster for tetanus, diphtheria, and pertussis; universal use of hepatitis A vaccine; rotavirus vaccine; human papillomavirus vaccine; and a routine recommendation for influenza vaccination for children 6 to 59 months of age have been added to the routine immunization recommendations in the United States. These new vaccines have great potential to reduce the burden of diseases preventable through vaccination, but their use requires a large investment of resources, infrastructure development, and public and provider education.

An economic evaluation of the impact of seven vaccines—diphtheria-tetanus-acellular pertussis (DTaP); tetanus; *Haemophilus influenzae* type b (Hib); polio; measles-mumps-rubella; hepatitis B; and varicella routinely given as part of the childhood immunization schedule—found them to be enormously effective. Routine childhood vaccination with these vaccines, which prevent nearly 14 million cases of disease and more than 33,000 deaths over the lifetime of children born in any given year, resulted in an annual cost saving of US$ 9.9 billion in direct medical cost and an additional US$ 33.4 billion in savings in indirect costs.

Childhood vaccination coverage rates are at record high levels for every vaccine and for all vaccination series measures, and have generally improved since 2000. In 2000, 73% of children aged 19–35 months had received four doses of DTP vaccine, three doses of polio vaccine, one dose of measles-containing vaccine, and three doses of Hib and hepatitis B vaccine. In 2004 this combined coverage improved to 81%. Vaccine coverage also has greatly improved for some new vaccines. During the 1990s, approximately 11,000 hospitalizations and 100 deaths occurred annually due to **varicella**. Great progress was made in educating health care providers and the public about the benefits of varicella vaccine, and coverage in 2004 reached 88%.

Unfortunately, the burden from vaccine-preventable diseases among adults in the United States remains high. **Pneumonia** and **influenza** were the fifth leading cause of death in all persons aged 65 and older, based on 2000 national mortality data. Although vaccines are available for adults against these two diseases, in 2004 only 65% of persons 65 years of age and older reported having had an influenza vaccination, and 57% of persons 65 years of age and older reported having a pneumococcal vaccination. A critical challenge in the United States is extending the successes in childhood immunization to adults.

Diseases Preventable by Blood Screening

Before being released for use in patients, blood donations are screened for hepatitis B and C viruses; human immunodeficiency virus (HIV 1 and 2); human T-lymphotropic virus, types I and II; and the bacterium that causes syphilis.

Intestinal Infectious Diseases

Foodborne diseases cause an estimated 76 million illnesses, 325,000 hospitalizations, and 5,000 deaths in the United States each year. Known pathogens account for an estimated 14 million illnesses, 60,000 hospitalizations, and 1,800 deaths. Three pathogens, *Salmonella, Listeria*, and *Toxoplasma*, are responsible for 1,500 deaths each year, more than 75% of those caused by known pathogens; unknown agents account for the remaining 62 million illnesses, 265,000 hospitalizations, and 3,200 deaths.

Escherichia coli O157:H7 is estimated to cause 73,000 illnesses in the United States annually. From 1982 to 2002, 49 states reported 350 outbreaks, representing 8,598 cases, 1,493 hospitalizations, 354 hemolytic uremic syndrome cases, and 40 deaths. The transmission route for 183 of the cases was foodborne, 74 unknown, 50 person to-person, 31 waterborne, 11 animal contact, and 1 laboratory-related. The food vehicle for 75 foodborne outbreaks was ground beef; produce was responsible for 38 outbreaks.

In the United States, contaminated drinking water in homes and businesses is usually a result of water main breaks or other emergency situations. Parasites cause the majority of problems. During 1999–2000, 39 outbreaks associated with drinking water were reported by 25 states. These outbreaks caused illness among an estimated 2,068 persons and were linked to 2 deaths. Of the 39 outbreaks, 28 (71.8%) were linked to groundwater sources, and 18 (64.3%) of those were associated with private or non-community wells that were not regulated by the United States Environmental Protection Agency.

Chronic Communicable Diseases

In 2000, 16,309 new **tuberculosis** (TB) cases were reported, for a rate of 5.8 new cases per 100,000 population. By 2004, new tuberculosis cases had dropped to 14,517, for a rate of 4.9 per 100,000. Although tuberculosis disease rates continued to decline between 2000 and 2004, TB continues to be an important endemic disease in the United States. Most cases were among younger and middle-aged adults. In 2004, 34% of the cases were among 25–44-year-olds and 29% among 45–64-year-olds; only 11% were in children under 15 years old. Moreover, between 2000 and 2004 the number of cases among U.S.-born persons decreased from 53% of all cases to 46%, while the number of cases among the foreign-born population increased from 47% of all cases to 54%. Because the U.S.-born and the foreign-born population both increased, new tuberculosis cases had a net decrease from 2000 to 2004 among both populations, from 3.5 to 2.6 new cases per 100,000 for the U.S.-born population and from 25.3 to 22.8 per 100,000 among the foreign-born. In 2004, California, New York, and Texas accounted for 42% of the overall national case total. The District of Columbia, Hawaii, California, Texas, New York, and Alaska had the highest rates, followed by southern states. As did tuberculosis incidence rates, tuberculosis death rates also declined through the early 2000s. In 2000 the tuberculosis-specific death rate was 0.3 per 100,000 population; according to preliminary data, by 2003, this rate had dropped to 0.2 per 100,000.

The decline in tuberculosis rates has been attributed to increased efforts to identify and promptly treat cases and to ensure treatment compliance, to improved infection controls in institutional settings, to a decrease in the incidence of AIDS, and to the declining frequency of multi-drug resistant cases.

Leprosy remains relatively uncommon in the United States. In 2002, 96 cases were reported in the country.

Acute Respiratory Infections

Pneumonia and influenza were two of the leading causes of death in the United States in the early 2000s. The age-adjusted death rate for **influenza** and **pneumonia** was 21.8 per 100,000 population in 2003. Although influenza vaccine is provided widely to the public during flu season, production delays have led to vaccine shortfalls in three of the last five influenza seasons (2000–2001 through 2004–2005).

HIV/AIDS and Other Sexually Transmitted Infections

At the end of 2004, there were more than 944,305 cumulative AIDS cases and 529,113 AIDS deaths in the country. Approximately 415,193 persons were living with AIDS by the end of 2004.

AIDS incidence and mortality rates were both higher in men, with males accounting for 73% of all adult and adolescent HIV/AIDS cases in 2004. From 2001 to 2004, the estimated number of HIV/AIDS cases decreased 2% among males and 15% among females. During this period, the estimated number of HIV/AIDS cases increased among men who have sex with men and decreased among injection drug users, heterosexual adults, adolescents, and children. Women were especially at risk of acquiring HIV infection through heterosexual sex and subsequently developing AIDS, since it is easier for women to sexually acquire HIV from male partners than for males to acquire it from female partners. An estimated 10,410 women became newly infected with HIV in 2004; approximately 68% of them were African-American, 16% were White, and 15% were Hispanic. An estimated three-quarters of all infected women were infected with HIV through heterosexual contact, and the majority of the remaining women were infected through injection drug use. Among men and women who inject heroin and cocaine, sharing HIV-infected needles is the primary means of transmission. HIV-infected women who inject drugs are more likely to develop AIDS from their infection than are their male counterparts with the same HIV concentration in their blood.

New pediatric AIDS cases have been declining steadily since 1994 when the government issued guidelines recommending testing and treatment of pregnant women and neonates to reduce perinatal HIV transmission. The vast majority of AIDS cases occur through perinatal exposure. In 2003, about 150 new AIDS cases were reported among children under age 13, compared with more than 700 cases in 1990.

AIDS is not uniformly distributed geographically: rates continued to be high in metropolitan areas in the country's Northeast, which had the second highest rate of any region in the U.S. This reflected the differential distribution between urban and rural areas—northeastern cities lie within the major drug-trade corridor that follows Interstate 95 and have disproportionately higher percentages of injection drug users. The South had the highest AIDS rates in the country in 2000–2004, which is attributable primarily to those areas with the greater concentrations of poverty, such as inner cities and the rural South.

Sexually transmitted infections take an especially heavy toll on women's health. Each year an estimated one million women in the United States suffer a symptomatic episode of **pelvic inflammatory disease**.

Every 7–10 years, drops in **syphilis** in the country have been followed by epidemics. The rate of primary and secondary syphilis reported in the United States decreased during the 1990s, and in 2000 was the lowest since reporting began in 1941. However, the rate of reported primary and secondary syphilis has increased each year since 2001, primarily among men. In 2004, reported primary and secondary syphilis cases increased to 7,980, from 7,177 in 2003, an increase of 11.2%. The number of reported cases in women increased for the first time in over a decade, though only slightly. Cases of congenital syphilis continued to decline; 353 cases were reported in 2004, down from 432 in 2003.

Reported **chlamydia** rates continued to increase from 2000 to 2004. In 2004, 929,462 cases of genital *Chlamydia trachomatis* were reported, an increase of 5.9% compared with the 2003 rate. These trends are probably due to continued expansion of screening programs for chlamydia, the use of improved diagnostic tests that have greater sensitivity, and improved surveillance systems for this disease. There were 330,132 cases of **gonorrhea** reported in the United States in 2004. Since 2000, the reported gonorrhea rate has decreased 15.2%, after a plateau in 1998 and 1999. Chlamydia was the most common of the three sexually transmit-

ted infections, with reported rates of 319.6 cases per 100,000 population in 2004; gonorrhea ranked second, with 113 per 100,000; and syphilis was a distant third, with 2.7 per 100,000.

About 6.2 million Americans get a new genital **human papillomavirus** (HPV) infection each year. Approximately 10 of the 30 identified genital HPV types can lead, in rare cases, to development of cervical cancer. Research has shown that for most women (90%), cervical HPV infection becomes undetectable within two years. Although only a small proportion of women have persistent infection, persistent infection with "high-risk" types of HPV is the main risk factor for cervical cancer.

Sexually transmitted infection rates are disproportionately high among ethnic minorities, a disparity that is associated with these groups' higher levels of poverty and lack of access or failure to access health services.

Zoonoses

In 2001, 49 states, the District of Columbia, and Puerto Rico reported 7,437 cases of **rabies** in animals and no cases in humans to the Centers for Disease Control and Prevention (Hawaii is the only state that has never reported an indigenously acquired rabies case in humans or animals). The total number of reported cases increased by 0.92% from those reported in 2000 (7,369 cases). Wild animals accounted for 93% of reported cases of rabies in 2001. Raccoons continued to be the most frequently reported rabid wildlife species (37.2% of all animal cases during 2001), followed by skunks (30.7%), bats (17.2%), foxes (5.9%), and other wild animals, including rodents and lagomorphs (0.7%). Reported cases in raccoons and foxes decreased 0.4% and 3.5%, respectively, from the totals reported in 2000. Reported cases in skunks and bats increased 2.6% and 3.3%, respectively, from the totals reported in 2000.

NONCOMMUNICABLE DISEASES

Nutritional and Metabolic Diseases

In the 2000s, the country has continued to face an epidemic of **obesity**. In 1988–1994, the percentage of the adult population that was obese was 22.3%; by 2003–2004 the percentage had increased to 32.2%. An additional 34.1% of adults were overweight in the latter two years. The proportion of adults who are obese varies widely by state (Figure 4). Among children and adolescents aged 2–19 years, 34.8% were at risk of overweight in 2003–2004. A reported 27% of adults did not engage in any physical activity and only one-quarter consumed the recommended fruits and vegetables five or more times daily. Excessively overweight persons have higher mortality rates than those not overweight, being at higher risk for diabetes, cardiovascular disease, and certain cancers. Each year an estimated 300,000 adults in the country die prematurely of causes related to obesity. The total cost of obesity-related illness in the United States is about US$ 100 billion per year.

FIGURE 4. Obesity^a trends among adults, United States of America, 1991, 1996, and 2004.

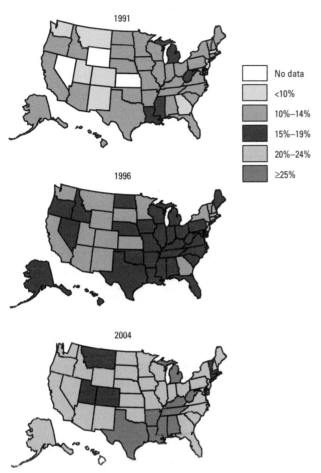

1991

1996

2004

No data
<10%
10%–14%
15%–19%
20%–24%
≥25%

Source: U.S. Department of Health and Human Services, Centers for Disease Control and Prevention, National Center for Chronic Disease Prevention and Health Promotion, Behavioral Risk Factor Surveillance System (BRFSS).
^aBMI ≥30, or about 30 lb overweight for a 5'4" person.

The proportion of the adult population with **diabetes** rose from 8.4% in 1988–1994 to 9.4% in 1999–2002. The rapid increase in obesity, an important risk factor for Type 2 diabetes, is an important factor in this increase. Rates of childhood diabetes also are increasing rapidly, due in part to increasing levels of childhood obesity. The direct and indirect costs associated with diabetes are estimated to be US$ 132 billion per year.

Cardiovascular Diseases

Cardiovascular disease, mainly heart disease and stroke, is a major cause of death in the country, accounting for 36.9% of all deaths in 2003. More than 24 million people in the United States are estimated to have some form of cardiovascular disease. In 2003, an estimated 6.8 million inpatient cardiovascular operations and procedures were performed in the United States. In

2006 the estimated direct and indirect costs of cardiovascular disease were estimated at US$ 403.1 billion.

Cardiovascular disease rates are not uniform across the United States. After adjusting for age, cardiovascular disease rates were highest in the South in 2003. Because cardiovascular disease rates increase with age and proportionately there are more elderly women than elderly men, the death rate from this disease was higher among women.

Malignant Neoplasms

Approximately one-quarter of all deaths in the country are due to cancer. The 2003 annual health care and loss-of-productivity costs of cancer morbidity and mortality are estimated at US$ 192 billion.

In 2006, it was estimated that 1.4 million new cases of invasive cancer, excluding skin cancer and carcinoma in situ, were diagnosed in the United States. Over 100,000 in situ cancers, primarily breast and melanoma, were estimated for the same year. Among men, the most common cancers diagnosed in 2006 were **prostate, lung and bronchus**, and **colon and rectum**. Prostate cancers represented one-third of all new cancers in men. Among women, the most common cancers diagnosed were **breast, lung and bronchus**, and **colon and rectum**; these cancer sites combined represented more than half of all cancers diagnosed in women. On average, there was a one-in-two chance that a man would develop invasive cancer over his lifetime, and a one-in-three chance for a woman.

The overall incidence of cancer was relatively stable between 1992 and 2003, although trends for women have shown a small annual increase of 0.3% since 1987. Breast cancer incidence rates increased slowly throughout the 1990s, but remained level during 2001–2003. Rates for colon and rectum cancers began to decline in the mid-1980s for both men and women, with decreases reported in the last ten years for most racial and ethnic populations. Lung and bronchus cancer incidence rates have declined for men for more than 20 years but continue to increase for women, though more slowly during the past decade. Prostate cancer incidence has increased since the mid-1990s.

Lung cancer was the leading cause of cancer deaths among men and women, and is primarily caused by smoking tobacco. In 2006, an estimated 90,330 men and 72,130 women died of lung cancer. Breast cancer deaths were second for women at 40,970, and prostate cancer was second for men at 27,350 deaths. There was an estimated total of 564,830 cancer deaths in the United States in 2006, with 291,270 occurring in men and 273,560 in women.

OTHER HEALTH PROBLEMS OR ISSUES

Disasters

The United States experienced a variety of natural disasters throughout the reporting period. Hurricanes on the Atlantic coast, the Gulf of Mexico, and the Pacific coast; earthquakes near the San Andreas fault and other fault lines, especially on the Pacific coast; tornadoes in the Plains states; and floods in every section of the country have left in their wake loss of life, injuries, major disruptions in daily life, and extensive property damage. As was the case with many sectors, the public and private health care sectors were challenged to respond.

In 2005, 48 major disasters were declared. Winter storms caused major disasters to be declared in seven states. Puerto Rico and 20 states suffered seasonal storms, including tropical storms, and/or flooding, all leading to major disasters being declared. Three states declared major disasters due to tornadoes and 11 states sustained destruction due to fires. Major disasters were declared in American Samoa due to a cyclone and in the Northern Mariana Islands due to a typhoon. Hurricanes led to major disaster declarations in six states. Hurricane Katrina, a strong category 3 hurricane on the Saffir-Simpson scale, was one of the strongest storms to strike the United States coast in the last 100 years and ranks among the worst natural disasters in the country's history. The hurricane caused the city of New Orleans to be evacuated, marking the first time a major American city has been completely evacuated. Inland effects included high winds and some flooding in several states and widespread destruction in the states of Alabama, Florida, Louisiana, and Mississippi. The damage to individuals and to families torn apart by the hurricane was immeasurable, with estimates of over 1,800 deaths directly and indirectly due to Katrina—the highest total death count in the country due to a disaster since the 1928 major hurricane in southern Florida. Katrina's damage was compounded when Hurricane Rita made landfall soon after near the Texas-Louisiana border. The impact of these hurricanes highlighted the myriad of challenges posed by natural disasters, and the response to this disaster will help guide future public health and medical emergency preparedness response efforts. The importance of this cannot be underestimated since the Atlantic Basin is predicted to have an active hurricane phase during the next 10–20 years.

Violence and Other External Causes

In the United States, the home is the second most common site of unintentional fatal injuries; motor vehicles on the road is the first. More than 18,000 people in the United States die each year from unintentional injuries that occur in the home. Falls account for one-third of unintentional injury deaths in the home. Males experience substantially more fatal unintentional injuries at home than females. However, females experience slightly more nonfatal home injuries than males. Older adults experience the highest rates of unintentional home injury deaths among all ages, with persons at least 80 years of age experiencing injury death rates more than 20 times greater than their younger counterparts.

Victims of more severe injuries are seen in hospital emergency departments. In 2004, there were more than 41 million injury-related visits to emergency departments in the United States. Almost 21% of all injuries seen in hospital emergency departments in 2004 were the result of falls. Motor vehicle crashes accounted for almost 11% of injury-related emergency department visits. There were 2.3 million violence-related injury visits to emergency departments in 2004, with more than 75% of those resulting from an assault and about 23% of the violence-related visits resulting from self-inflicted injuries.

Violence is a significant problem in the United States. From infants to the elderly, it affects people in all stages of life. In 2003, 17,732 people died as a result of homicide and 31,484 died by suicide. The number of violent deaths tells only part of the story. Many more survive violence and are left with permanent physical and emotional scars. Violence also erodes communities by reducing productivity, decreasing property values, and disrupting social services.

In 2004, U.S. residents age 12 or older experienced an estimated 5.2 million violent crimes (rape/sexual assault, robbery, aggravated assault, and simple assault). For violent crimes overall, aggregated rates declined by 9% from 2001–2002 to 2003–2004. Taken together, the one-year (2003–2004) and two-year (2001–2002 to 2003–2004) change estimates indicate that crime rates remain stabilized at the lowest levels experienced since 1973. Of all violent crimes reported by victims in 2004, approximately 4.6 million were aggravated or simple assault, 600,000 were robbery, and 200,000 were rape/sexual assault. Males and youths—those who historically have been the most vulnerable to violent victimization—continued to be victimized at higher rates than others in 2004. During 2004, armed offenders were involved in 22% of all violent crime incidents. The presence of a weapon was related to the type of crime. For example, rape and sexual assault incidents (8%) were less likely than robberies (46%) to be committed by an armed offender. The type of weapon also varied by the type of violence: 19% of robbery incidents occurred with a firearm present, compared to 5% of assault incidents. The rate of firearm violence declined significantly from 1993 to 2004 (from 5.9 to 1.4 victimizations per 1,000 people aged 12 or older).

In 2003, the year for which the most comprehensive data are available, the FBI reported a total of 16,500 murders or nonnegligent manslaughters, a 1.7% increase from 2002. Although the rate of homicide changes year to year, the relationship between the victim's characteristics and the homicide tends to remain the same. In 2003, 78% of murder victims were male. When the race of the victim was known, just under 49% were White and the same number were Black, and less than 3% were other races. Murder is generally perpetrated between persons of the same race. Offenders were most often male (90%) and adult (92%). When information on the victim/offender relationship was available, 78% of the offenders were known to the victim; 29% of murders were triggered by an argument. Firearms were used in 71% of homicides.

The average annual number of rape victimizations for 2003–2004 was 65,510, a decrease of 27.9% from 2001–2002. Nationwide, almost 63 per 100,000 females reported being raped in

2000. Metropolitan areas had rates of 65 forcible rapes per 100,000, while rural counties had rates of 43. Cities saw an increase in reported rapes of 1.5% between 1999 and 2000, while suburban areas saw a decline of almost 1%. Rates in rural counties were virtually unchanged. Of all forcible rapes, 12% were perpetrated by juveniles.

There was a decline in the frequency of aggravated assaults reported to law enforcement in 2004. Non-metropolitan counties had the lowest rate of aggravated assaults, at 171 offenses per 100,000 inhabitants; cities had the highest, with 344; and suburbs ranked in the middle, with 234.

Oral Health

The nation's oral health is the best it has ever been, yet oral diseases remain common in the United States. The nation spends an estimated US$ 60 billion annually on dental services, including approximately 500 million visits to dental offices. Those who suffer the most from oral health problems include poor Americans, especially children and the elderly. Members of racial and ethnic groups also experience a disproportionate level of oral health problems. Those with disabilities and complex health conditions are also at greater risk for oral diseases, which may further complicate their health.

Most adults show some sign of gum disease. Severe gum disease affects about 14% of adults aged 45–54 years. More than one-third of adults living below the poverty level (18 years and older) have at least one untreated decayed tooth, compared to 16% of adults living above the poverty level. Older Americans who are economically disadvantaged, disabled, homebound, or institutionalized or lack insurance tend to have a greater risk for poor oral health.

Dental decay is one of the most common chronic infectious diseases among U.S. children. Among low-income children, almost 30% of tooth decay remains untreated. More than twice as many children and adolescents from low-income families had untreated decay (20%) as those from families with higher incomes (8%).

Each year, more than 30,000 new cases of cancer of the oral cavity and pharynx are diagnosed, and approximately 7,400 persons die of these diseases.

Emerging and Reemerging Health Threats

Emerging and reemerging infectious diseases pose a continuing threat in the United States. Although modern advances have conquered some diseases, outbreaks of severe acute respiratory syndrome (SARS) and monkeypox in 2003, and an observed increase in antimicrobial resistance, particularly of methicillin-resistant *Staphylococcus aureus* (MRSA), are recent reminders of the extraordinary ability of microbes to adapt and evolve.

During the 2003 outbreak of SARS, eight people in the United States had laboratory evidence of SARS caused by a new coronavirus (SARS-CoV). All of them had traveled to the U.S. from other parts of the world. That same year, there were 37 confirmed and 10 probable human cases of monkeypox in the country. Most of them got sick after having had contact with pet prairie dogs that were sick with monkeypox. This was the first time that there had been an outbreak of monkeypox in the United States.

In a recent study, almost 60% of skin infections in adult patients at emergency departments in 11 U.S. cities were caused by MRSA, and invasive MRSA infections (associated with health care facilities or spread within the community) are increasing in communities where these numbers are being tracked. Data suggests that 8% to 20% of clinical MRSA isolates are community-associated.

Global threats also have emerged, including the possibility of a highly pathogenic avian influenza that is capable of infecting humans through direct contact with infected birds. This influenza strain, influenza A (H5N1), first appeared in humans in Hong Kong in 1997 and, since then, has infected more than 200 people in the Eastern Hemisphere, with a mortality rate of over 50%. The threat of influenza A (H5N1) or another novel influenza virus causing an influenza pandemic has led the United States to undertake significant preparedness efforts aimed at preventing or slowing a potential pandemic.

Morbidity and mortality caused by chemical, biological, radiological, and nuclear agents also have emerged as health threats in the United States. In October 2001, the first inhalational anthrax case in the United States since 1976 was identified in a media company worker in Florida. A national investigation was initiated to identify additional cases and determine possible exposures to *Bacillus anthracis*. Surveillance was enhanced to identify cases, which were defined as clinically compatible illness with laboratory-confirmed *B. anthracis* infection. From October 4 to November 20, 2001, 22 cases of anthrax (11 inhalational, 11 cutaneous) were identified; 5 of the inhalational cases were fatal. Twenty (91%) case-patients were either mail handlers or were exposed to worksites where contaminated mail was processed or received. *B. anthracis* isolates from four powder-containing envelopes, 17 specimens from patients, and 106 environmental samples were indistinguishable by molecular subtyping. Illness and death occurred not only at targeted worksites, but also along the path of mail and in other settings. Since this incident, the United States has undertaken significant efforts to increase surveillance and develop and acquire countermeasures for threats from chemical, biological, radiological, and nuclear agents.

RESPONSE OF THE HEALTH SECTOR

Health Policies and Plans

There were no fundamental system-wide health reforms in the late 1990s, but there were some major adjustments and new commitments made to meet evolving needs.

Starting in 2006, Medicare beneficiaries were offered coverage for prescription drugs; by May 2006, 90% of Medicare enrollees were receiving the coverage. Most people pay a monthly premium for this coverage, which is helping to lower prescription drug costs and helps protect against higher costs in the future. Medicare Prescription Drug Coverage is an insurance plan: private companies provide the coverage and beneficiaries choose the drug plan and pay a monthly premium.

In 2005, Congress and the Department of Health and Human Services took steps to address the rising cost of long-term care for people with disabilities (including the elderly). While the majority of those with long-term care needs rely on unpaid care from relatives and friends, the average cost for a private room in a nursing home is US$ 70,000 per year. The largest public payer for long-term care in the U.S. is the Medicaid program, a federal-state partnership that covers institutional and community-based care for low-income elderly and disabled persons. Medicaid long-term care expenditures were US$ 47.3 billion in 2004. Medicare, the health insurance program for the elderly and disabled, generally does not cover long-term care, with the exception of some time limited post-acute stays. A relatively new source of financing for long-term care is private long-term care insurance. Approximately 9.2 million long-term care policies were sold from 1987 through 2002, and nearly US$ 5.6 billion in benefits were paid out in 2004. Because Congress enacted several key reforms to encourage Americans to plan ahead for the possibility of needing long-term care (for example, by purchasing long-term care insurance), the number of private policy holders is increasing at a rapid rate.

Following the terrorist attacks of September 11, 2001, and reinforced by the hurricanes of 2005, emergency preparedness has become a critical area of focus at the federal, state, and community levels, and much progress has been made. In 2004 and 2005, the U.S. Department of Health and Human Services provided more than US$ 2 billion to states, territories, and localities to strengthen their capacity to respond to terrorism and other public health emergencies. The funds will be used to support the National Response Plan to upgrade infectious disease surveillance and investigation, enhance the readiness of hospitals and the health care system to deal with large numbers of casualties, expand public health laboratory and communications capacities, and improve connectivity between hospitals and local and state health departments to enhance disease reporting.

In 2003, the first-ever federal privacy standards to protect patients' medical records and other health information provided to health plans, doctors, hospitals, and other providers took effect. Developed by the Department of Health and Human Services, these new standards provide patients with access to their medical records and more control over how their personal health information is used and disclosed. They represent a uniform, federal level of privacy protection for consumers across the country by limiting the ways that health plans, pharmacies, hospitals, and other covered entities can use patients' personal medical information. Regulations protect medical records and other individually identifiable health information, whether it is on paper, in computers, or communicated orally. The law creating these privacy protections also encourages electronic transactions.

Finally, there is increasing recognition, in both the public and private sectors, that significant improvements in health care quality, continuity of care, and efficiency of care may be realized through implementation of health information technology. Several activities have been initiated to support its adoption. In April 2004, the President signed an Executive Order recognizing the need to develop and implement a nationwide interoperable health information technology infrastructure and establishing the position of the National Coordinator for Health Information Technology in the Department of Health and Human Services. It is anticipated that the new infrastructure will be developed as a joint public/private effort and that it will be decentralized by standards and address a variety of privacy and security issues.

Organization of the Health System

The United States' health system is actually a cluster of health systems of diverse complexity. Federal, state, and local governments have defined, often in concert with one another, their roles in protecting the public's health. State public health departments are not under the jurisdiction of federal health agencies and administrations, and, in many states, city and county local public health departments are not under the jurisdiction of state public health departments. As a rule, direct health care services are provided by the private sector. Many of these governmental and nongovernmental services share public funds, technical advice, regulatory standards, and health research provided by federal, state, and local governments.

The federal government manages various programs; oversees research; and provides technical advice and direction, training, funding, and other public health resources, mainly through the Department of Health and Human Services. The Department often works through state and local government programs and with other partners. Many other federal government organizations outside the Department's jurisdiction, such as the Environmental Protection Agency, the Social Security Administration, the Department of Agriculture, the Department of Transportation, and the Department of Homeland Security, also are active in securing the population's safety and health.

Responsibility for individual health care issues is much more decentralized. The government provides health insurance to highly vulnerable groups, such as some families in poverty, the disabled, and the elderly. Most persons, however, acquire private health insurance coverage through their employers or on their own.

Direct health care services, including primary, secondary, and tertiary care, are provided primarily by thousands of private-sector hospitals and clinics throughout the country. The federal government directly funds additional hospitals and clinics that care for military personnel and veterans and for American Indians and Alaskan Natives.

The Burden of the Obesity Epidemic

The United States is in the midst of an obesity and overweight epidemic. Between the two survey periods 1976–1980 and 2003–2004, the prevalence of obesity in adults and in children 2–5 years old more than doubled. Among 6–11-year-olds and 12–19-year-olds, it more than tripled. One of the health objectives set in the Government's Healthy People 2010 initiative is to reduce the prevalence of obesity among adults to below 15%, and the Steps Program is one of the most promising initiatives in the effort to achieve this goal. This program will provide grants to communities to implement chronic disease prevention and health promotion activities designed to address such issues as obesity, diabetes, physical inactivity, and poor nutrition.

Public Health Services

Universally available services such as potable water and municipal solid waste disposal are generally managed or regulated by local and state governments. Health issues that cross local and state boundaries—such as air pollution, food safety, and food supplementation for vulnerable populations—are typically regulated by federal and state governments. Quality of health care and credentialing of health professionals are generally the responsibility of nongovernmental, nonprofit organizations and state governments.

Among many other regulatory, administrative, and advisory roles, state and local governments have adopted responsibility for disease surveillance, drug safety regulations, device safety, workplace safety, air and water contamination standards, and safety behaviors such as seatbelt use and adherence to speed limits. The federal, state, and local governments also respond to disease outbreaks and other health emergencies, such as natural or human-caused disasters.

Health Promotion

The federal government continues to pursue its ambitious health promotion and disease prevention campaign. "Healthy People 2010" sets a comprehensive, nationwide agenda designed to improve the health of everyone in the United States during the first decade of the 21st century. "Healthy People 2010" is committed to promoting health and preventing illness, disability, and premature death. The initiative has two overarching goals: to help persons of all ages increase the quality and the number of years of healthy life, and to eliminate health differences, be they differences by gender, race or ethnicity, education or income, disability, geographic location, or sexual orientation.

"Healthy People 2010" encompasses nearly 500 objectives clustered in 28 focus areas. Many objectives focus on interventions designed to reduce or eliminate illness, disability, or premature death; others deal with broader issues such as improving access to quality health care, strengthening public health services, and improving the availability of health-related information. The campaign enlists communities, the nonprofit and for-profit private sectors, and government to reduce identified risk factors and enhance protective factors to decrease the incidence of unhealthy conditions and disease.

Human Resources

In 2004, there were more than 17 million jobs in the health sector or in health occupations outside the health sector, accounting for nearly 12% of the total U.S. workforce. Among these were approximately 2.4 million registered nurses, 1.45 million nursing aides, 1.3 million personal care or home health aides, 567,000 physicians, 230,000 pharmacists, and 150,000 dentists.

Noting that health care is the fastest growing employment sector in the country, the U.S. Bureau of Labor Statistics projected that between 2004 and 2014, the health care sector will grow by more than 27%, compared to a growth under 12% for all other employment sectors. Within health care, jobs in home health care and offices of health practitioners, particularly physician offices, are projected to grow the fastest. The health occupations projected to add the most new jobs over the 10-year period are registered nurses (703,000 new jobs), home health aides (350,000 new jobs), and nursing aides (325,000 new jobs). More than 200,000 physicians and 100,000 new pharmacists will also be needed to fill new jobs as well as replace those who leave existing positions.

Most sources acknowledge a serious nursing shortage, which may become more severe as the population continues to age. Reimbursement issues, working conditions, and regulatory requirements are cited as contributing factors.

Research and Technological Development in Health

The government and the private sector devote extensive human and financial resources to direct and indirect research on health, including such topics as biomedicine, pharmaceuticals, health systems and policies, food and product safety, and agricultural and environmental health. This work cuts across numerous governmental agencies, as well as the nonprofit and corporate sectors.

In 2005, the U.S. Department of Health and Human Services spent more than US$ 30 billion on research, demonstration, and evaluation, including investments for medical research, public health, and food and drug safety. The National Institutes of Health invests more than US$ 27 billion annually in medical research, 80% of which is awarded through almost 50,000 competitive grants to more than 212,000 researchers at more than 2,800 universities, medical schools, and other research institutions in every state and around the world. Another 10% of the Institutes' budget supports projects conducted in its own laboratories by nearly 6,000 scientists.

Within the Department of Health and Human Services, the Centers for Disease Control and Prevention (CDC) spends more than US$ 650 million on research to meet health and safety challenges, including public health research on emerging infectious diseases, environmental threats, the aging population, and lifestyle choices. Another Department component, the Food and Drug Administration (FDA), conducts research and carries out regulatory activities to ensure the safety of food, drugs, devices, and cosmetics. FDA spends over US$ 140 million on research. Other major areas of research within the Department of Health and Human Services include health care quality, aging, and mental health services.

Although basic research is conducted by the government, most pharmaceutical and medical device research is paid for by the companies that produce these products. A private organization representing the country's leading pharmaceutical research and biotechnology companies estimated that, industry-wide, research and investment reached US$ 51.3 billion in 2005.

Health Sector Expenditures and Financing

The U.S. spent US$ 1.9 trillion on health care in 2004. The health spending share of GDP grew 0.1%, to 16% in 2004. This was a smaller share increase than experienced in recent years, as economic growth in 2004 was the fastest since 1989. Per capita health expenditures increased from an annual US$ 4,539 in 2000 to US$ 6,280 in 2004. Health spending rose 7.9% in 2004, slower than the 8.2% growth in 2003 and 9.1% in 2002.

Although private spending continued to represent the lion's share of health spending in 2004 (US$ 1.03 trillion compared to total federal/state US$ 847 billion), federal and state spending for health care rose 8.2% in 2004. Public spending was dominated by Medicare (US$ 309 billion in 2004), with Medicaid spending close behind (US$ 291 billion).

The government provides health insurance coverage to qualified populations living in poverty (primarily through Medicaid) and to those 65 years and older (primarily through Medicare), as well as to the military. In 2004, about 88% of persons covered by private health insurance were on some kind of employment-based plan.

The proportion of the population with government health insurance coverage increased from 24.7% in 2000 to 27.3% in 2005. This change in government coverage was primarily due to the increase in the percentage of the population with Medicaid coverage, which rose from 10.6% in 2000 to 13.0%, or 38.1 million persons, in 2005. Medicare coverage for the elderly remained relatively stable throughout the reporting period, with 42.5 million beneficiaries in 2005. About nine million members of the U.S. military receive health care through the military health program, TRICARE.

In 2004, private payers played a greater role in slowing spending than public payers. Private spending growth slowed to 7.6% in 2004, compared with 8.6% in 2003. Out-of-pocket payments grew 5.5% in 2004, slower than aggregate health spending growth and slower than private insurance premiums, both in aggregate and on a per-enrollee basis. In 2004, the per-enrollee private health insurance premium grew by 8.4%, compared to 2002 growth of 11.5% and 2003 growth of 10.4%.

The share of personal health spending growth associated with prescription drugs has declined since 2000, coincident with a higher share of spending growth for hospital services. Prescription drugs accounted for a 23% share of personal health spending growth between 1997 and 2000, but accounted for only 14% by 2002–2004. Hospital spending, however, accounted for 28% of personal health spending growth between 1997 and 2000, but rose to 38% by 2002–2004.

Hospital spending represented nearly one-third of national health expenditures; the 2004 growth in hospital spending accounted for 33% of the overall increase in health spending. Spending for prescription drugs increased 8.2% in 2004, compared to a growth of 10.2% in 2003 and 14.3% in 2000–2002. In 2004, spending on prescription drugs accounted for nearly 11% of health spending. Spending for physician services constituted 21% of health spending in 2004. Total costs for long-term care of the elderly were US$ 211.4 billion in 2004.

URUGUAY

0   50   100 Miles

Artigas

Salto

Rivera

Paysandú

Tacuarembó

Cerro Largo

Río Negro

Durazno

Treinta y Tres

Soriano

Flores

Florida

Lavalleja

Rocha

Colonia

San José

Canelones

Maldonado

Montevideo

★ **Montevideo**

The Eastern Republic of Uruguay is bordered on the west by Argentina, on the north and northeast by the Federative Republic of Brazil, and on the east and south by the Atlantic Ocean and the Río de la Plata. It has a land area of 176,215 km^2 and a maritime area of 125,057 km^2. It has uneven terrain, with an average elevation of 117 m and a maximum of 514 m, and fertile lowlands along the coast. The climate is temperate, with four seasons during which there is occasional frost and hail, strong winds, droughts, and floods.

GENERAL CONTEXT AND HEALTH DETERMINANTS

The population is 3,241,003 (1) and is largely concentrated in the capital of Montevideo (41%). Males comprise 48.3% of the population, and 51.7% is female.

Uruguay is a representative democracy, with elections every five years. The country is divided into 19 departments, governed by Departmental Councils (31 members) and an Intendant. The national government is made up of the Executive Branch, consisting of the President and 13 ministers; the Legislative Branch, which has two houses—the Senate and the Chamber of Deputies; and the Judicial Branch, comprised of the Supreme Court of Justice and other courts. The 2004 national elections were won by a leftist coalition, for the first time in the history of the country, and the new government took office on March 1, 2005.

Social, Political, and Economic Determinants

Uruguay has a Human Development Index (HDI) of 0.838 and ranks 46th in the world (2). During 2000–2004, the economy went through a recession, and in 2002 suffered a severe economic crisis with a decline in employment and serious consequences to the financial system. The per capita gross domestic product (GDP) went from US$ 6,043 in 2000 to its lowest level in 2003 at US$ 3,309, and by 2005 was at US$ 5,081. The unemployment rate was 12.6% in 2000, rose to 16.9% in 2002, and was 12.2% in 2005. The fall of the GDP, the increase of the unemployment rate, and the indebting in dollars of the urban and rural population have made the situation of poverty more acute throughout the country. In 1999, 15.3% of the population lived below the poverty line, a level which rose to 32.1% by 2004, concentrated largely among children (56.5% of boys and girls between 0 and 5 years lived below the poverty line in 2004) (3, 4). The increase in poverty and the subsequent loss of social security generated direct impacts on the health system of the country. The population seeking care in the public sector increased without a corresponding increase in spending by sector type (either public or private). Approximately 5.4% of the population lives in informal settlements. Montevideo is the department that has the highest concentration of these informal settlements (10.1% of the population). The distribution by age of the population living in these settlements differs from the general distribution of the population: 26% of the population of these settlements is between the ages of 0 and 9 years, and 64% are adolescents or youth (1).

The economic crisis has also worsened international emigration, with many youth and adults emigrating to other countries, as shown in Figure 1. Between 1996 and 2004, 122,000 persons emigrated, representing one fifth of the average number of total annual births in that period.

In 2004, 27.1% of persons in the lowest income quintile had between 0 and 3 years of formal education, while 7.5% in the highest quintile had achieved the same number of years of education. In the lowest quintile, only 2.0% of people had finished 13 years or more of education, while 38% in the highest quintile reached this level (5).

Since 2003 it has been obligatory to complete 10 years of education (seven years of primary school and three of secondary school or technical education). According to 2004 data from the National Institute of Statistics (INE), the proportion of persons between 14 and 15 years of age who completed six years of study was 62.9% among men and 95.8% among women. Among those aged 20 and 21 years, the percentages who completed 12 years of education were lower: 32.3% of men and 42.7% of women.

Illiteracy (quantified by the National Expanded Household Survey, 2006) (6) is 2.3% of the total population of the country (2.7% of men and 2.0% of women). However, in Montevideo, illiteracy is somewhat less than 2.0%, and in the smallest communities and rural areas it is almost at 4.0%. Illiterate men outnumber women in all ages, with the greatest difference in persons aged 65 years and older (5.6% of men and 4.4% of women).

FIGURE 1. Structure of the population emigrating from Uruguay, 1996–2004.

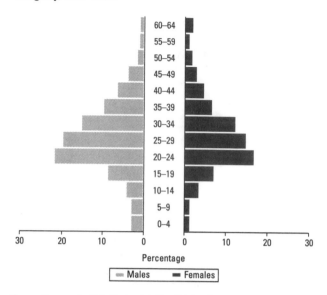

Source: Uruguay, Instituto Nacional de Estadisística, Censo 2004, Fase 1. Summary of results for the entire country.

FIGURE 2. Population structure, by age, sex, and geographic area, Uruguay, 2004.

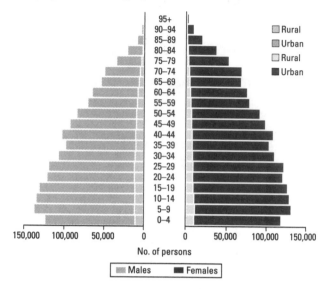

Source: Uruguay, Instituto Nacional de Estadística. Censo 2004, Fase I, Síntesis de resultados.

Illiteracy among men who live in informal settlements is 6.1% while among women it is 4.7%.

While women have more years of education than men, the situation is completely the inverse in terms of their insertion in the workforce and remuneration. The rate of employment in urban areas in 2004 was 62.9% for men and 40.6% for women.

Demographics, Mortality, and Morbidity

The annual rate of demographic growth for the entire country (2005) was 0.6%. Ninety-two percent of the Uruguayan population lives in urban areas, and 8.0% live in rural areas. The urban population grows at an annual rate of 4.3% per 1,000 inhabitants, while the rural population decreases at an intercensal mean annual rate of 11.2 per 1,000 population.

By age distribution, persons aged 65 years and older constitute 13.4% of the population. As shown in Figure 2, those 80 years and older represent 3.2% of the total population in Uruguay.

In effect, the aging of the population is a demographic characteristic and the population pyramid (2004) takes the form of a spindle. Such aging is accompanied by a simultaneous decrease in births. The oldest population grows at an average annual rate of 8.5 per 1,000 while the rest of the age groups grow at a rate of 2.4 per 1,000.

As seen in Figure 3, the period 2001–2004 shows a decline in the number of births. The total rate of fertility dropped to 2.5 children per woman in 1996 to 2.1 children per woman in 2004. Adolescent pregnancies show clear differences based on the so-

cioeconomic status of the mother. While in Montevideo (where 38% of all people are born) 4.8% of women of high socioeconomic level have their first child before turning 18 years of age, 30.7% of women of low socioeconomic level have their first child before turning 18. The crude birth rate was 15.1 live births per 1,000 population in 2004, which represents a decrease compared to previous years. Life expectancy at birth is 75.3 years on average for both sexes, with a difference of more than 7 years between the sexes: 78.9 years for women and 71.6 years for men.

A national death registry exists, under the oversight of the Civil Registry Office, with data collected by the Ministry of Public Health. All death certificates must be signed by a physician (Law No. 5453, May 1942). In 1997, Uruguay began using the International Classification of Diseases, Tenth Edition (ICD-10). Approximately 65% of all deaths occur in hospitals or in other health institutions.

The crude mortality rate was 9.76 per 1,000 population in 2004 (32,220 deaths). According to available data from 2003 (7), 80% of the deaths were due to the following largest groups of causes (ICD-10): diseases of the circulatory system (33.6%); tumors (neoplasms) (23.4%); diseases of the respiratory system (9.4%); symptoms, signs, and abnormal clinical and laboratory findings, not elsewhere classified (8.2%); and external causes (5.7%).

In 2005, the infant mortality rate was 12.7 per 1,000 live births, with a neonatal mortality rate of 7.1 per 1,000 live births and a post-neonatal mortality rate of 5.6 per 1,000 live births (8).

The rate of infant mortality dropped from 29.4 per 1,000 live births in 1985 to 12.7 per 1,000 live births in 2005. This decrease

FIGURE 3. Registered births and crude birth rate, Uruguay, 1990–2004.

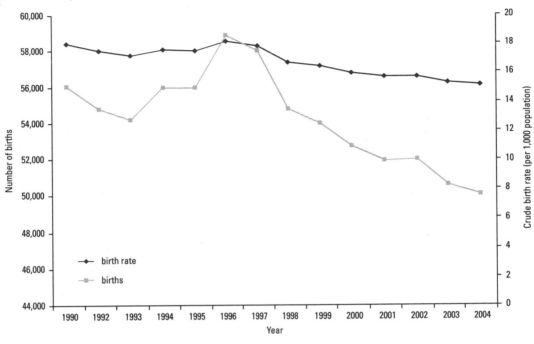

Source: INE. Censo 2004, Fase 1, synthesis of results.

(56.8%) is principally due to the decrease in infant mortality of children receiving care in public sector health institutions (which decreased two-thirds, while in the public sector institutions infant mortality rate decreased one third). Between 1986 and 2001, the infant mortality rate decreased 44.3% in Montevideo, while in the rest of the country it decreased 53.9%. While the rates of infant mortality declined between 1997 and 2002, differences exist among the different departments: the highest rate of infant mortality was registered in the northeastern parts of the country (Rivera, Cerro Largo, Tacuarembó), while those located south of the Rio Negro presented lower rates (9). In Montevideo, those neighborhoods with poorer housing conditions, such as makeshift or precarious housing with poor access to sanitation facilities and maternal-child care, had higher rates of infant mortality.

HEALTH OF POPULATION GROUPS

Children under 5 Years Old

Since 1996, there has been a decrease in the number of births, with 50,051 births in 2004 (the crude birth rate declined from 18.2 per 1,000 in 1996 to 15.2 per 1,000 in 2004). Of births in 2004, 37.0% were in Montevideo and 63.0% in the rest of the country. Low-birthweight infants (less than 2,500 grams) comprised 8.6% of the newborns. Among children less than one year of age, congenital malformations were the principal cause of

death (24.0%). The second most important cause of death was intrauterine hypoxia and other difficulties or respiratory conditions of newborns (13.0%), and bacterial sepsis was the third leading cause (9.0%). The number of cases of congenital syphilis notified and confirmed in 2005 in Uruguay was 29 (rate of 0.6 per 1,000 live births). It should be noted that there is an unquantified underregistration of cases. In the population of children 1–4 years of age, the three principal causes of death were accidents and adverse effects (23.9%), congenital anomalies (13.8%), and acute respiratory infections and pneumonia (11.0%).

Children 5–9 Years Old

In 2004, accidents were the cause of 39.5% of the deaths in this age group, followed by deaths due to tumors (17.3%). In 1999 the three pediatric departments of the School of Medicine of the University of the Republic incorporated into the curriculum a strategy on Integrated Management of Childhood Illness (AIEPI) for undergraduates in medical studies. In 2001, the Ministry of Public Health and the School of Medicine signed an agreement for its joint implementation into all primary care for the country. While several workshops and training courses have been conducted, so far the direct impact has not been measured to determine what they might have contributed to the decline in most common childhood illnesses.

Adolescents 10–19 Years Old

As with children between 5 and 9 years of age, in 2004, accidents were the principal cause of death for the group between 10 and 19 years of age (33.2% of the deaths in this group). The second most common cause was suicides (12.5%), followed by tumors (9.5%) and violence or homicides (9.1%). Adolescent pregnancy constituted 16.5% of the total number of pregnancies in 2001.

Adults 20–59 Years Old

Of the 32,220 deaths in 2004, 15% occurred in this age group. Sixty-nine percent of these deaths were due to three principal causes: tumors (30.0%), diseases of the circulatory system (20.0%), and external causes (19.0%).

In terms of maternal mortality, in 2005, 11 deaths were registered, four of those due to complications from abortion, for a maternal mortality rate of 23.3 per 100,000 live births.

Older Adults 60 Years Old and Older

The principal causes of death in this age group were diseases of the circulatory system (2,274 per 100,000 persons 60 years and older), tumors (1,405 per 100,000), and chronic diseases of the lower respiratory system, acute respiratory infections, and pneumonia (620 per 100,000).

Persons with Disabilities

The first National Survey of People with Disabilities was conducted between September 2003 and August 2004 (10). The principal results show a prevalence of disabilities of 7.6% in the general population (estimated 210,400 disabled persons). No significant differences in prevalence were found between the capital and the rest of the country. Women have a higher prevalence (8.2%) than men (7.0%). More than half of the persons with at least one disability (50.8%) were 65 years or older, followed by persons aged 50 to 64 years (18.4%) and by persons aged 30–49 years (12.9%). There is an increase in the prevalence of disability with age, with one of every four older adults developing a disability. The majority of the population with disabilities (66.0%) has only one disability, independent of gender. The survey participants attributed their disability in 51.0% of the cases to an illness, 21.0% to birth, 18.0% to aging, and 9.0% to an accident. Twenty-one percent of the disabled reported that they needed help in caring for themselves and 40.0% required assistance to leave their homes.

The main disabilities reported were difficulties in walking (33%), vision (25%), and hearing (13.6%). The proportion of persons with a disability with a low level of education (37.0%) is much higher than those who are not disabled (12.6%). Only 16.5% of economically active persons with a disability are employed, versus 53.4% of those without a disability.

HEALTH CONDITIONS AND PROBLEMS

COMMUNICABLE DISEASES

Vector-borne Diseases

One potential problem is the reintroduction of the *Aedes aegypti* mosquito, along with the possible appearance of cases of **dengue**, which was newly detected in 1997 after being absent since its eradication in 1958. Through a rigorous prevention plan, infestation is limited to certain geographic zones (basically to three cities: Salto, Mercedes, and Fray Bentos). No native cases of dengue have been notified (since August 2006), although some have been found in neighboring countries.

Uruguay has controlled **Chagas' disease** to a large extent. Its main vector, *Triatoma infestans*, was present in two thirds of the national territory, but by 1997, the specific vector control program, integrated in the Southern Cone Chagas Control Initiative, had managed to eliminate or minimize household infestation. Successive international evaluations in 1998, 1999, and 2000 certified this accomplishment, and Uruguay is the first endemic country to interrupt transmission. Surveillance and control currently continue in an effort to completely eliminate *T. infestans*.

The pulmonary syndrome of **hantavirus** was first seen in the country in 1997, and since then has maintained a low annual incidence (0.22 cases per 100,000 population) in the entire southern region of the country. Its average lethality was 24%, and 72% of the cases were among men (2006). The most important risk factor is living or working in rural areas. The wild rodent involved is the *Oligorzomys flavescens*.

The prevalence rate of **leprosy** for all of Uruguay in 2005 was 0.04 per 10,000 population. The highest rates were registered in two departments of the northeast coast, Artigas (0.53 per 10,000) and Río Negro (0.19 per 10,000). Montevideo had a rate of 0.01 per 10,000. The number of notified and confirmed annual cases of leprosy in Uruguay dropped from 628 in 1989 to 15 in 2002. Between 10 and 20 cases are notified and confirmed annually throughout the entire country.

Vaccine-preventable Diseases

Since the beginning of the 1980s, no cases of **poliomyelitis, neonatal tetanus,** or **diphtheria** have been found. In 1999, the last cases of **measles** were registered, and currently eradication is in process. No cases of **rubella** have been found since 2002 either. In 2005, an outbreak of **infectious parotitis (mumps)** in Montevideo occurred, largely affecting youth between 18 and 24 years of age, who had received only one dosage of the vaccine. More than 2,500 cases occurred, but no deaths were reported. Obligatory vaccination against **chickenpox** began in 1999.

Between 2002 and 2005, the vaccination coverage among children less than one year of age was greater than 95% for all the different vaccines included in the Expanded Immunization Program (EIP) (11), which in 2006 were: diphtheria, hepatitis b, parotitis, poliomyelitis, rubella, measles, tetanus, whopping cough, tuberculosis, chickenpox, meningitis, and other infections such as *Haemophilus influenzae* type b.

The number of notified and confirmed cases of **viral hepatitis A** during 2005 was 2,877 (88.7 cases per 100,000 population); San José (633 cases per 100,000), Artigas (608 per 100,000), Canelones (89.9 per 100,000), and Montevideo (34.2 per 100,000) were the departments with the most cases.

Chronic Communicable Diseases

Since the mid-1990s, the incidence of **tuberculosis** cases has not shown substantial changes, with an average of 650 new cases being registered annually (annual rate of 20.0 per 100,000 population). However, 729 cases were registered in 2004 and 723 cases were registered in 2005 (rate of 22.3 per 100,000 population).

HIV infection has brought about an increase in the number of tuberculosis cases. On average, during 1994–2004, 10% of the cases of tuberculosis were among HIV/AIDS patients, and 12% of the cases registered in 2005 were carriers of the infection. The co-infected patients with tuberculosis and HIV/AIDS are largely young adults, especially between 25 and 34 years. A significantly larger number of patients with biologically unconfirmed pulmonary tuberculosis exists in relation to the HIV-negative tuberculosis population. The rate of abandonment of treatment is greater among HIV-negative patients. Until 2005, no major tendency in the development of TB drug resistance was seen in the Uruguayan population. Another unique situation is overpopulation of detention centers where more than 600 cases of TB per 100,000 are registered in some centers, which is a rate 30 times greater than in the general population.

HIV/AIDS and Other Sexually Transmitted Infections

As of 2005, the HIV/AIDS epidemic was largely driven by sexual transmission (71%; prevalence of 1,975 cases in that year), particularly through heterosexual transmission (63%). Transmission through infected blood was responsible for 25.4% of the cases (prevalence of 706 cases in 2005) and perinatal transmission was responsible for 3.6% of the cases (prevalence of 101 cases in 2005). Sentinel studies in 2000 showed the HIV prevalence to be 0.23% of the population, rising to 0.45% in 2004. In 2005, it was found that 78.3% of persons living with HIV/AIDS were from Montevideo, and 21.7% were found in the rest of the country.

From 1983 to 2006 a total of 6,463 cases of HIV-positive patients were registered, and 2,895 cases of AIDS (total number of accumulated cases) were registered. Of the persons with AIDS, 1,467 have died (mortality rate of 51%). As of June 2006 it is estimated Uruguay has 7,890 persons living with HIV or with AIDS, and that of those approximately 1,700 are on treatment. The rest, approximately 6,190 persons identified as living with HIV/AIDS, are not receiving treatment for different reasons: personal abandonment of indicated treatment, choice of alternative treatments (without antiretrovirals), or, in some cases, lack of in-

dication by the physician. However, according to the last sentinel study (2004), approximately 5,000 people living with HIV/AIDS have not been identified as such.

Of the total number of cases up to 2005, 67.0% of those HIV positive are male. The most affected are those between 15 and 44 years, with a maximum incidence in those 25 to 34 years. The male/female ratio dropped from 8.9 in 1989 to 2.2 in 2005.

In 1991 Uruguay passed a law that establishes that the provision of treatment is compulsory to all persons living with HIV/AIDS. In 1996 100% treatment coverage was achieved for all those living with HIV/AIDS requiring treatment as indicated by their physicians. Since 1997, all health centers are required by law to offer HIV testing to all pregnant women at their prenatal visits. In 1998, the National Consensus Commission was created to standardize treatment protocols. In 2002, the National Fund to Fight AIDS was created to finance antiretroviral treatment and corresponding paraclinical exams; the Fund is financed through a 3% tax on insurance policies, and taxes on the sale of football players to foreign teams.

Zoonoses

Uruguay was declared free of **foot-and-mouth-disease (FMD)** without vaccination in 1999. However, in 2000 the virus was reintroduced in the department of Rivera, and the pertinent recommendations of the World Organization for Animal Health (OIE) were implemented. In 2001, another reemergence of the disease occurred on the eastern coast, and since then bovine vaccination was reinitiated. A bivalent OA vaccination was chosen over a trivalent OAC vaccination, as there has been no trace of the virus in the Southern Cone for several years.

Very few cases of **brucellosis** (five cases in 2005) and **anthrax** (four cases in 2005) have been found in rural workers since 2000, as both zoonotic diseases are on the decline.

Leptospirosis is an occupational and epizootic disease found in specific areas dedicated to dairy farming and the cultivation of rice and sugar cane. Since 2002, there has been a greater awareness of the importance of this disease, leading to an increase in outbreak notifications. The outbreaks have been largely brought on by the floods and recent growth in the informal suburban settlements. In 2000, 23 cases were notified, while in 2002, 247 cases were notified (*12*).

Hydatidosis or cystic echinococcosis is a highly endemic parasitosis that, with intervention by the National Honorary Commission to Fight Hydatidosis, has been drastically reduced in terms of prevalence among children, real and operative incidence in men, and prevalence in canines (definite host), ovines, and bovines (intermediate hosts). In 1993, 367 cases were operated on nationwide (39.8% of them coming from Montevideo); and, in 2002, 139 patients were operated on (31.7% of them coming from Montevideo). On the basis of this national experience, the Southern Cone Subregional Project of Surveillance and Control of Hydatidosis was formed in 2004 (Argentina, Brazil, Chile, and

Uruguay), with the Technical Secretariat of the Pan American Health Organization (PAHO)/Pan American Foot and Mouth Disease Center (PANAFTOSA) and the Food and Agriculture Organization of the United Nations (FAO).

Prevention, surveillance, and control of zoonotic diseases and other illnesses transmitted by arthropods has been reorganized by law and the National Honorary Commission to Fight Hydatidosis was transformed into the National Commission of Zoonosis, in charge of handling these pathologies and responsible for the coordination of all programs in this area.

NONCOMMUNICABLE DISEASES

Metabolic and Nutritional Diseases

The major nutritional problems in Uruguay are **obesity** and **protein energy malnutrition**; the prevalence of **nutritional anemia** and **vitamin A deficiency** is unknown. A survey conducted in 2000 revealed that 51% of Uruguayans are **overweight** and 17% are obese (*13*). According to 2005 figures, the greatest proportion of obese children is found in those less than 1 year (7.8%), and malnutrition is highest among children age 1 (11.8%), measured by weight and height (*14*).

School-based censuses of children in the first grade in public schools (approximately 85% of the total child population attends public schools) reveal that 19.7%, 18.1%, and 22.9% of children had a height deficiency in 1987, 1990, and 2002, respectively. Data from 2002 suggest that the nutritional status of children has shown deterioration according to international standards (National Center for Health Statistics, CDC) since it was expected that the height deficiency that year would be 15.9% (*2*).

Cardiovascular Diseases

Diseases of the circulatory system have been the leading cause of death for nearly 50 years, accounting for 33.0% of all deaths in 2004. The mortality rate for these diseases was 330 per 100,000 population in 1999 and 328 per 100,000 in 2004.

The most common are **cerebrovascular diseases**, with a mortality rate of 114 per 100,000 population, and **ischemic diseases**, with a mortality rate of 86 per 100,000 population. Cerebrovascular diseases have a greater mortality rate among women than among men (128 vs. 98 per 100,000), while the opposite is true for ischemic disease, which is more frequent in men (101 and 72 per 100,000 population, respectively).

Malignant Neoplasms

Malignant neoplasms represented 23.5% of all deaths in Uruguay in 2004. A hospital-based morbidity study conducted in the first part of 2005 by the Ministry of Health among private health institutions found that tumors represented 9.6% of hospital discharges, with malignant tumors comprising 66% of the total. The rates of hospital discharge for this cause did not show a

significant difference between men and women (3.47 and 3.77 per 1,000 persons, respectively). More than 90% of the cases corresponded to persons aged 45 and older. In the general population, the most frequent types of tumors were, first, breast cancer, followed by cancer of the trachea, bronchus, and lung; and thirdly cancer of the colon. In men, cancer of the trachea, bronchus and lung predominated followed by cancer of the prostate and then cancer of the bladder, while among women, breast cancer led with 27% of the cases, followed by non-Hodgkins lymphoma and colon cancer. The average hospital stay for neoplasms is 10 days.

OTHER HEALTH PROBLEMS OR ISSUES

Mental Health

In 2005 the rate of mortality due to suicide was 20.6 per 100,000 population, and it was higher in men (77%) and in the interior of the country (70.9%). Of all persons treated in ambulatory mental health facilities in the country, 54% were women and 11% were children or adolescents. The average number of contacts per person is 3.3 per year. The most common diagnoses for admission to psychiatric hospitals were schizophrenia (44%) and changes in mood (20%).

Oral Health

Through decree by Executive Order, production and obligatory sale of fluoridated salts was initiated throughout the country in 1999. During that year, the last DMFT (decayed, missing, and filled teeth) survey among 12 year olds was taken, with an index of 2.47.

RESPONSE OF THE HEALTH SECTOR

Health Policies and Plans

The Constitution establishes that the State will legislate on all questions or issues related to health and public hygiene in order to achieve physical, moral, and social improvement of the Uruguayan population. The State will provide free preventive care and assistance only to indigents or those lacking sufficient resources. The Ministry of Public Health (MSP) was created in 1934 by Law No. 9.202, and is the organization responsible for establishing norms and regulating the sector, developing preventive programs, and administrating their assistance services.

In order to respond to the increasing poverty that was identified particularly after 2002, the Ministry of Social Development (MIDES) was created by Law No. 17.866 (*15*) in March of 2005. One of its principal policies is the National Plan for Social Emergencies (PANES) that consists of monthly transfers of a sum of money by the State to those households that are below the poverty line and whose incomes per person do not surpass the amount for a basic basket of food (*16*). In return for the money, persons are requested to provide some compensation, such as carrying out community work, ensuring that their children attend school, and that they care for their health. The program will be carried out for two years, followed by an evaluation to determine the results.

The Child, Adolescent and Family Program (Infamilia) (*17*), operating within the framework of the Ministry of Social Development, aims to improve the living conditions and social insertion of boys and girls and their families through specific policies, many of which are linked to health and poverty. The Program supports the promotion of integrated development and the growth of boys and girls from 0 to 4 years through the support of the Plan CAIF (Child and Family Care Centers), which provides care to 13,800 children throughout the country through 210 care centers. The Infamilia Program also works with the Ministry of Public Health to develop activities regarding sexual and reproductive health, including the accompanying of adolescent mothers and fathers during the first year following birth; the training of youth promoters; and the creation of specialized spaces for adolescent care. In 2005, more than 50 socio-educational agents accompanied more than 1,500 adolescent mothers and fathers, and training for health professionals in sexual and reproductive health was also conducted.

Health Strategies and Programs

In 2000 the Ministry of Public Health established a program to strengthen the Collective Health Care Institutions, with financing from the Inter-American Development Bank, which had a partial impact particularly on a group of private institutions located in Montevideo. The debt situation and other structural causes were the reason for the closure of many Collective Health Care Institutions, which declined in number from 50 in 2000 to 41 in 2005. Several institutions remain at risk, and the health authority has to play an active role in the evaluation of the fulfillment of their responsibilities as well as in control of their economic-financial management. Beginning in March 2005, the new government proposed that, given the critical situation of the sector, profound changes must be made to the models of health care, finance, and management. It hopes to achieve this through the construction of a National Integrated Health System and a National Insurance program to finance it. Therefore, a comprehensive strategy and inter-institutional coordination with other areas such as food, education, housing, and social security, among others, are considered absolutely necessary (*18*).

The health system is currently very fragmented and inequitable: the population covered by the public assistance services is largely younger, mostly female, and further below the income and education level than the population covered by the private sector. At the same time, the private sector has three times the amount of resources per beneficiary than the private sector. With the crisis in 2002, the utilization of the public sector has grown due to reduced employment opportunities, and those unemployed lost health coverage through social security. The lack of a corresponding increase in the resources assigned to the public sector has resulted in a worsening of the inequities in quality and access.

Organization of the Health System

In March of 2005 the government proposed a global reform to the health sector (*18*), with a principal objective of contributing to equity in access to health services, through changes to the model of care and the application of a Primary Health Strategy, prioritizing the needs and rights of citizens through disease prevention, education, and health promotion, with an emphasis on active development of healthy behaviors and social participation. The reform also proposes changes to the management model, with an emphasis on democratization, transparency, efficacy, and efficiency to improve quality of care, as well as to the financing model, through the creation of a National Health Insurance program, proposing that resources be assigned and distributed to the health sector to meet the needs of the population. In the proposed insurance scheme, the users would contribute to the system based on family income and would obtain access to integrated coverage for health services. Public and private businesses would contribute an amount proportional to the number of employed workers. The institutions providing health services would receive income that would make it possible for them to achieve a reasonable balance between the number of enrollees and the cost of their care, based on the level of risk and expected expense for the population covered. This implies charging different costs through risk premiums based on sex, age, and other variables. The participating private health care institutions would follow the guidelines, norms, and controls that are defined as a condition for them to be financed by the insurance. The proposal includes a universal salary, regardless of where one works, as well as an overall cap on remunerations. The administration of the National Health Insurance program would be in the office of a Health Superintendent. The financial control and the quality of the core proposed services are the main components of the proposal.

In 2006 one of the first legal instruments designed by the Ministry of Public Health, and currently under discussion in the Parliament, was the Law of Administrative Decentralization of the State Health Services Administration, that separates the Administration from the structure of the Ministry of Public Health and converts it into an autonomous organization. The new organization would be directed by three delegates of the Executive Branch, a representative from the beneficiaries, and a representative from the workers of the State Health Services Administration. The purpose of this project is to complete the decentralization process begun in 1987 and to allow the Ministry of Public Health to concentrate on its steering role of the health sector.

The health system (*19–22*) has been historically characterized by a high level of fragmentation in the public and private sectors and by significant involvement of the private sector.

Various institutions make up the public sector providing health services. The network of the State Health Services Administration establishments is the largest in the country, and it includes hospitals, health centers, polyclinics, and family physicians. It provides coverage to the low-income population and is estimated to cover approximately 1,400,000 persons, approximately 40% of the total population. The State Health Services Administration provides 8,000 beds. The Armed Forces Health Services has its own hospital infrastructure in Montevideo with 450 beds and nursing services in the military units in the rest of the country. It provides coverage to approximately 165,000 people (active duty military, retirees, and their dependents). The Police Health Service has a hospital infrastructure of 132 beds in Montevideo, and in the interior of the country contracts services from the State Health Services Administration and private providers. It provides coverage to 70,000 (active duty police, retirees, and their dependents). The Scientific Hospital of the University of the Republic covers the same population as the State Health Services Administration and has 450 functioning beds. The Maternal-Child Service of the Social Welfare Bank has its own centers and provides coverage to couples and the children of beneficiaries of the Illness Insurance program who do not have private coverage. The State Insurance Fund provides direct care through its own 160-bed hospital in Montevideo and contracts services in the interior of the country. It covers occupational accidents and illness for the private sector. The Autonomous Entity Services and the Decentralized Services provide coverage to their workers, and in some cases, former employees and their families. The medical services of the 19 departments have varying levels of development, all providing primary health care and covering the low-income population.

The Collective Health Care Institutions are located in the private sector, with 41 medical centers with prepaid comprehensive services, 12 of which have their base in Montevideo and the rest in the interior of the country. It is a tightly regulated sector, and prices are subject to administrative control by the Ministry of Economics and Finance. Furthermore, the Ministry of Public Health determines which services it must provide and controls its aspects of care, as well as its economic and financial aspects. The majority of these organizations have their own inpatient services and their beneficiaries number 1,400,000. The institutions have between 3,000 and 240,000 affiliates. Private insurance plans are comprised of private businesses, largely commercial in nature, which provide care services through prepayment. This subsector includes institutions that provide total coverage (similar to the Collective Health Care Institutions), as well as partial. Starting in 2000, the State began to tighten its control over these organizations, particularly for those that are competition for the Ministry of Public Health. There are six companies which offer private insurance plans, including comprehensive coverage, and provide care to 55,000 subscribers. The mobile emergency systems are made up of a particular type of private

partial coverage insurance, which includes domiciliary ambulatory coverage in case of emergency. Most of the subscribers to these insurance plans have double coverage, and they complement their public or private comprehensive insurance plan with these services. The Institutes of Highly Specialized Medicine are also care-providing organizations, and they sell high-technology services. There are also a large number of private businesses, sanatoriums, and clinics that sell ambulatory services or inpatient care.

Public Health Services

On February 20, 2004, within the framework of strengthening the Epidemiological Surveillance of the Ministry of Public Health (Decree 64/004), the National Code on the Required Notification of Disease and Health Events was put into place, which includes a listing of notifiable diseases and events and the definition of a suspicious case, of a confirmed case, and the corresponding prevention and control methods. At the same time, the organization and functioning of the ministerial units in charge of communicable disease surveillance, chronic disease, environmental health, accidents, and nutrition were redesigned. In the area of maternal-child health, the Ministry of Public Health has required prevention activities in the polyclinics throughout the departments, and it also has incorporated, through the health reform process, measures to ensure greater equity, such as free prenatal care.

Also through this framework, the organization and functioning of the National Public Health Laboratory have been redesigned (Decrees 384/999 and 241/000). The goals include technical assistance and supervision of the National Network of Clinical Analysis Laboratories (public and private), epidemiological surveillance, the development of diagnostic norms and protocols, the quality control of reagents, procedures, and techniques, and outside evaluation. In March 2006 the Ministry of Public Health designed a National Contingency Plan for Pandemic Influenza (which includes avian influenza). The Ministry of Public Health is also working with other sectors, particularly with the Ministry of Livestock, Agriculture and Fisheries, to prevent avian influenza among producers.

The coverage of potable water services is 98% for the total population living in formal or regular settlements. A technical renovation and expansion of potable water service coverage continues to be developed, which was started during the 1990s by the Public Sanitation Office (official agency). The country continues to face the challenge of providing potable water coverage to the population residing in informal settlements around the outskirts of Montevideo, which represents 10.1% of the population of the capital. Sanitation services only reach approximately 80% of the population in the urban area of Montevideo, with more than 50% receiving services through the national sanitation network. In the urban interior of the country, 30% of the population receives services through the sanitation network, and approximately 50%

of the urban population in the interior of the country disposes of their own waste water (through septic tanks).

Traditionally, Uruguay has maintained a high level of food safety. The national responsibilities for food safety fall to the Ministry of Public Health, while the direct execution of food in-oculation activities corresponds to the municipal authorities. Other actors in this area are the Technological Laboratory of Uruguay (LATU), the Ministry of Agriculture, Livestock and Fishery, consumer protection organizations, and the industrial and food services business associations. Several departments have their own comprehensive food safety programs as a strategy to protect health, production, and the local labor market. Work continues through the System for Epidemiological Surveillance of Food-Borne Disease, coordinated by the Ministry of Public Health at the national level. The municipal authorities conduct bromatological controls and the Consumer Defense Area (ADECO) of the Ministry of Economy is responsible for product quality control, among other duties.

Individual Care Services

Blood donation in Uruguay is voluntary according to national norms. Some 35,000 Uruguayans receive transfusions every year. Eighty-seven blood banks exist in Uruguay: 45 public and 42 in the private sector. One hundred percent of blood is screened for the following diseases: syphilis, viral hepatitis B (superficial antigen and "anticore" antibody), viral hepatitis C, HIV (anti HTLV-1 and 2), and Chagas' disease. Based on the pre-donation questionnaire, 17% of would-be donors are rejected, and 4.7% of blood samples are discarded after screening (23).

Health Promotion

As a way to address community health, the Ministry of Public Health has begun a "productive and health communities" strategy in certain at-risk rural and suburban areas, with the goal of including comprehensive health activities in the development of production and local work. It has supported cooperative projects and small and mid-sized community businesses, based on the production of foodstuffs, artisan goods, and other local/regional products. The Ministry of Public Health and the Ministry of Agriculture, Livestock and Fishery programs have played an active role in these activities.

Uruguay ratified the Framework Convention on Tobacco Control. In 2006 the country enacted a national law that made all public spaces, workplaces, bars and restaurants smoke-free and made Uruguay a pioneer in the Region in the battle against tobacco.

Health Supplies

A broad legal framework exists to regulate the importation, production, distribution, sales, and propaganda of pharmaceuti-cals. The Ministry of Public Health controls the requirements to authorize the sanitary registration of pharmaceuticals considered necessary, efficacious, safe, and under conditions that guarantee quality and compliance with the norms of the production laboratories. The Ministry of Public Health depends on the evaluation and registry units; inspection of manufacturers, importers, distributors, and places of sale and usage; and on laboratory analysis to control the quality of medications.

The control includes all areas of production (licensure of manufacturer, sanitary registration of products, and good manufacturing practices) and of distribution (outfitting and inspection of establishments and compliance with best practices).

Norms require an obligatory common *vade mecum* (reference book) for all the Collective Health Care Institutions, and a separate one exists for all the public services. Some of the goals defined by the new administration since 2005 include: approve the Law of Generic Drugs; provide guaranteed access and availability to medications as soon as they are approved for the Sole Therapeutic Drug Formulary for the entire health system; strengthen drug surveillance; stimulate national production through competition and with adequate quality controls; and promote the rational use of drugs.

Decree 165/99 establishes that the manufacturing, registration, importation, commercialization, use, and control of diagnostic reagents, medical equipment, and therapeutic devices are the exclusive domain of the Department of Medical Technology, of the Division of Health Products, belonging to the General Directorate of Health of the Ministry of Public Health. The Ministry of Industry and Energy, through the Directorate of Nuclear Technology, has responsibility for all equipment that emits ionizing radiation. Since 2004 it has coordinated with the Department of Medical Technology on the registration of this type of equipment (Decree 43/004).

In 2004 the first National Census of Medical Equipment was completed with the objective of undertaking a diagnostic review of the medical equipment being used throughout the country, with the goal of planning for the rational introduction of new technologies. It should be noted that a high percentage of equipment is obsolete or in very precarious maintenance condition, which has resulted in the regulation of maintenance services for medical equipment.

Through the framework of implementing the Comprehensive National Health System since 2005, the government considered it necessary to create an Information System on Medical Technology, with the goal of systematically gathering information on the habilitation, organization, functioning, and use of medical equipment.

With regard to the functioning of manufacturing companies and importers of medical products, Good Manufacturing Practice Inspections were begun, as required by MERCOSUR norm 4/95, and the goal is to require this certification for all national companies.

Human Resources

Medical doctors must be professional university graduates with a diploma granted by an officially recognized institution, must register with the Ministry of Public Health to practice as a professional, and must register with the Retirement and Pension Office for University Professionals. For foreign professionals to be able to practice in Uruguay they must have an authorized diploma from a university or institution recognized by the Ministry of Education and Culture.

As of December 31, 2005, Uruguay had 13,390 physicians (41.3 per 10,000 population). The supply of physicians is characteristically a specialized workforce in which, on average, every professional holds more than two jobs (24). In terms of the workforce overview, a study has confirmed (25) that medical work is spread among a relatively important number of sources of employment. The average number of jobs is higher than two jobs per professional, but it varies depending on how many years the professional has been working as a medical doctor and the concentration of work in the private sector. Human resources in health are shown in Table 1.

The system for human resources training, from the point of view of the programs and based on the number of graduated professionals and technicians, does not take into consideration the health needs of the population based on demographic and epidemiological parameters when planning. Similarly, the identification of human resources for the sector also has not been a priority area for action on the part of health authorities. In 2005, the implementation of an information system on available health resources in the public and private health services was begun, including data on the quantity and type of positions, level of care where they work, and remunerations and quantity of medical interventions, which demonstrate advancement in the characterization of such resources.

Furthermore, the Ministry of Public Health and the School of Medicine are developing other joint activities with an agenda linked to the Medical Residency Programs and other areas related to human resources.

TABLE 1. Health professionals in Uruguay.

Profession	Total number	Ratio per 10,000 population
Physicians	13,390	41.3
Dentists	4,308	13.3
Licensed nurses	3,543	10.9
Pharmacists	1,476	4.6
Midwives	579	1.8

Source: Calculated with data from the Retirement and Pension Office for University Professionals.

Health Sector Expenditures and Financing

Studies have shown a trend in health expenditures increasing from 1994 until 2000, and decreasing from 2000 until 2004. The relationship between health expenditure and gross domestic product (GDP) can be seen in Table 2.

As shown in Table 3, the resources for the health sector come from both the public and private sectors. The public sector spends approximately US$ 12 per person per month, while the private sector spends US$ 32 per person per month. Although the coverage of care is almost evenly split between the public and private sectors, there is a large and historical difference in expenditures between the two sectors.

Public financing is comprised largely of taxes, contributions to social security, and tariffs for services on some companies. National and municipal taxes exist that finance health expenditures, and the General Budget for Expenses and Investment is the instrument by which the resources are assigned to the public agencies on the national level. The resources available for the Ministry of Public Health correspond largely to the budget of the State Health Services Administration. The municipal taxes are collected by the departmental governments, which, in function of their own budgetary assignments, contribute to the system to finance the provision of health services to the population of the department, as well as to finance the coverage of their own employees. According to the 1975 Law 14.407, the employees and employers in a private activity should contribute 3% and 5%, respectively, to the Illness Insurance program of the Social Welfare Bank. The law also provides for the possibility of not contributing the aforementioned support to the Health Insurance program, given that the employer and the employees agree that the support for coverage will be financed through other insurance plans. According to the 1995 Law 16.713, the right to coverage through the Illness Insurance program is given to those pensioners below a certain predetermined income level; those who opt for this arrangement contribute 3% of their pension. Teachers and judicial employees in the public sector have obtained the right to supported coverage through the Social Welfare Bank. This coverage, as well as the deficit of the actively employed and those retired, is financed through the transferences from the Central Government to social security.

Some of the public agencies (the National Administration of Combustibles, Alcohol, and Cement; and three banks (Banco República, Banco Hípotecario, and Banco de Seguros) finance the health coverage of their employees, and those funds come from the fees charged for their services. Private financing is largely comprised of out-of-pocket expenses by those persons who have voluntary or private providers.

The sources of financing of the health system are made up of organizations that have the securing and administering of funds for the purchase of services (such as the Illness Insurance program of the BPS) as their specific function, as well as other organizations whose principal function is the provision of services.

TABLE 2. Trends in health expenditures, Uruguay, 1994–2004.

Year	Population (thousands)	Health expenditures (millions US$)	GDP (millions US$)	Expenditure in health as a percentage of GDP (%)	Per capita expenditure in health (US$)
1994	3,195	1,590	17,518	9.1	498
1995	3,218	1,781	19,318	9.2	553
1997	3,265	2,163	21,695	10.0	662
1998	3,289	2,292	22,371	10.2	697
1999	3,303	2,238	20,912	10.7	678
2000	3,322	2,182	20,042	10.9	657
2004	3,241	1,184	13,215	9.0	365

Source: Cuentas Nacionales en Salud 2004 y Cuentas de Gasto y Financiamiento, 1990–2000.

TABLE 3. Sources of health financing, Uruguay, 2000 and 2004.

Sources of financing	2000 (%)	2004 (%)
General taxes	21.9	20.2
Local taxes	0.3	1.7
Parastatal and public corporations	2.3	2.3
Social security		
Employer contributions	9.6	11.9
Contributions of the employee/pensioner	4.6	5.8
Transfers of the government to social security	3.3	7.7
Health expenditures with private financing	53.4	49.6
Health expenditures financed externally	0.0	0.0
Debt	4.5	0.8
General total	100.0%	100.0%
(millions of US$)	(2,182)	(1,184)

Beginning with the social security contributions and the transfers of the government the comprehensive care for approximately 600,000 workers and retired people are financed and covered, which form part of the care providers of the private sector.

The National Fund of Resources, a non-State public institution whose objective is to finance a group of high-cost, low-frequency providers, is also an institutional agent of financing. Its funds are derived largely from the payment of the Illness Insurance program of the Social Welfare Bank, by the actively employed and pensioners who are covered; out-of-pocket payments from all persons voluntarily affiliated with a Collective Health Care Institution; payment for services from the General Revenue for the coverage of those receiving services from the State Health Services Administration; and specific taxes. The National Fund of Resources contracts public and private providers (named by the Institutes of Highly Specialized Medicine) for the coverage of high-technology care. Other organizations such as the State Health Services Administration, the Military Health System of the National Ministry of Defense, the Police Health System of the Ministry of the Interior, the Municipal Intendancies, and the State Insurance Fund, are financial agents that also receive funds through public financing and provide care.

At the private level the Collective Health Care Institutions and the private health insurance plans fulfill a double role as financing agent and provider of services.

Technical Cooperation and External Financing

The majority of the projects begun in the 1990s financed by the World Bank were completed by the end of 2000. The Strengthening Project of the Collective Health Care Institutions, developed during that same year, was funded by the Inter-American Development Bank (IDB).

Beginning in 2005, new lines of support from the World Bank began, largely linked to the social area, including the reform of the health sector. The technical cooperation of the Pan American Health Organization (PAHO)/World Health Organization (WHO) continues working to comply with the resolutions of the Governing Bodies and the national and departmental health authorities. From December 2000 to July 2006, the Ministry of Public Health,

Response to Deepening Poverty

In 2002 Uruguay suffered a severe economic crisis with a decline in employment and serious consequences for the financial system. The increase in unemployment and the debt in dollars of the urban and rural population have made poverty more acute. In 1999, 15.3% of the population lived below the poverty line, with the figure rising to 32.1% by 2004, concentrated largely among children (56.5% of boys and girls between 0 and 5 years lived below the poverty line in 2004).

As a response, the Ministry of Social Development (MIDES) was created in March 2005. One of its main policies is the National Plan for Social Emergencies (PANES) that consists of monthly government cash transfers to households below the poverty line whose per capita incomes do not exceed the cost of a basic basket of food. The cash transfers are contingent on the beneficiaries performing community work, and ensuring that their children attend school and go for medical checkups. The program will last for two years, followed by an evaluation of the results. MIDES also operates the Child, Adolescent and Family Program (Infamilia), which aims to improve the living conditions and social integration of children and their families through specific policies, several of which are linked to health and poverty. The Program supports the promotion of comprehensive development and growth among boys and girls from 0 to 4 years and, together with the Ministry of Health, it carries out actions for sexual and reproductive education, including support for teenage parents for the first year following the birth of a child, training for youth promoters, and the creation of specialized spaces to assist adolescents.

with support from PAHO and financing from the IDB, developed a project on oral health that included a cost-effectiveness study on the technique or practice of the atraumatic restoration (PRAT). This research is simultaneously being conducted in other countries in the Region. As a consequence of the research, the Ministry of Public Health and the Intendancy of Canelones signed a framework agreement of complementary work, known as the Departmental Health Plan. One of its lines of work in primary health care includes oral health.

In 2004, the Memorandum of Understanding between the governments of Uruguay and Italy was approved by law for a credit of 15 million Euros to acquire new equipment for the public health sector. This represents the largest investment in health of the current administration.

References

1. Uruguay, Instituto Nacional de Estadística. Censo 2004. Total del país. Síntesis de resultados. Montevideo: INE; 2005. Available at: http://www.ine.gub.uy/fase1new/TotalPais/divulgacion _TotalPais.asp.
2. United Nations Development Programme. Informe del desarrollo humano en Uruguay. Montevideo: PNUD; 2005. Available at: http://www.undp.org.uy/.
3. Calvo JJ. Las necesidades básicas insatisfechas en Uruguay. Montevideo: Universidad de la República; 2005.
4. Uruguay, Instituto Nacional de Estadísticas. Estimaciones de pobreza por método de ingreso. Montevideo: INE; 2004.
5. Uruguay, Instituto Nacional de Estadística. Indicadores de género 2001–2004. Montevideo: INE; 2006.
6. Uruguay, Instituto Nacional de Estadística. Encuesta Nacional de Hogares Ampliada. Montevideo: INE; 2006. Available at: http://www.ine.gub.uy/enha2006/enha.asp.
7. Uruguay, Ministerio de Salud Pública, Departamento de Información Poblacional. Mortalidad por edad, causa, sexo y departamento, 2003. Available at: http://www.msp.gub.uy/ noticia_219_1.html.
8. Uruguay, Ministerio de Salud Pública, Departamento de Información Poblacional. Mortalidad infantil, 2003. Available at: http://www.msp.gub.uy/subcategoria_4_1_1.html.
9. Uruguay, Instituto Nacional de Estadística. Uruguay en cifras 2002. Población. Montevideo: INE. Available at: www.ine.gub. uy/biblioteca/uruguayencifras/poblacion.pdf.
10. Uruguay, Instituto Nacional de Estadística. Encuesta Nacional de Discapacidad 2004. Montevideo: INE; 2004.
11. Uruguay, Ministerio de Salud Pública, Departamento de Epidemiología. Programa Ampliado de Inmunizaciones; 2002–2005.
12. Uruguay. Ministerio de Salud Pública. Available at: http:// www.msp.gub.uy/index_1.html.
13. Pisabarro R, Irrazába E, Recalde A. Primera Encuesta Nacional de Sobrepeso y Obesidad (ENSO I). Rev Med Uruguay. 2000; 16(1):31–8.

14. Uruguay, Ministerio de Salud Pública, Programa Nacional de Nutrición. Manual para la promoción de prácticas saludables de alimentación en la población uruguaya. Montevideo: MSP; 2005. Available at: http://www.msp.gub.uy/imgnoticias/2111.pdf.

15. Uruguay. Ley N° 17.866. Foundation of the Ministry of Social Development. Available at: http://www.mides.gub.uy/normativa/index.html.

16. Uruguay, Ministerio de Desarrollo Social. Presentación del Plan de Emergencia y Políticas Sociales. Montevideo: MIDES; 2005. Available at: http://www.mides.gub.uy/archivo_doc/index.html.

17. Uruguay, Ministerio de Desarrollo Social. Programa Infancia, Adolescencia y Familia, Infamilia. Available at: http://infamilia.gub.uy.

18. Encuentro Progresista-Frente Amplio. Programa de salud del gobierno del Encuentro Progresista; March 2005.

19. Uruguay, Administración de los Servicios de Salud del Estado. Planificación de la Red Asistencial de la Administración de los Servicios de Salud del Estado. Montevideo: ASSE; 2002.

20. Portillo J, Buglioli M, Lazarov L. Servicios de salud en el Uruguay [capítulo]. En: Los sistemas de salud en Iberoamérica de cara al siglo XXI. Guadalajara: Universidad de Guadalajara; Pan American Health Organization; 2004.

21. Uruguay, Ministerio de Salud Pública. Cuentas Nacionales de Gasto y Financiamiento 1999-2000. Montevideo: MSP; 2002.

22. Uruguay, Ministerio de Salud Pública. Cuentas Nacionales en Salud 2004. Montevideo: MSP; abril 2006. Available at: http://www.msp.gub.uy/noticia_523_1.html.

23. Uruguay, Servicio Nacional de Sangre. La transfusión de sangre en Uruguay. informe 2003. Montevideo: SNS; 2003.

24. Uruguay, Caja de Jubilaciones y Pensiones Profesionales del Uruguay. Available at: http://www.cjppu.org.uy/info_interes_estadistica_2005.htm.

25. Uruguay, Equipos Mori. Encuesta Médica Nacional 2004. Sindicato Médico del Uruguay, Federación Médica del Interior. Available at: http://www.smu.org.uy/gremiales/documentos/estadistica/informefenc2004.pdf.

VENEZUELA

Saint Lucia

Aruba

Netherlands
Antilles

Barbados

Grenada

Trinidad and
Tobago

Falcón

Caracas

Zulia

Lara

7

6

5

4

2

3

Sucre

9

8

Monagas

Anzoá-
tegui

Delta
Amacuro

10

Guárico

Colombia

11

Barinas

12

Apure

Bolívar

Guyana

Amazonas

Brazil

1 Nueva Esparta
2 Vargas
3 Miranda
4 Capital District
5 Aragua
6 Carabobo
7 Yaracuy
8 Cojedes
9 Trujillo
10 Portuguesa
11 Mérida
12 Táchira

0   100   200 Miles

The Bolivarian Republic of Venezuela is a federation organized into 23 states, a capital district, and federal dependencies distributed in 335 municipalities. It has a land area covering 916,446 km^2 and a population estimated at 26,577,423 in 2005—49.7% women (*1*)—with a density of 29 people per km^2 and an annual average growth rate of 1.7% (*2*).

GENERAL CONTEXT AND HEALTH DETERMINANTS

Social, Political, and Economic Determinants

The gross domestic product (GDP) grew by approximately 19% in 2004 and by 9% in 2005 (*2*), mainly owing to oil revenues. The poverty level, measured by income, rose from 39.1% in 2001 to 42.4% in 2005 and extreme poverty climbed from 14.2% to 17% (*1*). In 2003, according to the Human Development Report (*3*), the country ranked 14th out of 81 countries in development (11th place in 2001). The Gini coefficient fell from 0.48 in 1998 to 0.46 in the first half of 2004. The poorest 20% obtains 4.7% of the country's income and the wealthiest 20% obtains 52.3%.

Inflation grew from 12.5% in 2001 to 21.8% in 2004. As of December 2005, 65.4% of the population was economically active, 49.5% of whom were women (*2*). The employment rate was 91.1% (15.9% in the public sector and 84.1% in the private sector) and 47.6% of jobs were in the informal sector. The net activity rate, which refers to the capacity to engage in productive economic activities, was 65.3% in 2001, and 68.8% in 2004 (*2*), and the trend indicates that the percentage of people able to engage in economic activities in the country continues to grow.

Table 1 shows Venezuela's classification in social territories (units of analysis composed of a group of people who share similar sociocultural and economic profiles but do not necessarily correspond to existing geopolitical boundaries) and Figure 1 shows that life expectancy has increased in the more developed territories.

In 2004, public investment in education as a percentage of GDP was 4.9% (*2*). For the 2004–2005 school year, the net enrollment rate by age group was 51.7% in preschool; 90.7% in primary school; and 30.6% in secondary, upper secondary, and vocational school (*2*). In 2001, the illiteracy rate was 6.4% (*2*). On 28 October 2005, Venezuela declared itself "illiteracy free" in the wake of the Robinson Mission, which was an initiative to teach more than 1 million Venezuelans around the country to read and write.

In 2004, the housing shortage in Venezuela was about 1.1 million units, and the qualitative shortage was 1.8 million; 68% of occupied housing is located in shantytowns and public housing projects built by the government (*4*).

To combat poverty, include excluded groups, and respond to the commitments to achieve the Millennium Development Goals (MDGs), the national government has implemented large-scale, rapid social programs known as "missions." The *Misión Barrio Adentro* and the *Misión Milagro* stand out in the field of health care. Other missions promote education, culture, employment, food access, sustainable development, research, and other human development areas.

Demographics, Mortality, and Morbidity

In 2005, 31.2% of the population was under 15 years of age and 7.5% was 60 and over (*1*). In 2004, the birth rate was 24.4 per 1,000 population; the general fertility rate was 2.69 children per woman, and the mortality rate per 1,000 people was 4.5 (6.1 for men and 3.9 for women) (*1, 2*). This situation has produced a population pyramid with an increasingly narrow base (Figure 2). According to the most recent census (2001), 87.1% of the population is urban; 57% lives in the coastal area, 22% in border areas, and 21% in the central region (*1*).

Life expectancy at birth was 72.7 years (76.6 for women and 69.8 for men) in 2002 and 73.2 years (76.2 for women and 70.3 for men) in 2005 (*2*). In 2004, there was a life expectancy gap of 9.4 years between the population living in the most developed and the least developed states (74.6 years in the Capital District and 65.2 years in Delta Amacuro) (*1*).

In 2004, the 10 leading groups of causes of death, expressed as unadjusted rates per 100,000 people, were heart disease (93); cancer (67); suicides, homicides, and other violent deaths (57.2); accidents of all kinds (32.1); cerebrovascular disease (31.7); diabetes (27.3); conditions originating in the perinatal period (20.1); chronic lower respiratory diseases (12.1); influenza and pneumonia (11); and liver disease (8.5). The differences by sex in violent deaths (100.4 in men and 10 in women) and accidents of all kinds (49.1 in men and 14.9 in women) are striking (*5*). Deaths due to violence were the leading cause of potential years of life lost in the country. Underreporting of mortality is between 10% and 15%.

TABLE 1. Classification of Venezuela in social territories, 2002.

Social territory 1 (least developed)	Social territory 2	Social territory 3	Social territory 4	Social territory 5 (most developed)
Amazonas	Yaracuy	Lara	Nueva Esparta	Capital District
Delta Amacuro	Sucre	Falcón	Aragua	Miranda
Guárico	Trujillo	Monagas	Anzoátegui	
	Portuguesa	Mérida	Bolívar	
	Barinas	Táchira	Carabobo	
	Apure	Cojedes	Zulia	

Source: Data obtained from the Human Development Index and Context in Venezuela. INE-UNDP, 2002. Strata defined by per capita income using purchasing power parity.

FIGURE 1. Life expectancy at birth, by social territory, Venezuela, 2002.

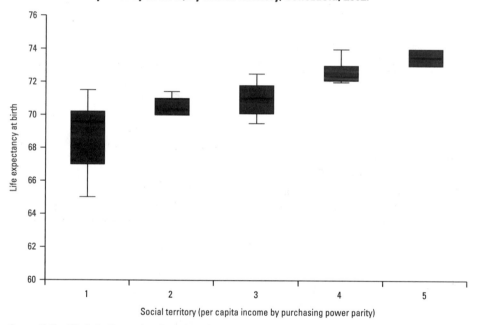

Source: National Statistics Bureau. http://www.ine.gob.ve.

HEALTH OF POPULATION GROUPS

Children under 5 Years Old

In 2005, children under 1 year of age accounted for 2.2% of the general population (51.2% were boys). The prevalence of low birthweight fell from 12% in 1999 to 8% in 2002 (*1*). The infant mortality rate has steadily decreased in recent decades (Figure 3). Infant mortality expressed as the rate per 1,000 live births was 25.8 in 1990, 17.7 in 2000, and 17.5 in 2004 (*5*). Projections of this trend using the ARIMA method indicate that the country will have a rate of 10.7 deaths per 1,000 live births by 2015, which is close to the MDG of 8.5. Social territory 2 (Table 1) has the highest rate (21.7) and social territory 5 the lowest (14.6).

The deaths among children under 1 as a proportion of total deaths fell from 14.2% in 1990–1994 to 8.4% in 2000–2004. In 2004, 66.5% of deaths in children under 1 occurred in the neonatal period and 33.5% in the postneonatal period (*5*). The proportional contribution of the five leading causes of death was: certain conditions originating in the perinatal period 56.7%, congenital defects 16.2%, intestinal infectious diseases 8.1%, influenza and pneumonia 4.6%, and accidents of all kinds 3.5% (*5*).

In 2005, the 1- to 4-year age group made up 8.4% of the population (51.4% were boys) (*1*). In 2004, mortality from all causes expressed as the rate per 100,000 boys and girls between the ages of 1 and 4 was 73.7 (76.6 for boys and 70.7 for girls). The leading five causes of death were: accidents of all kinds (16.6), intestinal infectious diseases (13.8), influenza and pneumonia (12), congenital defects (10.7), and nutritional deficiencies (9.8) (*5*).

FIGURE 2. Population structure by age and sex, Venezuela, 2005.

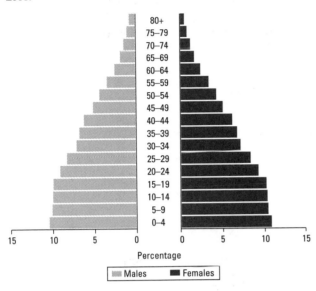

Children 5–9 Years Old

In 2005, the 5- to 9-year age group accounted for 10.2% of the total population (51.1% were boys) (*1*). In 2004, mortality from all causes expressed as the rate per 100,000 boys and girls in this age group was 34.4 (40.9 for boys and 27.6 for girls). The five leading causes of death were: accidents of all kinds (12.2), cancer (4.4), congenital defects (2.7), infant cerebral paralysis (1.7), and influenza and pneumonia (1.2). The difference between the sexes in deaths caused by accidents of all kinds stands out (16.8 for boys and 7.3 for girls) (*5*).

Adolescents 10–14 and 15–19 Years Old

In 2005, the 10- to 19-year age group accounted for 20.1% of the total population (50.9% were males). In 2004, the specific fertility rate among girls between the ages of 15 and 19 was estimated as 91.7 per 1,000 population (*1*).

In 2002, the Ministry of Health reported 98,099 births in the 10- to 19-year age group (22.4% of all births), with percentages higher than the national average in the following states: Apure (31.2% of total births), Guárico (27.8%), Cojedes (27.2%), Portuguesa (26.9%), and Barinas (25.7%). The prevalence of low birthweight for babies born to mothers between the ages of 10 and 14 was 12.6%, and it was 9.2% for mothers between the ages of 15 and 19 (8% for mothers of all ages) (*6*).

In 2004, the mortality rate for adolescents between 10 and 14 years old was 44 per 100,000 (52.0 for males and 35.0 for females) and for adolescents between 15 and 19 years of age it was 158.0 per 100,000 (253.0 for males and 59.0 for females) (*1*). Violence was the main cause of death in adolescent males between the ages of 15 and 19 years (*5*).

Adults 20–59 Years Old

In 2005, the 20- to 59-year age group made up 51.3% of the population, with one half being males (*1*). In 2004, the five lead-

FIGURE 3. Infant mortality, Venezuela, 1940–2003.

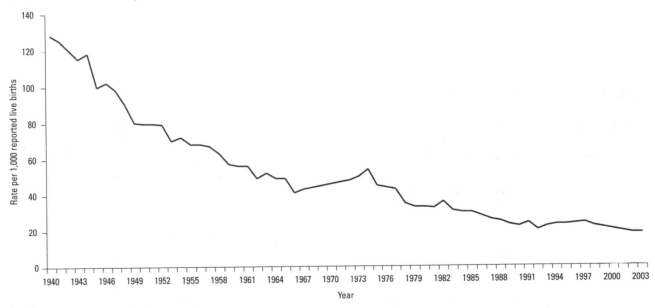

Source: Ministry of Health, National Epidemiology Directorate, 2006, Venezuela.

FIGURE 4. Maternal mortality, Venezuela, 1940–2003.

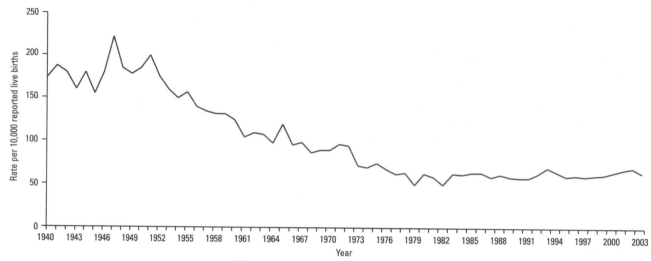

Source: Ministry of Health, National Epidemiology Directorate, 2006, Venezuela.

ing causes of death (rate per 100,000 population) were: 82.3, violent events (153.4 for men and 11.1 for women); 57.3, cancer (47.7 for men and 67.0 for women); 49.2, heart disease (68.6 for men and 29.9 for women); 45.3, accidents of all kinds (76.1 for men and 14.5 for women); and 13.8, diabetes (15.9 for men and 11.7 for women) (5).

Maternal mortality fell steadily until the end of the 1970s. Since then, the level has remained stable, with slight variations (Figure 4), but inequalities persist among the social territories. In 2004, the maternal mortality rate was 59.9 per 100,000 live births. Maternal deaths in 2000–2004 averaged 331 a year (5). In 2004, the proportional contribution of the leading five causes of maternal deaths was 28.6% from edema, proteinuria, and hypertension; 22.6% from other obstetrical complications; 20.8% from pregnancies ended by abortion; 13.8% from complications related to labor and delivery; and 10.1% from complications in the puerperium (5). In 2004, institutional coverage of care during delivery was 98% and coverage of prenatal checkups in Ministry of Health establishments was 25.5% (1).

Older Adults 60 Years Old and Older

In 2005, the group aged 60 and up accounted for 7.6% of the population, 47.1% of whom were males (1). In 2004, the proportional distribution of the leading causes of death was 19.1% from heart disease, 10.5% from cancer, 6.8% from cerebrovascular diseases, 5.1% from diabetes, and 2.8% from chronic lower respiratory diseases (5). In 2005, the main causes of morbidity were arterial hypertension (17.2%), visual disorders (13.9%), respiratory disorders (12.7%), diabetes (11.3%), and osteoarthrosis and osteoarthritis (10%) (7).

Workers

Occupational risks over the last decade have tended to increase as a consequence of informal employment, the use of unsuitable premises, and the use of homes as production centers. In 2004, the National Occupational Accident Prevention, Health, and Safety Administration (INPSASEL) reported 1,339 cases of muscular-skeletal disorders (68.6%), pathologies related to chemical risks (9.9%), psychosocial disorders (5.7%), respiratory disorders (4.9%), voice pathologies (4.3%), skin conditions (3.1%), occupational deafness (2.5%), exposure to extreme temperatures (0.4%), work-related zoonoses (brucellosis) (0.4%), and radiation disorders (0.3%) (8). Significant underreporting is assumed and the real figures for work-related disabilities and deaths are unknown.

Persons with Disabilities

According to the 2001 census, 4.2% of the population had a disability of some kind, for a total of 927,397 people (0.13% blindness, 0.15% deafness, 0.38% retardation, 0.15% loss of the upper limbs, 0.31% loss of the lower limbs, and 3.1% other causes) (1), although underreporting is assumed. *Misión Barrio Adentro* launched a process to strengthen comprehensive rehabilitation services.

Ethnic Groups

The indigenous population represents 2.3% of the total (532,743 people) (1) and is distributed among 36 ethnic groups who live in 10 states. The diseases that prevail in this population are tuberculosis, malaria, hepatitis, intestinal parasitosis, malnutrition, onchocerciasis, and respiratory and digestive disorders. The Amazon Tropical Disease Research and Control Center (CAICET) reported that the incidence of tuberculosis among the Yanomami was 10 times higher than for the nonindigenous population. In the states of Amazonas and Bolívar, the four leading causes of death in this ethnic group are malaria (40.1% of reported mortality), malnutrition, hepatitis B, and intestinal infections (gastroenteritis, amoebic dysentery, and helminthiasis). The indigenous population, in particular the Yanomami and Añú, are highly vulnerable to sexually transmitted infections owing to their contact with miners and tourists (9).

HEALTH CONDITIONS AND PROBLEMS

COMMUNICABLE DISEASES

Vector-borne Diseases

In 2002, three cases of **yellow fever** were reported in Zulia, with the start of an outbreak that lasted until 2003; of the total of 34 cases, 21 were in Zulia (with 9 deaths), 11 in Táchira (with 5 deaths), and 2 in Portuguesa. Also, the surveillance system in Zulia reported 9 cases (with 6 deaths) among people from northern Santander in Colombia. In 2004, a total of 5 cases were reported, with 2 in Mérida (with 1 death) and 3 in Monagas (with 2 deaths); in 2005, there were 12 cases with 8 deaths in the country, with 3 in Mérida (with 2 deaths), 1 in Apure (with 1 death), 1 in Bolívar (with 1 death), and 7 in Portuguesa (with 4 deaths) (10).

In 2003, an unconventional surveillance system was introduced, which identified the disease in primates in Apure, Barinas, Monagas, Sucre, Guárico, and Portuguesa in 2004 and 2005. In response to the outbreak, 953 samples were processed for viral isolation between 2003 and 2005, with three isolations in humans and four in primates (11). Also, in 2004, the Anatomical-Pathological Institute of the Central University of Venezuela introduced the immunohistochemical technique. Up to 2005, 121 tests had been performed (85 in humans and 36 in primates), with 8 humans and 3 Araguato monkeys testing positive for yellow fever (12).

American cutaneous **leishmaniasis** has been diagnosed in different parts of the country even though there is no national surveillance system. For the states that keep statistics, the largest number of cases have been reported in Lara (288 human cases in 2005), Nueva Esparta (13 in 2001 and 21 in 2005, with a prevalence in dogs estimated at 15% to 20%), and Sucre (6 in 2003 and 3 in 2004) (13).

The risk zone for **Chagas' disease** covers 164 municipalities in 18 states located in the Andean foothills, the coast, the north central region, and the plains; 80% of the population at risk lives in rural communities with no basic services. In 2000, 16,670 houses were examined for the presence of contaminated vectors, with

859 of them positive for *Rhodnius prolixus* and 51 for *Trypanosoma cruzi*. In 2004, 5,746 houses were examined and 135 were positive for *R. prolixus* and 26 for *T. cruzi*. Based on the proportion of positive cases out of the total number of samples, seroprevalence for *T. cruzi* was calculated as 8.1% in 2000 and 5.8% in 2005 (14).

The population at risk of contracting **malaria** (i.e., people living in municipalities where the disease has been transmitted during two consecutive years) fell from 36% in 2000 to just under 20% in 2004. However, the incidence of the disease nearly tripled in that same period, from 0.3% in 2000 to 0.9% in 2004. Most cases were caused by *Plasmodium vivax* (90% in 2004) (15). In 2003, 31,719 cases were reported, for a rate of 611 per 100,000 people in the at-risk population and 121 per 100,000 people in the total population. The state with the highest incidence was Amazonas, with 7,131 cases per 100,000 people, and the state with the lowest incidence was Zulia, with 15 cases per 100,000 people. In 2004, 46,655 cases were reported (899 per 100,000 people in the at-risk population and 179 per 100,000 people in the total population). The parasite formula in December 2003 was 82.6% for *P. vivax*, 16.7% for *P. falciparum*, 0.6% mixed (*P. falciparum* and *P. vivax*), and 0.1% for *P. malariae* (16).

The annual parasite index (API) has risen since 2001, and in 2004 it was 8.99 per 1,000 people for all areas. The API for *P. falciparum* fell in 2004 compared with the previous year (0.89 versus 1.07), but it remained far higher than in 2001 and 2002. The API for *P. vivax* rose steadily from 2.38 in 2001 to 8.08 in 2004 (15). The Ministry of Health has begun to use an artesunate-mefloquine combination to treat uncomplicated malaria (17).

Classic **dengue fever** and **dengue hemorrhagic fever** are endemo-epidemic in the country, with four virus types circulating. The year with the highest incidence was 2001, when there were 85,262 cases, for a rate of 446.15 per 100,000 population (77,344 classic dengue and 7,918 hemorrhagic dengue). The number of cases fell gradually until 2004, when 30,693 cases were reported (28,707 classic dengue and 1,987 hemorrhagic). There was an increase in 2005, with 42,217 cases reported (39,536 classic and 2,681 hemorrhagic) (18). The progressive reduction in the number of deaths from hemorrhagic dengue in the period is worth noting: from 50 in 2001 to 19 in 2004 (5).

In 2005, the population at risk of **onchocerciasis** in Venezuela accounted for 22% of the total in the Americas. There are 625 endemic communities reported in three areas: northeast, north-central, and south; 74.4% of the cases are in the northeast. The susceptible population eligible to receive treatment with ivermectin is 99,484 people and between 2003 and 2005 coverage rates exceeded 85% (19).

Vaccine-preventable Diseases

In 2004 and 2005, coverage with routine vaccinations for children under 1 year of age was over 90% for BCG (96% and 95%, respectively) and for yellow fever vaccine (94% both years), while coverage with the other vaccines remained between 80% and 90% in 2005 (80% OPV3, 87% DPT3, 87% Hib, 88% Hep B, and 76% MMR). Coverage with the pentavalent vaccine (DPT, hepatitis B, and *Haemophilus influenzae* type b) rose from 37% in 2004, when it was introduced in the country, to 80% in 2005 (*20*). To increase coverage, in 2004 the Ministry of Health implemented the National Vaccination Plan which, in addition to coverage for the population under 5 years with the vaccines included in the national vaccination model, provides vaccinations against hepatitis B and yellow fever for the at-risk adult population.

The progress made with yellow fever vaccinations for children over 1 year after the outbreak in 2003 should be emphasized. By 2005, over 15 million doses had been applied, mainly vaccinating the population over 1 year that lives in 140 high-risk municipalities in nine states, with an estimated population of 7,756,921. In those municipalities, general coverage of 90% has been achieved. Also, the yellow fever vaccine is administered regularly as part of the Expanded Immunization Program (PAI), to children 1 year of age, with coverage rates exceeding 90% in the last three years (*20*). Venezuela has participated actively in the Americas Vaccination Week (SVA) since 2003 and has used this initiative to strengthen its regular program and conduct campaigns.

With regard to the epidemiological behavior of vaccine-preventable diseases, in 2005 the country remained free from confirmed cases of **poliomyelitis** (the last case was reported in 1989). In the same year, one confirmed case of neonatal **tetanus** was reported (the last case was in 2001) and one of **diphtheria** (last case in 1992). The number of cases of **whooping cough** rose from 286 in 2002 to 367 in 2003 and to 715 in 2004. On the other hand, there was a marked drop in the number of cases of **rubella** confirmed clinically and in the laboratory: 2,724 in 2003 and 2,885 in 2004 compared to 4,047 reported in 2002 and 9,996 in 2001 (*6*).

The country was affected by an outbreak of **measles** from week 36 of 2001 to week 46 of 2002, with a total of 2,501 cases distributed among 17 of the 24 states, with 84% of the cases in Zulia, which was hardest hit. The outbreak mainly affected the under-5-year age group, particularly children under 1, with 699 cases and a rate of 122.5 per 100,000. Young adults, mainly between the ages of 20 and 34 years, also had high incidence rates. The virus that caused the outbreak was imported by a traveler from Europe who went to the municipality of Zamora in the state of Falcón and was not opportunely detected. The disease spread to the rest of the state and then to the rest of the country. Thanks to intensive control activities, the outbreak lasted only 14 months and the event is considered to be the last presentation of the measles virus (D9), which is widely endemic in the Americas.

Intestinal Infectious Diseases

Mortality in children under 5 years caused by intestinal infectious diseases expressed in rates per 100,000 people was 37.3 in

2002 (*21*) and 35.3 in 2004, with approximately 70% of those deaths among children under 1 year (*22*). There were 1,213,460 cases of **diarrhea** reported in children under 5 in 2004 and 1,214,461 in 2005 (*23*).

Chronic Communicable Diseases

Venezuela has been classified since 2004 among the group of countries in the Americas with a moderate burden of **tuberculosis** (TB). In 2004, 6,519 new cases of TB in all its forms were reported, for a rate of 25.1 per 100,000 people; the highest incidences were in Delta Amacuro (111.9), the Capital District (66.2), Amazonas (44.0), Monagas (43.9), Portuguesa (33.9), and Vargas (31.2). The pulmonary form accounted for 84.4% of all the new cases of TB that were reported, with 68.6% of them bacilliferous; 51.3% presented in the 15- to 44-year age group; 8.9% were in children under 15 years; and 15.3% were in people 65 years of age and over. The tubercular meningitis rate in the 0- to 4-year group was 0.2 per 100,000. AIDS/TB coinfection continues to rise and the association is present in 5% of new cases of TB and in 3.5% of reported relapses. The total number of relapses reported was 425, and 68% of them were confirmed bacteriologically. The country uses passive case detection and therefore underdiagnosis is assumed (*24*).

In 2004, the national prevalence rate of **leprosy** was 0.54 per 10,000 people; however, rates above 1.0 persist in the states of Cojedes, Portuguesa, Barinas, and Apure. New cases are more frequent with advancing age and in males, predominating in rural zones and unconsolidated urban settlements. The multibacillary form is the most prevalent. The detection rate was 0.27 per 10,000 people (*25*).

Acute Respiratory Infections

Mortality in children under 5 years from acute respiratory infections, expressed in rates per 100,000 people, was 24.5 in 2002 (*21*) and 27.2 in 2004, with 60% of them in children under 1 year. (*22*). Preliminary figures report 6,694,002 acute respiratory infections in 2004 and 6,716,211 in 2005 (*23*).

HIV/AIDS and Other Sexually Transmitted Infections

Between 1982 and 2005, 53,465 cases of AIDS were reported with 6,372 deaths. The epidemic is considered theoretically concentrated, with a prevalence in the population from 15 to 49 years of 0.7% and an estimated 110,000 cases of HIV infection. It should be kept in mind that AIDS was reported in only 13 of the 24 states, which suggests the existence of underreporting that has still not been estimated. The trend observed through the detection of people with the infection is an increase in heterosexual transmission and feminization of the epidemic. The male-to-female ratio fell from 9.8:1 in 1990–1994 to 3:1 in 2000–2004. The Ministry of Health offers universal access, free of charge, to antiretroviral drugs, diagnostic tests, and immunological and virological monitoring. Antiretroviral treatment rose from 52% in 2004 to 100% in December 2005 (26).

Zoonoses

Coordination of actions between the Ministry of Health and the Ministry of Agriculture and Land has been stepped up. Through regular meetings of the National Zoonoses Committee, it has been possible to effectively implement joint projects from the planning to the action stages.

The geographic distribution of **rabies** in dogs was reduced from 11 states in 1991 to 1 state (Zulia) in 2001. The annual number of cases of canine rabies in Zulia has risen continually, from 82 cases in 2001 to 181 in 2004. However, intervention by local authorities made it possible to improve the structure of the vaccination campaigns carried out in mid-2004 and to reduce the incidence by 57% in 2005 (76 cases) (27). In 2003, there were two cases of human rabies transmitted by dogs, while, in 2004, five cases of human rabies were reported, three of them transmitted by dogs in Zulia and two by hematophagous bats in Sucre; no human cases were reported in 2005 (6).

With regard to **equine encephalitis**, the Ministry of Health and the Ministry of Agriculture and Land maintain a joint vaccination program of equines in high- and moderate-risk municipalities. In 2004, 297,046 doses were applied and 303,211 in 2005. In 2004, 29 outbreaks of the disease were reported, with 13 being eastern equine encephalitis (EEE), 9 Venezuelan equine encephalitis (EEV), and 7 with positive serology for both viruses. In 2005, 5 outbreaks were reported, 4 caused by EEE and 1 by EEV (28). In 2005, a national surveillance program was carried out for West Nile virus to monitor its possible entry into the country.

In 2000, 419 cases of **leptospirosis** were reported in the wake of the floods in Vargas (29), with the number dropping gradually to 98 cases in 2004 (30). The 2005 floods caused an outbreak with 90 suspected cases and 6 deaths (31).

With regard to birds, the country has been historically free from all the viruses that cause **avian influenza**, which was corroborated through sampling at the end of 2005, with negative results for the commercially raised bird population consisting of about 78 million birds (31). A permanent surveillance system is being implemented for commercial and backyard birds, and migratory birds are being monitored.

In 2003, an epidemic of **foot-and-mouth disease** affected 63 farms; the incidence fell to 13 farms in 2005, predominantly in the western part of the country. **Vesicular stomatitis** fell from 22 outbreaks reported in 2003 to 12 farms affected in 2005, and its incidence continues to be low (27).

As for **brucellosis**, in 2003 new regulations were approved for diagnostic tests and for the destination of animals that tested positive. This led to an increase in serological tests from 504,310 in 2003 to 1,197,636 in 2005. The prevalence of the disease in an-

imals was 8 per 1,000 in the field in 2005. Vaccinations increased from 273,448 in 2004 to 478,182 in 2005 (6).

NONCOMMUNICABLE DISEASES

Metabolic and Nutritional Diseases

The prevalence of the nutritional anthropometric deficit in children under 5 was low (weight/age <10%, height/age <20%, and weight/height <5%). The main problem was low height for age (12.5%); low weight for age was 5.2% and acute nutritional deficit was 4.1%. The prevalence of overweight was 3.1%.

Of 78,405 hospital pediatric admissions (<13 years) for all causes in 24 sentinel hospitals in 2004, 1.4% had serious malnutrition, with a predominance of marasmus, with children under 1 year being the hardest hit. The highest rates for pathologies linked to malnutrition were for diarrhea (3.4%), helminthiasis (1.5%), bronchitis (1.3%), anemia (1.2%), and pneumonia (0.4%) (32).

OTHER HEALTH PROBLEMS OR ISSUES

Disasters

The torrential rains of 2002 and 2005 almost everywhere in the country, which caused flooding and mudslides, stand out: 300,000 people were left homeless and there were 98 deaths. A large number of health centers were affected (33). In 2005, 90 accidents were reported in the oil industry, which indicated a pressing need to promote or recover safety margins in the country's oil and petrochemical industries (34). The Civil Protection and Disaster Management Law was promulgated in 2003 and the Risk Management Law in 2005. In 2005, the Ministry of Health created the Emergency and Disaster Coordination Office and the Health Department of Metropolitan Caracas established a Health Risk Management Unit.

The Ministry of Health prepared the National Plan for Surveillance, Prevention, and Control to address a possible avian influenza pandemic and the National Surveillance System for Acute Respiratory Infections, Pneumonia, and Influenza was strengthened by implementing an epidemiological investigation file for acute respiratory infections (35).

Violence and Other External Causes

The Interministerial Commission for Road Awareness, Accident Prevention, and Education (CIAPEV) was established in 2003. In 2004, the Ministry of Health's National Accident and Other Violent Events Program was reactivated. In 2004, 117,227 deaths were reported, with 5,437 caused by traffic accidents (21% women), 7,348 homicides (6.2% women), and 1,034 suicides (19.4% women), with the number of deaths from accidents and violence totaling 13,819 (36).

Between 2000 and 2004, an average of 4,000 domestic violence complaints were reported each year. More than 40% of the complaints involved physical or psychological violence. In the aggressor-victim relationship, more than 80% of acts of violence are performed by the partner or former partner (*37*).

Addictions

Smoking by people more than 15 years old declined from 40% in 1984 (*38*) to 28% in 2005, according to studies conducted by the Central University of Venezuela and the National Anti-Smoking Office (*39*), which had national coverage. This drop was accompanied by a reduction in per capita consumption of cigarettes from 2,100 in 1984 to 900 in 2005. In the population under 15 years, the percentage of smokers increased from 2.7% in 1984 to 13% in 2000 (*40*). These results indicate that the policies to combat smoking implemented in the country have mainly had an impact on adults and have been less effective among youths. Resolutions of the Ministry of Health that ban tobacco advertising and restrict access to tobacco products by minors, which were approved in March 2006, constitute a strategy to reduce consumption by youths. The resolutions in question and the regulations governing tobacco products and their packaging place Venezuela among the most advanced countries in policies to control and prevent tobacco use.

In 2000, **alcohol consumption** was a factor in 50% of homicides and suicides and in 40% of traffic accidents (*39*). In 2003, a survey on alcohol consumption conducted by the National Commission to Combat Illegal Drug Use (*41*) reported that 31% of the respondents were regular alcohol users; 36.7% started between the ages of 10 and 14 years; and 48.2% started between the ages of 15 and 19. Since 1979, the country has had an Alcohol and Alcoholic Beverages Revenue Law that regulates the sale, production, taxation, and advertising of alcohol. Advertising was prohibited on radio and television between 1979 and 2004, when beer, wine, and liquor advertising was reauthorized in the media, but it was restricted again in 2005. It is also prohibited to sell alcohol to youths under 18 years and there is a tax on the sale of domestic and imported alcoholic beverages to the public.

Drug consumption in the country is moderate, according to the National Commission to Combat Illegal Drug Use. In 2005, the prevalence among people over age 15 who had tried drugs of some kind was 2.2% (4% men and 0.7% women). The age group with the highest consumption was between 20 and 39 years (3% of the population). The most widely used drug was marijuana, followed by cocaine and crack. For all of them, consumption is higher among men, except for ecstasy, where the figure for women was 5.4%, compared to 1.1% for men. The parts of the country where prevalence is highest are Vargas (4.5%), the Capital District (4.2%), and Miranda (4.1%) (*39*).

Environmental Pollution

Twenty-five deaths were reported from accidental poisoning and pesticide exposure in 2002 (*21*) and 24 deaths in 2004 (*22*).

Preliminary figures indicate that there were 4,028 cases of pesticide poisoning in 2004 and 3,572 in 2005 (*23*).

RESPONSE OF THE HEALTH SECTOR

Health Policies and Plans

The Constitution of the Bolivarian Republic of Venezuela, approved in a referendum in 1999, proposes a process of legislation and institutional reform and new strategies to bring about the necessary changes. It lays the groundwork for developing the legal nature and the organizational model for Venezuela's health sector. Article 83 establishes that health is a fundamental social right, an integral part of the right to life, and an obligation of the State. To guarantee the right to health, article 84 orders the creation of a National Public Health System (SPNS) that is intersectoral in nature, decentralized and participatory, and integrated into the National Social Security System. It is governed by the principles of gratuitousness, universality, comprehensiveness, equity, social integration, and solidarity. Article 85 establishes that its financing is an obligation of the State. Article 86 establishes that everyone has the right to social security as a not-for-profit public service that guarantees health and assures protection from different contingencies. In 2002, the National Assembly passed the Social Security System Organic Law and is in the process of drafting a Health Organic Law, which compiles policies and establishes the rules governing the sector's new institutional framework.

The Ministry of Health is the lead agency in the health sector and is responsible for regulating, formulating, designing, evaluating, controlling, and monitoring health policies, programs, and plans. Through the primary care strategy known as *Misión Barrio Adentro*, implemented under an agreement with the Republic of Cuba, it is in charge of integrating the sources of financing and allocating resources to establish the SPNS and providing comprehensive health care for all population groups, particularly low-income sectors.

During the period 2001–2005, 68 resolutions, 14 decrees, 7 laws, 3 agreements, and 1 directive were issued in the field of health. The most important are: regulation of the second-level access and medical care program, known as the Community Clinics Network, where the changes in the SPNS's care services are apparent; the requirement that the SPNS health establishments are allowed to purchase only the drugs that appear on the national basic list of essential medications; and the Workplace Accident Prevention, Conditions, and Environment Organic Law.

Health Strategies and Programs

With a view to attaining MDGs 4 and 5 by 2015, the Venezuelan government has established *Proyecto Madre*, with a vision of comprehensive and intersectoral care, whose objective is to reduce maternal and child mortality. The project is a strategy designed and promoted by the Ministry of Health to improve the health of children under 5 years of age and of pregnant women. It incorporates a strong disease prevention and health promotion component, which is intended to strengthen knowledge about healthy habits and lifestyles in families and communities, and the practice of care and assistance for pregnant women and children under 5 in the home, as a way of contributing to the growth and full development of all family members (42).

Organization of the Health System

The health services system has been marked by complicated and segmented organization and functioning. It is composed of the public and private subsectors and many players that regulate, finance, insure, and deliver services.

In the 1990s, the health system began a process of decentralizing the services of the then Ministry of Health and Social Welfare to the state level, which took place in 17 states. However, the process was not consolidated and therefore the health sector has both decentralized and centralized services.

At the end of 2005, the Ministry of Health reported that there were 4,804 public ambulatory establishments on the primary level, 4,605 (96%) of which belong to the ministry, in addition to the ambulatory network of the *Misión Barrio Adentro* with approximately 8,600 consultation points. There are 296 public hospitals, with 214 reporting to the Ministry of Health or the state governments, 33 to the Venezuelan Social Insurance Administration (IVSS), 29 to the National Geriatrics Administration (INAGER), 13 to the Armed Forces Social Protection Administration (IPSFA), 3 to Petróleos de Venezuela (PDVSA), 2 to the Corporación Venezolana de Guyana (CVG), 1 to the municipality of Miranda, and 1 to the Municipal Police Force of Caracas. The private sector has 344 health centers (315 for profit and 29 benevolent institutions). In 2003, the public sector had 23,858 beds in hospitals (9.2 beds per 10,000 people) (1).

The treatment capability of the system has improved with the introduction of the *Misión Barrio Adentro* and waiting times for surgery and specialized ambulatory care have been reduced under an agreement with the Cuban government to treat patients in that country, particularly through *Misión Milagro*, which offers eye surgery.

Public Health Services

Misión Barrio Adentro is a primary care strategy that consists of organizing structures, programs, and human, technical, and financial resources, with the goal of gradually extending services and expanding comprehensive health care actions to strengthen the SPNS. In 2003, the *Misión* received US$ 169.4 million from Petróleos de Venezuela (PDVSA) to build up the primary health care network, which was administered directly by the Ministry of Health through a trust with the Economic and Social Development Bank. The agreement between the Ministry of Health and

the PDVSA also included construction of 100 primary care modules by the PDVSA.

The National Network of Public Health Laboratories is coordinated by the Rafael Rangel National Hygiene Institute and its main objective is to strengthen cooperation between the states to monitor, prevent, and control communicable diseases in the country and detect congenital hypothyroidism and phenylketonuria in neonates.

The network's most important achievements include: strengthening the capacity to diagnose and monitor communicable diseases on the national level, with a significant increase in the number of diagnostic tests processed in the network's laboratories, which rose from 123,483 in 2001 to 463,465 in 2005; expansion of diagnostic coverage of the different health programs countrywide, with the goal of providing a rapid and timely response for decision making (Caicara in Orinoco, Santa Elena in Uairén, Tumeremo, Güiria, Santa Bárbara in Zulia, and Altagracia in Orituco); the establishment and consolidation of diagnostic tests for congenital metabolic diseases, which led to an increase in the number of tests from 40,442 in 2001 to 293,186 in 2005; strengthening the program to prevent the vertical transmission of HIV, which means that all the regional laboratories screen pregnant women for HIV in addition to hepatitis B and hepatitis C; and the establishment of an information system to obtain up-to-date data on the incidence or seroprevalence of communicable diseases throughout the country. It was also ensured that the population would have access to those services free of charge (43).

Regular annual public investments in the water and sanitation sector did not exceed 0.2% of GDP between 2000 and 2005. In 2001 a national sanitation plan was consolidated, with additional funds of US$ 88.9 million, which meant a budget increase of 26.7% for the sector. One factor that contributes to the sector's financial deficit is unbilled water, which amounts to about 63% (44).

Potable water coverage rose from 86% in 1998 to 91% in 2004 in urban zones. Areas without coverage correspond mainly to rural and unconsolidated urban areas and indigenous groups. The country has 151 treatment systems. There are shortcomings in monitoring and control of water quality in rural areas. In 2003, 66% of the rural population had household water connections (44). The population with adequate liquid waste disposal rose from 66% in 2000 to 77% in 2004 (44) and the shortfall is mainly in rural and unconsolidated urban areas and among indigenous groups.

In Venezuela, 24.3% of municipalities have controlled sanitary landfills and 59.2% use open air dumps (45). The country does not have secure disposal for hazardous materials, including hospital waste. The Solid Waste Law was promulgated in 2004 and guidelines were established for regional solid waste management plans. Trash collection in mid-sized and large cities and final disposal in general are serious problems, because the trash that is not collected is dumped into the environment without control. As a result, it becomes a risk factor for the exposed population, particularly people who work in contact with trash and who live close to final disposal sites.

The system for monitoring air quality is limited; only Caracas, Maracaibo, and Valencia have monitoring networks, mainly for particulate matter, but the information is not available and there are no published inventories of emissions. A study conducted in 2003 indicates that the average concentration of inhalable particles (PM_{10}) in Maracaibo is double the WHO guidelines (46). Leaded gasoline has not been sold in the country since August 2005.

The proliferation of sources of ionizing radiation, particularly in medical activities, led the Ministry of Health to draw up a register of public and private health centers that use radiation. The following shortcomings were found: 65% of the services do not have personal radiation detection kits, 40% present structural failures, and none of them perform environmental monitoring to control exposure (47).

Nutritional availability in 2004 was fully sufficient (>110%) in iron, thiamine, niacin, and vitamin C; only just sufficient (100%–110%) in riboflavin; insufficient (95%–100%) in vitamin A; and critically insufficient (<95%) in calories and proteins. In 2002, national production of calories, proteins, and fats was low, with the greatest vulnerability in the fats group. In 2005, the average value of a standard food basket was US$ 178, and the minimum wage was US$ 189.

Between 2000 and 2002, 31 outbreaks of food-borne diseases were reported in Venezuela (48). The country's food control model is based on interventions by various institutions with different legal frameworks, functions, and responsibilities that do not act in coordination (49).

Under the leadership of the Ministry of Health, an intersectoral committee was established to work on a project leading to implementation of the International Sanitary Regulation (ISR) in the country. Technical groups were set up to work on specific areas: regulatory framework, diagnosis, organization, warning and surveillance systems, and information systems. In view of WHO's request to voluntarily move ahead with the points in the ISR related to preparation for a possible avian influenza epidemic, the group that has made the most progress is the group on ports, airports, and overland border crossings, which already has a protocol for evaluating basic installed capacity.

Individual Care Services

During the first 18 months of *Misión Barrio Adentro*, 163 million free medical consultations took place (6.5 consultations per person), with 14.8 million dental checkups and 3.8 million eye examinations; 1.4 million pairs of glasses have been provided. Also, 567,000 emergency consultations and 1.1 million rehabilitation treatments were carried out. As a complement, the *Misión Milagro* was launched in mid-2004, which provided surgery in Cuba for 176,000 Venezuelans with eye problems (as of February 2006), while 8,500 patients from Latin American countries were operated on in Venezuela for the same difficulties.

The services system is composed of primary care clinics, comprehensive diagnostic centers, comprehensive rehabilitation facilities, high-technology centers, and hospitals. To operate them, regional technical committees were set up in the 24 states under *Misión Barrio Adentro*, composed of representatives of the state and municipal governments, prisons, the Ministry of Health's Regional Health Directorates, the Regional Directorates of the Ministry of Housing and Habitat, the Cuban Medical Mission, the Health Committees, the Francisco Miranda Front, the National Armed Forces, and joint public and private enterprises.

The goal was for each community clinic to cover 250 families or 1,250 individuals, which means that roughly 14,000 clinics would be required. At the end of 2005, about 640 primary care clinics were operating and 1,670 were in the process of being equipped under the coordination of the Ministry of Health. There are also about 6,900 consultation points that operate out of rooms in houses facilitated by families living in low-income areas, which will gradually be replaced by 4,600 primary care clinics. The infrastructure in operation could cover 11.4 million people. The clinics have 103 free drugs for treatment of the most prevalent diseases. There are also dental clinics (1 for every 4 medical clinics) and as of November 2005 close to 2,000 Venezuelan dentists had been incorporated into the system. In addition, 470 eye clinics are operating (1 for every 6 medical clinics) and approximately 1,450 will be needed to cover the public's requirements.

In March 2006, there were 100 comprehensive diagnostic centers around the country, which operate 24 hours a day year-round and provide emergency services and intermediate and intensive care. As of the same date, they had provided 4.1 million laboratory tests, 567,000 emergency consultations, 792,000 ultrasounds, 398,000 x-rays, 324,936 electrocardiograms, 1,108 surgeries, 59,000 endoscopies, and 1.1 million rehabilitation treatments. Also as of March 2006, there were 100 comprehensive rehabilitation rooms, providing the following services: electrotherapy, cervical-lumbar traction, thermotherapy, hydrotherapy, pediatric exercises, adult exercises, occupational therapy, natural medicine and acupuncture, speech therapy, phoniatrics, and podiatry. The high-technology centers were designed as centers for medical diagnosis based on noninvasive medical imaging.

In October 2005, the Ministry of Health began a process of consultation to identify the equipment that should be installed in its 214 hospitals. The National Health Technology Evaluation Committee (CONETS), jointly with a group of experts, prepared technical protocols to determine the technologies required for the optimum functioning of the public hospitals. Sixty percent of the country's beds and 50% of its operating rooms are concentrated in 43 hospitals belonging to the Ministry of Health, most of them located in the capitals of the 24 states (50).

The Ministry of Health is responsible for coordinating all aspects of the organization, operation, monitoring, and evaluation of the blood banks in the National Blood Banks Program (PNBS), through the national coordination office. The main objectives of

Training for Comprehensive-care, General Physicians through Social Programs Known as "Missions"

To combat poverty, achieve the inclusion of socially and economically excluded groups, and respond to the commitments made to achieve the Millennium Development Goals, the Government has implemented large-scale, rapid social programs known as "missions." The *Misión Barrio Adentro* and the *Misión Milagro* stand out in the field of health care, while *Misión Robinson* is designed to reduce illiteracy, and *Misión Mercal* to guarantee food security.

Undergraduate medical training takes a community approach and is carried out through *Misión Barrio Adentro* under an agreement with the Republic of Cuba. In the medium term, the international cooperants will gradually be replaced with Venezuelan personnel, to ensure the sustainability of the process from the technical and financial standpoints. It is a study/work program, with three days a week spent at the community clinics and two days in the classroom. The first cohort, which has been undergoing training since 2005, has 15,000 students and there are a further 2,500 students following the same program in Cuba. The goal is to train 25,000 Venezuelan doctors to replace the Cuban physicians.

the PNBS are to guarantee a safe blood supply and provide quality products and services tailored to the needs and specific rights of the population, which takes a gender and ethnic approach throughout the life cycle.

The network of blood banks is composed of 270 units, with 86 in the Ministry of Health, 28 in the Venezuelan Social Insurance Administration, 126 in private institutions, and 30 in other institutions. Transfusions are also performed in 1 community clinic and in 4 diagnostic centers (*51*).

Health Promotion

The Constitution establishes that health is a fundamental social right that forms part of the right to life, where many determining factors converge, including physical, biological, demographic, social, economic, and environmental factors. Accordingly, health policy forms part of a broader set of government policies that give priority to social factors. On the local level, priority is given to the policy on endogenous development nuclei through the social territories where institutional responses and community needs are coordinated.

Another constitutional mandate is participation by society in the implementation and control of public management and in the strategic development plans for local intervention. The Health Committees were established as entities for community organization and participation in solving health problems, and to date there are more than 8,000 of them around the country. In 2006, the Community Councils Law was passed to promote linkage and integration among different community organizations and permit the public to directly manage public policies and community projects. In that same year, the Ministry of Citizen Participation and Social Development was established by splitting the Ministry of Health and Social Development.

Health Supplies

The Ministry of Health regulates and oversees medications from their production to their use by patients. There are 4,347 registered pharmaceuticals that are currently sold; 33% of those products are classified as over-the-counter, while 67% need to be prescribed by a physician (*52, 53*). The most recent list of essential basic medications prepared by the National Therapeutic Committee of the Ministry of Health is composed of 328 active principles that are sold in 534 pharmaceutical presentations (*54*) and whose technical fiches are described in the National Therapeutic Form (*55*). The national market for drugs grew from US$ 1.86 billion in 2004 to US$ 2.10 billion in 2005, with 63% corresponding to multinational industries and 37% to national ones (*56*). The psychotropic drugs segment is represented by 10 active ingredients, with consumption in 2005 amounting to 1,073 kg. For narcotics, the segment is composed of 30 active ingredients, with national consumption in 2005 of 431 kg (*57*). As for pharmaceutical monitoring, the two executive centers (the National Pharmacological Monitoring Centre of the National Hygiene Institute and the Drug Monitoring Center of the Central University of Venezuela) processed 529 reports of adverse reactions to medications in 2004 and 533 in 2005, which were sent to the Uppsala Monitoring Center of Sweden (WHO Collaborating Center) (*56, 57*). In 2005, the distribution of four large groups of antimicrobials was restricted (quinolone, macrolides-lincosamides, third-generation cephalosporins, and drugs whose active principle is rifampicin) (*58*).

Human Resources

The Ministry of Health's staff totaled 150,263 in 2005, including professionals, 3.6% of whom were at the central level, 12.6% in the centralized states, 72.7% in decentralized states, and 11.2%

in reporting agencies. Of that total, 85.7% were permanent, 11% were contracted, and 3.3% were acting (*59*).

In 2003, the IVSS's hospital, ambulatory services, and central administration staff numbered 43,390, with 33,630 working in services and 9,770 in administration (*1*). In 2000, there were 20 physicians for every 10,000 people, with a marked contrast between the Capital District (42.2) and Sucre (11.5) (*59*). According to a census taken by the Venezuelan Medical Federation, in 2005 there were approximately 53,300 active physicians registered in Venezuela and about 1,100 of them work in *Misión Barrio Adentro* together with 15,000 Cuban doctors, and therefore in that year there were 25 doctors per 10,000 people. In 2000, there were 4.5 nurses per 10,000 people, with the highest percentage in Falcón (9.8) and the lowest in Nueva Esparta (2) (*59*). Training in general medicine is carried out in *Misión Barrio Adentro* under an agreement with the Republic of Cuba and takes the form of a study/work program. The purpose is, in the medium term, to gradually replace the international cooperants with Venezuelan personnel, to ensure the sustainability of the process from technical and financial standpoints. The first cohort that has been undergoing training in the country since 2005 has 15,000 students and a further 2,500 students are following the same program in Cuba. The goal is to train 25,000 Venezuelan doctors to replace the Cuban physicians.

Research and Technological Development in Health

With regard to scientific and technical information on health, in 2005, Venezuela's Virtual Health Library was made official (http://www.bvs.org.ve), whose executive secretariat is the Dr. Arnoldo Gabaldón Institute for Advanced Studies in Public Health, which reports to the Ministry of Health. SciELO Venezuela (http://www.scielo.org.ve) was consolidated and accredited and has 22 different journals in its collection.

Health Sector Expenditures and Financing

Public social investment as a percentage of GDP rose from 11% in 2000 to 12.1% in 2004. Real per capita social investment fell from US$ 516.80 in 2000 to US$ 226.90 in 2005. Public spending on health rose from 1.4% of GDP in 2000 to 1.6% in 2004 (*2*). Since 2000 public investment has increased and private investment has stabilized. The government sought to funnel part of its oil earnings to the excluded and impoverished population.

References

1. Venezuela, Instituto Nacional de Estadísticas. Available at: http://www.ine.gob.ve. Accessed 29 August 2006.
2. Venezuela, Sistema Integrado de Indicadores Sociales para Venezuela. Available at: http://www.sisov.mpd.gov.ve. Accessed 29 August 2006.
3. Programa de las Naciones Unidas para el Desarrollo. Informe sobre desarrollo humano 2005. La cooperación internacional ante una encrucijada: ayuda al desarrollo, comercio y seguridad en un mundo desigual. New York: PNUD; 2005. Available at: http://hdr.undp.org/reports/global/2005/espanol/. Accessed 24 August 2006.
4. Venezuela, Fundación Vivienda Popular. Situación habitacional en Venezuela. Available at: http://www.viviendaenred.com. Accessed 5 September 2006.
5. Venezuela, Ministerio de Salud y Desarrollo Social. Anuario de mortalidad 2004. Caracas: MSDS; 2005. Available at: http://www.msds.gov.ve/msds/documentos/Anuario.zip. Accessed 8 August 2006.
6. Venezuela, Ministerio de Salud y Desarrollo Social, Dirección General de Epidemiología y Análisis Estratégico. Archivos de 2001–2005.
7. Venezuela, Instituto Nacional de Geriatría. Proyección de la población de adultos mayores y sus principales causas de morbilidad y mortalidad. [Presentation by A. Capielo]. Caracas: INAGER; 2005.
8. Venezuela, Instituto Nacional de Prevención, Salud y Seguridad Laborales. Available at: http://www.inpsasel.gov.ve/. Accessed 25 September 2006.
9. Venezuela, Centro Amazónico de Investigación y Control de Enfermedades Tropicales "Simón Bolívar." Available at: http://www.innova.org.ve:8000/. Accessed in 2006.
10. Venezuela, Ministerio de Salud y Desarrollo Social. Reporte internacional periódico de vigilancia de fiebre amarilla, 2001–2005. Caracas: MSDS; 2005.
11. Universidad Central de Venezuela, Instituto Anatomopatológico. Archivos; 2005.
12. Venezuela, Ministerio de Salud y Desarrollo Social. Reunión Nacional de Zoonosis, 2006. Caracas: MSDS; 2006.
13. Venezuela, Ministerio de Ciencia y Tecnología, Instituto Nacional de Investigaciones Agrícolas; Centro Nacional de Investigaciones Agropecuarias, Laboratorio de Enfermedades Vesiculares, 2005.
14. Benítez J. Programa Nacional de Control de Chagas. Situación 2006. Caracas: Ministerio de Salud y Desarrollo Social; 2006.
15. Venezuela, Ministerio de Salud y Desarrollo Social, Programa de Malaria; 2003.
16. Organización Panamericana de la Salud. Malaria en Venezuela. Quito: OPS; 2006.
17. Villegas L. Paludismo en Venezuela. Caracas; 2004.
18. Venezuela, Ministerio de Salud y Desarrollo Social, Dirección de Vigilancia Epidemiológica. Informe anual de casos de dengue, 2004. Caracas: MSDS; 2005.
19. Venezuela, Ministerio de Salud y Desarrollo Social, Programa Nacional de Eliminación de la Oncocercosis; 2006.
20. Venezuela, Programa Ampliado de Inmunizaciones. Boletines. Caracas: PAI; 2006.
21. Venezuela, Ministerio de Salud y Desarrollo Social. Anuario de mortalidad, 2003. Caracas: MSDS; 2004.

22. Venezuela, Ministerio de Salud y Desarrollo Social. Anuario de mortalidad, 2005. Caracas: MSDS; 2006.
23. Venezuela, Ministerio de Salud y Desarrollo Social. Boletín Epidemiológico. Semana epidemiológica N° 52; diciembre de 2005.
24. Venezuela, Ministerio de Salud y Desarrollo Social, Programa Nacional de Tuberculosis y Otras Enfermedades Respiratorias; 2006.
25. Venezuela, Instituto de Biomedicina. Available at: http://www.biomedicina.org.ve/. Accessed 28 July 2006.
26. Venezuela, Ministerio de Salud y Desarrollo Social, Programa Nacional de Prevención de VIH/SIDA; 2006.
27. Centro Panamericano de Fiebre Aftosa. Sistema de Información Epidemiológica. Available at: http://siepi.panaftosa.org.br/Painel.aspx. Accessed 22 September 2006.
28. Venezuela, Servicio Autónomo de Sanidad Animal, División de Control Zoosanitario; 2005.
29. Venezuela, Ministerio de Salud y Desarrollo Social. Encuentro Nacional de Leptospirosis. Caracas: MSDS; 2005.
30. Venezuela, Ministerio de Salud y Desarrollo Social. Informe de la situación de leptospirosis en Venezuela. Caracas: MSDS; 2005
31. Venezuela, Servicio Autónomo de Sanidad Animal, Oficina de Apoyo y Vigilancia Epidemiológica; 2005.
32. Venezuela, Instituto Nacional de Nutrición, Sistema de Vigilancia Alimentaria y Nutricional; 2005.
33. Venezuela, Ministerio de Relaciones Interiores y Justicia, Dirección Nacional de Protección Civil; 2006. Available at: http://www.pcivil.gob.ve/. Accessed 11 September 2006.
34. Asociación Venezolana de la Industria Química y Petroquímica, 2006. Available at: http://www.asoquim.com/. Accessed 15 August 2006.
35. Venezuela, Ministerio de Salud y Desarrollo Social. Plan nacional de vigilancia, prevención y control ante una posible pandemia de influenza aviar. Caracas: MSDS; 2006.
36. Venezuela, Ministerio de Salud y Desarrollo Social. Perfil de país sobre accidentes y otros hechos violentos. Caracas: MSDS; 2005.
37. Venezuela, Ministerio del Interior y Justicia, Cuerpo de Investigaciones Científicas, Penales y Criminalísticas, 2005. Available at: http://www.cicpc.gov.ve/. Accessed 14 September 2006.
38. Venezuela, Ministerio de Sanidad y Asistencia Social. Estudio Nacional Antitabáquico; 1984.
39. Venezuela, Ministerio del Interior y Justicia, Oficina Nacional Antidrogas. Available at: http://www.ona.gob.ve. Accessed 15 August 2006.
40. Primer informe. Encuesta Mundial de Tabaquismo en Jóvenes. EMTAJOVEN Venezuela. Ministerio de Salud y Desarrollo Social; 2000.
41. Venezuela, Comisión Nacional Contra el Uso Indebido de las Drogas; Unión Europea. Informe Final. I Encuesta de Hogares sobre Consumo de Drogas en la República Bolivariana de Venezuela; 2006.
42. Venezuela, Ministerio de Salud y Desarrollo Social. Propuesta de alianza con universidades y sociedades científicas para fortalecimiento de Proyecto Madre; 2006.
43. Venezuela, Ministerio de Salud y Desarrollo Social. Red Nacional de Laboratorios de Salud Pública, 2001–2005.
44. Venezuela, Ministerio del Ambiente y de los Recursos Naturales. Informe de gestión del sector agua potable y saneamiento, 1999–2004. Caracas: MARN; 2005.
45. Organización Panamericana de la Salud. Informe de la evaluación regional de los servicios de manejo de residuos sólidos municipales en América Latina y el Caribe. Washington, DC: OPS; 2005.
46. Velásquez H, Molina B, Morales J, Cano Y, Romero A. Niveles de contaminación atmosférica por gases ácidos (SO2 y NO2) y partículas inhalables (PM10) en dos sitios de la ciudad de Maracaibo, Venezuela. Presented at I Congreso Internacional de Cuenca del Lago de Maracaibo, August 2006.
47. Venezuela, Ministerio de Salud y Desarrollo Social. Informe de los servicios de radiofísica sanitaria. Caracas: MSDS; 2004.
48. Organización Panamericana de la Salud, Organización Mundial de la Salud, Sistema Regional de Vigilancia de las Enfermedades Trasmitidas por Alimentos; 2006.
49. Organización Panamericana de la Salud; Instituto Interamericano de Cooperación para la Agricultura; Organización de las Naciones Unidas para la Agricultura y la Alimentación. Proyecto Sistema Nacional Integrado de Control de Alimentos; 2005.
50. Organización Panamericana de la Salud. Informe sobre la cooperación estratégica de país. Caracas; 2006.
51. Venezuela, Ministerio de Salud y Desarrollo Social, Coordinación Nacional de Bancos de Sangre. PowerPoint presentation.
52. Venezuela, Ministerio de Salud y Desarrollo Social. Lista básica nacional de medicamentos esenciales, 2003. Caracas: MSDS; 2005.
53. Venezuela, Ministerio de Salud y Desarrollo Social. Formulario Terapéutico Nacional, 2004. Caracas: MSDS; 2004.
54. Venezuela, Ministerio de Salud y Desarrollo Social, Dirección de Drogas, Medicamentos y Cosméticos, Departamento de Psicotrópicos y Estupefacientes. Archivos; 2005.
55. Venezuela, Centro Nacional de Vigilancia Farmacológica. Archivos, 2005.
56. Venezuela, Instituto Nacional de Higiene "Rafael Rangel." Archivos. Caracas; 2005.
57. Intercontinental Marketing Services-Health. Global pharmaceutical market forecasts: market reports. Available at: http://www.ims-global.com/insigth/report/global/report.htm. Accessed 21 September 2006.
58. Venezuela. Gaceta Oficial de la República Bolivariana de Venezuela; 2 de enero de 2006; (38.348):5–8.
59. Venezuela, Ministerio de Salud y Desarrollo Social. Indicadores básicos de salud de la República Bolivariana de Venezuela, 2004. Caracas: MSDS; 2005.

UNITED STATES–MEXICO BORDER AREA

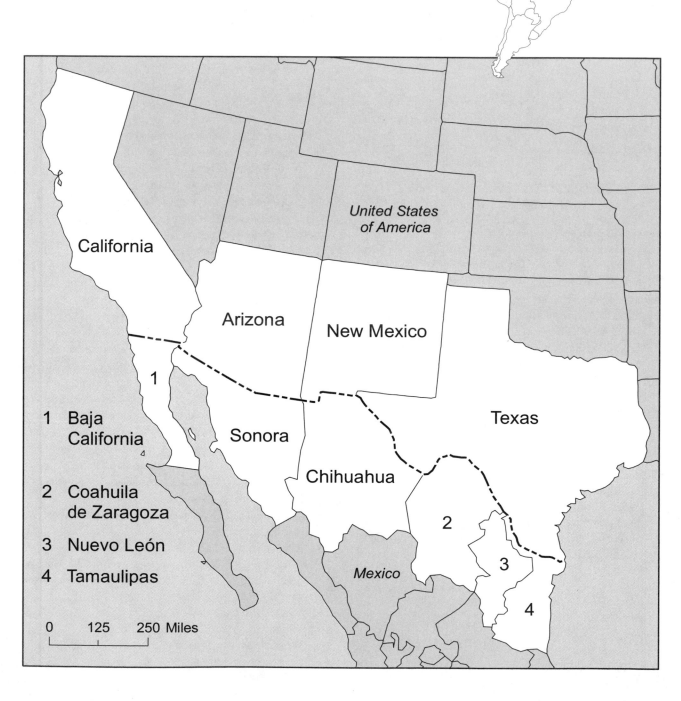

California

United States of America

Arizona

New Mexico

Texas

1

1 Baja California

Sonora

2 Coahuila de Zaragoza

Chihuahua

2

3 Nuevo León

Mexico

3

4 Tamaulipas

4

0   125   250 Miles

The United States–Mexico border extends for 1,952 miles (3,141 kilometers), stretching from the Gulf of Mexico to the Pacific Ocean. The 1983 La Paz Agreement—signed by the federal governments of the United States and Mexico for the protection, improvement, and conservation of the environment along the border—defines the border area as the land within 100 km (62.5 mi) on either side of the international boundary.

GENERAL CONTEXT AND HEALTH DETERMINANTS

Border areas in the two countries share environmental, social, economic, cultural, and epidemiological features with one another, but they operate under different policies, norms, and regulations.

The U.S.-Mexico border is made up of 10 states,[1] 48 United States counties, 80 Mexican municipalities, and 14 pairs of sister cities,[2] constituting a total population of slightly more than 13 million. As will be seen in the text ahead, in general—although clearly there are exceptions—health determinants on the Mexico side of the border show more positive conditions than in Mexico as a whole. The opposite is seen along the United States side of the border, where health determinants are generally worse than for the United States as a whole.

Social, Political, and Economic Determinants

The United States–Mexico border is the most traveled border in the world. According to the U.S. Immigration and Naturalization Service, in 2002, more than 190 million people entered the United States from Mexico through 24 official ports of entry. According to information published online by *Economic Development America*, in 2004, approximately 60% of the 500 million visitors admitted into the United States entered across the U.S.-Mexico border, as did 90 million cars and 4.3 million trucks; this human and vehicular traffic is a major contributor to the US$ 638 million in trade conducted along the border each day. Data

from the United States Department of Transportation's Bureau of Transportation Statistics showed that the number of trucks entering the U.S. in 2005 increased to 4.9 million, ranging from 40,042 (0.8% of all truck crossings) in New Mexico to 3,275,563 (66% of all truck crossings) in Texas.

Mexico is the United States' third leading business trading partner; the U.S. is Mexico's main trading partner. In 2003, Mexico's exports to the U.S. amounted to US$ 146.8 trillion, and its imports from the U.S. for the same period were US$ 105.7 trillion.

Mexico's *maquiladoras*—plants that import raw materials and components for processing or assembly by Mexican labor and then export the finished products—have become the largest component of U.S.-Mexico trade and are an engine of growth in the border area. Most *maquiladoras* are U.S.-owned and import most of their components from U.S. suppliers.

With the signing of the North American Free Trade Agreement (NAFTA) and the consequent lifting of most trade and investment barriers among Canada, Mexico, and the United States, the rate of industrial development along the border flourished further: in 1990, there were about 1,700 plants operating in Mexico; by 2001 they had more than doubled, to nearly 3,800 *maquiladora* plants, 2,700 of which were in the border states. In 2004, it is estimated that more than one million Mexicans were employed in the more than 3,000 *maquiladoras* located along the border.

Despite the extraordinary degree of cross-border interdependency, economic development along the border is uneven. For example, Mexico's border states have lower unemployment rates and higher wages compared to other regions of the country. Mexico's border states also have the lowest poverty rates and highest literacy rates in the country.

Conditions in the United States are the reverse: four of the seven poorest cities and five of the poorest counties in the United States are located in Texas along the Mexican border. Generally, counties on the U.S. side have experienced an increase in unemployment and a decrease in per capita income over the past 30 years. For example, in the city of El Paso, Texas, poverty is twice the national average and average income is one-third the national figure. The educational level of the population in U.S.

---

[1]On the Mexico side: Baja California, Chihuahua, Coahuila, Nuevo León, Sonora, and Tamaulipas. On the United States side: Arizona, California, New Mexico, and Texas.

[2]San Diego/Tijuana (California/Baja California), Calexico/Mexicali (California/Baja California), Yuma/San Luis (Arizona/Sonora), Nogales/Nogales (Arizona/Sonora), Naco/Naco (Arizona/Sonora), Douglas/Agua Prieta (Arizona/Sonora), Columbus/Puerto Palomas (New Mexico/Chihuahua), El Paso/Ciudad Juárez (Texas/Chihuahua), Presidio/Ojinaga (Texas/Chihuahua), Del Rio/Ciudad Acuña (Texas/Coahuila), Eagle Pass/Piedras Negras (Texas/Coahuila), Laredo/Nuevo Laredo (Texas/Tamaulipas), McAllen/Reynosa (Texas/Tamaulipas), and Brownsville/Matamoros (Texas/Tamaulipas).

border counties also is lower than elsewhere in the country. Nationwide, the percentage of persons without a middle-school education is 0.5%, compared to 22.1% in Luna, 21% in Presidio County, and 20.1% in Maverick.

The benefits of growing trade between Mexico and the United States notwithstanding, the boom has had its down sides. For example, growing trade between the two nations has brought with it an increase in freight vehicle traffic, potentially exacerbating the risk of environmental pollution and traffic-related injuries. Moreover, in addition to formal trade, there are cross-border networks of informal and even illegal trade. On the one hand there is drug trafficking: according to the United States Drug Enforcement Agency, 65% of the cocaine consumed in the United States enters through the Mexican border, and virtually 100% of the heroin produced in Mexico and South America targets U.S. markets. On the other hand, there is a booming market for used tires that accumulate by the millions in several waste piles in all Mexican border cities.

While economic growth clearly has contributed toward higher employment, the border area's infrastructure has not been able to keep pace. In addition, as millions of new residents from the interior of Mexico and elsewhere in Latin America flock to the border area, lured by the promise of jobs and a better life, already strained resources, including health resources, are further taxed.

Infectious diseases easily pass through the permeable border, as hundreds of thousands of persons trek back and forth across its boundary. And, whereas years back the border area was mainly rural, it is urbanizing rapidly, which brings on all the diseases of big cities caused by contamination, stress, and nutritional habits. Like many emerging nations, the U.S.-Mexico border must cope with the double burden of communicable diseases coupled with chronic illnesses.

Environmental health issues are by far the most pressing problems in the border area, including poor air quality, water scarcity and contamination, lead contamination, and improper waste disposal, to name but a few. Water is the most precious resource in a large portion of the border that is primarily arid. And air pollution ranks among the worst environmental problems: particulate matter levels continue to exceed standards during peak events, and many projects looking at the health effects of air pollution continue to be carried out in the region. Ozone pollution also threatens many communities, even though a relaxation in the standard (from a 1 hour average to an 8 hour average) has reduced the number of instances that exceed set limits.

Rural communities along the border are confronted with a host of environmental problems, including pollution from agricultural activities that threaten surface- and groundwater resources with contamination. Pesticide contamination poses a greater threat to areas with a high concentration of farming, such as the Imperial Valley and the Rio Grande Valley. Programs monitoring human exposure are scattered and not coordinated.

Demographics, Mortality, and Morbidity

The annual net flow of Mexican migration to the United States increased notably during the final three decades of the 20th century, spiking from an annual average of just under 30,000 people between 1961 and 1970 to close to 400,000 between 2001 and 2004. This continuously growing migratory flow has resulted in a large Mexican-origin community living in the United States. Clearly this enormous human movement has implications for family structure, employment, and health care, and it clearly begs for further exploration and study.

According to information for 2004 from the U.S.-Mexico Health Initiative, all four United States border states were among the 13 states in that country with more than 100,000 Mexican immigrants: in ascending order, New Mexico had 111,049 Mexican immigrants, Arizona had 618,105, Texas had 2,356,703, and California had 4,026,219. Together, the four U.S. border states had more than seven million Mexican immigrants living within their borders in 2005.

In 2001–2004, three-quarters of migrants lacked proper documentation to legally cross the border, an increase compared to less than half who lacked such documentation in 1993–1997.

A U.S. Government Accountability Office (GAO) report to the United States Senate on illegal immigration in August 2006 stated that border-crossing deaths have doubled since 1995. Data analysis showed that the annual number of border-crossing deaths increased from 241 deaths in 1999 to 472 in 2005, with most of the increase occurring in the Border Patrol's Tucson Sector, which includes much of the Arizona desert. Data from the National Center for Health Statistics (NCHS) for 1990–2003 show a major shift in the causes of migrant border-crossing deaths—traffic fatalities were the leading cause of migrant border-crossing deaths in the early 1990s, while from the late 1990s onward, heat exposure was the leading cause. The increase in deaths due to heat exposure over the last 15 years was attributed to a shift of migrant traffic from urban areas like San Diego and El Paso to the desert, as a result of the implementation of the Southwest Border Strategy in 1994. Because of their migratory nature, undocumented immigrants have less access to preventive and curative services.

Border communities are predominantly urban, with 83% of the population of San Diego, Pima, El Paso, Hidalgo, and Cameron counties in the United States living in urban settings. Hispanics account for 40% of the border states' population; 48% of the population in border counties is Hispanic.

More than 13 million people live in the border area, 53% of them on the United States side. If rapid population growth trends persist (more than twice that of the overall growth in each country), the total population is expected to reach 20 million by 2020. For the U.S., according to the 2000 census, overall growth was 0.92%, compared with an average 2.87% growth in border counties. In 2005, with annual growth rates ranging from 1.2% to 2.7%, the six Mexican border states (average 1.8%) registered faster growth than the country, which had a growth rate of 1.0%.

Nearly 95% of the border population lives in 14 pairs of sister cities. The Ciudad Juarez–El Paso sister city metropolis has more than two million inhabitants, making it the largest border community. According to the 2000 census, the fastest growing border communities, with population gains of almost 5% per year, were Hidalgo and Reynosa.

The population on both sides of the border is relatively young. In 2005, 29% of persons living on the Mexican side of the border were younger than 15 years of age, slightly less than the overall 30% figure for the nation. On the U.S. side, 23% of the population was younger than 15, compared to 21% for the country as a whole. In 2003, the fertility rate for U.S. border states taken together was 2.4, compared to 2.0 for the nation. The total fertility rate in Mexico's border states in 2005 was 2.1, on a par with the country's overall rate.

Life expectancy at birth for U.S. border states in 2003 ranged from 72.2 years (Arizona) to 77.2 years (Texas). Life expectancy at birth in 2005 for Mexican border states ranged from 75.8 years (Tamaulipas) to 76.6 years (Baja California), all higher than the national figure of 75.4 years. Women outlived men by 4.4 to 5.3 years.

In 2003, the crude mortality rate in the four U.S. border states was lower than the 842 deaths per 100,000 population figure for the United States as a whole—Texas, 700; California, 675; Arizona, 778; and New Mexico, 790. It should be noted that in 1992–1994, crude mortality rates in United States border states were 60% to 70% greater than their corresponding age-standardized rates using a world standard population. Based on a mortality rate evaluation, the population on the Mexican side of the border is younger than that on the U.S. side.

This trend is expected to hold in 2001–2005. In 2003, crude mortality rates per 100,000 population show that three border states on the Mexico side had higher rates than that country's national figure (470)—Coahuila (477), Chihuahua (540), and Sonora (506); the lowest rate was found in Tamaulipas, at 430.

In 1992–1994, age standardized rates among Mexico border states were 25%–37% higher than corresponding crude rates. This same general trend is expected for 2001–2005.

Health problems are similar on each side of the border, and affect similar populations. Six of the 10 leading causes of mortality are the same in both nations: heart disease, malignant neoplasms, cerebrovascular diseases, diabetes mellitus, liver disease and cirrhosis, and land transport accidents. Pulmonary tuberculosis and water- and food-borne diseases also are important infectious diseases along the border.

In 2003, the 10 leading causes of death in the four U.S. border states were all heart diseases (182–195 deaths per 100,000 population), malignant neoplasms (153–173), cerebrovascular diseases (41–50), accidents (30–65), chronic lower respiratory disease (34–50), influenza and pneumonia (16–23), diabetes (20–32), Alzheimer's disease (18–31), suicide (10–18), and chronic liver disease and cirrhosis (10–17). The five leading

causes were the same in 1992–1994. It is noteworthy that HIV/AIDS was not a leading cause in either time period.

In 2003, the leading causes of death for the six Mexican border states were ischemic heart disease (57–82 deaths per 100,000 population), malignant neoplasms (62–72), diabetes mellitus (48–79), cerebrovascular disease (23–29), liver disease and cirrhosis (15–19), chronic lower respiratory infections (11–19), certain diseases originating in the perinatal period (11–21), land transport accidents (8–18), acute respiratory infections (6–13), and diseases of the urinary system (9–13). The lowest mortality rates for six of the 10 leading causes were found in Baja California and four of the highest rates were found in Chihuahua.

A comparison of these disease categories with leading causes in 1992–1994 finds few differences, but the rates in the earlier period, except for heart disease, were about the same or lower—ischemic heart disease (54–67), malignant neoplasms (56–69), diabetes (33–46), cerebrovascular disease (25–28), and chronic liver disease and cirrhosis (12–20). Again, interestingly, AIDS was not one of the leading causes of death in either time period.

It is important to note that the range of diabetes mortality rates in 2003 was roughly twice as great in Mexico's border states as in U.S. border states. In 1992–1994, the ratio of diabetes mortality rates for 45–64-year-olds in Mexico's border areas to those in the U.S. border area of sister cities was 6.3 to 1.

Evidence suggests that sedentary lifestyles and poor nutritional habits have contributed to high rates of chronic disease on both sides of the border, though both populations are relatively young.

HEALTH OF POPULATION GROUPS

Children under 5 Years Old

In 2003, all four United States border states had lower infant morality rates than the national level (6.8 per 1,000 live births): 5.2 in California, 5.8 in New Mexico, 6.5 in Arizona, and 6.6 in Texas. The overall combined infant mortality rate for the four border states on the United States side in 2003 was lower than it was in 1992–1994.

Data published in 2004 in *Salud Pública de México* indicate that in 2003, two Mexican border states (Chihuahua and Baja California) had female infant mortality rates that were higher than the national figure (14.5 female infant deaths per 1,000 live female births), and Baja California, Chihuahua, and Sonora had higher male infant mortality rates than the overall national rate (18.4 male infant deaths per 1,000 live births).

In 1992–1994, infant mortality rates in Mexican border states doubled those of United States border states. The infant mortality rates in Mexican border states ranged from 12.6 infant deaths per 1,000 live births in Tamaulipas to 20.6 in Coahuila; Mexico's national rate was 17.7.

The four leading causes of infant deaths in 2003 in the U.S. border states were congenital anomalies, short gestation, SIDS, and maternal pregnancy complications.

The leading causes of infant mortality in the six Mexican border states in 2003 closely resembled those for Mexico as a whole. The 10 leading causes included certain conditions originating in the perinatal period, congenital malformations of the heart, lower acute respiratory infections, infectious intestinal diseases, protein calorie malnutrition, anencephaly and similar malformations, defects of the abdominal wall, Down's syndrome, lower acute respiratory infections, and spina bifida. The reported perinatal mortality rate was reported as 77.4 per 1,000 live births in 2003.

In 2003, the United States border states accounted for 25% of the 4,965 deaths among children 1–4 years of age in the country, with 557 deaths in California, 524 deaths in Texas, 134 deaths in Arizona, and 46 deaths in New Mexico. In 1992–1994, the United States border states accounted for 23% of the 20,630 deaths of children 1–4 years old in the United States, with 2,600 deaths in California, 1,634 deaths in Texas, 420 deaths in Arizona, and 167 deaths in New Mexico.

The leading four causes of death in children 1–4 years old in three United States border states (Arizona, California, and New Mexico) in 2003 were unintentional injuries, congenital anomalies, malignant neoplasms, and homicide; the pattern was similar in Texas, but there, homicide ranked as the fourth cause. Mortality rates among children 1–4 years old per 1,000 population in 1992–1994 ranged from 0.39 in California to 0.53 in Arizona, compared to the overall rate in the United States of 0.44.

In Mexico's border states in 2003, the leading causes of death in children 1–4 years old closely resembled those of the country as a whole: infectious intestinal diseases, lower acute respiratory infections, congenital malformations of the heart, motor vehicle accidents, accidental drowning and submersion, protein calorie malnutrition, leukemia, homicides, anemia, and epilepsy.

Among Mexico's border states in 1992–1994, rates ranged from 0.67 per 1,000 children 1–4 years old in Nuevo León to 1.1 in Chihuahua, compared to Mexico's overall rate of 1.2.

Adults

Maternal mortality rates for U.S. border states in 2003 showed Texas with the highest (15.9 maternal deaths per 100,000 live births); followed by California (15.0); and then by Arizona and New Mexico, each at 5.0. A review of maternal mortality for 2000–2003 showed that New Mexico has consistently had the lowest maternal mortality rate, while California had the highest rate in 2000, 2002, and 2003. In 2001, Texas had the highest rate at 11.0.

Maternal mortality rates for Mexico's border states in 2003 showed Baja California with the highest rate, at 62.8 per 100,000 live births, followed by Chihuahua (53.7), Tamaulipas (45.2), Coahuila (32.1), Sonora (29.3), and Nuevo León (15.9). With the exception of Baja California, all the other states had lower rates

than Mexico as a whole (62.6). Nuevo León consistently had the lowest rate throughout 2001–2003. Sonora registered the lowest rate in 2000. The national rate was higher than the state rates throughout 2000–2003.

In comparison with rates in 2003, maternal mortality rates for 1992–1994 ranged from 16.1 maternal deaths per 100,000 live births in Baja California and Tamaulipas to 38.3 in Sonora. The maternal mortality rates of Mexico's border states were all lower than rates for the country as a whole (47.7). In 1992–1994 the rates for the United States border states ranged from 3.4 in Arizona to 10.8 maternal deaths per 100,000 live births in New Mexico. The overall United States maternal mortality rate was 7.9 maternal deaths per 1,000 live births.

Data on early prenatal care (percentage of live births with early prenatal care) in the U.S. border states for 2001–2003 showed that California's rate, at 86.4%, is higher than the national rate (83.7%), whereas the other three states had lower rates of 80.6% (Texas), 76.6% (Arizona), and 68.9% (New Mexico). Prenatal care (number of visits for pregnant women) in 2004 for Mexico's border states ranged from 5.5 (Tamaulipas) to 6.2 (Baja California), both of which were higher than the national average (5.0). Visits for each state are 5.9 (Nuevo Leon) and 6.0 (Coahuila, Chihuahua, and Sonora).

The percentage of deliveries attended by trained personnel in Mexico's border states in 2004 ranged from a low of 63% (Chihuahua) to a high of 96.4% (Coahuila), indicating that coverage in five of the border states was higher than the national figure of 74.2%.

Indigenous Peoples

There are 26 U.S. federally recognized Native American tribes (ranging in size from 9 to 17,000 members) and 7 Mexican indigenous peoples in the border area. Some of these tribes and peoples share extensive family and cultural ties.

In May 2006, Arizona and Sonora created a health council to represent Arizona border communities in the Tohono O'odham Nation, Western Pima County, and the Northwest Sonora border communities of Caborca, Sonoyta, and Puerto Peñasco. The health council will be one of 13 other binational health councils located along the U.S.-Mexico border and the first trinational health council, encompassing the United States, Mexico, and the Tohono O'odham Nation.

Health inequities along the border particularly affect indigenous populations, who are especially vulnerable as a result of poverty and lack of health insurance. Health professionals in the area suggest that the number of indigenous people who leave their home area has increased in recent years, and these groups are the most vulnerable, given the linguistic and cultural barriers they face in order to access health services.

HEALTH CONDITIONS AND PROBLEMS

COMMUNICABLE DISEASES

Vector-borne Diseases

In 2005, 3,000 cases of **West Nile virus** were reported in the United States, and 40% of these were in the four U.S. border states: Arizona (113 cases and 5 deaths), California (880 cases and 19 deaths), New Mexico (33 cases and 2 deaths), and Texas (195 cases and 11 deaths). The 37 deaths represent 31% of the total deaths from West Nile virus reported in the U.S. in 2005.

Although there were no reported cases of West Nile virus in border states on Mexico's side from 2003 to 2005, the many cases reported in the U.S. along the border in 2005 suggest that West Nile virus may well be a health concern along both sides of the border.

Although there were only 61 indigenous cases of **dengue fever** reported in the United States during 1980–1999, dengue is a reemerging threat along the border. In 2005, on the Mexican side of the border, 4,333 dengue cases were reported in Tamaulipas during the first 41 weeks. Subsequently, the Border Infectious Diseases Surveillance (BIDS) program undertook active surveillance at participating clinics in the U.S. and identified 18 cases of dengue. One of these was a case of **dengue hemorrhagic fever**, the first locally acquired classic dengue hemorrhagic fever case in the continental United States.

There were no reported cases of dengue in the six Mexican border states in 2002 and 2003. In 2001, the six border states reported a total of 171 cases led by Tamaulipas (93 cases), followed by Nuevo León (76 cases), Baja California, and Coahuila (1 case each), while there were no cases reported in Chihuahua and Sonora. These six states accounted for 2.8% of the total reported 6,095 cases in Mexico.

Vaccine-preventable Diseases

Childhood immunization programs have been a success in both countries and in the border area. There have been record high vaccination coverage rates and vaccine-preventable diseases are at an all time low. **Measles** is no longer endemic and rubella control has been effective. **Poliomyelitis** had been eradicated in the Americas.

The United States National Infant Immunization Week and Vaccination Week in the Americas have been conducted jointly in the border area since 2004.

According to the United States Centers for Disease Control and Prevention, 2004 immunization coverage with a complete vaccine series (DPT/polio/MCV/Hib/HepB) in the United States overall is 81%. In the border states on the U.S. side, coverage was 71% in Arizona; 81% in California; 84% in New Mexico; and 73% in Texas.

Vaccination coverage in Mexico is very high. Data from Mexico's Instituto Nacional de Salud Pública indicate that in December 2004, immunization coverage of fully immunized children 1–4 years old in Mexico's border states (96%) was higher than the national average of 93%. Tamaulipas had the highest coverage in 2004.

Hepatitis A incidence has decreased substantially from that seen in 1987–1997, when all border states and most border counties reported incidence rates of ≥20 cases per 100,000 population each year. By 2004, only two border areas had rates of ≥20 per 100,000 population.

Data for Mexico for 2000–2004 indicate that in 2003, there were more than 15,000 cases of hepatitis A (the lowest in the period), increasing to 16,000 in 2004. There were 1,888 reported cases in the six Mexican border states, accounting for 12.3% of the total cases in Mexico in 2003. The highest number of cases occurred in different states each year, with Tamaulipas having the highest number of cases in 2001 (939), Nuevo León in 2002 (836), Baja California in 2003 (489), and Coahuila in 2004 (439).

The four U.S. border states accounted for 1,125 cases of hepatitis B, 20.5% of the 5,497 cases in the United States in 2005; the six Mexican border states accounted for 126 cases, 21.5% of the 587 cases in Mexico that same year.

Intestinal Infectious Diseases

The four U.S. border states accounted for 49 cases of **typhoid fever** in 2005, 80 in 2004, 91 in 2003, and 65 in 2002.

The six Mexican border states accounted for 11,544 cases of typhoid fever in 2005, indicating serious food and water sanitation problems. Reported cases increased between 2002 and 2004, with 2,725, 6,123, and 8,342 reported annual number of cases of typhoid, respectively. Tamaulipas has consistently had the highest number of cases since 2001, with the highest number of typhoid cases—5,837—reported in 2005.

Chronic Communicable Diseases

Tuberculosis (TB) continues to be a concern for border areas in both Mexico and the United States. Both countries report approximately 15,000 cases of all forms of tuberculosis on a yearly basis. In 2005, the tuberculosis incidence rate in Mexico was 15 per 100,000, while the United States reported a rate of 4.7 incident TB cases per 100,000 population. What is more troubling is that the U.S.-Mexico border states reported a tuberculosis incidence rate higher then the national average, with rates of 7.9 in U.S. border states and 26.3 in Mexican border states. Efforts to control tuberculosis in the United States–Mexico border are reflected in the 2005–2010 Strategic Plan of Ten against Tuberculosis, a binational initiative created by the health officers of the 10 U.S.-Mexico border states in June 1995.

In 2005, a total of 11,547 cases of tuberculosis were reported in the U.S. The four border states accounted for 3,560 (31%), broken down as follows: Arizona, 221; California, 2,034; New Mexico, 35; and Texas, 1,270.

In 2005, a total of 14,038 cases of tuberculosis were reported in Mexico, of which the six border states accounted for 4,277 (31%), ranging from 407 cases (Coahuila) to 1,172 (Baja California).

HIV/AIDS and Other Sexually Transmitted Infections

In 2005 Baja California ranked seventh in the nation and first among Mexico's border states in the number of new reported AIDS cases (160), approximately 4.5% of the total AIDS cases reported at the national level; Coahuila had 43 reported new cases (1.2%), the fewest along the border.

Data published in *Salud Pública de México* indicate that the highest male and female mortality from AIDS occurred in Baja California. In 2003, male mortality from AIDS per 100,000 males in Baja California (32.1) was twice the national figure for males (16.7), while female mortality, at 5.3 per 100,000 females, also is higher than the national figure for females (3.1). A review of mortality data due to AIDS during 2000–2003 shows that males had a consistently higher mortality rate due to AIDS than females.

In 1992–1994, mortality from AIDS was 0.9 per 100,000 in Mexico's sister cities, the same rate for Mexico as a whole. In comparing border states with Mexico, only Baja California had a rate (1.3) higher than the national rate; the remaining border states all had rates below 0.5 per 100,000 population. In 1992–1994 on the U.S. side of the border, mortality rates for AIDS in sister cities (1.6) almost doubled those of Mexican sister cities, but were half those for the United States as a whole (4.0).

Zoonoses

The four U.S. border states accounted for 47 reported human brucellosis cases in 2005. California had 26 cases, Texas had 17, New Mexico had 1, and Arizona had 3.

In 2005, the six Mexican border states accounted for 759 reported cases (38.2% of the total reported human cases of brucellosis in Mexico). From 2001 to 2005, the number of reported human cases of brucellosis ranged from 1,083 in 2002 to 1,988 in 2005. Coahuila had the highest number of cases among the six Mexican border states in 2003 (491 cases), in 2004 (618 cases), and in 2005 (311), while Nuevo León reported the highest numbers in 2001 (423 cases) and in 2002 (435 cases).

NONCOMMUNICABLE DISEASES

Metabolic and Nutritional Diseases

Diabetes is on the rise along the U.S.-Mexico border, with the number of persons with diabetes increasing at an alarming rate on both sides. In 2003, diabetes was the third leading cause of death in Mexican border states and the sixth leading cause of death on the U.S. side. Of the 14,513 deaths in U.S. border states that same year, California accounted for 7,093 deaths, or 20 deaths per 100,000 population, and New Mexico for 559, or 32 per

100,000. Arizona had 20.7 deaths per 100,000 population and Texas had 25.6 deaths per 100,000. In comparison, in 1992–1994, crude diabetes mellitus mortality rates for border states were 17.6 deaths per 100,000 in Arizona, 13.2 in California, 24.4 in New Mexico, and 23.1 in Texas.

In Mexican border states, mortality due to diabetes mellitus has been increasing for both males and females. Data published in *Salud Pública de México* indicate that the highest mortality from diabetes in 2003 was in Coahuila, with male mortality at 70.3 per 100,000 and female mortality at 89.2 per 100,000. The second highest was in Tamaulipas, with male and female mortality rates of 56.5 and 68.2, respectively. These rates are substantially higher than those seen a decade ago. In 1992–1994, the average annual male and female mortality rates in Coahuila for diabetes were 40.4 male deaths per 100,000 and 51.9 female deaths per 100,000 each year—about 30 per 100,000 less than in 2003. In Tamaulipas, the male rate was 35.7 and the female rate was 41.9 in 1992–1994—about 20 per 100,000 less than 2003.

In comparison, in 1992–1994 in United States sister cities, the diabetes mellitus crude mortality rate was 17.3 per 100,000 population, while in Mexico's sister cities, the rate was 2.5 times greater, at 43.6. Female rates were slightly higher than male rates on both sides of the border. Among Mexico's sister cities, the diabetes mellitus mortality rate for males was 40.4; for females, 46.6. On the United States side, the male diabetes mellitus mortality rate was 16.1; for females, 18.5.

A diabetes prevalence study was conducted from February 2001 to October 2002 on 4,027 individuals (1,905 on the United States side and 2,122 on Mexico's side) in 45 border communities (38 in Mexico and 16 in the U.S.). Initial results showed that approximately 1.2 million (15.7%) of the 7.5 million adults who live along the U.S.-Mexico border area have diabetes. Of these, roughly 500,000 live on the Mexican side of the border with the remaining 700,000 living on the U.S. side. It is estimated that pre-diabetes affects about 14% (645,000) of the total adult population residing on the United States side of the border.

In response to the diabetes problem, the U.S.-Mexico Border Diabetes Project was established to determine the prevalence of diabetes along the border and to develop and implement binational diabetes prevention and control programs targeted to the needs of the border population.

Obesity, too, is a serious problem affecting the population living along the border. According to the 2001–2002 U.S.-Mexico Border Diabetes Prevention and Control Project study, it is estimated that 5.3 million adults living along the Mexico border are overweight or obese. One million of them live on the Mexican side of the border, and 1.5 million live on the U.S. side. Obese individuals along the U.S. side of the border have 2.8 times greater risk of developing diabetes than individuals with normal weight, and on the Mexican side, the risk is 2.2 times greater. The rate for obese men is slightly higher on the U.S. side (37.7%), compared to men on the Mexico side (26.7%). The reverse holds true for obese women, whose rates are higher on the Mexico side (31.9%).

Cardiovascular Diseases

Heart disease continues to be the leading cause of death on both sides of the U.S.-Mexico border. In 2003, there were 124,932 deaths from heart disease in the U.S. border states, ranging from 3,402 deaths in New Mexico, for a crude rate of 181.5 deaths per 100,000 population, to 68,864 deaths in California, for a crude mortality rate of 194.1 per 100,000 population. The heart disease mortality rate in Arizona was 195.1 and in Texas it was 188.9.

In 2003, the mortality rate due to heart disease in the Mexican border states (62.6 deaths per 100,000 population) was higher than the national rate (45.4). The mortality rate ranged from 54.8 (Baja California) to 77.7 (Sonora).

For 1992–1994, the mortality rate from heart disease in Mexico's sister cities was about 1.4 times that of Mexico as a whole. Comparisons of rates at the state level with that of the national level showed Baja California's rate to be 1.4 times greater and Sonora 1.8 times greater than the overall rate for Mexico.

The main contribution to heart disease mortality in 2003 was mortality from ischemic heart disease, with crude rates among Mexico's border states that ranged from Baja California (56.8 per 100,000 population) to Nuevo León (102.0). In 1992–1994, ischemic heart disease rates ranged from 49.0 in Coahuila to 67.0 in Sonora.

Malignant Neoplasms

Malignant neoplasms continue to be the second leading cause of death in all four U.S. and all six Mexico border states.

In 2003, there were 100,916 deaths due to malignant neoplasms in the U.S. border states, ranging from 3,103 deaths in New Mexico, for a crude mortality rate of 166 deaths per 100,000 population, to 54,319 deaths in California, for a rate of 153 deaths per 100,000 population. Arizona and Texas had rates of 173 and 153, respectively. All fell under the crude mortality rate for the country as a whole, 192 deaths per 100,000 population.

In 1992–1994, mortality rates for malignant neoplasms were also greater in New Mexico (157 deaths per 100,000 population per year), California (163), Arizona (195), and Texas (171) than in the United States as a whole (205).

In 2000, five of the six Mexican border states had mortality rates for malignant neoplasms that were higher than Mexico's national figure (65.3 malignant neoplasm deaths per 100,000 population).

Malignant neoplasm of the cervix uteri is the most frequent type of cancer among women of reproductive age and the leading cause of death among women 25 years and older in the border states.

In Mexico in 2003, the mortality rate for malignant neoplasms of the cervix uteri was 16.2 deaths per 100,000 females. Two bor-

der states had similar, although slightly higher rates: Coahuila with 16.7 deaths per 100,000 females and Chihuahua, with 16.3.

Mortality rates for malignant neoplasm of the cervix uteri ranged from 6.7 per 100,000 females in Nuevo León to 10.9 in Coahuila in 2003. During 1992–1994, average annual malignant neoplasm death rates from cervix uteri ranged from 8.4 in Nuevo León to 12.8 in Tamaulipas; the rate for Mexico overall was 11.2. Only Nuevo León had a lower rate than the national rate among Mexico's border states.

Mortality rates for malignant neoplasm of the breast for 2001–2003 were consistently higher in Mexican border states than in the country overall, with a crude mortality rate of 8.0 per 100,000 females. In 2003, Baja California had the same rate for deaths from malignant neoplasm of the breast as did Mexico as a whole, 15.7 breast cancer deaths per 100,000 females.

Mortality rates for malignant neoplasm of the breast ranged from 8.3 deaths per 100,000 females in Baja California to 11.0 in Chihuahua in 2003. In 1992–1994, the rate ranged from 6.7 in Baja California to 10.7 in Nuevo León; the national rate was 11.2 deaths from malignant neoplasm of the breast per 100,000 women.

Mortality rates for malignant neoplasm of the prostate ranged from 7.3 deaths per 100,000 males in Tamaulipas to 10.5 in Sonora. In 1992–1994, the rate ranged from 5.7 in Baja California to 8.0 in Sonora; the national rate was 6.2 deaths due to prostate cancer per 100,000 males.

OTHER HEALTH CONDITIONS AND PROBLEMS

Disasters

In the past five years, the border area suffered natural disasters, including hurricanes, forest fires, and floods. In 2005, hurricanes Rita and Katrina hit East Texas and Tamaulipas. Forest fires also caused damage to all four United States border states. In 2006, floods resulting from sudden and severe rainfall occurring within a short period damaged El Paso, Las Cruces, and Ciudad Juarez. None of these cities were prepared for severe rainfall events nor had they adequate storm drainage systems. This led to many displaced persons and damages to houses and infrastructure. There were no fatalities reported as a direct result of the floods in either country.

Violence and Other External Causes

In 2003, violence ranked high among crude mortality rates in the border states, with Chihuahua having the highest rate at 16.9 violent deaths per 100,000 population and Nuevo León the lowest, at 3.3; similar patterns with slightly higher rates were found in 1992–1994. In 2003, males were 6.7 times more likely to die a violent death than females in Mexico's border states. In Baja California, 3.5% of total deaths in 2003 were due to homicides. On the U.S. side, border state homicide rates ranged from 7 to 9 homicides per 100,000 population in 2003, lower than the 10 to 13 per 100,000 population in 1992–1994.

Traffic along the border is huge, with an estimated 800,000 to 1 million border crossings each day. According to the United States National Center for Health Statistics (part of the Centers for Disease Control and Prevention), motor vehicle accidents were the eighth leading cause of death in 44 border counties on the U.S. side in 2000, resulting in about 1,000 deaths. For Hispanics, motor vehicle crashes were the fifth leading cause of death, compared to a rank of ninth for non-Hispanic whites. Using the years of potential life lost (YPLL) measure, motor vehicle crashes were the third leading cause of death for Hispanics living on the border (the fifth leading cause for white non-Hispanics living there). When broken down by age group, data showed that motor vehicle crashes are the leading cause of death for age groups 1–4, 5–14, 15–24, and 25–34 at the national, border state, and border county levels.

Data from Mexico for 2003 showed that observed mortality rates due to traffic accidents (deaths per 100,000 population) for males ranged from a high of 25.1 in Chihuahua, to 24.9 in Tamaulipas, 22.3 in Sonora, 18.4 in Nuevo León, 16.7 in Coahuila, and a low of 11.3 in Baja California. Female morality rates were highest in Chihuahua (7.9), followed by Sonora (6.7); the pattern followed the same trend as for males in 2003.

Mental Health and Addictions

Addiction, tobacco consumption, and mental health are public health problems of concern along the border. Adolescents are the most vulnerable population group, at high risk for addiction, including tobacco consumption; suicide; traffic-related injuries; and unwanted pregnancy.

In 2003, suicide was the ninth leading cause of death in U.S. border states, with a rate of 15.1 suicides per 100,000 population in Arizona and 18.3 per 100,000 in New Mexico. The suicide rate for the United States overall in 2003 was 10.8 suicides per 100,000 population. Suicide was the tenth leading cause of death in California (7.0 suicides per 100,000 population) and Texas (6.9). In 1992–1994, the average annual suicide rate in the United States was 12.0 per 100,000 population. Average annual suicide rates during 1992–1994 were higher than the 2003 rates in the U.S. border states, with Arizona at 18.1 per 100,000 population, California at 12.1, New Mexico at 18.4, and Texas at 12.7.

In 2003, suicide was the second leading cause of death for 10–14-year-olds in Arizona and New Mexico, and the second leading cause for 25–34-year-olds in Arizona, New Mexico, and Texas. Homicide was the second leading cause of death among 15–24-year-olds throughout the U.S. border area, as well as for 25–34-year-olds in Texas.

According to information from Mexico's National Statistics, Geography, and Informatics Institute (Instituto Nacional de Estadística, Geografía e Informática, INEGI), the State of Baja California registered the highest frequency of suicide in youths 18–25 years old on a per capita basis nationwide. Among men of all ages, Baja California Sur ranked sixth in the nation in suicides in 2003. In response, the State launched a telephone "hotline" campaign in 2004 to provide suicide, drug, and domestic violence counseling. In Coahuila there were 120 recorded suicides in 2003. The male to female suicide ratio approached 3 to 1.

The suicide rates in the six Mexico border states in 1992–1994 were Baja California at 3.0 per 100,000 population, Sonora at 4.2, Chihuahua at 4.0, Coahuila at 2.7, Nuevo León at 2.9, and Tamaulipas at 4.7. In the same period, Mexico's national suicide rate was 2.7 per 100,000 population.

In 2003, injuries (intentional and unintentional) were the second leading cause of death in Mexico's border states.

Environmental Pollution

The most persistent and pervasive pollutants found in the sister cities are ozone and particulate matter (PM10, or particulate matter 10μ in diameter or less). From 2001 to 2005, concentrations of ozone were higher than the binational standard of 0.08 ppm in Mexicali/Imperial Valley and Tijuana/San Diego. Ozone concentrations in Ciudad Juarez/El Paso improved during the past five years, staying below established standards in 2004 and 2005. Ozone concentrations in the Lower Rio Grande Valley also were below established standards. Annual mean concentrations of PM10 (mean for year of interest with the two prior years) from 2001 to 2005 in the Lower Rio Grande Valley were lower than the binational annual standard of 50 $\mu g/m^3$. Concentrations in the other four border monitoring areas exceeded the set limit, with the highest concentrations observed in Mexicali/Imperial Valley.

RESPONSE OF THE HEALTH SECTOR

Health Policies and Plans

The United States-Mexico Border Health Commission (BHC), which was created in 2000, is charged with providing international leadership to optimize health and quality of life along the border. The binational Commission has 26 members, comprising federal secretaries of health, chief health officers of the 10 border states, and prominent community health professionals from both nations; it is headed by the secretaries of health of both countries. The BHC operates on an independent budget, defines the binational health agenda, and presides over the administration of health services along the border.

In response to the terrorist attacks of September 11, 2001, the United States and Mexico signed the U.S.-Mexico Border Alliance, reiterating their commitment to cooperate towards achieving a safe, orderly border through specific actions designed to strengthen their common interests in matters of security, economic development, and tourism during the coming years. Preparedness against bioterrorism attacks has been given a higher

Opening a Window to Health

Next to solving environmental problems, ensuring that people have adequate access to health services is the leading challenge for the U.S.–Mexico border. More than 13 million souls live along the border, and between 250 million to 400 million persons crisscross the border each year. Communicable diseases take a particularly heavy toll along the border. Of the West Nile virus cases seen in the United States in 2005, 40% occurred in the four U.S. Border States. The border also experienced a dengue epidemic and there was at least one case of dengue hemorrhagic fever reported on the United States. The "Ventana a la Salud" program attempts to bring access to health care to difficult to reach populations. Through the program, Mexico's consular system, in partnership with local health advocacy and health service organizations, and sometimes with U.S. Government co-financing, has set up "health windows" in several Consulate Offices. Bilingual and bicultural staff provide health assessments, referrals, information on patient rights, and linkages to available services.

priority in border states through various initiatives, including the establishment of the Early Warning Infectious Disease Surveillance (EWIDS) program by the U.S.-Mexico Border Health Commission in 2004.

In addition to having epidemiological and laboratory functions, the program aims to strengthen cross-border activities in early detection, identification, and reporting of infectious diseases associated with potential bioterrorism agents.

After the signing of the North American Free Trade Agreement, Canada, Mexico, and the United States created the Commission for Environmental Cooperation (CEC) of North America to address regional environmental concerns, help prevent potential trade and environmental conflicts, and promote the effective enforcement of environmental law. In addition, Mexico and the United States created the Border Environment Cooperation Commission (BECC) and the North American Development Bank (NADB). BECC identifies, evaluates, and certifies environmental infrastructure projects; the Bank, a binational financial institution capitalized equally by both countries, finances environmental projects certified by the BECC. Both institutions work together with communities and project sponsors in both countries to develop and finance infrastructure necessary for a clean and healthy environment for border residents.

Since 2002, the Border Legislative Conference has met several times each year to find shared solutions to problems along the border. The Conference consists of state legislators of Mexico and United States border states, who gather to consider common problems, exchange information, and develop joint programs wherever appropriate.

Health Strategies and Programs

Working through the Border Health Commission, the United States and Mexico governments define health priorities for the border area. To this end, during the Commission's second meeting in 2001, they issued the Healthy Border 2010 Program, which sets a binational agenda of health promotion and disease prevention. The Program's two central objectives are: 1) to improve the quality of life and increase years of healthy life, and 2) to eliminate health disparities. The goals of the Healthy Border 2010 Program are channeled along 11 areas, each with its own specific aims. The areas and their respective goals are: 1) access to health care, by ensuring access to primary health care services; 2) cancer, by reducing breast and cervical cancer deaths; 3) diabetes, by reducing mortality and hospitalization due to the disease; 4) environmental health, by improving household access to sewage and drainage and reducing hospitalizations from acute pesticide poisoning; 5) HIV/AIDS, by reducing the incidence of HIV/AIDS; 6) immunization and communicable diseases, by broadening the scope of vaccinations for children and lessening the incidence of hepatitis and tuberculosis; 7) injury prevention, by reducing mortality from motor vehicle accidents as well as mortality from unintended injuries among children; 8) maternal and child health, by reducing infant mortality from birth defects, improving prenatal care, and bringing down pregnancy rates among adolescents; 9) mental health, by reducing suicide mortality; 10) oral health, by improving access to oral health services; and 11) respiratory diseases, by reducing the rate of hospitalization from asthma. Health problems or conditions such as cardiovascular diseases, tobacco use, substance abuse, gastrointestinal diseases, nutrition and obesity, lack of physical activity, and bioterrorism preparedness will be incorporated into the Program in the future.

As a way to address the border area's most pressing environmental and environmentally related problems, in 2003 representatives from the U.S.-Mexico border gathered to launch the Border 2012 Program, a 10-year working plan whose mission is to protect the environment and public health along the border, consistent with principles of sustainable development. This latest incarnation of a multi-year, binational environmental initiative represents a collaborative effort among federal, state, and local governments and agencies from both nations, as well as the active participation of U.S. tribal governments. The Border 2012 Program's six goals are: to reduce water contamination; to reduce air pollution; to reduce land contamination; to improve environmental health; to reduce exposure to chemicals as a result of accidental chemical releases or acts of terrorism; and to improve environmental performance through compliance, enforcement, pollution prevention, and promotion of environmental stewardship. To measure the Program's results, implementation reports will be prepared every two years to review progress, a five-year progress report will be issued in 2007, and a final report will be released in 2012. The Program is working on a strategy to control the used-tire piles in the future and clean up existing ones.

Organization of the Health System

In the United States, the health care system is characterized by a demand model, and health care is delivered on a fee-for-service system. Health services are provided by nonprofit institutions or by private entities. In 2000, 65% of the population of the U.S. border states was covered by private insurance and 25.6% by government insurance.

According to data from statehealthfacts.org (a website that is part of The Henry J. Kaiser Family Foundation), in 2004–2005, 51% of the population of the border states on the U.S. side was covered by private insurance (individual employer and Medicaid individual), 27% was covered by government insurance (Medicare, Medicaid, and other public Medicare), and 22% had no insurance. In general, the percentage of persons without private or public health insurance in U.S. border communities was higher than the national figure (22% versus 17%).

In Mexico, health care is considered a constitutional right. Various institutions provide health care services. The social security subsystem provides coverage to employed persons and their dependents, and is complemented by services provided by the government to unemployed persons, known as the "open population." There also are private health care services available, either through payment for medical insurance or through direct payment to providers. Beginning in 2002, an additional avenue of access to health care became available as part of the national health plan, known as *seguro popular* (people's insurance), which now covers approximately one million families.

In 2000, Mexico's border communities generally enjoyed greater social security coverage (59%) than the national average (43%). The greatest social security coverage occurred in the most industrialized border communities. Data for 2005 from the National Institute of Statistics, Geography, and Informatics (INEGI) showed that the percentage of border-state population covered by insurance (Social Security Institute insurance [IMSS], state employees insurance [ISSSTE], government provided insurance for government and state oil industry [ISSSTE/PEMEX], Armed

Forces insurance [SDN], the *seguro popular* created in 2001, and other insurance venues) was higher than the national figure. In 2005, Nuevo León had the highest health insurance coverage (69.2%), and Baja California and Tamaulipas had the lowest (56.2%). Coverage for other states in the same year was 58.4% in Chihuahua, 64.7% in Tamaulipas, 66% in Sonora, and 69% in Coahuila.

Public Health Services

The United States' and Mexico's health care systems have various programs and projects in place to promote health along the border. On the Mexican side, the Department of Health has health promotion offices in each of the 13 largest border cities, each of which has state-level support. On the U.S. side, some local health departments have health promotion sections that address specific needs. In late 2003, a Binational Border Health Promotion Plan began to be created.

The Binational Health Week that began in California in 2001 is one of the largest combined mobilization efforts (federal and state government agencies, community based organizations, and volunteers) designed to improve the health and well-being of the underserved Latino population living in Canada, Mexico, and the United States. Health-promotion and health-education activities are held throughout the border during this week.

The launching of a health station (*Ventanilla de Salud*) at the Mexican Consulate in El Paso in April 2006 marks the fourth such station in an initiative operating throughout the United States–Mexico border, along with those in San Diego (California), McAllen (Texas), and Tucson (Arizona). The *Ventanilla de Salud* program is a partnership among local health advocacy and health services organizations and the Mexican consular network designed to incorporate bilingual, bicultural, and highly trained health educators and advocates as part of Mexican consular services in the United States to counsel clients on eligibility for government-funded health insurance, other primary care services, and, when appropriate, various legal issues.

Based on the 2000 census, access to piped water within the house is 90% or higher in U.S. border communities. In Mexico's border communities, access is lower, ranging from a low of 66% in Acuña to a high of 85% in Ciudad Juarez and Piedras Negras.

Human Resources

According to data published online in statehealthfacts.org (a website that is part of The Henry J. Kaiser Family Foundation), in 2004 all four U.S. border states had fewer than the overall United States average of non-federal physicians (28.1 per 10,000 population). There were fewer physicians per 10,000 population in each of the four border states than in the U.S. as a whole, by as much as 22% in Texas and as little as 7% in California. The same is true for registered nurses: the ratio of registered nurses per

10,000 population in the four U.S. border states is approximately 20% lower than the national rate of 28 per 10,000 population. Border counties in Arizona and California have the same number of physicians, nurses, and dentists per 10,000 population as the United States as a whole, while border counties in New Mexico and Texas have lower health worker ratios than the national or state average.

In 2004, the distribution of human resources in Mexico's border states was comparable to the national figures of 11 physicians per 10,000 population and 19 nurses per 10,000 population. According to information from the secretaries of health in Mexican border states, the ratio of physicians per 10,000 population in Baja California was 8 and in Tamaulipas, 15; the figures for social security ranged from 9 in Baja California and Chihuahua to 14 in Tamaulipas. The number of nurses per 10,000 population ranged from 17 in Baja California and Chihuahua to 24 in Coahuila.

Research and Technology

At the border health research agenda council meeting in February 2002, four research areas of interest were identified—disease control and prevention; health and the environment; health care systems, services, and human resource development; and health, society, and development.

PAHO's United States-Mexico Border Field Office began to engage in activities designed to facilitate the use of appropriate technology, including providing training to border institutions on the use of the geographic information system software, SIGEPI, and on the use of other communications software.

The information and knowledge management center at the El Paso Field Office houses online databases of periodicals and/or journals and provides access to courses as a way to develop competence in information search. It also distributes bibliographic material and produces various technical documents on public health issues in various formats.

Health Sector Expenditures and Financing

The United States and Mexico finance health in vastly different ways. The percentages presented in this section are intended for in-country comparisons only.

In the United States border states in 2004, total health expenditures as a percentage of the gross state product (GSP) ranged from 11% in California, to 12% in Arizona and Texas, to 13% in New Mexico. At the national level, total health expenditures as a percentage of the gross domestic product were 13%.

In Mexico's border states, public expenditure in health as a percentage of GDP (public expenditure) in 2004 ranged from 2.1% in Nuevo León to 3.3% in Sonora, compared to the national level of 3%. Public expenditure in health as a percentage of the total public expenditure ranged from 16.5% in Tamaulipas to 26.9% in Nuevo León, compared to the national level of 17.4%.

Technical Cooperation and External Financing

The United States Agency for International Development (USAID) provides funds and technical assistance to strengthen epidemiological surveillance systems and deal with chronic diseases, tuberculosis, and disaster mitigation on the border.

The Pan American Health Organization (PAHO) has had a field office on the U.S.-Mexico border since 1942. The field office currently contributes to meeting the objectives of Healthy Border 2010, Border 2012, and other border health initiatives, within the framework of the Strategic Plan of the Pan American Sanitary Bureau, 2003–2007, and the Millennium Development Goals. The Organization will continue to provide technical cooperation and services.

Other local, national, and international institutions also work along the border. There are also coalitions, agencies, associations, foundations, academic institutions, and government and nongovernmental organizations that provide funding for health-related activities on both sides of the border.

Bibliography

Albertorio-Díaz JR, Notzon FS. Diabetes at the border: a profile of hospitalization rates along the US-Mexico border region; 2006. Presentation at the 63rd Annual Meeting of the United States-Mexico Border Health Association.

Ambriz L. Information and Knowledge Management Report. El Paso: Pan American Health Organization United States-Mexico Border Field Office; 2006: 13.

Border Health Research Agenda Council. Border Health Research Agenda Council Meeting Report. Edinburg (Texas); 2002. Available from: http://www.fep.paho.org/english/Alianzas/BHRAC%20Report%20English.pdf.

Bruns A. Maquilas or bust. Site Selection Online 2004;42(2): 88–90.

Cheryl W. Cancer deaths, California 2000–2003. California Department of Health Services; 2005.

Daniel C. Diabetes deaths in California, 2004. California Department of Health Services; 2006.

Erik S. Brucellosis cases in Texas (2000–2005). Texas Department of State Health Services; 2006.

Group USCSW. 1999–2002 Incidence and Mortality Web-based Report. Atlanta: United States Department of Health and Human Services; Centers for Disease Control and Prevention; National Cancer Institute; 2005.

Henry J. Kaiser Family Foundation. State Health Facts 2005. Menlo Park (California); 2005.

Hereford J. The U.S.-Mexico Border: Integrated Economies: Economic Development America (EDA); 2006.

International Boundary and Water Commission. International Boundary and Water Commission, Its Mission, Organization and Procedures for Solution of Boundary and Water Problems. 2006. Available from: http://www.ibwc.state.gov/html/about_us.html. Accessed 25 September 2006.

Mariana M. New lab ready to help solve Juarez crimes. The Houston Chronicle. 2006 Sept 22; Sect. A. Page 22. Available from: http://www.chron.com/.

Mathews TJ. Infant mortality statistics from the 2001 period linked birth/infant death data set. Hyattsville (Maryland); 2003.

México, Consejo Nacional de Población. Proyecciones de la población en México. CONAPO; 2002.

México, Instituto Nacional de Estadística Geográfica e Informática. XII Censo General de Población y Vivienda 2000. 2000.

México, Instituto Nacional de Estadística Geográfica e Informática. Anuario Estadístico: Baja California Sur, Edición 2003. México, DF: INEGI; Gobierno del Estado de Baja California Sur; 2004. Pág. 410.

México, Instituto Nacional de Salud Pública. Encuesta Nacional de Salud: 2003.

México, Secretaría de Salud, Dirección General de Epidemiología. Anuarios de morbilidad. SSA; 2005.

México, Secretaría de Salud, Dirección General de Epidemiología. Vigilancia Epidemiológica. Semana 1, 2005. SSA; 2005.

México, Secretaría de Salud. Las 20 primeras causas de mortalidad, jurisdiccional y por municipio. Ciudad Juárez; 2002.

México, Secretaría de Salud. Mortality in women; 2002.

México, Secretaría de Salud. Principal causes of infant mortality. SSA; 2002.

Nalder SN. Cases of brucellosis in New Mexico (2000–2005). 2006.

Pan American Health Organization. Basic Indicators 2003. Health Situation of the United States-Mexico Border. El Paso: PAHO; 2003.

Pan American Health Organization. Basic Indicators 2003. Washington, DC: PAHO; 2003.

Pan American Health Organization. Boletín Epidemiológico; 2002–2005.

Pan American Health Organization. U.S.-Mexico Border Diabetes Prevention and Control Project: First Report of Results. PAHO; 2005.

Sandy F. California's infant mortality rate, 2003. Sacramento: California Department of Health Services; 2005.

Steven S. Human Immunodeficiency Virus Disease Deaths California, 2000–2003. California Department of Health Services; 2005.

Sun B. Brucellosis cases in California (2000–2005). California Department of Health Services; 2006.

United Nations Development Program. Human Development Report. New York: Oxford University Press; 2005.

United States, Arizona Department of Health Services. Arizona Health Status and Vital Statistics; 2006.

United States, Arizona Department of Health Services, Office of Border Health. 2006. Available from: http://www.azdhs.gov/phs/borderhealth/index.htm. Accessed 22 August 2006.

United States, Arizona Public Health Association. Health Disparities in Arizona's Racial and Ethnic Minority Populations. 2005.

United States, Bureau of the Census. [Computer data]. 2000. Available from: http://www.census.gov/.

United States, California Department of Health Services. Deaths and Age-Adjusted Death Rates for Leading Causes of Death by Sex, California, 2000–2003. Report No. VSCA 05-07. May 2004.

United States, California Department of Health Services. Death, Percent of Deaths, Death Rates, and Age-Adjusted Death Rates for Leading Causes of Death: 2005.

United States, Centers for Disease Control and Prevention. Behavioral Risk Factor Surveillance System. Atlanta: CDC; 2003.

United States, Central Intelligence Agency. The World Fact Book. Washington, DC: CIA; 2005.

United States, Department of Health and Human Services; Centers for Disease Control and Prevention; National Center for Health Statistics. Health, United States, 2005. With Chartbook on Trends in the Health of Americans. Hyattsville, Maryland: National Center for Health Statistics; 2005.

United States, Environmental Protection Agency. Border 2012: U.S.-Mexico environmental program: response summary report, 2002. Washington, DC: EPA; 2003: 59 pp.

United States, Environmental Protection Agency. U.S.-Mexico Border 2012 Framework. EPA; 2003.

United States, Government Accountability Office. Illegal Immigration: United States. GAO; 2006.

United States-Mexico Border Health Commission. Healthy Border 2010: an agenda for improving health on the United States-Mexico border. El Paso: United States-Mexico Border Health Commission; 2003.

United States-Mexico Border Health Commission. Inauguration of the Ventanilla de Salud in El Paso. 2006.

United States, Texas Department of State Health Services. Texas resident life expectancy at birth for selected years. 2006.

Wasem RE. Congressional Research Service (CRS) Report for Congress. Unauthorized Aliens in the United States: Estimates since 1986. Washington, DC; 2006.

William FA. Cases of brucellosis in Arizona (2000–2005). 2006.

World Bank, International Economics Department Development Data Group. World Development Indicators. Washington, DC: International Bank for Reconstruction and Development; 2003.

World Bank. World Development Report. New York: Oxford University Press. 1997–2006.

World Health Organization. Global Initiative on Children's Environmental Health. Pilot Projects. WHO; 2006: 2.

World Health Organization. Preventing chronic diseases: a vital investment: WHO global report. WHO; 2005.

World Health Organization; Public Health Agency of Canada. Ottawa; 2005.

Zuniga E, Wallace SP, Berumen S, Castaneda X, et al. Mexico-United States Migration: Health Issues. Mexico, DF: Consejo Nacional de Población; 2005.

ACRONYMS

ACT	Amazon Cooperation Treaty Organization
ADC	Andean Development Corporation
AIDIS	Inter-American Association of Sanitary and Environmental Engineering
AIDS	Acquired immunodeficiency syndrome
ALAESP	Latin American and Caribbean Association of Public Health Education
API	Annual parasite index
BCIE	Central American Bank for Economic Integration
BIREME	Latin American and Caribbean Center on Health Sciences Information (PAHO)
BMI	Body mass index
CAN	Andean Community of Nations
CAREC	Caribbean Epidemiology Center (PAHO)
CARICOM	Caribbean Community
CCA	Common Country Assessments (NU)
CDB	Caribbean Development Bank
CDC	Centers for Disease Control and Prevention (USA)
CEHI	Caribbean Environmental Health Institute
CELADE	Latin American and Caribbean Demographic Center (ECLAC)
CEPIS	Pan American Center for Sanitary Engineering and Environmental Sciences (PAHO)
CERSSO	Regional Center for Occupational Safety and Health
CFNI	Caribbean Food and Nutrition Institute (PAHO)
CHRC	Caribbean Health Research Council
CIDA	Canadian International Development Agency
CIOMS	Council for International Organizations of Medical Sciences
COHRED	Council on Health Research for Development
COLABIOCLI	Latin American Confederation of Clinical Biochemistry
COPICHAS	Confederation of Indigenous Peoples of the South American Chaco Region
CPC	Caribbean Program Coordination (PAHO)
CPI	Consumer price index
CRICS	Regional Congress on Health Sciences Information
DAC	Development Assistance Committee (OECD)
DALY	Disability-adjusted life years
DANIDA	Danish International Development Agency
DOTS	Directly observed treatment, short course
EAP	Economically active population
ECLAC	Economic Commission for Latin America and the Caribbean (UN)
EPA	Environmental Protection Agency (USA)
EPI	Expanded Program on Immunization
FAO	Food and Agriculture Organization of the United Nations
FCTC	Framework Convention on Tobacco Control (WHO)
FIOCRUZ	Oswaldo Cruz Foundation
GAVI	Global Alliance for Vaccines and Immunization
GDP	Gross domestic product
GEF	Global Environment Facility
GFATM	Global Fund to Fight AIDS, Tuberculosis, and Malaria
GIVS	Global Immunization Vision and Strategies

GMP	Good manufacturing practices
GNI	Gross national income
GNP	Gross national product
GTZ	German Technical Cooperation Agency
HACCP	Hazard analysis critical control point
HDI	Human development index (UNDP)
HINARI	Health InterNetwork Access to Research Initiative
HIPC	Heavily Indebted Poor Countries Initiative (IMF/World Bank)
HIV	Human immunodeficiency virus
HPSRI	Health-Promoting Schools Regional Initiative
IACHR	Inter-American Commission on Human Rights
IAEA	International Atomic Energy Agency
IAM	Amazon Malaria Initiative
IBRD	International Bank for Reconstruction and Development (World Bank)
IBWC	International Boundary and Water Commission
ICOH	International Commission on Occupational Health
ICPD	International Conference on Population and Development
ICRC	International Committee of the Red Cross
IDA	International Development Association (World Bank)
IDB	Inter-American Development Bank
IFRC	International Federation of Red Cross and Red Crescent Societies
IHR	International Health Regulations
ILO	International Labor Organization
IMCI	Integrated Management of Childhood Illnesses
IMF	International Monetary Fund
INCAP	Institute of Nutrition of Central America and Panama (PAHO)
IOM	International Organization for Migration
IPCC	United Nations Intergovernmental Panel on Climate Change
IRET	Regional Institute for the Study of Toxic Substances
ISCA	Central American Health Initiative
IUHPE	International Union for Health Promotion and Education
JICA	Japan International Cooperation Agency
JMP	Joint Monitoring Program (WHO/UNICEF)
LAMM	Latin American and Caribbean Initiative for Maternal Mortality Reduction
LILACS	Latin American and Caribbean Literature on Health Sciences (PAHO)
MDG	Millennium development goals
MERCOSUR	Southern Common Market
NAFTA	North American Free Trade Agreement
NGO	Nongovernmental organization
OAS	Organization of American States
OCHA	Office for the Coordination of Humanitarian Affairs (NU)
ODA	Official development assistance
OECD	Organisation for Economic Co-operation and Development
OECS	Organization of Eastern Caribbean States
OEPA	Onchocerciasis Elimination Program for the Americas
OIE	World Organization for Animal Health
ORAS-CONHU	Andean Health Agency-Hipólito Unánue Agreement
OREALC	Regional Office for Education in Latin America and the Caribbean (UNESCO)
PAHEF	Pan American Health and Education Foundation
PAHO	Pan American Health Organization

PANAFTOSA	Pan American Foot-and-Mouth Disease Center (PAHO)
PANCAP	Pan Caribbean Partnership Against HIV/AIDS
PANDRH	Pan American Network for Drug Regulatory Harmonization
PASB	Pan American Sanitary Bureau
PHAC	Canadian Public Health Agency
PHEFA	Hemispheric Program for the Eradication of Foot-and-Mouth Disease
PLAGSALUD	Occupational and Environmental Aspects of Exposure to Pesticides in the Central American Isthmus
PPP	Purchasing power parity
RAVREDA	Amazon Network for the Surveillance of Antimalarial Drug Resistance
RBM	Roll Back Malaria
RECACER	Central American Network for the Prevention and Control of Emerging and Reemerging Diseases
RELAB	Latin American Biology Network
RELAC	Latin American and Caribbean Network of Environmental Laboratories
REMSAA	Meeting of Andean Area Health Ministers
REPAMAR	Pan American Environmental Waste Management Network
REPIDISCA	Pan American Network of Information and Documentation in Sanitary
RESSCAD	Meeting of the Health Sector of Central America and the Dominican Republic
RICTSAL	Network of Science and Technology Health Indicators
RICYT	Network of Science and Technology Indicators
RIMSA	Inter-American Meeting at Ministerial Level on Health and Agriculture
SARS	Severe Acute Respiratory Syndrome
SciELO	Scientific Electronic Library Online
ScienTI	International Network of Information and Knowledge Sources for Sciences, Technology and Innovation Management
SICA	Central American Integration System
SIDA	Swedish International Development Cooperation Agency
SIREVA	Regional System of Vaccines (PAHO)
TCC	Technical cooperation among countries
UN	United Nations
UNAIDS	Joint United Nations Program on HIV/AIDS
UNASUR	Union of South American Nations
UNDAF	United Nations Development Assistance Framework
UNDG	United Nations Development Group
UNDP	United Nations Development Programme
UNEP	United Nations Environment Programme
UNESCO	United Nations Educational, Scientific, and Cultural Organization
UNFPA	United Nations Fund for Population Activities
UNGASS	United Nations General Assembly Special Session
UNHCR	United Nations High Commissioner for Refugees
UNICEF	United Nations Children's Fund
UNIFEM	United Nations Development Fund for Women
UNSCEAR	United Nations Scientific Committee on the Effects of Atomic Radiation
VHL	Virtual Health Library
VIVSALUD	Inter-American Healthy Housing Network
VWA	Vaccination week in the Americas
WFP	World Food Program
WHO	World Health Organization
WTO	World Trade Organization